Register
Access

M000313003

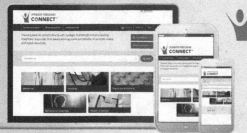

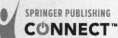

Your print purchase of *APRN and PA's Complete Guide to Prescribing Drug Therapy 2022* **includes online access to the contents of your book**—increasing accessibility, portability, and searchability!

Access today at:
http://connect.springerpub.com/content/reference-book/978-0-8261-7935-7
or scan the QR code at the right with your smartphone. Log in or register, then click "Redeem a voucher" and use the code below.

EMYXF87W

Scan here for quick access.

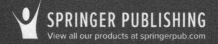

SPRINGER PUBLISHING
View all our products at springerpub.com

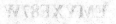

The APRN and PA's Complete Guide to Prescribing Drug Therapy

2022

Mari J. Wirfs, PhD, MN, RN, APRN, ANP-BC, FNP-BC, CNE, began her career with an ASN (1968, Dekalb College), and subsequently completed a BSN (1970, Georgia State University), MS (1975, Emory University), Post-Masters Certificates in Primary Care of the Adult (1997) and Family (1997, LSU Health Sciences Center), and PhD in Higher Education Administration and Leadership (1991, University of New Orleans). She is a nationally certified Adult Nurse Practitioner (1997, American Nurses Credentialing Center), Family Nurse Practitioner (1998, American Academy of Nurse Practitioners), and Certified Nurse Educator (2008, National League for Nursing). Her career spans 50+ years inclusive of collegiate undergraduate and graduate nursing education and clinical practice in critical care, pediatrics, psychiatric–mental health nursing, and advanced practice primary care nursing. During her academic career, she has achieved the rank of professor with tenure in two university systems.

Dr. Wirfs was a founding member of the medical staff in the establishment of Baptist Community Health Services, a community-based nonprofit primary care clinic founded post-hurricane Katrina in the New Orleans Lower Ninth Ward. Since 2002, Dr. Wirfs has served as clinical director and primary care provider at the Family Health Care Clinic, serving faculty, staff, students, and their families at New Orleans Baptist Theological Seminary (NOBTS). She is also adjunct graduate faculty, teaching neuropsychology and psychopharmacology, in the NOBTS Guidance and Counseling program. She is a long-time member of the National Organization of Nurse Practitioner Faculties (NONPF), Sigma Theta Tau International Honor Society of Nursing, and several other academic honor societies.

Dr. Wirfs has completed, published, and presented six quantitative research studies focusing on academic leadership, nursing education, and clinical practice issues, including one for the Army Medical Department conducted during her 8 year reserve service in the US Army Nurse Corps. Her publications include co-authored family primary care certification review books and study materials. Her first prescribing guide, *Clinical Guide to Pharmacotherapeutics for the Primary Care Provider*, was published by Advanced Practice Education Associates (APEA) from 1999 to 2014. *The APRN's Complete Guide to Prescribing Drug Therapy* (launched in 2016), *The APRN's Complete Guide to Prescribing Pediatric Drug Therapy* (launched in 2017), and *The PA's Complete Guide to Prescribing Drug Therapy* (launched in 2017) are published by Springer Publishing Company.

The APRN's Complete Guide to Prescribing Pediatric Drug Therapy 2018 was awarded second place, **Book of the Year 2017** in the Child Health Category, by the *American Journal of Nursing (AJN)*, official publication of the **American Nurses Association (ANA)**. The panel of judges included the co-founder of the nurse practitioner role and first nurse practitioner program, Dr. Loretta C. Ford, Professor Emerita. Dr. Wirfs was the recipient of the **2018 AANP Nurse Practitioner State Award for Excellence from Louisiana** by the **American Association of Nurse Practitioners (AANP)**.

The APRN and PA's Complete Guide to Prescribing Drug Therapy

2022

Mari J. Wirfs, PhD, MN, RN,
APRN, ANP-BC, FNP-BC, CNE

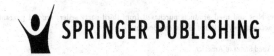

SPRINGER PUBLISHING

Copyright © 2022 Springer Publishing Company, LLC

Springer Publishing Company, LLC
11 West 42nd Street
New York, NY 10036
www.springerpub.com

Acquisitions Editor: Rachel X. Landes
Composition: Exeter Premedia Services Private Ltd.

ISBN: 978-0-8261-8551-8
e-book ISBN: 978-0-8261-8549-5
DOI: 10.1891/9780826185495

21 22 23 24 / 5 4 3 2

This book is a quick reference for healthcare providers practicing in primary care settings. The information has been extrapolated from a variety of professional sources and is presented in condensed and summary form. It is not intended to replace or substitute for complete and current manufacturer prescribing information, current research, or knowledge and experience of the user. For complete prescribing information, including toxicities, drug interactions, contraindications, and precautions, the reader is directed to the manufacturer's package insert and the published literature. The inclusion of a particular brand name neither implies nor suggests that the author or publisher advises or recommends the use of that particular product or considers it superior to similar products available by other brand names. Neither the author nor the publisher makes any warranty, expressed or implied, with respect to the information, including any errors or omissions, herein.

Library of Congress Cataloging-in-Publication Data
Names: Wirfs, Mari J., author.
Title: The APRN and PA's complete guide to prescribing drug therapy 2020 / Mari J. Wirfs.
Description: New York, NY: Springer Publishing Company, LLC, [2020] | Includes bibliographical references and index.
Identifiers: LCCN 2017008900| ISBN 9780826179333 | ISBN 9780826179340 (ebook)
Subjects: | MESH: Drug Therapy—nursing | Advanced Practice Nursing—methods | Handbooks
Classification: LCC RM301 | NLM WY 49 | DDC 615.1—dc23
LC record available at https://lccn.loc.gov/2017008900

Printed in the United States of America.

◯ CONTENTS

xiv ■ Contents

SECTION II: APPENDICES

---

*Online only; available at connect.springerpub.com/content/reference-book/978-0-8261-7935-7/section/
sectionII/appendix.

---

*Online only; available at connect.springerpub.com/content/reference-book/978-0-8261-7935-7/section/
sectionII/appendix.

---

*Online only; available at connect.springerpub.com/content/reference-book/978-0-8261-7935-7/section/sectionII/appendix.

---

*Online only; available at connect.springerpub.com/content/reference-book/978-0-8261-7935-7/section/sectionII/appendix.

Kelley M. Anderson, PhD, FNP
Assistant Professor of Nursing, Georgetown University School of Nursing and Health Studies,
Washington, DC

Kathleen Bradbury-Golas, DNP, RN, FNP-C, ACNS-BC
Associate Clinical Professor, Drexel University, Philadelphia, Pennsylvania; Family Nurse
Practitioner, Virtua Medical Group, Hammonton and Linwood, New Jersey

Lori Brien, MS, ACNP-BC
Instructor, Advanced Practice Nursing Department, Georgetown University School of Nursing
and Health Studies, Washington, DC

Jill Cash, MSN, APN, CNP
Nurse Practitioner, Logan Primary Care, West Frankfort, Illinois

Catherine M. Concert, DNP, RN, FNP-BC, AOCNP, NE-BC, CNL, CGRN
Nurse Practitioner-Radiation Oncology, Laura and Isaac Perlmutter Cancer Center, New York
University Langone Medical Center; Clinical Assistant Professor, Pace University Lienhard
School of Nursing, New York, New York

Kate DeMutis, MSN, CRNP
Senior Lecturer, Adult-Gerontology Primary Care Nurse Practitioner Program, Centralized
Clinical Site Coordinator-Primary Care, University of Pennsylvania School of Nursing,
Philadelphia, Pennsylvania

Gaye M. Douglas, DNP, MEd, APRN-BC
Assistant Professor of Nursing, Francis Marion University, Florence, South Carolina

Brenda Douglass, DNP, APRN, FNP-C, CDE, CTTS
Coordinator of Clinical Faculty, Assistant Clinical Professor, Drexel University College of
Nursing and Health Professions, Philadelphia, Pennsylvania

Aileen Fitzpatrick, DNP, RN, FNP-BC
Clinical Assistant Professor, Pace University Lienhard School of Nursing, New York, New York

Nancy M. George, PhD, RN, FNP-BC, FAANP
Director of DNP Program, Associate Clinical Professor, Wayne State University College of
Nursing, Detroit, Michigan

Tracy P. George, DNP, APRN-BC, CNE
Assistant Professor of Nursing, Amy V. Cockcroft Fellow 2016-2017, Francis Marion
University, Florence, South Carolina

Cheryl Glass, MSN, WHNP, RN-BC
Clinical Research Specialist, KePRO, TennCare's Medical Solutions Unit, Nashville, Tennessee

Kathleen Gray, DNP, FNP-C
Assistant Professor, Georgetown School of Nursing and Health Studies, Washington, DC

Norma Stephens Hannigan, DNP, MPH, FNP-BC, DCC, FAANP
Clinical Professor of Nursing, Coordinator, Accelerated Second Degree (A2D) Program/
Sophomore Honors Program, Hunter College, CUNY Hunter-Bellevue School of Nursing,
New York, New York

Ella T. Heitzler, PhD, WHNP, FNP, RNC-OB
Assistant Professor, Georgetown University School of Nursing and Health Studies,
Washington, DC

Mary T. Hickey, EdD, RN
Clinical Professor of Nursing, Hunter College, CUNY Hunter-Bellevue School of Nursing,
New York, New York

Deborah L. Hopla, DNP, APRN-BC
Assistant Professor of Nursing, Director MSN/FNP Track, Amy V. Cockcroft Fellow, Francis
Marion University, Florence, South Carolina

Julia M. Hucks, MN, APRN-BC
Assistant Professor of Nursing, Family Nurse Practitioner, Francis Marion University,
Florence, South Carolina

Honey M. Jones, DNP, ACNP-BC
Acute Care Nurse Practitioner, Duke University Medical Center; Clinical Associate Faculty,
MSN Program, Duke University School of Nursing, Durham, North Carolina

Melissa H. King, DNP, FNP-BC, ENP-BC
Director of Advanced Practice Providers, Director of TelEmergency, Department of
Emergency Medicine, University of Mississippi Medical Center, Jackson, Mississippi

Brittany M. Newberry, PhD, MSN, MPH, APRN, ENP, FNP
Board Certified Emergency and Family Nurse Practitioner; Vice President Education and
Professional Development of Hospital MD; Chair, Practice Committee of American Academy
of Emergency Nurse Practitioners; Adjunct Faculty, Emory University School of Nursing,
Atlanta, Georgia

Andrea Rutherfurd, MS, MPH, FNP-BC
Clinical Faculty Advisor, Adjunct Instructor, FNP Program, Georgetown University School of
Nursing and Health Studies, Washington, DC

Samantha Venable, MSN, RN, FNP
Family Nurse Practitioner, Correctional Nursing, Trabuco Canyon, California

Michael Watson, DNP, APRN, FNP-BC
Lead Family Nurse Practitioner, Wadley Regional Medical Center, Emergency Department,
Texarkana, Texas

The APRN and PA's Complete Guide to Prescribing Drug Therapy 2022 is a prescribing reference intended for use by healthcare providers in all clinical practice settings who are involved in the primary care management of patients with acute, episodic, and chronic health problems and needs for health promotion and disease prevention. It is organized in a concise and easy-to-read format. Comments are interspersed throughout, including such clinically useful information as laboratory values to be monitored, patient teaching points, and safety information. If pediatric indications for a drug have not been established or a drug is not recommended for a pediatric subgroup, this information is noted accordingly.

This reference is divided into two major sections. **Section I** presents drug treatment regimens for over 600 clinical diagnoses. Each drug is listed alphabetically by generic name, followed by: FDA pregnancy category (A, B, C, D, X); over-the-counter availability (OTC); DEA schedule (I, II, III, IV, V); generic availability (G); dosing regimens; brand/trade name(s); dose forms; whether tablets, caplets, or chew tabs are single scored (*), cross-scored (**), or tri-scored (***); flavors of chewable, sublingual, buccal, and liquid forms; and information regarding additives (i.e., dye-free, sugar-free, preservative-free or preservative type, alcohol-free or alcohol content). Non-pharmaceutical products and drugs that received initial FDA approval on or after June 30, 2015, do not have an FDA pregnancy letter designation. For information regarding special populations, including pregnant and breastfeeding females, refer to the manufacturer's package insert or visit https://www.accessdata.fda.gov/scripts/cder/daf/ to view the product label online. Visit https://www.drugs.com/pregnancy-categories.html to view the FDA Pregnancy and Lactation Labeling Final Rule (PLLR) and new label format.

Section II presents clinically useful information organized in table format, including: the JNC-8 and ASH recommendations for hypertension management, childhood immunization recommendations, brand/trade name drugs (with contents) for the management of common respiratory symptoms, anti-infectives by classification, pediatric dosing by weight for liquid forms, glucocorticosteroids by potency and route of administration, and contraceptives by route of administration and estrogen and/or progesterone content. An alphabetical cross-reference index of drugs by generic and brand/trade name, with FDA pregnancy category and controlled drug schedule, facilitates quick identification of drugs by alternate names and page location(s).

Selected diseases and diagnoses (e.g., angina, ADHD, growth failure, glaucoma, Parkinson's disease, multiple sclerosis, cystic fibrosis) and selected drugs (e.g., antineoplastics, antipsychotics, antiarrhythmics, anti-HIV drugs, anticoagulants) are included because patients are frequently referred to primary care providers by specialists for follow-up monitoring and on-going management. Further, the shifting healthcare paradigm is such that with expanding roles and patient empowerment through education, initial diagnosis and initiation of treatment is increasing in primary care with measurable increases in access to quality healthcare and improved patient self-care. Several diseases are included that may not be prevalent in North America but have been identified in other parts of the world. Endemic diseases for which there is no FDA-approved drug treatment are also included with known transmission and treatment interventions. Accordingly, this guide serves primary care providers internationally. Today's healthcare providers are in an era of rapidly expanding knowledge in the field of genomics, and thus, each new edition of this prescribing guide contains new drug classes and new FDA-approved drugs.

For quick reference to pediatric weight-based dosing of a drug, the user is directed to the dose-by-weight table for that drug in the appendices. Potential safe, efficacious, prescribing and monitoring of drug therapy regimens requires adequate knowledge about (a) the pharmacodynamics and pharmacokinetics of drugs, (b) concomitant therapies, and (c) individual characteristics of the patient (e.g., age, weight, current and past medical history, physical examination findings, hepatic and renal function, and co-morbidities, and risk factors). Users of this clinical guide are encouraged to utilize the manufacturer's package insert, recommendations and guidance of specialists, standard-of-practice protocols, and the current research literature for more comprehensive information about specific drugs (e.g., special precautions, drug-drug and drug-food interactions, risk versus benefit, age-related considerations, potential adverse reactions, and appropriate patient-centered care.

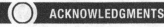

ACKNOWLEDGMENTS

This publication, which we consider to be a "must have" for students, academicians, and practicing clinicians represents the culmination of Springer Publishing Company's collaborative team effort. The production team at Exeter Premedia Services, on behalf of Springer Publishing Company, managed the complex files as content was updated and cross-referenced for the final product. The work of reviewers from academia and clinical practice was essential to the process, and their contributions are greatly appreciated. I am proud of my association with these dedicated professionals, and I thank them on behalf of the healthcare community worldwide for supporting the end goal of quality healthcare for all people.

Sincerely, Dr. Mari J. Wirfs

ACE-Is and **ARBs** are contraindicated in the 2nd and 3rd trimesters of pregnancy. Addition of a daily ACE-I or ARB is strongly recommended for renal protection in patients with hypertension and/or diabetes. The "ACE inhibitor cough," a dry cough, is an adverse side effect produced by an accumulation of bradykinins that occurs in 5% to 10% of the population and resolves within days of discontinuing the drug.

Alcohol is contraindicated with concomitant **narcotic analgesics, benzodiazepines, SSRIs, antihistamines, TCAs,** and other sedating agents due to risk of over-sedation.

Alpha-1 blockers have a potential adverse side effect of sudden hypotension, especially with first dose. Alert the patient regarding this "first-dose effect" and recommend the patient sit or lie down to take the first dose. Usually start at lowest dose and titrate upward.

Antidepressant monotherapy should be avoided until any presence of (hypo) mania or positive family history for bipolar spectrum disorder has been ruled out as antidepressant monotherapy can induce mania in the bipolar patient.

For patients 65 years-of-age and older, consult the **May 2017 Beers Criteria** for Potentially Inappropriate Medication (PIM) Use in Older Adults, to help improve the safety of prescribing medications for older adults, presented in table format at: https://www.priorityhealth.com/provider/clinical-resources/medication-resources/~/media/documents/pharmacy/cms-high-risk-medications.pdf

Aspirin is contraindicated in children and adolescents with *Varicella* or other viral illness, and 3rd trimester of pregnancy.

Beta-blockers, by all routes of administration, are generally contraindicated in severe COPD, history of or current bronchial asthma, sinus bradycardia, and 2nd or 3rd degree AV block. Use a cardio-specific beta blocker where appropriate in these cases.

A **biosimilar** product is one that has been FDA-approved based on data demonstrating that it is highly similar to a previously FDA-approved biological product, known as the reference product. Accordingly, the FDA has determined that there are no clinically meaningful differences between the biosimilar product and the reference product (e.g., **Cyltezo** [*adalimumab-adbm*] is biosimilar to **Humira** [*adalimumab*]). A biosimilar product has been demonstrated for the condition(s) of use (e.g. indication(s), dosing regimen(s)), strength(s), dosage form(s), and route(s) of administration described in its full prescribing information in the manufacturer's package insert.

The FDA **Breakthrough Therapy Designation (BTD)** is intended to expedite the development and review of a drug candidate that is planned for use, alone or in combination with one or more other drugs, to treat a serious or life-threatening disease or condition when preliminary clinical evidence indicates that the drug may demonstrate substantial improvement over existing therapies on one or more clinically significant endpoints. The benefits of Breakthrough Therapy Designation include the same benefits as Fast Track Designation (FTD), plus an organizational commitment involving the FDA's senior managers with more intensive guidance from the FDA (e.g., *Zulresso [brexanolone]*) received the FDA Breakthrough Therapy Designation for treatment of post-partum depression.

Calcium channel blockers may cause the adverse side effect of pedal edema (feet, ankles, lower legs) that resolves with discontinuation of the drug.

Codeine is known to be excreted in breast milk: <12 years, not recommended; 12-<18, use extreme caution; not recommended for children and adolescents with asthma or other chronic breathing problem. The FDA and the European Medicines Agency (EMA) are investigating the safety of using *codeine*-containing medications to treat pain, cough, and colds in children 12-<18 years because of the potential for serious side effects, including slowed or difficult breathing.

Check **drug interactions** at https://www.drugs.com/drug_interactions.php

Check FDA **drug recalls, market withdrawals, and safety alerts** (http://www.fda.gov/Safety/Recalls/default.htm).

Contraceptives that are estrogen-progesterone combinations and **progesterone-only** are contraindicated in pregnancy (pregnancy category X).

Corticosteroids increase blood sugar in patients with diabetes and decrease immunity; therefore, consider risk versus benefit in susceptible patients, use lowest effective dose, and taper gradually to discontinue.

Diclofenac is contraindicated with *aspirin* allergy and, as with all other NSAIDs, should be avoided in late pregnancy (≥30 weeks) because it may cause premature closure of the ductus arteriosus.

Erythromycin may increase INR with concomitant warfarin, as well as increase serum level of digoxin, benzodiazepines, and statins.

Finasteride, a 5-alpha reductase inhibitor, is associated with low but increased risk of high-grade prostate cancer. Pregnant females should not touch broken tablets.

Fluoroquinolones and **quinolones** are contraindicated <18 years-of-age, pregnancy, and breastfeeding. *Exception:* in the case of anthrax, *ciprofloxacin* is indicated for patients <18 years-of-age and dosed based on mg/kg body weight. Risk of tendonitis or tendon rupture (ex: *ciprofloxacin, gemifloxacin, levofloxacin, moxifloxacin, norfloxacin, ofloxacin*).

Fluoroquinolones can increase the risk of aortic dissection or aortic aneurysm rupture and should not be used in patients at increased risk (including patients with peripheral artery disease, hypertension, Marfan syndrome, Ehlers-Danlos syndrome, and older adults) unless there is no other available treatment option.

The U.S. Preventive Services Task Force (USPSTF) recommends against using **hormone replacement therapy (HRT)** for primary prevention of chronic conditions among post-menopausal women. The harms associated with combined use of estrogen and a progestin, such as increased risks of invasive breast cancer, venous thromboembolism, and coronary heart disease, far outweigh the benefits.

Ibuprofen is contraindicated in children <6 months of age and in the 3rd trimester of pregnancy.

Live vaccines are contraindicated in patients who are immunosuppressed or receiving immunosuppressive therapy, including immunosuppressive levels of corticosteroid therapy.

Metronidazole and *tinidazole* are contraindicated in the 1st trimester of pregnancy. Alcohol is contraindicated during treatment with oral forms and for 72 hours after therapy due to a possible *disulfiram*-like reaction (nausea, vomiting, flushing, headache).

When prescribing **opioid analgesics**, presumptive urine **drug testing** (UDT) should be performed when opioid therapy for chronic pain is initiated, along with subsequent use as adherence monitoring, using in-office point of service testing to identify patients who are non-compliant or abusing prescription drugs or illicit drugs. American Society of Interventional Pain Physicians (ASIPP)

Orphan Drug designation means the drug is a first-in-class and/or the drug is for treatment of a rare disease and/or the drug is a first and only treatment for a disease and the application for FDA approval has received priority review as incentive to assist and encourage the development of drugs for rare diseases.

Oral **PDE5 inhibitors** are contraindicated in patients taking nitrates due to risk of hypotension or syncope (ex: *avanafil, sildenafil, tadalafil, vardenafil*).

Chronic long-term **proton pump inhibitor (PPI)** use carries a risk to renal function (consider risk-benefit and alternative treatment). PPIs should be discontinued, and should not be initiated, in patients with acute kidney injury (AKI) and chronic kidney disease (CKD).

Statins are strongly recommended as adjunctive therapy for patients with diabetes, with **or** without abnormal lipids.

Sulfonamides (ex: *sulfamethoxazole, trimethoprim*) are not recommended in pregnancy or lactation. CrCl 15-30 mL/min: reduce dose by 1/2; CrCl <15 mL/min: not recommended. Contraindicated with G6PD deficiency. A high fluid intake is indicated during sulfonamide therapy to avoid crystallization in the kidneys.

Tetracyclines are contraindicated in children <8 years-of-age, pregnancy, and breastfeeding (discolors developing tooth enamel). A side effect may be photo-sensitivity (photophobia). Do not take with antacids, calcium supplements, milk or other dairy, or within 2 hours of taking another drug (ex: *doxycycline, minocycline*).

Tramadol is known to be excreted in breast milk. The FDA and the European Medicines Agency (EMA) are investigating the safety of using *tramadol*-containing medications to treat pain in children 12-18 years because of the potential for serious side effects, including slowed or difficult breathing.

The **Transmucosal Immediate Release Fentanyl (TIRF) Risk Evaluation and Mitigation Strategy (REMS)** program is an FDA-required program designed to ensure informed risk-benefit decisions before initiating treatment, and while patients are treated to ensure appropriate use of TIRF medicines. The purpose of the TIRF REMS Access program is to mitigate the risk of misuse, abuse, addiction, overdose, and serious complications due to medication errors with the use of TIRF medicines. You must enroll in the TIRF REMS Access program to prescribe, dispense, **or** distribute TIRF medicines. To register, call the TIRF REMS Access program at 1-866-822-1483 **or** register online at https://www.tirfremsaccess.com/TirfUI/rems/home.action

The APRN and PA's Complete Guide to Prescribing Drug Therapy

2022

SECTION I

DRUG THERAPY BY CLINICAL DIAGNOSIS

ACETAMINOPHEN OVERDOSE

ANTIDOTE/CHELATING AGENT

▷ *acetylcysteine* (B)(G) *Loading Dose:* 150 mg/kg administered over 15 minutes;
Maintenance: 50 mg/kg administered over 4 hours; then 100 mg/kg administered over 16 hours
Pediatric: same as adult
    Acetadote *Vial: soln for IV infusion after dilution:* 200 mg/ml (30 ml; dilute in D₅W (preservative-free)
    Comment: *Acetaminophen* overdose is a medical emergency due to the risk of irreversible hepatic injury. An IV infusion of *acetylcysteine* should be started as soon as possible and within 24 hours if the exact time of ingestion is unknown. Use a serum *acetaminophen* nomogram to determine need for treatment. Extreme caution is needed if used with concomitant hepatotoxic drugs.

ACNE ROSACEA

Comment: All acne rosacea products should be applied sparingly to clean, dry skin as directed. Avoid use of topical corticosteroids.

▷ *ivermectin* (C)(G) apply bid
    Soolantra *Crm:* 1% (30 gm)
    Comment: **Soolantra** is a macrocyclic lactone. Exactly how it works to treat rosacea is unknown.

TOPICAL ALPHA-1A ADRENOCEPTOR AGONIST

▷ *oxymetazoline hcl* (B) apply a pea-sized amount once daily in a thin layer covering the entire face (forehead, nose, cheeks, and chin) avoiding the eyes and lips; wash hands immediately
Pediatric: <18 years: not recommended; ≥18 years: same as adult
    Rhofade *Crm* 1% (30 gm tube)
    Comment: **Rhofade** acts as a vasoconstrictor. Use with caution in patients with cerebral <u>or</u> coronary insufficiency, Raynaud's phenomenon, thromboangiitis obliterans, scleroderma, <u>or</u> Sjögren's syndrome. **Rhofade** may increase the risk of angle closure glaucoma in patients with narrow-angle glaucoma. Advise patients to seek immediate medical care if signs and symptoms of potentiation of vascular insufficiency <u>or</u> acute angle closure glaucoma develop.

TOPICAL ALPHA-2 AGONIST

▷ *brimonidine* (B) apply to affected area once daily
Pediatric: <18 years: not recommended; ≥18 years: same as adult
    Mirvaso
    Gel: 0.33% (30, 45 gm tube; 30 gm pump)
    Comment: **Mirvaso** is indicated for persistent erythema; *brimonidine* constricts dilated facial blood vessels to reduce redness.

TOPICAL ANTIMICROBIALS

▷ *azelaic acid* (B)(G) apply to affected area bid
    Azelex *Crm:* 20% (30, 50 gm)
    Finacea *Gel:* 15% (30 gm); *Foam:* 15% (50 gm)
▷ *metronidazole* (B) apply to clean dry skin
    MetroCream apply bid
      Emol crm: 0.75% (45 gm)
    MetroGel apply once daily
      Gel: 1% (60 gm tube; 55 gm pump)
    MetroLotion apply bid
      Lotn: 0.75% (2 oz)

▷ *minocycline* topical foam apply to affected areas once daily; gently rub into the skin

    Pediatric: <9 years: not recommended; ≥9 years: same as adult

      Amzeeq *Aerosol can:* 4% (30 gm)

      Comment: **Amzeeq** *(minocycline)* is a tetracycline-class drug indicated to treat inflammatory lesions of non-nodular moderate-to-severe acne vulgaris in patients >9 years-of-age. The propellant in **Amzeeq** is flammable. Instruct the patient to avoid fire, flame, and smoking during and immediately following application. Use of tetracycline-class of drugs orally during the second and third trimesters of pregnancy, infancy and childhood up to the age of 8 years may cause permanent discoloration of the teeth (yellow-gray-brown) and reversible inhibition of bone growth. If *Clostridium difficile*-associated diarrhea occurs, discontinue **Amzeeq**. If liver injury is suspected, discontinue **Amzeeq**. Patients who are on anticoagulant therapy may require downward adjustment of their anticoagulant dosage. Avoid co-administration with penicillins. **Amzeeq** may cause fetal harm when when used during pregnancy. Breastfeeding is not recommended while using **Amzeeq**.

▷ *sodium sulfacetamide* (C)(G) apply 1-3 x daily

      Klaron *Lotn:* 10% (2 oz)

▷ *sodium sulfacetamide+sulfur* (C)

      Clenia Emollient Cream apply 1-3 x daily

        Wash: sod sulfa 10%+sulfur 5% (10 oz)

      Clenia Foaming Wash wash affected area once or twice daily

        Wash: sod sulfa 10%+sulfur 5% (6, 12 oz)

      Rosula Gel apply 1-3 x daily

        Gel: sod sulfa 10%+sulfur 5% (45 ml)

      Rosula Lotion apply tid

        Lotn: sod sulfa 10%+sulfur 5% (45 ml) (alcohol-free)

      Rosula Wash wash bid

        Clnsr: sod sulfa 10%+sulfur 5% (335 ml)

ORAL ANTIMICROBIALS

▷ *doxycycline* (D)(G) 40-100 mg bid

    Pediatric: <8 years: not recommended; ≥8 years, <100 lb: 2 mg/lb on first day in 2 divided doses, followed by 1 mg/lb/day in 1-2 divided doses; ≥8 years, ≥100 lb: same as adult; *see Appendix CC.19. doxycycline* (Vibramycin Syrup/Suspension) *for dose by weight*

      Acticlate *Tab:* 75, 150**mg

      Adoxa *Tab:* 50, 75, 100, 150 mg ent-coat

      Doryx *Tab:* 50, 75, 100, 150, 200 mg del-rel

      Doxteric *Tab:* 50 mg del-rel

      Monodox *Cap:* 50, 75, 100 mg

      Oracea *Cap:* 40 mg del-rel

      Vibramycin *Tab:* 100 mg; *Cap:* 50, 100 mg; *Syr:* 50 mg/5 ml (raspberry-apple) (sulfites); *Oral susp:* 25 mg/5 ml (raspberry)

      Vibra-Tab *Tab:* 100 mg film-coat

▷ *minocycline* (D)(G) 200 mg on first day; then 100 mg q 12 hours x 9 more days

    Pediatric: <8 years: not recommended; ≥8 years, <100 lb: 2 mg/lb on first day in 2 divided doses, followed by 1 mg/lb q 12 hours x 9 more days; ≥8 years, ≥100 lb: same as adult

      Dynacin *Cap:* 50, 100 mg

      Minocin *Cap:* 50, 75, 100 mg; *Oral susp:* 50 mg/5 ml (60 ml) (custard) (sulfites, alcohol 5%)

ACNE VULGARIS

ORAL CONTRACEPTIVES

see Appendix H. Contraceptives
see Appendix H.4. Progesterone-Only Oral Contraceptives ("Mini-Pill")

Comment: In their 2016 published report, researchers concluded different hormonal contraceptives have significantly varied effects on acne. Women (n = 2,147) who were using a hormonal contraceptive at the time of their first consultation for acne comprised the study sample. Participants completed an assessment at baseline to report how the contraceptive affected their acne. Then the researchers used the Kruskal-Wallis test and logistic regression analysis to compare the outcomes by contraceptive type. On average, the vaginal ring and combined oral contraceptives (COCs) improved acne, whereas depot injections, subdermal implants, and hormonal intrauterine devices worsened acne. In the COC categories, *drospirenone* was the most helpful in improving acne, followed by *norgestimate* and *desogestrel*, and then *levonorgestrel* and *norethindrone*. Although triphasic progestin dosage had a positive effect on acne, estrogen dosage did not.

TOPICAL ANDROGEN RECEPTOR INHIBITOR

▷ *clascoterone* apply a thin layer to affected area twice daily (morning and evening)
  Pediatric: <12 years: not recommended; ≥12 years: same as adult
    Winlevi *Crm:* 1%
    Comment: Winlevi is a first-in-class topical androgen receptor inhibitor for the treatment of acne vulgaris. Hypothalmic-pituitary-adrenal (HPA) axis suppression may occur during or after treatment with *clascoterone*. Attempt to withdraw use if HPA suppression occurs. Pediatric patients may be more susceptible to systemic toxicity. Elevated potassium level has been observed in some subjects during clinical trials. The most common adverse reactions (incidence 7-12%) have been erythema, reddening, pruritis, and scaling/dryness. Additionally, edema, stinging, and burning has occurred in >3% of patients and were reported in a similar percentage of patients treated with vehicle. There are no available data on Winlevi cream use in pregnant females to evaluate for an associated risk of major birth defects, miscarriage, or adverse maternal or fetal outcomes. There are no data regarding the presence of *clascoterone* or its metabolite in human milk or effects on the breastfed infant.

TOPICAL ANTIMICROBIALS

Comment: All topical antimicrobials should be applied sparingly to clean, dry skin.
▷ *azelaic acid* (B)(G) apply to affected area bid
    Azelex *Crm:* 20% (30, 50 gm)
    Finacea *Gel:* 15% (30 gm); *Foam:* 15% (50 gm)
▷ *benzoyl peroxide* (C)(G)
  Comment: *Benzoyl peroxide* may discolor clothing and linens.
    Benzac-W initially apply to affected area once daily; increase to bid-tid as tolerated
      Gel: 2.5, 5, 10% (60 gm)
    Benzac-W Wash wash affected area bid
      Wash: 5% (4, 8 oz); 10% (8 oz)
    Benzagel apply to affected area one or more x/day
      Gel: 5, 10% (1.5, 3 oz) (alcohol 14%)
    Benzagel Wash wash affected area bid
      Gel: 10% (6 oz)

Desquam X⁵ wash affected area bid
Wash: 5% (5 oz)
Desquam X¹⁰ wash affected area bid
Wash: 10% (5 oz)
Triaz apply to affected area daily bid
Lotn: 3, 6, 9% (bottle), 3% (tube); *Pads:* 3, 6, 9% (jar)
ZoDerm apply once or twice daily
Gel: 4.5, 6.5, 8.5% (125 ml); *Crm:* 4.5, 6.5, 8.5% (125 ml); *Clnsr:* 4.5, 6.5, 8.5% (400 ml)

▷ *clindamycin* topical **(B)** apply to affected area bid
Pediatric: <12 years: not recommended; ≥12 years: same as adult
Cleocin T *Pad:* 1% (60/pck; alcohol 50%); *Lotn:* 1% (60 ml); *Gel:* 1% (30, 60 gm); *Soln w. applicator:* 1% (30, 60 ml) (alcohol 50%)
Clindagel *Gel:* 1% (42, 77 gm)
Evoclin Foam: 1% (50, 100 gm) (alcohol)

▷ *clindamycin+benzoyl peroxide* topical **(C)** apply to affected area once daily
Pediatric: <12 years: not recommended; ≥12 years: same as adult
Acanya (G) apply to affected area once daily-bid
Gel: clin 1.2%+benz 2.5% (50 gm)
BenzaClin (G) apply to affected area bid
Gel: clin 1%+benz 5% (25, 50 gm)
Duac apply daily in the evening
Gel: clin 1%+benz 5% (45 gm)
Onexton Gel (G) apply to affected area once daily
Gel: clin 1.2%+benz 3.75% (50 gm pump) (alcohol-free) (preservative-free)

▷ *dapsone* topical **(C)(G)** apply to affected area bid
Pediatric: <12 years: not recommended; ≥12 years: same as adult
Aczone *Gel:* 5, 7.5% (30, 60, 90 gm pump)

▷ *erythromycin+benzoyl peroxide* **(C)** initially apply to affected area once daily; increase to bid as tolerated
Benzamycin Topical Gel *Gel:* eryth 3%+benz 5% (46.6 gm/jar)

▷ *minocycline* topical foam apply to affected areas once daily; gently rub into the skin
Pediatric: <9 years: not recommended; ≥9 years: same as adult
Amzeeq *Aerosol can:* 4% (30 gm)
Comment: Amzeeq *(minocycline)* is a tetracycline-class drug indicated to treat inflammatory lesions of non-nodular moderate-to-severe acne vulgaris in patients >9 years-of-age. The propellant in **Amzeeq** is flammable. Instruct the patient to avoid fire, flame, and smoking during and immediately following application. Use of tetracycline-class of drugs orally during the second and third trimesters of pregnancy, infancy and childhood up to the age of 8 years may cause permanent discoloration of the teeth (yellow-gray-brown) and reversible inhibition of bone growth. If *Clostridioides difficile*-associated diarrhea occurs, discontinue **Amzeeq**. If liver injury is suspected, discontinue **Amzeeq**. Patients who are on anticoagulant therapy may require downward adjustment of their anticoagulant dosage. Avoid co-administration with penicillins. **Amzeeq** may cause fetal harm when when used during pregnancy. Breastfeeding is not recommended while using **Amzeeq**.

▷ *sodium sulfacetamide* **(C)(G)** apply tid
Klaron *Lotn:* 10% (2 oz)

ORAL ANTIMICROBIALS

▷ *doxycycline* **(D)(G)** 100 mg bid
Pediatric: <8 years: not recommended; ≥8 years, <100 lb: 2 mg/lb on first day in 2 divided doses, followed by 1 mg/lb/day in 1-2 divided doses; ≥8 years, ≥100 lb:

same as adult; *see Appendix CC.19. doxycycline* (Vibramycin Syrup/Suspension) *for dose by weight*

Acticlate *Tab*: 75, 150**mg

Adoxa *Tab*: 50, 75, 100, 150 mg ent-coat

Doryx *Tab*: 50, 75, 100, 150, 200 mg del-rel

Doxteric *Tab*: 50 mg del-rel

Monodox *Cap*: 50, 75, 100 mg

Oracea *Cap*: 40 mg del-rel

Vibramycin *Tab*: 100 mg; *Cap*: 50, 100 mg; *Syr*: 50 mg/5 ml (raspberry-apple) (sulfites); *Oral susp*: 25 mg/5 ml (raspberry)

Vibra-Tab *Tab*: 100 mg film coat

▷ *erythromycin base* **(B)(G)** 250 mg qid, 333 mg tid or 500 mg bid x 7-10 days; then taper to lowest effective dose

Pediatric: <45 kg: 30-50 mg in 2-4 divided doses x 7-10 days; ≥45 kg: same as adult

Ery-Tab *Tab*: 250, 333, 500 mg ent-coat

PCE *Tab*: 333, 500 mg

▷ *erythromycin ethylsuccinate* **(B)(G)** 400 mg qid x 7-10 days

Pediatric: 30-50 mg/kg/day in 4 divided doses x 7-10 days; may double dose with severe infection; max 100 mg/kg/day; *see Appendix CC.21. erythromycin ethylsuccinate* (E.E.S. Suspension, Ery-Ped Drops/Suspension) *for dose by weight*

EryPed *Oral susp*: 200 mg/5 ml (100, 200 ml) (fruit); 400 mg/5 ml (60, 100, 200 ml) (banana); *Oral drops*: 200, 400 mg/5 ml (50 ml) (fruit); *Chew tab*: 200 mg wafer (fruit)

E.E.S. *Oral susp*: 200, 400 mg/5 ml (100 ml) (fruit)

E.E.S. Granules *Oral susp*: 200 mg/5 ml (100, 200 ml) (cherry)

E.E.S. 400 Tablets *Tab*: 400 mg

▷ *minocycline* **(D)(G)** initially 50-200 mg/day in 2 divided doses; reduce dose to once daily after improvement

Pediatric: <8 years: not recommended; ≥8 years: same as adult

Dynacin *Cap*: 50, 100 mg

Minocin *Cap*: 50, 75, 100 mg; *Oral susp*: 50 mg/5 ml (60 ml) (custard) (sulfites, alcohol 5%)

Minolira *Tab*: 105, 135 mg ext-rel

Solodyn *Tab*: 55, 65, 80, 105, 115 mg ext-rel

Comment: Once-daily dosing of **Minolira** or **Solodyn,** extended-release *minocyclines*, is approved for inflammatory lesions of non-nodular moderate-to-severe acne vulgaris for patients ≥12 years-of-age. The recommended dose of **Solodyn** is 1 mg/kg once daily x 12 weeks.

▷ *sarecycline* one tab daily based with or without food; <9 years: not recommended; ≥9 years: *33-54 kg*: 60 mg; *55-84 kg*: 100 mg; *85-136 kg*: 150 mg

Seysara *Tab*: 60, 100, 150 mg

Comment: **Seysara** is a first-in-class, *tetracycline*-derived, once daily treatment for inflammatory lesions of non-nodular moderate-to-severe acne. Efficacy of **Seysara** beyond 12 weeks and safety beyond 12 months have not been established. **Seysara** has not been evaluated in the treatment of infections. To reduce the development of drug-resistant bacteria as well as to maintain the effectiveness of other antibacterial drugs, **Seysara** should be used only as indicated. If *Clostridioides difficile*-associated diarrhea (antibiotic-associated colitis) occurs, discontinue **Seysara**. Central nervous system side effects, including light-headedness, dizziness, or vertigo, have been reported with *tetracycline* use. Patients who experience these symptoms should be cautioned about driving vehicles or using hazardous machinery. These symptoms may disappear during therapy and may disappear when the drug is discontinued. **Seysara** may cause intracranial hypertension;

discontinue **Seysara** if symptoms occur. Photosensitivity can occur with **Seysara**; minimize or avoid exposure to natural or artificial sunlight. *tetracycline* is contraindicated <8 years-of-age, in pregnancy, and lactation (discolors developing tooth enamel). A side effect may be photo-sensitivity (photophobia). Avoid co-administration with retinoids and penicillin. Decrease anticoagulant dosage as appropriate. Monitor for toxicities of drugs that may require dosage reduction (e.g., P-glycoprotein substrates) and monitor for toxicities. Do not take with antacids, calcium supplements, iron preparations, milk or other dairy, or within two hours of taking another drug.

▷ *tetracycline* (D)(G) initially 1 gm/day in 2-4 divided doses; after improvement, 125-500 mg daily
  Pediatric: <8 years: not recommended; ≥8 years, <100 lb: 25-50 mg/kg/day in 2-4 divided doses; ≥8 years, ≥100 lb: same as adult; *see* Appendix CC.31. *tetracycline* (Sumycin Suspension) *for dose by weight*
    Achromycin V *Cap:* 250, 500 mg
    Sumycin *Tab:* 250, 500 mg; *Cap:* 250, 500 mg; *Oral susp:* 125 mg/5 ml (100, 200 ml) (fruit) (sulfites)

TOPICAL RETINOIDS

Comment: Wash affected area with a soap-free cleanser; pat dry and wait 20 to 30 minutes; then apply sparingly to affected area; use only once daily in the evening. Avoid applying to eyes, ears, nostrils, and mouth.

▷ *adapalene* (C) apply once daily at HS
  Pediatric: <12 years: not recommended; ≥12 years: same as adult
    Differin *Crm:* 0.1% (45 gm); *Gel:* 0.1, 0.3% (45 gm) (alcohol-free); *Pad:* 0.1% (30/pck) (alcohol 30%); *Lotn:* 0.1% (2, 4 oz)
▷ *tazarotene* (X)(G) apply to affected area once daily at HS
  Pediatric: <12 years: not recommended; ≥12 years: same as adult
    Arazlo *Tube:* **0.045% (45 gm)**
    Commment: **Arazlo** *(tazarotene)* is a lotion formulation of retinoid *tazarotene* approved for the topical treatment of acne vulgaris in patients ≥9 years-of-age.
    Avage Cream *Crm:* 0.1% (30 gm)
    Tazorac Cream *Crm:* 0.05, 0.1% (15, 30, 60 gm)
    Tazorac Gel *Gel:* 0.05, 0.1% (30, 100 gm)
▷ *tretinoin* (C)(G) apply sparingly to affected area once or twice daily
  Comment: Dryness, pain, erythema, irritation, and exfoliation may occur during treatment. Avoid paranasal creases and mucous membranes. Minimize exposure to sunlight and sunlamps. Use sunscreen and protective clothing when sun exposure cannot be avoided. Use with caution if allergic to fish due to potential for allergenicity to fish protein.
  Pediatric: <12 years: not recommended; ≥12 years: same as adult
    Altreno *Lotn:* 0.05% (45 gm tube)
    Comment: **Altreno** is indicated for children >9 years-of-age. Apply a thin film to affected area bid.
    Atralin Gel *Gel:* 0.05% (45 gm)
    Avita *Crm:* 0.025% (20, 45 gm); *Gel:* 0.025% (20, 45 gm)
    Retin-A Cream *Crm:* 0.025, 0.05, 0.1% (20, 45 gm)
    Retin-A Gel *Gel:* 0.01, 0.025% (15, 45 gm) (alcohol 90%)
    Retin-A Liquid *Soln:* 0.05% (alcohol 55%)
    Retin-A Micro Gel *Gel:* 0.04, 0.08, 0.1% (20, 45 gm)
    Tretin-X Cream *Crm:* 0.075% (35 gm) (parabens-free, alcohol-free, propylene glycol-free)
▷ *trifarotene 0.005% cream* apply a thin layer to the affected areas of the face chest, shoulders, and/or back once daily, in the evening, to clean and dry skin; avoid

contact with the eyes, lips, paranasal creases, and mucous membranes
Pediatric: <9 years: not recommended; ≥9 years: same as adult
  Aklief *Pump:* 30, 45, 70 gm

TOPICAL RETINOID+ANTIMICROBIAL COMBINATIONS

Comment: Wash affected area with a soap-free cleanser; pat dry and wait 20-30 minutes; then apply sparingly to affected area; use only once daily in the evening. Avoid eyes, ears, nostrils, and mouth.

▷ *adapalene+benzoyl peroxide* (C)(G) apply a thin film once daily
Pediatric: <18 years: not recommended
  Epiduo Gel *Gel:* adap 0.1%+benz 2.5% (45 gm)
  Epiduo Forte Gel *Pump gel:* adap 0.3%+benz 2.5% (15, 30, 45, 60 gm)
▷ *tretinoin+clindamycin* (C)(G) apply a thin film once daily
Pediatric: <18 years: not recommended
  Ziana *Gel:* tret 0.025%+clin 1.2% (30, 60 gm)

ORAL RETINOID

Comment: Oral retinoids are indicated only for severe recalcitrant nodular acne unresponsive to conventional therapy including systemic antibiotics.

▷ *isotretinoin* (X) initially 0.5-1 mg/kg/day in 2 divided doses; maintenance 0.5-2 mg/kg/day in 2 divided doses x 4-5 months; repeat only if necessary 2 months following cessation of first treatment course
Pediatric: <12 years: not recommended; ≥12 years: same as adult
  Accutane *Cap:* 10, 20, 40 mg (parabens)
  Amnesteem *Cap:* 10, 20, 40 mg (soy)
Comment: *Isotretinoin* is highly teratogenic and, therefore, female patients should be counseled prior to initiation of treatment as follows: Two negative pregnancy tests are required prior to initiation of treatment and monthly thereafter. Not for use in females who are or who may become pregnant or who are breastfeeding. Two effective methods of contraception should be used for 1 month prior to, during, and continuing for 1 month following completion of treatment. Low-dose *progestin* (mini-pill) may be an *inadequate* form of contraception. No refills; a new prescription is required every 30 days and prescriptions must be filled within 7 days. Serum lipids should be monitored until response is established (usually initially and again after 4 weeks). Bone growth, serum glucose, ESR, RBCs, WBCs, and liver enzymes should be monitored. Blood should not be donated during, or for 1 month after, completion of treatment. Avoid the sun and artificial UV light. *isotretinoin* should be discontinued if any of the following occurs: visual disturbances, tinnitus, hearing impairment, rectal bleeding, pancreatitis, hepatitis, significant decrease in CBC, hyperlipidemia (particularly hypertriglyceridemia).

 ACROMEGALY

GROWTH HORMONE RECEPTOR ANTAGONIST

▷ *pegvisomant* (B) *Loading dose:* 40 mg SC; *Maintenance:* 10 mg SC daily; titrate by 5 mg (increments or decrements, based on IGF-1 levels) every 4 to 6 weeks; max 30 mg/day
Pediatric: <12 years: not recommended; ≥12 years: same as adult
  Somavert *Inj:* 10, 15, 20 mg
Comment: Prior to initiation of *pegvisomant*, patients should have baseline fasting serum glucose, HgbA1c, serum K$^+$ and Mg^{++}, liver function tests (LFTs), EKG, and gall bladder ultrasound.

CYCLOHEXAPEPTIDE SOMATOSTATIN

▷ **pasireotide (C)** administer SC in the thigh or abdomen; initial dose is 0.6 mg or 0.9 mg bid; titrate dose based on response and tolerability; for patients with moderate hepatic impairment *(Child-Pugh Class B)*, the recommended initial dosage is 0.3 mg twice daily and max dose 0.6 mg twice daily; avoid use in patients with severe hepatic impairment *(Child-Pugh Class C)*

Pediatric: <12 years: not recommended; ≥12 years: same as adult

Signifor LAR *Amp:* 0.3, 0.6, 0.9 mg/ml, single-dose, long-act rel (LAR) susp for inj

SOMATOSTATIN ANALOG

▷ *octreotide acetate*

Comment: *octreotide acetate* is indicated for reduction of growth hormone (GH) and insulin-like growth factor 1 (IGF-1) (somatomedin C) in adult patients with acromegaly who have had inadequate response to or cannot be treated with surgical resection, pituitary irradiation, and bromocriptine mesylate at maximally tolerated doses. Monitor patients treated with *octreotide acetate* for cholelithiasis. Glucose monitoring is recommended and antidiabetic treatment may need adjustment. Hypothyroidism may occur; monitor thyroid levels periodically. Bradycardia, arrhythmia, or conduction abnormalities may occur; use with caution in at-risk patients. Common adverse side effects may include diarrhea, cholelithiasis, abdominal pain, flatulence. Advise pre-menopausal females of the potential for an unintended pregnancy.

PARENTERAL FORMS

▷ *octreotide acetate*

Bynfezia Pen initiate at 50 mcg SC 3 x/day; typical dose is 100 mcg SC 3 x/day

Prefilled Pen: 2.5 mg/ml (2500 mcg/ml) 2.8 ml, single-patient-use

Sandostatin initiate at 50 mcg SC 3 x/ day; IGF-I (somatomedin C) levels every 2 weeks can be used to guide titration; goal is to achieve growth hormone levels <5 ng/mL or IGF-I (somatomedin C) levels <1.9 unit/mL (males) and <2.2 unit/mL (females); most common effective dose is 100 mcg SC 3 x/day; some patients require up to 500 mcg SC 3 x/day for maximum effectiveness; >300 mcg/day seldom results in additional biochemical benefit; if dose increase fails to provide additional benefit, the dose should be reduced; IGF-I (somatomedin C) or growth hormone levels should be re-evaluated at 6-month intervals

Vial: 200, 1000 mcg/5 ml, multidose; *Amp:* 50, 100, 500 mcg/ml

Comment: **Sandostatin** should be withdrawn yearly for approximately 4 weeks from patients who have received irradiation to assess disease activity. If growth hormone or IGF-I (somatomedin C) levels increase and signs and symptoms recur, **Sandostatin** therapy may be resumed.

Sandostatin LAR Depot after administering **Sandostatin** 50 mcg SC 3 x/day for 2 weeks, initiate Sandostatin LAR Depot suspension 20 mg IM intragluteally every 4 weeks for 3 months

Vial: 10, 20, 30 mg/6 ml, single-use

Comment: **Sandostatin LAR Depot** is indicated for treatment in patients with acromegaly who have first responded to **Sandostatin** with achievement of growth hormone levels <5 ng/mL or IGF-I (somatomedin C) levels <1.9 unit/mL (males) and <2.2 unit/mL (females).

ORAL FORM

▷ **Mycapssa** initiate at 40 mg daily, as 20 mg twice daily; titrate in increments of 20 mg; max 80 mg/day; monitor insulin-like growth factor 1 (IGF-1) levels and patient's signs and symptoms every two weeks during the dose titration or as indicated once the maintenance dose is achieved, monitor IGF-1 levels and patient's signs and symptoms monthly or as indicated; *ESRD*: initiate at 20 mg once daily; titrate and adjust maintenance dose based on IGF-1 levels, signs and symptoms, and tolerability (take with a glass of water on an empty stomach, at least 1 hour before a meal or at least 2 hours after a meal

    Cap: 20 mg del-rel

Comment: Mycapssa is an oral form of *octreotide* indicated for long-term maintenance treatment of patients with acromegaly who have responded to and tolerated treatment with parental *octreotide* or *lanreotide*. Most common adverse reactions (incidence >10%) are nausea, diarrhea, headache, arthralgia, asthenia, hyperhidrosis, peripheral swelling, blood glucose increased, vomiting, abdominal discomfort, dyspepsia, sinusitis, and osteoarthritis. Concomitant use of Mycapssa with other drugs mainly metabolized by CYP3A4 that have a narrow therapeutic index (e.g., *quinidine*) should be used with caution.

ACTINIC KERATOSIS (AK)

▷ *aminolevulinic acid 10%* clean and prepare all lesions prior to applying gel 1 mm thick and include 5 mm of the surrounding skin; max application area 20 cm² and max 2 gm per treatment; apply an occlusive dressing x 3 hours; photodynamic therapy involves preparation of lesions, application of the Ameluz, occlusion, and illumination with BF-RhodoLED only by a qualified healthcare provider; remove remaining gel at the end of the treatment; may re-treat in 3 months after the initial treatment; BF-RhodoLED user manual for detailed lamp safety and operating instructions.

Pediatric: <18 years: not recommended; ≥18 years: same as adult

    Ameluz *Gel*: 10% (2 gm tube) 100 mg/gm of *aminolevulinic acid hcl* (equivalent to 78 mg/gm *aminolevulinic acid*) (xanthan gum, soybean phosphatidylcholine, polysorbate 80, medium-chain triglycerides, dibasic sodium phosphate, monobasic sodium phosphate, propylene glycol, sodium benzoate, isopropal alcohol)

    Comment: Ameluz (*aminolevulinic acid*) 10% gel, a porphyrin precursor, in combination with photodynamic therapy using BF-RhodoLED lamp, is indicated for the lesion-directed and field-directed treatment of actinic keratoses of mild-to-moderate severity on the face and scalp. The most common adverse reactions (incidence ≥10%) have been application site erythema, pain/burning, irritation, edema, pruritus, exfoliation, scab formation, induration, and vesicles. Concomitant use of other photosensitizing agents may increase the risk of phototoxic reaction to photodynamic therapy (e.g., St. John's wort, *griseofulvin*, thiazide diuretics, sulfonylureas, phenothiazines, sulfonamides, quinolones, and tetracyclines). Patient and healthcare provider must wear protective eyewear before and during operation of the BF-RhodoLED lamp. Treated lesions should be protected from sunlight exposure for 48 hours posttreatment. Special care should be taken to avoid bleeding during lesion preparation in patients with inherited or acquired a coagulation disorder. Avoid direct contact of Ameluz with the eyes and mucous membranes. There are no human or animal reproductive studies of Ameluz use in pregnancy to inform a drug-associated risk. Systemic absorption of *aminolevulinic acid* is negligible. No data are available regarding the presence of *aminolevulinic acid* in human milk or effects on the breastfed infant; however, breastfeeding is not expected to result in infant exposure to the drug due to negligible systemic absorption.

▷ *diclofenac sodium 3%* (C; D ≥30 wks)(G) apply to lesions bid x 60-90 days

Pediatric: <12 years: not established; ≥12 years: same as adult

    Solaraze Gel *Gel*: 3% (50 gm) (benzyl alcohol)

Comment: *Diclofenac* is contraindicated with **aspirin** allergy. As with other NSAIDs, **Solaraze Gel** should be avoided in late pregnancy (≥30 weeks) because it may cause premature closure of the ductus arteriosus.

> **Voltaren Gel** apply qid; avoid non-intact skin
> *Gel:* 1% (100 gm)

▷ *fluorouracil* (X)(G) apply to lesion(s) daily-bid until erosion occurs, usually 2-4 weeks

Pediatric: <12 years: not recommended; ≥12 years: same as adult
> **Carac** *Crm:* 0.5% (30 gm)
> **Efudex** (G) *Crm:* 5% (25 gm); *Soln:* 2, 5% (10 ml w. dropper)
> **Fluoroplex** *Crm:* 1% (30 gm); *Soln:* 1% (30 ml w. dropper)

▷ *imiquimod* (B)(G)

Pediatric: <18 years: not recommended; ≥18 years: same as adult
> **Aldara** (G) rub into lesions before bedtime and remove with soap and water 8 hours later; treat 2 times per week; max 16 weeks
> *Crm:* 5% (single-use pkts/carton)
> **Zyclara** rub into lesions before bedtime and remove with soap and water 8 hours later; treat for 2-week cycles separated by a 2-week no-treatment cycle; max 2 packs per application; max one treatment course per area
> *Crm:* 3.75% (single-use pkts; 28/carton) (parabens)

▷ *ingenol mebutate* (C) limit application to one contiguous skin area of about 25 cm^2 using one unit dose tube; allow treated area to dry for 15 minutes; wash hands immediately after application; may remove with soapy water after 6 hours; *Face and Scalp*: apply 0.015% gel to lesions daily x 3 days; *Trunk and Extremities*: apply 0.05% gel to lesions daily x 2 days

Pediatric: <18 years: not recommended; ≥18 years: same as adult
> **Picato** *Gel:* 0.015% (3 single-use tubes), 0.05% (2 single-use tubes)

Src KINASE AND TUBULIN POLYMERIZATION INHIBITOR

▷ *tirbanibulin* apply to the treatment field on the face or scalp once daily for 5 consecutive days using 1 single-dose packet per application

Pediatric: <18 years: not established; ≥18 years: same as adult
> **Klisyri** *Oint:* 1%, single-dose pkts (25 mg/pkt)
> Comment: **Klisyri** *(tirbanibulin)* is a first-in-class dual Src Kinase and tubulin polymerization inhibitor for the topical treatment of actinic keratosis on the face or scalp. The most common adverse reactions (incidence ≥2%) have been local skin reactions, application site pruritus, and application site pain.

⬤ ADRENOCORTICAL INSUFFICIENCY

CORTICOSTEROID

▷ *hydrocortisone granules* individualize the dose, using the lowest possible dosage; *Recommended Starting Replacement Dose:* 8 to 10 mg/m^2 daily (higher doses may be needed based on patient's age and symptoms of the disease; lower starting doses may be sufficient in patients with residual but decreased endogenous cortisol production; round the dose to the nearest 0.5 mg or 1 mg. More than one capsule may be needed to supply the required dose; divide the total daily dose into 3 doses and administer 3 times daily; older patients may have their daily dose divided by 2 and administered twice daily; do not swallow the capsule; do not chew or crush the granules; see the mfr pkg insert for full prescribing information and for detailed administration instructions.

> **Alkindi Sprinkle** *Cap:* 0.5 mg, 1 mg, 2 mg, 5 mg oral granules
> Comment: **Alkindi Sprinkle** is indicated as replacement therapy in pediatric patients with adrenocortical insufficiency. Use the minimum dosage to achieve desired clinical response. Common adverse reactions

for corticosteroids include fluid retention, alteration in glucose tolerance, elevation in blood pressure, behavioral and mood changes, increased appetite, and weight gain. Corticosteroids decrease bone formation and increase bone resorption, which may lead to inhibition of bone growth and development of osteoporosis. Use may be associated with severe psychiatric adverse reactions, such as euphoria, mania, psychosis with hallucinations, and delirium or depression. Symptoms typically emerge within a few days or weeks of starting the treatment. Most reactions resolve after either dose reduction or withdrawal. Cataracts, glaucoma, and central serous chorioretinopathy have been reported with prolonged use of high doses. Monitor patients for blurred vision or other visual disturbances. Prolonged use with supraphysiologic doses may cause Cushing's syndrome. Monitor patients for signs and symptoms of Cushing's syndrome every 6 months, pediatric patients under one year of age may require more frequent monitoring. Long-term use in excessive doses may cause growth retardation; monitor the patient's growth. Excessive doses may increase the risks of new infections or exacerbation of latent infections with any pathogen, including viral, bacterial, fungal, protozoan, or helminthic infections. Monitor patients for signs and symptoms of infections. Treat all infections seriously and initiate stress dosing of corticosteroids early. Undertreatment or sudden discontinuation of therapy may lead to adrenocortical insufficiency, adrenal crisis, and death. Increase the dose during periods of stress. Switch patients who are vomiting, severely ill, or unable to take oral medications to parenteral corticosteroid formulations.

ALCOHOL DEPENDENCE, DETOXIFICATION/ALCOHOL WITHDRAWAL SYNDROME

ALCOHOL WITHDRAWAL SYNDROME

Comment: Total length of time of a given detoxification regimen and/or length of time of treatment at any dose reduction level may be extended based on patient-specific factors, including potential or actual seizure, hallucinosis, and increased sympathetic nervous system activity (severe anxiety, unwanted elevation in vital signs). If any of these symptoms are anticipated or occur, revert to an earlier step in the dosing regimen to stabilize the patient, extend the detoxification timeline, and consider appropriate adjunctive drug treatments (e.g., anticonvulsants, antipsychotic agents, antihypertensive agents, sedative hypnotics agents).

▷ *clorazepate* (D)(IV)(G) in the following dosage schedule: *Day 1:* 30 mg initially, followed by 30-60 mg in divided doses; *Day 2:* 45-90 mg in divided doses; *Day 3:* 22.5-45 mg in divided doses; *Day 4:* 15-30 mg in divided doses; Thereafter, gradually reduce the daily dose to 7.5-15 mg; then discontinue when patient's condition is stable; max dose 90 mg/day

  Pediatric: <18 years: not recommended; ≥18 years: same as adult

   Tranxene *Tab:* 3.75, 7.5, 15 mg

   Tranxene T-Tab *Tab:* 3.75*, 7.5*, 15*mg

▷ *chlordiazepoxide* (D)(IV)(G)

  Pediatric: <18 years: not recommended; ≥18 years: same as adult

   Librium 50-100 mg q 6 hours x 24-72 hours; then q 8 hours x 24-72 hours; then q 12 hours x 24-72 hours; then daily x 24-72 hours

    Cap: 5, 10, 25 mg

   Librium Injectable 50-100 mg IM or IV; then 25-50 mg IM tid-qid prn; max 300 mg/day

    Inj: 100 mg

▷ *diazepam* (D)(IV)(G) 2-10 mg q 6 hours x 24-72 hours; then q 8 hours x 24-72 hours; then q 12 hours x 24-72 hours; then daily x 24-72 hours

Pediatric: <18 years: not recommended; ≥18 years: same as adult
> **Diastat** *Rectal gel delivery system:* 2.5 mg
> **Diastat Acu Dial** *Rectal gel delivery system:* 10, 20 mg
> **Valium** *Tab:* 2*, 5*, 10*mg
> **Valium Injectable** *Vial:* 5 mg/ml (10 ml); *Amp:* 5 mg/ml (2 ml); *Prefilled syringe:* 5 mg/ml (5 ml)
> **Valium Intensol Oral Solution** *Conc oral soln:* 5 mg/ml (30 ml w. dropper) (alcohol 19%)
> **Valium Oral Solution** *Oral soln:* 5 mg/5 ml (500 ml) (wintergreen-spice)

▷ **oxazepam** (C) 10-15 mg tid-qid x 24-72 hours; decrease dose <u>and/or</u> frequency every 24-72 hours; total length of therapy 5-14 days; max 120 mg/day
Pediatric: <18 years: not recommended; ≥18 years: same as adult
> *Cap:* 10, 15, 30 mg

ABSTINENCE THERAPY
GABA Taurine Analog

▷ **acamprosate** (C)(G) 666 mg tid; begin therapy during abstinence; continue during relapse; *CrCl 30-50-mL/min:* max 333 mg tid; *CrCl <30 mL/min:* contraindicated
Pediatric: <18 years: not recommended; ≥18 years: same as adult
> **Campral** *Tab:* 333 mg ext-rel
> Comment: **Campral** does <u>not</u> eliminate <u>or</u> diminish alcohol withdrawal symptoms.

AVERSION THERAPY

▷ **disulfiram** (X)(G)
Pediatric: <18 years: not recommended; ≥18 years: same as adult
> **Antabuse** 500 mg once daily x 1-2 weeks; then 250 mg once daily
> *Tab:* 250, 500 mg; *Chew tab:* 200, 500 mg
Comment: *Disulfiram* use requires informed consent. Contraindications: severe cardiac disease, psychosis, concomitant use of *isoniazid, phenytoin, paraldehyde,* and topical and systemic alcohol-containing products. Approximately 20% remains in the system for 1 week after discontinuation.

 ALLERGIC REACTION: GENERAL

Oral Second Generation Antihistamines *see* Appendix AA. Drugs for the Management of Allergy, Cough, and Cold Symptoms online at https://connect.springerpub.com/content/reference-book/978-0-8261-7935-7/back-matter/part02/back-matter/bmatter27
Topical Corticosteroids *see* Appendix K. Topical Corticosteroids by Potency
Parenteral Corticosteroids *see* Appendix M. Parenteral Corticosteroids
Oral Corticosteroids *see* Appendix L. Oral Corticosteroids

FIRST GENERATION PARENTERAL ANTIHISTAMINE

▷ **diphenhydramine** (C)(G) 25-50 mg IM immediately; then q 6 hours prn
Pediatric: <12 years: *See mfr pkg insert:* 1.25 mg/kg up to 25 mg IM x 1 dose; then every 6 hours prn
> **Benadryl Injectable** *Vial:* 50 mg/ml (1 ml single-use); 50 mg/ml (10 ml multi-dose); *Amp:* 10 mg/ml (1 ml); *Prefilled syringe:* 50 mg/ml (1 ml)

FIRST GENERATION ORAL ANTIHISTAMINES

▷ **diphenhydramine** (B)(G) 25-50 mg q 6-8 hours; max 100 mg/day
Pediatric: <2 years: not recommended; 2-6 years: 6.25 mg q 4-6 hours; max 37.5 mg/day; >6-12 years: 12.5-25 mg q 4-6 hours; max 150 mg/day; >12 years: same as adult

Benadryl (OTC) *Chew tab:* 12.5 mg (grape) (phenylalanine); *Liq:* 12.5 mg/5 ml (4, 8 oz); *Cap:* 25 mg; *Tab:* 25 mg; *Dye-free soft gel:* 25 mg; *Dye-free liq:* 12.5 mg/5 ml (4, 8 oz)

▷ *hydroxyzine* **(C)(G)** 50-100 mg qid; max 600 mg/day
Pediatric: <6 years: 50 mg/day divided qid; ≥6 years: 50-100 mg/day divided qid
Atarax *Tab:* 10, 25, 50, 100 mg; *Syr:* 10 mg/5 ml (alcohol 0.5%)
Vistaril *Cap:* 25, 50, 100 mg; *Oral susp:* 25 mg/5 ml (4 oz) (lemon)

ALLERGIES: MULTI-FOOD

Comment: Eight food-types cause about 90% of food allergy reactions—*Milk* (mostly in children), *Eggs, Peanuts, Tree nuts*, (e.g., walnuts, almonds, pine nuts, brazil nuts, and pecans), *Soy, Wheat* (and other grains with gluten, including barley, rye, and oats), *Fish* (mostly in adults), *Shellfish* (mostly in adults). Combining *omalizumab* with oral immunotherapy (OIT) significantly improves the effectiveness of OIT in children with multiple food allergies, according to the results of a recent study. Researchers conducted a blinded, phase 2 clinical trial including children aged 4 to 15 years who had multi-food allergies validated by double-blind, placebo-controlled food challenges. Participants were randomly assigned (3:1) to either receive *omalizumab* with multi-food oral immunotherapy or placebo. *omalizumab* and placebo were administered for 16 weeks, with oral immunotherapy beginning at 8 weeks. Overall, at week 36, a significantly greater proportion of the *omalizumab*-treated participants passed double-blind, placebo-controlled food challenges, compared with placebo (83% vs 33%). No serious or severe adverse events were reported. In multi-food allergic patients, *omalizumab* improves the efficacy of multi-food oral immunotherapy and enables safe and rapid desensitization.

IGE BLOCKER (IGG1K MONOCLONAL ANTIBODY)

▷ *omalizumab* **(B)** 150-375 mg SC every 2-4 weeks based on body weight and pre-treatment serum total IgE level; max 150 mg/injection site; approved for patient self-administration after education by a qualified healthcare provider
Pediatric: <12 years: not recommended; 30-90 kg + IgE >30-100 IU/ml 150 mg q 4 weeks; 90-150 kg + IgE >30-100 IU/ml or 30-90 kg + IgE >100-200 IU/ml or 30-60 kg + IgE >200-300 IU/ml 300 mg q 4 hours; >90-150 kg + IgE >100-200 IU/ml or >60-90 kg + IgE >200-300 IU/ml or 30-70 kg + IgE >300-400 IU/ml 225 mg q 2 weeks; >90-150 kg + IgE >200-300 IU/ml or >70-90 kg + IgE >300-400 IU/ml or 30-70 kg + IgE >400-500 IU/ml or 30-60 kg + IgE >500-600 IU/ml or 30-60 kg + IgE >600-700 IU/ml 375 mg q 2 weeks; ≥12 years: same as adult
Xolair *Vial:* 150 mg, single-dose, pwdr for SC injection after reconstitution
Prefilled syringe: 75 mg/0.5 ml, 150 mg/1 ml single-dose (preservative-free)

ALPHA-1 ANTITRYPSIN (AAT) DEFICIENCY

Comment: Alpha-1 antitrypsin (AAT, a major circulating serine protease inhibitor) deficiency is a common genetic (autosomal co-dominant) condition characterized by low serum levels of AAT. Absence of deficiency of AAT accelerates lung tissue degradation and increases the risk for development of COPD and early onset emphysema, particularly in smokers. Extrapulmonary complications of ATT deficiency include liver disease (onset as early as childhood), granulomatosis with polyangitis (GPA, previously known as Wegener's granulomatosis), vasculitis, and necrotizing panniculitis. Management of symptomatic AAT and exacerbations includes bronchodilators (LABA/LAMA) and inhaled corticosteroids in line with the management of COPD symptoms and exacerbations (Global Initiative for Chronic Obstructive Lung Diaease [GOLD]). Management of ATT includes smoking cessation; avoidance of environmental pollutants; immunizations against influenza, pneumonia, and hepatitis; antibiotic therapy as needed (with *amoxicillin* or a macrolide); and management in a critical care setting for acute respiratory distress/failure. Pharmacologic management of AAT deficiency may also include AAT infusion therapy (with alpha-1 proteinase inhibitor, the only treatment to slow disease progression). *Brand names:* **Aralasp**, **Glassia**, **Prolastin**, **Prolastin-C**, **Zemaira**.

▷ *alpha-1 proteinase inhibitor (human)* (C)(G) recommended dosage of **Aralast** is 60 mg/kg administered once weekly via IV infusion, by a qualified healthcare provider, at a rate not to exceed 0.08 ml/kg; if any adverse event occurs, the rate should be reduced or the infusion interrupted until the symptoms subside; the infusion may then be resumed at a rate tolerated; refer to mfr pkg insert for detailed preparation directions and administration protocol.

Pediatric: safety and effectiveness in pediatric patients have not been established.

> **Aralast** *Vial:* 25 ml/0.5 gm, 50 ml/1 gm (1 single-use vial of product + 1 single-use vial of diluent + 1 double-ended transfer needle and 1-20 micron filter; sterile, stable, lyophilized preparation of preservative-free purified human alpha1-proteinase inhibitor (a1-PI), also known as alpha1-antitrypsin, for reconstitution with diluent provided; do not administer or mix with other agents or diluting solutions; when reconstituted, concentration of a1-PI is not less than 16 mg/ml and the specific activity is not less than 0.55 mg active a1-PI/mg total protein; refrigerate; do not freeze; administer within 3 hours after the reconstituted product is warmed to room temperature; discard partially used vials.

Comment: Alpha 1-Proteinase Inhibitor (Human), **Aralast**, is indicated for chronic augmentation therapy in patients having congenital deficiency of a1-PI with clinically evident emphysema. Clinical and biochemical studies have demonstrated that with such therapy, **Aralast** is effective in maintaining target serum a1-PI trough levels and increasing a1-PI levels in epithelial lining fluid (ELF). Clinical data demonstrating the long-term effects of chronic augmentation or replacement therapy of individuals with **Aralast** are not available. **Aralast** is not indicated as therapy for lung disease patients in whom congenital a1-PI deficiency has not been established. **Aralast** is contraindicated in individuals with selective IgA deficiencies (IgA level <15 mg/dl) who have known antibody against IgA, since they may experience a severe reactions, including anaphylaxis, to IgA which may be present. **Aralast** is prepared from large pools of human plasma by using the Cohn-Oncley cold alcohol fractionation process, followed by purification steps including polyethylene glycol and zinc chloride precipitations and ion exchange chromatography. To reduce the risk of viral transmission, the manufacturing process includes treatment with a solvent detergent (SD) mixture (tri-n-butyl phosphate and polysorbate 80) to inactivate enveloped viral agents, such as HIV and Hepatitis B and C. In addition, a nano-filtration step is incorporated prior to final sterile filtration to reduce the risk of transmission of non-enveloped viral agents. It is not known whether **Aralast** can cause fetal harm when administered to pregnant females or can affect reproductive capacity. It is not known whether alpha1-proteinase inhibitor is excreted in human milk.

 ALZHEIMER'S DISEASE

NUTRITIONAL SUPPLEMENT

▷ *l-methylfolate calcium (as metafolin)+methylcobalamin+n-acetyl cysteine* take 1 cap once daily

> **Cerefolin** *Cap:* metafo 5.6 mg+methyl 2 mg+n-ace cys 600 mg (gluten-free, yeast-free, lactose-free)

Comment: **Cerefolin** is indicated in the dietary management of patients treated for early memory loss, with emphasis on those at risk for neurovascular oxidative stress, hyperhomocysteinemia, mild- to- moderate cognitive impairment with or without vitamin B12 deficiency, vascular dementia, or Alzheimer's disease.

REVERSIBLE ANTICHOLINESTERASE INHIBITORS (RAIs)

Comment: The RAI drugs do not halt disease progression. They are indicated for early-stage disease; not effective for severe dementia. If treatment is stopped for more than several days, re-titrate from lowest dose. Side effects include nausea, anorexia, dyspepsia, diarrhea, headache, and dizziness. Side effects tend to resolve with continued treatment. Peak cognitive improvements are seen 12 weeks into therapy (increased spontaneity, reduced apathy, lessened confusion, and improved attention, conversational language, and performance of daily routines).

▷ *donepezil* (C)(G) initially 5 mg q HS, increase to 10 mg after 4-6 weeks as needed; max 23 mg/day

    Aricept *Tab:* 5, 10, 23 mg

    Aricept ODT *ODT tab:* 5, 10 mg orally-disint

▷ *galantamine* (B) initially 4 mg bid x at least 4 weeks; usual maintenance 8 mg bid; max 16 mg bid

    Razadyne *Tab:* 4, 8, 12 mg

    Razadyne ER *Tab:* 8, 16, 24 mg ext-rel

    Razadyne Oral Solution *Oral soln:* 4 mg/ml (100 ml w. calib pipette)

▷ *rivastigmine* (B)(G)

    Exelon initially 1.5 mg bid, increase every 2 weeks as needed; max 12 mg/day; take with food

        Cap: 1.5, 3, 4.5, 6 mg

    Excelon Oral Solution initially 1.5 mg bid; may increase by 1.5 mg bid at intervals of at least 2 weeks; usual range 6-12 mg/day; max 12 mg/day; if stopped, restart at lowest dose and re-titrate; may take directly from syringe or mix with water, fruit juice, or cola

        Oral soln: 2 mg/ml (120 ml w. dose syringe)

    Excelon Patch initially apply 4.6 mg/24 hr patch; if tolerated, may increase to 9.5 mg/24 hr patch after 4 weeks; max 13.3 mg/24 hr; change patch daily; apply to clean, dry, hairless, intact skin; rotate application site; allow 14 days before applying new patch to same site

        Patch: 4.6, 9.5, 13.3 mg/24 hr trans-sys (30/carton)

▷ *tacrine* (C) initially 10 mg qid, increase 40 mg/day q 4 weeks as needed; max 160 mg/day

    Cognex *Cap:* 10, 20, 30, 40 mg

Comment: Transaminase levels should be checked every 3 months while taking Cognex.

N-METHYL-D-ASPARTATE (NMDA) RECEPTOR ANTAGONIST

▷ *memantine* (B)(G)

    Namenda initially 5 mg once daily; titrate weekly in 5 mg/day increments; *Week 2:* 5 mg bid; *Week 3:* 5 mg AM and 10 mg PM; *Week 4:* 10 mg bid; *CrCl 5-29 mL/min:* max 5 mg bid

        Tab: 5, 10 mg

    Namenda Oral Solution initially 5 mg once daily; titrate weekly in 5 mg increments administered bid

        Oral soln: 2 mg/ml (360 ml) (peppermint) (sugar-free, alcohol-free)

    Namenda Titration Pak

        Cap: 7 x 7 mg, 7 x 14 mg, 7 x 21 mg, 7 x 28 mg/pck

Namenda XR initially 7 mg once daily; titrate in 7 mg increments weekly; max 28 mg once daily; do <u>not</u> divide doses
Cap: 7, 14, 21, 28 mg ext-rel
Comment: *Memantine* does <u>not</u> halt disease progression. It is indicated for moderate-to-severe dementia.

N-METHYL-D-ASPARTATE (NMDA) RECEPTOR ANTAGONIST+ ACETYLCHOLIN-ESTERASE INHIBITOR COMBINATION

▷ *memantine+donepezil* (C)(G) initiate one 28/10 dose daily in the evening after stabilized on *memantine* and *donepezil* separately; start the day after the last dose of *memantine* and *donepezil* taken separately; swallow whole <u>or</u> open cap and sprinkle on applesauce; *CrCl 5-29 ml/min:* take one 14/10 dose once daily in the evening
Namzaric
Cap: **Namzaric 7/10** mem 7 mg+done 10 mg
Namzaric 14/10 mem 14 mg+done 10 mg
Namzaric 21/10 mem 21 mg+done 10 mg
Namzaric 28/10 mem 28 mg+done 10 mg

ERGOT ALKALOID (DOPAMINE AGONIST)

▷ *ergoloid mesylate* (C) 1 mg tid
Hydergine *Tab:* 1 mg
Hydergine LC *Cap:* 1 mg
Hydergine Liquid *Liq:* 1 mg/ml (100 ml w. calib dropper) (alcohol 28.5%)

◯ AMEBIASIS

AMEBIASIS (INTESTINAL)

▷ *diiodohydroxyquin (iodoquinol)* (C)(G) 650 mg tid pc x 20 days
Pediatric: <6 years: 40 mg/kg/day in 3 divided doses pc x 20 days; max 1.95 gm; 6-12 years: 420 mg tid pc x 20 days
Tab: 210, 650 mg
▷ *metronidazole* (**not for use in 1st; B in 2nd, 3rd**)(G) 750 mg tid x 5-10 days
Pediatric: 35-50 mg/kg/day in 3 divided doses x 10 days
Flagyl *Tab:* 250*, 500*mg
Flagyl 375 *Cap:* 375 mg
Flagyl ER *Tab:* 750 mg ext-rel
▷ *tinidazole* (C) 2 gm daily x 3 days; take with food
Pediatric: <3 years: not recommended; ≥3 years: 50 mg/kg daily x 3 days; take with food; max 2 gm/day
Tindamax *Tab:* 250*, 500*mg
Comment: Other than for use in the treatment of *giardiasis* and *amebiasis* in pediatric patients older than 3 years-of-age, safety and effectiveness of *tinidazole* in pediatric patients have <u>not</u> been established. *tinidazole* is excreted in breast milk in concentrations similar to those seen in serum and can be detected in breast milk for up to 72 hours following administration. Interruption of breastfeeding is recommended during *tinidazole* therapy and for 3 days following the last dose.
▷ *paromomycin* 25-35 mg/kg/day in 3 divided doses x 5-10 days
Pediatric: same as adult
Humatin *Cap:* 250 mg

AMEBIASIS (EXTRA-INTESTINAL)

▷ *chloroquine phosphate* (C)(G) 1 gm PO daily x 2 days; then 500 mg daily x 2 to 3 weeks <u>or</u> 200-250 mg IM daily x 10-12 days (when oral therapy is impossible); use with intestinal amebicide

Pediatric: see mfr pkg insert
    Aralen *Tab:* 500 mg; *Amp:* 50 mg/ml (5 ml)

AMEBIC LIVER ABSCESS

ANTI-INFECTIVES

▷ *metronidazole* (C)(G) 250 mg tid <u>or</u> 500 mg bid <u>or</u> 750 mg daily x 7 days
    Pediatric: <12 years: not recommended; ≥12 years: same as adult
      Flagyl *Tab:* 250*, 500*mg
      Flagyl 375 *Cap:* 375 mg
      Flagyl ER *Tab:* 750 mg ext-rel
▷ *tinidazole* (C) 2 gm once daily x 3-5 days; take with food
    Pediatric: <3 years: not recommended; ≥3 years: 50 mg/kg once daily x 3-5 days;
    take with food; max 2 gm/day
      Tindamax *Tab:* 250*, 500*mg
Comment: Other than for use in the treatment of *giardiasis* and *amebiasis* in
pediatric patients older than 3 years-of-age, safety and effectiveness of *tinidazole*
in pediatric patients have <u>not</u> been established. *Tinidazole* is excreted in breast
milk in concentrations similar to those seen in serum and can be detected in breast
milk for up to 72 hours following administration. Interruption of breastfeeding is
recommended during *tinidazole* therapy and for 3 days following the last dose.

AMENORRHEA: SECONDARY

▷ *estrogen+progesterone* (X)
    Premarin (*estrogen*) 0.625 mg daily x 25 days; then 5 days off; repeat monthly
    Provera (*progesterone*) 5-10 mg last 10 days of cycle; repeat monthly
▷ *estrogen replacement* (X)
    see **Menopause**
▷ *human chorionic gonadotropin* 5,000-10,000 units IM x 1 dose following last dose
    of menotropins
      Pregnyl *Vial:* 10,000 units (10 ml) w. diluent (10 ml)
▷ *medroxyprogesterone* (X) *Monthly:* 5-10 mg last 5-10 days of cycle; begin on the
    16th <u>or</u> 21st day of cycle; repeat monthly; *One-time only:* 10 mg once daily x 10
    days
      Amen *Tab:* 10 mg
      Provera *Tab:* 2.5, 5, 10 mg
▷ *norethindrone* (X) 2.5-10 mg daily x 5-10 days
      Aygestin *Tab:* 5 mg
▷ *progesterone, micronized* (X)(G) 400 mg q HS x 10 days
      Prometrium *Cap:* 100, 200 mg
Comment: Administration of *progesterone* induces optimum secretory
transformation of the *estrogen*-primed endometrium. Administration of
progesterone is contraindicated with breast cancer, undiagnosed vaginal
bleeding, genital cancer, severe liver dysfunction <u>or</u> disease, missed abortion,
thrombophlebitis, thromboembolic disorders, cerebral apoplexy, and pregnancy.

AMYOTROPHIC LATERAL SCLEROSIS (ALS, LOU GEHRIG'S DISEASE)

PYRAZOLONE FREE RADICAL SCAVENGER

▷ *edaravone* recommended dosage is 60 mg as an IV infusion administered over
    60 minutes; Initial treatment cycle: daily dosing for 14 days, followed by a 14-day
    drug-free period; Subsequent treatment cycles: daily dosing for 10 days out of
    14-day periods, followed by 14-day drug-free periods

Radicava *IV soln:* 30 mg/100 ml single-dose polypropylene bag for IV infusion (sodium bisulfite)

Comment: Most common adverse reactions (at least 10%) are confusion, gait disturbance, and headache. There are no adequate data on the developmental risk associated with the use of **Radicava** in pregnancy. There are no data on the presence of *edaravone* in human milk or the effects on the breastfed infant. However, based on animal data, may cause embryo/fetal harm.

GLUTAMATE INHIBITOR

▷ *riluzole* 50 mg twice daily; take at least 1 hour before or 2 hours after a meal; measure serum aminotransferases before and during treatment

Exservan *Oral film:* 50 mg

Comment: **Exservan** *(riluzole)* an oral film formulation of the approved glutamate Inhibitor *riluzole* for the treatment of patients with amyotrophic lateral sclerosis (ALS) who have difficulty swallowing. Use of **Exservan** is not recommended in patients with baseline elevations of serum aminotransferase >5 times upper limit of normal (ULN); discontinue **Exservan** if there is evidence of liver dysfunction. Monitor patient for signs and symptoms of neutropenia and advise patients to report any febrile illness. Discontinue **Exservan** if interstitial lung disease develops. Co-administration of strong-to-moderate CYP1A2 inhibitors may increase **Exservan**-associated adverse reactions. Co-administration of strong to moderate CYP1A2 inducers may result in decreased **Exservan** efficacy. **Exservan**-treated patients who take other hepatotoxic drugs may be at increased risk for hepatotoxicity. Most common adverse reactions (incidence ≥5% and greater than placebo) have been oral hypoesthesia, asthenia, nausea, decreased lung function, hypertension, and abdominal pain. Based on animal data, **Exservan** may cause fetal harm. Decreased embryo/fetal viability, growth, and functional development was observed at clinically relevant doses. Women should be advised of a possible risk to the fetus associated with use of **Exservan** during pregnancy. There are no data on the presence of *riluzole* in human milk or effects on the breastfed infant. *riluzole* or its metabolites have been detected in milk of lactating animals. Developmental and health benefits of breastfeeding should be considered along with the mother's clinical need for **Exservan** and any potential adverse effects on the breastfed infant from **Exservan** or from the underlying maternal condition.

 ANAPHYLAXIS

Parenteral Corticosteroids *see* Appendix M. Parenteral Corticosteroids
Oral Corticosteroids *see* Appendix L. Oral Corticosteroids

▷ *epinephrine* (C)(G) 0.3-0.5 mg (0.3-0.5 ml of a 1:1000 soln) SC q 20-30 minutes as needed up to 3 doses
Pediatric: <2 years: 0.05-0.1 ml; 2-6 years: 0.1 ml; ≥6-12 years: 0.2 ml; All: q 20-30 minutes as needed up to 3 doses; ≥12 years: same as adult

ANAPHYLAXIS EMERGENCY TREATMENT KITS

▷ *epinephrine* (C) 0.3 ml IM or SC in thigh; may repeat if needed
Pediatric: 0.01 mg/kg SC or IM in thigh; may repeat if needed; <15 kg: not established; 15-30 kg: 0.15 mg; >30 kg: same as adult

Adrenaclick *Auto-injector:* 0.15, 0.3 mg (1 mg/ml; 1, 2/carton) (sulfites)
Auvi-Q *Auto-injector:* 0.15, 0.3 mg (1 mg/ml; 1/pck w. 1 non-active training device) (sulfites)
EpiPen *Auto-injector:* 0.3 mg (*epi* 1:1000, 0.3 ml (1, 2/carton) (sulfites)

EpiPen Jr *Auto-injector:* 0.15 mg (*epi* 1:2000, 0.3 ml) (1, 2/carton) (sulfites)
Symjepi *Prefilled syringe:* 0.3 mg (0.3 ml) single-dose for manual injection
Comment: Each **Symjepi** syringe is over-filled for stability purposes. More than half the solution remains in the syringe after use (and the syringe cannot be re-used).

Twinject *Auto-injector:* 0.15, 0.3 mg (epi 1:1000) (1, 2/carton) (sulfites)

▷ *epinephrine* plus *chlorpheniramine* (C) *epinephrine* 0.3 ml SC or IM *plus* 4 tabs *chlorpheniramine* by mouth
Pediatric: infants to 2 years: 0.05-0.1 ml SC or IM; ≥2-6 years: 0.15 ml SC or IM plus 1 tab chlor; ≥6-12 years: 0.2 ml SC or IM plus 2 tabs chlor; ≥12 years: same as adult

Ana-Kit: *Prefilled injector:* 0.3 ml epi 1:1000 for self-injection plus 4 x chlor 2 mg chew tabs

ANEMIA: BETA THALASSEMIA-ASSOCIATED

ERYTHROID MATURATION AGENT (EMA)

Comment: Reblozyl *(luspatercept-aamt)* is a first-in-class erythroid maturation agent (EMA) indicated for the treatment of beta thalassemia-associated anemia in adult patients who require regular red blood cell (RBC) transfusions. **Reblozyl** is not indicated for use as a substitute for RBC transfusions in patients who require immediate correction of anemia.

▷ *luspatercept-aamt* recommended starting dose is 1 mg/kg SC once every 3 weeks into the upper arm, abdomen, or thigh; divide doses requiring >1.2 ml reconstituted volume into separate similar volume injections and inject into separate sites; if multiple injections are required, use a new syringe and needle for each injection; review hemoglobin (Hgb) results prior to each administration; if the patient does not achieve a reduction in RBC transfusion burden after at least 2 consecutive doses (6 weeks) at the 1 mg/kg starting dose, increase the **Reblozyl** dose to 1.25 mg/kg; do not increase the dose beyond the maximum dose of 1.25 mg/kg; if an RBC transfusion occurs prior to dosing, the pre-transfusion Hgb must be considered for dosing purposes; if a planned administration of **Reblozyl** is delayed or missed, administer **Reblozyl** as soon as possible and continue dosing as prescribed, with at least 3 weeks between doses; if the pre-dose Hgb is ≥11.5 gm/dL, and the Hgb level is not influenced by recent transfusion, delay dosing until the Hgb is ≤11 gm/dL; if the patient experiences a response followed by a lack of, or loss of, response to **Reblozyl**, initiate a search for causative factors (e.g., a bleeding event); if typical causes for a lack or loss of hematologic response are excluded, follow dosing recommendations therapy (see mfr pkg insert) for management of patients with an insufficient response to **Reblozyl**; if the patient does not experience a decrease in transfusion burden after 9 weeks of treatment (administration of 3 doses) at the maximum dose level or if unacceptable toxicity occurs at any time, *discontinue* **Reblozyl**
Pediatric: safety and efficacy not established

Reblozyl *Vial:* 25, 75 mg, single-dose; pwdr for reconstitution and SC administration (see mfr pkg insert for reconstitution directions)
Comment: There is increased risk of thrombosis/thromboembolism in patients with beta thalassemia. Monitor patients receiving **Reblozyl** for signs and symptoms of thromboembolic events and institute treatment promptly. Monitor blood pressure (BP) during treatment and initiate antihypertensive treatment if necessary. The most common adverse reactions (incidence >10%) in patients with beta thalassemia have been headache, bone pain, arthralgia, fatigue, cough, abdominal pain, diarrhea, and dizziness. There are no available

data on **Reblozyl** use in pregnant females to inform a drug-associated risk of major birth defects, miscarriage, or adverse maternal or fetal outcomes. In animal reproduction studies, administration of *luspatercept-aamt* in pregnancy during the period of organogenesis resulted in adverse developmental outcomes, including embryo/fetal mortality, alterations to growth, and structural abnormalities at exposures (based on area under the curve [AUC]) above those occurring at the maximum recommended human dose (MRHD). Advise pregnant females of the potential embryo/fetal risk. Advise females of reproductive potential of the potential risk of embryo/fetal toxicity and to use effective contraception. Advise patient not to breastfeed. *luspatercept-aamt* has been detected in milk of lactating rats. When a drug is present in animal milk, it is likely that the drug will be present in human milk. There are no data on the presence of **Reblozyl** in human milk or effects on the breastfed infant. Because of the potential for serious adverse reactions, advise patients that breastfeeding is not recommended during treatment with **Reblozyl** and for 3 months after the last dose.

ANEMIA OF CHRONIC KIDNEY DISEASE (CKD)/ ANEMIA OF CHRONIC RENAL FAILURE (CRF)

PHOSPHATE BINDER

▶ **ferric citrate** *Iron Deficiency Anemia in Chronic Kidney Disease Not on Dialysis:* starting dose is 1 tablet 3 x/day with meals; adjust dose as needed to achieve and maintain hemoglobin goal, up to max 12 tabs/day; *Hyperphosphatemia in Chronic Kidney Disease on Dialysis:* starting dose is 2 tabs orally 3 x/day with meals; adjust dose by 1 to 2 tabs as needed to maintain serum phosphorus at target levels, up to max 12 tabs/day; dose can be titrated at 1 week or longer intervals
Pediatric: <18 years: not recommended; ≥18 years: same as adult

Aurexia *Tab:* 210 mg *ferric iron* (equivalent to 1 gm *ferric citrate*)
Comment: Aurexia is a phosphate binder indicated for the control of serum phosphorus levels in patients ≥18 years-of-age with chronic kidney disease (CKD) on dialysis. Ferric iron binds dietary phosphate in the GI tract and precipitates as ferric phosphate. This compound is insoluble and is excreted in the stool. **Aurexia** is also an iron replacement product indicated for the treatment of iron deficiency anemia in patients >18 years-of-age with chronic kidney (CKD) not on dialysis. Ferric iron is reduced from the ferric to the ferrous form by ferric reductase in the GI tract. After transport through the enterocytes into the blood, oxidized ferric iron circulates bound to the plasma protein transferrin, for incorporation into hemoglobin. **Aurexia** is contraindicated in iron overload syndromes (e.g., hemochromatosis). Monitor ferritin and TSAT. When clinically significant drug interactions are expected, consider separation of the timing of administration. Consider monitoring clinical responses or blood levels of the concomitant medication. The most common adverse reactions (incidence ≥5%) are discolored feces, diarrhea, constipation, nausea, vomiting, cough, abdominal pain, and hyperkalemia. There are no available data on **Aurexia** use in pregnancy to inform a drug-associated risk of major birth defects and miscarriage; however, an overdose of iron may carry a risk for spontaneous abortion, gestational diabetes and fetal malformation. There are no human data regarding effects of **Aurexia** on the breastfed infant. Accidental overdose of iron-containing products is a leading cause of fatal poisoning in children under 6 years-of-age. Keep this product out of reach of children. In case of accidental overdose, contact poison control center immediately and transfer to emergency care.

ERYTHROPOIESIS STIMULATING AGENTS (ESAS)

▷ **darbepoetin alpha** (erythropoiesis stimulating protein) (**C**) administer IV or SC q 1-2 weeks; do not increase more frequently than once per month; *Not currently receiving epoetin alpha:* initially 0.75 mcg/kg once weekly; adjust based on Hgb levels (target not to exceed 12 gm/dL); reduce dose if Hgb increases more than 1 gm/dL in any 2-week period; suspend therapy if polycythemia occurs; *Converting from* **epoetin alpha** *and for dose titration:* see mfr pkg insert

Pediatric: <12 years: not recommended; ≥12 years: same as adult

  Aranesp *Vial:* 25, 40, 60, 100, 150, 200, 300, 500 mcg/ml (single-dose) for IV or SC administration (preservative-free, albumin [human] or polysorbate 80)

  Aranesp Singleject, Aranesp Sureclick Singleject *Prefilled syringe:* 25, 40, 60, 100, 150, 200, 300, 500 mcg (single-dose) for IV or SC administration (preservative-free, albumin [human] or polysorbate 80)

▷ **peginesatide** (**C**) use lowest effective dose; initiate when Hgb <10 gm/dL; do not increase dose more often than every 4 weeks; if Hgb rises rapidly (i.e., >1 gm/ dL in 2 weeks or >2 gm/dL in 4 weeks), reduce dose by 25% or more; if Hgb approaches or exceeds 11 gm/dL, reduce or interrupt dose and then when Hgb decreases, resume dose at approximately 25% below previous dose; if Hgb does not increase by >1 gm/dL after 4 weeks, increase dose by 25%; if response is inadequate after a 12-week escalation period, use lowest dose that will maintain Hgb sufficient to reduce need for RBC transfusion; discontinue if response does not improve; *Not currently on ESA:* initially 0.04 mg/kg as a single IV or SC dose once monthly; *Converting from* **epoetin alfa:** administer first dose 1 week after last **epoetin alfa;** *Converting from* **darbepoetin alfa:** administer first dose at next scheduled dose of **darbepoetin alfa**

Pediatric: <12 years: not established; ≥12 years: use lowest effective dose

  Omontys *Vial, single-use:* 2, 3, 4, 5, 6 mg (0.5 ml) (preservative-free); *Vial, multi-use:* 10, 20 mg (2 ml) (preservatives); *Prefilled syringe:* 2, 3, 4, 5, 6 mg (0.5 ml) (preservative-free)

ERYTHROPOIETIN HUMAN, RECOMBINANT

▷ **epoetin alpha** (**C**) individualize; initially 50-100 units/kg 3 x/week; IV (dialysis or nondialysis) or SC (nondialysis); usual max 200 units/kg 3 x/week (dialysis) or 150 units/kg 3 x/week (non-dialysis); target Hct 30-36%

Pediatric: <1 month: not recommended; ≥1 month: individualize; *Dialysis:* initially 50 units/kg 3 x/week IV or SC; target Hct 30-36%

  Epogen *Vial:* 2,000, 3,000, 4,000, 10,000, 40,000 units/ml (1 ml) single-use for IV or SC administration (albumin [human]; preservative-free)

  Epogen Multidose *Vial:* 10,000 units/ml (2 ml); 20,000 units/ml, (1 ml) for IV or SC administration (albumin [human]; benzoyl alcohol)

  Procrit *Vial:* 2,000, 3,000, 4,000, 10,000, 40,000 units/ml (1 ml) single-use for IV or SC administration (albumin [human]) (preservative-free)

  Procrit Multidose *Vial:* 10,000 units/ml (2 ml); 20,000 units/ml, (1 ml) for IV or SC administration (albumin [human]; benzoyl alcohol)

▷ **epoetin alfa-epbx** evaluate iron status before and during treatment and maintain iron repletion; correct or exclude other causes of anemia before initiating treatment *Patients with CKD: Initial dose (infants ≥1 month and children):* 50 units/kg 3 x/week; *Initial dose (≥18 years-of-age):* 50-100 units/kg 3 x/week; individualize maintenance dose; intravenous route recommended for patients on hemodialysis; *Patients on Zidovudine due to HIV-infection:* 100 units/kg 3 x/ week; *Patients with Cancer on Chemotherapy:* 40,000 units once weekly or 150 units/kg 3 x weekly (adults); 600 Units/kg IV once weekly (pediatric patients >5 years); *Surgery Patients:* 300 units/kg once daily for 15 days or 600 units/kg once weekly

Retacrit *Vial:* 2,000, 3,000, 4,000, 10,000, 40,000 units/ml (1 ml), single-dose, for SC <u>or</u> IV infusion

Comment: **Retacrit** *(epoetin alfa-epbx)* is the first FDA-approved biosimilar to **Epogen/Procrit** *(epoetin alfa)* for the SC <u>or</u> IV infusion treatment of anemia caused by chronic kidney disease (CKD), chemotherapy, <u>or</u> *zidovudine* treatment for human immunodeficiency virus infection. **Retacrit** is also approved for use before and after surgery to reduce the potential need for blood transfusions due to blood loss during surgery. Common reported adverse side effects with **Retacrit** include high blood pressure, joint pain, muscle spasm, fever, and dizziness. Contraindications to **Retacrit** include uncontrolled hypertension, pure red cell aplasia (PRCA) that begins after treatment with **Retacrit** <u>or</u> other erythropoietin protein drugs, and serious allergic reactions to **Retacrit** <u>or</u> other *epoetin alfa* products. BBW: ESAs increase the risk of myocardial infarction, stroke, venous thromboembolism, thrombosis of vascular access, and tumor progression <u>or</u> recurrence, and death (see mfr pkg insert for the full BBW). Therefore, use the lowest **Retacrit** dose sufficient to reduce the need for red blood cell (RBC) transfusions and DVT prophylaxis is recommended. The limited available data on *epoetin alfa* use in pregnancy are insufficient to determine a drug-associated risk of adverse developmental outcomes. There is no information regarding the presence of *epoetin alfa* products in human milk <u>or</u> effects on the breastfed infant. Safety and effectiveness in pediatric patients <1 month-of age have <u>not</u> been established.

ANEMIA: FOLIC ACID DEFICIENCY

▷ *folic acid* (A)(OTC) 0.4-1 mg once daily
Comment: *Folic acid (vitamin B9)* 400 mcg daily is recommended during pregnancy to prevent neural tube defects. Women who have had a baby with a neural tube defect should take 400 mcg every day, even when <u>not</u> planning to become pregnant, and if planning to become pregnant should take 4 mg daily during the month before becoming pregnant until at least the 12th week of pregnancy.

ANEMIA: IRON DEFICIENCY (ADA)

Comment: Hemochromatosis and hemosiderosis are contraindications to iron therapy. **Iron** supplements are best absorbed when taken between meals and with **vitamin C**-rich foods. Excessive *iron* may be extremely hazardous to infants and young children. All vitamin and mineral supplements should be kept out of the reach of children. Untreated iron deficiency anemia (IDA) in pregnancy is associated with adverse maternal outcomes such as postpartum anemia. Adverse pregnancy outcomes associated with IDA include increased risk for preterm delivery and low birth weight.

IRON PREPARATIONS

▷ *ferrous gluconate* (A)(G) 1 tab once daily
   Pediatric: <12 years: not recommended; ≥12 years: same as adult
   Fergon (OTC)
      Tab: iron 27 mg (240 mg as gluconate)
▷ *ferric maltol* 30 mg twice daily on an empty stomach (1 hour before <u>or</u> 2 hours after a meal); continue as long as necessary to replenish body iron stores; do <u>not</u> open, break, <u>or</u> chew
   Pediatric: safety and efficacy not established
   Accrufer *Cap:* 30 mg

Comment: Accrufer *(ferric maltol)*, formerly **Feraccru**, is a non-salt formulation of ferric iron for the treatment of iron deficiency in adults. **Accrufer** is not absorbed systemically as an intact complex following oral administration. Maternal use in pregnancy is not expected to result in fetal exposure and breastfeeding is not expected to result in exposure of the infant.

▷ *ferrous sulfate* (A)(G)

Feosol Tablets (OTC) 1 tab tid-qid pc and HS
Pediatric: <6 years: use elixir; ≥6-12 years: 1 tab tid pc
  Tab: iron 65 mg (200 mg as sulfate)

Feosol Capsules (OTC) 1-2 caps daily
Pediatric: not recommended
  Cap: iron 50 mg (169 mg as sulfate) sust-rel

Feosol Elixir (OTC) 5-10 ml tid between meals
Pediatric: <1 year: not recommended; >1-11 year: 2.5-5 ml tid between meals; ≥12 years: same as adult
  Elix: iron 44 mg (220 mg as sulfate) per 5 ml

Fer-In-Sol (OTC) 5 ml daily
Pediatric: <4 years, use drops; ≥4 years: 5 ml once daily
  Syr: iron 18 mg (90 mg as sulfate) per 5 ml (480 ml)

Fer-In-Sol Drops (OTC)
Pediatric: <4 years: 0.6 ml daily; ≥4 years: use syrup
  Oral drops: iron 15 mg (75 mg as sulfate) per 5 ml (50 ml)

ANEMIA: PERNICIOUS/MEGALOBLASTIC

Comment: Signs of **vitamin B12** deficiency include megaloblastic anemia, glossitis, paresthesias, ataxia, spastic motor weakness, and reduced mentation.

▷ *vitamin B12 (cyanocobalamin)* (A)(G) 500 mcg intranasally once a week; may increase dose if serum B-12 levels decline; adjust dose in 500 mcg increments
Nascobal Nasal Spray *Intranasal gel:* 500 mcg/0.1 ml (1.3 ml, 4 doses) (citric acid, benzalkonium chloride)
Comment: **Nascobal Nasal Spray** is indicated for maintenance of hematologic remission following IM B-12 therapy without nervous system involvement. Must be primed before each use.

ANESTHESIA: PROCEDURAL SEDATION

▷ *remimazolam* individualize and titrate **Byfavo** to desired clinical effect; 2.5 mg to 5 mg IV over 1-minute; if necessary, administer supplemental doses of 1.25 mg to 2.5 mg IV over 15 seconds; wait at least 2 minutes before administration of any supplemental dose; may be administered only by a qualified HCP who is trained in the administration of conscious sedation, who is not involved in the conduct of the diagnostic or therapeutic procedure, in an appropriate healthcare setting, equipped with supportive and resuscitative supplies and equipment
Pediatric: <18 years: not recommended; ≥18 years: same as adult
Byfavo *Vial:* 20 mg, single-patient, pwdr for reconstitution and intravenous push (IVP) administration
Comment: **Byfavo** *(remimazolam)* is an ultra-short-acting intravenous *benzodiazepine* sedative/anesthetic for the induction and maintenance of procedural sedation in adults undergoing procedures lasting 30 minutes or less. The administering personnel must be trained in the detection and management of airway obstruction, hypoventilation, and apnea, including the maintenance of a patent airway, supportive ventilation, and cardiovascular resuscitation. **Byfavo** has been associated with hypoxia, bradycardia, and hypotension. Continuously monitor vital signs during sedation and through the recovery

period. Resuscitative drugs, and age- and size-appropriate equipment for bag/valve/mask-assisted ventilation must be immediately available during administration of **Byfavo**. Concomitant use of benzodiazepines with opioid analgesics may result in profound sedation, respiratory depression, coma, and death. The sedative effect of intravenous **Byfavo** can be accentuated by concomitantly administered CNS depressant medications, including other benzodiazepines and *propofol*. Continuously monitor patients for respiratory depression and depth of sedation. Sedating drugs, such as **Byfavo**, may cause confusion and over-sedation in the elderly; elderly patients generally should be observed closely. *Severe Hepatic Impairment:* reduced dosage may be indicated; titrate carefully to effect. Infants born to mothers using benzodiazepines during the later stages of pregnancy have been reported to experience symptoms of sedation. Although there are no data on the effects of **Byfavo** use in pregnant females, available data from published observational studies of pregnant females exposed to other benzodiazepines have not established a drug-associated risk of major birth defects, miscarriage, or adverse maternal or embryo/fetal outcomes. Breastfeeding females may pump and discard breast milk for 5 hours after treatment with **Byfavo**.

ANGINA PECTORIS: STABLE

▷ *aspirin* (D) 325 mg (range 75-325 mg) once daily
Comment: Daily *aspirin* dose is contingent upon whether the patient is also taking an anticoagulant or antiplatelet agent.

CALCIUM ANTAGONISTS

Comment: Calcium antagonists are contraindicated with history of ventricular arrhythmias, sick sinus syndrome, 2nd or 3rd degree heart block, cardiogenic shock, acute myocardial infarction, and pulmonary congestion.

▷ *amlodipine* (C)(G) 5-10 mg daily
Pediatric: <12 years: not recommended; ≥12 years: same as adult
Norvasc *Tab:* 2.5, 5, 10 mg

▷ *amlodipine benzoate* recommended starting dose 5 mg orally once daily; max 10 mg once daily; small stature, fragile, or elderly patients, or patients with hepatic insufficiency may be started on 2.5 mg once daily
Pediatric: <6 years: not studied; ≥6 years: starting dose: 2.5-5 mg once daily
Katerzia *Oral susp:* 1 mg/ml (150 ml), keep refrigerated
Comment: **Katerzia** *(amlodipine benzoate)* is a calcium channel blocker in an oral suspension formulation indicated for the treatment of hypertension in adults and children ≥6 years-of-age, to lower blood pressure. Lowering blood pressure reduces the risk of fatal and nonfatal cardiovascular events, primarily strokes and myocardial infarctions. **Katerzia** is also indicated for adult patients with Coronary Artery Disease (CAD), Chronic Stable Angina (CSA), Vasospastic Angina (Prinzmetal's or Variant Angina), Angiographically Documented Coronary Artery Disease in patients without heart failure or an ejection fraction <40%, at the same dose as for blood pressure management (2.5-10 mg once daily).

▷ *diltiazem* (C)(G)
Pediatric: <12 years: not recommended; ≥12 years: same as adult
Cardizem initially 30 mg qid; may increase gradually every 1-2 days; max 360 mg/day in divided doses
Tab: 30, 60, 90, 120 mg
Cardizem CD initially 120-180 mg daily; adjust at 1- to 2-week intervals; max 480 mg/day
Cap: 120, 180, 240, 300, 360 mg ext-rel

Cardizem LA initially 180-240 mg daily; titrate at 2 week intervals; max 540 mg/day

    Tab: 120, 180, 240, 300, 360, 420 mg ext-rel

Cartia XT initially 180 mg <u>or</u> 240 mg once daily; max 540 mg once daily

    Cap: 120, 180, 240, 300 mg ext-rel

Dilacor XR initially 180 mg <u>or</u> 240 mg once daily; max 540 mg once daily

    Cap: 180, 240 mg ext-rel

Tiazac initially 120-180 mg daily; max 540 mg/day

    Cap: 120, 180, 240, 300, 360, 420 mg ext-rel

▷ *nicardipine* (C)(G) initially 20 mg tid; adjust q 3 days; max 120 mg/day

Pediatric: not recommended

    Cardene *Cap:* 20, 30 mg

▷ *nifedipine* (C)(G)

Pediatric: <12 years: not recommended; ≥12 years: same as adult

Adalat CC initially 30 mg once daily; usual range 30-60 mg tid; max 90 mg/day

    Tab: 30, 60, 90 mg ext-rel

Procardia initially 10 mg tid; titrate over 7-14 days: max 30 mg/dose and 180 mg/day in divided doses

    Cap: 10, 20 mg

Procardia XL initially 30-60 mg daily; titrate over 7-14 days; max dose 90 mg/day

    Tab: 30, 60, 90 mg ext-rel

▷ *verapamil* (C)(G)

Pediatric: <12 years: not recommended; ≥12 years: same as adult

Calan 80-120 mg tid; increase daily <u>or</u> weekly if needed

    Tab: 40, 80*, 120*mg

Calan SR initially 120 mg once daily; increase weekly if needed

    Tab: 120, 180, 240 mg

Covera HS initially 180 mg q HS; titrate in steps to 240 mg; then to 360 mg; then to 480 mg if needed

    Tab: 180, 240 mg ext-rel

Isoptin SR initially 120-180 mg in the AM; may increase to 240 mg in the AM; then 180 mg q 12 hours <u>or</u> 240 mg in the AM and 120 mg in the PM; then 240 mg q 12 hours

    Tab: 120, 180*, 240*mg sust-rel

BETA-BLOCKERS

Comment: Beta-blockers are contraindicated with history of sick sinus syndrome (SSS), 2nd <u>or</u> 3rd degree heart block, cardiogenic shock, pulmonary congestion, asthma, moderate-to-severe COPD with FEV1 <50% predicted, patients with chronic bronchodilator treatment.

▷ *atenolol* (D)(G) initially 25-50 mg daily; increase weekly if needed; max 200 mg daily

Pediatric: <12 years: not recommended; ≥12 years: same as adult

Tenormin *Tab:* 25, 50, 100 mg

▷ *metoprolol succinate* (C)

Pediatric: <12 years: not recommended; ≥12 years: same as adult

    Toprol-XL initially 100 mg in a single dose once daily; increase weekly if needed; max 400 mg/day

    Tab: 25*, 50*, 100*, 200*mg ext-rel

▷ *metoprolol tartrate* (C)

Pediatric: <12 years: not recommended; ≥12 years: same as adult

    Lopressor (G) initially 25-50 mg bid; increase weekly if needed; max 400 mg/day

    Tab: 25, 37.5, 50, 75, 100 mg

▷ **nadolol** (C)(G) initially 40 mg daily; increase q 3-7 days; max 240 mg/day
  Pediatric: not recommended
    Corgard *Tab:* 20*, 40*, 80*, 120*, 160*mg
▷ **propranolol** (C)(G)
  Pediatric: <12 years: not recommended; ≥12 years: same as adult
    Inderal LA initially 80 mg daily in a single dose; increase q 3-7 days; usual
    range 120-160 mg/day; max 320 mg/day in a single dose
      Cap: 60, 80, 120, 160 mg sust-rel
    InnoPran XL initially 80 mg q HS; max 120 mg/day
      Cap: 80, 120 mg ext-rel

NITRATES

Comment: Use a daily nitrate dosing schedule that provides a dose-free period of
14 hours or more to prevent tolerance. *aspirin* and *acetaminophen* may relieve
nitrate-induced headache. *Isosorbide* is not recommended for use in MI and/or
CHF. Nitrate use is a contraindication for using phosphodiesterase type 5 inhibitors:
sildenafil (**Viagra**), *tadalafil* (**Cialis**), *vardenafil* (**Levitra**).
▷ **isosorbide dinitrate** (C)
  Pediatric: <12 years: not recommended; ≥12 years: same as adult
    Dilatrate-SR 40 mg once daily; max 160 mg/day
      Cap: 40 mg sust-rel
    Isordil Titradose initially 5-20 mg q 6 hours; maintenance 10-40 mg q 6 hours
      Tab: 5, 10, 20, 30, 40 mg
▷ **isosorbide mononitrate** (C)
  Pediatric: <12 years: not recommended; ≥12 years: same as adult
    Imdur initially 30-60 mg q AM; may increase to 120 mg daily; max 240 mg/
    day
      Tab: 30*, 60*, 120 mg ext-rel
    Ismo 20 mg upon awakening; then 20 mg 7 hours later
      Tab: 20*mg
▷ **nitroglycerin** (C)(G)
  Pediatric: <12 years: not recommended; ≥12 years: same as adult
    Nitro-Bid Ointment initially 1/2 inch q 8 hours; titrate in 1/2 inch increments
      Oint: 2% (20, 60 gm)
    Nitrodisc initially one 0.2-0.4 mg/Hr patch for 12-14 hours/day
      Transdermal disc: 0.2, 0.3, 0.4 mg/hour (30, 100/carton)
    Nitrolingual Pump Spray 1-2 sprays on or under tongue; max 3 sprays/15
    minutes
      Spray: 0.4 mg/dose (14.5 gm, 200 doses)
    Nitromist 1-2 sprays at onset of attack, on or under the tongue while sitting;
    may repeat q 5 minutes as needed; max 3 sprays/15 minutes; may use
    prophylactically 5-10 minutes prior to exertion; do not inhale spray; do not
    rinse mouth for 5-10 minutes after use
      Lingual aerosol spray: 0.4 mg/actuation (230 metered sprays)
    Nitrostat 1 tab SL; may repeat q 5 minutes x 3
      SL tab: 0.3 (1/100 gr), 0.4 (1/150 gr), 0.6 (1/4 gr) mg
    Transderm-Nitro initially one 0.2 mg/hour or 0.4 mg/hour patch for 12-14
    hours/day
      Transdermal patch: 0.1, 0.2, 0.4, 0.6, 0.8 mg/hour

NON-NITRATE PERIPHERAL VASODILATOR

▷ **hydralazine** (C)(G) initially 10 mg qid x 2-4 days; then increase to 25 mg qid for
remainder of first week; then increase to 50 mg qid; max 300 mg/day
  Pediatric: <12 years: not recommended; ≥12 years: same as adult
    Tab: 10, 25, 50, 100 mg

NITRATE+PERIPHERAL VASODILATOR COMBINATION

▶ *isosorbide+hydralazine HCl* (C) initially 1 tab tid; max 2 tabs tid
　Pediatric: <12 years: not established; ≥12 years: same as adult
　　Bidil *Tab:* isosorb 20 mg+hydral 37.5 mg

NON-NITRATE ANTI-ANGINAL

▶ *ranolazine* (C) initially 500 mg bid; may increase to max 1 gm bid
　Pediatric: <12 years: not recommended; ≥12 years: same as adult
　　Ranexa *Tab:* 500, 1000 mg ext-rel
　　Comment: **Ranexa** is indicated for the treatment chronic angina that is
　　inadequately controlled with other antianginals. Use with *amlodipine*, beta-
　　blocker, or nitrate.

ANOREXIA/CACHEXIA

APPETITE STIMULANTS

▶ *cyproheptadine* (B)(G) initially 4 mg tid prn; then adjust as needed; usual range
　12-16 mg/day; max 32 mg/day
　Pediatric: <2 years: not recommended; ≥2-6 years: 2 mg bid-tid prn; max 12 mg/
　day; 7-14 years: 4 mg bid-tid prn; max 16 mg/day; >14 years: same as adult
　　Periactin *Tab:* cypro 4*mg; *Syr:* cypro 2 mg/5 ml
▶ *dronabinol* (cannabinoid) (B)(III)
　Pediatric: safety and efficacy not established; younger patients may be more
　sensitive to neurological and psychoactive effects of *dronabinol;* **Syndros** contains
　dehydrated alcohol and 5.5% (w/w) propylene glycol; ethanol competitively
　inhibits the metabolism of propylene glycol, which may lead to elevated
　concentrations of propylene glycol; preterm neonates may be at increased
　risk of propylene glycol associated adverse events due to diminished ability to
　metabolize it, thereby, leading to accumulation; avoid use with preterm infants in
　the immediate postnatal period
　　Marinol initially 2.5 mg bid before lunch and dinner; may reduce to 2.5 mg q
　　HS or increase to 2.5 mg before lunch and 5 mg before dinner; max 20 mg/day
　　in divided doses
　　　Cap: 2.5, 5, 10 mg (sesame oil)
　　Syndros take each dose with 6-8 oz water
　　Anorexia/cachexia associated with weight loss in patients with AIDS: intially
　　2.1 mg twice daily 1 hour before lunch and dinner; if elderly, or severe or
　　persistent CNS effects occur, reduce dose to 2.1 mg once daily 1 hour before
　　dinner or at bedtime; if tolerated, may gradually increase to 2.1 mg 1 hour
　　before lunch and dinner or at bedtime as tolerated; max 8.4 mg twice daily
　　Nausea/vomiting associated with chemotherapy: recommended starting dosage
　　is 4.2 mg/m², administered 1 to 3 hours prior to chemotherapy; then, every 2
　　to 4 hours after chemotherapy for a total 4-6 doses/day; administer the first
　　dose on an empty stomach at least 30 minutes prior to eating; subsequent
　　doses can be taken without regard to meals
　　Oral soln: 5 mg/ml (50% w/w dehydrated alcohol, 5.5% w/w propylene glycol)
　　Comment: *Dronabinol* is contraindicated within 14 days before and 7 days
　　after taking *disulfiram* or *metronidazole. dronabinol* is highly protein-bound.
　　Therefore, there is potential for displacement of other drugs from plasma
　　proteins. Monitor for adverse reactions to concomitant narrow therapeutic index
　　drugs (e.g., *warfarin, cyclosporine, amphotericin B*) when initiating or increasing
　　the dosage of *dronabinol.* Delta-9-THC has been measured in the cord blood
　　of some infants whose mothers reported prenatal use of cannabis, suggesting
　　dronabinol may cross the placenta to the fetus during pregnancy. Effects of delta-
　　9-THC on the fetus are not known. There are limited data on the presence of

dronabinol in human milk and effects on the breastfed infant. The reported effects of inhaled cannabis transferred to the breastfeeding infant have been inconsistent and insufficient to establish causality. Because of the possible adverse effects from *dronabanol* on the breastfed infant, advise females with nausea/vomiting associated with cancer chemotherapy not to breastfeed during treatment with *dronabinol* and for 9 days after the last chemotherapy dose.

▷ *megestrol* (progestin) (X)(G) 40 mg qid
Pediatric: <12 years: not recommended; ≥12 years: same as adult
  Megace *Tab:* 20*, 40*mg
  Megace ES *Oral susp (concentrate):* 125 mg/ml; 625 mg/5 ml (5 oz) (lemon-lime)
  Megace Oral Suspension *Oral susp:* 40 mg/ml (8 oz); 820 mg/20 ml) (lemon-lime)
  Megestrol Acetate Oral Suspension (G) 125 mg/ml
  Comment: *Megestrol* is indicated for the treatment of anorexia, cachexia, or an unexplained, significant weight loss in patients with a diagnosis of AIDS.

 ANTHRAX (*BACILLUS ANTHRACIS*)

POSTEXPOSURE PROPHYLAXIS OF INHALATIONAL ANTHRAX AND TREATMENT OF INHALED AND CUTANEOUS ANTHRAX INFECTION

Comment: *B. anthracis* spores are resistant to destruction, are easily spread by release into the air, and cause irreversible tissue damage and death. The most lethal form is inhalational anthrax. Even with the most aggressive treatment, the mortality rate is about 45%. People at risk are those who work in slaughterhouses, tanneries, and wood mills who are exposed to infected animals.

Comment: All 14 members of the Advisory Committee on Immunization Practices (ACIP) voted to approve the anthrax vaccine recommendations for 2018-2019 at their meeting. The recommendations to the committee sought to optimize the use of Anthrax Vaccine Adsorbed (AVA) in postexposure prophylaxis (PEP) in the event of a wide-area release of *B anthracis* spores. In this event, a mass vaccination effort would be undertaken, requiring expedited administration of AVA. ACIP now recommends that the intramuscular administration may be used over the traditional subcutaneous approach if there are any operational or logistical challenges that delay effective vaccination. Another recommendation from ACIP would allow two full-doses or three half-doses of AVA to be used to expand vaccine coverage for PEP in the event there is an inadequate vaccine supply. The committee also recommended that AbxPEP, an antimicrobial, be stopped 42 days after the first dose of AVA or 2 weeks after the last dose. The committee's recommendations will be used by the CDC to inform state and local health departments to better prepare for an emergency response to a wide-area release of *B anthracis* spores. The committee's recommendations must be approved by the CDC's director before they are considered official recommendations.

Immune Globulin

▷ *bacillus anthracis immune globulin intravenous (human)* administer via IV infusion at a maximum rate of 2 ml/min; dose is weight-based as follows, but may be doubled in severe cases if weight >5 kg:
Pediatric: <16 years: not established; 5-<10 kg: 1 vial; 10-<18 kg: 2 vials; 18-<25 kg: 3 vials; 25-<35 kg: 4 vials; 35-<50 kg: 5 vials; 50-<60 kg: 6 vials; ≥60 kg: 7 vials
  Anthrasil *Vial:* (60 units) sterile solution of purified human immune globulin gm (IgG) containing polyclonal antibodies that target the anthrax toxins of *Bacillus anthracis* for IV infusion
  Comment: **Anthrasil** is indicated for the emergent treatment of inhaled anthrax, in combination with appropriate antibacterial agents

MONOCLONAL ANTIBODIES

Comment: *Obiltoxaximab* and *raxibacumab* have no antibacterial activity; rather, they are monoclonal antibodies that neutralize toxins produced by *B. anthracis* by binding to the bacterium's protective antigen, preventing intracellular entry of key enzymatic toxin components. *Obiltoxaximab* (**Anthim**) and *raxibacumab* are indicated for treatment of inhalational anthrax, in combination with appropriate antibacterial drugs, and for prophylaxis of inhalational anthrax when alternative therapies are unavailable or inappropriate. Vials must be refrigerated and protected from light. Do not shake the vials. Pre-medicate the patient with *diphenhydramine*.

▷ *obiltoxaximab* 16 mg/kg diluted in 0.9% NS via IV infusion over 90 minutes
   Pediatric: see mfr pkg insert for dosing based on kilograms body weight
      Anthim *Vial:* 600 mg in 6 ml (100 mg/ml) single-use, for dilution in 0.9% NS
      and IV infusion

▷ *raxibacumab* (B)(G) 40 mg/kg diluted in 0.45% NS or 0.9% NS via IV infusion
   over 2 hours and 15 minutes; see mfr pkg insert for recommended volume of
   dilution according to weight-based dose
   Pediatric: ≤15 kg: 80 mg/kg; >15-50 kg: 60 mg/kg; >50 kg: same as adult
      Vial: 1700 mg/34 ml (50 mg/ml), single-use, for dilution and IV infusion

ANTIBACTERIAL AGENTS

▷ *ciprofloxacin* (C) 500 mg (or 10-15 mg/kg/day) q 12 hours for 60 days (start as
   soon as possible after exposure)
   Pediatric: <18 years: 20-40 mg/kg/day divided q 12 hours; ≥18 years: same as
   adult
      Cipro (G) *Tab:* 250, 500, 750 mg; *Oral susp:* 250, 500 mg/5 ml (100 ml)
      (strawberry)
      Cipro XR *Tab:* 500, 1000 mg ext-rel
      ProQuin XR *Tab:* 500 mg ext-rel
   Comment: *Ciprofloxacin* is usually contraindicated <18 years-of-age, and during
   pregnancy and lactation, a fluoroquinolone. Risk/benefit must be assessed in the
   case of anthrax.

▷ *doxycycline* (D)(G) 100 mg daily bid
   Pediatric: <8 years: usually contraindicated ≥8 years, <100 lb: 2 mg/lb on first day
   in 2 divided doses, followed by 1 mg/lb/day in a single or divided doses; ≥8 years,
   ≥100 lb: same as adult; *see Appendix CC.19. doxycycline* (Vibramycin Syrup/
   Suspension) *for dose by weight*
      Acticlate *Tab:* 75, 150**mg
      Adoxa *Tab:* 50, 75, 100, 150 mg ent-coat
      Doryx *Tab:* 50, 75, 100, 150, 200 mg del-rel
      Doxteric *Tab:* 50 mg del-rel
      Monodox *Cap:* 50, 75, 100 mg
      Oracea *Cap:* 40 mg del-rel
      Vibramycin *Tab:* 100 mg; *Cap:* 50, 100 mg; *Syr:* 50 mg/5 ml (raspberry-apple)
      (sulfites); *Oral susp:* 25 mg/5 ml (raspberry)
      Vibra-Tab *Tab:* 100 mg film-coat
   Comment: *Doxycycline,* a tetracycline, is usually contraindicated <8 years-of-age,
   in pregnancy, and lactation (discolors developing tooth enamel). Risk/benefit
   must be assessed in the case of anthrax.

▷ *minocycline* (D)(G) 2 mg/lb on first day in 2 divided doses, followed by 1 mg/lb
   every 12 hours x 9 more days; ≥8 years, >100 mg: 100 mg every 12 hours
   Pediatric: usually not recommended; ≥8 years, <100 lb: same as adult
      Dynacin *Cap:* 50, 100 mg
      Minocin *Cap:* 50, 75, 100 mg; *Oral susp:* 50 mg/5 ml (60 ml) (custard)
      (sulfites, alcohol 5%)

Comment: *Minocycline,* a tetracycline, is usually contraindicated <8 years-of-age, in pregnancy, and lactation (discolors developing tooth enamel). Risk/benefit must be assessed in the case of anthrax.

TREATMENT OF GI AND OROPHARYNGEAL ANTHRAX

▷ *ciprofloxacin* (C) 400 mg IV q 12 hours (start as soon as possible); then, switch to 500 mg PO q 12 hours for total 60 days; infuse dose over 60 minutes
Pediatric: <18 years: usually not recommended; 10-15 mg/kg IV q 12 hours (start as soon as possible); then switch to 10-15 mg/kg PO q 12 hours for 60 days
  Cipro (G) *Tab:* 250, 500, 750 mg; *Oral susp:* 250, 500 mg/5 ml (100 ml) (strawberry); *IV conc:* 10 mg/ml after dilution (20, 40 ml); *IV premix:* 2 mg/ml (100, 200 ml)
  Cipro XR *Tab:* 500, 1000 mg ext-rel
  ProQuin XR *Tab:* 500 mg ext-rel
  Comment: *Ciprofloxacin* is usually contraindicated <18 years-of-age, and during pregnancy and lactation, a fluoroquinolone, risk/benefit must be assessed in the case of anthrax.

▷ *doxycycline* (D)(G) 100 mg daily bid
Pediatric: <8 years: not recommended ≥8 years, <100 lb: 2 mg/lb on first day in 2 divided doses, followed by 1 mg/lb/day in a single or divided doses; ≥8 years, ≥100 lb: same as adult; *see Appendix CC.19. doxycycline* (Vibramycin Syrup/ Suspension) *for dose by weight*
  Acticlate *Tab:* 75, 150**mg
  Adoxa *Tab:* 50, 75, 100, 150 mg ent-coat
  Doryx *Tab:* 50, 75, 100, 150, 200 mg del-rel
  Doxteric *Tab:* 50 mg del-rel
  Monodox *Cap:* 50, 75, 100 mg
  Oracea *Cap:* 40 mg del-rel
  Vibramycin *Tab:* 100 mg; *Cap:* 50, 100 mg; *Syr:* 50 mg/5 ml (raspberry-apple) (sulfites); *Oral susp:* 25 mg/5 ml (raspberry)
  Vibra-Tab *Tab:* 100 mg film-coat
  Comment: *Doxycycline* is usually contraindicated <8 years-of-age, in pregnancy, and lactation, a tetracycline, risk/benefit must be assessed in the case of anthrax.

▷ *minocycline* (D)(G) 100 mg q 12 hours
Pediatric: <8 years: usually not recommended; ≥8 years, <100 lb: 2 mg/lb on first day in 2 divided doses, followed by 1 mg/lb q 12 hours x 9 more days; ≥8 years, ≥100 lb: same as adult
  Dynacin *Cap:* 50, 100 mg
  Minocin *Cap:* 50, 75, 100 mg; *Oral susp:* 50 mg/5 ml (60 ml) (custard) (sulfites, alcohol 5%)
  Comment: *Minocycline* is usually contraindicated <8 years-of-age, in pregnancy, and lactation, a tetracycline, risk/benefit must be assessed in the case of anthrax.

ANXIETY DISORDER: GENERALIZED (GAD), ANXIETY DISORDER: SOCIAL (SAD)

FIRST GENERATION ORAL ANTIHISTAMINES

▷ *diphenhydramine* (B)(G) 25-50 mg q 6-8 hours; max 100 mg/day
Pediatric: <2 years: not recommended; 2-6 years: 6.25 mg q 4-6 hours; max 37.5 mg/day; >6-12 years: 12.5-25 mg q 4-6 hours; max 150 mg/day; ≥12 years: same as adult
  Benadryl (OTC) *Chew tab:* 12.5 mg (grape) (phenylalanine); *Liq:* 12.5 mg/5 ml (4, 8 oz); *Cap:* 25 mg; *Tab:* 25 mg; *Dye-free soft gel:* 25 mg; *Dye-free liq:* 12.5 mg/5 ml (4, 8 oz)

▷ *hydroxyzine* (C)(G) 50-100 mg qid; max 600 mg/day
   Pediatric: <6 years: 50 mg/day divided qid; ≥6 years: 50-100 mg/day divided qid
    Atarax *Tab:* 10, 25, 50, 100 mg; *Syr:* 10 mg/5 ml (alcohol 0.5%)
    Vistaril *Cap:* 25, 50, 100 mg; *Oral susp:* 25 mg/5 ml (4 oz) (lemon)
   Comment: *Hydroxyzine* is contraindicated in early pregnancy and in patients
with a prolonged QT interval. It is not known whether this drug is excreted in
human milk; therefore, *hydroxyzine* should not be given to nursing mothers.

AZAPIRONE

▷ *buspirone* (B) initially 7.5 mg bid; may increase by 5 mg/day q 2-3 days; max 60
mg/day
   Pediatric: <6 years: not recommended; ≥6 years: same as adult
    BuSpar *Tab:* 5, 10, 15*, 30*mg

BENZODIAZEPINES

Comment: If possible when considering a benzodiazepine to treat anxiety, a
short-acting benzodiazepines should be used only prn to avert intense anxiety
and panic for the least time necessary while a different non-addictive antianxiety
regimen (e.g., SSRI, SNRI, TCA, *buspirone*, and beta-blocker) is established
and effective treatment goals achieved. Benzodiazepines have a high addiction
potential when they are chronically used and are common drugs of abuse.
Benzodiazepine withdrawal syndrome may include restlessness, agitation, anxiety,
insomnia, tachycardia, tachypnea, diaphoresis, and may be potentially life
threatening, depending on the benzodiazepine and the length of use. Symptoms
of withdrawal from short-acting benzodiazepines, such as *alprazolam* (Xanax),
oxazepam, *lorazepam* (Ativan), *triazolam* (Halcion), usually appear within 6-8
hours after the last dose and may continue 10-14 days. Symptoms of withdrawal
from long-acting benzodiazepines, such as *diazepam* (Valium), *clonazepam*
(Klonopin), *chlordiazepoxide* (Librium), usually appear within 24-96 hours
after the last dose and may continue from 3-4 weeks to 3 months. People who are
heavily dependent on benzodiazepines may experience *protracted withdrawal
syndrome* (PAWS), random periods of sharp withdrawal symptoms months after
quitting. A closely monitored medical detoxification regimen may be required for
a safe withdrawal and to prevent PAWS. Detoxification includes gradual tapering
of the benzodiazepine along with other medications to manage the withdrawal
symptoms.

Short-Acting Benzodiazepines

▷ *alprazolam* (D)(IV)(G)
   Pediatric: <18 years: not recommended; ≥18 years:
    Niravam initially 0.25-0.5 mg tid; may titrate every 3-4 days; max 4 mg/day
     Tab: 0.25*, 0.5*, 1*, 2*mg orally-disint
    Xanax initially 0.25-0.5 mg tid; may titrate every 3-4 days; max 4 mg/day
     Tab: 0.25*, 0.5*, 1*, 2*mg
    Xanax XR initially 0.5-1 mg once daily, preferably in the AM; increase at
    intervals of at least 3-4 days by up to 1 mg/day. Taper no faster than 0.5 mg
    every 3 days; max 10 mg/day. When switching from immediate-release
    alprazolam, give total daily dose of immediate-release once daily.
     Tab: 0.5, 1, 2, 3 mg ext-rel
▷ *oxazepam* (C)(IV)(G) 10-15 mg tid-qid for moderate symptoms; 15-30 mg tid-
qid for severe symptoms
   Pediatric: <12 years: not recommended; ≥12 years: same as adult
   Cap: 10, 15, 30 mg

Intermediate-Acting Benzodiazepines

▷ *lorazepam* (D)(IV)(G) 1-10 mg/day in 2-3 divided doses
  Pediatric: <12 years: not recommended; ≥12 years: same as adult
     Ativan *Tab:* 0.5, 1*, 2*mg
     Lorazepam Intensol *Oral conc:* 2 mg/ml (30 ml w. graduated dropper)

Long-Acting Benzodiazepines

▷ *chlordiazepoxide* (D)(IV)(G)
  Pediatric: <6 years: not recommended; ≥6 years: 5 mg bid-qid; increase to 10 mg
  bid-tid
     Librium 5-10 mg tid-qid for moderate symptoms; 20-25 mg tid-qid for severe
     symptoms
        Cap: 5, 10, 25 mg
     Librium Injectable 50-100 mg IM or IV; then 25-50 mg IM tid-qid prn; max
     300 mg/day
        Inj: 100 mg
▷ *chlordiazepoxide+clidinium* (D)(IV) 1-2 caps tid-qid: max 8 caps/day
  Pediatric: not recommended
     Librax *Cap:* chlor 5 mg+clid 2.5 mg
▷ *clonazepam* (D)(IV)(G) initially 0.25 mg bid; increase to 1 mg/day after 3 days
  Pediatric: <18 years: not recommended; ≥18 years: same as adult
     Klonopin *Tab:* 0.5*, 1, 2 mg
     Klonopin Wafers dissolve in mouth with or without water
        Wafer: 0.125, 0.25, 0.5, 1, 2 mg orally-disint
▷ *clorazepate* (D)(IV)(G) 30 mg/day in divided doses; max 60 mg/day
  Pediatric: <9 years: not recommended; ≥9 years: same as adult
     Tranxene *Tab:* 3.75, 7.5, 15 mg
     Tranxene SD do not use for initial therapy
        Tab: 22.5 mg ext-rel
     Tranxene SD Half Strength do not use for initial therapy
        Tab: 11.25 mg ext-rel
     Tranxene T-Tab *Tab:* 3.75*, 7.5*, 15*mg
▷ *diazepam* (D)(IV)(G) 2-10 mg bid to qid
  Pediatric: <12 years: not recommended; ≥12 years: same as adult
     Diastat *Rectal gel delivery system:* 2.5 mg
     Diastat AcuDial *Rectal gel delivery system:* 10, 20 mg
     Valium *Tab:* 2*, 5*, 10*mg
     Valium Injectable *Vial:* 5 mg/ml (10 ml); *Amp:* 5 mg/ml (2 ml); *Prefilled
     syringe:* 5 mg/ml (5 ml)
     Valium Intensol Oral Solution *Conc oral soln:* 5 mg/ml (30 ml w. dropper)
     (alcohol 19%)
     Valium Oral Solution *Oral soln:* 5 mg/5 ml (500 ml) (wintergreen spice)

TRICYCLIC ANTIDEPRESSANTS (TCAs)

Comment: Co-administration of TCAs with SSRIs requires extreme caution.
▷ *amitriptyline* (C)(G) 10-20 mg q HS
  Pediatric: <12 years: not recommended; ≥12 years: same as adult
     Tab: 10, 25, 50, 75, 100, 150 mg
▷ *amoxapine* (C) initially 50 mg bid-tid; after 1 week may increase to 100 mg bid-
  tid; usual effective dose 200-300 mg/day; if total dose exceeds 300 mg/day, give in
  divided doses (max 400 mg/day); may give as a single bedtime dose (max 300 mg
  q HS)
  Pediatric: <12 years: not recommended; ≥12 years: same as adult
     Tab: 25, 50, 100, 150 mg

▷ *clomipramine* (C)(G) initially 25 mg daily in divided doses; gradually increase to 100 mg during first 2 weeks; max 250 mg/day; total maintenance dose may be given at HS
Pediatric: <10 years: not recommended; 10-<16 years: initially 25 mg daily in divided doses; gradually increase; max 3 mg/kg or 100 mg, whichever is smaller; ≥16 years: same as adult
    Anafranil *Cap:* 25, 50, 75 mg

▷ *desipramine* (C)(G) 100-200 mg/day in single or divided doses; max 300 mg/day
Pediatric: <12 years: not recommended; ≥12 years: same as adult
    Norpramin *Tab:* 10, 25, 50, 75, 100, 150 mg

▷ *doxepin* (C)(G) usual optimum dose 75-150 mg/day; elderly lower initial dose and therapeutic dose; max single dose 150 mg; max 300 mg/day in divided doses
Pediatric: <12 years: not recommended; ≥12 years: same as adult
    Sinequan
    Cap: 10, 25, 50, 75, 100, 150 mg; *Oral conc:* 10 mg/ml (4 oz w. dropper)
Comment: Glaucoma, urinary retention, and bipolar disorder are contraindications to *doxepin*. Separate from MAOIs by at least 14 days. Separate from *fluoxetine* by at least 5 weeks. Avoid abrupt cessation. *doxepin* is potentiated by CYP2D6 inhibitors (e.g., *cimetidine*, SSRIs, phenothiazines, type 1C antiarrhythmics).

▷ *imipramine* (C)(G)
Pediatric: <12 years: not recommended; ≥12 years: same as adult
Tofranil initially 75 mg daily (max 200 mg); adolescents initially 30-40 mg daily (max 100 mg/day); if maintenance dose exceeds 75 mg daily, may switch to **Tofranil PM** for divided or bedtime dose
    Tab: 10, 25, 50 mg
Tofranil PM initially 75 mg daily 1 hour before HS; max 200 mg
    Cap: 75, 100, 125, 150 mg

▷ *nortriptyline* (D)(G) initially 25 mg tid-qid; max 150 mg/day
Pediatric: <12 years: not recommended; ≥12 years: same as adult
    Pamelor *Cap:* 10, 25, 50, 75 mg; *Oral soln:* 10 mg/5 ml (16 oz)

▷ *protriptyline* (C) initially 5 mg tid; usual dose 15-40 mg/day in 3-4 divided doses; max 60 mg/day
Pediatric: <12 years: not recommended; ≥12 years: same as adult
    Vivactil *Tab:* 5, 10 mg

▷ *trimipramine* (C) initially 75 mg/day in divided doses; max 200 mg/day
Pediatric: <12 years: not recommended; ≥12 years: same as adult
    Surmontil *Cap:* 25, 50, 100 mg

PHENOTHIAZINES

▷ *prochlorperazine* (C)(G)
Pediatric: <12 years: not recommended; ≥12 years: same as adult
    Compazine 5 mg tid-qid
        Tab: 5 mg; *Syr:* 5 mg/5 ml (4 oz) (fruit); *Rectal supp:* 2.5, 5, 25 mg
    Compazine Spansule 15 mg q AM or 10 mg q 12 hours
        Spansule: 10, 15 mg sust-rel

▷ *trifluoperazine* (C)(G) 1-2 mg bid; max 6 mg/day; max 12 weeks
Pediatric: <12 years: not recommended; ≥12 years: same as adult
    Stelazine *Tab:* 1, 2, 5, 10 mg

SELECTIVE SEROTONIN REUPTAKE INHIBITORS (SSRIs)

Comment: Co-administration of SSRIs with TCAs requires extreme caution. Concomitant use of MAOIs and SSRIs is absolutely contraindicated. Avoid St. John's wort and other serotonergic agents. A potentially fatal adverse event is *serotonin syndrome*, caused by serotonin excess. Milder symptoms require HCP intervention to avert severe symptoms that can be rapidly fatal without urgent/emergent medical care. Symptoms include restlessness, agitation, confusion, tachycardia, hypertension, dilated pupils, muscle twitching, muscle rigidity, loss of muscle coordination, diaphoresis, diarrhea, headache, shivering, piloerection, hyperpyrexia, cardiac arrhythmias, seizures, loss of consciousness, coma, and death. Common symptoms of the *serotonin discontinuation syndrome* include flu-like symptoms (nausea, vomiting, diarrhea, headaches, diaphoresis); sleep disturbances (insomnia, nightmares, constant sleepiness); mood disturbances (dysphoria, anxiety, agitation); cognitive disturbances (mental confusion, hyperarousal); and sensory and movement disturbances (imbalance, tremors, vertigo, dizziness, electric-shock-like sensations in the brain often described by sufferers as "brain zaps").

➤ *citalopram* (C)(G) initially 20 mg once daily; may increase after week to 40 mg once daily; max 40 mg
  Pediatric: 12 years: not recommended; ≥12 years: same as adult
    Celexa *Tab:* 10, 20, 40 mg; *Oral soln:* 10 mg/5 ml (120 ml) (peppermint) (sugar-free, alcohol-free, parabens)

➤ *escitalopram* (C)(G) initially 10 mg daily; may increase to 20 mg daily after 1 week; *Elderly* or hepatic impairment, 10 mg once daily
  Pediatric: <12 years: not recommended; 12-17 years: initially 10 mg once daily; may increase to 20 mg once daily after 3 weeks
    Lexapro *Tab:* 5, 10*, 20*mg
    Lexapro Oral Solution *Oral soln:* 1 mg/ml (240 ml) (peppermint) (parabens)

➤ *fluoxetine* (C)(G)
    Prozac initially 20 mg daily; may increase after 1 week; doses >20 mg/day may be divided into AM and noon doses; max 80 mg/day
    Pediatric: <8 years: not recommended; 8-17 years: initially 10-20 mg once daily; start lower weight children at 10 mg once daily; if starting at 10 mg once daily, may increase after 1 week to 20 mg once daily
      Cap: 10, 20, 40 mg; *Tab:* 30*, 60*mg; *Oral soln:* 20 mg/5 ml (4 oz) (mint)
    Prozac Weekly following daily *fluoxetine* therapy at 20 mg/day x 13 weeks, may initiate **Prozac Weekly** 7 days after the last 20 mg *fluoxetine* dose
    Pediatric: <12 years: not recommended; ≥12 years: same as adult
      Cap: 90 mg ent-coat del-rel pellets

➤ *paroxetine maleate* (D)(G)
  Pediatric: <12 years: not recommended; ≥12 years: same as adult
    Paxil initially 10-20 mg daily in AM; may increase by 10 mg/day at weekly intervals as needed; max 60 mg/day
      Tab: 10*, 20*, 30, 40 mg
    Paxil CR initially 12.5-25 mg daily in AM; may increase by 12.5 mg at weekly intervals as needed; max 62.5 mg/day
      Tab: 12.5, 25, 37.5 mg ent-coat cont-rel
    Paxil Suspension initially 10-20 mg daily in AM; may increase by 10 mg/day at weekly intervals as needed; max 60 mg/day
      Oral susp: 10 mg/5 ml (250 ml) (orange)

➤ *paroxetine mesylate* (D)(G) initially 7.5 mg daily in AM; may increase by 10 mg/day at weekly intervals as needed; max 60 mg/day
  Pediatric: <12 years: not recommended; ≥12 years: same as adult
    Brisdelle *Cap:* 7.5 mg

➤ *sertraline* (C) initially 50 mg daily; increase at 1 week intervals if needed; max 200 mg daily
  Pediatric: <6 years: not recommended; 6-12 years: initially 25 mg daily; max 200 mg/day; 13-17 years: initially 50 mg daily; max 200 mg/day
    Zoloft *Tab:* 15*, 50*, 100*mg; *Oral conc:* 20 mg per ml (60 ml [dilute just before administering in 4 oz water, ginger ale, lemon-lime soda, lemonade, or orange juice]) (alcohol 12%)

SEROTONIN-NOREPINEPHRINE REUPTAKE INHIBITORS (SNRIs)

▷ *desvenlafaxine* (C)(G) swallow whole; initially 50 mg once daily; max 120 mg/day
  Pediatric: <18 years: not recommended; ≥18 years: same as adult
    Pristiq *Tab:* 50, 100 mg ext-rel

▷ *duloxetine* (C)(G) swallow whole; initially 30 mg once daily x 1 week; then,
  increase to 60 mg once daily; max 120 mg/day
  Pediatric: <12 years: not recommended; ≥12 years: same as adult
    Cymbalta *Cap:* 20, 30, 40, 60 mg del-rel

▷ *venlafaxine* (C)(G)
    Effexor initially 75 mg/day in 2-3 divided doses; may increase at 4-day
    intervals in 75 mg increments to 150 mg/day; max 225 mg/day
    Pediatric: <18 years: not recommended; ≥18 years: same as adult
      Tab: 37.5, 75, 150, 225 mg

    Effexor XR initially 75 mg q AM; may start at 37.5 mg daily x 4-7 days; then
    increase by increments of up to 75 mg/day at intervals of at least 4 days; usual
    max 375 mg/day
    Pediatric: <18 years: not recommended; ≥18 years: same as adult
      Tab: Cap: 37.5, 75, 150 mg ext-rel

COMBINATION AGENTS

▷ *chlordiazepoxide+amitriptyline* (D)(G)
  Pediatric: <12 years: not recommended; ≥12 years: same as adult
    Limbitrol 3-4 tabs/day in divided doses
      Tab: chlor 5 mg+amit 12.5 mg
    Limbitrol DS 3-4 tabs/day in divided doses; max 6 tabs/day
      Tab: chlor 10 mg+amit 25 mg

▷ *perphenazine+amitriptyline* (C)(G) 1 tab bid-qid
  Pediatric: <12 years: not recommended; ≥12 years: same as adult
    Tab: **Etrafon 2-10** perph 2 mg+amit 10 mg
      Etrafon 2-25 perph 2 mg+amit 25 mg
      Etrafon 4-25 perph 4 mg+amit 25 mg

ⓘ APHASIA, EXPRESSIVE: STROKE-INDUCED

Comment: In a case report published in NEJM, a 52-year-old right-handed woman who sustained an ischemic stroke 3 years prior, the areas of infarction included the left insula, putamen, and superior temporal gyrus. Her stroke resulted in expressive aphasia, leaving her with no intelligible words, but with intact full language comprehension. *zolpidem* 10 mg was prescribed for insomnia. In repeated measures, it was found that the patient consistently demonstrated dramatic speech improvement, durable until HS, and return of the expressive aphasia in the AM. Subsequent single-photon-emission computed tomography (SPECT) scanning of this patient indicated that *zolpidem* increases flow in the Broca area of the brain, an area intimately involved with speech. From these observations, the authors concluded that a select subgroup of patients with aphasia, perhaps with subcortical lesions and spared but hypometabolic cortical structures, might benefit from this treatment. It may be worth trying *zolpidem* in patients who have been labeled with otherwise refractory chronic expressive aphasia. This finding raises the questions, could this intervention help patients earlier in the course, patients with milder disease, <u>and/or</u> patients with other ischemic central nervous system syndromes?

▷ *zolpidem* oral solution spray (imidazopyridine hypnotic) (C)(IV)(G) 2 actuations
  (10 mg) immediately before bedtime; *Elderly, debilitated,* <u>or</u> *hepatic impairment:* 2
  actuations (5 mg); max 2 actuations (10 mg)

Pediatric: <18 years: not recommended; ≥18 years: same adult

ZolpiMist *Oral soln spray:* 5 mg/actuation (60 metered actuations) (cherry)
Comment: The lowest dose of *zolpidem* in all forms is recommended for persons >50 years-of-age and women as drug elimination is slower than in men.

▷ *zolpidem* tabs (pyrazolopyrimidine hypnotic) **(B)(IV)(G)** 5-10 mg or 6.25-12.5 extrel q HS prn; max 12.5 mg/day x 1 month; do not take if unable to sleep for at least 8 hours before required to be active again; delayed effect if taken with a meal
Pediatric: <18 years: not recommended; ≥18 years: same adult

Ambien *Tab:* 5, 10 mg
Ambien CR *Tab:* 6.25, 12.5 mg ext-rel
Comment: The lowest dose of *zolpidem* in all forms is recommended for persons >50 years-of-age and women as drug elimination is slower than in men.

▷ *zolpidem* sublingual tabs **(C)(IV)** (imidazopyridine hypnotic) dissolve 1 tab under the tongue; allow to disintegrate completely before swallowing; take only once per night and only if at least 4 hours of bedtime remain before planned time for awakening
Pediatric: <18 years: not recommended; ≥18 years: same adult

Edluar *SL Tab:* 5, 10 mg
Intermezzo *SL Tab:* 1.75, 3.5 mg
Comment: **Edluar** is indicated for the treatment of insomnia when a middle-of-the-night awakening is followed by difficulty returning to sleep. The lowest dose of *zolpidem* in all forms is recommended for persons >50 years-of-age and women as drug elimination is slower than in men.

APHTHOUS STOMATITIS (MOUTH ULCER, CANKER SORE)

Comment: Aphthous ulcers are very painful sores with an inflamed base and non-viable tissue in the center that appears bacterial or viral. Although the sores are usually neither bacterial nor viral, herpetiform ulcers are most prevalent among the elderly). The sores may be single round/ovoid or several may be coalesced to form larger lesions, and located under the lip, on the buccal membrane, and/or on the tongue. Poor oral hygiene or an underlying immunity impairment can predispose the patient to ulcer formation (e.g., chronic illness, chemotherapy, poor nutrition, vitamin and mineral deficiencies, allergies, local trauma, stress, tobacco use, and inflammatory bowel disease). They are frequently the result of local trauma (e.g., orthodontic-ware, chipped tooth) or allergy/irritation to a toothpaste or mouthwash ingredient (e.g. sodium lauryl sulfate). Changing toothpaste and applying dental wax to sharp edges are recommended until dental care is accessed. Debridement of the nonviable tissue by the direct application of salt (osmotic pulling pressure) for a few minutes, thus leaving a healthy tissue crater, speeds healing. Relief of the offending source of tissue trauma and application of a 5 mg prednisone tablet directly to the debrided ulcer are other remedies with reported success. These sores usually first appear in childhood or adolescence. Family history may have a role in the formation of recurrent aphthous stomatitis (RAS). When cases tend to occur in the same family (est 25-40% of the time), the ulcers are earlier and with greater severity.

ANTI-INFLAMMATORY AGENTS

▷ *dexamethasone* elixir **(B)** 5 ml swish and spit q 12 hours
Pediatric: <12 years: not recommended; ≥12 years: same as adult
Elix: 0.5 mg/ml

▷ *triamcinolone acetonide* 0.1% dental paste **(G)** press (do not rub) a thin film onto lesion at bedtime and, if needed, 2-3 x daily after meals; re-evaluate if no improvement in 7 days
Pediatric: <12 years: not recommended; ≥12 years: same as adult
Oralone *Dental paste:* 0.1% (5 gm)

▷ *triamcinolone* 1% in **Orabase (B)** apply 1/4 inch to each ulcer bid-qid until ulcer heals

 Pediatric: <12 years: not recommended; ≥12 years: same as adult

  Kenalog in Orabase *Crm:* 1% (15, 60, 80 gm)

TOPICAL ANESTHETICS

▷ *benzocaine* topical gel **(C)(G)** apply tid-qid

▷ *benzocaine* topical spray **(C)(G)** 1 spray to painful area every 2 hours as needed; retain for 15 seconds, then spit

  Cepacol Spray (OTC), Chloraseptic Spray (OTC)

▷ *lidocaine* viscous soln **(B)(G)** 15 ml gargle <u>or</u> swish, then spit; repeat after 3 hours; max 8 doses/day

 Pediatric: <3 years: not recommended; 3-11 years: 1.25 ml; apply with cotton-tipped applicator; may repeat after 3 hours; max 8 doses/day; ≥12 years: same as adult

  Xylocaine Viscous Solution *Viscous soln:* 2% (20, 100, 450 ml)

▷ *triamcinolone* **(Kenalog)** in **Orabase (C)** apply with swab

DEBRIDING AGENT/CLEANSER

▷ *carbamide peroxide 10%* **(OTC)** apply 10 drops to affected area; swish x 2-3 minutes, then spit; do <u>not</u> rinse; repeat treatment qid

 Pediatric: <3 years: not recommended; ≥3 years: same as adult

  Gly-Oxide *Liq:* 10% (50, 60 ml squeeze bottle w. applicator)

ANTI-INFECTIVES

▷ *minocycline* **(D)(G)** swish and spit 10 ml susp (50 mg/5 ml) <u>or</u> 1 x 100 mg cap <u>or</u> 2 x 50 mg caps dissolved in 180 ml water, bid x 4-5 days

 Pediatric: <8 years: not recommended; ≥8 years: same as adult

  Dynacin *Cap:* 50, 100 mg

  Minocin *Cap:* 50, 75, 100 mg; *Oral susp:* 50 mg/5 ml (60 ml) (custard) (sulfites, alcohol 5%)

▷ *tetracycline* **(D)** swish and spit 10 ml susp (125 mg/5 ml) <u>or</u> one 250 mg tab/cap dissolved in 180 ml water qid x 4-5 days

 Pediatric: <8 years: not recommended; ≥8 years: same as adult; *see Appendix CC.31.*

 tetracycline (Sumycin Suspension) *for dose by weight*

  Achromycin V *Cap:* 250, 500 mg

  Sumycin *Tab:* 250, 500 mg; *Cap:* 250, 500 mg; *Oral susp:* 125 mg/5 ml (100, 200 ml) (fruit) (sulfites)

◯   ASPERGILLOSIS, BLASTOMYCOSIS, HISTOPLASMOSIS

INVASIVE INFECTION

▷ *isavuconazonium* **(C)** swallow cap whole; *Loading dose:* 372 mg q 8 hours x 6 doses (48 hours); *Maintenance:* 372 mg once daily starting 12-24 hours after last loading dose

 Pediatric: <18 years: not established; ≥18 years: same as adult

  Cresemba *Cap:* 186 mg; *Vial:* 372 mg pwdr for reconstitution (7/blister pck) (preservative-free)

  Comment: Cresemba is indicated for the treatment of invasive aspergillus and mucormycosis in patients >18-years-old who are at high risk due to being severely compromised.

▷ *itraconazole* take with food; do <u>not</u> break, crush, <u>or</u> chew; 130 mg (2 x 65 mg caps) once daily; if no obvious improvement <u>or</u> there is evidence of progressive fungal disease, the dose should be increased in 65 mg increments to a maximum of

260 mg/day [130 mg [2 x 65 mg capsules] twice daily); doses >130 mg/day should be administered in two divided doses; *Treatment of Life-saving Situations:* although clinical studies did <u>not</u> provide for a loading dose, it is recommended, based on pharmacokinetic data, that a loading dose should be used; a loading dose of 130 mg (2 x 65 mg capsules) 3 x/day (390 mg/day) is recommended to be administered for the first 3 days, followed by the appropriate recommended dosing based on indication; treatment should be continued for a minimum of 3 months and until clinical parameters and laboratory tests indicate that the active fungal infection has subsided; an inadequate period of treatment may lead to recurrence of active infection

Tolsura *Gelcap:* 65 mg

Comment: **Tolsura** is <u>not</u> interchangeable <u>or</u> substitutable with other *itraconazole* products. **Tolsura** is <u>not</u> indicated for the treatment of onychomycosis. **Tolsura** is an azole antifungal indicated for the treatment of blastomycosis (pulmonary and extrapulmonary), histoplasmosis (including chronic cavitary pulmonary disease and disseminated, non-meningeal histoplasmosis) and aspergillosis (pulmonary and extrapulmonary, in patients who are intolerant of <u>or</u> who are refractory to ***amphotericin B*** therapy). These serious infections most commonly occur in vulnerable <u>or</u> immunocompromised patients, for example, hose with a history of cancer, transplants (solid organ <u>or</u> bone marrow), HIV/AIDS, <u>or</u> chronic rheumatic disorders, and are often associated with high mortality rates <u>or</u> long-term health issues. Most common adverse reactions (incidence ≥1%) are nausea, rash, vomiting, edema, headache, diarrhea, fatigue, fever, pruritus, hypertension, abnormal hepatic function, abdominal pain, dizziness, hypokalemia, anorexia, malaise, decreased libido, somnolence, albuminuria, and impotence. *itraconazole* is mainly metabolized through CYP3A4.

▷ *posaconazole* **(D)(G)** *Oral Therapy:* take with food; swallow tab whole; *Day 1:* 300 mg bid; then 300 mg once daily x 13 days; *IV Infusion Therapy:* must be administered through an in-line filter over approximately 90 minutes via a central venous line. <u>Never</u> administer **Noxafil** as an IV bolus injection; *Loading Dose:* a single 300 mg IV infusion; *Maintenance Dose: a single* 300 mg IV infusion once daily for duration of treatment (e.g., resolution of neutropenia <u>or</u> immunosuppression)

Pediatric: <13 years: not recommended; ≥13 years: same as adult

Noxafil *Tab:* 100 mg ext-rel; *Oral susp:* 40 mg/ml (105 oz w. dosing spoon) (cherry); *Vial:* 300 mg/16.7 ml (18 mg/ml) soln for IV infusion

Comment: **Noxafil** is indicated as prophylaxis for invasive aspergillus and candida infections in patients >13-years-old who are at high risk due to being severely compromised.

▷ *voriconazole* **(D)(G)** *PO:* <40 kg: 100 mg q 12 hours; may increase to 150 mg q 12 hours if inadequate response; >40 kg: 200 mg q 12 hours; may increase to 300 mg q 12 hours if inadequate response; *IV:* 6 mg/kg q 12 hours x 2 doses; then 4 mg/kg q 12 hours; max rate 3 mg/kg/hour over 1-2 hours

Pediatric: <12 years: not recommended; ≥12 years: same as adult

Vfend *Tab:* 50, 200 mg

Vfend I.V. for Injection *Vial:* 200 mg pwdr for reconstitution (preservative-free)

Vfend *Oral susp:* 40 mg/ml pwdr for reconstitution (75 ml) (orange)

 ASTHMA

Parenteral Corticosteroids *see* Appendix M. Parenteral Corticosteroids
Oral Corticosteroids *see* Appendix L. Oral Corticosteroids

EPINEPHRINE INHALATION AEROSOL (BRONCHODILATOR)

▷ *epinephrine inhalation aerosol* (C)(OTC) shake and spray one time into the air prior to each inhalation; after 1 inhalation, wait 1 minute; if inadequate relief, may repeat; 1-2 inhalations constitutes one dose; wait at least 4 hours between doses; max 8 inhalations/24 hours

Pediatric: <12 years: safety and efficacy not established; ≥12 years: same as adult

Primatene MIST Pump inhal: *0.125 mg per inhalation spray* (160 sprays) (no sulfites; dehydrated alcohol 1%, hydrofluoroalkane [HFA-134a], polysorbate 80, thymol)

Comment: **Primatene Mist** *(epinephrine inhalation aerosol)* is indicated for the temporary relief of mild symptoms of intermittent asthma (wheezing, chest tightness, shortness of breath), and is delivered by a metered-dose inhaler (MDI) with a non-chorofluorocarbon (CFC) propellant. After every 20 sprays, the spray indicator resets (160, 140, 120...20, 0). The spray indicator cannot be manually reset.

INHALED RACEPINEPHRINE (BRONCHODILATOR)

Comment: Inhalation racemic epinephrine is indicated for urgent/emergent acute bronchospasm rescue (e.g., acute asthma attack, laryngospasm, croup, epiglottitis, acute inflammation causing airway obstruction). Inhalational racemic epinephrine is only recommended for use during pregnancy when there are no alternatives and benefit outweighs risk.

▷ *racepinephrine* (C)(OTC)(G) for atomized (nebulizer) treatment.

Pediatric: <4 years: not recommended; ≥4 years: same as adult

Asthmanefrin *Starter kit:* 10 x 0.5 ml vials 2.25% solution for atomized inhalation w. EZ Breathe Atomizer; *Refills:* 30 x 0.5 ml vials 2.25% solution for atomized inhalation

INHALED BETA-2 AGONISTS (BRONCHODILATORS)

▷ *albuterol sulfate* (C)(G)

AccuNeb Inhalation Solution 1 unit-dose vial tid-qid prn by nebulizer; ages 2-12 years only; not for adult

Pediatric: <2 years: not recommended; 2-12 years: initially 0.63 mg or 1.25 mg tid-qid; 6-12 years: with severe asthma, or >40 kg, or 11-12 years: initially 1.25 mg tid-qid

Inhal soln: 0.63, 1.25 mg/3 ml (3 ml, 25/carton) (preservative-free)

Albuterol Inhalation Solution (G) not recommended for adults

Pediatric: <2 years: not recommended; ≥2 years: 1 vial via nebulizer over 5-15 minutes

Inhal soln: 0.63 mg/3 ml (0.021%); 1.25 mg/3 ml (0.042%) (25/carton)

Albuterol Inhalation Solution 0.5% (G) not recommended

Pediatric: <4 years: not recommended; ≥4 years: same as adult

Inhal soln: 0.083% (25/carton)

Albuterol Nebules (G) 2.5 mg (0.5 ml of 5% diluted to 3 ml with sterile NS or 3 ml of 0.083%) tid-qid

Pediatric: use <12 years: other forms; ≥12 years: same as adult

Inhal soln: 0.083% (25/carton)

ProAir Digihaler *Inhal pwdr* 117 mcg/actuation (0.65 gm, 200 inh)

Pediatric: <4 years: not established; ≥4 years: same as adult

Comment: **ProAir Digihaler is** the first and only digital inhaler, with built-in sensors that detect inhaler use and measure inspiratory flow. The data is sent to the companion mobile app using Bluetooth Wireless Technology for patients and health-care professionals to review over time. **ProAir Digihaler** is indicated for the treatment or prevention of bronchospasm in reversible obstructive airway disease and for the prevention of exercise-induced bronchospasm.

Proair HFA Inhaler 1-2 inhalations q 4-6 hours prn; 2 inhalations 15 minutes before exercise as prophylaxis for exercise-induced asthma (EIA)
Pediatric: <4 years: not established; ≥4 years: same as adult
    Inhaler: 90 mcg/actuation (0.65 gm, 200 inh) (CFC-free)
Proair RespiClick 1-2 inhalations q 4-6 hours prn; 2 inhalations 15-30 minutes before exercise as prophylaxis for exercise-induced asthma (EIA)
Pediatric: <12 years: not established; ≥12 years: same as adult
    Inhaler: 90 mcg/actuation (8.5 gm, 200 inh)
Proventil HFA Inhaler 1-2 inhalations q 4-6 hours prn; 2 inhalations 15 minutes before exercise as prophylaxis for exercise-induced asthma (EIA)
Pediatric: <4 years: use syrup; ≥4 years: same as adult
    Inhaler: 90 mcg/actuation with a dose counter (6.7 gm, 200 inh)
Proventil Inhalation Solution 2.5 mg diluted to 3 ml with normal saline tid-qid prn by nebulizer
Pediatric: use syrup
    Inhal soln: 0.5% (20 ml w. dropper); 0.083% (3 ml; 25/carton)
Ventolin Inhaler 2 inhalations q 4-6 hours prn; 2 inhalations 15 minutes before exercise as prophylaxis for exercise-induced asthma
Pediatric: <2 years: not recommended; 2-4 years: use syrup; ≥4 years: same as adult
    Inhaler: 90 mcg/actuation (17 gm, 220 inh)
Ventolin Rotacaps 1-2 cap inhalations q 4-6 hours prn; 2 inhalations 15 minutes before exercise as prophylaxis for exercise-induced asthma (EIA)
Pediatric: <4 years: not recommended; ≥4 years 1-2 caps q 4-6 hours prn
    Rotacaps: 200 mcg/rotacap dose (100 doses)
Ventolin 0.5% Inhalation Solution
Pediatric: <2 years: not recommended; ≥2 years: initially 0.1-0.15 mg/kg/dose tid-qid prn; 10-15 kg: 0.25 ml diluted to 3 ml with normal saline by nebulizer tid-qid prn; >15 kg: 0.5 ml diluted to 3 ml with normal saline by nebulizer tid-qid prn
    Inhal soln: 20 ml w. dropper
Ventolin Nebules
Pediatric: <2 years: not recommended; ≥2 years: initially 0.1-0.15 mg/kg/ dose tid-qid prn; 10-15 kg: 1.25 mg <u>or</u> 1/2 nebule tid-qid prn; >15 kg: 2.5 mg <u>or</u> 1 nebule tid-qid prn
    Inhal soln: 0.083% (3 ml; 25/carton)
▷ *isoproterenol* (B) *Rescue:* 1 inhalation prn; repeat if no relief in 2-5 minutes; *Maintenance:* 1-2 inhalations q 4-6 hours
Pediatric: <12 years: not recommended; ≥12 years: same as adult
    Medihaler-1SO *Inhaler:* 80 mcg/actuation (15 ml, 30 inh)
▷ *levalbuterol tartrate* (C)(G) initially 0.63 mg tid q 6-8 hours prn by nebulizer; may increase to 1.25 mg tid at 6-8 hour intervals as needed
Pediatric: <12 years: not recommended; ≥12 years: same as adult
    Xopenex *Inhal soln:* 0.31, 0.63, 1.25 mg/3 ml (24/carton) (preservative-free)
    Xopenex HFA *Inh:* 45 mg (15 gm, 200 inh) (preservative-free)
    Xopenex Concentrate *Vial:* 1.25 mg/0.5 ml (30/carton) (preservative-free)
▷ *metaproterenol* (C)(G)
    Alupent 2-3 inhalations tid-qid prn; max 12 inhalations/day
    Pediatric: <6 years: use syrup; ≥6 years: via nebulizer 0.1-0.2 ml diluted with normal saline to 3 ml, up to q 4 hours prn
      Inhaler: 0.65 mg/actuation (14 gm, 200 doses)
    Alupent Inhalation Solution 5-15 inhalations tid-qid prn; q 4 hours prn for acute attack
    Pediatric: <6 years: use syrup ≥6 years: via nebulizer 0.1-0.2 ml diluted with normal saline to 3 ml, up to q 4 hours prn
      Inhal soln: 5% (10, 30 ml w. dropper)

▶ *pirbuterol* (C) 1-2 inhalations q 4-6 hours prn; max 12 inhalations/day
  Pediatric: <12 years: not recommended; ≥12 years: same as adult
    Maxair *Autohaler:* 200 mcg/actuation (14 gm, 400 inh); *Inhaler:* 200 mcg/
    actuation (25.6 gm, 300 inh)
▶ *terbutaline* (B) 2 inhalations q 4-6 hours prn
  Pediatric: <12 years: not recommended; ≥12 years: same as adult
    Inhaler: 0.2 mg/actuation (10.5 gm, 300 inh)

INHALED ANTICHOLINERGICS
▶ *ipratropium bromide* (C)(G)
  Pediatric: <12 years: not established; ≥12 years: same as adult
    Atrovent 2 inhalations qid; additional inhalations as required; max 12
    inhalations/day
    Inhaler: 18 mcg/actuation (14 gm, 200 inh)
    Atrovent Inhalation Solution 500 mcg tid-qid prn by nebulizer
    Inhal soln: 0.02% (500 mcg in 2.5 ml; 25/carton)

INHALED CORTICOSTEROIDS
Comment: Inhaled corticosteroids are not for primary (rescue) treatment of acute
asthma attack. After every inhalation of a steroid or steroid-containing medication
treatment, rinse mouth to reduce risk of oral candidiasis. Inhaled corticosteroids
are not for primary (rescue) treatment of acute asthma attack. For twice daily
dosing, allow 12 hours between doses.
▶ *beclomethasone dipropionate* (C)(G) *Previously using only bronchodilators:*
  initiate 40-80 mcg bid; max 320 mcg bid; *Previously using inhaled corticosteroid:*
  initiate 40-160 mcg bid; max 320 mcg/day; *Previously taking a systemic
  corticosteroid:* attempt to wean off the systemic drug after approximately 1 week
  after initiating; rinse mouth after use
  Pediatric: <12 years: not recommended; ≥12 years: same as adult
    Qvar *Inhal aerosol:* 40, 80 mcg/metered dose actuation (8.7 gm, 120 inh)
    metered dose inhaler (chlorofluorocarbon [CFC]-free)
▶ *budesonide* (B)
    Pulmicort Flexhaler initially 180-360 mcg bid; max 360 mcg bid; rinse mouth
    after use
    Pediatric: <6 years: not recommended; ≥6 years: 1-2 inhalations bid
      Flexhaler: 90 mcg/actuation (60 inh); 180 mcg/actuation (120 inh)
    Pulmicort Respules (G) adults and ≥8 years: use flexhaler
    Pediatric: <12 months: not recommended; 12 months-8 years: *Previously using
    only bronchodilators:* initiate 0.5 mg/day once daily or in 2 divided doses; may
    start at 0.25 mg daily; *Previously using inhaled corticosteroids:* initiate 0.5 mg
    once daily or in 2 divided doses; max 1 mg/day; *Previously taking oral
    corticosteroids:* initiate 1 mg/day daily or in 2 divided doses; ≥8 years: use
    flexhaler; rinse mouth after use
      Inhal susp: 0.25, 0.5, 1 mg/2 ml (30/carton)
▶ *ciclesonide* (C) initially 80 mcg bid; max 320 mcg/day; rinse mouth after use;
  Previously on inhaled corticosteroid: initially 80 mcg bid; *Previously on oral steroid:*
  320 mg bid
  Pediatric: <12 years: not recommended; ≥12 years: same as adult
    Alvesco *Inhal aerosol:* 80, 160 mcg/actuation (6.1 gm, 60 inh)
▶ *flunisolide* (C) rinse mouth after use
    AeroBid, AeroBid-M initially 2 inhalations bid; max 8 inhalations/day; rinse
    mouth after use
    Pediatric: <6 years: not recommended; 6-15 years: 2 inhalations bid; ≥15 years:
    same as adult
      Inhaler: 250 mcg/actuation (7 gm, 100 inh)

Aerospan HFA initially 160 mcg bid; max 320 mcg bid
Pediatric: <6 years: not recommended; 6-11 years: 80 mcg bid; max 160 mcg bid; ≥12 years: same as adult
Inhaler: 80 mcg (5.1 gm, 60 doses; 80 mcg, 120 doses)

▷ *fluticasone furoate* (C) *currently not on inhaled corticosteroid:* usually initiate at 100 mcg once daily at the same time each day; may increase to 200 mcg once daily if inadequate response after 2 weeks; max 200 mcg/day; rinse mouth after use
Pediatric: <12 years: not established; ≥12 years: same as adult
Arnuity Ellipta *Inhal:* 100, 200 mcg/dry pwdr per inhalation (30 doses)
Comment: **Arnuity Ellipta** is not for primary treatment of status asthmaticus or acute asthma episodes. **Arnuity Ellipta** is contraindicated with severe hypersensitivity to milk proteins.

▷ *fluticasone propionate* (C)
ArmorAir 1 inhalation bid (12 hours apart); initially 55 mcg bid; *Previously using an inhaled corticosteroid:* see mfr pkg insert; if insufficient response after 2 weeks, may increase the bid dose; max 232 mcg bid; after stability achieved, titrate to lowest effective dose; do not use with spacer or volume-holding chamber
Pediatric: <12 years: not established; ≥12 years: same as adult
Inhaler: 55, 113, 232 mcg/actuation (60 inh)
Flovent, Flovent HFA initially 88 mcg bid; *Previously using an inhaled corticosteroid:* initially 88-220 mcg bid; *Previously taking an oral corticosteroid:* 880 mcg bid; rinse mouth after use
Pediatric: <11 years: use **Flovent Diskus** ≥12 years: same as adult
Inhaler: 44 mcg/actuation (7.9 gm, 60 inh; 13 gm, 120 inh); 110 mcg/actuation (13 gm, 120 inh); 220 mcg/actuation (13 gm, 120 inh)
Flovent Diskus initially 100 mcg bid; max 500 mcg bid; *Previously using an inhaled corticosteroid:* initially 100-250 mcg bid; max 500 mcg bid; *Previously taking an oral corticosteroid:* 1000 mcg bid
Pediatric: <4 years: not recommended; 4-11 years: initially 50 mcg bid; max 100 mcg bid; rinse mouth after use; ≥12 years: same as adult
Diskus: 50, 100, 250 mcg/inh dry pwdr (60 blisters w. diskus)

▷ *mometasone furoate* (C) 220-440 mcg once daily or bid; max 880 mcg/day; rinse mouth after use
Asmanex HFA *Inhaler:* 100, 200 mcg/actuation (13 gm, 120 inh)
Pediatric: <12 years: not established; ≥12 years: same as adult
Asmanex Twisthaler *Inhaler:* 110 mcg/actuation (30 inh), 220 mcg/actuation (30, 60, 120 inh)
Pediatric: <4 years: not recommended; 4-11 years: 110 mcg once daily in the PM; >12 years: may use **Asmanex HFA**; rinse mouth after use

▷ *triamcinolone* (C)
Azmacort 2 inhalations tid-qid or 4 inhalations bid; rinse mouth after use
Pediatric: <6 years: not recommended; 6-12 years: 1-2 inhalations tid or 2-4 inhalations bid; >12 years: same as adult
Inhaler: 100 mcg/actuation (20 gm, 240 inh)

LEUKOTRIENE RECEPTOR ANTAGONISTS (LRAS)

Comment: The LRAs are indicated for prophylaxis and chronic treatment, only. Not for primary (rescue) treatment of acute asthma attack.

▷ *montelukast* (B)(G) 10 mg once daily in the PM; for EIB, take at least 2 hours before exercise; max 1 dose/day
Pediatric: <12 months: not recommended; 12-23 months: one 4 mg granule pkt daily; 2-5 years: one 4 mg chew tab or granule pkt daily; 6-14 years: one 5 mg chew tab daily; ≥15 years: same as adult
Singulair *Tab:* 10 mg

Singulair Chewable *Chew tab:* 4, 5 mg (cherry) (phenylalanine)
Singulair Oral Granules *Granules:* 4 mg/pkt; take within 15 minutes of
opening pkt; may mix with applesauce, carrots, rice, or ice cream

▷ *zafirlukast* (B) 20 mg bid, 1 hour ac or 2 hours pc
  Pediatric: <7 years: not recommended; 7-11 years: 10 mg bid 1 hour ac or 2 hours
  pc; ≥12 years: same as adult
    Accolate *Tab:* 10, 20 mg
▷ *zileuton* (C)(G)
  Pediatric: <12 years: not recommended; ≥12 years: same as adult
    Zyflo 1 tab qid (total 2400 mg/day)
    Tab: 600 mg
    Zyflo CR 2 tabs bid (total 2400 mg/day)
    Tab: 600 mg ext-rel

IGE BLOCKER (IGG1K MONOCLONAL ANTIBODY)

▷ *omalizumab* (B) 150-375 mg SC every 2-4 weeks based on body weight and
  pretreatment serum total IgE level; max 150 mg/injection site; approved for
  patient self-administration after education by a qualified healthcare provider
  Pediatric: <12 years: not recommended; 30-90 kg + IgE >30-100 IU/ml 150 mg
  q 4 weeks; 90-150 kg + IgE >30-100 IU/ml or 30-90 kg + IgE >100-200 IU/ml
  or 30-60 kg + IgE >200-300 IU/ml 300 mg q 4 hours; >90-150 kg + IgE >100-
  200 IU/ml or >60-90 kg + IgE >200-300 IU/ml or 30-70 kg + IgE >300-400 IU/
  ml 225 mg q 2 weeks; >90-150 kg + IgE >200-300 IU/ml or >70-90 kg + IgE
  >300-400 IU/ml or 30-70 kg + IgE >400-500 IU/ml or 30-60 kg + IgE >500-600
  IU/ml or 30-60 kg + IgE >600-700 IU/ml 375 mg q 2 weeks
    Xolair *Vial:* 150 mg, single-dose, pwdr for SC injection after reconstitution;
    Prefilled syringe: 75 mg/0.5 ml, 150 mg/1 ml single-dose (preservative-free)

INHALED MAST CELL STABILIZERS (PROPHYLAXIS)

Comment: IMCSs are for prophylaxis and chronic treatment, only. Not for primary
(rescue) treatment of acute asthma attack.

▷ *cromolyn sodium* (B)(G)
    Intal 2 inhalations qid; 2 inhalations up to 10-60 minutes before precipitant as
    prophylaxis; rinse mouth after use
    Pediatric: <2 years: not recommended; 2-5 years: use inhal soln via nebulizer;
    >5 years: 2 inhalations qid via inhaler
      Inhaler: 0.8 mg/actuation (8.1, 14.2 gm; 112, 200 inh)
    Intal Inhalation Solution 20 mg by nebulizer qid; 20 mg up to 10-60 minutes
    before precipitant as prophylaxis
    Pediatric: <2 years: not recommended; ≥2 years: same as adult
      Inhal soln: 20 mg/2 ml (60, 120/carton)

▷ *nedocromil sodium* (B)
    Tilade 2 sprays qid; rinse mouth after use
    Pediatric: <6 years: not recommended; ≥6 years: 2 sprays qid
      Inhaler: 1.75 mg/spray (16.2 gm; 104 sprays)
    Tilade Nebulizer Solution 0.5% 1 amp qid by nebulizer
    Pediatric: <2 years: not recommended; ≥2 years: initially 1 amp qid by
    nebulizer; 2-5 years: initially 1 amp tid by nebulizer; ≥5 years: same as adult
      Inhal soln: 11 mg/2.2 ml (2 ml; 60, 120/carton)

INHALED LONG-ACTING ANTICHOLINERGIC

▷ *tiotropium (as bromide monohydrate)* (C) 2 inhalations once daily using
  inhalation device; do not swallow caps

Pediatric: <12 years: not recommended; ≥12 years: same as adult

Spiriva HandiHaler *Inhal device:* 18 mcg/cap pwdr for inhalation (5, 30, 90 caps w. inhalation device)

Spiriva Respimat *Inhal device:* 1.25, 2.5 mcg/actuation cartridge w. inhalation device (4 gm, 60 metered actuations) (benzylkonian chloride)

Comment: *Tiotropium* is for prophylaxis and chronic treatment, <u>only</u>. <u>Not</u> for primary (rescue) treatment of acute attack. Avoid getting powder in eyes. Caution with narrow-angle glaucoma, BPH, bladder neck obstruction, and pregnancy. Contraindicated with allergy to *atropine* <u>or</u> its derivatives (e.g., *ipratropium*).

INHALED ANTICHOLINERGIC+BETA-2 AGONIST

▷ *ipratropium bromide+albuterol sulfate* (C) 2 inhalations qid
Pediatric: <12 years: not recommended; ≥12 years: same as adult

Combivent 2 inhalations qid; additional inhalations as required; max 12 inhalations/day

Inhaler: ipra 18 mcg+albu 90 mcg/actuation (14.7 gm, 200 inh)

Duoneb 1 vial via nebulizer 4-6 times daily prn

Inhal soln: ipra 0.5 mg (0.017%)+albu 2.5 mg (0.083%) per 3 ml (23/carton)

INHALED LONG-ACTING BETA-2 AGONIST (LABA)

Comment: LABA agents are <u>not</u> for primary (rescue) treatment of acute asthma attack. For twice daily dosing, allow 12 hours between doses.

▷ *arformoterol* (C) 15 mcg bid via nebulizer
Pediatric: <12 years: not recommended; ≥12 years: same as adult

Brovana *Inhal soln:* 15 mcg/2 ml (2 ml; 30/carton)

Comment: *Arformoterol* is indicated for the treatment of COPD but is used off-label for the treatment of asthma. It is used for prophylaxis and chronic treatment, <u>only</u>. <u>Not</u> for primary (rescue) treatment of acute attack.

▷ *formoterol fumarate* (C)

Foradil Aerolizer 12 mcg q 12 hours
Pediatric: <5 years: not recommended; ≥5 years: same as adult

Inhaler: 12 mcg/cap (12, 60 caps w. device)

Perforomist 20 mcg q 12 hours
Pediatric: <12 years: not recommended; ≥12 years: same as adult

Inhal soln: 20 mcg/2 ml (60/carton)

Comment: *Formoterol* is for prophylaxis and chronic treatment, <u>only</u>. <u>Not</u> for primary (rescue) treatment of acute attack. Do <u>not</u> mix *formoterol* with other drugs. Use of *formoterol* is off-label for asthma.

▷ *olodaterol* (C) 12 mcg q 12 hours
Pediatric: <12 years: not established; ≥12 years: same as adult

Striverdi Respimat

Inhal soln: 2.5 mcg/cartridge (metered actuation) (40 gm, 60 metered actuations) (benzalkonium chloride)

Comment: **Striverdi Respimat** is contraindicated in persons with asthma without concomitant use of long-term control medication.

▷ *salmeterol* (C)(G) 2 inhalations q 12 hours prn; 2 inhalations at least 30-60 minutes before exercise as prophylaxis for exercise-induced asthma; do <u>not</u> use extra doses for exercise-induced bronchospasm if already using regular dose
Pediatric: <4 years: not recommended; 4-<12 years: 1 inhalation q 12 hours prn; 1 inhalation at least 30-60 minutes before exercise as prophylaxis for exercise-induced asthma; do <u>not</u> use extra doses for exercise-induced bronchospasm if already using regular dose; ≥12 years: same as adult

Serevent Diskus *Diskus (pwdr):* 50 mcg/actuation (60 doses/diskus)

INHALED CORTICOSTEROID+LONG-ACTING BETA-2 AGONIST (LABA)

Comment: Inhaled corticosteroids and LABA agents are not for primary (rescue) treatment of acute asthma attack. For twice daily dosing, allow 12 hours between doses. After every inhalation of a steroid or steroid-containing medication treatment, rinse mouth to reduce risk of oral candidiasis.

▷ *budesonide+formoterol* (C) 1 inhalation bid; rinse mouth after use

Pediatric: <12 years: not established; ≥12 years: same as adult

Symbicort 80/4.5 *Inhaler:* bud 80 mcg+for 4.5 mcg

Symbicort 160/4.5 *Inhaler:* bud 160 mcg+for 4.5 mcg

▷ *fluticasone propionate+salmeterol* (C)

Advair HFA *Not previously using inhaled steroid:* start with 2 inh 45/21 or 115/21 bid; if insufficient response after 2 weeks, use next higher strength; max 2 inh 230/50 bid; allow 12 hours between doses; *Already using inhaled steroid;* see mfr pkg insert

Advair HFA 45/21 1 inhalation bid; rinse mouth after use

Pediatric: <12 years: not recommended; ≥12 years: same as adult

Inhaler: flu pro 45 mcg+sal 21 mcg/actuation (CFC-free)

Advair HFA 115/21 1 inhalation bid; rinse mouth after use

Pediatric: <12 years: not established; ≥12 years: same as adult

Inhaler: flu pro 115 mcg+sal 21 mcg/actuation (CFC-free)

Advair HFA 230/21 1 inhalation bid; rinse mouth after use

Pediatric: <12 years: not established; ≥12 years: same as adult

Inhaler: flu pro 230 mcg+sal 21 mcg/actuation (CFC-free)

Advair Diskus (G) *Not previously using inhaled steroid:* start with 1 inh 100/50 bid; *Already using inhaled steroid:* see mfr pkg insert; rinse mouth after use

Advair Diskus (G) 100/50 1 inhalation bid; rinse mouth after use

Pediatric: <4 years: not recommended; 4-11 years: 1 bid; >11 years: 1 inhalation bid

Diskus: flu pro 100 mcg+sal 50 mcg/actuation (60 blisters)

Advair Diskus (G) 250/50 1 inhalation bid; rinse mouth after use

Pediatric: <4 years: not recommended; 4-12 years: use 100/50 strength; >12 years: same as adult

Diskus: flu pro 250 mcg+sal 50 mcg/actuation (60 blisters)

Advair Diskus (G) 500/50 1 inhalation bid; rinse mouth after use

Pediatric: <4 years: not recommended; 4-12 years: use 100/50 strength; >12 years: same as adult

Diskus: flu pro 500 mcg+sal 50 mcg/actuation (60 blisters)

AirDuo RespiClick pwdr for oral inhalation; *Not previously using an inhaled steroid:* 1 inh 55/14 bid; *Already using an inhaled steroid:* see mfr pkg insert; if insufficient response after 2 weeks, titrate with a higher strength; max inh 232/14 bid

Pediatric: <12 years: not established; ≥12 years: same as adult

AirDuo RespiClick 55/14 flu pro 55 mcg+sal (as xinafoate) 14 mcg dry pwdr/actuation (60 actuations)

AirDuo RespiClick 113/14 flu pro 113 mcg+sal (as xinafoate) 14 mcg dry pwdr/actuation (60 actuations)

AirDuo RespiClick 232/14 flu pro 232 mcg+sal (as xinafoate) 14 mcg dry pwdr/actuation (60 actuations)

▷ *fluticasone furoate+vilanterol* (C) 1 inhalation 100/25 once daily at the same time each day

Pediatric: <17 years: not established; ≥17 years: same as adult

Breo Ellipta

Breo Ellipta 100/25 flu 100 mcg+vil 25 mcg dry pwdr per inhalation (30 doses)

       Breo Ellipta 200/25 flu 200 mcg+vil 25 mcg dry pwdr per inhalation
(30 doses)
Comment: **Breo Ellipta** is contraindicated with severe hypersensitivity to
milk proteins.

▷ *mometasone furoate+formoterol fumarate* (C) 2 inhalations bid; rinse mouth after
use
Pediatric: <12 years: not established; ≥12 years: same as adult
    Dulera
      Dulera 100/5 *Inhaler:* mom 100 mcg/for 5 mcg (HFA)
      Dulera 200/5 *Inhaler:* mom 200 mcg/for 5 mcg (HFA)
    Comment: **Dulera** is <u>not</u> a rescue inhaler.

INHALED ANTICHOLINERGIC+LONG-ACTING BETA-2 AGONIST (LABA)

▷ *glycopyrrolate+formoterol fumarate* (C) 2 inhalations bid (AM & PM)
Pediatric: <18 years: not established; ≥18 years: same as adult
    Bevespi Aerosphere 9/4.8 *Metered dose inhaler:* gly 9 mcg+for 4.8 mcg/
inhalation (10.7 gm, 120 inh)

INHALED CORTICOSTEROID+ANTICHOLINERGIC+LONG-ACTING BETA-2 AGONIST (LABA) COMBINATION

▷ *Trelegy Ellipta* one inhalation once daily
Pediatric: not established
    furo 100 mcg/umec 62.5 mcg/vilan 25 mcg dry
Comment: **Trelegy Ellipta** is maintenance therapy for patients with asthma
and/or COPD, who are receiving fixed-dose *furoate* and *vilanterol* for airflow
obstruction and to reduce exacerbations, <u>or</u> receiving *umeclidinium* and a fixed-
dose combination of *fluticasone furoate* and *vilanterol*. **Trelegy Ellipta** is the first
FDA-approved once-daily single-dose inhaler that combines *fluticasone furoate*, a
corticosteroid, *umeclidinium*, a long-acting muscarinic antagonist, and *vilantero*,
a long-acting beta-2 adrenergic agonist. Common adverse reactions reported with
Trelegy Ellipta have included headache, back pain, dysgeusia, diarrhea, cough,
oropharyngeal pain, and gastroenteritis. **Trelegy Ellipta** has been found to increase
the risk of pneumonia in patients with COPD, and increase the risk of asthma-related
death. **Trelegy Ellipta** is <u>not</u> indicated for the treatment of acute bronchospasm.

ORAL BETA-2 AGONISTS (BRONCHODILATORS)

▷ *albuterol* (C)
    Albuterol Syrup (G) *Adult:* 2-4 mg tid-qid; may increase gradually; max 8 mg
qid; *Elderly:* initially 2-3 mg tid-qid; may increase gradually; max 8 mg qid
Pediatric: <2 years: not recommended; ≥2-6 years: 0.1 mg/kg tid; initially max
2 mg tid; may increase gradually to 0.2 mg/kg tid; max 4 mg tid; >6-12 years: 2
mg tid-qid; may increase gradually; max 6 mg qid; ≥12 years: same as adult
    Syr: 2 mg/5 ml
    Proventil 2-4 mg tid-qid prn
Pediatric: <6 years: not recommended; ≥6 years: same as adult
    Tab: 2, 4 mg
    Proventil Repetabs 4-8 mg q 12 hours prn
Pediatric: use syrup
    Repetab: 4 mg sust-rel
    Proventil Syrup 5-10 ml tid-qid prn; may increase gradually; max 20 ml qid prn
Pediatric: <2 years: not recommended; ≥2-6 years: 0.1 mg/kg tid prn; max
initially 5 ml tid prn; may increase gradually to 0.2 mg/kg tid prn; max 10 ml tid;
>6-14 years: 5 ml tid-qid prn; may increase gradually; max 60 ml/day in divided
doses; >14 years: same as adult
    Syr: 2 mg/5 ml

Ventolin 2-4 mg tid-qid prn; may increase gradually; max 8 mg qid
Pediatric: <2 years: not recommended; ≥2-6 years: 0.1 mg/kg tid prn; max
initially 2 mg tid prn; may increase gradually to 0.2 mg/kg tid; max 4 mg tid;
>6-14 years: 2 mg tid-qid prn; may increase gradually; max 6 mg tid
   Tab: 2, 4 mg; *Syr:* 2 mg/5 ml (strawberry)
VoSpire ER 4-8 mg q 12 hours prn; max 32 mg/day divided q 12 hours;
swallow whole; do not crush or chew
Pediatric: <6 years: not recommended; ≥6-12 years: 4 mg q 12 hours; max 24
mg/day q 12 hours; >12 years: same as adult
   Tab: 4, 8 mg ext-rel
▷ *metaproterenol* (C) 20 mg tid-qid prn
Pediatric: <6 years: not recommended (doses of 1.3-2.6 mg/kg/day have been used);
≥6-9 years (<60 lb): 10 mg tid-qid prn; >9-12 years (>60 lb): 20 mg tid-qid prn; >12
years: same as adult
   Alupent *Tab:* 10, 20 mg; *Syr:* 10 mg/5 ml

METHYLXANTHINES

Comment: Check serum theophylline level just before 5th dose is administered.
Therapeutic theophylline level: 10-20 mcg/ml.
▷ *theophylline* (C)(G)
   Theo-24 initially 300-400 mg once daily at HS; after 3 days, increase to 400-
600 mg once daily at HS; max 600 mg/day
Pediatric: <45 kg: initially 12-14 mg/kg/day; max 300 mg/day; increase after 3
days to 16 mg/kg/day to max 400 mg; after 3 more days increase to 30 mg/kg/
day to max 600 mg/day; ≥45 kg: same as adult
   Cap: 100, 200, 300, 400 mg ext-rel
Theo-Dur initially 150 mg bid; increase to 200 mg bid after 3 days; then to 300
mg bid after 3 more days
Pediatric: <6 years: not recommended; 6-15 years: initially 12-14 mg/kg/day
in 2 divided doses; max 300 mg/day; then increase to 16 mg/kg in 2 divided
doses; max 400 mg/day; then to 20 mg/kg/day in 2 divided doses; max 600 mg/
day; ≥15 years: same as adult
   Tab: 100, 200, 300 mg ext-rel
Theolair-SR
Pediatric: not recommended
   Tab: 200, 250, 300, 500 mg sust-rel
Uniphyl 400-600 mg daily with meals
Pediatric: not recommended
   Tab: 400*, 600*mg cont-rel

METHYLXANTHINE+EXPECTORANT COMBINATION

▷ *dyphylline+guaifenesin* (C) 1 tab qid
   Lufyllin GG *Tab:* dyphy 200 mg+guaif 200 mg; *Elix:* dyphy 100 mg+guaif 100 mg
per 15 ml

INTERLEUKIN-4 RECEPTOR ALPHA ANTAGONIST

▷ *dupilumab* administer SC into the upper arm, abdomen, or thigh; rotate sites;
initially 600 mg (2 x 300 mg injections at different sites), followed by 300 mg SC
once every other week; may use with or without topical corticosteroids; may use
with calcineurin inhibitors, but reserve only for problem areas (e.g., face, neck,
intertriginous, and genital areas); avoid live vaccines.
Pediatric: <12 years: not recommended; ≥12 years: same as adult
   Dupixent *Prefilled syringe:* 300 mg/2 ml (2/pck without needle)
(preservative-free)

Comment: *Dupilumab* is a human monoclonal IgG4 antibody that inhibits interleukin-4 (IL-4) and interleukin-13 (IL-13) signaling by specifically binding to the IL4Ra subunit shared by the IL-4 and IL-13 receptor complexes, thereby inhibiting the release of pro-inflammatory cytokines, chemokines, and IgE. *dupilumab* is indicated as an add-on maintenance therapy for patients ≥12 years-of-age with moderate-to-severe asthma with an eosinophilic subtype or with oral corticosteroid-dependent asthma.

HUMANIZED INTERLEUKIN-5 ANTAGONIST MONOCLONAL ANTIBODY

▷ **mepolizumab** 100 mg SC once every 4 weeks in upper arm, abdomen, or thigh
   Pediatric: <12 years: not recommended; ≥12 years: same as adult
   Nucala *Vial:* 100 mg pwdr for reconstitution, single-use (preservative-free)
   Comment: **Nucala** is an add-on maintenance treatment for severe asthma. There is a pregnancy exposure registry that monitors pregnancy outcomes in women exposed to **Nucala** during pregnancy. Healthcare providers can enroll patients or encourage patients to enroll themselves by calling 1-877-311-8972 or visiting www.mothertobaby.org/asthma.

INTERLEUKIN-4 RECEPTOR ALPHA ANTAGONIST

▷ **dupilumab** administer SC into the upper arm, abdomen, or thigh; rotate sites;
   Initial Dose: 400 mg (2 x 200 mg SC in different sites); then, 200 mg SC every other week or *Initial Dose:* 600 mg (2 x 300 mg SC in different sites); then, 300 mg SC every other week (this dosing regimen is for patients requiring concomitant oral corticosteroids or with co-morbid moderate-to-severe atopic dermatitis for which **Dupixent** is indicated
   Pediatric: <12 years: not recommended; ≥12 years: same as adult
   Dupixent *Prefilled syringe:* 200 mg/1.14 ml, 300 mg/2 ml, single-dose (2/pck without needle) (preservative-free)
   Comment: *Dupilumab* is a human monoclonal IgG4 antibody that inhibits interleukin-4 (IL-4) and interleukin-13 (IL-13) signaling by specifically binding to the IL4Ra subunit shared by the IL-4 and IL-13 receptor complexes, thereby inhibiting the release of pro-inflammatory cytokines, chemokines, and IgE. *dupilumab* is indicated as an add-on maintenance therapy for patients ≥12 years-of-age with moderate-to-severe asthma with an eosinophilic subtype or with oral corticosteroid-dependent asthma. **Dupixent** is also indicated, at different dosing regimens, for patients ≥12 years-of-age with atopic dermatitis, and adult patients with chronic rhinosinusitis with nasal polyposis (CRSwNP). Avoid live vaccines.

⬤ ASTHMA-COPD OVERLAP SYNDROME (ACOS)

Comment: An estimated 16% of patients with asthma or COPD have asthma-COPD overlap syndrome (ACOS), a poorly understood disease with an increasing morbidity and mortality. PROSPRO (Prospective Study to Evaluate Predictors of Clinical Effectiveness in Response to Omalizumab), a 48-week, prospective, multicenter, observational study, included patients (n = 806) who were 12 years-of-age and older who were initiating *omalizumab* treatment for moderate-to-severe allergic asthma, including patient with co-morbid COPD (n = 78). Researchers reported that *omalizumab* (**Xolair**) decreased asthma exacerbations and improved symptom control to a similar extent in patients with ACOS as seen in patients with asthma but no COPD. While patients with COPD typically experience annual declines in lung function, at least some of the ACOS patients in this study, which included one of the largest observational cohorts to date of patients with ACOS, showed preserved lung function after 48 weeks of *omalizumab* treatment (as demonstrated by improved post-bronchodilator FEV_1 at end of stud and asthma exacerbations numbers reduced from baseline though month 12, from 3 or more exacerbations in both ACOS and non-ACOS groups to 1.1 or less.

IGE BLOCKER (IGG1K MONOCLONAL ANTIBODY)

▷ *omalizumab* (B) 150-375 mg SC every 2-4 weeks based on body weight and pretreatment serum total IgE level; max 150 mg/injection site; approved for patient self-administration after education by a qualified healthcare provider
Pediatric: <12 years: not recommended; 30-90 kg + IgE >30-100 IU/ml 150 mg q 4 weeks; 90-150 kg + IgE >30-100 IU/ml or 30-90 kg + IgE >100-200 IU/ml or 30-60 kg + IgE >200-300 IU/ml 300 mg q 4 hours; >90-150 kg + IgE >100-200 IU/ml or >60-90 kg + IgE >200-300 IU/ml or 30-70 kg + IgE >300-400 IU/ml 225 mg q 2 weeks; >90-150 kg + IgE >200-300 IU/ml or >70-90 kg + IgE >300-400 IU/ml or 30-70 kg + IgE >400-500 IU/ml or 30-60 kg + IgE >500-600 IU/ml or 30-60 kg + IgE >600-700 IU/ml 375 mg q 2 weeks
   Xolair *Vial:* 150 mg, single-dose, pwdr for SC injection after reconstitution; *Prefilled syringe:* 75 mg/0.5 ml, 150 mg/1 ml, single-dose (preservative-free)

INHALED CORTICOSTEROID+ANTICHOLINERGIC+LONG-ACTING BETA-2 AGONIST (LABA) COMBINATION

▷ *Trelegy Ellipta* one inhalation once daily
Pediatric: not established
   furo 100 mcg/umec 62.5 mcg/vilan 25 mcg dry
Comment: **Trelegy Ellipta** is maintenance therapy for patients with asthma and/or COPD, who are receiving fixed-dose *furoate* and *vilanterol* for airflow obstruction and to reduce exacerbations, or receiving *umeclidinium* and a fixed-dose combination of *fluticasone furoate* and *vilanterol*. **Trelegy Ellipta** is the first FDA-approved once-daily single-dose inhaler that combines *fluticasone furoate*, a corticosteroid, *umeclidinium*, a long-acting muscarinic antagonist, and *vilantero*, a long-acting beta-2 adrenergic agonist. Common adverse reactions reported with **Trelegy Ellipta** have included headache, back pain, dysgeusia, diarrhea, cough, oropharyngeal pain, and gastroenteritis. **Trelegy Ellipta** has been found to increase the risk of pneumonia in patients with COPD, and increase the risk of asthma-related death. **Trelegy Ellipta** is not indicated for the treatment of acute bronchospasm.

ASTHMA: SEVERE, EOSINOPHILIA; HYPEREOSINOPHILIA SYNDROMES (HES)

Comment: Currently available therapies for patients with severe eosinophilia asthma and hypereosinophilia syndromes (HES) include anti-IgE therapy (*omalizumab [Xolaiir]*), antiinterleukin monoclonal antibodies *mepolizumab* (Nucala), *reslizumab* (Cinqair), *benralizumab* (Fasenra), and interleukin receptor antagonist *dupilumab* (Dupixent). The data on pregnancy exposure from the clinical trials are insufficient to inform on drug-associated risk. Monoclonal antibodies are transported across the placenta in a linear fashion as pregnancy progresses; therefore, potential effects on a fetus are likely to be greater during the second and third trimester of pregnancy. IgG is known to be present in human milk; however, effects on the breastfed infant are unknown.

INTERLEUKIN-4 RECEPTOR ALPHA ANTAGONIST

▷ *dupilumab* administer SC into the upper arm, abdomen, or thigh; rotate sites; *Initial Dose:* 400 mg (2 x 200 mg SC in different sites); then, 200 mg SC every other week or *Initial Dose:* 600 mg (2 x 300 mg SC in different sites); then, 300 mg SC every other week (this dosing regimen is for patients requiring concomitant oral corticosteroids or with co-morbid moderate-to-severe atopic dermatitis for which **Dupixent** is indicated

Pediatric: <12 years: not recommended; ≥12 years: same as adult

Dupixent *Prefilled syringe:* 200 mg/1.14 ml, 300 mg/2 ml, single-dose (2/pck without needle) (preservative-free)

Comment: *Dupilumab* is a human monoclonal IgG4 antibody that inhibits interleukin-4 (IL-4) and interleukin-13 (IL-13) signaling by specifically binding to the IL4Ra subunit shared by the IL-4 and IL-13 receptor complexes, thereby inhibiting the release of pro-inflammatory cytokines, chemokines, and IgE. *dupilumab* is indicated as an add-on maintenance therapy for patients ≥12 years-of-age with moderate-to-severe asthma with an eosinophilic subtype or with oral corticosteroid-dependent asthma. **Dupixent** is also indicated, at different dosing regimens, for patients ≥12 years-of-age with atopic dermatitis, and adult patients with chronic rhinosinusitis with nasal polyposis (CRSwNP). Avoid live vaccines.

HUMANIZED INTERLEUKIN-5 ANTAGONIST MONOCLONAL ANTIBODY

Interleukin-5 Antagonist Monoclonal Antibody (IgG1 Kappa)

▷ *mepolizumab* *Severe Asthma:* 100 mg SC once every 4 weeks; *HES/EGPA:* 300 mg as 3 separate 100-mg SC injections once every 4 weeks; administer in the arm, abdomen, or thigh.

Pediatric: <6 years, not established; 6-11 years, *Severe Asthma:* 40 mg SC once every 4 weeks; ≥12 years, *Severe Asthma:* 100 mg SC once every 4 weeks; ≥12 years, *HES for ≥6 months Without an Identifiable Non-Hematologic Secondary Cause:* 300 mg as 3 separate 100-mg SC injections once every 4 weeks. *EGPA,* ≥18 years: same as adult

Nucala *Vial:* 100 mg pwdr for reconstitution, single-use *Prefilled syringe:* 100 mg/ml (1 ml) single-dose; Prefilled autoinjector: 100 mg/ml (1 ml) (preservative-free) (natural rubber latex-free)

Comment: **Nucala** is an interleukin-5 antagonist monoclonal antibody (IgG1 kappa). It is an add-on maintenance treatment for patients ≥12 years-of-age with severe asthma and with an eosinophilic phenotype and hypereosinophilia syndromes (HES). **Nucala** is also indicated for the treatment of patients ≥18 years-of-age with eosinophilic granulomatosis with polyangiitis (EGPA). **Nucala** is not for relief of acute bronchospasm or status asthmaticus. Hypersensitivity reactions (e.g., anaphylaxis, angioedema, bronchospasm, hypotension, urticaria, and rash) have occurred after administration of **Nucala**; discontinue **Nucala** in the event of a hypersensitivity reaction. Herpes zoster infections have occurred in patients receiving **Nucala**. Consider vaccination if medically appropriate. Do not discontinue systemic or inhaled corticosteroids abruptly upon initiation of therapy with **Nucala**. Decrease corticosteroids gradually, if appropriate. Treat patients with pre-existing parasitic helminth infections before therapy with **Nucala**. If patients become infected while receiving treatment with **Nucala** and do not respond to anti-helminth treatment, discontinue **Nucala** until parasitic infection resolves. The most common adverse reactions (incidence ≥5%) include headache, injection site reaction, back pain, and fatigue. Formal drug interaction trials have not been performed with **Nucala**. The data on pregnancy exposure are insufficient to inform on drug-associated risk. Monoclonal antibodies, such as *mepolizumab*, are transported across the placenta in a linear fashion as pregnancy progresses; therefore, potential effects on a fetus are likely to be greater during the second and third trimester of pregnancy. There is a pregnancy exposure registry that monitors pregnancy outcomes in patients exposed to **Nucala** during pregnancy. Healthcare providers can enroll patients or encourage patients to enroll themselves by calling 1-877-311-8972 or visiting www.mothertobaby.org/asthma. There is no information regarding the presence of *mepolizumab* in human milk or effects on the breastfed infant.

Interleukin-5 Antagonist Monoclonal Antibody (IgG4 Kappa)

▷ *resilumab* should be administered by a qualified healthcare professional and, in line with clinical practice, monitoring of patients after administration of biologic agents is recommended; recommended dose is 3 mg/kg once every 4 weeks via IV infusion over 20-50 minutes; do not administer as an IV push (IVP) or bolus
Pediatric: <18 years: not established; ≥18 years: same as adult

Cinqair *Vial:* 100 mg/10 ml (10 mg/ml) soln single-use (preservative-free)
Comment: Cinqair is an interleukin-5 antagonist monoclonal antibody (IgG4 kappa). It is an add-on maintenance treatment for patients ≥18 years-of-age with severe asthma and with an eosinophilic phenotype. **Cinqair** is also indicated for the treatment of patients >18 years-of-age with eosinophilic granulomatosis with polyangiitis (EGPA). **Cinqair** is not for relief of acute bronchospasm or status asthmaticus. Hypersensitivity reactions (e.g., anaphylaxis, angioedema, bronchospasm, hypotension, urticaria, and rash) have occurred after administration of **Cinqair**; discontinue **Cinqair** in the event of a hypersensitivity reaction. Herpes zoster infections have occurred in patients receiving **Cinqair**. Consider vaccination if medically appropriate. Do not discontinue systemic or inhaled corticosteroids abruptly upon initiation of therapy with **Cinqair**. Decrease corticosteroids gradually, if appropriate. Treat patients with pre-existing parasitic helminth infections before therapy with **Cinqair**. If patients become infected while receiving treatment with **Cinqair** and do not respond to anthelminth treatment, discontinue **Cinqair** until parasitic infection resolves. The most common adverse reactions (incidence ≥5%) include headache, injection site reaction, back pain, and fatigue. Formal drug interaction trials have not been performed with **Cinqair**. The data on pregnancy exposure are insufficient to inform on drug-associated risk. Monoclonal antibodies, such as *resilumab*, are transported across the placenta in a linear fashion as pregnancy progresses; therefore, potential effects on a fetus are likely to be greater during the second and third trimester of pregnancy. There is a pregnancy exposure registry that monitors pregnancy outcomes in patients exposed to **Cinqair** during pregnancy. Healthcare providers can enroll patients or encourage patients to enroll themselves by calling 1-877-311-8972 or visiting www.mothertobaby.org/asthma. There is no information regarding the presence of *resilumab* in human milk or effects on the breastfed infant.

IGE BLOCKER (IGG1K MONOCLONAL ANTIBODY)

▷ *omalizumab* (B) 150-375 mg SC every 2-4 weeks based on body weight and pretreatment serum total IgE level; max 150 mg/injection site; approved for patient self-administration after education by a qualified healthcare provider
Pediatric: <12 years: not recommended; >12 years: 30-90 kg + IgE >30-100 IU/ml 150 mg q 4 weeks; 90-150 kg + IgE >30-100 IU/ml or 30-90 kg + IgE >100-200 IU/ml or 30-60 kg + IgE >200-300 IU/ml 300 mg q 4 hours; >90-150 kg + IgE >100-200 IU/ml or >60-90 kg + IgE >200-300 IU/ml or 30-70 kg + IgE >300-400 IU/ml 225 mg q 2 weeks; >90-150 kg + IgE >200-300 IU/ml or >70-90 kg + IgE >300-400 IU/ml or 30-70 kg + IgE >400-500 IU/ml or 30-60 kg + IgE >500-600 IU/ml or 30-60 kg + IgE >600-700 IU/ml 375 mg q 2 weeks

Xolair *Vial:* 150 mg, single-dose, pwdr for SC injection after reconstitution; *Prefilled syringe:* 75 mg/0.5 ml, 150 mg/1 ml, single-dose (preservative-free)

INTERLEUKIN-5 RECEPTOR ALPHA-DIRECTED CYTOLYTIC MONOCLONAL ANTIBODY (IGG1,KAPPA)

▷ *benralizumab* should be administered by a qualified healthcare professional and, in line with clinical practice, monitoring of patients after administration of biologic agents is recommended; recommended dose is 30 mg SC every 4 weeks for the first 3 doses; then, once every 8 weeks thereafter; inject SC into the upper

arm, abdomen, or thigh. Store in refrigerator; do not freeze; prior to administration, warm **Fasenra** by leaving carton at room temperature for about 30 minutes. Administer within 24 hours or discard into sharps container.
Pediatric: <12 years: not established; ≥12 years: same as adult

Fasenra *Prefilled syringe:* 30 mg/ml soln, single-dose (preservative-free)
Comment: *Benralizumab* is an interleukin-5 receptor alpha-directed cytolytic monoclonal antibody (IgG1, kappa) produced in Chinese hamster ovary cells by recombinant DNA technology. **Fasenra** is indicated for the add-on maintenance treatment of patients with severe asthma ≥12 years-of-age, and with an neosinophilic phenotype. It is not for treatment of other eosinophilic conditions: Discontinue systemic or inhaled corticosteroids abruptly upon initiation of therapy with **Fasenra**; decrease corticosteroids gradually, if appropriate. Treat patients with pre-existing parasitic helminth infection before therapy with **Fasenra**. If patients become infected while receiving **Fasenra** and do not respond to anti-helminth treatment, discontinue **Fasenra** until the parasitic infection resolves. The most common adverse reactions (incidence ≥5%) include headache and pharyngitis. No formal drug interaction studies have been conducted. The data on pregnancy exposure from the clinical trials are insufficient to inform on drug-associated risk. Monoclonal antibodies such as *benralizumab* are transported across the placenta during the third trimester of pregnancy; therefore, potential effects on a fetus are likely to be greater during the third trimester of pregnancy. In women with poorly or moderately controlled asthma, evidence demonstrates that there is an increased risk of preeclampsia in the mother and neonate prematurity, low birth weight, and small for gestational age. The level of asthma control should be closely monitored in pregnant females and treatment adjusted as necessary to maintain optimal control. There is no information regarding the presence of *benralizumab* in human or animal milk, and the effects of *benralizumab* on the breastfed infant and on milk production are not known.

 ATROPHIC VAGINITIS

Oral Estrogens *see Menopause*

VAGINAL ESTROGEN PREPARATIONS

➢ *estradiol* (X)(G)
 Vagifem Vaginal Tablet 1 tab intravaginally daily x 2 weeks; then 1 tab intravaginally twice weekly
  Vag tab: 10 mcg (15 tabs w. applicators)
 Yuvafem Vaginal Tablet 1 tab intravaginally daily x 2 weeks; then 1 tab intravaginally twice weekly
  Vag tab: 10 mcg (15 tabs w. applicators)
➢ *estradiol* (X)(G)
 Estrace Vaginal Cream 2-4 gm daily x 1-2 weeks; then gradually reduce to 1/2 initial dose x 1-2 weeks; then maintenance dose of 1 gm 1-3 x/week
  Vag crm: 0.01% (1 oz tube w. calib applicator)
➢ *estrogens, conjugated* (X)
 Premarin Cream 2 gm/day intravaginally
  Vag crm: 1.5 oz w. applicator marked in 1/2 gm increments to max 2 gm
➢ *estropipate* (X)
 Ogen Cream 2-4 gm intravaginally daily x 3 weeks; discontinue 4th week; continue in this cyclical pattern
  Vag crm: 1.5 mg/gm (42.5 gm w. calib applicator)

ATTENTION DEFICIT HYPERACTIVITY DISORDER (ADHD)

SELECTIVE NOREPINEPHRINE REUPTAKE INHIBITORS (SNRIs)

▷ *atomoxetine* (C)(G) take one dose daily in the morning or in two divided doses in the morning and late afternoon or early evening; initially 40 mg/kg; increase after at least 3 days to 80 mg/kg; then after 2-4 weeks may increase to max 100 mg/day
Pediatric: <6 years: not recommended; ≥6 years, <70 kg: initially 0.5 mg/kg/day: increase after at least 3 days to 1.2 mg/kg/day; max 1.4 mg/kg/day or 100 mg/day (whichever is less); ≥6 years, >70 kg: same as adult

Strattera *Cap:* 10, 18, 25, 40, 60, 80, 100 mg

Comment: **Strattera** is not associated with stimulant or euphoric effects. May discontinue without tapering. Common adverse effects associated with *atomoxetine* in children and adolescents included upset stomach, decreased appetite, nausea or vomiting, dizziness, tiredness, and mood swings. For adult patients, the most common adverse side effects included constipation, dry mouth, nausea, decreased appetite, sexual side effects, problems passing urine, and dizziness. Other adverse effects associated with *atomoxetine* included severe liver damage and potential for serious cardiovascular events. In addition, *atomoxetine* increases the risk of suicidal ideation in children and adolescents. Healthcare providers should monitor patients taking this medication for clinical worsening, suicidality, and unusual changes in behavior, particularly within the first few months of initiation or during dose changes.

STIMULANTS

▷ *amphetamine, mixed salts of single entity amphetamine* (C)(II)
Adzenys ER initially 12.5 mg (10 ml) once daily in the morning; take with or without food; individualize the dosage according to the therapeutic needs and response
Pediatric: <6 years: not recommended; 6-17 years: take with or without food; individualize the dosage according to the therapeutic needs and response; 6-12 years: initially 6.3 mg (5 ml) once daily in the morning; max dose 18.8 mg (15 ml); 13-17 years:12.5 mg (10 ml) once daily in the morning; ≥17 years: same as adult

Oral susp: 125 mg/ml ext-rel (450 ml) (orange)

Comment: Patients taking **Adderall XR** may be switched to **Adzenys ER** at the equivalent dose taken once daily; switching from any other amphetamine products (e.g., **Adderall** immediate-release), discontinue that treatment, and titrate with **Adzenys ER** using the titration schedule (see mfr pkg insert). To avoid substitution errors and overdosage, do not substitute for other amphetamine products on a mg-per-mg basis because of different amphetamine salt compositions and differing pharmacokinetic profiles. No dosage adjustments for renal or hepatic insufficiency are provided in the manufacturer's labeling.

Adzenys XR-ODT take with or without food; individualize the dosage according to the therapeutic needs and response; initially 12.5 mg once daily; max recommended dose 18.8 mg once daily
Pediatric: <6 years: not recommended; ≥6 years: take with or without food; individualize the dosage according to the therapeutic needs and response; 6-12 years: initially 6.3 mg once daily in the morning; increase in increments of 3.1 mg or 6.3 mg at weekly intervals; max recommended dose 18.8 mg once daily; ≥13 years: 12.5 mg (10 ml) once daily in the morning

Comment: Patients taking **Adderall XR** may be switched to **Adzenys XR-ODT** at the equivalent dose taken once daily; switching from any other amphetamine products (e.g., **Adderall** immediate-release), discontinue that treatment, and titrate with **Adzenys XR-ODT** using the titration schedule (see mfr pkg insert). To avoid substitution errors and overdosage, do <u>not</u> substitute for other amphetamine products on a mg-per-mg basis because of different amphetamine salt compositions and differing pharmacokinetic profiles. No dosage adjustments for renal <u>or</u> hepatic insufficiency are provided in the manufacturer's labeling.

Dyanavel XR Oral Suspension <6 years: not recommended; ≥6 years: initially 2.5 mg <u>or</u> 5 mg once daily in the morning; may increase in increments of 2.5 mg to 5 mg per day every 4-7 days; max 20 mg per day; shake bottle prior to administration

> *Oral susp:* 2.5 mg/ml (464 ml) ext-rel

Evekeo <3 years: <u>not</u> recommended; ≥3-5 years: initially 2.5 mg once <u>or</u> twice daily at the same time(s) each day; may increase by 2.5 mg/day at weekly intervals; max 40 mg/day; >5 years: initially 5 mg once <u>or</u> twice daily at the same time(s) each day; may increase by 5 mg/day at weekly intervals; max 40 mg/day

> *Tab:* 5, 10 mg

Mydayis initially 12.5 mg once daily in the morning; may titrate at weekly intervals; max 50 mg/day

Pediatric: <13 years: not recommended; 13-17 years: initially 12.5 mg once daily in the morning; may titrate at weekly intervals; max 25 mg/day; >17 years: same as adult

> *Cap:* 12.5, 25, 37.5, 50 mg ext-rel

▷ *dexmethylphenidate* (C)(II)(G) <u>not</u> indicated for adults

Focalin <6 years: <u>not</u> established; ≥6 years: initially 2.5 mg bid; allow at least 4 hours between doses; may increase at 1 week intervals; max 20 mg/day

> *Tab:* 2.5, 5, 10*mg (dye-free)

Focalin ER <6 years: <u>not</u> established; ≥6 years: initially 5 mg weekly; usual dose 10-30 mg/day

> *Cap:* 15, 30 mg ext-rel

Focalin XR <6 years: <u>not</u> established; ≥6 years: initially 5 mg weekly; usual dose 10-30 mg/day

> *Cap:* 5, 10, 15, 20, 25, 30, 35, 40 mg ext-rel

▷ *dextroamphetamine sulfate* (C)(II)(G) initially start with 10 mg daily; increase by 10 mg at weekly intervals if needed; may switch to daily dose with sust-rel spansules when titrated

Pediatric: <3 years: not recommended; ≥3-5 years: 2.5 mg daily; may increase by 2.5 mg daily at weekly intervals if needed; 6-12 years: initially 5 mg daily <u>or</u> bid; may increase by 5 mg/day at weekly intervals; usual max 40 mg/day; >12 years: initially 10 mg daily; may increase by 10 mg/day at weekly intervals; max 40 mg/day

> **Dexedrine** *Tab:* 5*mg (tartrazine)
> **Dexedrine Spansule** *Cap:* 5, 10, 15 mg ext-rel
> **Dextrostat** *Tab:* 5, 10 mg (tartrazine)

▷ *dextroamphetamine saccharate+dextroamphetamine sulfate+amphetamine aspartate+amphetamine sulfate* (C)(II)(G) <u>not</u> indicated for adults

Adderall initially 10 mg daily; may increase weekly by 10 mg/day; usual max 60 mg/day in 2-3 divided doses; first dose on awakening; then q 4-6 hours prn

Pediatric: <6 years: not indicated; ≥6-12 years: initially 5 mg daily; may increase by 5 mg/day at weekly intervals; >12 years: same as adult

> *Tab:* 5**, 7.5**, 10**, 12.5**, 15**, 20**, 30**mg

Adderall XR 20 mg by mouth once daily in AM; may increase by 10 mg/day at weekly intervals; max: 60 mg/day

Pediatric: <6 years: not recommended; ≥6 years: initially 10 mg daily in the AM; may increase by 10 mg/day at weekly intervals; max 30 mg/day; 13-17

years: 10-20 mg by mouth daily in the AM; may increase by 10 mg/day at
weekly intervals; max 40 mg/day; Do not chew; may sprinkle on apple sauce
  Cap: 5, 10, 15, 20, 25, 30 mg ext-rel

▷ *lisdexamfetamine dimesylate* (C)(II) 30 mg once daily in the AM; may increase
by 10-20 mg/day at weekly intervals; max 70 mg/day
Pediatric: <6 years: not recommended; ≥6 years: same as adult
  Vyvanse *Cap:* 20, 30, 40, 50, 60, 70 mg
  Comment: May dissolve **Vyvanse** capsule contents in water; take immediately.

▷ *methylphenidate (regular-acting)* (C)(II)(G)
  Methylin, Methylin Chewable, Methylin Oral Solution usual dose 20-30 mg/
  day in 2-3 divided doses 30-45 minutes before a meal; max 60 mg/day
  Pediatric: <6 years: not recommended; ≥6 years: initially 5 mg bid ac (breakfast
  and lunch); may increase 5-10 mg/day at weekly intervals; max 60 mg/day
    Tab: 5, 10*, 20*mg; *Chew tab:* 2.5, 5, 10 mg; (grape) (phenylalanine); *Oral
    soln:* 5, 10 mg/5 ml (grape)
  Ritalin 10-60 mg/day in 2-3 divided doses 30-45 minutes ac; max 60 mg/day
  Pediatric: <6 years: not recommended; ≥6 years: initially 5 mg bid ac
  (breakfast and lunch); may increase by 5-10 mg at weekly intervals as needed;
  max 60 mg/day
    Tab: 5, 10*, 20*mg

▷ *methylphenidate (long-acting)* (C)(II)
  Concerta initially 18 mg q AM; may increase in 18 mg increments as needed;
  max 54 mg/day; do not crush or chew
  Pediatric: <6 years: not recommended; ≥6-12 years: initially 18 mg daily; max
  54 mg/day; ≥13-17 years: initially 18 mg daily; max 72 mg/day or 2 mg/kg,
  whichever is less
    Tab: 18, 27, 36, 54 mg sust-rel
  Cotempla XR-ODT take consistently with or without food in the morning
  Pediatric: <6 years: not recommended; 6-17 years: initially 8.6 mg; may
  increase as needed and tolerated by 8.6 mg/day; daily dosage >51.8 mg is not
  recommended.
    ODT: 8.6, 17.3, 25.9 mg ext-rel orally-disint
  Jornay PM 20 mg daily in the evening; adjust the timing of administration
  between 6:30 PM and 9:30 PM to optimize the tolerability and the efficacy the
  next morning and throughout the day; dose may be increased weekly in 20
  mg per day increments; max 100 mg once daily; administer consistently either
  with or without food; swallow caps whole or open and sprinkle the entire dose
  onto applesauce
  Pediatric: <6 years: not established; ≥6 years: same as adult
    Cap: 20, 40, 60, 80, 100 mg del-rel/ext-rel
  Comment: **Jornay PM** is a proprietary drug therapy platform that consists
  of two functional film coatings. The first layer delays the initial drug release
  for up to 10 hours. The second layer helps control the release rate of the
  active ingredient throughout the day. Do not substitute **Jornay PM** for other
  methylphenidate product on a milligram-per-milligram basis.
  Metadate CD (G) 1 cap daily in the AM; may sprinkle on food; do not crush
  or chew
  Pediatric: <6 years: not recommended; ≥6 years: initially 20 mg daily; may
  gradually increase by 20 mg/day at weekly intervals as needed; max 60 mg/day
    Cap: 10, 20, 30, 40, 50, 60 mg immed- and ext-rel beads
  Metadate ER 1 tab daily in the AM; do not crush or chew
  Pediatric: <6 years: not recommended; ≥6 years: use in place of regular-acting
  methylphenidate when the 8-hour dose of **Metadate-ER** corresponds to the
  titrated 8-hour dose of regular-acting *methylphenidate*
    Tab: 10, 20 mg ext-rel (dye-free)

QuilliChew ER (G) initially 1 x 10 mg chew tab once daily in the AM
Pediatric: <6 years: not recommended; initially 10 mg daily; may gradually
increase by 20 mg/day at weekly intervals as needed; max 60 mg/day
   Chew tab: 20*, 30*40 mg ext-rel
Quillivant XR (G) initially 20 mg once daily in the AM, with or without
food; may be titrated in increments of 10-20 mg/day at weekly intervals; daily
doses above 60 mg have not been studied and are not recommended; shake
the bottle vigorously for at least 10 seconds to ensure that the correct dose is
administered
Pediatric: <6 years: not recommended; ≥6 years: same as adult
   Bottle: 5 mg/ml, 25 mg/5 ml pwdr for reconstitution; 300 mg (60 ml), 600
   mg (120 ml), 750 mg (150 ml), 900 mg (180 ml)
Comment: **Quillivant XR** must be reconstituted by a pharmacist, not by the
patient or caregiver.
Ritalin LA (G) 1 cap daily in the AM
Pediatric: <6 years: not recommended; ≥6 years: use in place of regular-
acting *methylphenidate* when the 8-hour dose of **Ritalin LA** corresponds to
the titrated 8-hour dose of regular-acting *methylphenidate*; max 60 mg/day
   Cap: 10, 20, 30, 40 mg ext-rel (immed- and ext-rel beads)
Ritalin SR 1 cap daily in the AM
Pediatric: <6 years: not recommended; ≥6 years: use in place of regular-acting
methylphenidate when the 8-hour dose of **Ritalin SR** corresponds to the
titrated 8-hour dose of regular-acting *methylphenidate*; max 60 mg/day
   Tab: 20 mg sust-rel (dye-free)
▷ *methylphenidate* transdermal patch (C)(II)(G)
Pediatric: <6 years: not recommended; ≥6-17 years: initially 10 mg patch applied
to hip 2 hours before desired effect daily in the AM; may increase by 5-10 mg at
weekly intervals; max 60 mg/day; >17 years: not applicable
   Daytrana *Transdermal patch:* 10, 15, 20, 30 mg
▷ *pemoline* (B)(IV) 18.75-112.5 mg/day; usually start with 37.5 mg in AM; may
increase 18.75 mg/day at weekly intervals; max 112.5 gm/day
Pediatric: <6 years: not recommended; ≥6 years: same as adult
   Cylert *Tab:* 18.75*, 37.5*, 75*mg
   Cylert Chewable *Chew tab:* 37.5*mg
Comment: Check baseline serum ALT and monitor every 2 weeks thereafter.
▷ *serdexmethylphenidate+dexmethylphenidate* (II) Starting dose: 39.2 mg/7.8 mg
once daily in the morning. *After one week:* increase to 52.3 mg/10.4 mg once
daily; swallow whole or open capsule and sprinkle onto applesauce or add to
water, do not crush or chew
Pediatric: 6-12 years: *Starting dose:* is 39.2 mg/7.8 mg once daily in the morning;
After one week: may increase to 52.3 mg/10.4 mg once daily or decrease to 26.1
mg/5.2 mg once daily; max 52.3 mg/10.4 mg once daily; 13-17 years: same as
adult; swallow whole or open capsule and sprinkle onto applesauce or add to
water, do not crush or chew
   Azstarys 1 tab once daily; titrate individual components
   Cap: **Azstarys 26.1 mg/5.2 mg** serdex 26.1 mg+dexmeth 5.2 mg
        Azstarys 39.2 mg/7.8 mg serdex 39.2 mg+dexmeth 7.8 mg
        Azstarys 52.3 mg/10.4 mg serdex 52.3 mg+dexmeth 10.4 mg

CENTRAL ALPHA-2 AGONIST

▷ *guanfacine* (B)(G)
Pediatric: <6 years: not recommended; ≥6-17 years: initially 1 mg once daily;
may increase by 1 mg/day at weekly intervals; usual max 4 mg/day; >17 years:
not applicable
   Intuniv *Tab:* 1, 2, 3, 4 mg ext-rel

Comment: Take **Intuniv** with water, milk, or other liquid. Do not take with a high-fat meal. Withdraw gradually by 1 mg every 3-7 days.

SELECTIVE NOREPINEPHRINE REUPTAKE INHIBITOR (SNRI)

▷ *viloxazine*

Pediatric: <6 years: not established; 6-11 years: Recommended starting dose is 100 mg once daily; may titrate in increments of 100 mg weekly to max 400 mg once daily; 12-17 years: Recommended starting dose is 200 mg once daily; may titrate after 1 week, by an increment of 200 mg to max 400 mg once daily; Capsules may be swallowed whole or opened and the entire contents sprinkled onto applesauce; Do not bite crush, or chew capsuled or capsule contents; *Hepatic Impairment*: not recommended. *Severe Renal Impairment*: max 200 mg once daily.

Qelbree *Cap*: 100, 150, 200 mg ext-rel

Comment: **Qelbree** *(viloxazine)* is a selective norepinephrine reuptake inhibitor (SNRI) for the treatment of attention deficit hyperactivity disorder (ADHD) in pediatric patients 6 to 17 years-of-age. The most commonly observed adverse reactions to **Qelbree** (≥5% and at least twice the rate of placebo) have been somnolence, decreased appetite, fatigue, nausea, vomiting, insomnia, and irritability. Black Box Warning (BBW): In clinical trials, higher rates of suicidal thoughts and behavior were reported in pediatric patients treated with Qelbree than in patients treated with placebo. Closely monitor for worsening and emergence of suicidal thoughts and behavior. Contraindictions to **Qelbree** are (1) concomitant administration of monoamine oxidase inhibitors (MAOIs) or dosing within 14 days after discontinuing an MAOI and (2) concomitant administration of sensitive CYP1A2 substrates or CYP1A2 substrates with a narrow therapeutic range. Moderate sensitive CYP1A2 substrates are not recommended for co-administration with **Qelbree**; dose reduction may be warranted. **Qelbree** may cause maternal harm in pregnancy; discontinue when pregnancy is recognized. Available data from case series with *viloxazine* use in pregnant women are insufficient to determine a drug-associated risk of major birth defects, miscarriage or adverse maternal outcomes. There is a pregnancy exposure registry that monitors pregnancy outcomes in women exposed **Qelbree** during pregnancy. Healthcare providers are encouraged to register patients by calling the National Pregnancy Registry for Psychiatric Medications at 1-866-961-2388 or visiting HYPERLINK "http://www.womensmentalhealth.org/preg" www.womensmentalhealth.org/preg. There are no data on the presence of *viloxazine* in human milk or effects on the breastfed infant. However, it is likely that *viloxazine* is present in human milk.

TRICYCLIC ANTIDEPRESSANTS (TCAS)

see **Depression**

OTHER AGENTS

▷ *clonidine* (C)(G)

Catapres 4-5 mcg/kg/day

Pediatric: <12 years: not recommended; ≥12 years: same as adult

Tab: 0.1*, 0.2*, 0.3*mg

Catapres-TTS <12 years: not recommended; ≥12 years: initially 0.1 mg patch weekly; increase after 1-2 weeks if needed; max 0.6 mg/day

Patch: 0.1, 0.2 mg/day (12/carton); 0.3 mg/day (4/carton)

Kapvay not indicated for adults

Pediatric: <6 years: not recommended; ≥6-12 years: initially 0.1 mg at bedtime x 1 week; then 0.1 mg bid x 1 week; then 0.1 mg AM and 0.2 mg PM x 1 week; then 0.2 mg bid; withdraw gradually by 0.1 mg/day at 3-7 day intervals

Tab: 0.1, 0.2 mg ext-rel

Nexiclon XR initially 0.18 mg (2 ml) suspension or 0.17 mg tab once daily; usual max 0.52 mg (6 ml suspension) once daily
Pediatric: <12 years: not recommended; ≥12 years: same as adult
  Tab: 0.17, 0.26 mg ext-rel; *Oral susp:* 0.09 mg/ml ext-rel (4 oz)

AMINOKETONES (FOR THE TREATMENT OF ADHD)

➤ *bupropion HBr* (C)(G) initially 100 mg bid for at least 3 days; may increase to 375 or 400 mg/day after several weeks; then after at least 3 more days, 450 mg in 4 divided doses; max 450 mg/day, 174 mg/single dose
Pediatric: <18 years: not recommended; ≥18 years: Safety and effectiveness in the pediatric population have not been established. When considering the use of **Aplenzin** in a child or adolescent, balance the potential risks with the clinical need
  Aplenzin *Tab:* 174, 348, 522 mg

➤ *bupropion HCl* (C)(G)
Forfivo XL do not use for initial treatment; use immediate-release *bupropion* forms for initial titration; switch to **Forfivo XL** 450 mg once daily when total dose/day reaches 450 mg; may switch to **Forfivo XL** when total dose/day reaches 300 mg for 2 weeks and patient needs 450 mg/day to reach therapeutic target; swallow whole, do not crush or chew
  Pediatric: <18 years: not recommended; >18 years: same as adult; Safety and effectiveness of long-acting and extended-release *bupropion* in the pediatric population have not been established. When considering the use of **Forfivo XL** in a child or adolescent, balance the potential risks with the clinical need
  Tab: 450 mg ext-rel

Wellbutrin initially 100 mg bid for at least 3 days; may increase to 375 or 400 mg/day after several weeks; then after at least 3 more days, 450 mg in 4 divided doses; max 450 mg/day, 150 mg/single dose
Pediatric: <12 years: not recommended; ≥12 years: same as adult
  Tab: 75, 100 mg

Wellbutrin SR initially 150 mg in AM for at least 3 days; may increase to 150 mg bid if well tolerated; usual dose 300 mg/day; max 400 mg/day
Pediatric: <12 years: not recommended; ≥12 years: same as adult
  Tab: 100, 150 mg sust-rel

Wellbutrin XL initially 150 mg in AM for at least 3 days; increase to 150 mg bid if well tolerated; usual dose 300 mg/day; max 400 mg/day
Pediatric: <12 years: not recommended; ≥12 years: same as adult
  Tab: 150, 300 mg sust-rel

◯ BACTERIAL ENDOCARDITIS: PROPHYLAXIS

Comment: Bacterial endocarditis prophylaxis is appropriate for persons with a history of previous infective endocarditis, persons with a prosthetic cardiac valve or prosthetic material used for valve repair, cardiac transplant patients who develop cardiac valvulopathy, congenital heart disease (CHD), unrepaired cyanotic CHD including palliative shunts and conduits, completely repaired congenital heart defect(s) with prosthetic material or device, whether placed by surgery or by catheter intervention, during the first 6 months after the procedure, repaired CHD with residual defects at the site or adjacent to the site of a prosthetic patch or prosthetic device (which may inhibit endothelialization), or any other condition deemed to place a patient at high risk.

DENTAL, ORAL, RESPIRATORY TRACT, ESOPHAGEAL PROCEDURES
➤ *amoxicillin* (B)(G) 2 gm PO 30-60 minutes before procedure as a single dose or 3 gm 1 hour before procedure and 1.5 gm 6 hours later

Pediatric: 50 mg/kg as a single dose <u>or</u> 50 mg/kg (max 3 gm) 1 hour before procedure and (max 1.5 gm) 25 mg/kg 6 hours later; ≥40 kg: same as adult; *see* Appendix CC.3. *amoxicillin* (Amoxil Suspension, Trimox Suspension) *for dose by weight*

> **Amoxil** *Cap:* 250, 500 mg; *Tab:* 875*mg; *Chew tab:* 125, 200, 250, 400 mg (cherry-banana-peppermint) (phenylalanine); *Oral susp:* 125, 250 mg/5 ml (80, 100, 150 ml) (strawberry); 200, 400 mg/5 ml (50, 75, 100 ml) (bubble gum); *Oral drops:* 50 mg/ml (30 ml) (bubble gum)

> **Trimox** *Tab:* 125, 250 mg; *Cap:* 250, 500 mg; *Oral susp:* 125, 250 mg/5 ml (80, 100, 150 ml) (raspberry-strawberry)

▷ *ampicillin* (B)(G) 2 gm PO/IM/IV 30-60 minutes before procedure
Pediatric: <12 years: 50 mg/kg PO/IM/IV 30-60 minutes before procedure; ≥12 years: same as adult

> **Omnipen, Principen** *Cap:* 250, 500 mg; *Oral susp:* 125, 250 mg/5 ml (100, 150, 200 ml) (fruit)

> **Unasyn** *Vial:* 1.5, 3 gm

▷ *azithromycin* (B)(G) 500 mg 30-60 minutes before procedure
Pediatric: <12 years: 15 mg/kg 30-60 minutes before procedure; max 500 mg; *see* Appendix CC.7. *azithromycin* (Zithromax Suspension, Zmax Suspension) *for dose by weight*; ≥12 years: same as adult

> **Zithromax** *Tab:* 250, 500, 600 mg; *Oral susp:* 100 mg/5 ml (15 ml); 200 mg/5 ml (15, 22.5, 30 ml) (cherry)

▷ *cefazolin* (B) 1 gm IM/IV 30-60 minutes before procedure
Pediatric: <12 years: 25 mg/kg IM/IV 30-60 minutes before procedure; ≥12 years: same as adult

> **Ancef** *Vial:* 250, 500 mg; 1, 5 gm

> **Kefzol** *Vial:* 500 mg; 1 gm

▷ *ceftriaxone* (B)(G) 1 gm IM/IV as a single dose
Pediatric: <12 years: 50 mg/kg IM/IV as a single dose; ≥12 years: same as adult

> **Rocephin** *Vial:* 250, 500 mg; 1, 2 gm

▷ *cephalexin* (B)(G) 2 gm as a single dose 30-60 minutes before procedure
Pediatric: 50 mg/kg as a single dose 30-60 minutes before procedure; *see* Appendix CC.15. *cephalexin* (Keflex Suspension) *for dose by weight*

> **Keflex** *Cap:* 250, 333, 500, 750 mg; *Oral susp:* 125, 250 mg/5 ml (100, 200 ml) (strawberry) w

▷ *clarithromycin* (C)(G) 500 mg <u>or</u> 500 mg ext-rel as a single dose 30-60 minutes before procedure
Pediatric: 15 mg/kg as a single dose 30-60 minutes before procedure; *see* Appendix CC.16. *clarithromycin* (Biaxin Suspension) *for dose by weight*

> **Biaxin** *Tab:* 250, 500 mg

> **Biaxin Oral Suspension** *Oral susp:* 125, 250 mg/5 ml (50, 100 ml) (fruit-punch)

> **Biaxin XL** *Tab:* 500 mg ext-rel

▷ *clindamycin* (B)(G) 600 mg PO as a one-time single-dose <u>or</u> 300 mg 30-60 minutes before procedure and 150 mg 6 hours later; take with a full glass of water
Pediatric: <12 years: 20 mg/kg (max 300 mg) 1 hour before procedure and 10 mg/kg (max 150 mg) 6 hours later; take with a full glass of water; *see* Appendix CC.17. *clindamycin* (Cleocin Pediatric Granules) *for dose by weight*; ≥12 years: same as adult

> **Cleocin** (G) *Cap:* 75 (tartrazine), 150 (tartrazine), 300 mg; *Vial:* 150 mg/ml (2, 4 ml) (benzyl alcohol)

> **Cleocin Pediatric Granules** (G) *Oral susp:* 75 mg/ml (100 ml)(cherry)

▷ *erythromycin estolate* (B)(G) 1 gm 1 hour before procedure; then 500 mg 6 hours later
Pediatric: <12 years: 20 mg/kg 1 hour before procedure; then 10 mg/kg 6 hours later; *see Appendix CC.20. erythromycin* estolate (Ilosone Suspension) *for dose by weight*; ≥12 years: same as adult

> **Ilosone** *Pulvule:* 250 mg; *Tab:* 500 mg; *Liq:* 125, 250 mg/5 ml (100 ml)

▷ **penicillin v potassium** (B)(G) 2 gm 1 hour before procedure; then 1 gm 6 hours later or 2 gm 1 hour before procedure; then 1 gm q 6 hours x 8 doses
Pediatric: <12 years, <60 lb: 1 gm 1 hour before procedure; then 500 mg 6 hours later or 1 gm 1 hour before procedure; then 500 mg q 6 hours x 8 doses; *see* Appendix CC.29. penicillin v potassium (Pen-Vee K Solution, Veetids Solution) *for dose by weight;* ≥12 years: same as adult
　　Pen-Vee K *Tab:* 250, 500 mg; *Oral soln:* 125 mg/5 ml (100, 200 ml); 250 mg/5 ml (100, 150, 200 ml)

BACTERIAL VAGINOSIS (BV, *GARDNERELLA VAGINALIS*)

PROPHYLAXIS AND RESTORATION OF VAGINAL ACIDITY

▷ **acetic acid+oxyquinolone** (C) one full applicator intravaginally bid for up to 30 days
Pediatric: <12 years: not recommended; ≥12 years: same as adult
　　Relagard *Gel:* acet acid 0.9%+oxyq 0.025% (50 gm tube w. applicator)
　　Comment: The following treatment regimens for *bacterial vaginosis* are published in the **2015 CDC Sexually Transmitted Diseases Treatment Guidelines.** Treatment regimens are presented by generic drug name first, followed by information about brands and dose forms. BV is associated with adverse pregnancy outcomes, including premature rupture of the membranes, preterm labor, preterm birth, intra-amniotic infection, and postpartum endometritis. Therefore, treatment is recommended for all pregnant females with symptoms or positive screen.

RECOMMENDED REGIMENS

Regimen 1
▷ **metronidazole** 500 mg bid x 7 days or **metronidazole** ext-rel 750 mg once daily x 7 days

Regimen 2
▷ **metronidazole** gel 0.75% one applicatorful (5 gm) once daily x 5 days

Regimen 3
▷ **clindamycin** cream 2% one full applicatorful (5 gm) intravaginally once daily at bedtime x 5 days

ALTERNATE REGIMENS

Regimen 1
▷ **tinidazole** 2 gm once daily x 2 days

Regimen 2
▷ **tinidazole** 1 gm once daily x 5 days

Regimen 3
▷ **clindamycin** 300 mg bid x 7 days

Regimen 4
▷ **clindamycin** ovules 100 mg intravaginally once daily at bedtime x 3 days

Regimen 5
▷ **secnidazole** one 2 gm packet as a single dose

Drug Brands and Dose Forms

▷ **clindamycin** (B)
　　Cleocin (G) *Cap:* 75 (tartrazine), 150 (tartrazine), 300 mg
　　Cleocin Pediatric Granules (G) *Oral susp:* 75 mg/5 ml (100 ml) (cherry)

Cleocin Vaginal Cream *Vag crm:* 2% (21, 40 gm tubes w. applicator)
Cleocin Vaginal Ovules *Vag supp:* 100 mg
▷ *metronidazole* (not for use in 1st; B in 2nd, 3rd)
   Flagyl *Tab:* 250*, 500*mg
   Flagyl 375 *Cap:* 375 mg
   Flagyl ER *Tab:* 750 mg ext-rel
   MetroGel-Vaginal, Vandazole *Vag gel:* 0.75% (70 gm w. applicator) (parabens)
   Nuvessa 1.3% one single-dose, pre-filled disposable applicatorful,
   administered once intravaginally at bedtime.
      Prefilled disposable applicator: 1.3% (65 mg/5 gm, 1 applicator/carton),
      single-dose
   Comment: Nitroimidazole antimicrobials are indicated for the treatment of
   bacterial vaginosis in females ≥12 years-of-age. Breastfeeding is not
   recommended; discontinue breastfeeding for 2 days after use. Concomitant
   use of *disulfiram*, or within 2 weeks of *disulfiram*, and concomitant use of
   alcohol are contraindications to *metronidazole* use.
▷ *secnidazole*
   Solosec *Oral granules:* 2 gm/pkt
   Comment: Solosec is a nitromidazole antimicrobial. Do not dissolve Solosec
   in liquid. Sprinkle contents onto applesauce, yogurt, or pudding. Consume
   within 30 mins without chewing or crunching. May follow with a glass of
   water. Potential adverse side effects are vulvovaginal pruritus, vulvovaginal
   candidiasis, headache, nausea, dysgeusia, vomiting, diarrhea, and abdominal
   pain. Whereas *metronidazole* and *tinidazole* are contraindicated during the
   first trimester of pregnancy, no adverse developmental outcomes have been
   found in animal reproductive studies and the labeling for *senidazole* does not
   include a restriction for use in pregnancy. Breastfeeding is not recommended
   during and for 96 hours after dose; may pump and discard milk during this
   time period.
▷ *tinidazole* (C)
   Tindamax *Tab:* 250*, 500*mg
   Comment: Other than for use in the treatment of *giardiasis* and *amebiasis* in
   pediatric patients >3 years-of-age, safety and effectiveness of *tinidazole* in
   pediatric patients have not been established. *Tinidazole* is excreted in breast milk
   in concentrations similar to those seen in serum and can be detected in breast
   milk for up to 72 hours following administration. Interruption of breastfeeding is
   recommended during *tinidazole* therapy and for 3 days following the last dose.

BALDNESS: MALE PATTERN

TYPE II 5-ALPHA-REDUCTASE SPECIFIC INHIBITOR
▷ *finasteride* (X)(G) 1 mg daily
   Propecia *Tab:* 1 mg
   Comment: Pregnant females should not touch broken *finasteride* tabs. Use of
   Propecia, a 5-alpha reductase inhibitor, is associated with low but increased risk
   of high-grade prostate cancer.

PERIPHERAL VASODILATOR
▷ *minoxidil* topical soln (C)(G) 1 ml from dropper or 6 sprays bid
   Pediatric: <18 years: not recommended; ≥18 years: same as adult
   Rogaine for Men (OTC) *Regular soln:* 2% (60 ml w. applicator) (alcohol 60%);
      Extra strength soln: 5% (60 ml w. applicator) (alcohol 30%)
   Rogaine for Women (OTC) Regular soln: 2% (60 ml w. applicator) (alcohol
      60%); *Topical aerosol:* 5%
   Comment: Do not use *minoxidil* on abraded or inflamed scalp.

BELL'S PALSY

▷ *prednisone* (C)(G) 80 mg once daily x 3 days; then 60 mg daily x 3 days; then 40 mg daily x 3 days; then 20 mg x 1 dose; then discontinue
Pediatric: <18 years: oral suspension options by weight
    Deltasone *Tab:* 2.5*, 5*, 10*, 20*, 50*mg

BENIGN ESSENTIAL TREMOR

ANTI-PARKINSON'S AGENT

▷ *amantadine* (C)(G) 200 mg daily <u>or</u> 100 mg bid; 4 tsp of syrup once daily <u>or</u> 2 tsp bid
    Gocovri *Cap:* 68.5, 37 mg ext-rel
    Symmetrel *Tab:* 100 mg; *Syr:* 50 mg/5 ml (raspberry)

BETA-BLOCKER

▷ *propranolol* (C)(G)
    Inderal initially 40 mg bid; usual range 160-240 mg/day
        Tab: 10*, 20*, 40*, 60*, 80*mg
    Inderal LA initially 80 mg once daily in a single dose; increase q 3-7 days; usual range 120-160 mg/day; max 320 mg/day in a single dose
        Cap: 60, 80, 120, 160 mg sust-rel
    InnoPran XL initially 80 mg q HS; max 120 mg/day
        Cap: 80, 120 mg ext-rel

BENIGN PROSTATIC HYPERPLASIA (BPH)

ALPHA-1 BLOCKERS

Comment: Educate patient regarding potential side effect of hypotension, especially with the first dose. Usually start at lowest dose and titrate upward.
▷ *doxazosin* (C)
    Cardura initially 1 mg daily; may double dose every 1-2 weeks; max 8 mg/day
        Tab: 1*, 2*, 4*, 8*mg
    Cardura XL initially 4 mg once daily with breakfast; may titrate after 3-4 weeks; max 8 mg/day
        Tab: 4, 8 mg ext-rel
▷ *silodosin* (B)(G) 8 mg once daily; *CrCl 30-50 mL/min:* 4 mg once daily
    Rapaflo *Cap:* 4, 8 mg
▷ *terazosin* (C)(G) initially 1 mg q HS; titrate up to 10 mg once daily; max 20 mg/day
    Hytrin *Cap:* 1, 2, 5, 10 mg

ALPHA-1A BLOCKERS

▷ *alfuzosin* (B)(G) 10 mg once daily taken immediately after the same meal each day
    UroXatral *Tab:* 10 mg ext-rel
▷ *tamsulosin* (B)(G) initially 0.4 mg once daily; may increase to 0.8 mg daily after 2-4 weeks if needed
    Flomax *Cap:* 0.4 mg
    Comment: May take **Flomax** 0.4 mg <u>plus</u> **Imitrex** 0.5 mg once daily as combination therapy.

TYPE II 5-ALPHA-REDUCTASE INHIBITOR

Comment: Pregnant females and females of childbearing age should <u>not</u> handle *finasteride*. Monitor for potential side effects of decreased libido <u>and/or</u> impotence. Low, but increased risk of being diagnosed with high-grade prostate cancer.

▷ *finasteride* (X) 5 mg once daily
    Proscar *Tab:* 5 mg

TYPES I AND II 5-ALPHA-REDUCTASE INHIBITOR

Comment: Pregnant females and females of childbearing age should not handle *dutasteride*. Monitor for potential side effects of decreased libido and/or impotence. Low, but increased risk of being diagnosed with high-grade prostate cancer.

▷ *dutasteride* (X)(G) 0.5 mg once daily
    Avodart *Cap:* 0.5 mg
    Comment: May take **Avodart** 0.5 mg with **Flomax** 0.4 mg once daily as combination therapy.

TYPE I AND II 5-ALPHA-REDUCTASE INHIBITOR+ALPHA-1A BLOCKER

▷ *dutasteride+tamsulosin* (X)(G) take 1 cap once daily after the same meal each day
    Jalyn *Cap:* duta 0.5 mg+tam 0.4 mg

PHOSPHODIESTERASE TYPE 5 (PDE5) INHIBITORS, CGMP-SPECIFIC

Comment: Oral PDE5 inhibitors are contraindicated in patients taking nitrates. Caution with history of recent MI, stroke, life-threatening arrhythmia, hypotension, hypertension, cardiac failure, unstable angina, retinitis pigmentosa, CYP3A4 inhibitors (e.g., *cimetidine*, the azoles, *erythromycin*, grapefruit juice), protease inhibitors (e.g., *ritonavir*), CYP3A4 inducers (e.g., *rifampin*, *carbamazepine*, *phenytoin*, *phenobarbital*), alcohol, antihypertensive agents. Side effects include headache, flushing, nasal congestion, rhinitis, dyspepsia, and diarrhea.

▷ *tadalafil* (B)(G) 5 mg once daily at the same time each day; *CrCl 30-50 mL/ min:* initially 2.5 mg; *CrCl <30 mL/min:* not recommended; *Concomitant alpha blockers:* not recommended
    Cialis *Tab:* 2.5, 5, 10, 20 mg

 BILE ACID DEFICIENCY

BILE ACID

▷ *ursodiol* (B)
    Dissolution of radiolucent non-calcified gallstones <20 mm diameter: 8-10 mg/ kg/day in 2-3 divided doses; *Prevention:* 13-15 mg/kg/day in 4 divided doses
    Pediatric: <12 years: not recommended; ≥12 years: same as adult
    Actigall *Cap:* 300 mg
    Comment: *Ursodiol* decreases the amount of cholesterol produced by the liver and absorbed by the intestines. It helps break down cholesterol that has formed into stones in the gallbladder. *Ursodiol* increases bile flow in patients with primary biliary cirrhosis. It is used to treat small gallstones in people who cannot have cholecystectomy surgery and to prevent gallstones in overweight patients undergoing rapid weight loss. *Ursodiol* is not for treating gallstones that are calcified.

BINGE EATING DISORDER

CENTRAL NERVOUS SYSTEM (CNS) STIMULANT

▷ *lisdexamfetamine dimesylate* (C)(II) swallow whole or may open and mix/dissolve contents of cap in yogurt, water, orange juice and take immediately; 30 mg once daily in the AM; may adjust in increments of 20 mg at weekly intervals; target dose 50-70 mg/day; max 70 mg/day; *GFR 15-<30 mL/min:* max 50 mg/day; *GFR <15 mL/min, ESRD:* max 30 mg/day

Pediatric: <18 years: not established; ≥18 years: same as adult
Vyvanse *Cap:* 10, 20, 30, 40, 50, 60 70 mg
Comment: **Vyvanse** is not approved or recommended for weight loss treatment
of obesity.

BIPOLAR DISORDER

Comment: Bipolar I Disorder is characterized by one or more manic episodes
that last at least a week or require hospitalization. Severe mania may manifest
symptoms of psychosis. Bipolar II Disorder is characterized by one or more
depressive episodes accompanied by at least one hypomanic episode. When one
parent has Bipolar Disorder, the risk to each child of developing the disorder
is estimated to be 15-30%. When both parents have the disorder, the risk to
each child increases to 50-75%. Symptoms of mood disorders may be difficult
to diagnose in children and adolescents because they can be mistaken for
age-appropriate emotions and behaviors or overlap with symptoms of other
conditions such as ADHD. However, since anxiety and depression in children
may be precursers to Bipolar Disorder, these behaviors should be carefully
monitored and evaluated. The cornerstone of treatment for Bipolar Disorder is
mood-stabilizers (*lithium* and *valproate*). Common adjunctive agents include
antiepileptics, antipsychotics, and combination agents. Mounting evidence
suggests that antidepressants aren't effective in the treatment of bipolar
depression. A major study funded by the National Institute of Mental Health
(NIMH) showed that adding an antidepressant to a mood stabilizer was no
more effective in treating bipolar depression than using a mood stabilizer alone.
Another NIMH study found that antidepressants work no better than placebo. If
antidepressants are used at all, they should be combined with a mood stabilizer
such as *lithium* or *valproic acid*. Antidepressants, without a concomitant mood
stabilizer, can increase the frequency of mood cycling and trigger a manic
episode. Many experts believe that over time, antidepressant use as monotherapy
(i.e., without a mood stabilizer) in people with Bipolar Disorder has a mood
destabilizing effect, increasing the frequency of manic and depressive episodes.
Drugs and conditions that can mimic Bipolar Disorder include thyroid disorders,
corticosteroids, antidepressants, adrenal disorders (e.g., Addison's disease,
Cushing's syndrome), antianxiety drugs, drugs for Parkinson's disease, vitamin
B12 deficiency, neurological disorders (e.g., epilepsy, multiple sclerosis).

MOOD STABILIZERS
Lithium Salts Mood Stabilizer
▷ *lithium carbonate* (D)(G) swallow whole; *Usual maintenance:* 900-1200 mg/day
in 2-3 divided doses
Pediatric: <12 years: not recommended; ≥12 years: same as adult
Lithobid *Tab:* 300 mg slow-rel
Comment: Signs and symptoms of *lithium* toxicity can occur below 2 mEq/L and
include blurred vision, tinnitus, weakness, dizziness, nausea, abdominal pains,
vomiting, diarrhea to (severe) hand tremors, ataxia, muscle twitches, nystagmus,
seizures, slurred speech, decreased level of consciousness, coma, and death.

Valproate Mood Stabilizer
▷ *divalproex sodium* (D)(G) take once daily; swallow ext-rel form whole; initially
25 mg/kg/day in divided doses; max 60 mg/kg/day; *Elderly:* reduce initial dose
and titrate slowly
Pediatric: <12 years: not recommended; ≥12 years: same as adult
Depakene *Cap:* 250 mg; *Syr:* 250 mg/5 ml (16 oz)
Depakote *Tab:* 125, 250 mg

Depakote ER *Tab:* 250, 500 mg ext-rel
Depakote Sprinkle *Cap:* 125 mg

ANTIEPILEPTICS

▷ *carbamazepine* (D) ext-rel oral forms should be swallowed whole; may open caps and sprinkle on applesauce (do <u>not</u> crush <u>or</u> chew beads); initially 400 mg/day in 2 divided doses; adjust in increments of 200 mg/day; max 1.6 gm/day. *Elderly:* reduce initial dose and titrate slowly; oral doses are preferred; IV administration is recommended when the patient is unable to swallow an oral form (see **Carnexiv**)

Pediatric: <12 years: not recommended; ≥12 years: same as adult

    Carbatrol (G) *Cap:* 200, 300 mg ext-rel

    Carnexiv *Vial:* 10 mg/ml (20 ml)

    Comment: The total daily dose of **Carnexiv** is 70% of the total daily oral *carbamazepine* dose (see mfr pkg insert for dosage conversion table). The total daily dose should be equally divided into four 30-minute infusions, separated by 6 hours. Must be diluted prior to administration. Patients should be switched back to oral *carbamazepine* at their previous total daily oral dose and frequency of administration as soon as clinically appropriate. The use of **Carnexiv** for more than 7 consecutive days has <u>not</u> been studied.

    Equetro (G) *Cap:* 100, 200, 300 mg ext-rel

    Tegretol (G) *Tab:* 200*mg; *Chew tab:* 100*mg; *Oral susp:* 100 mg/5 ml (450 ml; citrus-vanilla)

    Tegretol XR (G) *Tab:* 100, 200, 400 mg ext-rel

    Comment: *Carbamazepine* is indicated in mixed episodes in bipolar I disorder.

▷ *lamotrigine* (C)(G) <u>Not</u> *taking an enzyme-inducing antiepileptic drug (EIAED) (e.g., phenytoin, carbamazepine, phenobarbital, primidone, valproic acid):* 25 mg once daily x 2 weeks; then 50 mg once daily x 2 weeks; then 100 mg once daily x 2 weeks; then target dose 200 mg once daily; *Concomitant valproic acid:* 25 mg every other day x 2 weeks; then 25 mg once daily x 2 weeks; then 50 mg once daily x 1 week; then target dose 100 mg once daily; *Concomitant EIAED, not valproic acid:* 50 mg once daily x 2 weeks; then 100 mg daily in divided doses; then increase weekly by 100 mg in divided doses to target dose 400 mg/day in divided doses daily.

Pediatric: <12 years: not recommended; ≥12 years: same as adult

    Lamictal *Tab:* 25*, 100*, 150*, 200*mg

    Lamictal Chewable Dispersible Tab *Chew tab:* 2, 5, 25, 50 mg (black current)

    Lamictal ODT *ODT:* 25, 50, 100, 200 mg

    Lamictal XR *Tab:* 25, 50, 100, 200 mg ext-rel

    Comment: *Lamotrigine* is indicated for maintenance treatment of bipolar I disorder. See mfr pkg insert for drug interactions, interactions with contraceptives and hormone replacement therapy, and discontinuation protocol.

ANTIPSYCHOTICS

Comment: Common side effects of antipsychotic drugs include drowsiness, weight gain, sexual dysfunction, dry mouth, constipation, and blurred vision. *Neuroleptic Malignant Syndrome* (NMS) and *Tardive Dyskinesia* (TD) are adverse side effects (ASEs) most often associated with the older antipsychotic drugs. Risk is decreased with the newer "atypical" antipsychotic drugs. However, these syndromes can develop, although much less commonly, after relatively brief treatment periods at low doses. Given these considerations, antipsychotic drugs should be prescribed in a manner that is most likely to minimize the occurrence. NMS, a potentially fatal symptom complex, is characterized by hyperpyrexia, muscle rigidity, altered mental status and evidence of autonomic instability (irregular pulse <u>or</u> blood pressure, tachycardia, diaphoresis, and cardiac dysrhythmia). Additional signs may include elevated creatine phosphokinase (CPK), myoglobinuria (rhabdomyolysis), and acute renal failure (ARF). TD is a syndrome consisting of potentially irreversible, involuntary, dyskinetic movements that can develop in patients with antipsychotic drugs. Characteristics include repetitive involuntary movements, usually of the jaw, lips, and tongue, such as grimacing, sticking out the tongue, and smacking the lips. Some affected people also experience involuntary movement of the extremities or difficulty breathing. The syndrome may remit, partially or completely, if antipsychotic treatment is withdrawn. If signs and symptoms of NMS and/or TD appear in a patient, management should include immediate discontinuation of antipsychotic drugs and other drugs not essential to concurrent therapy, intensive symptomatic treatment, medical monitoring, and treatment of any concomitant serious medical problems. The risk of developing NMS and/or TD, and the likelihood that either syndrome will become irreversible, is believed to increase as the duration of treatment and the total cumulative dose of antipsychotic drugs administered to the patient increase. The first and only FDA-approved treatment for TD is **valbenazine (Ingrezza)** (*see* Tardive Dyskinesia)

▷ *aripiprazole* (C)(G) initially 15 mg once daily; may increase to max 30 mg/day
  Pediatric: <10 years: not recommended; ≥10-17 years: initially 2 mg/day in a single dose for 2 days; then increase to 5 mg/day in a single dose for 2 days; then increase to target dose of 10 mg/day in a single dose; may increase by 5 mg/day at weekly intervals as needed to max 30 mg/day
    Abilify *Tab:* 2, 5, 10, 15, 20, 30 mg
    Abilify Discmelt *Tab:* 15 mg orally-disint (vanilla) (phenylalanine)
    Abilify Maintena *Vial:* 300, 400 mg ext-rel pwdr for IM injection after reconstitution; 300, 400 mg single dose prefilled dual-chamber syringes w. supplies
    Comment: **Abilify** is indicated for acute and maintenance treatment of mixed episodes in bipolar I disorder, as monotherapy or as adjunct to *lithium* or *valproic acid.*

▷ *asenapine* (C)(G) allow SL tab to dissolve on tongue; do not split, crush, chew, or swallow; do not eat or drink for 10 minutes after administration; *Monotherapy:* 10 mg bid; *Adjunctive therapy:* 5 mg bid; may increase to max 10 mg bid
  Pediatric: <10 years: not established; 10-17 years: *Monotherapy:* initially 2.5 mg bid; may increase to 5 mg bid after 3 days; then to 10 mg bid after 3 more days; max 10 mg bid
    Saphris *SL tab:* 2, 5, 5, 10 mg (black cherry)
    Comment: **Saphris** is indicated for acute treatment of manic or mixed episodes in bipolar I disorder, as monotherapy or as adjunct to *lithium* or *valproic acid.*

▷ *cariprazine* initially 1.5 mg once daily; recommended therapeutic dose 3-6 mg/day
  Pediatric: <12 years: not established; ≥12 years: same as adult
    Vraylar *Cap:* 1.5, 3, 4.5, 6 mg; 7-count (1 x 1.5 mg, 6 x 3 mg) mixed blister pck
    Comment: **Vraylar** is an atypical antipsychotic with partial agonist activity at D2 and 5-HT1A receptors and antagonist activity at 5-HT2A receptors. It is indicated for acute treatment of mixed episodes in bipolar I disorder. There is a **Vraylar** pregnancy exposure registry that monitors pregnancy outcomes in women exposed to **Vraylar** during pregnancy. For more information, contact the National Pregnancy Registry for Atypical Antipsychotics at 1-866-961-2388 or visit https://womensmentalhealth.org/clinical-and-research-programs/pregnancyregistry. Safety and effectiveness in pediatric patients have not been established.

▷ *lurasidone* (B)(G) initially 20 mg once daily; usual range 20 to max 120 mg/day; take with food; *CrCl <50 mL/min, moderate hepatic impairment (Child-Pugh 7-9):* max 80 mg/day; *Child-Pugh 10-15):* max 40 mg/day
  Pediatric: <10 years: not established; 10-17 years: initially 20 mg once daily; may titrate up to max 80 mg/day; >17 years: same as adult

Latuda *Tab:* 20, 40, 60, 80, 120 mg

Comment: **Latuda** is indicated for major depressive episodes associated with bipolar I disorder as monotherapy and as adjunctive therapy with *lithium* or *valproic* acid. Contraindicated with concomitant strong CYP3A4 inhibitors (e.g., *ketoconazole, voriconazole, clarithromycin, ritonavir*) and inducers (e.g., *phenytoin, carbamazepine, rifampin, St. John's wort*); see mfr pkg insert if patient taking moderate CYP3A4 inhibitors (e.g., *diltiazem, atazanavir, erythromycin, fluconazole, verapamil*). The efficacy of **Latuda** in the treatment of mania associated with bipolar disorder has not been established.

▷ *quetiapine fumarate* (C)(G)

SeroQUEL initially 25 mg bid, titrate q 2nd or 3rd day in increments of 25-50 mg bid-tid; usual maintenance 400-600 mg/day in 2-3 divided doses
Pediatric: <10 years: not recommended; ≥10-17 years: initially 25 mg bid, titrate q 2nd or 3rd day in increments of 25-50 mg bid-tid; max 600 mg/day in 2-3 divided doses
Tab: 25, 50, 100, 200, 300, 400 mg

SeroQUEL XR swallow whole; administer once daily in the PM; *Day 1:* 50 mg; *Day 2:* 100 mg; *Day 3:* 200 mg; *Day 4:* 300 mg; usual range 400-600 mg/day
Pediatric: <18 years: not recommended; ≥18 years: same as adult
Tab: 50, 150, 200, 300, 400 mg ext-rel

▷ *risperidone* (C) *Tab:* initially 2-3 mg once daily; may adjust at 24 hour intervals by 1 mg/day; usual range 1-6 mg/day; max 6 mg/day; *Oral soln:* do not take with cola or tea; *M-tab:* dissolve on tongue with or without fluid; *Consta:* administer deep IM in the deltoid or gluteal; give with oral *risperidone* or other antipsychotic x 3 weeks; then stop oral form; 25 mg IM every 2 weeks; max 50 mg every 2 weeks

Risperdal
Pediatric: <5 years: not established; 5-10 years: initially 0.5 mg once daily at the same time each day adjust at 24 hour intervals by 0.5-1 mg to target dose 1-2.5 mg/day; usual range 1-6 mg/day; max 6 mg/day; >10 years: same as adult
Tab: 0.25, 0.5, 1, 2, 3, 4 mg; *Oral soln:* 1 mg/ml (100 ml)

Risperdal Consta
Pediatric: <18 years: not established; ≥18 years: same as adult
Vial: 12.5, 25, 37.5, 50 mg pwdr for long-acting IM inj after reconstitution, single-use, w. diluent and supplies

Risperdal M-Tab
Pediatric: <10 years: not established; ≥10 years: same as adult
Tab: 0.5, 1, 2, 3, 4 mg orally-disint (phenylalanine)

Comment: **Risperdol** tabs, oral solution, and M-tabs are indicated for the short-term monotherapy of acute mania or mixed episodes associated with bipolar I disorder, or in combination with *lithium* or *valproic acid* in adults

Risperdol Consta is indicated as monotherapy or adjunctive therapy to *lithium* or *valproic acid* for the maintenance treatment of mania and mixed episodes in bipolar I disorder.

▷ *ziprasidone* (C)(G) *Adult:* take with food; initially 40 mg bid; on day 2, may increase to 60-80 mg bid; *Elderly:* lower initial dose and titrate slowly
Pediatric: <12 years: not recommended; ≥12 years: same as adult
Geodon *Cap:* 20, 40, 60, 80 mg

Comment: **Geodon** is indicated for acute and maintenance treatment of mixed episodes in bipolar I disorder, as monotherapy or as adjunct to *lithium* or *valproic acid.*

COMBINATION AGENTS

Thienobenzodiazepine+Selective Serotonin Reuptake Inhibitor (SSRI) Combinations

▷ *olanzapine+fluoxetine* (C) initially 1 x 6/25 cap once daily in the PM; titrate; max 1 x 12/50 cap once daily in the PM

Pediatric: <10 years: not recommended; 10-17 years: initially 1 x 3/25 cap once daily in the PM; max 1 x 12/50 cap once daily in the PM

Symbyax

> *Cap:* **Symbyax 3/25** olan 3 mg+fluo 25 mg
> **Symbyax 6/25** olan 6 mg+fluo 25 mg
> **Symbyax 6/50** olan 6 mg+fluo 50 mg
> **Symbyax 12/25** olan 12 mg+fluo 25 mg
> **Symbyax 12/50** olan 12 mg+fluo 50 mg

Comment: **Symbyax** is indicated for the treatment of depressive episode associated with bipolar I disorder and treatment-resistant depression (TRD).

◯ BITE: CAT

TETANUS PROPHYLAXIS

▷ *tetanus toxoid* vaccine (C) 0.5 ml IM x 1 dose if previously immunized; *see* **Tetanus** for patients not previously immunized
    Vial: 5 Lf units/0.5 ml (0.5, 5 ml); *Prefilled syringe:* 5 Lf units/0.5 ml (0.5 ml)

ANTI-INFECTIVES

▷ *amoxicillin+clavulanate* (B)(G)
    Augmentin 500 mg tid or 875 mg bid x 10 days
    Pediatric: 40-45 mg/kg/day divided tid x 10 days or 90 mg/kg/day divided bid x 10 days *see* Appendix CC.4. *amoxicillin+clavulanate* (Augmentin Suspension) *for dose by weight*
        Tab: 250, 500, 875 mg; *Chew tab:* 125, 250 mg (lemon-lime); 200, 400 mg (cherry-banana) (phenylalanine); *Oral susp:* 125 mg/5 ml (banana), 250 mg/5 ml (75, 100, 150 ml) (orange); 200, 400 mg/5 ml (50, 75, 100 ml) (orange) (phenylalanine)
    Augmentin ES-600 not recommended for adults
    Pediatric: <3 months: not recommended; ≥3 months, <40 kg: 90 mg/kg/day in 2 divided doses x 10 days; ≥40 kg: not recommended
        Oral susp: 42.9 mg/5 ml (50, 75, 100, 125, 150, 200 ml) (strawberry cream) (phenylalanine)
    Augmentin XR 2 tabs q 12 hours x 10 days
    Pediatric: <16 years: use other forms; ≥16 years: same as adult
        Tab: 1000*mg ext-rel
▷ *doxycycline* (D)(G) 100 mg bid day 1; then 100 mg daily x 10 days
    Pediatric: <8 years: not recommended ≥8 years, <100 lb: 2 mg/lb on first day in 2 divided doses, followed by 1 mg/lb/day in 1-2 divided doses; *see Appendix CC.19. doxycycline* (Vibramycin Syrup/Suspension) for dose by weight; ≥8 years, ≥100 lb: same as adult
        Acticlate *Tab:* 75, 150**mg
        Adoxa *Tab:* 50, 75, 100, 150 mg ent-coat
        Doryx *Tab:* 50, 75, 100, 150, 200 mg del-rel
        Doxteric *Tab:* 50 mg del-rel
        Monodox *Cap:* 50, 75, 100 mg
        Oracea *Cap:* 40 mg del-rel
        Vibramycin *Tab:* 100 mg; *Cap:* 50, 100 mg; *Syr:* 50 mg/5 ml (raspberry-apple) (sulfites); *Oral susp:* 25 mg/5 ml (raspberry)
        Vibra-Tab *Tab:* 100 mg film-coat
▷ *penicillin v potassium* (B)(G) 500 mg PO qid x 3 days
    Pediatric: <12 years: 15-50 mg/kg/day in 3-6 divided doses x 3 days; *see* Appendix CC.29. *penicillin v potassium* (Pen-Vee K Solution, Veetids Solution) *for dose by weight;* ≥12 years: same as adult

Pen-Vee K *Tab:* 250, 500 mg; *Oral soln:* 125 mg/5 ml (100, 200 ml); 250 mg/5 ml (100, 150, 200 ml)

◯ BITE: DOG

TETANUS PROPHYLAXIS

▷ *tetanus toxoid* vaccine (C) 0.5 ml IM x 1 dose if previously immunized; *see Tetanus* for patients not previously immunized
   Vial: 5 Lf units/0.5 ml (0.5, 5 ml); *Prefilled syringe:* 5 Lf units/0.5 ml (0.5 ml)

ANTI-INFECTIVES

▷ *amoxicillin+clavulanate* (B)(G)
   Augmentin 500 mg tid or 875 mg bid x 10 days
   Pediatric: 40-45 mg/kg/day divided tid x 10 days or 90 mg/kg/day divided bid x 10 days *see* Appendix CC.4. *amoxicillin+clavulanate* (Augmentin Suspension) *for dose by weight*
      Tab: 250, 500, 875 mg; *Chew tab:* 125, 250 mg (lemon-lime); 200, 400 mg (cherry-banana) (phenylalanine); *Oral susp:* 125 mg/5 ml (banana), 250 mg/5 ml (75, 100, 150 ml) (orange); 200, 400 mg/5 ml (50, 75, 100 ml) (orange) (phenylalanine)
   Augmentin ES-600 not recommended for adults
   Pediatric: <3 months: not recommended; ≥3 months, <40 kg: 90 mg/kg/day in 2 divided doses x 10 days; ≥40 kg: not recommended
      Oral susp: 42.9 mg/5 ml (50, 75, 100, 125, 150, 200 ml) (strawberry cream) (phenylalanine)
   Augmentin XR 2 tabs q 12 hours x 10 days
   Pediatric: <16 years: use other forms; ≥16 years: same as adult
      Tab: 1000*mg ext-rel
▷ *clindamycin* (B) (administer with fluoroquinolone in adult and TMP-SMX in children) 300 mg qid x 10 days
   Pediatric: 8-16 mg/kg/day in 3-4 divided doses x 10 days; *see* Appendix CC.17. *clindamycin* (Cleocin Pediatric Granules) *for dose by weight*
      Cleocin (G) *Cap:* 75 (tartrazine), 150 (tartrazine), 300 mg
      Cleocin Pediatric Granules (G) *Oral susp:* 75 mg/5 ml (100 ml) (cherry)
▷ *doxycycline* (D)(G) 100 mg bid
   Pediatric: <8 years: not recommended ≥8 years, <100 lb: 2 mg/lb on first day in 2 divided doses, followed by 1 mg/lb/day in 1-2 divided doses; ≥8 years, ≥100 lb: same as adult; *see Appendix CC.19. doxycycline* (Vibramycin Syrup/Suspension) *for dose by weight*
      Acticlate *Tab:* 75, 150**mg
      Adoxa *Tab:* 50, 75, 100, 150 mg ent-coat
      Doryx *Tab:* 50, 75, 100, 150, 200 mg del-rel
      Doxteric *Tab:* 50 mg del-rel
      Monodox *Cap:* 50, 75, 100 mg
      Oracea *Cap:* 40 mg del-rel
      Vibramycin *Tab:* 100 mg; *Cap:* 50, 100 mg; *Syr:* 50 mg/5 ml (raspberry-apple) (sulfites); *Oral susp:* 25 mg/5 ml (raspberry)
      Vibra-Tab *Tab:* 100 mg film-coat
▷ *penicillin v potassium* (B)(G) 500 mg PO qid x 3 days
   Pediatric: 50 mg/kg/day in 4 divided doses x 3 days; ≥12 years: same as adult; *see* Appendix CC.29. *penicillin v potassium* (Pen-Vee K Solution, Veetids Solution) *for dose by weight*

Pen-Vee K *Tab:* 250, 500 mg; *Oral soln:* 125 mg/5 ml (100, 200 ml); 250 mg/5 ml (100, 150, 200 ml)

◯ BITE: HUMAN

TETANUS PROPHYLAXIS

▷ *tetanus toxoid* vaccine (C) 0.5 ml IM x 1 dose if previously immunized; *see Tetanus* for patients <u>not</u> previously immunized
    Vial: 5 Lf units/0.5 ml (0.5, 5 ml); *Prefilled syringe:* 5 Lf units/0.5 ml (0.5 ml)

ANTI-INFECTIVES

▷ *amoxicillin+clavulanate* (B)(G)
    Augmentin 500 mg tid <u>or</u> 875 mg bid x 10 days
    Pediatric: 40-45 mg/kg/day divided tid x 10 days <u>or</u> 90 mg/kg/day divided bid x 10 days *see* Appendix CC.4. *amoxicillin+clavulanate* (Augmentin Suspension) *for dose by weight*
        Tab: 250, 500, 875 mg; *Chew tab:* 125, 250 mg (lemon-lime); 200, 400 mg (cherry-banana) (phenylalanine); *Oral susp:* 125 mg/5 ml (banana), 250 mg/5 ml (75, 100, 150 ml) (orange); 200, 400 mg/5 ml (50, 75, 100 ml) (orange) (phenylalanine)
    Augmentin ES-600 not recommended for adults
    Pediatric: <3 months: not recommended; ≥3 months, <40 kg: 90 mg/kg/day in 2 divided doses x 10 days; ≥40 kg: not recommended
        Oral susp: 42.9 mg/5 ml (50, 75, 100, 125, 150, 200 ml) (strawberry cream) (phenylalanine)
    Augmentin XR 2 tabs q 12 hours x 10 days
    Pediatric: <16 years: use other forms; ≥16 years: same as adult
        Tab: 1000*mg ext-rel
▷ *cefoxitin* (B) 80-160 mg/kg/day IM in 3-4 divided doses x 10 days; max 12 gm/day
    Pediatric: <3 months: not recommended; ≥3 months: same as adult
    Mefoxin Injectable *Vial:* 1, 2 g
▷ *ciprofloxacin* (C) 500 mg bid x 10 days
    Pediatric: <18 years: not recommended; ≥18 years: same as adult
    Cipro (G) *Tab:* 250, 500, 750 mg; *Oral susp:* 250, 500 mg/5 ml (100 ml) (strawberry)
    Cipro XR *Tab:* 500, 1000 mg ext-rel
    ProQuin XR *Tab:* 500 mg ext-rel
▷ *erythromycin base* (B)(G) 250 mg qid x 10 days
    Pediatric: <45 kg: 30-40 mg/kg/day in 4 divided doses x 10 days; ≥45 kg: same as adult
    Ery-Tab *Tab:* 250, 333, 500 mg ent-coat
    PCE *Tab:* 333, 500 mg
▷ *erythromycin ethylsuccinate* (B)(G) 400 mg qid x 10 days
    Pediatric: 30-50 mg/kg/day in 4 divided doses x 10 days; may double dose with severe infection; max 100 mg/kg/day; *see Appendix CC.21. erythromycin ethylsuccinate* (E.E.S. Suspension, Ery-Ped Drops/Suspension) *for dose by weight*
    EryPed *Oral susp:* 200 mg/5 ml (100, 200 ml) (fruit); 400 mg/5 ml (60, 100, 200 ml) (banana); *Oral drops:* 200, 400 mg/5 ml (50 ml) (fruit); *Chew tab:* 200 mg wafer (fruit)
    E.E.S. *Oral susp:* 200, 400 mg/5 ml (100 ml) (fruit)
    E.E.S. Granules *Oral susp:* 200 mg/5 ml (100, 200 ml) (cherry)
    E.E.S. 400 Tablets *Tab:* 400 mg
▷ *trimethoprim+sulfamethoxazole* (TMP-SMX)(D)(G) bid x 10 days
    Pediatric: <2 months: not recommended; ≥2 months: 40 mg/kg/day of *sulfamethoxazole* in 2 divided doses bid x 10 days; *see Appendix C.33.*

trimethoprim+sulfamethoxazole (Bactrim Suspension, Septra Suspension) *for dose by weight*

> **Bactrim, Septra** 2 tabs bid x 10 days
> *Tab:* trim 80 mg+sulfa 400 mg*
> **Bactrim DS, Septra DS** 1 tab bid x 10 days
> *Tab:* trim 160 mg+sulfa 800 mg*
> **Bactrim Pediatric Suspension, Septra Pediatric Suspension**
> *Oral susp:* trim 40 mg+sulfa 200 mg per 5 ml (100 ml) (cherry) (alcohol 0.3%)

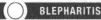
BLEPHARITIS

OPHTHALMIC AGENTS

➤ *erythromycin* ophthalmic ointment (B) apply 1/2 inch bid-qid x 14 days; then q HS x 10 days
Pediatric: same as adult
> **Ilotycin** *Oint:* 5 mg/gm (1/2 oz)

➤ *polymyxin b+bacitracin* ophthalmic ointment (C) apply 1/2 inch bid-qid x 14 days; then q HS
Pediatric: same as adult
> **Polysporin** *Oint:* poly b 10,000 U+baci 500 U (3.75 gm)

➤ *polymyxin b+bacitracin+neomycin* ophthalmic ointment (C) apply 1/2 inch bid-qid x 14 days; then q HS
Pediatric: same as adult
> **Neosporin** *Oint:* poly b 10,000 U+baci 400 U+neo 3.5 mg/gm (3.75 gm)

➤ *sodium sulfacetamide* (C)
> **Bleph-10 Ophthalmic Solution** 2 drops q 4 hours x 7-14 days
> *Pediatric:* <2 years: not recommended; ≥2 years: 1-2 drops q 2-3 hours during the day x 7-14 days
> *Ophth soln:* 10% (2.5, 5, 15 ml) (benzalkonium chloride)
> **Bleph-10 Ophthalmic Ointment** apply 1/2 inch qid and HS x 7-14 days
> *Pediatric:* <2 years: not recommended; ≥2 years: same as adult
> *Ophth oint:* 10% (3.5 gm) (phenylmercuric acetate)

SYSTEMIC AGENTS

➤ *tetracycline* (D)(G) 250 mg qid x 7 days
Pediatric: <8 years: not recommended; ≥8 years, <100 lb: 25-50 mg/kg/day in 2-4 divided doses x 7-10 days; ≥100 lb: same as adult; *see Appendix CC.31. tetracycline* (Sumycin Suspension) *for dose by weight*
> **Achromycin V** *Cap:* 250, 500 mg
> **Sumycin** *Tab:* 250, 500 mg; *Cap:* 250, 500 mg; *Oral susp:* 125 mg/5 ml (100, 200 ml) (fruit) (sulfites)

BLEPHAROPTOSIS, ACQUIRED (DROOPY EYELID)

DIRECT-ACTING ALPHA-ADRENERGIC RECEPTOR AGONIST

➤ *oxymetazoline hydrochloride ophthalmic solution, 0.1%* instill one drop into one <u>or</u> both ptotic eye(s) once daily
Pediatric: not established
> **Upneeq** *Ophth soln:* 0.1% (0.3 ml; 15, 30 single patient-use containers in a foil-pouch within a child-resistant zipper bag/carton)
> Comment: **Upneeq** *(oxymetazoline hydrochloride ophthalmic solution, 0.1%)* is a novel, once-daily ophthalmic formulation of *oxymetazoline*. The most common adverse reactions (incidence 1-5%) have been punctate keratitis, conjunctival hyperemia, dry eye, blurred vision, instillation site

pain, eye irritation, and headache. Alpha-adrenergic agonists as a class may impact blood pressure. Advise patients with cardiovascular disease, orthostatic hypotension, and/or uncontrolled hypertension or hypotension to seek medical care if their condition worsens. Use with caution in patients with cerebral or coronary insufficiency or Sjögren's syndrome and advise patients to seek medical care if signs and symptoms of potentiation of vascular insufficiency develop. Advise patients to seek immediate medical care if pain, redness, blurred vision, and photophobia occur (signs and symptoms of acute angle closure). There are no available data on **Upneeq** in pregnant females to inform a drug-associated risk for major birth defects and miscarriage. No clinical data are available to assess the amount of *oxymetazoline* present in human breastmilk post-dose. Developmental and health benefits of breastfeeding should be considered along with the mother's clinical need for **Upneeq** and any potential adverse effects on the breastfed infant.

BOWEL RESECTION WITH PRIMARY ANASTOMOSIS

▷ *alvimopan* (B) administer 12 mg 30 minutes to 5 hours prior to surgery; then, 12 mg bid for up to 7 days; max 15 doses
Pediatric: <18 years: not established; ≥18 years: same as adult

Entereg *Cap:* 12 mg
Comment: **Entereg** is a peripherally acting μ-opioid receptor antagonist indicated to accelerate the time to upper and lower gastrointestinal recovery following partial large or small bowel resection surgery with primary anastomosis. Therapeutic doses of opioids for more than 7 consecutive days prior to **Entereg** is contraindicated. A higher number of myocardial infarctions was reported in patients treated with *alvimopan* 0.5 mg twice daily, compared with placebo in a 12-month study in patients treated with opioids for chronic pain, although a causal relationship has not been established. **Entereg** is not recommended for patients with severe hepatic impairment and end stage renal disease (ESRD). Dosage adjustment is not required in patients with mild to severe renal impairment but they should be monitored for adverse effects. The most common adverse reactions (incidence ≥3%) in patients undergoing bowel resection were anemia, dyspepsia, hypokalemia, back pain, and urinary retention. **Entereg** is available only for short-term (15 doses) use in hospitalized patients and only hospitals that have registered in and met all of the requirements for the ENTEREG Access Support and Education (E.A.S.E.) program may use **Entereg**.

BRONCHIOLITIS

Inhaled Beta-2 Agonists (Bronchodilators) *see Asthma*
Oral Beta-2 Agonists (Bronchodilators) *see Asthma*
Inhaled Corticosteroids *see Asthma*
Parenteral Corticosteroids *see* Appendix M. Parenteral Corticosteroids
Oral Corticosteroids *see* Appendix L. Oral Corticosteroids

BRONCHITIS: ACUTE & ACUTE EXACERBATION OF CHRONIC BRONCHITIS (AECB)

Comment: Antibiotics are seldom needed for treatment of acute bronchitis because the etiology is usually viral.
Inhaled Beta-2 Agonists (Bronchodilators) *see Asthma*
Oral Beta-2 Agonists (Bronchodilators) *see Asthma*

Decongestants *see* Appendix AA. Drugs for the Management of Allergy, Cough, and Cold Symptoms online at https://connect.springerpub.com/content/reference-book/978-0-8261-7935-7/back-matter/part02/back-matter/bmatter27

Expectorants *see* Appendix AA. Drugs for the Management of Allergy, Cough, and Cold Symptoms online at https://connect.springerpub.com/content/reference-book/978-0-8261-7935-7/back-matter/part02/back-matter/bmatter27

Antitussives *see* Appendix AA. Drugs for the Management of Allergy, Cough, and Cold Symptoms online at https://connect.springerpub.com/content/reference-book/978-0-8261-7935-7/back-matter/part02/back-matter/bmatter27

ANTI-INFECTIVES FOR SECONDARY BACTERIAL INFECTION

▷ *amoxicillin* (B)(G) 500-875 mg bid *or* 250-500 mg tid x 10 days
   Pediatric: <40 kg (88 lb): 20-40 mg/kg/day in 3 divided doses x 10 days *or* 25-45 mg/kg/day in 2 divided doses x 10 days; ≥40 kg: same as adult; *see* Appendix CC.3.
   amoxicillin (Amoxil Suspension, Trimox Suspension) *for dose by weight*
   Amoxil *Cap:* 250, 500 mg; *Tab:* 875*mg; *Chew tab:* 125, 200, 250, 400 mg (cherry-banana-peppermint) (phenylalanine); *Oral susp:* 125, 250 mg/5 ml (80, 100, 150 ml) (strawberry); 200, 400 mg/5 ml (50, 75, 100 ml) (bubble gum); *Oral drops:* 50 mg/ml (30 ml) (bubble gum)
   Moxatag *Tab:* 775 mg ext-rel
   Trimox *Tab:* 125, 250 mg; *Cap:* 250, 500 mg; *Oral susp:* 125, 250 mg/5 ml (80, 100, 150 ml) (raspberry-strawberry)
▷ *amoxicillin+clavulanate* (B)(G)
   Augmentin 500 mg tid *or* 875 mg bid x 7-10 days
   Pediatric: 40-45 mg/kg/day divided tid x 10 days *or* 90 mg/kg/day divided bid x 10 days *see* Appendix CC.4. *amoxicillin+clavulanate* (Augmentin Suspension) *for dose by weight*
      Tab: 250, 500, 875 mg; *Chew tab:* 125, 250 mg (lemon-lime); 200, 400 mg (cherry-banana) (phenylalanine); *Oral susp:* 125 mg/5 ml (banana), 250 mg/5 ml (75, 100, 150 ml) (orange); 200, 400 mg/5 ml (50, 75, 100 ml) (orange) (phenylalanine)
   Augmentin ES-600 not recommended for adults
   Pediatric: <3 months: not recommended; ≥3 months, <40 kg: 90 mg/kg/day in 2 divided doses x 7-10 days; ≥40 kg: not recommended
      Oral susp: 42.9 mg/5 ml (50, 75, 100, 125, 150, 200 ml) (strawberry cream) (phenylalanine)
   Augmentin XR 2 tabs q 12 hours x 7-10 days
   Pediatric: <16 years: use other forms; ≥16 years: same as adult
      Tab: 1000*mg ext-rel
▷ *ampicillin* (B) 250-500 mg qid x 10 days
   Pediatric: not recommended for bronchitis in children
      Omnipen, Principen *Cap:* 250, 500 mg; *Oral susp:* 125, 250 mg/5 ml (100, 150, 200 ml) (fruit)
▷ *azithromycin* (B)(G) 500 mg x 1 dose on day 1, then 250 mg daily on days 2-5 *or* 500 mg once daily x 3 days *or* 2 gm in a single dose
   Pediatric: not recommended for bronchitis in children
      Zithromax *Tab:* 250, 500, 600 mg; *Oral susp:* 100 mg/5 ml (15 ml); 200 mg/5 ml (15, 22.5, 30 ml) (cherry); *Pkt:* 1 gm for reconstitution (cherry-banana)
      Zithromax Tri-pak *Tab:* 3 x 500 mg tabs/pck
      Zithromax Z-pak *Tab:* 6 x 250 mg tabs/pck
      Zmax *Oral susp:* 2 gm ext-rel for reconstitution (cherry-banana) (148 mg Na⁺)
▷ *cefaclor* (B)(G)
      Ceclor 250 mg tid *or* 375 mg bid 3-10 days
      Pediatric: <1 month: not recommended; 1 month-12 years: 20-40 mg/kg divided bid or q 12 hours x 3-10 days; max 1 gm/day; see Appendix CC.8.
      cefaclor (Ceclor Suspension) *for dose by weight*; >12 years: same as adult

Tab: 500 mg; *Cap:* 250, 500 mg; *Susp:* 125 mg/5 ml (75, 150 ml)
(strawberry); 187 mg/5 ml (50, 100 ml) (strawberry); 250 mg/5 ml (75, 150
ml) (strawberry); 375 mg/5 ml (50, 100 ml) (strawberry)

Ceclor Extended Release 375-500 mg bid x 3-10 days
Pediatric: <16 years: ext-rel not recommended; ≥16 years: same as adult
Tab: 375, 500 mg ext-rel

▷ *cefadroxil* (B) 1-2 gm in 1-2 divided doses x 10 days
Pediatric: 30 mg/kg/day in 2 divided doses x 10 days; *see* Appendix CC.9. *cefadroxil*
(Duricef Suspension) *for dose by weight*

Duricef *Tab:* 1 gm; *Cap:* 500 mg; *Oral susp:* 250 mg/5 ml (100 ml); 500 mg/5
ml (75, 100 ml) (orange-pineapple)

▷ *cefdinir* (B) 300 mg bid x 5-10 days <u>or</u> 600 mg daily x 10 days
Pediatric: <6 months: not recommended; 6 months-12 years: 14 mg/kg/day
in 1-2 divided doses x 10 days; ≥12 years: same as adult; *see* Appendix CC.10.
cefdinir (Omnicef Suspension) *for dose by weight*

Omnicef *Cap:* 300 mg; *Oral susp:* 125 mg/5 ml (60, 100 ml) (strawberry)

▷ *cefditoren pivoxil* (B) 400 mg bid x 10 days
Pediatric: <12 years: not recommended; ≥12 years: same as adult

Spectracef *Tab:* 200 mg

Comment: **Spectracef** is contraindicated with milk protein allergy <u>or</u> carnitine
deficiency.

▷ *cefixime* (B)(G)
Pediatric: <6 months: not recommended; ≥6 months-12 years, <50 kg: 8 mg/kg/day
in 1-2 divided doses x 10 days; ≥12 years, >50 kg: same as adult; *see* Appendix CC.11.
cefixime (Suprax Oral Suspension) *for dose by weight*

Suprax *Tab:* 400 mg; *Cap:* 400 mg; *Oral susp:* 100, 200, 500 mg/5 ml (50, 75,
100 ml) (strawberry)

▷ *cefpodoxime proxetil* (B) 200 mg bid x 10 days
Pediatric: <2 months: not recommended; ≥2 months-12 years: 10 mg/kg/day
(max 400 mg/dose) <u>or</u> 5 mg/kg/day bid (max 200 mg/dose) x 10 days; >12 years:
same as adult; *see* Appendix CC.12. *cefpodoxime proxetil* (Vantin Suspension) *for
dose by weight*

Vantin *Tab:* 100, 200 mg; *Oral susp:* 50, 100 mg/5 ml (50, 75, 100 ml) (lemon
creme)

▷ *cefprozil* (B) 500 mg q 12 hours x 10 days
Pediatric: <2 years: not recommended; 2-12 years: 15 mg/kg q 12 hours x 10 days;
see Appendix CC.13. *cefprozil* (Cefzil Suspension) *for dose by weight;* >12 years:
same as adult

Cefzil *Tab:* 250, 500 mg; *Oral susp:* 125, 250 mg/5 ml (50, 75, 100 ml) (bubble
gum) (phenylalanine)

▷ *ceftibuten* (B) 400 mg daily x 10 days
Pediatric: 9 mg/kg daily x 10 days; max 400 mg/day; *see* Appendix CC.14. *ceftibuten*
(Cedax Suspension) *for dose by weight*

Cedax *Cap:* 400 mg; *Oral susp:* 90 mg/5 ml (30, 60, 90, 120 ml); 180 mg/5 ml
(30, 60, 120 ml) (cherry)

▷ *ceftriaxone* (B)(G) 1-2 gm IM daily continued 2 days after signs of infection have
disappeared; max 4 gm/day
Pediatric: 50 mg/kg IM daily and continued 2 days after clinical stability

Rocephin *Vial:* 250, 500 mg; 1, 2 gm

▷ *cephalexin* (B)(G) 250-500 mg qid <u>or</u> 500 mg bid x 10 days
Pediatric: 25-50 mg/kg/day in 4 divided doses x 10 days; ≥12 years: same as adult;
see Appendix CC.15. *cephalexin* (Keflex Suspension) *for dose by weight*

Keflex *Cap:* 250, 333, 500, 750 mg; *Oral susp:* 125, 250 mg/5 ml (100, 200 ml)
(strawberry)

▷ *clarithromycin* (C)(G) 500 mg bid <u>or</u> 500 mg ext-rel once daily x 7 days
  Pediatric: <6 months: not recommended; ≥6 months: 7.5 mg/kg bid x 7 days; *see
  Appendix CC.17. clindamycin* (Cleocin Pediatric Granules) *for dose by weight;*
  ≥12 years: same as adult
    Biaxin *Tab:* 250, 500 mg
    Biaxin Oral Suspension *Oral susp:* 125, 250 mg/5 ml (50, 100 ml)
    (fruit-punch)
    Biaxin XL *Tab:* 500 mg ext-rel
▷ *dirithromycin* (C)(G) 500 mg daily x 7 days
  Pediatric: <12 years: not recommended; ≥12 years: same as adult
    Dynabac *Tab:* 250 mg
▷ *doxycycline* (D)(G) 100 mg bid x 10 days
  Pediatric: <8 years: not recommended; ≥8 years, <100 lb: 2 mg/lb on first day in
  2 divided doses, followed by 1 mg/lb/day in 1-2 divided doses; ≥8 years, ≥100 lb:
  same as adult; *see Appendix CC.19. doxycycline* (Vibramycin Syrup/Suspension)
  for dose by weight
    Acticlate *Tab:* 75, 150**mg
    Adoxa *Tab:* 50, 75, 100, 150 mg ent-coat
    Doryx *Tab:* 50, 75, 100, 150, 200 mg del-rel
    Doxteric *Tab:* 50 mg del-rel
    Monodox *Cap:* 50, 75, 100 mg
    Oracea *Cap:* 40 mg del-rel
    Vibramycin *Tab:* 100 mg; *Cap:* 50, 100 mg; *Syr:* 50 mg/5 ml (raspberry-apple)
    (sulfites); *Oral susp:* 25 mg/5 ml (raspberry)
    Vibra-Tab *Tab:* 100 mg film-coat
▷ *erythromycin ethylsuccinate* (B)(G) 400 mg qid x 7 days
  Pediatric: 30-50 mg/kg/day in 4 divided doses x 7 days; may double dose
  with severe infection; max 100 mg/kg/day; *see Appendix CC.21. erythromycin
  ethylsuccinate* (E.E.S. Suspension, Ery-Ped Drops/Suspension) *for dose by
  weight*
    EryPed *Oral susp:* 200 mg/5 ml (100, 200 ml) (fruit); 400 mg/5 ml (60, 100,
    200 ml) (banana); *Oral drops:* 200, 400 mg/5 ml (50 ml) (fruit); *Chew tab:*
    200 mg wafer (fruit)
    E.E.S. *Oral susp:* 200, 400 mg/5 ml (100 ml) (fruit)
    E.E.S. Granules *Oral susp:* 200 mg/5 ml (100, 200 ml) (cherry)
    E.E.S. 400 Tablets *Tab:* 400 mg
▷ *gemifloxacin* (C) 320 mg daily x 5 days
  Pediatric: <18 years: not recommended; ≥18 years: same as adult
    Factive *Tab:* 320*mg
▷ *levofloxacin* (C) *Uncomplicated:* 500 mg daily x 7 days; *Complicated:* 750 mg daily
  x 7 days
  Pediatric: <18 years: not recommended; ≥18 years: same as adult
    Levaquin *Tab:* 250, 500, 750 mg
▷ *loracarbef* (B) 200-400 mg bid x 7 days
  Pediatric: 30 mg/kg/day in 2 divided doses x 7 days; ≥12 years: same as adult;
  see Appendix CC.27. *loracarbef* (Lorabid Suspension) *for dose by weight*
    Lorabid *Pulvule:* 200, 400 mg; *Oral susp:* 100 mg/5 ml (50, 100 ml);
    200 mg/5 ml (50, 75, 100 ml) (strawberry bubble gum)
▷ *moxifloxacin* (C)(G) 400 mg daily x 5 days
  Pediatric: <18 years: not recommended; ≥18 years: same as adult
    Avelox *Tab:* 400 mg; IV soln: 400 mg/250 ml (latex-free, preservative-free)
▷ *ofloxacin* (C)(G) 400 mg bid x 10 days
  Pediatric: <18 years: not recommended; ≥18 years: same as adult
    Floxin *Tab:* 200, 300, 400 mg

▷ **telithromycin (C)** 800 mg once daily x 7-10 days; *Severe renal impairment including dialysis:* 600 mg once daily; *Severe renal impairment with coexisting hepatic impairment:* 400 mg once daily.
Pediatric: <18 years: not recommended; ≥18 years: same as adult
    Ketek *Tab:* 400, 500 mg
Comment: *Telithromycin* is a ketolide indicated for the treatment of mild-to-moderate CAP). Fatal acute liver injury has been reported; discontinue immediately if signs and symptoms of hepatitis occur. There is increased risk for ventricular arrhythmias, including ventricular tachycardia and *torsades de pointes* with fatal outcomes; avoid use in patients with known QT prolongation, hypokalemia, and with class IA and III antiarrhythmics. Fatalities with *colchicine*, rhabdomyolysis with HMG-CoA reductase inhibitors (statins), and hypotension with calcium channel blockers (CCBs) have been reported; therefore, avoid concomitant use. Monitor for toxicity and consider dose reduction of the concomitant medication, if concomitant use is unavoidable. Evaluate for *C. difficile* if diarrhea occurs. Contraindications include myasthenia gravis, concomitant *cisapride* or *pimozide*, and history of hepatitis or jaundice with any macrolide.

▷ **tetracycline (D)(G)** 250-500 mg qid x 7 days
Pediatric: <8 years: not recommended; ≥8 years, <100 lb: 25-50 mg/kg/day in 2-4 divided doses x 7 days; ≥8 years, ≥100 lb: same as adult; *see Appendix CC.31.*
tetracycline (Sumycin Suspension) *for dose by weight*
    Achromycin V *Cap:* 250, 500 mg
    Sumycin *Tab:* 250, 500 mg; *Cap:* 250, 500 mg; *Oral susp:* 125 mg/5 ml (100, 200 ml) (fruit) (sulfites)

▷ **trimethoprim+sulfamethoxazole (TMP-SMX)(D)(G)** bid x 10 days
Pediatric: <2 months: not recommended; ≥2 months: 40 mg/kg/day of *sulfamethoxazole* in 2 divided doses bid x 10 days; *see Appendix CC.33.*
trimethoprim+sulfamethoxazole (Bactrim Suspension, Septra Suspension) *for dose by weight;* ≥12 years: same as adult
    Bactrim, Septra 2 tabs bid x 10 days
      Tab: trim 80 mg+sulfa 400 mg*
    Bactrim DS, Septra DS 1 tab bid x 10 days
      Tab: trim 160 mg+sulfa 800 mg*
    Bactrim Pediatric Suspension, Septra Pediatric Suspension
      Oral susp: trim 40 mg+sulfa 200 mg per 5 ml (100 ml) (cherry) (alcohol 0.3%)

BRONCHITIS: CHRONIC/CHRONIC OBSTRUCTIVE PULMONARY DISEASE (COPD)

Oral Beta-2 Agonists (Bronchodilators) *see Asthma*
Inhaled Corticosteroids *see Asthma*
Parenteral Corticosteroids *see* Appendix M. Parenteral Corticosteroids
Oral Corticosteroids *see* Appendix L. Oral Corticosteroids
Inhaled Beta-2 Agonists (Bronchodilators) *see Asthma*

LONG-ACTING INHALED BETA-2 AGONIST (LABA)

▷ **indacaterol (C)** inhale contents of one 75 mcg cap daily
Pediatric: <12 years: not recommended; ≥12 years: same as adult
    Arcapta Neohaler *Neohaler Device/Cap:* 75 mcg pwdr for inhalation (5 blister cards, 6 caps/card)
Comment: Remove cap from blister cap immediately before use. For oral inhalation with **Neohaler** device only. *indacaterol* is indicated for the long-term maintenance treatment of bronchoconstriction in patients with COPD.

Not indicated for treating asthma, for primary treatment of acute symptoms, or for acute deterioration of COPD.

▷ **indacaterol+glycopyrrolate** (C) inhale the contents of one cap twice daily
Pediatric: <18 years: not recommended; ≥18 years: same as adult
    Utibron Neohaler *Neohaler Device/Cap:* inda 27.5 mcg+glyco 15.6 mcg pwdr for inhalation (1, 10 blister cards, 6 caps/card)

▷ **olodaterol** (C) 12 mcg q 12 hours
Pediatric: <12 years: not recommended; ≥12 years: same as adult
    Striverdi Respimat *Inhal soln:* 2.5 mcg/cartridge (metered actuation) (40 gm, 60 metered actuations) (benzalkonium chloride)

▷ **salmeterol** (C)(G) 1 inhalation q 12 hours
Pediatric: <4 years: not recommended; ≥4 years: same as adult
    Serevent Diskus *Diskus (pwdr):* 50 mcg/actuation (60 doses/diskus)

INHALED ANTICHOLINERGICS

▷ **glycopyrrolate inhalation solution** (C)
Lonhala Magnair administer the contents of one vial via Magnair handset
    Vial: 25 mcg/ml (1 ml) unit dose for use with Magnair handset; Starter Kit: 60 unit-dose vials w. Magnair handset;
    Refill Kit: 60 unit-dose vials w. Magnair handset
Comment: For oral inhalation only. Do not swallow **Lonhala** solution. Only use **Lonhala** vials with **Magnair**. Do not initiate in acutely deteriorating COPD or to treat acute symptoms. If paradoxical bronchospasm occurs, discontinue **Lonhala Magnair** immediately and institute alternative therapy. Worsening of narrow-angle glaucoma may occur; use with caution in patients with narrow-angle glaucoma and instruct patients to contact a physician immediately if symptoms occur. Worsening of urinary retention may occur. Use with caution in patients with prostatic hyperplasia (BPH) or bladder neck obstruction (BNO) and instruct patients to consult a physician immediately if symptoms occur. Avoid administration with other anticholinergic drugs. Consider risk versus benefit in patients with severe renal impairment. Most common adverse reactions (incidence ≥ 2.0%) are dyspnea and urinary tract infection. There are no adequate and well-controlled studies in pregnancy. **Lonhala Magnair** should only be used during pregnancy if the expected benefit to the patient outweighs the potential risk to the fetus. There are no data on the presence of **glycopyrrolate** or its metabolites in human milk or effects on the breastfed infant. The developmental and health benefits of breastfeeding should be considered along with the mother's clinical need for **Lonhala Magnair** and any potential adverse effects on the breastfed infant from **Lonhala Magnair** or from the underlying maternal condition.
Seebri Neohaler (C) inhale the contents of 1 capsule twice daily at the same time of day, AM and PM, using the Neohaler; do not swallow caps
    Pediatric: not indicated
    Inhal cap: 15.6 mcg (60/blister pck) dry pwdr for inhalation w. 1 Neo-haler device (lactose)

▷ **ipratropium bromide** (B)(G)
Pediatric: <12 years: not recommended; ≥12 years: same as adult
    Atrovent 2 inhalations qid; max 12 inhalations/day
    Inhaler: 14 gm (200 inh)
    Atrovent Inhalation Solution 500 mcg by nebulizer tid-qid
    Inhal soln: 0.02% (2.5 ml)
Comment: *Ipratropium bromide* is contraindicated with severe hypersensitivity to milk proteins.

▷ **umeclidinium** (C) 1 inhalation once daily at the same time each day
Pediatric: <12 years: not recommended; ≥12 years: same as adult

Incruse Ellipta *Inhal pwdr:* 62.5 mcg/inhalation (30 doses) (lactose)
Comment: **Incruse Ellipta** is contraindicated with allergy to *atropine* or its derivatives.

INHALED LONG-ACTING ANTI-CHOLINERGICS (LAA) (ANTIMUSCARINICS)

Comment: Inhaled LAAs are for prophylaxis and chronic treatment, only. Not for primary (rescue) treatment of acute attack. Avoid getting powder in eyes. Caution with narrow-angle glaucoma, BPH, bladder neck obstruction, and pregnancy. Contraindicated with allergy to atropine or its derivatives (e.g., *ipratropium*). Avoid other anticholinergic agents.

▷ *aclidinium bromide* (C) 1 inhalation twice daily using inhaler
  Pediatric: <12 years: not recommended; ≥12 years: same as adult
    Tudorza Pressair *Inhal device:* 400 mcg/actuation (60 doses per inhalation device)

▷ *glycopyrrolate inhalation solution* (C) administer the contents of one vial twice daily at the same times of day, AM and PM, via the **Magnair** neb inhal device; do not swallow solution; do not use **Magnair** with any other medicine; length of treatment is 2-3 minutes; do not use 2 vials/treatment or more than 2 vials/day
  Pediatric: not indicated
    Lonhala Magnair *Vial:* 25 mcg/ml (1 ml) unit dose for use with **Magnair** handset; *Starter Kit:* 60 unit-dose vials w. **Magnair** handset; *Refill Kit:* 60 unit-dose vials (low-density polyethylene [LDPE]) w. **Magnair** handset (preservative-free)
    Comment: **Lonhala Magnair** is the first nebulizing long-acting muscarinic antagonist (LAMA) approved for the treatment of COPD in the United States. Its approval was based on data from clinical trials in the Glycopyrrolate for Obstructive Lung Disease via Electronic Nebulizer (GOLDEN) program, including GOLDEN-3 and GOLDEN-4, 2 Phase 3, 12-week, randomized, double-blind, placebo-controlled, parallel-group, multicenter study. Do not initiate **Lonhala Magnair** in acutely deteriorating COPD or to treat acute symptoms. If paradoxical bronchospasm occurs, discontinue **Lonhala Magnair** immediately and institute alternative therapy. Worsening of narrow-angle glaucoma may occur; use with caution in patients with narrow-angle glaucoma and instruct patients to contact a physician immediately if symptoms occur. Worsening of urinary retention may occur. Use with caution in patients with prostatic hyperplasia (BPH) or bladder neck obstruction (BNO) and instruct patients to seek medical care immediately if symptoms occur. Avoid administration with other anticholinergic drugs. Consider risk versus benefit in patients with severe renal impairment. Most common adverse reactions (incidence ≥ 2.0%) have been dyspnea and urinary tract infection. There are no adequate and well-controlled studies in pregnancy. **Lonhala Magnair** should only be used during pregnancy if the expected benefit to the patient outweighs the potential risk to the fetus. There are no data on the presence of *glycopyrrolate* or its metabolites in human milk or effects on the breastfed infant. The developmental and health benefits of breastfeeding should be considered along with the mother's clinical need for **Lonhala Magnair** and any potential adverse effects on the breastfed infant from **Lonhala Magnair** or from the underlying maternal condition.

▷ *revefenacin inhalation solution* administer the contents of one vial via nebulizer once daily at the same times of day; do not swallow solution; do not use more than 1 vial/day; do not use **Yupelri** with any other medicine
  Pediatric: not indicated
    Yupelri *Vial:* 175 mcg/3 ml (3 ml) unit-dose solution for nebulizer

Comment: **Yupelri** is the first and only long-acting muscarinic antagonist (LAMA) solution for once daily nebulized administration. **Yupelri** is indicated for maintenance treatment of moderate-to-severe COPD. Do not initiate **Yupelri** in acutely deteriorating COPD or to treat acute symptoms. If paradoxical bronchospasm occurs, discontinue **Yupelri** immediately and institute alternative therapy. Worsening of narrow-angle glaucoma may occur; use with caution in patients with narrow-angle glaucoma and instruct patients to contact a healthcare provider immediately if symptoms occur. Use with caution in patients with prostatic hyperplasia or bladder-neck obstruction and instruct patients to contact a healthcare provider immediately if symptoms occur. May interact additively with other concomitantly used anticholinergic medications; avoid administration of **Yupelri** with other anticholinergic-containing drugs. Co-administration of **Yupelri** with OATP1B1 and OATP1B3 inhibitors (e.g. rifampicin, cyclosporine) may lead to an increase in exposure of the active metabolite; co-administration with **Yupelri** is not recommended. Avoid use of **Yupelri** in patients with hepatic impairment. Most common adverse reactions (incidence ≥2%) include cough, nasopharyngitis, upper respiratory tract infection, headache, and back pain. There are no adequate and well-controlled studies with **Yupelri** in pregnancy and no information regarding the presence of *revefenacin* in human milk or effects on the breastfed infant.

▷ *tiotropium (as bromide monohydrate)* (C) 1 inhalation daily using inhaler; do not swallow caps

　　Pediatric: <12 years: not recommended; ≥12 years: same as adult

　　Spiriva HandiHaler *Inhal device:* 18 mcg/cap (5, 30, 90 caps w. inhalation device)

INHALED LONG-ACTING MUSCARINIC ANTAGONIST (LAMA)+LONG-ACTING BETA-2 AGONIST (LABA) COMBINATION

▷ *aclidinium bromide+formoterol fumarate* one breath-actuated oral inhalation twice daily (morning and evening)

　　Duaklir Pressair *Inhal pwdr:* aclid brom 400 mcg+foro fum 12 mcg per actuation (30, 60 single-use metered doses/Pressair inhaler); remove the Pressair inhaler from the storage bag immediately before use and store the Pressair inhaler inside the sealed bag; discard the bag (and the desiccant sachet inside) and the Pressair inhaler after the marking "0" with a red background is visible in the middle of the dose indicator, when the device is empty and locks out, or 2 months after the date the sealed bag that the inhaler comes in was open, whichever comes first.

　　Comment: **Duaklir Pressair** *(aclidinium bromide+formoterol fumarate)* is a long-acting muscarinic antagonist (LAMA) and long-acting beta-2 agonist (LABA) fixed-dose combination maintenance bronchodilator for the treatment of COPD. **Duaklir Pressair** is not indicated for relief of acute bronchospasm or treatment of asthma. There are no adequate and well-controlled studies of **Duaklir Pressair** or its individual components in pregnancy to inform drug-associated embryo/fetal risks, and there are no available data on presence in human milk or effects on the breastfed infant.

▷ *ipratropium/albuterol* (C) 1 inhalation qid; max 6 inhalations/day
　　Pediatric: <12 years: not established; ≥12 years: same as adult

　　Combivent Respimat *Inhal soln:* ipra 20 mcg+alb 100 mcg per inhalation (4 gm, 120 inhal)

　　Comment: **Combivent Respimat** is contraindicated with *atropine* allergy.

▷ *tiotropium+olodaterol* (C) 2 inhalations once daily at the same time each day; max 2 inhalations/day
　　Pediatric: <12 years: not recommended; ≥12 years: same as adult

Stiolto Respimat *Inhal soln:* tio 2.5 mcg+olo 2.5 mcg per actuation (4 gm, 60 inh) (benzalkonium chloride)

Comment: **Stiolto Respimat** is not for treating asthma, acute bronchospasm, or acutely deteriorating COPD.

▷ *umeclidinium+vilanterol* (C) 1 inhalation once daily at the same time each day
Pediatric: <12 years: not recommended; ≥12 years: same as adult
    Anoro Ellipta *Inhal soln:* ume 62.5 mcg+vila 25 mcg per inhalation (30 doses)
    Comment: **Anoro Ellipta** is contraindicated with severe hypersensitivity to milk proteins.

INHALED CORTICOSTEROID+LONG-ACTING BETA-2 AGONIST (LABA) COMBINATION

▷ *fluticasone furoate+vilanterol* (C) 1 inhalation 100/25 once daily at the same time each day
Pediatric: <17 years: not recommended; ≥17 years: same as adult
    Breo Ellipta 100/25 *Inhal pwdr:* flu 100 mcg+vil 25 mcg dry pwdr per inhalation (30 doses)
    Breo Ellipta 200/25 *Inhal pwdr:* flu 200 mcg+vil 25 mcg dry pwdr per inhalation (30 doses)
    Comment: **Breo Ellipta** is contraindicated with severe hypersensitivity to milk proteins.

INHALED CORTICOSTEROID+ANTICHOLINERGIC+LONG-ACTING BETA-2 AGONIST (LABA) COMBINATION

▷ *budesonide+glycopyrrolate +fometerol fumarate* one inhalation twice daily
    Breztri Aerosphere *Metered Dose Inhal:* fixed-dose aerosol containing budes 160 mcg+glyco 9 mcg+fom fum4.8 mcg per inhalation
    Comment: **Breztri Aerosphere** is maintenance therapy for patients with COPD. Breztri is not indicated relief of acute bronchospasm or for the treatment of asthma. The most common adverse reactions (incidence ≥2%) have been URI, pneumonia, back pain, oral candidiasis, influenza, muscle spasm, UTI, cough, sinusitis, and diarrhea. If paradoxical bronchospasm occurs, discontinue **Breztri Aerosphere** and institute alternative therapy. Use with caution in patients with convulsive disorders, thyrotoxicosis, diabetes mellitus, and ketoacidosis. Be alert for hypokalemia and hyperglycemia. Use with caution in patients with cardiovascular disorders because of beta-adrenergic stimulation. Assess for decrease in bone mineral density initially and periodically thereafter. Glaucoma and cataracts may occur with long-term use of ICS. Worsening of narrow-angle glaucoma may occur; use with caution in patients with narrow-angle glaucoma and instruct patients to contact a healthcare provider immediately if symptoms occur. Consider referral to an ophthalmologist in patients who develop ocular symptoms or who use **Breztri Aerosphere** long term. Worsening of urinary retention may occur; use with caution in patients with prostatic hyperplasia or bladder-neck obstruction and instruct patients to contact a healthcare provider immediately if symptoms occur. *Candida albicans* infection of the mouth and pharynx may occur; advise patients to rinse mouth with water without swallowing after inhalation. Potential worsening of infections (e.g., existing tuberculosis; fungal, bacterial, viral, or parasitic infection; ocular herpes simplex); use with caution in patients with these infections. More serious or even fatal course of chickenpox or measles can occur in susceptible patients. There is risk of impaired adrenal function when transferring from systemic corticosteroids. Taper patients slowly from systemic corticosteroids if transferring to **Breztri Aerosphere**. Hypercorticism and adrenal suppression may occur with very high doses or at the regular dose in susceptible persons. *Budesonide* and **formoterol fumarate** systemic exposure may increase

in patients with severe hepatic impairment. In patients with severe renal impairment, use should be considered only if the potential benefit of the treatment outweighs the risk.

▷ *fluticasone furoate+umeclidinium+vilanterol* one inhalation once daily
   Trelegy Ellipta flutic furo 100 mcg+umec 62.5 mcg+vilan 25 mcg dry pwdr
   Comment: **Trelegy Ellipta** is maintenance therapy for patients with COPD, including chronic bronchitis and emphysema, who are receiving fixed-dose *furoate* and *vilanterol* for airflow obstruction and to reduce exacerbations, or receiving *umeclidinium* and a fixed-dose combination of *fluticasone furoate* and *vilanterol*. **Trelegy Ellipta** is the first FDA-approved once-daily single-dose inhaler that combines *fluticasone furoate*, a corticosteroid, *umeclidinium*, a long-acting muscarinic antagonist, and *vilantero*, a long-acting beta-2 adrenergic agonist. Common adverse reactions reported with **Trelegy Ellipta** included headache, back pain, dysgeusia, diarrhea, cough, oropharyngeal pain, and gastroenteritis. **Trelegy Ellipta** has been found to increase the risk of pneumonia in patients with COPD and increase the risk of asthma-related death in patients with asthma. **Trelegy Ellipta** is not indicated for the treatment of acute bronchospasm.

METHYLXANTHINES

Comment: Check serum theophylline level just before 5th dose is administered.
Therapeutic theophylline level: 10-20 mcg/ml.

▷ *theophylline* (C)(G)
   Theo-24 initially 300-400 mg once daily at HS; after 3 days, increase to 400-600 mg once daily at HS; max 600 mg/day
   Pediatric: <45 kg: initially 12-14 mg/kg/day; max 300 mg/day; increase after 3 days to 16 mg/kg/day to max 400 mg; after 3 more days increase to 30 mg/kg/day to max 600 mg/day; ≥45 kg: same as adult
      Cap: 100, 200, 300, 400 mg ext-rel
   Theo-Dur initially 150 mg bid; increase to 200 mg bid after 3 days; then increase to 300 mg bid after 3 more days
   Pediatric: <6 years: not recommended; ≥6-15 years: initially 12-14 mg/kg/day in 2 divided doses; max 300 mg/day; then increase to 16 mg/kg in 2 divided doses; max 400 mg/day; then to 20 mg/kg/day in 2 divided doses; max 600 mg/day
      Tab: 100, 200, 300 mg ext-rel
   Theolair-SR
   Pediatric: <12 years: not recommended; ≥12 years: same as adult
      Tab: 200, 250, 300, 500 mg sust-rel
   Uniphyl 400-600 mg daily with meals
   Pediatric: <12 years: not recommended; ≥12 years: same as adult
      Tab: 400*, 600*mg cont-rel

METHYLXANTHINE+EXPECTORANT COMBINATION

▷ *dyphylline+guaifenesin* (C)
   Lufyllin GG 1 tab qid or 15-30 ml qid
      Tab: dyphy 200 mg+guaif 200 mg; *Elix:* dyphy 100 mg+guaif 100 mg per 15 ml

SELECTIVE PHOSPHODIESTERASE 4 (PDE4) INHIBITOR

▷ *roflumilast* (C)(G) 500 mcg once daily
   Pediatric: <12 years: not recommended; ≥12 years: same as adult
      Daliresp *Tab:* 500 mcg
   Comment: *Roflumilast* is indicated to reduce the risk of COPD exacerbations in severe COPD patients with chronic bronchitis and a history of exacerbations.

LONG-ACTING MUSCARINIC ANTAGONISTS (LAMA)

▷ *glycopyrrolate* (C)
Comment: There are no data on the safety of *glycopyrrolate* use in pregnancy or presence of *glycopyrrolate* or its metabolites in human milk or effects on the breastfed infant.

Lonhala Magnair inhale the contents of 1 vial twice daily at the same times of day, AM and PM, via Magnair neb inhal device; do not swallow solution; do not use **Magnair** with any other medicine; length of treatment is 2-3 minutes; do not use 2 vials/treatment or more than 2 vials/day
Pediatric: not indicated for use in children

Neb soln: Vial: 25 mcg/1 ml single-dose for administration with Magnair neb inhal device; *Starter Kit:* 30 day supply (2 vials/pouch, 30 foil pouches/carton), and 1 complete MAGNAIR Nebulizer System; *Refill Kit:* (2 vials/pouch, 30 foil pouches/carton) and 1 complete MAGNAIR refill handset
Comment: **Lonhala Magnair** is the first nebulizing long-acting muscarinic antagonist (LAMA) approved for the treatment of COPD in the United States. Its approval was based on data from clinical trials in the Glycopyrrolate for Obstructive Lung Disease via Electronic Nebulizer (GOLDEN) program, including GOLDEN-3 and GOLDEN-4, 2 Phase 3, 12-week, randomized, double-blind, placebo-controlled, parallel-group, multicenter study.
Seebri Neohaler inhale the contents of 1 capsule twice daily at the same time of day, AM and PM, using the neohaler; do not swallow caps
Pediatric: not indicated for use in children

Inhal cap: 15.6 mcg (60/blister pck) dry pwdr for inhalation w. 1 Neohaler device (lactose)

BULIMIA NERVOSA

SELECTIVE SEROTONIN REUPTAKE INHIBITOR (SSRI)

▷ *fluoxetine* (C)(G)
Prozac initially 20 mg daily; may increase after 1 week; doses >20 mg/day may be divided into AM and noon doses; usual daily dose 60 mg; max 80 mg/day
Pediatric: <8 years: not recommended; 8-17 years: initially 10-20 mg/day; start lower weight children at 10 mg/day; if starting at 10 mg daily, may increase after 1 week to 20 mg daily; >17 years: same as adult

Cap: 10, 20, 40 mg; *Tab:* 30*, 60*mg; *Oral soln:* 20 mg/5 ml (4 oz) (mint)
Prozac Weekly following daily *fluoxetine* therapy at 20 mg/day for 13 weeks, may initiate **Prozac Weekly** 7 days after the last 20 mg *fluoxetine* dose
Pediatric: <12 years: not recommended; ≥12 years: same as adult

Cap: 90 mg ent-coat del-rel pellets

BURN: MINOR

▷ *silver sulfadiazine* (C)(G) apply topically to burn 1-2 x daily
Pediatric: <12 years: not recommended; ≥12 years: same as adult
Silvadene *Crm:* 1% (20, 50, 85, 400, 1000 gm jar; 20 gm tube)
Comment: *Silver sulfadiazine* is contradicted in sulfa allergy.

TOPICAL AND TRANSDERMAL ANESTHETICS

Comment: *Lidocaine* should not be applied to non-intact skin.
▷ *lidocaine* cream (B) apply to affected area bid prn
Pediatric: <12 years: not recommended; ≥12 years: same as adult
LidaMantle *Crm:* 3% (1, 2 oz)

Lidoderm *Crm:* 3% (85 gm)

ZTlido *lidocaine* topical system 1% (30/carton)

Comment: Compared to **Lidoderm** (*lidocaine* patch 5%) which contains 700 mg/patch, **ZTlido** only requires 35 mg per topical system to achieve the same therapeutic dose.

▷ *lidocaine* lotion (B) apply to affected area bid prn
Pediatric: <12 years: not recommended; ≥12 years: same as adult
LidaMantle *Lotn:* 3% (177 ml)

▷ *lidocaine* 5% patch (B)(G) apply up to 3 patches at one time for up to 12 hours/24-hour period (12 hours on/12 hours off); patches may be cut into smaller sizes before removal of the release liner; do not re-use
Pediatric: <12 years: not recommended; ≥12 years: same as adult
Lidoderm *Patch:* 5% (10x14 cm; 30/carton)

▷ *lidocaine+dexamethasone* (B)
Pediatric: <12 years: not recommended; ≥12 years: same as adult
Decadron Phosphate with Xylocaine *Lotn:* dexa 4 mg+lido 10 mg per ml (5 ml)

▷ *lidocaine+hydrocortisone* (B)(G) apply to affected area bid prn
Pediatric: <12 years: not recommended; ≥12 years: same as adult
LidaMantle HC *Crm:* lido 3%+hydro 0.5% (1, 3 oz); *Lotn:* (177 ml)

▷ *lidocaine* 2.5%+prilocaine 2.5% apply sparingly to the burn bid-tid prn
Pediatric: <12 years: not recommended; ≥12 years: same as adult
Emla Cream (B) 5, 30 gm/tube

 BURSITIS

Acetaminophen for IV Infusion *see Pain*
NSAIDs *see* NSAIDs online at https://connect.springerpub.com/content/reference-book/978-0-8261-7935-5/back-matter/part02/back-matter/bmatter10
Opioid Analgesics *see Pain*
Topical & Transdermal Analgesics *see Pain*
Parenteral Corticosteroids *see* Appendix M. Parenteral Corticosteroids
Oral Corticosteroids *see* Appendix L. Oral Corticosteroids
Topical Analgesic and Anesthetic Agents *see* Appendix I. Anesthetic Agents for Local Infiltration and Dermal/Mucosal Membrane Application online at https://connect.springerpub.com/content/reference-book/978-0-8261-7935-5/back-matter/part02/back-matter/bmatter9

 CANCER: BASAL CELL CARCINOMA (BCC)

PROGRAMMED DEATH RECEPTOR-1 (PD-1) BLOCKING ANTIBODY

▷ *cemiplimab-rwlc* 350 mg as an intravenous infusion over 30 minutes every 3 weeks
Pediatric: safety and efficacy not established
Libtayo *Vial:* 350 mg/7 ml (50 mg/ml), single-dose, soln for dilution and IV infusion

Comment: **Libtayo** is indicated for the treatment of (1) patients with locally advanced BCC (laBCC) previously treated with a hedgehog pathway inhibitor or for whom a hedgehog pathway inhibitor is not appropriate and (2) patients with metastatic BCC (mBCC) previously treated with a hedgehog pathway inhibitor or for whom a hedgehog pathway inhibitor is not appropriate. The most common adverse reactions (incidence ≥15%) have been musculoskeletal pain, fatigue, rash, and diarrhea. The most common Grade 3-4 laboratory abnormalities (incidence ≥2%) have been lymphopenia, hyponatremia, hypophosphatemia, increased aspartate aminotransferase, anemia, and hyperkalemia. For infusion-related reactions, interrupt, slow the rate of infusion, or permanently discontinue based on severity of the reaction. Immune-mediated adverse reactions, which may be severe or fatal, can occur in any organ system or tissue, including the following: immune-mediated pneumonitis, immune-mediated colitis, immune-mediated hepatitis, immune-mediated endocrinopathies, immune-mediated dermatologic adverse reactions, immune-mediated nephritis and renal dysfunction, and solid organ transplant rejection. Monitor for early identification and management. Evaluate liver enzymes, creatinine, and thyroid function at baseline and periodically during treatment. Withhold or permanently discontinue **Libtayo** based on the severity of reaction. Fatal and other serious complications can occur in patients who receive allogeneic hematopoietic stem cell transplantation (HSCT) before or after being treated with a PD-1/PD-L1 blocking antibody. Based on its mechanism of action, **Libtayo** can cause embryo/fetal harm when administered to a pregnant female. Animal studies have demonstrated that inhibition of the PD-1/PD-L1 pathway can lead to increased risk of immune-mediated rejection of the developing fetus resulting in fetal death. Advise women of the potential risk and advise males females of reproductive potential to use effective contraception during treatment with **Libtayo** and for at least 4 months after the last dose. There is no information regarding the presence of *cemiplimab-rwlc* in human milk or its effects on the breastfed infant. Because of the potential for serious adverse reactions in breastfed infants, advise mothers not to breastfeed during treatment and for at least 4 months after the last dose.

 CANCER: BLADDER, URETHRAL

NECTIN-4-DIRECTED ANTIBODY AND MICROTUBULE INHIBITOR CONJUGATE

▷ *enfortumab vedotin-ejfv* 1.25 mg/kg (max 125 mg) via IV infusion over 30 minutes on Days 1, 8, and 15 of a 28-day cycle until disease progression or unacceptable toxicity; for IV infusion only. Do not administer as an IV push or bolus. Do not mix with, or administer as an infusion with, other medicinal products; *Moderate/Severe Hepatic Impairment:* avoid use

Padcev Vial: 20, 30 mg, single-dose, pwdr for reconstitution, dilution, and IV infusion

Comment: Padcev is indicated for the treatment of adult patients with locally advanced or metastatic urothelial cancer who have previously received a programmed death receptor-1 (PD-1) or programmed death-ligand 1 (PD-L1) inhibitor, and a platinum-containing chemotherapy in the neoadjuvant/adjuvant, locally advanced or metastatic setting. This indication is approved under accelerated approval based on tumor response rate. Continued approval for this indication may be contingent upon verification and description of clinical benefit in confirmatory trials. Concomitant use of strong CYP3A4 inhibitors with **Padcev** may increase the exposure to monomethyl auristatin E (MMAE). The most common adverse reactions (incidence ≥20%) have been fatigue, peripheral neuropathy, decreased appetite, rash, alopecia, nausea, dysgeusia, diarrhea, dry eye, pruritus, and dry skin. Diabetic ketoacidosis (DKA) may occur in patients with and without pre-existing diabetes mellitus, which may be fatal. Closely monitor blood glucose (BG) levels in patients with, or at risk for, diabetes mellitus, or hyperglycemia. Withhold **Padcev** if BG >250 mg/dL. Monitor patients for new or worsening peripheral neuropathy and consider dose interruption, dose reduction, or discontinuation of **Padvev** as appropriate. Consider prophylactic artificial tears for dry eyes and treatment with ophthalmic topical steroids after an ophthalmic exam. Monitor for ocular disorders, including vision changes, and consider dose interruption or dose reduction of **Padcev** when symptomatic ocular disorders occur. Skin reactions may occur; if severe, withhold **Padcev** until improvement or resolution. Ensure adequate venous access prior to beginning the infusion and monitor the infusion site. Stop the infusion immediately for suspected extravasation. **Padcev** can cause embryo/fetal harm; therefore, advise women to use effective contraception. Because of the potential for serious adverse reactions in the breastfed infant, advise women not to breastfeed during treatment with **Padcev** and for at least 3 weeks after the last dose.

 CANCER: BREAST

NONSTEROIDAL ANTI-ESTROGEN AGENTS

▷ *fulvestrant* (D)(G) 250 mg IM once monthly; administer 2.5 ml IM in each buttock concurrently
  Faslodex *Prefilled syringe:* 50 mg/ml (2 x 2.5 ml, 1 x 5 ml)
▷ *letrozole* (D)(G) 2.5 mg daily
  Femara *Tab:* 2.5 mg film-coat

PROGRAMMED DEATH RECEPTOR-1 (PD-1)-BLOCKING ANTIBODY

▷ *pembrolizumab* 200 mg via IV infusion over 30 minutes every 3 weeks or 400 mg via IV infusion over 30 minutes every 6 weeks
  Keytruda *Vial:* 100 mg/4 ml (25 mg/ml) single-dose, soln for dilution and IV infusion
  Comment: **Keytruda** is indicated, in combination with chemotherapy, for the treatment of patients with locally recurrent unresectable or metastatic triple negative breast cancer (TNBC). **Keytruda** can cause fetal harm. Advise females of the potential embryo/fetal risk and to use effective method of contraception. Advise not to breastfeed. See mfr pkg insert for prescribing details.

KINASE INHIBITORS

▷ *abemaciclib* Starting dose in combination with *fulvestrant* or an aromatase inhibitor: 150 mg twice daily; *Starting dose as monotherapy:* 200 mg twice daily; dosing interruption and/or dose reductions may be required based on individual safety and tolerability
  Pediatric: <18 years: not recommended; >18 years: same as adult
  Verzenio *Tab:* 50, 100, 150, 200 mg
  Comment: **Verzenio** *(abemaciclib)* is indicated (1) in combination with an aromatase inhibitor as initial endocrine-based therapy for the treatment of postmenopausal women with hormone receptor (HR)-positive, human epidermal growth factor receptor 2 (HER2)-negative advanced or metastatic breast cancer, (2) in combination with *fulvestrant* for the treatment of women with hormone receptor (HR)-positive, human epidermal growth factor receptor 2 (HER2)-negative advanced or metastatic breast cancer with disease progression following endocrine therapy, and (3) as monotherapy for the treatment of adult patients with HR-positive, HER2-negative advanced or metastatic breast cancer with disease progression following endocrine therapy and prior chemotherapy in the metastatic setting. **Verzenio** can cause embryo/fetal harm. Advise patients of potential risk to a fetus and to use effective contraception. There are no data on the presence of *abemaciclib* in human milk or its effects on the breastfed infant. However, breastfeeding is not recommended. Reduce the dosing frequency when administering **Verzenio** to patients with severe hepatic impairment (Child-Pugh Class C). The most common adverse reactions (incidence ≥20%) have been diarrhea, neutropenia, nausea, abdominal pain, infections, fatigue, anemia, leukopenia, decreased appetite, vomiting, headache, alopecia, and thrombocytopenia.

▷ *alpelisib* recommended dose is 300 mg (2 x 150 mg tablets) as a single dose once daily; take with food

Pediatric: safety and efficacy not established

Piqray *Tab:* 50, 150, 200 mg film-coat

Comment: Piqray *(alpelisib)* is a kinase inhibitor indicated in combination with fulvestrant for the treatment of postmenopausal women, and men, with hormone receptor (HR)-positive, human epidermal growth factor receptor 2 (HER2)-negative, PIK3CA-mutated, advanced, or metastatic breast cancer as detected by an FDA-approved test following progression on or after an endocrine-based regimen. Piqray *(alpelisib)* is the first FDA-approved PI3K inhibitor for breast cancer treatment. The most common adverse reactions, including laboratory abnormalities (all grades, incidence ≥20%), have been increased sGLU and sCr, decreased lymphocyte count, increased GGTand ALT, decreased hemoglobin, increased lipase, stomatitis, loss of appetite, nausea, vomiting, diarrhea, weight loss, fatigue, decreased calcium, prolonged aPTT, and alopecia. For adverse reactions, consider dose interruption, dose reduction, or discontinuation. For a severe hypersensitivity reaction, permanently discontinue Piqray and promptly initiate appropriate treatment. Severe cases of pneumonitis and interstitial lung disease have been reported. Do not initiate treatment in patients with a history of SJS, EM, or Toxic Epidermal Necrolysis (TEN) and permanently discontinue Piqray if SJS, EM, or TEN is confirmed. Safety of Piqray in patients with Type 1 or uncontrolled Type 2 diabetes has not been established. Before initiating treatment, test fasting plasma glucose (FPG) and HbA1c, and optimize sGLU. Avoid co-administration of Piqray with strong CYP3A4 inducers and BCRP Inhibitors. Closely monitor when Piqray is co-administered with CYP2C9 substrates as these drugs may reduce Piqray activity. Piqray is used in combination with *fulvestrant*. Verify the pregnancy status in females of reproductive potential prior to initiating treatment with Piqray and *fulvdxtrant* and advise females of reproductive potential to use effective contraception during treatment and for 1 week after the last dose. Advise male patients with female partners of reproductive potential to use condoms and effective contraception during treatment and for 1 week after the last dose. There are no data on the presence of *alpelisib* in human milk or effects on the breastfed infant. Advise lactating women to not breastfeed during treatment with Piqray and for 1 week after the last dose.

▷ *sodium neratinib*

Antidiarrheal Prophylaxis: initiate *loperamide* with the first dose of Nerlynx and continue during the first 56 days of treatment; after day 56, use *loperamide* to maintain 1-2 bowel movements per day

Extended Adjuvant Treatment of Early Stage Breast Cancer: 240 mg (6 tablets) once daily, with food, continuously until disease recurrence for up to 1 year

Advanced or Metastatic Breast Cancer: 240 mg (6 tablets) once daily with food on Days 1-21 of a 21-day cycle plus *capecitabine* (750 mg/m² twice daily) on Days 1-14 of a 21-day cycle until disease progression or unacceptable toxicity Dose interruptions and/or dose reductions are recommended based on individual safety and tolerability

Hepatic Impairment: reduce starting dose to 80 mg

Pediatric: safety and efficacy not established

Nerlynx *Tab:* 40 mg

Comment: Nerlynx *(neratinib)* is a tyrosine kinase inhibitor (TKI) indicated (a) as a single agent, for the extended adjuvant treatment of adult patients with early stage HER2-positive breast cancer, to follow adjuvant trastuzumab-based therapy and (b) in combination with *capecitabine*, for the treatment of adult patients with advanced or metastatic HER2-positive breast cancer who have received two or more prior anti-HER2-based regimens in the metastatic setting. The most common adverse reactions (incidence ≥5%) have been (a) *Nerlynx as a single agent*: diarrhea, nausea, abdominal pain, fatigue, vomiting, rash, stomatitis, decreased appetite, muscle spasms, dyspepsia, AST or ALT increased, nail disorder, dry skin, abdominal distention, epistaxis, weight decreased, and urinary tract infection and (b) *Nerlynx in combination with capecitabine*: diarrhea, nausea, vomiting, decreased appetite, constipation, fatigue/asthenia, weight decreased, dizziness, back pain, arthralgia, urinary tract infection, upper respiratory tract infection, abdominal distention, renal impairment, and muscle spasms.

▷ *tucatinib* 300 mg twice daily; *Severe Hepatic Impairment:* 200 mg twice daily; take with or without food

   Pediatric: safety and efficacy not established

   Tukysa *Tab:* 50, 150 mg

   Comment: Tukysa *(tucatinib)* is a potent tyrosine kinase inhibitor for the treatment of patients with locally advanced or metastatic HER2-positive breast cancer. The most common adverse reactions (incidence ≥20%) have been diarrhea, palmar-plantar erythrodysesthesia, nausea, fatigue, hepatotoxicity, vomiting, stomatitis, decreased appetite, abdominal pain, headache, anemia, and rash. Severe diarrhea, including dehydration, acute kidney injury, and death have been reported. Administer antidiarrheal treatment as clinically indicated. Severe hepatotoxicity has been reported. Monitor ALT, AST, and bilirubin prior to starting **Tukysa**, every 3 weeks during treatment and as clinically indicated. Based on adverse reaction severity, interrupt dose and then re-start at reduced dose, or permanently discontinue **Tukysa** as indicated. Avoid concomitant use of strong CYP3A Inducers or moderate CYP2C8 Inducers. Avoid concomitant use of strong CYP2C8 Inhibitors; reduce **Tukysa** dose if concomitant use cannot be avoided. Avoid concomitant use of **Tukysa** with CYP3A substrates, where minimal concentration changes may lead to serious or life-threatening toxicities. Consider reducing the dose of P-gp substrates, where minimal concentration changes may lead to serious or life-threatening toxicities. **Tukysa** can cause fetal harm. Advise patients of potential risk to a fetus and to use effective contraception. Advise not to breastfeed and for at least 1 week after last **Tukysa** dose. Refer to the respective *trastuzumab* and *capecitabine* mfr pkg inserts for adverse reactions, drug interactions, and pregnancy, contraception, and breastfeeding information.

POLY ADP-RIBOSE POLYMERASE (PARP) INHIBITOR

▷ *olaparib* 400 mg twice daily; with or without food; continue treatment until disease progression or unacceptable toxicity;

   ASEs: consider dose interruption or dose reduction. *CrCl 31-50 mL/min:* 300 mg twice daily

   Pediatric: safety and efficacy not established

   Lynparza *Tab:* 100, 150 mg; *Cap:* 50 mg

   Comment: **Lynparza** is indicated for the treatment of adult patients with deleterious or suspected deleterious gBRCAm, HER2-negative metastatic breast cancer who have been treated with chemotherapy in the neoadjuvant, adjuvant, or metastatic setting. Patients with hormone receptor (HR)-positive breast cancer should have been treated with a prior endocrine therapy or be considered inappropriate for endocrine therapy. Select patients for therapy based on an FDA-approved companion diagnostic for Lynparza. Myelodysplastic Syndrome/Acute Myeloid Leukemia (MDS/AML) has occurred in <1.5% of patients exposed to **Lynparza** monotherapy and the majority of events had a fatal outcome. Monitor patients for hematological toxicity at baseline and monthly thereafter. Discontinue if MDS/AML is confirmed. Pneumonitis has occurred in <1% of patients exposed to **Lynparza**, and some cases have been fatal. Interrupt treatment if pneumonitis is suspected and discontinue if pneumonitis is confirmed. Avoid concomitant use of strong or moderate CYP3A inhibitors. If the inhibitor cannot be avoided, reduce the dose. Avoid concomitant use of strong or moderate CYP3A inducers as decreased efficacy can occur. The most common adverse reactions (incidence ≥20%) in clinical trials have been anemia, nausea, fatigue (including asthenia), vomiting, nasopharyngitis/ upper respiratory tract infection/influenza, diarrhea, arthralgia/myalgia, dysgeusia, headache, dyspepsia, decreased appetite, constipation, and stomatitis. The most common laboratory abnormalities (incidence ≥25%) have been decrease in Hgb, increase MCV, decrease in lymphocytes, decrease in leukocytes, decrease in absolute neutrophil count, increase in serum Cr, and decrease in platelets. **Lynparza** can cause embryo/fetal harm. Exclude pregnancy prior to initiation and advise females of reproductive potential to use effective contraception during and for 6 months after the last dose. Males with female partners should use effective contraception and <u>not</u> donate sperm during and for 3 months after last dose. Advise women <u>not</u> to breastfeed during and for 1 month after the last dose.

▷ *talazoparib* recommended dose 1 mg once daily with unacceptable toxicity occurs; for adverse reactions, consider dose interruption or dose reduction CrCl 30-59 mL/min: 0.75 mg once daily without food; treat until disease progression
Pediatric: <18 years: not recommended; >18 years: same as adult
  Talzenna *Cap:* 0.25, 1 mg
  Comment: **Talzenna** *(talazoparib)* is a poly (ADP-ribose) polymerase (PARP) inhibitor indicated for the treatment of adult patients with deleterious or suspected deleterious germline BRCA-mutated (*gBRCAm*) HER2-negative locally advanced or metastatic breast cancer. Select patients for therapy based on an FDA-approved companion diagnostic for **Talzenna.** Most common (incidence ≥20%) adverse reactions of any grade were fatigue, anemia, nausea, neutropenia, headache, thrombocytopenia, vomiting, alopecia, diarrhea, and decreased appetite. Most common laboratory abnormalities (incidence ≥25%) were *decreases* in hemoglobin, platelets, neutrophils, lymphocytes, leukocytes, and calcium and *increases* Increases in glucose, alanine aminotransferase, aspartate aminotransferase, and alkaline phosphatase. Reduce **Talzenna** dose with certain P-gp inhibitors. Monitor for potential increased adverse reactions with concomitant BCRP Inhibitors. There are no available data on **Talzenna** use in pregnant females to inform drug-associated embryo/fetal risk. However, animal studies have demonstrated embryo/fetal harm. Breastfeeding is <u>not</u> advisable.

HER2/NEU RECEPTOR ANTAGONISTS

▷ *margetuximab-cmkb Initial Dose:* 15 mg/kg via IV infusion over 120 minutes; then, 15 mg/kg via IV infusion over a minimum of 30 minutes every 3 weeks
  Margenza *Vial:* 250 mg/10 ml (25 mg/ml) single-dose
  Comment: **Margenza** *(margetuximab-cmkb)* is indicated, in combination with chemotherapy, for the treatment of adult patients with metastatic HER2- positive breast cancer who have received two or more prior anti-HER2 regimens, at least one of which was for metastatic disease. **Margenza** is an Fc-engineered, monoclonal antibody that targets the HER2 oncoprotein. HER2 is expressed by tumor cells in breast, gastroesophageal and other solid tumors. Similar to *trastuzumab*, *margetuximab-cmkb* inhibits tumor cell proliferation, reduces shedding of the HER2 extracellular domain, and mediates antibody-dependent cellular cytotoxicity (ADCC). The most common adverse drug reactions (incidence ≥10%) with **Margenza,**

in combination with chemotherapy, have beeen fatigue/asthenia, nausea, diarrhea, vomiting, constipation, headache, pyrexia, alopecia, abdominal pain, peripheral neuropathy, arthralgia/myalgia, cough, decreased appetite, dyspnea, infusion-related reactions (IRRs), palmar-plantar erythrodysesthesia, and extremity pain. **Margenza** can cause IRRs. Symptoms may include fever, chills, arthralgia, cough, dizziness, fatigue, nausea, vomiting, headache, diaphoresis, tachycardia, hypotension, pruritus, rash, urticaria, and dyspnea. Monitor patients during and after **Margenza** infusion. Have medications and emergency equipment to treat IRRs available for immediate use. In patients experiencing mild-to-moderate IRRs, decrease rate of infusion and consider pre-medications, including antihistamines, corticosteroids, and atipyretics. Monitor patients until symptoms completely resolve. Interrupt **Margenza** infusion in patients experiencing dyspnea or clinically significant hypotension and intervene with supportive medical therapy as needed. Permanently discontinue **Margenza** in all patients with severe or life-threatening IRRs. **Margenza** use may lead to reductions in left ventricular ejection fraction (LVEF). Evaluate cardiac function prior to and during treatment. **Margenza** has not been studied in patients with a pretreatment LVEF value of <50%, a prior history of myocardial infarction or unstable angina within 6 months, or congestive heart failure NYHA class II-IV. Withhold **Margenza** for ≥16% absolute decrease in LVEF from pretreatment values or LVEF below institutional limits of normal (or 50% if no limits available) and ≥10% absolute decrease in LVEF from pretreatment values. Permanently discontinue **Margenza** if LVEF decline persists greater than 8 weeks, or dosing is interrupted more than 3 times due to LVEF decline. Evaluate cardiac function within 4 weeks prior to, and every 3 months during, and upon completion of treatment. Conduct thorough cardiac assessment, including history, physical examination, and determination of LVEF by echocardiogram or MUGA scan. Monitor cardiac function every 4 weeks if **Margenza** is withheld for significant left ventricular cardiac dysfunction. Based on findings in animal studies and mechanism of action, **Margenza** can cause fetal harm when administered to a pregnant female. Postmarketing studies of other HER-2 directed antibodies during pregnancy resulted in cases of oligohydramnios and oligohydramnios sequence manifesting as pulmonary hypoplasia, skeletal abnormalities, and neonatal death. Verify pregnancy status of women of reproductive potential prior to initiation of **Margenza**. Advise pregnant females and females of reproductive potential that exposure to **Margenza** during pregnancy, or within 4 months prior to conception, can result in embryo/fetal harm. Advise women of reproductive potential to use effective contraception during treatment and for 4 months following the last dose of **Margenza**. Advise not to breastfeed.

Trastuzumab Products

Comment: Exposure to *trastuzumab* products during pregnancy can result in embryo/fetal toxicity including oligohydramnios, in some cases complicated by pulmonary hypoplasia and neonatal death. Verify the pregnancy status of females prior to initiation. Advise patients of these risks and the need for effective contraception. There is no information regarding the presence of *trastuzumab* products in human milk or effects on the breastfed infant. Treatment with a *trastuzumab* product can result in subclinical and clinical cardiac failure manifesting as CHF, and decreased LVEF, with greatest risk when administered concurrently with anthracyclines. Evaluate cardiac function prior to and during treatment. Discontinue for cardiomyopathy, anaphylaxis, angioedema, interstitial pneumonitis, or acute respiratory distress syndrome (ARDS). Monitor patient for exacerbation of chemotherapy-induced neutropenia (CIN). Do not substitute a *trastuzumab* product for or with **Kadcyla** (*ado-trastuzumab emtansine*). *Adjuvant*

Breast Cancer Treatment ASEs: most common incidence (incidence ≥5%) are headache, diarrhea, nausea, and chills. *Metastatic Breast Cancer Treatment ASEs:* most common (incidence ≥10%) are fever, chills, headache, infection, congestive heart failure, insomnia, cough, and rash.

Dosing of *trastuzumab* Products:
> *Adjuvant Treatment of HER2-Overexpressing Breast Cancer:* Administer initial dose of 4 mg/kg over 90 minutes via IV infusion; then, 2 mg/kg over 30 minutes via IV infusion once weekly x 12 weeks (with *paclitaxel* or *docetaxel*) or x 18 weeks (with *docetaxel* and *carboplatin*); then, one week after the last weekly dose of the *trastuzument* product, administer 6 mg/kg via IV infusion over 30 to 90 minutes once every 3 weeks to complete a total of 52 weeks of therapy
> or
> Administer initial dose of 8 mg/kg over 90 minutes via IV infusion, then, 6 mg/kg over 30 to 90 minutes via IV infusion once every 3 weeks x 52 weeks *Treatment of Metastatic HER2-Overexpressing Breast Cancer:* Administer initial dose of 4 mg/kg over 90 minutes via IV infusion; then, once weekly doses of 2 mg/kg via 30 minute IV infusions

▷ *trastuzumab*
    Herceptin for Injection *Vial:* 150 mg, single-dose; 420 mg multidose, pwdr for reconstitution, dilution, and IV infusion
▷ *trastuzumab-anns*
    Kanjinti *Vial:* 420 mg, multidose, (21 mg/ml) pwdr for reconstitution, dilution, and IV infusion infusion
    Comment: **Kanjinti** is biosimilar to **Herceptin** *(trastuzumab).* See **Trastuzumab Products** above for prescribing information.
▷ *trastuzumab-dkst*
    Ogivri for Injection *Vial:* 420 mg, multidose, pwdr for reconstitution, dilution, and IV infusion
    Comment: **Ogivri** is biosimilar to **Herceptin** *(trastuzumab).* See **Trastuzumab Products** above for prescribing information.
▷ *trastuzumab-dttb*
    Ontruzant for Injection *Vial:* 150 mg single-dose; 420 mg multidose; pwdr for reconstitution, dilution, and IV infusion
    Comment: **Ontruzant** is biosimilar to **Herceptin** *(trastuzumab).* See **Trastuzumab Products** above for prescribing information.
▷ *trastuzumab-pkrb*
    Herzuma *Vial:* 420 mg, multidose, pwdr for reconstitution, dilution, and IV infusion
    Comment: **Herzuma** is biosimilar to **Herceptin** *(trastuzumab).* See **Trastuzumab Products** above for prescribing information.
▷ *trastuzumab-qyyp*
    Adjuvant Treatment of HER2-Overexpressing Breast Cancer:
    Administer either:
    Initial dose of 4 mg/kg via IV infusion over 90 minutes; then, 2 mg/kg via IV infusion over 30 minutes once weekly x 12 weeks (with *paclitaxel* or *docetaxel*) or 18 weeks (with *docetaxel* and *carboplatin*); 1 week after the last weekly dose of **Trazimera**, administer 6 mg/kg via IV infusion over 30 to 90 minutes once every 3 weeks to complete a total of 52 weeks of therapy
    or
    Initial dose of 8 mg/kg via IV infusion over 90 minutes; then, 6 mg/kg via IV infusion over 30-90 minutes once every 3 weeks for a total of 52 weeks of therapy

Metastatic HER2-Overexpressing Breast Cancer:
   Initial dose of 4 mg/kg via IV infusion over 90 minute, followed by subsequent
   once weekly doses of 2 mg/kg via IV infusions over 30 minutes
Metastatic HER2-Overexpressing Gastric Cancer:
   Initial dose of 8 mg/kg via IV infusion over 90 minutes, followed by 6 mg/kg
   via IV infusion over 30-90 minutes once every 3 weeks
Pediatric: safety and efficacy not established
   Trazimera *Vial:* 420 mg, multidose, pwdr for reconstitution and IV infusion
   Comment: Trazimera is biosimilar to **Herceptin** (*trastuzumab*) indicated for the
   treatment of HER2-overexpressing breast cancer, and the treatment of HER2-
   overexpressing metastatic gastric or gastroesophageal junction adenocarcinoma.
   Do not substitute **Trazimera** (*trastuzumab-qyyp*) for or *with ado-trastuzumab
   emtansine. Trastuzumab* products can cause embryo/fetal harm when
   administered during pregnancy. Verify pregnancy status and advise females of
   reproductive potential to use effective contraception during treatment and for 7
   months following the last dose.

HER2/NEU RECEPTOR ANTAGONIST+ENDOGLYCOSIDASE COMBINATION

▷ *trastuzumab*+*hyaluronidase*
Pediatric: safety and efficacy not established
   Herceptin Hylecta administer a single-dose (600/10,000 in 5 ml) SC over 3-5
   minutes once every 3 weeks
   Vial: trastuzumab 600 mg+hyaluronidase 10,000 units/5 ml single-dose soln
   Comment: Herceptin Hylecta (*trastuzumab+hyaluronidase-oysk*) is a
   combination of the approved HER2/neu receptor antagonist *trastuzumab*
   (**Herceptin**) and *recombinant human hyaluronidase PH20* (an enzyme that
   helps to deliver *trastuzumab* under the skin) indicated for the treatment of
   HER2-overexpressing breast cancer. **Hercedptin Hylecta** has different dosage
   and administration instructions than intravenous trastuzumab products. Do
   not administer **Herceptin Hylecta** intravenously. Do not substitute **Herceptin
   Hylecta** for or with *ado-trastuzumab emtansine* or any other *trastuzumab*
   product. Most common ASEs in the treatment of *Adjuvant Breast Cancer*
   (incidence ≥10%) are fatigue, arthralgia, diarrhea, injection site reaction,
   upper respiratory tract infection, rash, myalgia, nausea, headache, edema,
   flushing, pyrexia, cough, and pain in extremity. Most common ASEs in the
   treatment of *Metastatic Breast Cancer* are based on intravenous *trastuzumab*)
   are (incidence ≥10%) are fever, chills, headache, infection, congestive heart
   failure, insomnia, cough, and rash. Exposure to **Herceptin Hylecta** during
   pregnancy can result in embryo/fetal toxicity (oligohydramnios, in some
   cases complicated by pulmonary hypoplasia and neonatal death). Verify the
   pregnancy status of females of reproductive potential prior to initiation and
   advise patients of these risks and the need for effective contraception. There
   is no information regarding the presence of *trastuzumab* or hyaluronidase in
   human milk or effects on the breastfed infant (consider the *trastuzumab* wash
   out period is 7 months).

HER2-DIRECTED ANTIBODY+ TOPOISOMERASE INHIBITOR CONJUGATE

▷ *fam-trastuzumab deruxtecan-nxki Recommended Dose:* 5.4 mg/kg via IV infusion
   once every 3 weeks (21-day cycle) until disease progression or unacceptable
   toxicity
   Enhertu *Vial:* 100 mg pwdr, single-dose, for reconstitution and IV infusion
   Comment: Enhertu (*fam-trastuzumab deruxtecan-nxki*) is an HER2-directed
   antibody and topoisomerase inhibitor conjugate indicated for the treatment
   of adult patients with unresectable or metastatic HER2-positive breast cancer

who have received two or more prior anti-HER2-based regimens in the metastatic setting. This indication is approved under accelerated approval based on tumor response rate and duration of response. Continued approval for this indication may be contingent upon verification and description of clinical benefit in a confirmatory trial. Do not substitute **Enhertu** for or with *trastuzumab* or *adotrastuzumab emtansine*. For intravenous infusion only. Do not administer as an IV push or bolus. Do not use Sodium Chloride Injection, USP. Management of adverse reactions to **Enhertu** (ILD, neutropenia, or left ventricular dysfunction) may require temporary interruption, dose reduction, or discontinuation. Neutropenia may develop. Monitor CBC prior to initiation of and prior to each dose of **Enhertu**, and as clinically indicated. Manage through treatment interruption or dose reduction. Assess LVEF prior to initiation of **Enhertu** and at regular intervals during treatment as clinically indicated and manage through treatment interruption or discontinuation. Permanently discontinue **Enhertu** in patients with symptomatic CHF. Interstitial lung disease (ILD) and pneumonitis, including fatal cases, have been reported with **Enhertu**. Monitor for, and promptly investigate, signs and symptoms including cough, dyspnea, fever, and other new or worsening respiratory symptoms. Permanently discontinue **Enhertu** in all patients with Grade 2 or higher ILD/pneumonitis. Advise patients of the risk and to immediately report symptoms. Verify pregnancy status of females prior to initiation of **Enhertu** as exposure to **Enhertu** during pregnancy can cause embryo/fetal harm. Advise patients of these risks and the need for effective contraception. There are no data regarding the presence of *fam-trastuzumab deruxtecan-nxki* in human milk or effects on the breastfed infant. Because of the potential for serious adverse reactions in the breastfed infant, advise women not to breastfeed during treatment with **Enhertu** and for 7 months after the last dose.

TROP-2-DIRECTED ANTIBODY+TOPOISOMERASE INHIBITOR CONJUGATE

▷ *sacituzumab govitecan-hziy* 10 mg/kg via IV infusion once weekly on Days 1 and 8 of continuous 21-day treatment cycles until disease progression or unacceptable toxicity; monitor patients during the infusion and for at least 30 minutes after completion of infusion; treatment interruption and/or dose reduction may be needed to manage adverse reactions

Pediatric: safety and efficacy not established

Trodelvy *Vial:* 180 mg, single-dose, pwdr for reconstitution, dilution, and IV infusion

Comment: **Trodelvy** *(sacituzumab govitecan-hziy)* is a Trop-2-directed antibody and topoisomerase inhibitor conjugate indicated for the treatment of adult patients with metastatic triple-negative breast cancer (mTNBC) who have received at least two prior therapies for metastatic disease. This indication is approved under accelerated approval based on tumor response rate and duration of response. Continued approval for this indication may be contingent upon verification and description of clinical benefit in confirmatory trials. Do not substitute **Trodelvy** for or use with other drugs containing irinotecan or its active metabolite SN-38. For intravenous infusion only. Avoid concomitant use of **Trodelvy** with UGT1A1 inhibitors or inducers. Do not administer as an intravenous push or bolus. Premedication for prevention of infusion reactions and prevention of chemotherapy-induced nausea and vomiting is recommended. The most common adverse reactions (incidence >25%) in patients with mTNBC are nausea, neutropenia, diarrhea, fatigue, anemia, vomiting, alopecia, constipation, rash, decreased appetite, and abdominal pain. Hypersensitivity reactions including severe anaphylactic reactions have been observed. Monitor patients for infusion-related reactions and permanently discontinue **Trodelvy** if a severe or lifethreatening reaction occurs. Use anti-emetic preventive treatment and withhold **Trodelvy** for patients with Grade 3 nausea or Grade 3-4 vomiting at the time of scheduled treatment. Patients who are homozygous for the uridine diphosphate-glucuronosyl transferase 1A1 (UGT1A1)*28 allele are at increased risk for neutropenia following initiation of **Trodelvy** treatment. **Trodelvy** can cause embryo/fetal harm. Advise females of potential embryo/fetal risk and to use effective contraception during treatment and for 6 months after last dose. Because of the potential for genotoxicity, advise male patients with female partners of reproductive potential to use effective contraception during treatment and for 3 months after the last dose. Advise females not to breastfeed during treatment and for one month after the last dose.

NONSTEROIDAL ANTI-ESTROGEN

▷ *tamoxifen citrate* (D)
 Ductal Carcinoma in Situ (DCIS): 20 mg once daily x 5 years
 Reduction in Breast Cancer Incidence in High Risk Women: 20 mg once daily x 5 years
  Tab: 10, 20 mg

Comment: *Tamoxifen citrate* is an orally administered nonsteroidal antiestrogen. *tamoxifen* is effective in the treatment of metastatic breast cancer in women and men. In females with ductal carcinoma in situ (DCIS), following breast surgery and radiation, *tamoxifen* is indicated to reduce the risk of developing invasive breast cancer. *tamoxifen* is indicated to reduce the incidence of breast cancer in females at high risk for breast cancer (high risk is defined as women at least 35 years-of-age with a 5-year predicted risk of breast cancer ≥1.67%, as calculated by the Gail Model). For pre-menopausal women with metastatic breast cancer, *tamoxifen* is an alternative to oophorectomy or ovarian irradiation. Available evidence indicates that patients whose tumors are estrogen receptor-positive are more likely to benefit from *tamoxifen* therapy. *tamoxifen* is indicated for the treatment of node-positive breast cancer in women following total mastectomy or segmental mastectomy, axillary dissection, and breast irradiation. In some *tamoxifen* adjuvant studies, most of the benefit to date has been in the subgroup with four or more positive axillary nodes. *tamoxifen* is indicated for the treatment of axillary node-negative breast cancer in women following total mastectomy or segmental mastectomy, axillary dissection, and breast irradiation. *tamoxifen* has demonstrated effectiveness in the palliative treatment of male breast cancer. *tamoxifen* reduces the occurrence of contralateral breast cancer in patients receiving adjuvant *tamoxifen* therapy for breast cancer. Reduction in recurrence and mortality has been greater in studies using *tamoxifen* for about 5 years than in those that used *tamoxifen* for a shorter period of therapy. Serious and life-threatening events associated with *tamoxifen* in the risk reduction setting (women at high risk for cancer and women with DCIS) include uterine malignancies, stroke, and pulmonary embolism. The benefits of *tamoxifen* outweigh its risks in women already diagnosed with breast cancer. The effects of age, gender, and race on the pharmacokinetics of *tamoxifen* have not been determined. Safety and efficacy of *tamoxifen* in girls aged 2 to 10 years with McCune-Albright Syndrome and precocious puberty have not been studied beyond one year of treatment. Effects of reduced liver function on the metabolism and pharmacokinetics of tamoxifen have not been determined. *In vitro* studies have shown that *erythromycin*, *cyclosporin*, *nifedipine,* and *diltiazem* competitively inhibited formation of

N-desmethyl tamoxifen. The clinical significance of these *in vitro* studies is unknown. **tamoxifen** is contraindicated in females who require concomitant coumarin-type anticoagulant therapy or in females with a history of deep vein thrombosis (DVT) or pulmonary embolus (PE). **tamoxifen** may cause fetal harm in pregnancy. Patients should be advised not to become pregnant while taking **tamoxifen** or within 2 months of discontinuation and should use barrier or non-hormonal contraceptive measures. **tamoxifen** does not cause infertility. Patients should be apprised of the potential risks to the fetus, including the potential long-term risk of a DES-like syndrome. For sexually active patients of child-bearing potential, **tamoxifen** should be initiated during menstruation. In patients with menstrual irregularity, a negative B-HCG immediately prior to the initiation of therapy is sufficient. **tamoxifen** has been reported to inhibit lactation. There are no data that address whether **tamoxifen** is excreted into human milk or effects on the breastfed infant. Because of the potential for serious adverse reactions in breastfed, patients taking tamoxifen should not breast feed. Although adverse reactions to **tamoxifen** are relatively mild and rarely severe enough to require discontinuation, loss of libido and impotence resulting in male discontinuation has been reported. In oligospermic males treated with **tamoxifen**, LH, FSH, testosterone, and estrogen levels were elevated. However, no significant clinical changes have been reported.

SELECTIVE ESTROGEN RECEPTOR MODULATOR (SERM)

▷ *toremifene* (D)(G) 60 mg once daily

Fareston *Tab:* 60 mg

Comment: **Fareston** *(toremifene)* is an estrogen agonist/antagonist indicated for the treatment of metastatic breast cancer (MBC) in postmenopausal women with estrogen-receptor positive or unknown tumors. Most common adverse reactions are hot flashes, sweating, nausea, and vaginal discharge. Fetal harm may occur when administered to a pregnant woman. Women should be advised not to become pregnant when taking **Fareston**. Females of childbearing potential should use effective non-hormonal contraception during **Fareston** therapy. Discontinue drug or nursing taking into account the importance of the drug to the mother.

CANCER: CERVICAL

VASCULAR ENDOTHELIAL GROWTH FACTOR (VEGF) INHIBITOR

▷ *bevacizumab-bvzr* administer 15 mg/kg every 3 weeks via IV infusion with *paclitaxel* and *cisplatin* or *paclitaxel* and *topotecan*; do not administer **Zirabev** for 28 days following major surgery and until the surgical wound is fully healed

Zirabev *Vial:* 100 mg/4 ml (25 mg/ml), 400 mg/16 ml (25 mg/ml), single-dose

Comment: **Zirabev** is biosimilar to **Avastin** *(bevacizumab)* with indications for the treatment of multiple types of cancer with *paclitaxel* and *cisplatin* or *paclitaxel* and *topotecan*.

PROGRAMMED DEATH RECEPTOR-1 (PD-1) BLOCKING ANTIBODY

▷ *pembrolizumab* 200 mg via IV infusion every 3 weeks or 400 mg via IV infusion every 6 weeks

Keytruda 100 mg/4 ml (25 mg/ml) soln, single-dose

Comment: **Keytruda** *(pembrolizumab)* is indicated for the treatment of multiple cancers, including recurrent or metastatic cervical cancer. **Keytruda** can cause fetal harm. Advise females of the potential embryo/fetal risk and to use effective method of contraception. Advise not to breastfeed. See mfr pkg insert for full prescribing information.

CANCER: COLORECTAL

PROGRAMMED DEATH RECEPTOR-1 (PD-1) BLOCKING ANTIBODY

▷ *pembrolizumab* 200 mg via IV infusion every 3 weeks **or** 400 mg via IV infusion every 6 weeks

Keytruda 100 mg/4 ml (25 mg/ml) soln, single-dose

Comment: **Keytruda** *(pembrolizumab)* is indicated for the treatment of multiple cancers, including recurrent **or** metastatic cervical cancer. **Keytruda** can cause fetal harm. Advise females of the potential embryo/fetal risk and to use effective method of contraception. Advise **not** to breastfeed. See mfr pkg insert for full prescribing information.

VASCULAR ENDOTHELIAL GROWTH FACTOR (VEGF) INHIBITOR

▷ *bevacizumab-bvzr Option 1:* 5 mg/kg via IV infusion every 2 weeks **with** bolus-IFL; *Option 2:* 10 mg/kg via IV infusion every 2 weeks **with** **FOLFOX4**; *Option 3:* 5 mg/kg via IV infusion every 2 weeks **or** 7.5 mg/kg every 3 weeks **with** *fluoropyrimidine-irinotecan-* **or** *fluoropyrimidine-oxaliplatin*-based chemotherapy, after progression on a first-line *bevacizumab* product-containing regimen; do **not** administer **Zirabev** for 28 days following major surgery and until surgical wound is fully healed

Zirabev *Vial:* 100 mg/4 ml (25 mg/ml), 400 mg/16 ml (25 mg/ml), single-dose

Comment: **Zirabev** is biosimilar to **Avastin** *(bevacizumab)*, with indications for the treatment of multiple types of cancer, including metastatic colorectal cancer, non-small cell lung cancer, glioblastoma, metastatic renal cell carcinoma, and cervical cancer, using diagnosis-specific dosing regimens. **Zirabev** is used to treat metastatic colorectal cancer, as a first- or second-line treatment, in combination with intravenous **fluorouracil**-based chemotherapy. **Zirabev** is also used to treat metastatic colorectal cancer, in combination with *fluoropyrimidine-irinotecan-* **or** *fluoropyrimidine-oxaliplatin*-based chemotherapy, for second-line treatment in patients who have progressed on a first-line *bevacizumab* product-containing regimen. **Zirabev** is **not** indicated for adjuvant treatment of colon cancer.

CANCER: CUTANEOUS SQUAMOUS CELL CARCINOMA (CSCC)

PROGRAMMED DEATH RECEPTOR-1 (PD-1) BLOCKING ANTIBODY

▷ *pembrolizumab* 200 mg via IV infusion every 3 weeks **or** 400 mg via IV infusion every 6 weeks

Keytruda 100 mg/4 ml (25 mg/ml) soln, single-dose

Comment: **Keytruda** *(pembrolizumab)* is indicated for the treatment of multiple cancers, including recurrent **or** metastatic cutaneous squamous cell carcinoma (cSCC) that is **not** curable by surgery **or** radiation. *Keytruda* can cause fetal harm. Advise females of the potential embryo/fetal risk and to use effective method of contraception. Advise **not** to breastfeed. See mfr pkg insert for full prescribing information.

CANCER: ENDOMETRIAL CARCINOMA

PROGRAMMED DEATH RECEPTOR-1 (PD-1)-BLOCKING ANTIBODY

▷ *dostarlimab-gxly Doses 1 through 4:* 500 mg via IV infusion every 3 weeks; *Beginning 3 weeks after Dose 4 (Dose 5 onwards):* 1,000 mg via IV infusion every 6 weeks

Pediatric: safety and efficacy not established

Jemperli *Vial:* 500 mg/10 ml (50 mg/ml), single-dose, soln for dilution and IV infusion

Comment: **Jemperli** is indicated for the treatment of adult patients with mismatch repair deficient (dMMR) recurrent or advanced endometrial cancer, as determined by an FDA-approved test, that has progressed on or following prior treatment with a platinum-containing regimen. The most common adverse reactions (incidence ≥20%) have been fatigue/asthenia, nausea, tissue, including the following: immune-mediated pneumonitis, immune-mediated colitis, immune-mediated hepatitis, immune-mediated endocrinopathies, immune-mediated nephritis, and immune-mediated, dermatologic adverse reactions. Monitor for signs and symptoms of immune-mediated adverse reactions. Evaluate clinical chemistries, including liver and thyroid function, at baseline and periodically during treatment. Withhold or permanently discontinue **Jemperli** and administer corticosteroids based on the severity of reaction. For infusion-related reactions, interrupt, slow the rate of infusion, or permanently discontinue **Jemperli** based on severity of reaction. Follow patients closely for evidence of transplant-related complications of allogeneic HSCT after PD-1/L-1–blocking antibody and intervene promptly. **Jemperli is** embryo-fetal toxic. Advise males and females of reproductive potential of the potential risk and to use effective contraception. Advise women not to breastfeed during treatment and for 4 months after the last dose.

▷ *pembrolizumab* 200 mg via IV infusion every 3 weeks or 400 mg via IV infusion every 6 weeks

Keytruda 100 mg/4 ml (25 mg/ml) soln, single-dose

Comment: **Keytruda** *(pembrolizumab)* is indicated for the treatment of multiple cancers, including advanced endometrial carcinoma, in combination with *lenvatinib*, that is not MSI-H or dMMR, with disease progression following prior systemic therapy, and the patient is not a candidate for curative surgery or radiation. **Keytruda** can cause fetal harm. Advise females of the potential embryo/fetal risk and to use effective method of contraception. Advise not to breastfeed. See mfr pkg insert for prescribing details.

CANCER: EPITHELIOID SARCOMA

▷ *tepotinib* Recommended dose: 450 mg once daily with food until disease progression or unacceptable toxicity.

Tepmetko *Tab:* 225 mg

Comment: **Tepmetko** is the first and only oral MET inhibitor for the treatment of patients with metastatic non-small cell lung cancer (NSCLC) harboring mesenchymal-epithelial transition (*MET*) exon 14 skipping alterations. The most common adverse reactions (incidence ≥20%) have been edema, fatigue, nausea, diarrhea, musculoskeletal pain, and dyspnea. The most common Grade 3 to 4 laboratory abnormalities (incidence ≥2%) have been decreased lymphocytes, decreased albumin, decreased sodium, increased gamma-glutamyltransferase, increased amylase, increased ALT, increased AST, and decreased hemoglobin. Avoid concomitant use of dual strong CYP3A inhibitors and P-gp inhibitors. Avoid concomitant use of certain P-gp substrates where minimal concentration changes may lead to serious or life-threatening toxicity. Immediately withhold **Tepmetko** in patients with suspected interstitial lung disease (ILD)/Pneumonitis. Permanently discontinue **Tepmetko** in patients diagnosed with ILD/pneumonitis of any severity. Monitor liver function tests and withhold, dose reduce, or permanently discontinue **Tepmetko** based on severity. **Tepmetko** is embryo-fetal toxic. Advise patients of reproductive potential of the risk and to use effective contraception. Advise not to breastfeed.

METHYLTRANSFERASE INHIBITOR

▷ *tazemetostat* 800 mg twice daily, with or without food, until disease progression or unacceptable toxicity; swallow tablets whole; if a dose is missed or vomiting occurs, do not take an additional dose, but continue with the next scheduled dose

Tazverik *Tab:* 200 mg, film-coat

Comment: Tazverik *(tazemetostat)* is indicated for the treatment of adults and pediatric patients ≥16 years-of-age with metastatic or locally advanced epithelioid sarcoma not eligible for complete resection. This indication is approved under accelerated approval based on overall response rate and duration of response. Continued approval for this indication may be contingent upon verification and description of clinical benefit in a confirmatory trial. Increases the risk of developing secondary malignancies, including T cell lymphoblastic lymphoma, myelodysplastic syndrome, and acute myeloid leukemia. The most common (incidence ≥20%) adverse reactions are pain, fatigue, nausea, decreased appetite, vomiting, and constipation. Recommended dose reductios of Tazverik for a first adverse reaction is 600 mg twice daily and for a second adverse reaction is 400 mg twice daily. Permanently discontinue Tazverik in patients who are unable to tolerate 400 mg twice daily. Avoid co-administration of strong and moderate CYP3A inhibitors with Tazverik. Reduce the dose of Tazverik if co-administration of moderate CYP3A inhibitors cannot be avoided. Avoid co-administration with of Tazverik with strong and moderate CYP3A inducers. Tazverik can cause embryo/fetal harm; therefore, advise patients of potential risk and to use effective non-hormonal contraception. Breastfeeding is not recommended during treatment and for 1 week after the last dose.

 CANCER: ESOPHAGEAL

PROGRAMMED DEATH RECEPTOR-1 (PD-1)-BLOCKING ANTIBODY

▷ *pembrolizumab* 200 mg via IV infusion every 3 weeks or 400 mg via IV infusion every 6 weeks

Keytruda 100 mg/4 ml (25 mg/ml) soln, single-dose

Comment: Keytruda *(pembrolizumab)* is indicated for the treatment of multiple cancers, including recurrent locally advanced or metastatic squamous cell carcinoma of the esophagus. Keytruda can cause fetal harm. Advise females of the potential embryo/fetal risk and to use an effective method of contraception. Advise not to breastfeed. See mfr pkg insert for prescribing details.

 CANCER: FALLOPIAN TUBE

POLY ADP-RIBOSE POLYMERASE (PARP) INHIBITOR

▷ *niraparib tosolate* 300 mg (3 x 100 mg) once daily, with or without food; continue treatment until disease progression or unacceptable adverse reaction; for adverse reactions, consider interruption of treatment, dose reduction, or dose discontinuation

Pediatric: safety and efficacy not established

Zejula *Cap:* 100 mg

Comment: Zejula *(niraparib)* is indicated for the maintenance treatment of adult patients with recurrent epithelial ovarian, fallopian tube, or primary peritoneal cancer who are in a complete or partial response to platinum-based chemotherapy, and for late-line treatment recurrent ovarian cancer. The most common adverse reactions (incidence ≥10%) have been anemia, thrombocytopenia, neutropenia, leukopenia, hypertension, palpitations, nausea, vomiting, abdominal pain/distention, diarrhea, constipation, mucositis/stomatitis, dry mouth, fatigue/asthenia, dyspepsia, decreased appetite, urinary tract infection, AST/ALT elevation, back pain, myalgia, arthralgia, headache, dizziness, dysgeusia, insomnia, anxiety, nasopharyngitis, dyspnea, cough, and rash. Monitor CBC weekly for the first month, monitor CBC monthly for the next 11 months, and then periodically thereafter. Monitor BP and HR monthly for the first year and periodically thereafter. Manage BP and HR with appropriate medication as indicated and adjust the **Zejula** dose if necessary. Because Myelodysplastic Syndrome/ Acute Myeloid Leukemia (MDS/AML) has occurred in patients exposed to **Zejula,** with some cases being fatal, monitor patients for hematological toxicity and discontinue **Zejula** if MDS/AML is confirmed. **Zejula** can cause embryo/fetal toxicity; therefore, advise females of reproductive potential of the potential risk and to use effective contraception. Advise women not to breastfeed during treatment with **Zejula** and for 1 month after receiving the final dose.

▷ *olaparib* 300 mg twice daily; with or without food; see the mfr pkg insert for recommended duration of treatment; *CrCl: 31-50 mL/min:* 200 mg twice daily
Pediatric: safety and efficacy not established

Lynparza *Tab:* 100, 150 mg

Comment: **Lynparza** is a first-class poly (ADP-ribose) polymerase (PARP) inhibitor indicated for:

(1) maintenance treatment of adult patients with deleterious or suspected deleterious germline or somatic BRCA-mutated advanced epithelial ovarian, fallopian tube or primary peritoneal cancer who are in complete or partial response to first-line platinum-based chemotherapy; select patients for therapy based on an FDA-approved companion diagnostic for **Lynparza;**

(2) maintenance treatment of adult patients with recurrent epithelial ovarian, fallopian tube, or primary peritoneal cancer, who are in complete or partial response to platinum-based chemotherapy;

(3) treatment of adult patients with deleterious or suspected deleterious germline BRCA-mutated (gBRCAm) advanced ovarian cancer who have been treated with three or more prior lines of chemotherapy. Select patients for therapy based on an FDA-approved companion diagnostic for **Lynparza;**

(4) first-line maintenance treatment with *bevacizumab* for HRD-positive advanced ovarian cancer

(5) treatment of adult patients with deleterious or suspected deleterious germline or somatic homologous recombination repair (HRR) gene-mutated metastatic castration-resistant prostate cancer (mCRPC) who have progressed following prior treatment with *enzalutamide* or *abiraterone;* select patients for therapy based on an FDA-approved companion diagnostic for **Lynparza.**

The most common adverse reactions (incidence ≥10%) in clinical trials have been nausea, fatigue (including asthenia), vomiting, abdominal pain, anemia, diarrhea, dizziness, neutropenia, leukopenia, nasopharyngitis/upper respiratory tract infection/influenza, respiratory tract infection, arthralgia/ myalgia, dysgeusia, headache, dyspepsia, decreased appetite, constipation, stomatitis, dyspnea, and thrombocytopenia. Avoid concomitant use of strong or moderate CYP3A inhibitors. If the inhibitor cannot be avoided, reduce the **Lynparza** dose. Avoid concomitant use of strong or moderate CYP3A inducers as decreased **Lynparza** efficacy can occur. The most common adverse reactions (incidence ≥20%) in clinical trials have been anemia, nausea, fatigue (including asthenia), vomiting, nasopharyngitis/ upper respiratory tract infection/influenza, diarrhea, arthralgia/myalgia, dysgeusia, headache, dyspepsia, decreased appetite, constipation, and stomatitis. The most common laboratory abnormalities (incidence ≥25%) have been decrease in Hgb, increase MCV, decrease in lymphocytes, decrease in leukocytes, decrease in absolute neutrophil count, increase in serum Cr, and decrease in platelets. **Lynparza** can cause embryo/fetal harm. Exclude pregnancy prior to initiation and advise females of reproductive potential to use effective contraception during and for 6 months after the last dose. Males with female partners should use effective contraception and <u>not</u> donate sperm during and for 3 months after last dose. Advise women <u>not</u> to breastfeed during and for 1 month after the last dose.

CANCER: GASTRIC/GASTROESOPHAGEAL

PROGRAMMED DEATH RECEPTOR-1 (PD-1)-BLOCKING ANTIBODY

➤ *pembrolizumab* administer 200 mg via IV infusion every 3 weeks <u>or</u> 400 mg via IV infusion every 6 weeks

Keytruda *Vial:* 100 mg/4 ml (25 mg/ml), single-dose, soln for IV infusion

Comment: The FDA granted accelerated approval to **Keytruda**, in combination with *trastuzumab*, *fluoropyrimidine* and *platinum-containing chemotherapy*, for the first-line treatment of patients with locally advanced unresectable <u>or</u> metastatic HER2-positive gastric <u>or</u> gastroesophageal junction (GEJ) adenocarcinoma. **Keytruda** can cause embryo/fetal harm. Advise females of the potential risk and to use effective method of contraception. Advise <u>not</u> to breastfeed. See mfr pkg insert for full prescribing information.

CANCER: GASTROINTESTINAL STROMAL TUMOR (GIST)

KINASE INHIBITOR

➤ *avapritinib* 300 mg once daily, on an empty stomach, at least 1 hour before <u>or</u> 2 hours after a meal

Ayvakit *Tab:* 100, 200, 300 mg

Comment: **Ayvakit** *(avapritinib)* is a kinase inhibitor indicated for the treatment of adults with unresectable or metastatic gastrointestinal stromal tumor (GIST) harboring a platelet-derived growth factor receptor alpha (PDGFRA) exon 18 mutation, including PDGFRA D842V mutations. Avoid co-administration of **Ayvakit** with strong and moderate CYP3A inhibitors; if co-administeration with a moderate inhibitor cannot be avoided, reduce the dose of **Ayvakit**. Avoid co-administration of **Ayvakit** with strong and moderate CYP3A inducers. CNS adverse reactions include cognitive impairment, dizziness, sleep disorders, mood disorders, speech disorders, and hallucinations. Depending on the severity, continue **Ayvakit** at same dose, withhold and then resume at same <u>or</u> reduced dose upon improvement, <u>or</u> permanently discontinue **Ayvakit**. The most common adverse reactions (incidence ≥20%) have been edema, nausea, fatigue/asthenia, cognitive impairment, vomiting, decreased appetite, diarrhea, hair color changes, increased lacrimation, abdominal pain, constipation, rash, and dizziness. **Ayvakit** can cause embryo/fetal harm. Verify the pregnancy status of females of reproductive potential prior to initiating **Ayvakit**. Advise females of reproductive potential of the potential risk and to use effective contraception. Breastfeeding is <u>not</u> recommended during treatment and for 2 weeks following the last Ayvakit dose.

▷ *ripretinib* 150 mg once daily, with or without food
Pediatric: safety and efficacy not established
    Qinlock *Tab:* 50 mg
    Comment: **Qinlock** *(ripretinib)* is a broad-spectrum KIT and PDGFRα
    inhibitor for the treatment of adult patients with advanced gastrointestinal
    stromal tumor (GIST) who have received prior treatment with three or
    more kinase inhibitors, including *imatinib*. The most common adverse
    reactions (incidence ≥20%) have been alopecia, fatigue, nausea, abdominal
    pain, constipation, myalgia, diarrhea, decreased appetite, palmarplantar
    erythrodysesthesia, and vomiting. The most common Grade 3 or 4 laboratory
    abnormalities (incidence ≥4%) have been increased lipase and decreased
    phosphate. Based on severity, withhold **Qinlock** and resume at same or reduced
    dose in the occurrence of Palmar-Plantar Erythrodysesthesia Syndrome
    (PPES). Monitor for new primary cutaneous malignancies when initiating
    Qinlock and routinely during treatment. Do not initiate **Qinlock** in patients
    with uncontrolled hypertension and monitor blood pressure during treatment.
    Assess ejection fraction by echocardiogram or MUGA scan prior to initiating
    Qinlock and during treatment, as clinically indicated. Permanently discontinue
    for Grade 3 or 4 left ventricular systolic dysfunction. There is risk of impaired
    wound healing with **Qinlock**. Therefore, withhold **Qinlock** for at least 1 week
    prior to elective surgery and do not administer for at least 2 weeks after major
    surgery and until adequate wound healing. Safe resumption of **Qinlock** after
    resolution of wound healing complications has not been established. Monitor
    more frequently for adverse reactions when co-administered with strong
    CYP3A Inhibitors. Avoid concomitant use of strong CYP3A inducers. **Qinlock**
    can cause fetal harm. There are no available data on **Qinlock** use in pregnant
    females to inform drug-associated risk. Therefore, verify pregnancy status in
    females of reproductive potential prior to initiating **Qinlock** and advise females
    of reproductive potential of the possible risk to the fetus and to use effective
    contraception. There are no data on the presence of *ripretinib* or its metabolites
    in human milk or effects on the breastfed infant. Because of the potential for
    serious adverse embryo/fetal effects, advise women not to breastfeed during
    treatment with **Retevmo** and for 1 week after the final dose.

CANCER: GLIOBLASTOMA MULTIFORME

VASCULAR ENDOTHELIAL GROWTH FACTOR (VEGF) INHIBITOR

▷ *bevacizumab-bvzr* 10 mg/kg via IV infusion every 2 weeks; do not administer
Zirabev for 28 days following major surgery and until the surgical wound is fully
healed
    Zirabev *Vial:* 100 mg/4 ml (25 mg/ml), 400 mg/16 ml (25 mg/ml), single-dose
    Comment: **Zirabev** is biosimilar to **Avastin** *(bevacizumab)* with indications
    for the treatment of multiple types of cancer, including metastatic colorectal
    cancer, non-small cell lung cancer, glioblastoma, metastatic renal cell
    carcinoma, and cervical cancer, using diagnosis-specific dosing regimens. See
    mfr pkg insert for prescribing information.

CANCER: HEAD AND NECK SQUAMOUS CELL CARCINOMA (HNSCC)

PROGRAMMED DEATH RECEPTOR-1 (PD-1)-BLOCKING ANTIBODY

▷ *pembrolizumab* 200 mg via IV infusion every 3 weeks or 400 mg via IV infusion
every 6 weeks
    Keytruda 100 mg/4 ml (25 mg/ml) soln, single-dose
    Comment: **Keytruda** *(pembrolizumab)* is indicated for the treatment of
    multiple cancers, including (1) first-line treatment of patients with metastatic

or with unresectable, recurrent head and neck squamous cell carcinoma (HNSCC) in combination with *platinum* and *fluorouracil* (FU), (2) as a single agent, for the first-line treatment of patients with metastatic or with unresectable, recurrent HNSCC whose tumors express PD-L1 (Combined Positive Score [CPS] ≥1) as determined by an FDA-approved test (see Dosage and Administration), and as a single agent, for patients with recurrent or metastatic HNSCC with disease progression on or after platinum-containing chemotherapy. **Keytruda** can cause fetal harm. Advise females of the potential embryo/fetal risk and to use effective method of contraception. Advise not to breastfeed. See mfr pkg insert for full prescribing information.

CANCER: HEPATOCELLULAR CARCINOMA

KINASE INHIBITOR

▷ *sorafenib* (G) 400 mg (2 x 200 mg) twice daily, without food
   Nexavar *Tab*: 200 mg
   Comment: **Nexavar** is indicated for the treatment of unresectable hepatocellular carcinoma. The most common adverse reactions (incidence ≥20%) have been diarrhea, fatigue, infection, alopecia, hand-foot skin reaction, rash, weight loss, decreased appetite, nausea, gastrointestinal and abdominal pains, hypertension, and hemorrhage. **Nexavar** in combination with *carboplatin* and *paclitaxel* is contraindicated in patients with squamous cell lung cancer. Avoid strong CYP3A4 inducers. Monitor ECG (for QT prolongation) and electrolytes in patients at increased risk for ventricular arrhythmias. Consider temporary or permanent discontinuation of **Nexavar** in the event of a cardiovascular event. Discontinue **Nexavar** if needed in the event of bleeding. Monitor the patient for hypertension, weekly during the first 6 weeks and periodically thereafter. Interrupt and/or decrease **Nexavar** for severe or persistent dermal reaction, and immediately disconue **Nexavar** if Stevens-Johnson syndrome or toxic epidermal necrolysis is suspected. Discontinue **Nexavar** in the event of gastrointestinal perforation. **Nexavar** may cause hepatotoxicity; monitor liver function tests regularly and discontinue for unexplained transaminase elevation. Monitor TSH monthly and adjust thyroid replacement therapy in patients with thyroid cancer. **Nexavar** may cause embryo/fetal harm; verify pregnancy status prior to initiating **Nexavar** and advise females and males of reproductive potential to use effective contraception. Advise women not to breastfeed.

PROGRAMMED DEATH RECEPTOR-1 (PD-1)-BLOCKING ANTIBODY

▷ *pembrolizumab* 200 mg via IV infusion every 3 weeks or 400 mg IV infusion every 6 weeks
   Keytruda 100 mg/4 ml (25 mg/ml) soln, single-dose
   Comment: **Keytruda** *(pembrolizumab)* is indicated for the treatment of multiple cancers, including hepatocellular carcinoma (HCC) previously treated with *sorafenib*. **Keytruda** can cause fetal harm. Advise females of the potential embryo/fetal risk and to use effective method of contraception. Advise not to breastfeed. See mfr pkg insert for full prescribing information.

CANCER: LEUKEMIA

ORAL NUCLEOSIDE METABOLIC INHIBITOR

▷ *azacytidine* 300 mg orally once daily on Days 1 through 14 of each 28-day cycle; administer an antiemetic before each dose for at least the first 2 cycles
   Onureg *Tab*: 200, 300 mg

Comment: Onureg *(azacitidine)* is an oral form of *azacytidine* indicated for the continued treatment of adult patients with AML who have achieved first complete remission (CR) or complete remission with incomplete blood count recovery (CRi) following intensive induction chemotherapy and are not able to complete intensive curative therapy. The indications and dosing regimen for Onureg differ from that of IV or SC forms of *azacytidine*; do not substitute Onureg for IV or SC forms. Monitor complete blood counts every other week for the first 2 cycles and prior to the start of each cycle thereafter. Increase monitoring to every other week for the 2 cycles after any dose reduction. Withhold, and then resume at the same or reduced dose or discontinue Onureg based on severity. Onureg can cause fetal harm; advise patients of the potential embryo/fetal risk and to use effective contraception. Advise not to breastfeed during treatment and for 1 week after the last dose.

PROGRAMMED DEATH RECEPTOR-1 (PD-1)-BLOCKING ANTIBODY

▷ *pembrolizumab* 200 mg via IV infusion every 3 weeks or 400 mg IV infusion every 6 weeks

Keytruda 100 mg/4 ml (25 mg/ml) soln, single-dose

Comment: Keytruda *(pembrolizumab)* is indicated for the treatment of multiple. Keytruda can cause fetal harm. Advise females of the potential embryo/fetal risk and to use effective method of contraception. Advise not to breastfeed. See mfr pkg insert for full prescribing information.

FOLATE ANALOG METABOLIC INHIBITOR

▷ *pemetrexed* for injection *Recommended dose, administered as a single agent or with cisplatin, in patients with CrCl ≥45 mL/min:* 500 mg/m2 via IV infusion over 10 minutes on Day 1 of each 21-day cycle; *Initiate Folic Acid:* 400 mcg to 1000 mcg orally once daily beginning 7 days prior to the first dose and continue until 21 days after the last dose; *Administer vitamin B12:* 1 mg IM 1 week prior to the first dose and every 3 cycles thereafter; *Administer dexamethasone:* 4 mg orally twice daily the day before, the day of, and the day after Pemfexy administration *Pediatric:* safety and efficacy not established

Pemfexy *Vial:* 500 mg/20 ml (25 mg/ml), single dose, for dilution and IV infusion

Comment: Pemfexy is a branded alternative to Alimta for the treatment of nonsquamous non-small cell lung cancer (NSCLC) and malignant pleural mesothelioma. Pemfexy is indicated: (1) in combination with *cisplatin*, for the initial treatment of patients with locally advanced or metastatic non-squamous, non-small cell lung cancer (NSCLC), (2) as a single agent for the maintenance treatment of patients with locally advanced or metastatic non-squamous NSCLC whose disease has not progressed after 4 cycles of *platinum-based first-line chemotherapy*, and (3) as a single agent for the treatment of patients with recurrent, metastatic non-squamous NSCLC after prior chemotherapy. Pemfexy is not indicated for the treatment of patients with squamous cell non-small cell lung cancer SCLC. Pemfexy can cause severe bone marrow suppression resulting in cytopenia and an increased risk of infection. Do not administer Pemfexy when the absolute neutrophil count is less than 1500 cells/mm^3 and platelets are <100,000 cells/mm^3. Initiate supplementation with oral folic acid and vitamin B12 IM to reduce the severity of hematologic and gastrointestinal toxicity. Pemfexy can cause severe, and sometimes fatal, renal failure. Do not administer when CrCl <45 mL/min. Permanently discontinue for severe and life-threatening bullous, blistering or exfoliating skin toxicity. Withhold for acute onset of new or progressive unexplained pulmonary symptoms and permanently discontinue if interstitial pneumonitis is confirmed. Radiation recall can occur in patients who received radiation weeks to years previously; permanently discontinue for signs of radiation recall. The most common adverse reactions (incidence ≥20%) of *pemetrexed*, when administered as a single agent have been fatigue, nausea, and anorexia. The most common adverse reactions (incidence ≥20%) of *pemetrexed* when administered with *cisplatin* have been vomiting, neutropenia, anemia, stomatitis/pharyngitis, thrombocytopenia, and constipation. **Pemfexy** is embryo/fetal toxic. Advise males and females of reproductive potential of the potential risk and to use effective contraception. Advise not to breastfeed.

CD20-DIRECTED CYTOLYTIC ANTIBODY

▷ *rituximab Recommended Dose:* 375 mg/m² via IV infusion the day prior to the initiation of *fludarabine* and *cyclophosphamide* (FC) chemotherapy; then, 500 mg/m² on Day 1 of cycles 2–6 (every 28 days); *First Infusion:* initiate at 50 mg/hr; in the absence of infusion toxicity, increase infusion rate by 50 mg/hr increments every 30 minutes, to max 400 mg/hr; *Subsequent Infusions: Standard Infusion:* initiate at 100 mg/hr; in the absence of infusion toxicity, increase by 100 mg/hr increments at 30-minute intervals, to max 400 mg/hr. Patients who have clinically significant cardiovascular disease or who have a circulating lymphocyte count ≥5000/mm³ before Cycle 2 should not be administered a 90-minute infusion; interrupt the infusion or slow the infusion rate for infusion-related reactions; continue the infusion at one-half the previous rate upon improvement of symptoms. **Rituxan** should only be administered by a qualified healthcare professional with appropriate medical support to manage severe infusion-related reactions that can be fatal if they occur
Pediatric: safety and efficacy not established
    Rituxan *Vial:* 100 mg/10 ml (10 mg/ml), 500 mg/50 ml (10 mg/ml), single-dose, soln for dilution and IV infusion (preservative-free)
    Comment: **Rituxan** is indicated for the treatment of adult patients with previously untreated and previously treated CD20-positive chronic lymphocytic Leukemia (CLL) in combination with *fludarabine* and *cyclophosphamide*. The most common adverse common reactions (incidence >25%) have been infusion-related reactions and neutropenia. For tumor lysis syndrome, administer aggressive IV hydration, anti-hyperuricemic agents, and monitor renal function. Monitor for infections; withhold **Rituxan** and institute appropriate anti-infective therapy. For cardiac adverse reactions, discontinue **Rituxan** infusions in case of serious or life-threatening events. Discontinue **Rituxan** in patients with rising serum creatinine or oliguria. Bowel obstruction and perforation can occur; consider and evaluate for abdominal pain, vomiting, or related symptoms. Live virus vaccinations prior to or during **Rituxan** treatment is not recommended. **Rituxan** is embryo/fetal toxic. Advise males and females of reproductive potential of the potential embryo/fetal risk and to use effective contraception. Advise women not to breastfeed during treatment and for at least 6 months after the last dose.

▷ *rituximab-arrx First Cycle:* 375 mg/m²; then, *Cycles 2 thru 6:* 500 mg/m² in combination with *fludarabine* and *phosphamide* FC administered every 28 days; administer all doses of **Riabni** in combination with glucocorticoids; **Riabni** should only be administered by a qualified healthcare professional with appropriate medical support to manage severe infusion-related reactions that can be fatal
    Riabni *Vial:* 100 mg/10 ml (10 mg/ml), 500 mg/50 ml (10 mg/ml) soln, single-dose
    Comment: **Riabni** *(rituximab-arrx)* is a biosimilar to **Rituxan** indicated for previously untreated and previously treated CD20-positive chronic lymphocytic leukemia (CLL) in combination with *fludarabine* and *cyclophosphamide* (FC). The most common adverse reactions in clinical trials with CLL (incidence ≥25%) have been infusion-related reactions and neutropenia. Monitor renal function. Discontinue **Riabni** in patients

with rising serum creatinine or oliguria. If tumor lysis syndrome (TLS) is suspected, administer aggressive IV hydration and anti-hyperuricemic agents. If infection occurs, withhold **Riabni** and institute appropriate anti-infective therapy. Bowel obstruction and perforation can occur; evaluate for abdominal pain, vomiting, and related symptoms. Live virus vaccine administration prior to or during treatment with **Riabni** is not recommended. **Riabni** can cause embryo/fetal harm. Advise females of reproductive potential of embryo/fetal risk and to use effective contraception. Advise not to breastfeed.

CD20-DIRECTED CYTOLYTIC ANTIBODY + ENDOGLYCOSIDASE

▷ *rituximab+hyaluronidase human* Administer 1,600 mg/26,800 Units (*rituximab* 1,400 mg and *hyaluronidase human* 23,400 Units) SC on Day 1 of Cycles 2–6 (every 28 days) for a total of 5 cycles following a single IV dose at Day 1, Cycle 1 (i.e., 6 cycles in total); *Pre-medicate:* with *acetaminophen* and antihistamine before each dose; consider pre-medication with glucocorticoids; **Rituxan Hycela** should only be administered by a qualified healthcare professional with appropriate medical support to manage severe infusion-related reactions that can be fatal if they occur.

Rituxan Hycela *Vial: rituximab* 1,400 mg +*hyaluronidase human* 23,400 Units per 11.7 ml (120 mg/2,000 Units per ml), single dose, soln for dilution and IV infusion; *rituximab* 1,600 mg +*hyaluronidase human* 26,800 Units per 13.4 ml (120 mg/2,000 Units per ml), single dose, soln for dilution and IV infusion

Comment: **Rytuxan Hycela** is a fixed 2-drug combination indicated for the treatment of chronic lymphacytic leukemia (CLL). The most common adverse reactions (incidence ≥20%) have been infections, neutropenia, nausea, thrombocytopenia, pyrexia, vomiting, and injection site erythema. There is risk of renal toxicity when **Rytuxin Hycela** is used in combination with **cisplatin**. Local cutaneous reactions may occur more than 24 hours after administration. Interrupt **Rytuxan Hycela** injections if severe reaction develops and administer aggressive IV hydration, anti-hyperuricemic agents, and monitor renal function. Monitor for infections; withhold and institute appropriate anti-infective therapy as appropriate. With cardiac adverse reactions, discontinue in case of serious or life-threatening events. Discontinue in patients with rising serum creatinine or oliguria. Bowel obstruction and perforation may occur; consider and evaluate for abdominal pain, vomiting, or related symptoms. Live virus vaccinations prior to or during treatment not recommended. **Rituxan Hycela** is embryo/fetal toxic. Advise males and females of reproductive potential of the potential embryo/fetal risk and to use effective contraception. Advise women not to breastfeed during treatment and for at least 6 months after the last dose.

 CANCER: LUNG

See **MESOTHELIOMA**

VASCULAR ENDOTHELIAL GROWTH FACTOR (VEGF) INHIBITOR

▷ *bevacizumab-bvzr* administer 15 mg/kg via IV infusion every 3 weeks with *carboplatin* and *paclitaxel*; do not administer **Zirabev** for 28 days following major surgery and until surgical wound is fully healed

Zirabev *Vial:* 100 mg/4 ml (25 mg/ml), 400 mg/16 ml (25 mg/ml), single-dose

Comment: **Zirabev** is biosimilar to **Avastin** (*bevacizumab*) with indications for the treatment of multiple types of cancer including non-small cell lung using diagnosis-specific dosing regimens. See mfr pkg insert for prescribing information. **Zirabev** is used, in combination with *carboplatin* and *paclitaxel*, for first-line treatment of unresectable, locally advanced, recurrent or metastatic non-squamous non-small cell lung cancer.

KINASE INHIBITORS

▷ *brigatinib* 90 mg once daily x 7 days; then, increase to 180 mg once daily; take with or without food; if a dose is missed or if the patient vomits after taking a dose, do not to repeat the dose, take the next dose at the regular time
Pediatric: safety and efficacy not established
   Alunbrig *Tab:* 30, 90, 180 mg film-coat
   Comment: **Alunbrig** *(brigatinib)* is an anaplastic lymphoma kinase (ALK) inhibitor for the treatment of patients with anaplastic lymphoma kinase (ALK)-positive metastatic non-small cell lung cancer (NSCLC) as detected by an FDA-approved test. The most common adverse reactions (incidence ≥25%) with **Alunbrig** have been diarrhea, fatigue, nausea, rash, cough, myalgia, headache, hypertension, vomiting, and dyspnea. Withhold **Alunbrig**, then consider dose reduction or permanent discontinuation, based on occurrence and/or severity of physiologic changes. Assess fasting serum glucose prior to starting **Alunbrig** and regularly during treatment. Monitor for new or worsening respiratory symptoms, particularly during the first week of treatment. Withhold **Alunbrig** for new or worsening respiratory symptoms and promptly evaluate for interstitial lung disease (ILD/pneumonitis. Monitor BP after 2 weeks and then at least monthly during treatment. Monitor heart rate regularly during treatment. Monitor CPK regularly during treatment and occurrence of muscle pain or weakness. Monitor lipase and amylase levels regularly during treatment. Monitor for hepatic impairment or renal impairment. **Alunbrig** can cause fetal harm. Verify pregnancy status in females of reproductive potential prior to initiating **Alunbrig**. Advise females of reproductive potential of the potential embryo/fetal risk and to use a non-hormonal method of effective contraception during treatment and for at least 4 months after the last dose. Advise not to breastfeed during treatment with **Alumbrig** and for 1 week after the last dose.

▷ *capmatinib* 400 mg twice daily with or without food
Pediatric: safety and efficacy not established
   Tabrecta *Tab:* 150, 200 mg
   Comment: **Tabrecta** *(capmatinib)* is indicated for the treatment of adult patients with metastatic non-small cell lung cancer (NSCLC), whose tumors have a mutation that leads to mesenchymal-epithelial transition (MET) exon 14 skipping, as detected by an FDA-approved test. The most common adverse reactions (incidence ≥ 20%) have been peripheral edema, nausea, fatigue, vomiting, dyspnea, and decreased appetite. Monitor for new or worsening pulmonary symptoms indicative of interstitial lung disease ILD/pneumonitis. Permanently discontinue **Tabrecta** in patients with ILD/pneumonitis. Monitor liver function tests. In the event of hepatotoxicity, withhold, reduce dose, or permanently discontinue **Tabrecta** based on severity. **Tabrecta** may cause photosensitivity reactions. Advise patients to limit direct ultraviolet exposure. **Tabrecta** can cause embryo/fetal harm. Advise patients of reproductive potential to use effective contraception. Advise not to breastfeed.

▷ *pralsetinib* 400 mg once daily; take on an empty stomach (no food for at least 2 hours before and at least 1 hour after taking the dose
Pediatric: safety and efficacy not established
   Gavreto *Cap:* 100 mg
   Comment: **Gavreto** *(pralsetinib)* is an oral selective RET kinase inhibitor for the treatment of adult patients with metastatic rearranged during transfection (RET) fusion-positive non-small cell lung cancer (NSCLC) as detected by an FDA approved test. This indication is approved under accelerated approval

based on overall response rate and duration of response. Continued approval for this indication may be contingent upon verification and description of clinical benefit in confirmatory trial(s). See the mfr pkginsert for prescribing information. There are no available data on **Gavreto** use in pregnant females to inform drug-associated risk. Based on findings from animal studies and its mechanism of action, **Gavreto** can cause embryo/fetal harm when administered to a pregnant female. There are no data on the presence of *pralsetinib* or its metabolites in human milk or their effects on the breastfed infant. Because of the potential for serious adverse reactions in breastfed children, advise women not to breastfeed during treatment with **Gavreto** and for 1 week after the final dose.

▷ *selpercatinib < 50 kg:* 120 mg twice daily; >50 kg: 160 mg twice daily; reduce dose in patients with severe hepatic impairment

Pediatric: <12 years: safety and efficacy not established; ≥12 years: same as adult

Retevmo *hgc:* 40, 80 mg

Comment: Retevmo *(selpercatinib)* is a kinase inhibitor indicated for adult patients with metastatic RET fusion-positive non-small cell lung cancer, adult and pediatric patients ≥12 years-of-age with advanced or metastatic RET-mutant medullary thyroid cancer (MTC) who require systemic therapy; adult and pediatric patients ≥12 years-of-age with advanced or metastatic RET fusion-positive thyroid cancer who require systemic therapy and who are radioactive iodine-refractory (if radioactive iodine is appropriate). The most common adverse reactions, including laboratory abnormalities, (incidence ≥ 25%) have been increased aspartate aminotransferase (AST), increased alanine aminotransferase (ALT), increased glucose, decreased leukocytes, decreased albumin, decreased calcium, dry mouth, diarrhea, increased creatinine, increased alkaline phosphatase, hypertension, fatigue, edema, decreased platelets, increased total cholesterol, rash, decreased sodium, and constipation. Monitor ALT and AST prior to initiating **Retevmo**, every 2 weeks during the first 3 months, then monthly thereafter and as clinically indicated. Do not initiate **Retevmo** in patients with uncontrolled hypertension; optimize BP prior to initiating **Retevmo** and monitor BP after 1 week, at least monthly thereafter and as clinically indicated. Monitor patients who are at significant risk of developing QTc prolongation. Assess QT interval, electrolytes and TSH at baseline and periodically during treatment. Monitor QT interval more frequently when **Retevmo** is concomitantly administered with strong and moderate CYP3A inhibitors or drugs known to prolong QTc interval. Permanently discontinue **Retevmo** in patients with severe or life-threatening hemorrhage. Withhold **Retevmo** and initiate corticosteroids in the occurrence of any hypersensitivity reaction and, upon resolution, resume at a reduced dose and increase dose by 1 dose level each week until reaching the dose taken prior to onset of hypersensitivity. Continue steroids until the patient reaches target dose of **Retevmo** and then taper. Withhold **Retevmo** for at least 7 days prior to elective surgery. Do not administer for at least 2 weeks following major surgery and until adequate wound healing. The safety of resumption of **Retevmo** after resolution of wound healing complications has not been established. Avoid co-administration with PPIs; if co-administration cannot be avoided, take **Retevmo** with food (with PPI) or modify its administration time (with H2 receptor antagonist or locally-acting antacid). Avoid co-administration strong and moderate CYP3A inhibitors; if co-administration cannot be avoided, reduce the **Retevmo** dose. Avoid co-administration with strong and moderate CYP3A inducers. Avoid co-administration with CYP2C8 and CYP3A substrates; if co-administration cannot be avoided, modify the substrate dosage as recommended in its product labeling. Based on findings from animal studies, and its mechanism of action, **Retevmo** can cause fetal harm. There are no available data on **Retevmo** use in pregnant women to inform drug-associated risk. Therefore, verify pregnancy status in females of reproductive potential prior to initiating **Retevmo** and advise females of reproductive potential of the possible risk to the fetus and to use effective contraception. There are no data on the presence of *selpercatinib* or its metabolites in human milk or effects on the breastfed infant. Because of the potential for serious adverse embryo/fetal effects, advise women not to breastfeed during treatment with **Retevmo** and for 1 week after the final dose.

▶ *tepotinib Recommended dose:* 450 mg once daily with food until disease progression or unacceptable toxicity.

Tepmetko *Tab:* 225 mg

Comment: **Tepmetko** is the first and only oral MET inhibitor for the treatment of patients with metastatic non-small cell lung cancer (NSCLC) harboring mesenchymal-epithelial transition (*MET*) exon 14 skipping alterations. The most common adverse reactions (incidence ≥20%) have been edema, fatigue, nausea, diarrhea, musculoskeletal pain, and dyspnea. The most common Grade 3 to 4 laboratory abnormalities (incidence ≥2%) have been decreased lymphocytes, decreased albumin, decreased sodium, increased gamma-glutamyltransferase, increased amylase, increased ALT, increased AST, and decreased hemoglobin. Avoid concomitant use of dual strong CYP3A inhibitors and P-gp inhibitors. Avoid concomitant use of certain P-gp substrates where minimal concentration changes may lead to serious or life-threatening toxicity. Immediately withhold **Tepmetko** in patients with suspected interstitial lung disease (ILD)/Pneumonitis. Permanently discontinue **Tepmetko** in patients diagnosed with ILD/pneumonitis of any severity. Monitor liver function tests and withhold, dose reduce, or permanently discontinue **Tepmetko** based on severity. **Tepmetko** is embryo-fetal toxic. Advise patients of reproductive potential of the risk and to use effective contraception. Advise not to breastfeed.

FOLATE ANALOG METABOLIC INHIBITOR

▶ *pemetrexed* for injection *Recommended dose, administered as a single agent or with cisplatin, in patients with CrCl ≥45 mL/min:* 500 mg/m2 via IV infusion over 10 minutes on Day 1 of each 21-day cycle; *Initiate Folic Acid:* 400 mcg to 1000 mcg orally once daily beginning 7 days prior to the first dose and continue until 21 days after the last dose; *Administer vitamin B12:* 1 mg IM 1 week prior to the first dose and every 3 cycles thereafter; *Administer dexamethasone:* 4 mg orally twice daily the day before, the day of, and the day after **Pemfexy** administration *Pediatric:* safety and efficacy not established

Pemfexy *Vial:* 500 mg/20 ml (25 mg/ml), single dose, for dilution and IV infusion

Comment: **Pemfexy** is a branded alternative to **Alimta** for the treatment of nonsquamous non-small cell lung cancer (NSCLC) and malignant pleural mesothelioma. **Pemfexy** is indicated: (1) in combination with *cisplatin* for the initial treatment of patients with locally advanced or metastatic non-squamous, non-small cell lung cancer (NSCLC), (2) as a single agent for the maintenance treatment of patients with locally advanced or metastatic non-squamous NSCLC whose disease has not progressed after 4 cycles of *platinum-based first-line chemotherapy*, and (3) as a single agent for the treatment of patients with recurrent, metastatic non-squamous NSCLC after prior chemotherapy. **Pemfexy** is not indicated for the treatment of patients with squamous cell non-small cell lung cancer SCLC. **Pemfexy** can cause severe bone marrow suppression resulting in cytopenia and an increased risk of infection. Do not administer **Pemfexy** when the absolute neutrophil count is less than 1500 cells/mm^3 and platelets are <100,000 cells/mm^3. Initiate supplementation with oral folic acid and vitamin B12 IM to reduce the severity of hematologic and gastrointestinal toxicity. **Pemfexy** can cause severe, and sometimes fatal, renal failure. Do not administer when CrCl <45 mL/min. Permanently discontinue for severe and life-threatening bullous, blistering or exfoliating skin toxicity. Withhold for acute onset of new or progressive unexplained pulmonary symptoms and permanently discontinue if interstitial pneumonitis is confirmed. Radiation recall can occur in patients who received radiation weeks to years previously; permanently discontinue for signs of radiation recall. The most common adverse reactions (incidence ≥20%) of *pemetrexed*, when administered as a single agent have been fatigue, nausea, and anorexia. The most common adverse reactions (incidence ≥20%) of *pemetrexed* when administered with *cisplatin* have been vomiting, neutropenia, anemia, stomatitis/pharyngitis, thrombocytopenia, and constipation. **Pemfexy** is embryo/fetal toxic. Advise males and females of reproductive potential of the potential risk and to use effective contraception. Advise not to breastfeed.

PROGRAMMED DEATH RECEPTOR-1 (PD-1) BLOCKING ANTIBODY

▷ *cemiplimab-rwlc* 350 mg as an intravenous infusion over 30 minutes every 3 weeks

Pediatric: safety and efficacy not established

Libtayo *Vial:* 350 mg/7 ml (50 mg/ml), single-dose, soln for dilution and IV infusion

Comment: **Libtayo** is indicated for the treatment of patients with metastatic cutaneous squamous cell carcinoma (mCSCC) or locally advanced CSCC (laCSCC) who are not candidates for curative surgery or curative radiation.

Comment: **Libtayo** is indicated for the first-line treatment of patients with NSCLC whose tumors have high PD-L1 expression (Tumor Proportion Score [TPS] ≥ 50%) as determined by an FDA-approved test, with no EGFR, ALK or ROS1 aberrations, and is (1) locally advanced where patients are not candidates for surgical resection or definitive chemoradiation or (2) metastatic. The most common adverse reactions (incidence ≥15%) have been musculoskeletal pain, fatigue, rash, and diarrhea. The most common Grade 3-4 laboratory abnormalities (incidence ≥2%) have been lymphopenia, hyponatremia, hypophosphatemia, increased aspartate aminotransferase, anemia, and hyperkalemia. For infusion-related reactions, interrupt, slow the rate of infusion, or permanently discontinue based on severity of the reaction. Immune-mediated adverse reactions, which may be severe or fatal, can occur in any organ system or tissue, including the following: immune-mediated pneumonitis, immune-mediated colitis, immune-mediated hepatitis, immune-mediated endocrinopathies, immune-mediated dermatologic adverse reactions, immune-mediated nephritis and renal dysfunction, and solid organ transplant rejection. Monitor for early identification and management. Evaluate liver enzymes, creatinine, and thyroid function at baseline and periodically during treatment. Withhold or permanently discontinue **Libtayo** based on the severity of reaction. Fatal and other serious complications can occur in patients who receive allogeneic hematopoietic stem cell transplantation (HSCT) before or after being treated with a PD-1/ PD-L1 blocking antibody. Based on its mechanism of action, **Libtayo** can cause embryo/fetal harm when administered to a pregnant female. Animal studies have demonstrated that inhibition of the PD-1/PD-L1 pathway can lead to increased risk of immune-mediated rejection of the developing fetus resulting in fetal death. Advise women of the potential risk and advise males females of reproductive potential to use effective contraception during treatment with **Libtayo** and for at least 4 months after the last dose. There is no information regarding the presence of *cemiplimab-rwlc* in human milk or its effects on the breastfed infant. Because of the potential for serious adverse reactions in breastfed infants, advise mothers not to breastfeed during treatment and for at least 4 months after the last dose.

▷ *pembrolizumab* 200 mg via IV infusion every 3 weeks or 400 mg via IV infusion every 6 weeks

Keytruda 100 mg/4 ml (25 mg/ml) soln, single-dose

Comment: **Keytruda** *(pembrolizumab)* is indicated for the treatment of multiple cancers, including: (1) metastatic **small cell lung cancer (SCLC)** with disease progression on or after *platinum*-based chemotherapy and at least one other prior line of therapy (this indication is approved under accelerated approval based on tumor response rate and durability of response; continued approval for this indication may be contingent upon verification and description of clinical benefit in confirmatory trials); (2) in combination with *pemetrexed* and *platinum* chemotherapy, for the first-line treatment of metastatic **non-squamous non-small cell lung cancer (NSCLC)**, with no EGFR or ALK genomic tumor aberrations; (3) in combination with *carboplatin* and either *paclitaxel* or *paclitaxel protein-bound* as a single agent, the treatment of patients with metastatic **NSCLC** whose tumors express PD-L1 (TPS ≥1%) as determined by an FDA-approved test; (4) as a single agent, for the first-line treatment of patients with **NSCLC** expressing PD-L1 (Tumor Proportion Score [TPS] ≥1%) as determined by an FDA-approved test, with no EGFR or ALK genomic tumor aberrations, metastatic or stage III where patients are not candidates for surgical resection or definitive chemoradiation; (5) as a single agent, is indicated for the treatment of metastatic **NSCLC** with tumors express PD-L1 (TPS ≥1%); as determined by an FDA-approved test, with disease progression on or after *platinum*-containing chemotherapy; patients with EGFR or ALK genomic tumor aberrations should have disease progression on FDA-approved therapy for these aberrations prior to receiving **Keytruda**. **Keytruda** can cause fetal harm. Advise females of the potential embryo/fetal risk and to use effective method of contraception. Advise not to breastfeed. See mfr pkg insert for full prescribing information.

CANCER: LYMPHOMA

KINASE INHIBITOR

▷ *umbralisib* 800 mg once daily with food

Pediatric: safety and efficacy not established

Ukoniq *Tab:* 200 mg

Comment: **Ukoniq** is an oral, once-daily, treatment of adult patients with (1) relapsed or refractory marginal zone lymphoma (MZL) who have received at least one prior anti-CD20-based regimen and (2) relapsed or refractory follicular lymphoma (FL) who have received at least 3 prior lines of systemic therapy. The most common (incidence ≥15%) adverse reactions, including laboratory abnormalities, have been increased creatinine, diarrhea-colitis, fatigue, nausea, neutropenia, transaminase elevation, musculoskeletal pain, anemia, thrombocytopenia, upper respiratory tract infection, vomiting, abdominal pain, decreased appetite, and rash. Manage toxicity using treatment interruption, dose reduction, or discontinuation. Monitor for fever and any new or worsening signs and symptoms of infection; evaluate promptly and treat as needed. Monitor blood counts during treatment. Monitor for the development of diarrhea or colitis and provide supportive care as appropriate. Monitor hepatic function. Withhold treatment, reduce dose, or discontinue treatment depending on severity and persistence of severe cutaneous reaction.

Ukoniq contains FD&C Yellow No. 5 (tartrazine) which may cause allergic-type reactions. Ukoniq is embryo/fetal toxic. Advise males and females of reproductive potential of the risk and to use effective contraception. Advise not to breastfeed during treatment and for 1 month after the last dose.

CD19-DIRECTED ANTIBODY AND ALKYLATING AGENT CONJUGATE

▷ *loncastuximab tesirine-lpyl* 0.15 mg/kg *via IV infusion* over 30 minutes on Day 1 of each 3-week cycle for the first 2 cycles; then, 0.075 mg/kg *via IV infusion* over 30 minutes every 3 weeks for subsequent cycles; *Premedicate:* with *dexamethasone* 4 mg orally or intravenously 2 x/daily for 3 days beginning the day before each infusion
Pediatric: safety and efficacy not established

Zynlonta *Vial:* 10 mg, single-dose, pwdr for reconstitution, dilution, and IV infusion

Comment: Zynlonta is indicated for the treatment of adult patients with relapsed or refractory large B-cell lymphoma after two or more lines of systemic therapy, including diffuse large B-cell lymphoma (DLBCL) not otherwise specified, DLBCL arising from low grade lymphoma, and high-grade B-cell lymphoma. The most common (incidence ≥20%) adverse reactions, including laboratory abnormalities, are thrombocytopenia, increased gamma-glutamyltransferase, neutropenia, anemia, hyperglycemia, transaminase elevation, fatigue, hypoalbuminemia, rash, edema, nausea, and musculoskeletal pain. Monitor patients for the development of pleural effusion, pericardial effusion, ascites, peripheral edema, and general edema; consider diagnostic imaging when symptoms develop or worsen. Monitor for myelosuppression. Withhold, reduce, or discontinue. Zynlonta based on severity. Monitor for infection and treat promptly. Monitor patients for new or worsening cutaneous reactions, including photosensitivity reactions; dermatologic consultation should be considered. Zynlonta is embryo-fetal toxic. Advise males and females of reproductive potential of the potential risk and to use effective contraception. Advise not to breastfeed during treatment and for 3 months after the last dose.

CHIMERIC ANTIGEN RECEPTOR (CAR) T-CELL THERAPY

▷ *lisocabtagene maraleucel* dosing is based on the number of chimeric antigen receptor (CAR)-positive viable T cells--50 to 110 × 106 CAR-positive viable T cells (consisting of CD8 and CD4 components); administer via IV infusion only; do not use a leukodepleting filter; *Before the infusion:* confirm availability of *tocilizumab*; administer a lymphodepleting regimen of *fludarabine* and *cyclophosphamide*; premedicate with *acetaminophen* and an H1 antihistamine; for autologous use only; must be administered in a certified healthcare facility
Pediatric: safety and efficacy not established

Breyanzi *Vial:* 50 to 110 × 106 CAR-positive viable T cells/5 ml (1.5 × 106 to 70 × 106 CAR-positive viable T cells/ml), single-dose, cell suspension for IV infusion; a single dose of contains 50 to 110 × 106 CAR-positive viable T cells consisting of 1:1 CAR-positive viable T cells of the CD8 and CD4 components, with each component supplied separately in 1-4 single-dose 5 ml vials.

Comment: Breyanzi is a CD19-directed genetically modified autologous T cell immunotherapy indicated for the treatment of adult patients with relapsed or refractory large B-cell lymphoma after two or more lines of systemic therapy, including diffuse large B-cell lymphoma (DLBCL) not otherwise specified (including DLBCL arising from indolent lymphoma), high-grade B-cell lymphoma, primary mediastinal large B-cell lymphoma, and follicular lymphoma grade 3B. The most common non-laboratory adverse reactions (incidence ≥20%) have been fatigue, cytokine release syndrome, musculoskeletal pain, nausea, headache, encephalopathy, infections (pathogen unspecified), decreased appetite, diarrhea, hypotension, tachycardia, dizziness, cough, constipation, abdominal pain, vomiting, and edema. Monitor for hypersensitivity reactions during infusion. Monitor patients for signs and symptoms of infection; treat appropriately. Patients may exhibit Grade 3 or higher cytopenias for several weeks following **Breyanzi** infusion. Monitor complete blood counts. Monitor and consider immunoglobulin replacement therapy. In the event that a secondary malignancy occurs after treatment with **Breyanzi**, contact Bristol-Myers Squibb at 1-888-805-4555. Advise patients to refrain from driving and engaging in hazardous occupations or activities, such as operating heavy or potentially dangerous machinery for at least 8 weeks after administration. There are no available data with **Breyanzi** use in pregnant females. No animal reproductive and developmental toxicity studies have been conducted with **Breyanzi** to assess whether it can cause embryo/fetal harm. It is not known if **Breyanzi** has the potential to be transferred to the fetus. Based on the mechanism of action, if the transduced cells cross the placenta, they may cause fetal toxicity including B-cell lymphocytopenia and hypogammaglobulinemia. Therefore, **Breyanzi** is not recommended for females who are pregnant. Pregnancy after **Breyanzi** infusion should be discussed with the treating physician. There is no information regarding the presence of **Breyanzi** in human milk or effect on the breastfed infant. The developmental and health benefits of breastfeeding should be considered along with the mother's clinical need for **Breyanzi** and any potential adverse effects on the breastfed infant from **Breyanzi** or from the underlying maternal condition.

FOLATE ANALOG METABOLIC INHIBITOR

▷ **pemetrexed** for injection *Recommended dose, administered as a single agent or with cisplatin, in patients with CrCl ≥45 mL/min:* 500 mg/m2 via IV infusion over 10 minutes on Day 1 of each 21-day cycle; *Initiate Folic Acid:* 400 mcg to 1000 mcg orally once daily beginning 7 days prior to the first dose and continue until 21 days after the last dose; *Administer vitamin B12:* 1 mg IM 1 week prior to the first dose and every 3 cycles thereafter; *Administer* **dexamethasone**: 4 mg orally twice daily the day before, the day of, and the day after **Pemfexy** administration
Pediatric: safety and efficacy not established

Pemfexy *Vial:* 500 mg/20 ml (25 mg/ml), single dose, for dilution and IV infusion

Comment: **Pemfexy** is a branded alternative to **Alimta** for the treatment of nonsquamous non-small cell lung cancer (NSCLC) and malignant pleural mesothelioma. **Pemfexy** is indicated: (1) in combination with *cisplatin* for the initial treatment of patients with locally advanced or metastatic non-squamous, non-small cell lung cancer (NSCLC), (2) as a single agent for the maintenance treatment of patients with locally advanced or metastatic non-squamous NSCLC whose disease has not progressed after 4 cycles of *platinum-based first-line chemotherapy*, and (3) as a single agent for the treatment of patients with recurrent, metastatic non-squamous NSCLC after prior chemotherapy. **Pemfexy** is not indicated for the treatment of patients with squamous cell non-small cell lung cancer SCLC. **Pemfexy** can cause severe bone marrow suppression resulting in cytopenia and an increased risk of infection. Do not administer **Pemfexy** when the absolute neutrophil count is less than 1500 cells/mm³ and platelets are <100,000 cells/mm³.
Initiate supplementation with oral folic acid and vitamin B12 IM to reduce the severity of hematologic and gastrointestinal toxicity. **Pemfexy** can cause severe, and sometimes fatal, renal failure. Do not administer when CrCl <45 mL/min. Permanently discontinue for severe and life-threatening

bullous, blistering or exfoliating skin toxicity. Withhold for acute onset of new or progressive unexplained pulmonary symptoms and permanently discontinue if interstitial pneumonitis is confirmed. Radiation recall can occur in patients who received radiation weeks to years previously; permanently discontinue for signs of radiation recall. The most common adverse reactions (incidence ≥20%) of *pemetrexed*, when administered as a single agent have been fatigue, nausea, and anorexia. The most common adverse reactions (incidence ≥20%) of *pemetrexed* when administered with *cisplatin* have been vomiting, neutropenia, anemia, stomatitis/pharyngitis, thrombocytopenia, and constipation. **Pemfexy** is embryo/fetal toxic. Advise males and females of reproductive potential of the potential risk and to use effective contraception. Advise not to breastfeed.

CD20-DIRECTED CYTOLYTIC ANTIBODY

▶ *rituximab* Rituxan should only be administered by a qualified healthcare professional with appropriate medical support to manage severe infusion-related reactions that can be fatal if they occur

Recommended Dose: 375 mg/m² via IV infusion according to the following schedules:
- Relapsed or Refractory, Low-Grade or Follicular, CD20-Positive, B-Cell NHL: Administer once weekly x 4 or 8 doses
- Re-treatment for Relapsed or Refractory, Low-Grade or Follicular, CD20-Positive, B-Cell NHL: Administer once weekly x 4 doses
- Previously Untreated, Follicular, CD20-Positive, B-Cell NHL Administer on Day 1 of each cycle of chemotherapy for up to 8 doses in patients with complete or partial response, initiate **Rituxan** maintenance 8 weeks following completion of a *rituximab* product in combination with chemotherapy; Administer **Rituxan** as a single agent every 8 weeks x 12 doses
- Non-progressing, Low-Grade, CD20-Positive, B-Cell NHL, after first-line CVP chemotherapy--Following completion of 6–8 cycles of CVP chemotherapy, administer **Rituxan** once weekly x 4 doses at 6-month intervals to maximum 16 doses
- Diffuse Large B-Cell NHL: Administer on Day 1 of each cycle of chemotherapy for up to 8 infusions.
- As a component of **Zevalin** therapeutic regimen for treatment of NHL: infuse 250 mg/m² in accordance with the **Zevalin** mfr pkg insert (refer to the **Zevalin** mfr pkg insert for full prescribing information regarding the **Zevalin** therapeutic regimen)

Rituxan should only be administered by a qualified healthcare professional with appropriate medical support to manage severe infusion-related reactions that can be fatal if they occur

Recommended Infusion Rate:
- *First Infusion:* initiate at 50 mg/hr; in the absence of infusion toxicity, increase infusion rate by 50 mg/hr increments every 30 minutes, to max 400 mg/hr
- *Subsequent Infusions: Standard Infusion:* initiate at 100 mg/hr; in the absence of infusion toxicity, increase by 100 mg/hr increments at 30-minute intervals, to max 400 mg/hr
- *Previously Untreated Follicular Non-Hodgekin's Lymphona (NHL) and Difuse Large B Cell Lymphoma (DLBCL):* if patients did not experience a Grade 3 or 4 infusion-related adverse event during Cycle 1, a 90-minute infusion can be administered in Cycle 2 with a glucocorticoid-containing chemotherapy regimen; initiate at a rate of 20% of the total dose given in the first 30 minutes and the remaining 80% of the total dose given over

the next 60 minutes; If the 90-minute infusion is tolerated in Cycle 2, the same rate can be used when administering the remainder of the treatment regimen (through Cycle 6 or 8)

- Patients who have clinically significant cardiovascular disease or who have a circulating lymphocyte count ≥5000/mm³ before Cycle 2 should not be administered a 90-minute infusion
- *Infusion-RelatedRreaction:* interrupt the infusion or slow the infusion rate for s; continue the infusion at one-half the previous rate upon improvement of symptoms

Pediatric: safety and efficacy not established

Rituxan *Vial:* 100 mg/10 ml (10 mg/ml), 500 mg/50 ml (10 mg/ml), single-dose, soln for dilution and IV infusion (preservative-free)

Comment: **Rituxan** is indicated for the treatment of adult patients with (1) relapsed or refractory, low grade or follicular, CD20-positive B-cell NHL, as a single agent therapy, (2) previously untreated follicular, CD20-positive, B-cell NHL, in combination with first line chemotherapy, and in patients achieving a complete or partial response to a *rituximab* product in combination with chemotherapy, as single-agent maintenance therapy, (3) non-progressing (including stable disease), low-grade, CD20 positive, B-cell NHL as a single agent after first-line *cyclophosphamide*, *vincristine*, and *prednisone* (CVP) chemotherapy, and (4) previously untreated diffuse large B-cell, CD20-positive NHL in combination with *cyclophosphamide*, *doxorubicin*, *vincristine*, and *prednisone* (CHOP) or other anthracycline-based chemotherapy regimen. In CLL patients older than 70 years of age, exploratory analyses suggest no benefit with the addition of **Rituxan** to FC. The most adverse common reactions (incidence >25%) have been infusion-related reactions, fever, lymphopenia, chills, infection and asthenia. For tumor lysis syndrome, administer aggressive IV hydration, anti-hyperuricemic agents, and monitor renal function. Monitor for infections; withhold **Rituxan** and institute appropriate anti-infective therapy. For cardiac adverse reactions, discontinue **Rituxan** infusions in case of serious or life-threatening events. Discontinue **Rituxan** in patients with rising serum creatinine or oliguria. Bowel obstruction and perforation can occur; consider and evaluate for abdominal pain, vomiting, or related symptoms. Live virus vaccinations prior to or during **Rituxan** treatment is not recommended. **Rituxan** is embryo/fetal toxic. Advise males and females of reproductive potential of the potential embryo/fetal risk and to use effective contraception. Advise women not to breastfeed during treatment and for at least 6 months after the last dose.

CD20-DIRECTED CYTOLYTIC ANTIBODY+ENDOGLYCOSIDASE

▷ *rituximab*+*hyaluronidase human* Administer 1,400 mg/23,400 Units (*rituximab* 1,400 mg and *hyaluronidase human* 23,400 Units) SC according to recommended schedule; *Pre-medicate:* with *acetaminophen* and antihistamine before each dose; consider pre-medication with glucocorticoids; patients must receive at least one full dose of a *rituximab* product via IV infusion before receiving **Rituxan Hycela** via SC injection; **Rituxan Hyclea** should only be administered by a qualified healthcare professional with appropriate medical support to manage severe infusion-related reactions that can be fatal if they occur

Administer via SC injection only:

- Relapsed or Refractory, Follicular Lymphoma: administer once weekly x 3 or 7 weeks following a full dose of a *rituximab* product by intravenous infusion at week 1 (i.e., 4 or 8 weeks in total)
- Re-treatment for Relapsed or Refractory, Follicular Lymphoma: administer once weekly x 3 weeks following a full dose of a **rituximab** product by intravenous infusion at week 1 (i.e., 4 weeks in total)

- Previously Un-treated, Follicular Lymphoma: administer on Day 1 of Cycles 2–8 of chemotherapy (every 21 days), for up to 7 cycles following a full dose of a *rituximab* product by IV infusion on Day 1 of Cycle 1 of chemotherapy (i.e., up to 8 cycles in total); for patients with complete or partial response: initiate maintenance treatment 8 weeks following completion of **Rituxan Hycela** in combination with chemotherapy; administer **Rituxan Hycela** as a single-agent every 8 weeks x 12 doses
- Non-progressing, Follicular Lymphoma after first line CVP chemotherapy: following completion of 6–8 cycles of CVP chemotherapy and a full dose of a *rituximab* product by IV infusion at week 1, administer once weekly x 3 weeks (i.e., 4 weeks in total) at 6-month intervals to max 16 doses
- Diffuse large B Cell Lymphoma: administer **Rituxan Hycela** 1,400 mg/23,400 Units via SC injection on Day 1 of Cycles 2–8 of CHOP chemotherapy for up to 7 cycles, following a full dose of a *rituximab* product via IV infusion at Day 1, Cycle 1 of CHOP chemotherapy (i.e., up to 6–8 cycles in total)

Rituxan Hycela *Vial: rituximab* 1,400 mg +*hyaluronidase human* 23,400 Units per 11.7 ml (120 mg/2,000 Units per ml), single dose, soln for dilution and IV infusion; *rituximab* 1,600 mg +*hyaluronidase human* 26,800 Units per 13.4 ml (120 mg/2,000 Units per ml), single dose, soln for dilution and IV infusion

Comment: **Rytuxan Hycela** is a fixed 2-drug combination indicated for the treatment of (1) relapsed or refractory follicular lymphoma as a single agent, (2) previously untreated follicular lymphoma in combination with first-line chemotherapy and, in patients achieving a complete or partial response to *rituximab* in combination with chemotherapy, as single agent maintenance therapy, (3) non-progressing (including stable disease) follicular lymphoma as a single agent after first-line *cyclophosphamide, vincristine,* and *prednisone* (CVP) chemotherapy, (4) Previously untreated diffuse large B-cell lymphoma (DLBCL) in combination with *cyclophosphamide, doxorubicin, vincristine, prednisone* (CHOP) or other anthracycline-based chemotherapy regimens. The most common adverse reactions (incidence ≥20%) have been (FL) infections, neutropenia, nausea, constipation, cough, and fatigue and (DLBCL) infections, neutropenia, alopecia, nausea, and anemia. There is risk of renal toxicity when **Rytuxin Hycela** is used in combination with **cisplatin**. Local cutaneous reactions may occur more than 24 hours after administration. Interrupt **Rytuxan Hycela** injections if severe reaction develops and administer aggressive IV hydration, anti-hyperuricemic agents, and monitor renal function. Monitor for infections; withhold and institute appropriate anti-infective therapy as appropriate. With cardiac adverse reactions, discontinue in case of serious or life-threatening events. Discontinue in patients with rising serum creatinine or oliguria. Bowel obstruction and perforation may occur; consider and evaluate for abdominal pain, vomiting, or related symptoms. Live virus vaccinations prior to or during treatment not recommended. **Rituxan Hycela** is embryo/fetal toxic. Advise males and females of reproductive potential of the potential embryo/fetal risk and to use effective contraception. Advise women not to breastfeed during treatment and for at least 6 months after the last dose.

▷ *rituximab-arrx* 375 mg/m² via IV infusion; administer all doses of **Riabni** in combination with glucocorticoids; **Riabni** should only be administered by a qualified healthcare professional with appropriate medical support to manage severe infusion-related reactions that can be fatal

Pediatric: safety and efficacy not established

Riabni *Vial:* 100 mg/10 ml (10 mg/ml), 500 mg/50 ml (10 mg/ml) soln for dilution and IV infusion, single-dose

Comment: **Riabni** *(rituximab-arrx)* is a biosimilar to **Rituxan** indicated for the treatment of adult patients with: (1) relapsed or refractory, low grade or follicular, CD20-positive B-cell NHL as a single agent (2) previously untreated follicular, CD20-positive, B-cell NHL in combination with first-line chemotherapy and, in patients achieving a complete or partial response to a *rituximab* product in combination with chemotherapy, as single-agent maintenance therapy (3) non-progressing (including stable disease), low-grade, CD20-positive, B-cell NHL as a single agent after first-line *cyclophosphamide*, *vincristine*, and *prednisone* (CVP) chemotherapy (4) previously untreated diffuse large B-cell, CD20-positive NHL in combination with *cyclophosphamide*, *doxorubicin*, *vincristine*, and *prednisone* (CHOP) or other *anthracycline*-based chemotherapy regimens. The most common adverse reactions in clinical trials with NHL (incidence ≥25%) have been infusion-related reactions, fever, lymphopenia, chills, infection, and asthenia. Monitor renal function. Discontinue **Riabni** in patients with rising serum creatinine or oliguria. If tumor lysis syndrome (TLS) is suspected, administer aggressive IV hydration and anti-hyperuricemic agents. If infection occurs, withhold **Riabni** and institute appropriate anti-infective therapy. Bowel obstruction and perforation can occur; evaluate for abdominal pain, vomiting, and related symptoms. Live virus vaccine administration prior to or during treatment with **Riabni** is not recommended. **Riabni** can cause embryo/fetal harm. Advise males and females of reproductive potential of embryo/fetal risk and to use effective contraception. Advise not to breastfeed.

CANCER: MELANOMA

PROGRAMMED DEATH RECEPTOR-1 (PD-1) BLOCKING ANTIBODY

▷ *pembrolizumab* 200 mg via IV infusion every 3 weeks or 400 mg via IV infusion every 6 weeks

Keytruda 100 mg/4 ml (25 mg/ml) soln, single-dose

Comment: **Keytruda** *(pembrolizumab)* is indicated for the treatment of multiple cancers, including unresectable or metastatic melanoma, and for the adjuvant treatment of melanoma with involvement of lymph node(s) following complete resection. **Keytruda** can cause fetal harm. Advise females of the potential embryo/fetal risk and to use effective method of contraception. Advise not to breastfeed. See mfr pkg insert for full prescribing information.

CANCER: MESOTHELIOMA

KINASE INHIBITOR

▷ *capmatinib* 400 mg twice daily with or without food

Tabrecta *Tab:* 150, 200 mg

Comment: **Tabrecta** *(capmatinib)* is a kinase inhibitor indicated for the treatment of adult patients with metastatic non-small cell lung cancer (NSCLC) whose tumors have a mutation that leads to mesenchymal-epithelial transition (MET) exon 14 skipping as detected by an FDA-approved test. The most common adverse reactions (incidence ≥ 20%) have been peripheral edema, nausea, fatigue, vomiting, dyspnea, and decreased appetite. Monitor for new or worsening pulmonary symptoms indicative of interstitial lung disease ILD/pneumonitis. Permanently discontinue **Tabrecta** in patients with ILD/pneumonitis. Monitor liver function tests. In the event of hepatotoxicity, withhold, reduce dose, or permanently discontinue **Tabrecta** based on severity. **Tabrecta** may cause photosensitivity reactions. Advise patients to limit direct ultraviolet exposure. **Tabrecta** can cause embryo/fetal harm. Advise patients of reproductive potential to use effective contraception. Advise <u>not</u> to breastfeed.

CANCER: MULTIPLE MYELOMA

PROTEASOME INHIBITOR

▷ *carfilzomib* see mfr pkg insert for recommended dosing regimens
  Pediatric: safety and efficacy not established
  Kyprolis *Vial:* 10, 30, 60 mg, single-dose, pwdr for reconstitution, dilution, and IV infusion
  Comment: **Kyprolis** *(carfilzomib)* is a indicated for the treatment of patients with relapsed <u>or</u> refractory multiple myeloma (1) who have received 1 to 3 lines of therapy in combination with *dexamethasone* <u>or</u> with *lenalidomide* <u>plus</u> *dexamethasone* <u>or</u> with *daratumumab* <u>plus</u> *dexamethasone* <u>or</u> (2) as a single agent for the treatment of patients with relapsed <u>or</u> refractory multiple myeloma who have received one <u>or</u> more lines of therapy. The most common adverse reactions (incidence 20%) in patients treated with **Kyprolis** (1) in the combination therapy trials have been anemia, diarrhea, fatigue, hypertension, pyrexia, URI, thrombocytopenia, cough, dyspnea, and insomnia and (2) in monotherapy trials have been fatigue, thrombocytopenia, nausea, pyrexia, dyspnea, diarrhea, headache, cough, and peripheral edema. See the mfr pkg insert for full prescribing information.

CD38-DIRECTED CYTOLYTIC ANTIBODY + ENDOGLYCOSIDASE

▷ *daratumumab+hyaluronidase-fihj* 1800 mg *daratumumab* + 30,000 units *hyaluronidase* administered subcutaneously (SC) into the abdomen over approximately 3-5 minutes according to recommended schedule (see mfr pkg insert); *Pre-medicate:* with a corticosteroid, *acetaminophen*, and a histamine-1 receptor antagonist; *Administer post-medications:* as recommended (see mfr pkg insert); must be administered by a qualified healthcare provider in an appropriate medical management setting
  Pediatric: safety and effficacy not established
  Darzalex Faspro *Vial:* 1800 mg *daratumumab* and 30,000 units *hyaluronidase-fihj* per 15 ml (120 mg and 2,000 units/ml) soln, single-dose
  Comment: **Darzalex Faspro** *(daratumumab+hyaluronidase-fihj)* is a combination of *daratumumab*, a CD38-directed cytolytic antibody, and *hyaluronidase-fihj*, an endoglycosidase, indicated for the treatment of adult patients with multiple myeloma:
  In combination with *bortezomib*, *melphalan*, and *prednisone* in newly diagnosed patients who are ineligible for autologous stem cell transplant;
  In combination with *lenalidomide* and *dexamethasone* in newly diagnosed patients who are ineligible for autologous stem cell transplant and in patients with relapsed <u>or</u> refractory multiple myeloma who have received at least one prior therapy;
  In combination with *bortezomib* and *dexamethasone* in patients who have received at least one prior therapy;
  As monotherapy, in patients who have received at least 3 prior lines of therapy, including a proteasome inhibitor (PI) and an immunomodulatory agent, <u>or</u> who are double-refractory to a PI and an immunomodulatory agent.
  The most common adverse reaction (incidence ≥20%) with **Darzalex Faspro** monotherapy has been URI. The most common adverse reactions (incidence ≥20%) with D-VMP have been URI, constipation, nausea, fatigue, pyrexia, peripheral sensory neuropathy, diarrhea, cough, insomnia, vomiting, and

back pain. The most common adverse reactions (incidence ≥20%) with
D-Rd have been fatigue, diarrhea, URI, muscle spasms, constipation, pyrexia,
pneumonia, and dyspnea. The most common hematology laboratory
abnormalities (incidence ≥40%) with **Darzalex Faspro** have been decreased
leukocytes, decreased lymphocytes, decreased neutrophils, decreased platelets,
and decreased hemoglobin. Permanently discontinue **Darzalex Faspro** for
life-threatening hypersensitivity or other administration reaction. Monitor
complete blood cell counts periodically during treatment. Monitor patients
with neutropenia for signs of infection. Consider withholding **Darzalex
Faspro** to allow recovery of neutrophils. Monitor for thrombocytopenia
periodically during treatment. Consider withholding **Darzalex Faspro** to
allow recovery of platelets. **Darzalex Faspro** may cause interference with
cross-matching and red blood cell antibody screening; therefore, type and
screen patients prior to starting treatment and inform blood banks that a
patient has received **Darzalex Faspro**. There are no available data on the use
of **Darzalex Faspro** in pregnancy to evaluate drug-associated risk of major
birth defects, miscarriage or adverse maternal or embryo/fetal outcomes
and animal reproduction studies have not been conducted. However, there
is potential for fetal harm. Assessment of potential risks with *daratumumab*
products are based on the mechanism of action and data from target antigen
CD38 knockout animal models. The combination of **Darzalex Faspro** and
lenalidomide is contraindicated in pregnancy, because *lenalidomide* may
cause birth defects and stillbirth. Advise females of reproductive potential
to use effective contraception during treatment and for 3 months after the
last dose Because immunoglobulin G1 (IgG1) monoclonal antibodies are
transferred across the placenta, and based on its mechanism of action,
Darzalex Faspro may cause depletion of fetal CD38 positive immune cells
and decreased bone density. Defer administering live vaccines to neonates
and infants exposed to *daratumumab* in utero until a hematology evaluation
is completed. There are no data on the presence of *daratumumab* and
hyaluronidase in human milk or effects on the breastfed infant. However,
because of the potential for serious adverse reactions in the breastfed infant
when administered with *lenalidomide* and *dexamethasone*, advise women not
to breastfeed during treatment.

B-CELL MATURATION ANTIGEN (BCMA)-DIRECTED ANTIBODY AND MICROTUBULE INHIBITOR CONJUGATE

▷ *belantamab mafodotin-blmf* 2.5 mg/kg via IV infusion over 30 minutes once
every 3 weeks

    Blenrep *Vial:* 100 mg, single-dose, pwdr for reconstitution, dilution, and IV
infusion

    Comment: **Blenrep** is indicated for the treatment of adult patients with
relapsed or refractory multiple myeloma who have received at least four
prior therapies including an anti-CD38 monoclonal antibody, a proteasome
inhibitor, and an immunomodulatory agent. This indication is approved
under accelerated approval based on response rate. Continued approval
for this indication may be contingent upon verification and description of
clinical benefit in confirmatory trial(s). The most common adverse reactions
(incidence ≥20%) are keratopathy (corneal epithelium change on eye
exam), decreased visual acuity, nausea, blurred vision, pyrexia, infusion-
related reactions, and fatigue. The most common grade 3 or 4 laboratory
abnormalities (incidence ≥5%) are decreased platelets, lymphocytes,
hemoglobin, and neutrophils, and increased creatinine and gamma-glutamyl
transferase. Obtain a baseline CBC prior to initiating therapy with **Blenrep**
and during therapy as clinically indicated. Monitor patients for infusion-

related reactions; interrupt and then reduce the rate or permanently discontinue based on the severity. **Blenrep** can cause embryo/fetal harm; advise females of reproductive potential of the potential risk and to use effective contraception. Advise not to breastfeed

ANTI-CANCER PEPTIDE-DRUG CONJUGATE

▷ *melphalan flufenamide Recommended dose:* 40 mg via IV infusion over 30 minutes on Day 1 of each 28-day treatment cycle, in combination with *dexamethasone*
Pediatric: safety and efficacy not established

Pepaxto *Vial:* 20 mg, single-dose, pwdr for reconstitution, dilution, and IV infusion

Comment: **Pepaxto** is an alkylating drug indicated, in combination with *dexamethasone*, for the treatment of adult patients with relapsed or refractory multiple myeloma who have received at least four prior lines of therapy and whose disease is refractory to at least one proteasome inhibitor, one immunomodulatory agent, and one CD38-directed monoclonal antibody. The most common adverse reactions (incidence >20%) have been fatigue, nausea, diarrhea, pyrexia and respiratory tract infection. The most common laboratory abnormalities (incidence ≥50%) have been decreased leukocytes, decreased platelets, decreased lymphocytes, decreased neutrophils, decreased hemoglobin, and decreased creatinine increase. Monitor these labs at baseline, during treatment, and as clinically indicated. **Pepaxto** is a genotoxic drug with risk of embryo/fetal harm. Advise females and males of reproductive potential for drug-associated embryo/fetal toxicity. Advise the use of effective contraception for 6 months after the last dose (females) and 3 months after the last dose (males). Breastfeeding is not recommended during treatment and for 1 week after the last dose.

CANCER: OVARIAN

POLY ADP-RIBOSE POLYMERASE (PARP) INHIBITOR

▷ *niraparib tosolate* 300 mg (3 x 100 mg) once daily, with or without food; continue treatment until disease progression or unacceptable adverse reaction; for adverse reactions, consider interruption of treatment, dose reduction, or dose discontinuation
Pediatric: safety and efficacy not established

Zejula *Cap:* 100 mg

Comment: **Zejula** *(niraparib)* is indicated for the maintenance treatment of adult patients with recurrent epithelial ovarian, fallopian tube, or primary peritoneal cancer who are in a complete or partial response to platinum-based chemotherapy, and for late-line treatment recurrent ovarian cancer. The most common adverse reactions (incidence ≥10%) have been anemia, thrombocytopenia, neutropenia, leukopenia, hypertension, palpitations, nausea, vomiting, abdominal pain/distention, diarrhea, constipation, mucositis/stomatitis, dry mouth, fatigue/asthenia, dyspepsia, decreased appetite, urinary tract infection, AST/ALT elevation, back pain, myalgia, arthralgia, headache, dizziness, dysgeusia, insomnia, anxiety, nasopharyngitis, dyspnea, cough, and rash. Monitor CBC weekly for the first month, monitor CBC monthly for the next 11 months, and then periodically thereafter. Monitor BP and HR monthly for the first year and periodically thereafter. Manage BP and HR with appropriate medication as indicated and adjust the **Zejula** dose if necessary. Because Myelodysplastic Syndrome/Acute Myeloid Leukemia (MDS/AML) has occurred in patients exposed to **Zejula,** with some cases being fatal, monitor patients for hematological toxicity and discontinue

Zejula if MDS/AML is confirmed. **Zejula** can cause embryo/fetal toxicity; therefore, advise females of reproductive potential of the potential risk and to use effective contraception. Advise women not to breastfeed during treatment with **Zejula** and for 1 month after receiving the final dose.

POLY (ADP-RIBOSE) POLYMERSE (PARP) INHIBITOR

▷ *rucaparib* 600 mg twice daily with or without food
   Pediatric: not established
     Rubraca *Tab*: 200, 250, 300 mg
     Comment: **Rubraca** *(rucaparib)* is indicated for maintenance treatment of adult patients with recurrent epithelial ovarian, fallopian tube, and primary peritoneal cancer who are in a complete or partial response to platinum-based chemotherapy and Treatment of adult patients with a deleterious BRCA mutation (germline and/or somatic)-associated epithelial ovarian, fallopian tube, or primary peritoneal cancer who have been treated with 2 or more chemotherapies. Select patients for therapy based on an FDA-approved companion diagnostic for **Rubraca**. Continue treatment until disease progression or unacceptable toxicity. For adverse reactions, consider interruption of treatment or dose reduction. The most common adverse reactions (incidence ≥20%) have been nausea, fatigue (including asthenia), vomiting, anemia, dysgeusia, AST/ALT elevation, constipation, decreased appetite, diarrhea, thrombocytopenia, neutropenia, stomatitis, nasopharyngitis/URI, rash, abdominal pain/distention, and dyspnea. The most common adverse reactions (incidence ≥20%) among patients with BRCA-mutated mCRPC have been fatigue (including asthenia), nausea, anemia, increased ALT/AST, decreased appetite, rash, constipation, thrombocytopenia, vomiting, and diarrhea. Myelodysplastic syndrome (MDS) and acute myeloid leukemia (AML) have occurred in patients exposed to **Rubraca**, and some cases have been fatal. Monitor patients for hematological toxicity at baseline and monthly thereafter. Discontinue **Rubraca** if MDS/AML is confirmed. Adjust the dosage of CYP1A2, CYP3A, CYP2C9, and CYP2C19 substrates if clinically indicated. **Rubraca** can cause embryo/fetal harm. Advise females of the potential embryo/fetal risk and to use effective contraception. Advise females not to breastfeed.

CANCER: PANCREATIC

POLY (ADP-RIBOSE) POLYMERASE (PARP) INHIBITOR

▷ *olaparib* 300 mg twice daily; with or without food; see the mfr pkg insert for recommended duration of treatment; *CrCl:31-50 mL/min:* 200 mg twice daily
   Pediatric: not studied
     Lynparza *Tab*: 100, 150 mg
     Comment: **Lynparza** is indicated for the maintenance treatment of adult patients with deleterious or suspected deleterious gBRCAm metastatic pancreatic adenocarcinoma whose disease has not progressed on at least 16 weeks of a first-line platinum-based chemotherapy regimen. Select patients for therapy based on an FDA-approved companion diagnostic for **Lynparza**. The most common adverse reactions (incidence ≥10%) in clinical trials have been nausea, fatigue (including asthenia), vomiting, abdominal pain, anemia, diarrhea, dizziness, neutropenia, leukopenia, nasopharyngitis/upper respiratory tract infection/influenza, respiratory tract infection, arthralgia/myalgia, dysgeusia, headache, dyspepsia, decreased appetite, constipation, stomatitis, dyspnea, and thrombocytopenia. Avoid concomitant use of strong or moderate CYP3A inhibitors. If the inhibitor cannot be avoided, reduce the **Lynparza** dose. Avoid concomitant use of strong or moderate CYP3A

inducers as decreased **Lynparza** efficacy can occur. The most common adverse reactions (incidence ≥20%) in clinical trials have been anemia, nausea, fatigue (including asthenia), vomiting, nasopharyngitis/ upper respiratory tract infection/influenza, diarrhea, arthralgia/myalgia, dysgeusia, headache, dyspepsia, decreased appetite, constipation, and stomatitis. The most common laboratory abnormalities (incidence ≥25%) have been decrease in Hgb, increase MCV, decrease in lymphocytes, decrease in leukocytes, decrease in absolute neutrophil count, increase in serum Cr, and decrease in platelets. **Lynparza** can cause embryo/fetal harm. Exclude pregnancy prior to initiation and advise females of reproductive potential to use effective contraception during and for 6 months after the last dose. Males with female partners should use effective contraception and <u>not</u> donate sperm during and for 3 months after last dose. Advise women <u>not</u> to breastfeed during and for 1 month after the last dose.

● CANCER: PERITONEAL

POLY ADP-RIBOSE POLYMERASE (PARP) INHIBITOR

▷ *niraparib tosolate* 300 mg (3 x 100 mg) once daily, with <u>or</u> without food; continue treatment until disease progression <u>or</u> unacceptable adverse reaction; for adverse reactions, consider interruption of treatment, dose reduction, <u>or</u> dose discontinuation
Pediatric: safety and efficacy not established
Zejula *Cap:* 100 mg
Comment: **Zejula** *(niraparib)* is indicated for the maintenance treatment of adult patients with recurrent epithelial ovarian, fallopian tube, <u>or</u> primary peritoneal cancer who are in a complete or partial response to platinum-based chemotherapy, and for late-line treatment recurrent ovarian cancer. The most common adverse reactions (incidence ≥10%) have been anemia, thrombocytopenia, neutropenia, leukopenia, hypertension, palpitations, nausea, vomiting, abdominal pain/distention, diarrhea, constipation, mucositis/stomatitis, dry mouth, fatigue/asthenia, dyspepsia, decreased appetite, urinary tract infection, AST/ALT elevation, back pain, myalgia, arthralgia, headache, dizziness, dysgeusia, insomnia, anxiety, nasopharyngitis, dyspnea, cough, and rash. Monitor CBC weekly for the first month, monitor CBC monthly for the next 11 months, and then periodically thereafter. Monitor BP and HR monthly for the first year and periodically thereafter. Manage BP and HR with appropriate medication as indicated and adjust the **Zejula** dose if necessary. Because Myelodysplastic Syndrome/Acute Myeloid Leukemia (MDS/AML) has occurred in patients exposed to **Zejula,** with some cases being fatal, monitor patients for hematological toxicity and discontinue **Zejula** if MDS/AML is confirmed. **Zejula** can cause embryo/fetal toxicity; therefore, advise females of reproductive potential of the potential risk and to use effective contraception. Advise women <u>not</u> to breastfeed during treatment with **Zejula** and for 1 month after receiving the final dose.

▷ *olaparib* 300 mg twice daily; with <u>or</u> without food; see the mfr pkg insert for recommended duration of treatment; *CrCl: 31-50 mL/min:* 200 mg twice daily
Pediatric: not established
Lynparza *Tab:* 100, 150 mg
Comment: **Lynparza** is a first-class poly (ADP-ribose) polymerase (PARP) inhibitor indicated for: (1) maintenance treatment of adult patients with deleterious <u>or</u> suspected deleterious germline <u>or</u> somatic BRCA-mutated advanced epithelial ovarian, fallopian tube <u>or</u> primary peritoneal cancer who are in complete <u>or</u> partial response to first-line platinum-based chemotherapy; select patients for therapy based on an FDA-approved companion diagnostic

for **Lynparza;** (2) maintenance treatment of adult patients with recurrent epithelial ovarian, fallopian tube, or primary peritoneal cancer who are in complete or partial response to platinum-based chemotherapy; (3) treatment of adult patients with deleterious or suspected deleterious germline BRCA-mutated (gBRCAm) advanced ovarian cancer who have been treated with three or more prior lines of chemotherapy. Select patients for therapy based on an FDA-approved companion diagnostic for **Lynparza;** (4) first-line maintenance treatment with ***bevacizumab*** for HRD-positive advanced ovarian cancer (5) treatment of adult patients with deleterious or suspected deleterious germline or somatic homologous recombination repair (HRR) gene-mutated metastatic castration-resistant prostate cancer (mCRPC) who have progressed following prior treatment with ***enzalutamide*** or ***abiraterone;*** select patients for therapy based on an FDA-approved companion diagnostic for **Lynparza**. The most common adverse reactions (incidence ≥10%) in clinical trials have been nausea, fatigue (including asthenia), vomiting, abdominal pain, anemia, diarrhea, dizziness, neutropenia, leukopenia, nasopharyngitis/upper respiratory tract infection/influenza, respiratory tract infection, arthralgia/myalgia, dysgeusia, headache, dyspepsia, decreased appetite, constipation, stomatitis, dyspnea, and thrombocytopenia. Avoid concomitant use of strong or moderate CYP3A inhibitors. If the inhibitor cannot be avoided, reduce the **Lynparza** dose. Avoid concomitant use of strong or moderate CYP3A inducers as decreased **Lynparza** efficacy can occur. The most common adverse reactions (incidence ≥20%) in clinical trials have been anemia, nausea, fatigue (including asthenia), vomiting, nasopharyngitis/ upper respiratory tract infection/influenza, diarrhea, arthralgia/myalgia, dysgeusia, headache, dyspepsia, decreased appetite, constipation, and stomatitis. The most common laboratory abnormalities (incidence ≥25%) have been decrease in Hgb, increase MCV, decrease in lymphocytes, decrease in leukocytes, decrease in absolute neutrophil count, increase in serum Cr, and decrease in platelets. **Lynparza** can cause embryo/fetal harm. Exclude pregnancy prior to initiation and advise females of reproductive potential to use effective contraception during and for 6 months after the last dose. Males with female partners should use effective contraception and not donate sperm during and for 3 months after last dose. Advise women not to breastfeed during and for 1 month after the last dose.

POLY (ADP-RIBOSE) POLYMERASE (PARP) INHIBITOR

▶ *rucaparib* 600 mg twice daily with or without food
    Pediatric: not established
    Rubraca *Tab:* 200, 250, 300 mg
    Comment: **Rubraca** *(rucaparib)* is indicated for maintenance treatment of adult patients with recurrent epithelial ovarian, fallopian tube, and primary peritoneal cancer who are in a complete or partial response to platinum-based chemotherapy and treatment of adult patients with a deleterious BRCA mutation (germline and/or somatic)-associated epithelial ovarian, fallopian tube, or primary peritoneal cancer who have been treated with two or more chemotherapies. Select patients for therapy based on an FDA-approved companion diagnostic for **Rubraca**. Continue treatment until disease progression or unacceptable toxicity. For adverse reactions, consider interruption of treatment or dose reduction. The most common adverse reactions (incidence ≥20%) have been nausea, fatigue (including asthenia), vomiting, anemia, dysgeusia, AST/ALT elevation, constipation, decreased appetite, diarrhea, thrombocytopenia, neutropenia, stomatitis, nasopharyngitis/URI, rash, abdominal pain/distention, and dyspnea. The most common adverse reactions (incidence ≥20%) among patients with

BRCA-mutated mCRPC have been fatigue (including asthenia), nausea, anemia, increased ALT/AST, decreased appetite, rash, constipation, thrombocytopenia, vomiting, and diarrhea. Myelodysplastic syndrome (MDS) and acute myeloid leukemia (AML) have occurred in patients exposed to **Rubraca**, and some cases have been fatal. Monitor patients for hematological toxicity at baseline and monthly thereafter. Discontinue **Rubraca** if MDS/AML is confirmed. Adjust the dosage of CYP1A2, CYP3A, CYP2C9, and CYP2C19 substrates if clinically indicated. **Rubraca** can cause embryo/fetal harm. Advise females of the potential embryo/fetal risk and to use effective contraception. Advise females not to breastfeed.

CANCER: PROSTATE

GONADOTROPIN-RELEASING HORMONE (GnRH) RECEPTOR ANTAGONIST

▷ *relugolix* Loading Dose: 360 mg on Day 1; then, 120 mg once daily ongoing; take at approximately the same time each day; If treatment with is interrupted for >7 days, resume administration with a 360 mg loading dose on the first day, followed by 120 mg once daily; take with or without food; swallow whole, do not crush or chew

Orgovyx Tab: 120 mg

Comment: **Orgovyx** *(relugolix)* is an oral gonadotropin-releasing hormone (GnRH) receptor antagonist indicated for the treatment of adult patients with advanced prostate cancer. The most common adverse reactions (incidence ≥10%) and laboratory abnormalities (incidence ≥15%) have been hot flush, glucose increased, triglycerides increased, musculoskeletal pain, hemoglobin decreased, alanine aminotransferase (ALT) increased, fatigue, aspartate aminotransferase (AST) increased, constipation, and diarrhea. Androgen deprivation therapy may prolong the QT interval. Avoid co-administration of **Orgovyx** with P-gp Inhibitors. If unavoidable, take **Orgovyx** first, separate dosing by at least 6 hours, and monitor patients more frequently for adverse reactions. Avoid co-administration of P-gp and Strong CYP3A Inducers. If unavoidable, increase the **Orgovyx** dose to 240 mg once daily. **Orgovyx** can cause fetal harm. Based on findings in animals and mechanism of action, **Orgovyx** can cause embryo/fetal harm and loss of pregnancy when administered to a pregnant female. There are no human data on the use of **Orgovyx** in pregnant females to inform the drug-associated risk. Advise males with female partners of reproductive potential to use effective contraception.

CYP17 INHIBITOR

▷ *abiraterone acetate*

Comment: Patients receiving treatment with *abiraterone acetate* should also receive a gonadotropin-releasing hormone (GnRH) analog concurrently or should have had a bilateral orchiectomy. Avoid concomitant strong CYP3A4 inducers; if a strong CYP3A4 must be co-administered, increase the *abiraterone acetate* dosing frequency. Avoid co-administration of *abiraterone acetate* with CYP2D6 substrates that have a narrow therapeutic index; if an alternative treatment cannot be used, exercise caution and consider a dose reduction of the CYP2D6 substrate. Hepatotoxicity can be severe and fatal. Do not initiate *abiraterone acetate* in patients with baseline severe hepatic impairment Child-Pugh Class C). *abiraterone acetate* should be discontinued if patients develop severe hepatotoxicity. Monitor liver function and modify, interrupt, or discontinue *Abiraterone acetate* dosing as recommended. Advise males with female partners of reproductive potential to use effective contraception during treatment and for 3 weeks after the last dose. Based on animal studies, *abiraterone acetate* may impair reproductive function and fertility in males of reproductive potential.

Yonsa 500 mg (4 x 125 mg tabs) administered once daily (in combination with *methylprednisolone* 4 mg administered orally twice daily); take with or without food; swallow whole with water; do not crush or chew

Tab: 125 mg

Comment: **Yonsa** is an ultramicrosize formulation of the oral CYP17 inhibitor *abiraterone acetate* (FDA-approved as **Zytiga**) used in combination with *methylprednisolone* for the treatment of metastatic castration-resistant prostate cancer (CRPC). The most common adverse side effects (incidence ≥10%) are fatigue, joint swelling or discomfort, edema, hot flush, diarrhea, vomiting, cough, hypertension, dyspnea, UTI, and confusion. The most common laboratory abnormalities (incidence >20%) are anemia, elevated alkaline phosphatase, hypertriglyceridemia, lymphopenia, hypercholesterolemia, hyperglycemia, elevated AST and ALT, hyperkalemia, and hypophosphatemia. Monitor for signs and symptoms of mineralocorticoid excess and adrenocortical insufficiency and treat as appropriate.

Zytiga *CRPC:* 1000 mg (4 x 250 mg or 2 x 500 mg tabs) administered once daily (in combination with *prednisone* 5 mg administered orally twice daily); *CSPC:* 1000 mg (4 x 250 mg or 2 x 500 mg tabs) administered once daily (in combination with *prednisone* 5 mg administered orally once daily); take on an empty stomach, at least 1 hour before or 2 hours after a meal; swallow whole with water; do not crush or chew

Tab: 250, 500 mg

Comment: **Zytiga** (*abiraterone acetate*) is an oral CYP17 inhibitor used in combination with *prednisone* for the treatment of metastatic castration-resistant prostate cancer (CRPC) and metastatic high-risk castration-sensitive prostate cancer (CSPC). The most common adverse reactions (incidence ≥10%) are fatigue, arthralgia, hypertension, nausea, edema, hypokalemia, hot flush, diarrhea, vomiting, upper respiratory infection, cough, and headache. The most common laboratory abnormalities (incidence ≥20%) are anemia, elevated alkaline phosphatase, hypertriglyceridemia, lymphopenia, hypercholesterolemia, hyperglycemia, and hypokalemia. Monitor for signs and symptoms of mineralocorticoid excess and adrenocortical insufficiency and treat as appropriate.

ANDROGEN RECEPTOR INHIBITOR (ARi)

▷ *apalutamide* administer 240 mg (4 x 60 mg tablets) once daily; swallow tablets whole, do not crush or chew; take with or without food.

Erleada *Tab:* 60 mg

Comment: **Erleada** (*apalutamide*) is the first FDA-approved treatment for non-metastatic, castration-resistant prostate cancer. Patients should also receive a gonadotropin-releasing hormone (GnRH) analog concurrently or should have had bilateral orchiectomy. Concomitant use of **Erleada** with medications that are sensitive substrates of CYP3A4, CYP2C19, CYP2C9, UGT, P-gp, BCRP, or OATP1B1 may result in loss of activity of these medications. The most common adverse reactions (incidence ≥10%) have been fatigue, hypertension, rash, diarrhea, nausea, weight decreased, arthralgia, fall, hot flush, decreased appetite, fracture, and peripheral edema. Falls (16%) and fractures (12%) have occurred in patients receiving **Erleada**. Evaluate patients for fall and fracture risk, and treat patients with bone-targeted agents according to established guidelines. Seizure has occurred in 0.2% of patients receiving **Erleada**. Permanently discontinue **Erleada** in patients who develop a seizure during treatment. Advise males with female partners of reproductive potential to use effective contraception.

▷ **darolutamide** 600 mg (2 x 300 mg tablets) twice daily; *Moderate Hepatic Impairment:* 300 mg twice daily; *Severe Renal Impairment (not on hemodialysis):* 300 mg twice daily; swallow whole, do <u>not</u> crush <u>or</u> chew; take with food

    Nubeqa *Tab:* 300 mg

    Comment: **Nubeqa** *(darolutamide)* is an androgen receptor inhibitor (ARi) indicated for the treatment of non-metastatic castration-resistant prostate cancer (nmCRPC). Patients taking **Nubeqa** should also receive a gonadotropin-releasing hormone (GnRH) analog concurrently <u>or</u> should have had bilateral orchiectomy. When **Nubeqa** is taken in combination with P-gp and Strong CYP3A Inhibitors, monitor patients more frequently for **Nubeqa** adverse reactions. Avoid concomitant use of P-gp and strong <u>or</u> moderate CYP3A inducers. Avoid concomitant use with drugs that are BCRP substrates where possible; if used together, monitor patients more frequently for adverse reactions and consider dose reduction of the BCRP substrate drug. The most common adverse reactions (incidence ≥2%) have been fatigue, pain in extremity, and rash. **Nubeqa** can cause embryo/fetal harm and loss of pregnancy. Advise males with female partners of reproductive potential to use effective contraception.

POLY ADP-RIBOSE POLYMERASE (PARP) INHIBITORS

▷ **niraparib tosolate** 300 mg (3 x 100 mg) once daily, with <u>or</u> without food

    Pediatric: safety and efficacy not established

    Zejula *Cap:* 100 mg

    Comment: **Zejula** *(niraparib)* is indicated for the maintenance treatment of adult patients with recurrent epithelial ovarian, fallopian tube, <u>or</u> primary peritoneal cancer who are in a complete or partial response to platinum-based chemotherapy, and for late-line treatment recurrent ovarian cancer. Continue treatment until disease progression <u>or</u> unacceptable adverse reaction; for adverse reactions, consider interruption of treatment, dose reduction, <u>or</u> dose discontinuation. The most common adverse reactions (incidence ≥10%) have been anemia, thrombocytopenia, neutropenia, leukopenia, hypertension, palpitations, nausea, vomiting, abdominal pain/distention, diarrhea, constipation, mucositis/stomatitis, dry mouth, fatigue/asthenia, dyspepsia, decreased appetite, urinary tract infection, AST/ALT elevation, back pain, myalgia, arthralgia, headache, dizziness, dysgeusia, insomnia, anxiety, nasopharyngitis, dyspnea, cough, and rash. Monitor CBC weekly for the first month, monitor CBC monthly for the next 11 months, and then periodically thereafter. Monitor BP and HR monthly for the first year and periodically thereafter. Manage BP and HR with appropriate medication as indicated and adjust the **Zejula** dose if necessary. Because myelodysplastic syndrome (MDS) and acute myeloid leukemia (AML) have occurred in patients exposed to **Zejula,** with some cases being fatal, monitor patients for hematological toxicity and discontinue **Zejula** if MDS/AML is confirmed. **Zejula** can cause embryo/fetal toxicity; therefore, advise females of reproductive potential of the potential risk and to use effective contraception. Advise women <u>not</u> to breastfeed during treatment with **Zejula** and for 1 month after receiving the final dose.

▷ **rucaparib** 600 mg twice daily with <u>or</u> without food

    Pediatric: safety and efficacy not established

    Rubraca *Tab:* 200, 250, 300 mg

    Comment: **Rubraca** *(rucaparib)* is indicated for the treatment of adult patients with a deleterious BRCA mutation (germline and/or somatic)-associated metastatic castration-resistant prostate cancer (mCRPC) who have been treated with androgen receptor-directed therapy and a taxane-based chemotherapy. This indication is approved under accelerated approval based on objective response rate and duration of response. Continued approval for this indication may be contingent upon verification and description of clinical benefit in confirmatory trials. Patients receiving **Rubraca** for mCRPC should also receive a gonadotropin-releasing hormone (GnRH) analog concurrently or should have had bilateral orchiectomy. Continue treatment until disease progression or unacceptable toxicity. For adverse reactions, consider interruption of treatment or dose reduction. The most common adverse reactions (incidence ≥20%) among patients with BRCA mutated mCRPC have been fatigue (including asthenia), nausea, anemia, increased ALT/AST, decreased appetite, rash, constipation, thrombocytopenia, vomiting, and diarrhea. Myelodysplastic syndrome (MDS) and acute myeloid leukemia (AML) have occurred in patients exposed to **Rubraca**, and some cases have been fatal. Monitor patients for hematological toxicity at baseline and monthly thereafter. Discontinue **Rubraca** if MDS/AML is confirmed. Adjust the dosage of CYP1A2, CYP3A, CYP2C9, and CYP2C19 substrates if clinically indicated.

 CANCER: RENAL CELL CARCINOMA (RCC)

KINASE INHIBITOR

▷ *sorafenib* (G) 400 mg (2 x 200 mg) twice daily, without food
   Nexavar *Tab:* 200 mg
   Comment: **Nexavar** is indicated for the treatment of advanced renal cell carcinoma. The most common adverse reactions (incidence ≥20%) have been diarrhea, fatigue, infection, alopecia, hand-foot skin reaction, rash, weight loss, decreased appetite, nausea, gastrointestinal, and abdominal pains, hypertension, and hemorrhage. **Nexavar** in combination with *carboplatin* and *paclitaxel* is contraindicated in patients with squamous cell lung cancer. Avoid strong CYP3A4 inducers. Monitor ECG (for QT prolongation) and electrolytes in patients at increased risk for ventricular arrhythmias. Consider temporary or permanent discontinuation of **Nexavar** in the event of a cardiovascular event. Discontinue **Nexavar** if needed in the event of bleeding. Monitor the patient for hypertension, weekly during the first 6 weeks and periodically thereafter. Interrupt and/or decrease **Nexavar** for severe or persistent dermal reaction, and immediately discontinue **Nexavar** if Stevens-Johnson syndrome or toxic epidermal necrolysis is suspected. Discontinue **Nexavar** in the event of gastrointestinal perforation. **Nexavar** may cause hepatotoxicity; monitor liver function tests regularly and discontinue for unexplained transaminase elevation. Monitor TSH monthly and adjust thyroid replacement therapy in patients with thyroid cancer. **Nexavar** may cause embryo/fetal harm; verify pregnancy status prior to initiating **Nexavar** and advise females and males of reproductive potential to use effective contraception. Advise women not to breastfeed.

VASCULAR ENDOTHELIAL GROWTH FACTOR (VEGF) INHIBITOR

▷ *bevacizumab-bvzr* 10 mg/kg via IV infusion every 2 weeks with *interferon alfa*; do not administer **Zirabev** for 28 days following major surgery and until the surgical wound is fully healed
   Zirabev *Vial:* 100 mg/4 ml (25 mg/ml), 400 mg/16 ml (25 mg/ml), single-dose
   Comment: **Zirabev** is biosimilar to **Avastin** *(bevacizumab)* with indications for the treatment of multiple types of cancer, including metastatic colorectal cancer, non-small cell lung cancer, glioblastoma, metastatic renal cell carcinoma, and cervical cancer, using diagnosis-specific dosing regimens. **Zirabev** is used to treat recurrent glioblastoma in adults. **Zirabev** is used to treat metastatic renal cell carcinoma in combination with *interferon alfa*.

PROGRAMMED DEATH LIGAND-1 (PD-L1) BLOCKING ANTIBODY

▷ *avelumab* 800 mg via IV infusion over 60 minutes every 2 weeks; pre-medicate for the first 4 infusions and subsequently as needed

Pediatric: <12 years: not established; ≥12 years: same as adult

Bavencio *Vial:* 200 mg/10 ml (20 mg/ml), single-dose, solution for IV infusion

Comment: Bavencio *(avelumab)* is indicated for treatment of patients with metastatic MCC. The most common adverse reactions (>20%) in patients treated for MCC have been fatigue, musculoskeletal pain, diarrhea, nausea, infusion-related reaction, rash, decreased appetite, and peripheral edema. Withhold **Bavencio** for moderate immune-mediated pneumonitis; permanently discontinue for severe, life-threatening, or recurrent moderate pneumonitis. Monitor LFTs for hepatotoxicity and immune-mediated hepatitis. Withhold **Bavencio** for moderate hepatitis; permanently discontinue for severe or life-threatening hepatitis. Withhold **Bavencio** for moderate or severe immune-mediated colitis and permanently discontinue for life-threatening or recurrent severe colitis. Immune-mediated endocrinopathies: Withhold **Bavencio** for severe or life-threatening endocrinopathies. Monitor renal function. Withhold **Bavencio** for moderate or severe nephritis and renal dysfunction and permanently discontinue for life-threatening nephritis or renal dysfunction. For infusion-related reactions, interrupt **Bavencio** or slow the rate of infusion for mild or moderate infusion-related reactions. Stop the infusion, and permanently discontinue **Bavencio**, for severe or life-threatening infusion-related reactions. Optimize management of cardiovascular risk factors. **Bavencio** can cause embryo/fetal harm. Advise females of reproductive potential of embryo/fetal risk potential and to use of effective contraception. There is no information regarding the presence of *avelumab* in human milk or effects on the breastfed infant. Advise not to breastfeed.

▷ *pembrolizumab* 200 mg via IV infusion every 3 weeks or 400 mg via IV infusion every 6 weeks

Keytruda 100 mg/4 ml (25 mg/ml) soln, single-dose

Comment: Keytruda *(pembrolizumab)* is indicated for the treatment of multiple cancers, including treatment of advanced renal cell carcinoma (RCC) in combination with *axitinib* as first-line treatment. **Keytruda** can cause fetal harm. Advise females of the potential embryo/fetal risk and to use effective method of contraception. Advise not to breastfeed. See mfr pkg insert for full prescribing information.

▷ *selpercatinib* < *50 kg:* 120 mg twice daily; >50 kg: 160 mg twice daily; reduce dose in patients with severe hepatic impairment

Pediatric: <12 years: not established; ≥12 years: same as adult

Retevmo *hgc:* 40, 80 mg

Comment: Retevmo *(selpercatinib)* is a kinase inhibitor indicated for adult patients with metastatic RET fusion-positive non-small cell lung cancer, adult and pediatric patients ≥12 years-of-age with advanced or metastatic RET-mutant medullary thyroid cancer (MTC) who require systemic therapy; adult and pediatric patients ≥12 years-of-age with advanced or metastatic RET fusion-positive thyroid cancer who require systemic therapy and who are radioactive iodine-refractory (if radioactive iodine is appropriate). The most common adverse reactions, including laboratory abnormalities, (incidence ≥ 25%) have been increased aspartate aminotransferase (AST), increased alanine aminotransferase (ALT), increased glucose, decreased leukocytes, decreased albumin, decreased calcium, dry mouth, diarrhea, increased creatinine, increased alkaline phosphatase, hypertension, fatigue, edema, decreased platelets, increased total cholesterol, rash, decreased sodium, and constipation. Monitor ALT and AST prior to initiating **Retevmo**, every 2 weeks during the first 3 months, then monthly thereafter and as clinically indicated.

Do not initiate **Retevmo** in patients with uncontrolled hypertension; optimize BP prior to initiating **Retevmo** and monitor BP after 1 week, at least monthly thereafter and as clinically indicated. Monitor patients who are at significant risk of developing QTc prolongation. Assess QT interval, electrolytes, and TSH at baseline and periodically during treatment. Monitor QT interval more frequently when **Retevmo** is concomitantly administered with strong and moderate CYP3A inhibitors or drugs known to prolong QTc interval. Permanently discontinue **Retevmo** in patients with severe or life-threatening hemorrhage. Withhold **Retevmo** and initiate corticosteroids in the occurrence of any hypersensitivity reaction and, upon resolution, resume at a reduced dose and increase dose by 1 dose level each week until reaching the dose taken prior to onset of hypersensitivity. Continue steroids until the patient reaches target dose of **Retevmo** and then taper. Withhold **Retevmo** for at least 7 days prior to elective surgery. Do not administer for at least 2 weeks following major surgery and until adequate wound healing. The safety of resumption of **Retevmo** after resolution of wound healing complications has not been established. Avoid co-administration with PPIs; if co-administration cannot be avoided, take **Retevmo** with food (with PPI) or modify its administration time (with H2 receptor antagonist or locally-acting antacid). Avoid co-administration strong and moderate CYP3A inhibitors; if co-administration cannot be avoided, reduce the **Retevmo** dose. Avoid co-administration with strong and moderate CYP3A inducers. Avoid co-administration with CYP2C8 and CYP3A substrates; if co-administration cannot be avoided, modify the substrate dosage as recommended in its product labeling. Based on findings from animal studies, and its mechanism of action, **Retevmo** can cause fetal harm. There are no available data on **Retevmo** use in pregnant women to inform drug-associated risk. Therefore, verify pregnancy status in females of reproductive potential prior to initiating **Retevmo** and advise females of reproductive potential of the possible risk to the fetus and to use effective contraception. There are no data on the presence of *selpercatinib* or its metabolites in human milk or effects on the breastfed infant. Because of the potential for serious adverse embryo/fetal effects, advise women not to breastfeed during treatment with **Retevmo** and for 1 week after the final dose.

CANCER: SQUAMOUS CELL CARCINOMA (SCC)

PROGRAMMED DEATH RECEPTOR-1 (PD-1) BLOCKING ANTIBODY

▷ *cemiplimab-rwlc* 350 mg as an intravenous infusion over 30 minutes every 3 weeks

Pediatric: safety and efficacy not established

Libtayo *Vial:* 350 mg/7 ml (50 mg/ml), single-dose, soln for dilution and IV infusion

Comment: **Libtayo** is indicated for the treatment of patients with metastatic cutaneous squamous cell carcinoma (mCSCC) or locally advanced CSCC (laCSCC) who are not candidates for curative surgery or curative radiation.

Comment: **Libtayo** is indicated for the treatment of patients with metastatic cutaneous squamous cell carcinoma (mCSCC) or locally advanced CSCC (laCSCC) who are not candidates for curative surgery or curative radiation. The most common adverse reactions (incidence ≥15%) have been musculoskeletal pain, fatigue, rash, and diarrhea. The most common Grade 3-4 laboratory abnormalities (incidence ≥2%) have been lymphopenia, hyponatremia, hypophosphatemia, increased aspartate aminotransferase, anemia, and hyperkalemia. For infusion-related reactions, interrupt, slow the rate of infusion, or permanently discontinue based on severity of the reaction.

Immune-mediated adverse reactions, which may be severe or fatal, can occur in any organ system or tissue, including the following: immune-mediated pneumonitis, immune-mediated colitis, immune-mediated hepatitis, immune-mediated endocrinopathies, immune-mediated dermatologic adverse reactions, immune-mediated nephritis and renal dysfunction, and solid organ transplant rejection. Monitor for early identification and management. Evaluate liver enzymes, creatinine, and thyroid function at baseline and periodically during treatment. Withhold or permanently discontinue **Libtayo** based on the severity of reaction. Fatal and other serious complications can occur in patients who receive allogeneic hematopoietic stem cell transplantation (HSCT) before or after being treated with a PD-1/ PD-L1 blocking antibody. Based on its mechanism of action, **Libtayo** can cause embryo/fetal harm when administered to a pregnant female. Animal studies have demonstrated that inhibition of the PD-1/PD-L1 pathway can lead to increased risk of immune-mediated rejection of the developing fetus resulting in fetal death. Advise women of the potential risk and advise males females of reproductive potential to use effective contraception during treatment with **Libtayo** and for at least 4 months after the last dose. There is no information regarding the presence of *cemiplimab-rwlc* in human milk or its effects on the breastfed infant. Because of the potential for serious adverse reactions in breastfed infants, advise mothers not to breastfeed during treatment and for at least 4 months after the last dose.

 CANCER: THYROID CARCINOMA

KINASE INHIBITOR

▷ *selpercatinib* < *50 kg*: 120 mg twice daily; >50 kg: 160 mg twice daily; reduce dose in patients with severe hepatic impairment

Pediatric: <12 years: not established; ≥12 years: same as adult

Retevmo *hgc*: 40, 80 mg

Comment: **Retevmo** *(selpercatinib)* is a kinase inhibitor indicated for adult patients with metastatic RET fusion-positive non-small cell lung cancer, adult and pediatric patients ≥12 years-of-age with advanced or metastatic RET-mutant medullary thyroid cancer (MTC) who require systemic therapy; adult and pediatric patients ≥12 years-of-age with advanced or metastatic RET fusion-positive thyroid cancer who require systemic therapy and who are radioactive iodine-refractory (if radioactive iodine is appropriate). The most common adverse reactions, including laboratory abnormalities (incidence ≥ 25%) have been increased aspartate aminotransferase (AST), increased alanine aminotransferase (ALT), increased glucose, decreased leukocytes, decreased albumin, decreased calcium, dry mouth, diarrhea, increased creatinine, increased alkaline phosphatase, hypertension, fatigue, edema, decreased platelets, increased total cholesterol, rash, decreased sodium, and constipation. Monitor ALT and AST prior to initiating **Retevmo**, every 2 weeks during the first 3 months, then monthly thereafter and as clinically indicated. Do not initiate **Retevmo** in patients with uncontrolled hypertension; optimize BP prior to initiating **Retevmo** and monitor BP after 1 week, at least monthly thereafter and as clinically indicated. Monitor patients who are at significant risk of developing QTc prolongation. Assess QT interval, electrolytes, and TSH at baseline and periodically during treatment. Monitor QT interval more frequently when **Retevmo** is concomitantly administered with strong and moderate CYP3A inhibitors or drugs known to prolong QTc interval. Permanently discontinue **Retevmo** in patients with severe or life-threatening hemorrhage. Withhold **Retevmo** and initiate corticosteroids in the occurrence of any hypersensitivity reaction and, upon resolution, resume at a reduced dose and increase dose by 1 dose level each week until reaching the dose taken prior to onset of hypersensitivity. Continue steroids until the patient reaches target dose of **Retevmo** and then taper. Withhold **Retevmo** for at least 7 days prior to elective surgery. Do not administer for at least 2 weeks following major surgery and until adequate wound healing. The safety of resumption of **Retevmo** after resolution of wound healing complications has not been established. Avoid co-administration with PPIs; if co-administration cannot be avoided, take **Retevmo** with food (with PPI) or modify its administration time (with H2 receptor antagonist or locally-acting antacid). Avoid co-administration strong and moderate CYP3A inhibitors; if co-administration cannot be avoided, reduce the **Retevmo** dose. Avoid co-administration with strong and moderate CYP3A inducers. Avoid co-administration with CYP2C8 and CYP3A substrates; if co-administration cannot be avoided, modify the substrate dosage as recommended in its product labeling. Based on findings from animal studies, and its mechanism of action, **Retevmo** can cause fetal harm. There are no available data on **Retevmo** use in pregnant women to inform drug-associated risk. Therefore, verify pregnancy status in females of reproductive potential prior to initiating **Retevmo** and advise females of reproductive potential of the possible risk to the fetus and to use effective contraception. There are no data on the presence of *selpercatinib* or its metabolites in human milk or effects on the breastfed infant. Because of the potential for serious adverse embryo/fetal effects, advise women not to breastfeed during treatment with **Retevmo** and for 1 week after the final dose.

▷ *sorafenib* (G) 400 mg (2 x 200 mg) twice daily, without food.
    Nexavar *Tab:* 200 mg
    Comment: **Nexavar** is indicated for the treatment of locally recurrent or metastatic, progressive, differentiated thyroid carcinoma refractory to radioactive iodine treatment. The most common adverse reactions (incidence ≥20%) have been diarrhea, fatigue, infection, alopecia, hand-foot skin reaction, rash, weight loss, decreased appetite, nausea, gastrointestinal and abdominal pains, hypertension, and hemorrhage. **Nexavar** in combination with *carboplatin* and *paclitaxel* is contraindicated in patients with squamous cell lung cancer. Avoid strong CYP3A4 inducers. Monitor ECG (for QT prolongation) and electrolytes in patients at increased risk for ventricular arrhythmias. Consider temporary or permanent discontinuation of **Nexavar** in the event of a cardiovascular event. Discontinue **Nexavar** if needed in the event of bleeding. Monitor the patient for hypertension, weekly during the first 6 weeks and periodically thereafter. Interrupt and/or decrease **Nexavar** for severe or persistent dermal reaction, and immediately disconue **Nexavar** if Stevens-Johnson syndrome or toxic epidermal necrolysis is suspected. Discontinue **Nexavar** in the event of gastrointestinal perforation. **Nexavar** may cause hepatotoxicity; monitor liver function tests regularly and discontinue for unexplained transaminase elevation. Monitor TSH monthly and adjust thyroid replacement therapy in patients with thyroid cancer. **Nexavar** may cause embryo/fetal harm; verify pregnancy status prior to initiating **Nexavar** and advise females and males of reproductive potential to use effective contraception. Advise women not to breastfeed.

CANCER: UROTHELIAL CARCINOMA

KINASE INHIBITOR

▷ *erdafitinib* recommended initial dosage is 8 mg orally once daily with a dose increase to 9 mg daily if criteria are met; swallow whole with or without food; prior to initiation of treatment, confirm the presence of FGFR genetic alterations in tumor specimens and confirm negative pregnancy

Pediatric: safety and effectiveness not established

Balversa *Tab:* 3, 4, 5 mg

Comment: **Balversa** *(erdafitinib)* is a kinase inhibitor indicated for the treatment of adult patients with locally advanced or metastatic urothelial carcinoma that has susceptible FGFR3 or FGFR2 genetic alterations and progressed during or following at least one line of prior platinum-containing chemotherapy including within 12 months of neoadjuvant or adjuvant platinum-containing chemotherapy. **Balversa** can cause central serous retinopathy/retinal pigment epithelial detachment (CSR/RPED). Perform monthly ophthalmological examinations during the first 4 months of treatment, every 3 months afterwards, and at any time for visual symptoms. Withhold **Balversa** when CSR/RPED occurs and permanently discontinue if it does not resolve within 4 weeks or if Grade 4 in severity. Increases in phosphate levels are a pharmacodynamic effect of **Balversa**. Monitor for hyperphosphatemia and manage with dose modifications when required. *Drug Interaction Precautions:* Avoid concomitant use of agents that can alter serum phosphate levels before the initial dose modification period. Avoid concomitant use of strong CYP2C9 or CYP3A4 inducers and consider alternative agents or monitor closely for adverse reactions. Increase **Balversa** dose up to 9 mg with concomitant use of moderate CYP2C9 or CYP3A4 inducers. Avoid concomitant use of CYP3A4 substrates with narrow therapeutic indices. Consider alternative agents or consider reducing the dose of OCT2 substrates based on tolerability; Separate **Balversa** administration by at least 6 hours before or after administration of P-gp substrates with narrow therapeutic indices. **Balversa** can cause fetal harm; advise females of reproductive potential, and their male partners, to use effective contraception during treatment with **Balversa** and for 1 month after the last dose. There are no data on the presence of *erdafitinib* in human milk or effects on the breastfed infant; advise mothers not to breastfeed.

PROGRAMMED DEATH RECEPTOR-1 (PD-1)-BLOCKING ANTIBODY

▷ *pembrolizumab* 200 mg via IV infusion over 30 minutes every 3 weeks or 400 mg via IV infusion over 30 minutes every 6 weeks

Keytruda *Vial:* 100 mg/4 ml (25 mg/ml) single-dose, soln for dilution and IV infusion

Comment: **Keytruda** is indicated for the treatment of multiple cancers including urothelial carcinoma. **Keytruda** can cause fetal harm. Advise females of the potential embryo/fetal risk and to use effective method of contraception. Advise not to breastfeed. See mfr pkg insert for full prescribing information.

⬤ CANDIDIASIS: ABDOMEN, BLADDER, ESOPHAGUS, KIDNEY

▷ *voriconazole* (D)(G) *PO:* <40 kg: 100 mg q 12 hours; may increase to 150 mg q 12 hours if inadequate response; ≥40 kg: 200 mg q 12 hours; may increase to 300 mg q 12 hours if inadequate; *IV:* 6 mg/kg q 12 hours x 2 doses; then 4 mg/kg q 12 hour; max rate 3 mg/kg/hour over 1-2 hours; response

Pediatric: <12 years: not recommended; ≥12 years: same as adult

Vfend *Tab:* 50, 200 mg

Vfend I.V. for Injection *Vial:* 200 mg pwdr for reconstitution (preservative-free)

Vfend *Oral susp:* 40 mg/ml pwdr for reconstitution (75 ml) (orange)

CANDIDIASIS: ORAL (THRUSH)

ORAL ANTIFUNGALS

▷ *clotrimazole* (C) *Prophylaxis:* 1 troche dissolved in mouth tid; *Treatment:* 1 troche dissolved in mouth 5 x/day x 10-14 days
  Pediatric: <3 years: not recommended; ≥3 years: same as adult
  Mycelex Troches *Troche:* 10 mg

▷ *fluconazole* (C) 200 mg x 1 dose first day; then 100 mg once daily x 13 days
  Pediatric: >2 weeks: 6 mg/kg x 1 day; then 3 mg/kg/day for at least 3 weeks; *see* Appendix CC.23. *fluconazole* (Diflucan Suspension) *for dose by weight*
  Diflucan *Tab:* 50, 100, 150, 200 mg; *Oral susp:* 10, 40 mg/ml (35 ml) (orange) (sucrose)

▷ *gentian violet* (G) apply to oral mucosa with a cotton swab tid x 3 days

▷ *itraconazole* (C)(G) 200 mg daily x 7-14 days
  Pediatric: 5 mg/kg daily x 7-14 days; max 200 mg/day; *see* Appendix CC.26. *itraconazole* (Sporanox Solution) *for dose by weight*
  Sporanox *Oral soln:* 10 mg/ml (150 ml) (cherry-caramel)

▷ *miconazole* (C) One buccal tab once daily x 14 days; apply to upper gum region; hold in place 30 seconds; do not crush, chew, or swallow
  Pediatric: <16 years: not recommended; ≥16 years: same as adult
  Oravig *Buccal tab:* 50 mg (14/pck)

▷ *nystatin* (C)(G)
  Mycostatin 1-2 pastilles dissolved slowly in mouth 4-5 x/day x 10-14 days; max 14 days
  Pediatric: same as adult
    Pastille: 200,000 units (30 pastilles/pck)
  Mycostatin Suspension 4-6 ml qid swish and swallow
  Pediatric: Infants: 1 ml in each cheek qid after feedings; *Older children:* same as adult
    Oral susp: 100,000 units/ml (60 ml w. dropper)

INVASIVE INFECTION

▷ *posaconazole* (D)(G) *Oral Therapy:* take with food; 100 mg bid on day one; then 100 mg once daily x 13 days; refractory, 400 mg bid x 13 days; *IV Infusion Therapy:* must be administered through an in-line filter over approximately 90 minutes via a central venous line. Never administer **Noxafil** as an IV bolus injection; *Loading Dose:* a single 300 mg IV infusion; *Maintenance Dose: a single* 300 mg IV infusion once daily; duration of therapy is based on recovery from neutropenia or immunosuppression.
  Pediatric: <13 years: not recommended; ≥13 years: same as adult
  Noxafil *Tab:* 100 mg ext-rel; *Oral susp:* 40 mg/ml (105 ml) (cherry); *Vial:* 300 mg/16.7 ml (18 mg/ml) soln for IV infusion
  Comment: Noxafil is indicated as prophylaxis for invasive aspergillus and candida infections in patients >13-years-old who are at high risk due to being severely compromised.

 CANDIDIASIS: SKIN

TOPICAL ANTIFUNGALS

▷ *butenafine* (B)(G) apply bid x 1 week or once daily x 4 weeks
  Pediatric: <12 years: not recommended; ≥12 years: same as adult
  Lotrimin Ultra (C)(OTC) *Crm:* 1% (12, 24 gm)
  Mentax *Crm:* 1% (15, 30 gm)

Comment: *Butenafine* is a benzylamine, not an azole. Fungicidal activity continues for at least 5 weeks after the last application.

▷ *ciclopirox* (B)

Loprox Cream apply bid; max 4 weeks
Pediatric: <10 years: not recommended; ≥10 years: same as adult
Crm: 0.77% (15, 30, 90 gm)

Loprox Lotion apply bid; max 4 weeks
Pediatric: <10 years: not recommended; ≥10 years: same as adult
Lotn: 0.77% (30, 60 ml)

Loprox Gel apply bid; max 4 weeks
Pediatric: <16 years: not recommended; ≥16 years: same as adult
Gel: 0.77% (30, 45 gm)

▷ *clotrimazole* (B) apply bid x 7 days
Pediatric: <12 years: not recommended; ≥12 years: same as adult
Lotrimin *Crm:* 1% (15, 30, 45 gm)
Lotrimin AF (OTC) *Crm:* 1% (12 gm); *Lotn:* 1% (10 ml); *Soln:* 1% (10 ml)

▷ *econazole* (C) apply bid x 14 days
Pediatric: <12 years: not recommended; ≥12 years: same as adult
Spectazole *Crm:* 1% (15, 30, 85 gm)

▷ *ketoconazole* (C) apply once daily x 14 days
Pediatric: <12 years: not recommended; ≥12 years: same as adult
Nizoral Cream *Crm:* 2% (15, 30, 60 gm)

▷ *miconazole* 2% (C) apply once daily x 2 weeks
Pediatric: <12 years: not recommended; ≥12 years: same as adult
Lotrimin AF Spray Liquid (OTC) *Spray liq:* 2% (113 gm) (alcohol 17%)
Lotrimin AF Spray Powder (OTC) *Spray pwdr:* 2% (90 gm) (alcohol 10%)
Monistat-Derm *Crm:* 2% (1, 3 oz); *Spray liq:* 2% (3.5 oz); *Spray pwdr:* 2% (3 oz)

▷ *nystatin* (C) dust affected skin freely bid-tid
Nystop Powder *Pwdr:* 100,000 U/gm (15 gm)

ORAL ANTIFUNGALS

▷ *amphotericin b* (B)
Fungizone *Oral susp:* 100 mg/ml (24 ml w. dropper)

▷ *ketoconazole* (C) 400 mg once daily x 1-2 weeks
Pediatric: <2 years: not recommended; ≥2 years: 3.3-6.6 mg/kg once daily
Nizoral *Tab:* 200 mg

INVASIVE INFECTION

▷ *posaconazole* (D)(G) *Oral Therapy:* take with food; 100 mg bid on day one; then 100 mg once daily x 13 days; refractory, 400 mg bid x 13 days *IV Infusion Therapy:* must be administered through an in-line filter over approximately 90 minutes via a central venous line. Never administer **Noxafil** as an IV bolus injection; *Loading Dose: a single* 300 mg IV infusion; *Maintenance Dose: a single* 300 mg IV infusion once daily; duration of therapy is based on recovery from neutropenia or immunosuppression.
Pediatric: <13 years: not recommended; ≥13 years: same as adult
Noxafil *Tab:* 100 mg ext-rel; *Oral susp:* 40 mg/ml (105 ml) (cherry); *Vial:* 300 mg/16.7 ml (18 mg/ml) soln for IV infusion
Comment: **Noxafil** is indicated as prophylaxis for invasive aspergillus and candida infections in patients >13 years old who are at high risk due to being severely compromised.

CANDIDIASIS: VULVOVAGINAL (MONILIASIS)

PROPHYLAXIS

▷ *acetic acid+oxyquinolone* (C) one full applicator intravaginally bid for up to 30 days

Pediatric: <12 years: not recommended; ≥12 years: same as adult

Relagard *Gel*: acetic acid 0.9%+oxyquin 0.025% (50 gm tube w. applicator)

Comment: The following treatment regimens for vulvovaginal candidiasis (VVC) are published in the **2015 CDC Sexually Transmitted Diseases Treatment Guidelines**. Treatment regimens are presented by generic drug name first, followed by information about brands and dose forms. Complicated VVC (recurrent, severe, non-albicans, or women with uncontrolled diabetes, debilitation, or immunosuppression) may require more intensive treatment and/or longer duration of treatment. VVC frequently occurs during pregnancy. Only topical azole therapies, applied for 7 days, are recommended during pregnancy.

RX ORAL AGENT

▷ *fluconazole* 150 mg in a single dose; complicated VVC, 150 mg x 3 doses on days 1, 4, 7 or weekly x 6 months

Rx INTRAVAGINAL AGENTS

Regimen 1

▷ *butoconazole* 2% cream (bioadhesive product) 5 gm intravaginally in a single dose

Regimen 2

▷ *nystatin* 100,000-unit vaginal tablet once daily x 14 days

Regimen 3

▷ *terconazole* 0.4% cream 5 gm intravaginally once daily x 7 days

Regimen 4

▷ *terconazole* 0.8% cream 5 gm intravaginally once daily x 3 days

Regimen 5

▷ *terconazole* 80 mg vaginal suppository intravaginally once daily x 3 days

OTC INTRAVAGINAL AGENTS

Regimen 1

▷ *butoconazole* 2% cream 5 gm intravaginally once daily x 3 days

Regimen 2

▷ *clotrimazole* 1% cream intravaginally once daily x 7-14 days

Regimen 3

▷ *clotrimazole* 2% cream intravaginally once daily x 3 days

Regimen 4

▷ *miconazole* 2% cream intravaginally once daily x 7 days

Regimen 5

▷ *miconazole* 4% cream intravaginally once daily x 3 days

Regimen 6

▷ **miconazole** 100 mg vaginal suppository intravaginally once daily x 7 days

Regimen 7

▷ **miconazole** 200 mg vaginal suppository intravaginally once daily x 3 days

Regimen 8

▷ **miconazole** 1,200 mg vaginal suppository intravaginally in a single application

Regimen 9

▷ **tioconazole** 6.5% ointment 5 gm intravaginally in a single application

DRUG BRANDS AND DOSE FORMS

▷ *butoconazole* cream 2% (C)
    Gynazole-12% Vaginal Cream *Prefilled vag applicator:* 5 g
    Femstat-3 Vaginal Cream (OTC) *Vag crm:* 2% (20 gm w. 3 applicators);
    Prefilled vag applicator: 5 gm (3/pck)

▷ *clotrimazole* (B)(OTC)
    Gyne-Lotrimin Vaginal Cream (OTC) *Vag crm:* 1% (45 gm w. applicator)
    Gyne-Lotrimin Vaginal Suppository (OTC) *Vag supp:* 100 mg (7/pck)
    Gyne-Lotrimin 3 Vaginal Suppository (OTC) *Vag supp:* 200 mg (3/pck)
    Gyne-Lotrimin Combination Pack (OTC) *Combination pck:* 7-100 mg supp
    <u>with</u> 7 gm 1% cream
    Gyne-Lotrimin 3 Combination Pack (OTC) *Combination pck:* 200 mg supp
    (7/pck) <u>plus</u> 1% cream (7 gm)
    Mycelex-G Vaginal Cream *Vag crm:* 1% (45, 90 gm w. applicator)
    Mycelex-G Vaginal Tab 1 *Tab:* 500 mg (1/pck)
    Mycelex Twin Pack *Twin pck:* 500 mg tab (7/pck) <u>with</u> 1% crm (7 gm)
    Mycelex-7 Vaginal Cream (OTC) *Vag crm:* 1% (45 gm w. applicator)
    Mycelex-7 Vaginal Inserts (OTC) *Vag insert:* 100 mg insert (7/pck)
    Mycelex-7 Combination Pack (OTC) *Combination pck:* 100 mg inserts
    (7/pck) <u>plus</u> 1% crm (7 gm)

▷ *fluconazole* (C)
    Diflucan *Tab:* 50, 100, 150, 200 mg; *Oral susp:* 10, 40 mg/ml (35 ml) (orange)

▷ *miconazole* (B)
    Monistat-3 Combination Pack (OTC) *Combination pck:* 200 mg supp (3/pck)
    <u>plus</u> 2% crm (9 gm)
    Monistat-7 Combination Pack (OTC) *Combination pck:* 100 mg supp (7/pck)
    <u>plus</u> 2% crm (9 gm)
    Monistat-7 Vaginal Cream (OTC) *Vag crm:* 2% (45 gm w. applicator)
    Monistat-7 Vaginal Suppositories (OTC) *Vag supp:* 100 mg (7/pck)
    Monistat-3 Vaginal Suppositories (OTC) *Vag supp:* 200 mg (3/pck)

▷ *nystatin* (C)
    Mycostatin *Vag tab:* 100,000 U (1/pck)

▷ *terconazole* (C)
    Terazol-3 Vaginal Cream *Vag crm:* 0.8% (20 gm w. applicator)
    Terazol-3 Vaginal Suppositories *Vag supp:* 80 mg supp (3/pck)
    Terazol-7 Vaginal Cream *Vag crm:* 0.4% (45 gm w. applicator)

▷ *tioconazole* (C)
    1-Day (OTC) *Vag oint:* 6.5% (prefilled applicator x 1)
    Monistat 1 Vaginal Ointment (OTC) *Vag oint:* 6.5% (prefilled applicator
    x 1)
    Vagistat-1 Vaginal Ointment (OTC) *Vag oint:* 6.5% (prefilled applicator
    x 1)

INVASIVE INFECTION

▷ *posaconazole* (D)(G) *Oral Therapy:* take with food; 100 mg bid on day 1; then 100 mg once daily x 13 days; refractory, 400 mg bid x 13 days; *IV Infusion Therapy:* must be administered through an in-line filter over approximately 90 minutes via a central venous line. Never administer **Noxafil** as an IV bolus injection; *Loading Dose: a single* 300 mg IV infusion; *Maintenance Dose: a single* 300 mg IV infusion once daily; duration of therapy is based on recovery from neutropenia or immunosuppression.
Pediatric: <13 years: not recommended; ≥13 years: same as adult
   Noxafil *Tab:* 100 mg ext-rel; *Oral susp:* 40 mg/ml (105 ml) (cherry); *Vial:* 300 mg/16.7 ml (18 mg/ml) soln for IV infusion
   Comment: **Noxafil** is indicated as prophylaxis for invasive aspergillus and candida infections in patients >13-years-old who are at high risk due to being severely compromised.

CANNABINOID HYPEREMESIS SYNDROME (CHS)

Comment: Cannabinoid hyperemesis syndrome (CHS) is indicated by recurrent episodes of refractory nausea and vomiting with vague diffuse abdominal pain (accompanied by compulsive, frequent, hot baths or showers for relief of abdominal pain; these behaviors are thought to be learned through their cyclical periods of emesis) in the setting of chronic cannabis use (at least weekly for >2 years. The nausea and vomiting typically do not respond to antiemetic medications. 5HT3 (e.g., *ondansetron*), D2 (e.g., *prochlorperazine*), H1 (e.g., *promethazine*), or neurokinin-1 receptor antagonists (e.g., *aprepitant*) can be tried, but these therapies often are ineffective. The recovery phase can last weeks to months despite continued cannabis use prior to returning to the hyperemetic phase. Symptoms that are worse in the morning, with normal bowel habits, and negative evaluation, including laboratory, radiography, and endoscopy. Resolution requires cannabis cessation from 1 to 3 months. Returning to cannabis use often results in the returning of CHS.

PHENOTHIAZINES

▷ *chlorpromazine* (C)(G) 10-25 mg PO q 4 hours prn or 50-100 mg rectally q 6-8 hours prn
Pediatric: <6 months: not recommended; ≥6 months: 0.25 mg/lb orally q 4-6 hours prn or 0.5 mg/lb rectally q 6-8 hours prn
   Thorazine *Tab:* 10, 25, 50, 100, 200 mg; *Spansule:* 30, 75, 150 mg sust-rel; *Syr:* 10 mg/5 ml (4 oz; orange custard); *Conc:* 30 mg/ml (4 oz); 100 mg/ml (2, 8 oz); *Supp:* 25, 100 mg
▷ *perphenazine* (C) 5 mg IM (may repeat in 6 hours) or 8-16 mg/day PO in divided doses; max 15 mg/day IM; max 24 mg/day PO
Pediatric: <12 years: not recommended; ≥12 years: same as adult
   Trilafon *Tab:* 2, 4, 8, 16 mg; *Oral conc:* 16 mg/5 ml (118 ml); *Amp:* 5 mg/ml (1 ml)
▷ *prochlorperazine* (C)(G) 5-10 mg tid-qid prn; usual max 40 mg/day
   Compazine
   Pediatric: <2 years or <20 lb: not recommended; 20-29 lb: 2.5 mg daily bid prn; max 7.5 mg/day; 30-39 lb: 2.5 mg bid-tid prn; max 10 mg/day; 40-85 lb: 2.5 mg tid or 5 mg bid prn; max 15 mg/day
   Tab: 5, 10 mg; *Syr:* 5 mg/5 ml (4 oz) (fruit)
   Compazine Suppository 25 mg rectally bid prn; usual max 50 mg/day

Pediatric: <2 years or <20 lb: not recommended; 20-29 lb: 2.5 mg daily-bid prn; max 7.5; mg/day; 30-39 lb: 2.5 mg bid-tid prn; max 10 mg/day; 40-85 lb: 2.5 mg tid or 5 mg bid prn; max 15 mg/day
Rectal supp: 2.5, 5, 25 mg
Compazine Injectable 5-10 mg tid or qid prn
Pediatric: <2 years or <20 lb: not recommended; ≥2 years or ≥20 lb: 0.06 mg/kg x 1 dose
Vial: 5 mg/ml (2, 10 ml)
Compazine Spansule 15 mg q AM prn or 10 mg q 12 hours prn usual max 40 mg/day
Pediatric: <12 years: not recommended; ≥12 years: same as adult
Spansule: 10, 15 mg sust-rel
▷ *promethazine* **(C)(G)** 25 mg PO or rectally q 4-6 hours prn
Pediatric: <2 years: not recommended; ≥2 years: 0.5 mg/lb or 6.25-25 mg q 4-6 hours prn
   Phenergan *Tab:* 12.5*, 25*, 50 mg; *Plain syr:* 6.25 mg/5 ml; *Fortis syr:* 25 mg/5 ml; *Rectal supp:* 12.5, 25, 50 mg
   Comment: *Promethazine* is contraindicated in children with uncomplicated nausea, dehydration, Reye's syndrome, history of sleep apnea, asthma, and lower respiratory disorders in children. *Promethazine* lowers the seizure threshold in children, may cause cholestatic jaundice, anticholinergic effects, extrapyramidal effects, and potentially fatal respiratory depression.

SUBSTANCE P/NEUROKININ 1 RECEPTOR ANTAGONIST

▷ *aprepitant* **(B)(G)** administer with 5HT-3 receptor antagonist; *Day 1:* 125 mg x 1 dose; *Starting Day 2:* 80 mg once daily in the morning
Pediatric: <6 months: years: not recommended; ≥6 months: use oral suspension (see mfr pkg insert for dose by weight
   Emend *Cap:* 40, 80, 125 mg (2 x 80 mg bi-fold pck; 1 x 25 mg/2 x 80 mg tri-fold pck); *Oral susp:* 125 mg pwdr for oral suspension, single-dose pouch w. dispenser; *Vial:* 150 mg pwdr for reconstitution and IV infusion

SEROTONIN (5HT-3) RECEPTOR ANTAGONISTS

▷ *dolasetron* **(B)** administer 100 mg IV over 30 seconds; max 100 mg/dose
Pediatric: <2 years: not recommended; 2-16 years: 1.8 mg/kg; >16 years: same as adult
   Anzemet *Tab:* 50, 100 mg; *Amp:* 12.5 mg/0.625 ml; *Prefilled carpuject syringe:* 12.5 mg (0.625 ml); *Vial:* 100 mg/5 ml (single-use); *Vial:* 500 mg/25 ml (multidose)
▷ *granisetron*
   Kytril (B) administer IV over 30 seconds; max 1 dose/week
   Pediatric: <2 years: not recommended; ≥2 years: 10 mcg/kg
      Tab: 1 mg; *Oral soln:* 2 mg/10 ml (30 ml) (orange); *Vial:* 1 mg/ml (1 ml single-dose) (preservative-free); 1 mg/ml (4 ml multidose) (benzyl alcohol)
   Sancuso (B) apply 1 patch; remove 24 hours (minimum) to 7 days (maximum)
   Transdermal patch: 3.1 mg/day
▷ *granisetron extended-release injection* administer SC over 20-30 seconds (due to drug viscosity) on Day 1 of chemotherapy and not more frequently than once every 7 days; *CrCl 30-59 mL/min:* repeat dose no more than every 14th day; *CrCl <30 mL/min:* not recommended; for patients receiving MEC, the recommended *dexamethasone* dosage is 8 mg IV on Day 1; for patients receiving AC combination chemotherapy regimens, the recommended *dexamethasone* dosage is 20 mg IV on Day 1, followed by 8 mg PO bid on Days 2, 3 and 4; if **Sustol** is administered with an NK₁ receptor antagonist, see that drug's mfr pkg insert for the recommended *dexamethasone* dosing

Pediatric: <12 years: not established; ≥12 years: same as adult

Sustol *Syringe:* 10 mg/0.4 ml ext-rel; prefilled single-dose/kit

Comment: At least 60 minutes prior to administration, remove the **Sustol** kit from refrigeration; activate a warming pouch and wrap the syringe in the warming pouch for 5-6 minutes to warm it to room temperature.

➤ *ondansetron* (C)(G) Oral Forms: 8 mg q 8 hours x 2 doses; then 8 mg q 12 hours
Pediatric: <4 years: not recommended; 4-11 years: 4 mg q 4 hours x 3 doses; then 4 mg q 8 hours

Zofran *Tab:* 4, 8, 24 mg

Zofran ODT *ODT:* 4, 8 mg (strawberry) (phenylalanine)

Zofran Oral Solution *Oral soln:* 4 mg/5 ml (50 ml) (strawberry) (phenylalanine); *Parenteral form:* see mfr pkg insert

Zofran Injection *Vial:* 2 mg/ml (2 ml single-dose); 2 mg/ml (20 ml muti-dose); 32 mg/50 ml (50 ml multi-dose); *Prefilled syringe:* 4 mg/2 ml, single-use (24/ carton)

Zuplenz Oral Soluble Film: 4, 8 mg oral-dis (10/carton) (peppermint)

Comment: The FDA has issued an updated warning against *ondansetron* use in pregnancy *ondansetron* is a 5-HT3 receptor antagonist approved by the FDA for preventing nausea and vomiting related to cancer chemotherapy and surgery. However, it has been used "off label" to treat the nausea and vomiting of pregnancy. The FDA has cautioned against the use of *ondansetron* in pregnancy in light of studies of *ondansetron* in early pregnancy and associated with congenital cardiac malformations and oral clefts (i.e., cleft lip and cleft palate). Further, there are potential maternal risks in pregnancy with electrolyte imbalance caused by severe nausea and vomiting (as with hyperemesis gravidarum). These risks include *serotonin syndrome* (a triad of cognitive and behavioral changes including confusion, agitation, autonomic instability, and neuromuscular changes). Therefore, *ondansetron* should <u>not</u> be taken during pregnancy.

➤ *palonosetron* (B)(G) administer 0.25 mg IV over 30 seconds; max 1 dose/week
Pediatric: <1 month: not recommended; 1 month to 17 years: 20 mcg/kg; max 1.5 mg/single dose; infuse over 15 minutes

Aloxi *Vial (single-use):* 0.075 mg/1.5 ml; 0.25 mg/5 ml (mannitol)

 CARCINOID SYNDROME DIARRHEA (CSD)

TRYPTOPHAN HYDROXYLASE

➤ *telotristat* take with food; 250 mg tid
Pediatric: <12 years: not established; ≥12 years: same as adult

Xermelo *Tab:* 250 mg (4 x 7 daily dose pcks/carton)

Comment: Take **Xermelo** in combination with somatostatin analog (SSA) therapy to treat patients inadequately controlled by SSA therapy. Breastfeeding females should monitor the infant for constipation.

CARDIOMYOPATHY OF TRANSTHYRETIN-MEDIATED AMYLOIDOSIS

TRANSTHYRETIN STABILIZERS

Comment: *Tafamidis* (**Vyndamax**) and *tafamidis meglumine* (**Vyndaqel**) are a transthyretin stabilizers indicated for the treatment of the cardiomyopathy of wild type <u>or</u> hereditary transthyretin-mediated amyloidosis in adults to reduce cardiovascular mortality and cardiovascular-related hospitalization. **Vyndamax** and **Vyndaqel** are <u>not</u> interchangeable <u>or</u> substitutable on a mg-per-mg basis. Although there are <u>no</u> contraindications to these drugs, animal studies have demonstrated potential for embryo/fetal harm. Consider pregnancy planning and prevention for females of reproductive potential. There are no available data on the presence of *tafamidis* in human milk <u>or</u> effects on the breastfed infant. Based on findings from animal studies, which suggest the potential for serious adverse reactions in the breastfed infant, breastfeeding is <u>not</u> recommended during treatment. Safety and efficacy of *tafamidis* has <u>not</u> been established in pediatric patients. No dosage adjustment is required patients ≥65 years-of-age.

▷ *tafamidis* 61 mg once daily
  Vyndamax *Cap*: 61 mg
▷ *tafamidis meglumine* 80 mg (4 x 20 mg) once daily
  Vyndaqel *Cap*: 20 mg

 CARPAL TUNNEL SYNDROME (CTS)

Acetaminophen for IV Infusion *see Pain*
NSAIDs *see* NSAIDs online at https://connect.springerpub.com/content/reference-book/978-0-8261-7935-7/back-matter/part02/back-matter/bmatter10
Opioid Analgesics *see Pain*
Topical & Transdermal Analgesics *see Pain*
Parenteral Corticosteroids *see* Appendix M. Parenteral Corticosteroids
Oral Corticosteroids *see* Appendix L. Oral Corticosteroids
Topical Analgesic and Anesthetic Agents *see* Appendix I. Anesthetic Agents for Local Infiltration and Dermal/Mucosal Membrane Application online at https://connect.springerpub.com/content/reference-book/978-0-8261-7935-7/back-matter/part02/back-matter/bmatter9

 CAT SCRATCH FEVER (*BARTONELLA* INFECTION)

Comment: Cat scratch fever is usually self-limited. Treatment should be limited to severe <u>or</u> debilitating cases.

ANTI-INFECTIVES

▷ *azithromycin* (B)(G) 500 mg x 1 dose on day 1, then 250 mg daily on days 2-5 <u>or</u> 500 mg daily x 3 days <u>or</u> **Zmax** 2 gm in a single dose
  Pediatric: 12 mg/kg/day x 5 days; max 500 mg/day; *see* Appendix CC.7.
  azithromycin (Zithromax Suspension, Zmax Suspension) *for dose by weight*
  Zithromax *Tab*: 250, 500, 600 mg; *Oral susp*: 100 mg/5 ml (15 ml); 200 mg/5 ml (15, 22.5, 30 ml) (cherry); *Pkt*: 1 gm for reconstitution (cherry-banana)
  Zithromax Tri-pak *Tab*: 3 x 500 mg tabs/pck
  Zithromax Z-pak *Tab*: 6 x 250 mg tabs/pck
  Zmax *Oral susp*: 2 gm ext-rel for reconstitution (cherry-banana) (148 mg Na⁺)
▷ *doxycycline* (D)(G) 100 mg daily bid
  Pediatric: <8 years: not recommended ≥8 years, <100 lb: 2 mg/lb on first day in 2 divided doses, followed by 1 mg/lb/day in 1-2 divided doses; ≥8 years, ≥100 lb: same as adult; *see Appendix CC.19.* doxycycline (Vibramycin Syrup/Suspension) *for dose by weight*
  Acticlate *Tab*: 75, 150**mg
  Adoxa *Tab*: 50, 75, 100, 150 mg ent-coat
  Doryx *Tab*: 50, 75, 100, 150, 200 mg del-rel
  Doxteric *Tab*: 50 mg del-rel
  Monodox *Cap*: 50, 75, 100 mg
  Oracea *Cap*: 40 mg del-rel
  Vibramycin *Tab*: 100 mg; *Cap*: 50, 100 mg; *Syr*: 50 mg/5 ml (raspberry-apple) (sulfites); *Oral susp*: 25 mg/5 ml (raspberry)
  Vibra-Tab *Tab*: 100 mg film-coat

▷ *erythromycin base* (B)(G) 500-1000 mg qid x 4 weeks
  Pediatric: <45 kg: 30-50 mg in 2-4 divided doses x 4 weeks; ≥45 kg: same as adult
   Ery-Tab *Tab:* 250, 333, 500 mg ent-coat
   PCE *Tab:* 333, 500 mg
▷ *erythromycin ethylsuccinate* (B)(G) 400 mg qid x 4 weeks
  Pediatric: 30-50 mg/kg/day in 4 divided doses x 4 weeks; may double dose with
  severe infection; max 100 mg/kg/day; *see Appendix CC.21. erythromycin*
  ethylsuccinate (E.E.S. Suspension, Ery-Ped Drops/Suspension) *for dose by weight*
   EryPed *Oral susp:* 200 mg/5 ml (100, 200 ml) (fruit); 400 mg/5 ml (60, 100,
   200 ml) (banana); *Oral drops:* 200, 400 mg/5 ml (50 ml) (fruit); *Chew tab:*
   200 mg wafer (fruit)
   E.E.S. *Oral susp:* 200, 400 mg/5 ml (100 ml) (fruit)
   E.E.S. Granules *Oral susp:* 200 mg/5 ml (100, 200 ml) (cherry)
   E.E.S. 400 Tablets *Tab:* 400 mg
▷ *trimethoprim+sulfamethoxazole (TMP-SMX)*(D)(G) bid x 10 days
  Pediatric: <2 months: not recommended; ≥2 months: 40 mg/kg/day of
  sulfamethoxazole in 2 divided doses bid x 10 days; *see Appendix CC.33.*
  trimethoprim+sulfamethoxazole (Bactrim Suspension, Septra Suspension) *for dose*
  by weight
   Bactrim, Septra 2 tabs bid x 10 days
    Tab: trim 80 mg+sulfa 400 mg*
   Bactrim DS, Septra DS 1 tab bid x 10 days
    Tab: trim 160 mg+sulfa 800 mg*
   Bactrim Pediatric Suspension, Septra Pediatric Suspension
    Oral susp: trim 40 mg+sulfa 200 mg per 5 ml (100 ml) (cherry) (alcohol
    0.3%)
Comment: Sulfonamides are contraindicated in the first trimester of pregnancy,
the final month of pregnancy, and infants <8 weeks-of-age. *CrCl 15-30 mL/min:*
reduce dose by 1/2; *CrCl <15 mL/min:* not recommended. Contraindicated with
G6PD deficiency. A high fluid intake is indicated during sulfonamide therapy to
avoid crystallization in the kidneys.

CELLULITE

COLLAGENASE CLOSTRIDIUM HISTOLYTICUM-AAES

▷ *collagenase clostridium histolyticum-aaes* a treatment area is defined as a single
  buttock receiving up to 12 injections, 0.3 ml each (up to a total of 3.6 ml); a
  treatment visit may consist of up to 2 treatment areas; treatment visits should be
  repeated every 21 days for 3 treatment visits; reconstitute **QWO** lyophilized
  powder with the supplied diluent prior to use; inject 0.84 mg per treatment area
  as 12 SC injections (0.3 ml administered as three 0.1 ml aliquots per injection)
  Pediatric: not established
   QWO *Vial:* 0.92, 1.84 mg, single dose, pwdr for reconstitution with provided
   diluent
   Comment: QWO *(collagenase clostridium histolyticum-aaes)* is a combination
   of bacterial collagenases indicated for the treatment of moderate-to-severe
   cellulite in the buttocks of adult women. The most common adverse reactions
   (incidence ≥1%) have been related to the injection site (bruising, pain,
   nodule, pruritus, erythema, discoloration, swelling, and warmth). Injection
   site bruising occurs frequently after **QWO** administration. Use with caution
   in patients with bleeding abnormalities <u>or</u> who are currently being treated
   with antiplatelet (<u>except</u> those taking ≤150 mg *aspirin* daily) <u>or</u> anticoagulant
   therapy. Serious hypersensitivity reactions, including anaphylaxis, may

occur with ***collagenase clostridium histolyticum***. If a serious hypersensitivity reaction occurs, initiate appropriate therapy. **QWO** must <u>not</u> be substituted for other injectable collagenase products. **QWO** is <u>not</u> indicated for the treatment of Peyronie's disease <u>or</u> Dupuytren's contracture. Following SC injection, the systemic concentrations for **QWO** have been below the bioanalytical assay limit of quantification. There are <u>no</u> available data on ***collagenase clostridium histolyticum*** use in pregnant women to evaluate for a drug-associated risk of major birth defects, miscarriage <u>or</u> adverse maternal <u>or</u> fetal outcomes. There are <u>no</u> data on the presence of ***collagenase clostridium histolyticum*** in human milk <u>or</u> effects on the breastfed infant.

CELLULITIS, ACUTE BACTERIAL SKIN AND SKIN STRUCTURE INFECTION (ABSSSI)

Comment: Duration of treatment should be 10-30 days. Obtain culture from site. Consider blood cultures.

ANTI-INFECTIVES

▶ *amoxicillin* **(B)(G)** 500-875 mg bid <u>or</u> 250-500 mg tid x 10 days
Pediatric: <40 kg (88 lb): 20-40 mg/kg/day in 3 divided doses x 10 days <u>or</u> 25-45 mg/kg/day in 2 divided doses x 10 days; ≥40 kg: same as adult; *see* Appendix CC.3.
amoxicillin (Amoxil Suspension, Trimox Suspension) *for dose by weight*
  Amoxil *Cap:* 250, 500 mg; *Tab:* 875*mg; *Chew tab:* 125, 200, 250, 400 mg (cherry-banana-peppermint) (phenylalanine); *Oral susp:* 125, 250 mg/5 ml (80, 100, 150 ml) (strawberry); 200, 400 mg/5 ml (50, 75, 100 ml) (bubble gum); *Oral drops:* 50 mg/ml (30 ml) (bubble gum)
  Moxatag *Tab:* 775 mg ext-rel
  Trimox *Tab:* 125, 250 mg; *Cap:* 250, 500 mg; *Oral susp:* 125, 250 mg/5 ml (80, 100, 150 ml) (raspberry-strawberry)
▶ *amoxicillin+clavulanate* **(B)(G)**
  Augmentin 500 mg tid <u>or</u> 875 mg bid x 7-10 days
  Pediatric: 40-45 mg/kg/day divided tid x 10 days <u>or</u> 90 mg/kg/day divided bid x 10 days *see* Appendix CC.4. *amoxicillin+clavulanate* (Augmentin Suspension) *for dose by weight*
  Tab: 250, 500, 875 mg; *Chew tab:* 125, 250 mg (lemon-lime); 200, 400 mg (cherry-banana) (phenylalanine); *Oral susp:* 125 mg/5 ml (banana), 250 mg/5 ml (75, 100, 150 ml) (orange); 200, 400 mg/5 ml (50, 75, 100 ml) (orange) (phenylalanine)
  Augmentin ES-600 not recommended for adults
  Pediatric: <3 months: not recommended; ≥3 months, <40 kg: 90 mg/kg/day in 2 divided doses x 7-10 days; ≥40 kg: not recommended
  Oral susp: 42.9 mg/5 ml (50, 75, 100, 125, 150, 200 ml) (strawberry cream) (phenylalanine)
  Augmentin XR 2 tabs q 12 hours x 7-10 days
  Pediatric: <16 years: use other forms; ≥16 years: same as adult
    Tab: 1000*mg ext-rel
▶ *azithromycin* **(B)(G)** 500 mg x 1 dose on day 1, then 250 mg daily on days 2-5 <u>or</u> 500 mg daily x 3 days <u>or</u> **Zmax** 2 gm in a single dose
  Pediatric: 12 mg/kg/day x 5 days; max 500 mg/day; *see* Appendix CC.7.
  azithromycin (Zithromax Suspension, Zmax Suspension) *for dose by weight*
  Zithromax *Tab:* 250, 500, 600 mg; *Oral susp:* 100 mg/5 ml (15 ml); 200 mg/5 ml (15, 22.5, 30 ml) (cherry); *Pkt:* 1 gm for reconstitution (cherry-banana)
  Zithromax Tri-pak *Tab:* 3 x 500 mg tabs/pck
  Zithromax Z-pak *Tab:* 6 x 250 mg tabs/pck
  Zmax *Oral susp:* 2 gm ext-rel for reconstitution (cherry-banana) (148 mg Na⁺)

▷ *cefaclor* (B)(G)

Ceclor 250 mg tid or 375 mg bid 3-10 days

Pediatric: <1 month: not recommended; 1 month-12 years: 20-40 mg/kg divided bid or q 12 hours x 3-10 days; max 1 gm/day; see Appendix CC.8. *cefaclor* (Ceclor Suspension) for *dose by weight;* >12 years: same as adult

Tab: 500 mg; *Cap:* 250, 500 mg; *Susp:* 125 mg/5 ml (75, 150 ml) (strawberry); 187 mg/5 ml (50, 100 ml) (strawberry); 250 mg/5 ml (75, 150 ml) (strawberry); 375 mg/5 ml (50, 100 ml) (strawberry)

Ceclor Extended Release 375-500 mg bid x 3-10 days

Pediatric: <16 years: ext-rel not recommended; ≥16 years: same as adult
Tab: 375, 500 mg ext-rel

▷ *cefpodoxime proxetil* (B) 400 mg bid x 7-14 days

Pediatric: <2 months: not recommended; ≥2 months-12 years: 10 mg/kg/day (max 400 mg/dose) or 5 mg/kg/day bid (max 200 mg/dose) x 7-14 days; see Appendix CC.12. *cefpodoxime proxetil* (Vantin Suspension) for *dose by weight;* >12 years: same as adult

Vantin *Tab:* 100, 200 mg; *Oral susp:* 50, 100 mg/5 ml (50, 75, 100 mg) (lemon creme)

▷ *cefprozil* (B) 500 mg q 12 hours x 10 days

Pediatric: <2 years: not recommended; 2-12 years: 15 mg/kg q 12 hours x 10 days; see Appendix CC.13. *cefprozil* (Cefzil Suspension) for *dose by weight;* >12 years: same as adult

Cefzil *Tab:* 250, 500 mg; *Oral susp:* 125, 250 mg/5 ml (50, 75, 100 ml) (bubble gum) (phenylalanine)

▷ *ceftaroline fosamil* (B) administer 600 mg once every 12 hours, by IV infusion over 5-60 minutes, x 5-14 days

Pediatric: <18 years: not established; ≥18 years: same as adult

Teflaro *Vial:* 400, 600 mg pwdr for reconstitution, single-use (10/carton)

Comment: Teflaro is indicated for the treatment of adults with acute bacterial skin and skin structures infection (ABSSSI).

▷ *ceftriaxone* (B)(G) 1-2 gm daily x 5-14 days IM; max 4 gm daily

Pediatric: 50-75 mg/kg IM in 1-2 divided doses x 5-14 days; max 2 gm/day
Rocephin *Vial:* 250, 500 mg; 1, 2 gm

▷ *cephalexin* (B)(G) 500 mg bid x 10 days

Pediatric: 25-50 mg/kg/day in 4 divided doses x 10 days; see Appendix CC.15. *cephalexin* (Keflex Suspension) for *dose by weight*

Keflex *Cap:* 250, 333, 500, 750 mg; *Oral susp:* 125, 250 mg/5 ml (100, 200 ml) (strawberry)

▷ *clarithromycin* (C)(G) 500 mg q 12 hours or 500 mg ext-rel once daily x 10 days

Pediatric: <6 months: not recommended; ≥6 months: 7.5 mg/kg bid x 10 days; see Appendix CC.16. *clarithromycin* (Biaxin Suspension) for *dose by weight*

Biaxin *Tab:* 250, 500 mg

Biaxin Oral Suspension *Oral susp:* 125, 250 mg/5 ml (50, 100 ml) (fruit-punch)

Biaxin XL *Tab:* 500 mg ext-rel

▷ *dalbavancin* (C) 1000 mg administered once as a single dose via IV infusion over 30 minutes or initially 1,000 mg once, followed by 500 mg 1 week later; infuse over 30 minutes; *CrCl* <30 *mL/min:* not receiving dialysis: initially 750 mg, followed by 375 mg 1 week later

Pediatric: <18 years: not established; ≥18 years: same as adult

Dalvance *Vial:* 500 mg pwdr for reconstitution, single-use (preservative-free)

Comment: Dalvance is a lipoglycopeptide indicated for the treatment of acute bacterial skin and skin structures infection (ABSSSI) caused by gram-positive bacteria.

▷ *delafloxacin* IV infusion: administer 300 mg every 12 hours over 60 minutes x 5-14 days; *Tablet:* 450 mg every 12 hours x 5-14 days; dosage for patients with renal impairment is based on eGFR (see mfr pkg insert)
Pediatric: <18 years: not recommended; ≥18 years: same as adult
  Baxdela *Tab:* 450 mg; *Vial:* 300 mg pwdr for reconstitution and IV infusion
  Comment: **Baxdela,** a fluoroquinolone, is indicated for the treatment of acute bacterial skin and skin structure infections (ABSSSI) caused by designated susceptible bacteria. Fluoroquinolones have been associated with disabling and potentially irreversible serious adverse reactions that have occurred together, including tendinitis and tendon rupture, peripheral neuropathy, and central nervous system effects. Discontinue **Baxdela** immediately and avoid the use of fluoroquinolones, including **Baxdela,** in patients who experience any of these serious adverse reactions. Fluoroquinolones may exacerbate muscle weakness in patients with myasthenia gravis. Therefore, avoid **Baxdela** in patients with known history of myasthenia gravis. Most common adverse reactions are nausea, diarrhea, headache, transaminase elevations, and vomiting. Closely monitor SCr in patients with severe renal impairment (eGFR 15-29 mL/min/1.73 m²) receiving intravenous *delafloxacin.* If SCr level increases occur, consider changing to oral *delafloxacin.* Discontinue **Baxdela** if eGFR decreases to <15 mL/min/1.73 m². The limited available data with **Baxdela** use in pregnant females are insufficient to inform a drug-associated risk of major birth defects and miscarriages. There are no data available on the presence of *delafloxacin* in human milk or effects on the breastfed infant.

▷ *dicloxacillin* (B)(G) 500 mg q 6 hours x 10 days
Pediatric: 12.5-25 mg/kg/day in 4 divided doses x 10 days; *see* Appendix CC.18. *dicloxacillin* (Dynapen Suspension) *for dose by weight*
  Dynapen *Cap:* 125, 250, 500 mg; *Oral susp:* 62.5 mg/5 ml (80, 100, 200 ml)

▷ *dirithromycin* (C)(G) 500 mg once daily x 5-7 days
Pediatric: <12 years: not recommended; ≥12 years: same as adult
  Dynabac *Tab:* 250 mg

▷ *erythromycin base* (B)(G) 250 mg qid or 333 mg tid or 500 mg bid x 7-10 days; then taper to lowest effective dose
Pediatric: <45 kg: 30-50 mg in 2-4 divided doses x 7-10 days; ≥45 kg: same as adult
  Ery-Tab *Tab:* 250, 333, 500 mg ent-coat
  PCE *Tab:* 333, 500 mg

▷ *erythromycin ethylsuccinate* (B)(G) 400 mg qid x 7-10 days
Pediatric: 30-50 mg/kg/day in 4 divided doses x 7-10 days; may double dose with severe infection; max 100 mg/kg/day; *see Appendix CC.21. erythromycin ethylsuccinate* (E.E.S. Suspension, Ery-Ped Drops/Suspension) *for dose by weight*
  EryPed *Oral susp:* 200 mg/5 ml (100, 200 ml) (fruit); 400 mg/5 ml (60, 100, 200 ml) (banana); *Oral drops:* 200, 400 mg/5 ml (50 ml) (fruit); *Chew tab:* 200 mg wafer (fruit)
  E.E.S. *Oral susp:* 200, 400 mg/5 ml (100 ml) (fruit)
  E.E.S. Granules *Oral susp:* 200 mg/5 ml (100, 200 ml) (cherry)
  E.E.S. 400 Tablets *Tab:* 400 mg

▷ *linezolid* (C)(G) 600 mg q 12 hours x 10-14 days
Pediatric: <5 years: 10 mg/kg q 8 hours x 10-14 days; 5-11 years: 10 mg/kg q 12 hours x 10-14 days; >11 years: same as adult
  Zyvox *Tab:* 400, 600 mg; *Oral susp:* 100 mg/5 ml (150 ml) (orange) (phenylalanine)
  Comment: *Linezolid* is indicated to treat susceptible vancomycin-resistant *E. faecium* infections of skin and skin structures, including diabetic foot without osteomyelitis.

▷ *loracarbef* (B) 200 mg bid x 10 days
Pediatric: 15 mg/kg/day in 2 divided doses x 10 days; *see* Appendix CC.27. *loracarbef* (Lorabid Suspension) *for dose by weight*

Lorabid *Pulvule:* 200, 400 mg; *Oral susp:* 100 mg/5 ml (50, 100 ml);
200 mg/5 ml (50, 75, 100 ml) (strawberry bubble gum)

▷ *moxifloxacin* (C)(G) 400 mg once daily x 5 days
Pediatric: <18 years: recommended; ≥18 years: same as adult

Avelox *Tab:* 400 mg; *IV soln:* 400 mg/250 mg (latex-free, preservative-free)

▷ *omadacycline* *before* oral dosing, fast x at least 4 hours and then take tablets with water; *after* oral dosing, no food or drink (except water) x 2 hours and no dairy products, antacids, or multivitamins x 4 hours; total treatment duration 7-14 days
OPTION 1, Loading Dose, Day 1: 200 mg via IV infusion over 60 minutes or 100 mg via IV infusion over 30 minutes twice; *Maintenance:* 100 mg via IV infusion over 30 minutes once daily or 300 mg orally once daily
OPTION 2 (tablets only): Day 1 and Day 2: 450 mg orally once daily; then, reduce dose to 300 mg orally once daily
Pediatric: <18 years: not recommended; ≥18 years: same as adult

Nuzyra *Tab:* 150 mg; *Vial:* 100 mg single dose for reconstitution, dilution, and IV infusion

Comment: **Nuzyra** *(omadacycline)* is an aminomethylcycline tetracycline antibiotic for the treatment of community-acquired bacterial pneumonia (CABP) and acute bacterial skin and skin structure infection (ABSSSI). The most common adverse reactions (incidence ≥2%) are nausea, vomiting, infusion site reactions, alanine aminotransferase (ALT) increased, aspartate aminotransferase (AST) increased, gamma-glutamyl transferase (GGT) increased, hypertension, headache, diarrhea, insomnia, and constipation. Like other tetracycline-class antibacterial drugs, **Nuzyra** may cause discoloration of deciduous teeth and reversible inhibition of bone growth when administered during the second and third trimester of pregnancy. The limited available data of **Nuzyra** use in pregnancy is insufficient to inform drug-associated risk of major birth defects and miscarriages. There is no information on the presence of *omadacycline* in human milk or effects on the breastfed infant.

▷ *oritavancin*
Comment: *Oritavancin* is a lipoglycopeptide antibacterial agent. There are two *oritavancin* products: **Kimyrsa** and **Orbactiv**. These have *differences* in dose strength, duration of infusion and preparation instructions, including reconstitution and dilution instructions and compatible diluents. Use of IV administered unfractionated *heparin sodium* is contraindicated for 120 hours (5 days) after *oritavancin* administration. *Oritavancin* has been shown to artificially prolong aPTT for up to 120 hours, and may prolong PT and INR for up to 12 hours and ACT for up to 24 hours. For patients who require aPTT monitoring within 120 hours of *Oritavancin* dosing, consider a non-phospholipid dependent coagulation test such as a Factor Xa (chromogenic) assay or an alternative anticoagulant not requiring aPTT. *Oritavancin* has been shown to artificially prolong PT/INR for up to 12 hours when administered concomitantly with *warfarin*; patients should be monitored for bleeding. Serious hypersensitivity reactions, including anaphylaxis, have been reported with the use of **oritavancin** products; discontinue infusion if signs of acute hypersensitivity occur. Carefully monitor patients with known hypersensitivity to glycopeptides. Infusion-related reactions have been reported with the glycopeptide class of antimicrobial agents. Stopping or slowing the infusion results in cessation of these reactions. *Clostridioides difficile*-associated diarrhea may develop; evaluate patients if diarrhea occurs. Institute appropriate alternate antibacterial therapy in patients with confirmed or suspected osteomyelitis. The most common adverse reactions (incidence ≥3%) in patients treated with *oritavancin* products have been headache, nausea, vomiting, limb and subcutaneous abscesses, and diarrhea. There are no available data on *oritavancin* use in pregnant females to evaluate for a drug-associated risk of major birth defects, miscarriage or adverse

maternal or embryo/fetal outcomes. In animal reproduction studies, no effects on embryo/fetal development or survival were observed throughout organogenesis. There are no data on the presence of *oritavancin* in human milk or the effects on the breastfed infant. In animal studies, *oritavancin* is present in breast milk. Developmental and health benefits of breastfeeding should be considered along with the mother's clinical need for *oritavancin* and any potential adverse effects on the breastfed infant from *oritavancin* or from the underlying maternal condition. **Kimyrsa** Administer 1,200 mg (1 vial) as a single dose via IV infusion over 1 hour; carefully follow the mfr pkg insert for full preparation, dilution, and infusion information

Pediatric: <18 years: safety and efficacy not established; ≥18 years: same as adult
> Vial: 1,200 mg, single-dose, pwdr for reconstitution, dilution, and IV infusion
Orbactiv Administer 1,200 mg (3 vials) as a single dose via IV infusion over 3 hours; carefully follow the mfr pkg insert for full preparation, dilution, and infusion information

Pediatric: <18 years: safety and efficacy not established; ≥18 years: same as adult
> Vial: 400 mg, single-dose, pwdr for reconstitution, dilution, and IV infusion

➤ *penicillin v potassium* (B) 250-500 mg q 6 hours x 5-7 days
Pediatric: <12 years: *see* Appendix CC.29. *penicillin v potassium* (Pen-Vee K Solution, Veetids Solution) *for dose by weight;* >12 years: same as adult
> **Pen-Vee K** *Tab:* 250, 500 mg; *Oral soln:* 125 mg/5 ml (100, 200 ml); 250 mg/5 ml (100, 150, 200 ml)

➤ *tedizolid phosphate* (C) administer 200 mg once daily x 6 days, via PO or IV infusion over 1 hour
Pediatric: <18 years: not established; ≥18 years: same as adult
> **Sivextro** *Tab:* 200 mg (6/blister pck)
> **Comment:** **Sivextro** is indicated for the treatment of adults with acute bacterial skin and skin structures infection (ABSSSI).

➤ *tigecycline* (D)(G) 100 mg as a single dose; then 50 mg q 12 hours x 5-14 days; with severe hepatic impairment (Child-Pugh Class C), 100 mg as a single dose; then 25 mg q 12 hours
Pediatric: <18 years: not recommended; ≥18 years: same as adult
> **Tygacil** *Vial:* 50 mg pwdr for reconstitution and IV infusion (preservative-free)
> **Comment:** **Tygacil** is contraindicated in pregnancy, and lactation (discolors developing tooth enamel). A side effect may be photo-sensitivity (photophobia). Do not give with antacids, calcium supplements, milk or other dairy, or within 2 hours of taking another drug.

CERUMEN IMPACTION

OTIC ANALGESIC

➤ *antipyrine+benzocaine+zinc acetate dihydrate* otic (C) fill ear canal with solution; then moisten cotton plug with solution and insert into meatus; may repeat every 1-2 hours prn
Pediatric: same as adult
> **Otozin** *Otic soln: antipyr* 5.4%+*benz* 1%+*zinc* 1% per ml (10 ml w. dropper)

CERUMINOLYTICS

➤ *triethanolamine* (OTC)(G) fill ear canal and insert cotton plug for 15-30 minutes before irrigating with warm water
> **Cerumenex** *Soln:* 10% (6, 12 ml)

➤ *carbamide peroxide* (OTC)(G) instill 5-10 drops in ear canal; keep drops in ear several minutes; then irrigate with warm water; repeat bid for up to 4 days
> **Debrox** *Soln:* 15, 30 ml squeeze bottle w. applicator

CHAGAS DISEASE (*AMERICAN TRYPANOSOMIASIS*)

Comment: Chagas Disease is a protozoal parasite (*Trypanosoma cruzi*) infection with increasing prevalence in the US attributed to immigration from *T. cruzi*-endemic areas of South and Central Latin America. Approximately 300,000 persons in the US have chronic Chagas Disease, and up to 30% of them will develop clinically evident cardiovascular and/or gastrointestinal disease. Chagas Disease is one of the five neglected parasitic infections (NPIs) targeted by CDC for public health action. Transmitted by the bite of the triatomine bug ("kissing bug"), which feeds on human blood, maternal-fetus vertical transmission, blood transfusion, consumption of contaminated food, and organ donation. A clinical marker is Romaña sign (periorbital swelling), chagoma (skin nodule), Schizotrypanides (nonpruritic morbilliform rash). Only two antiparasitic drugs, **benznidazole** and **nifurtimox**, have demonstrated effectiveness altering the progression of this chronic disease. These drugs are not FDA approved and are available only from CDC under investigational protocols. Treatment is indicated for all cases of acute or reactivated Chagas Disease and for chronic *Trypanosoma cruzi* infection in children ≤18. Congenital infections are considered acute disease. Treatment is strongly recommended up to 50 years old with chronic infection who do not already have advanced Chagas cardiomyopathy. For adults older than 50 years with chronic *T. cruzi* infection, the decision to treat with antiparasitic drugs should be individualized, weighing the potential benefits and risks for the patient. Patients taking either of these drugs should have a CBC and CMP at the start of treatment and then bi-monthly for the duration of treatment to monitor for rare bone marrow suppression. Contraindications for treatment include severe hepatic and/or renal disease. As safety for infants exposed through breastfeeding has not been documented, withholding treatment while breastfeeding is also recommended. For emergencies (for example, acute Chagas Disease with severe manifestations, Chagas Disease in a newborn, or Chagas Disease in an immunocompromised person) outside of regular business hours, call the CDC Emergency Operations Center (770-488-7100) and ask for the person on call for Parasitic Diseases. For more detailed information about screening, assessment, and treatment of this public health threat, see McDonald, J, & Mattingly, J. (November, 2016). Chagas disease: Creeping into family practice in the United States, *Clinician Reviews*, pp. 38-45, or call 404-718-4745 or e-mail questions to chagas@cdc.gov.

ANTI-PARASITIC AGENTS

▷ **benznidazole (G)** take with a meal to avoid GI upset; <2 years: not established; 2-12 years: 5-7.5 mg/kg/day divided bid x 60 days; >12 years: not established
  Comment: Common side effects of **benznidazole** are allergic dermatitis, peripheral neuropathy, insomnia, anorexia with weight loss. **beznidazole** is contraindicated in patients who have taken **disulfiram** within the previous 2 weeks because of potential for a psychotic reaction. Alcohol beverages, and any product containing propyline glycol, are contraindicated from 2 weeks before initiating the first dose of **beznidazole**, throughout treatment, and the first 3 days after the last dose of **beznidazole** to prevent a **disulfiram**-like reaction (e.g., flushing, headache, abdominal cramping, and nausea/vomiting.

▷ **nifurtimox (G)** take with a meal to avoid GI upset; ≤10 years: 15-20 mg/kg/day divided tid-qid x 90 days; 11-16 years: 12.5-15 mg/kg/day divided tid-qid x 90 days; ≥17 years: 8-10 mg/kg/day divided tid-qid x 90 days
  Comment: Common side effects of **nifurtimox** are anorexia and weight loss, nausea, vomiting, polyneuropathy, headache, dizziness or vertigo. **nifurtimox** is contraindicated in patients who have taken **disulfiram** within the previous 2

weeks because of potential for a psychotic reaction. Alcohol beverages, and any product containing propyline glycol, are contraindicated from 2 weeks before initiating the first dose of **nifurtimox**, throughout treatment, and the first 3 days after the last dose of **nifurtimox** to prevent a **disulfiram**-like reaction (e.g., flushing, headache, abdominal cramping, and nausea/vomiting).

Lampit *Weight-Based Dosing:* ≥40 kg: 8-10 mg/kg divided tid x 60 days; <40 kg: 10-20 mg/kg divided tid x 60 days; take with food; obtain a pregnancy test in females of reproductive potential prior to initiating treatment

    Tab: 30*, 120*mg

Comment: Lampit *(nifurtimox)* is a nitrofuran antiprotozoal indicated in pediatric patients (term newborn to <18 years-of-age and weighing at least 2.5 kg) for the treatment of Chagas disease *(American Trypanosomiasis)*, caused by *Trypanosoma cruzi*. The most frequently reported adverse reactions (≥5%) have been vomiting, abdominal pain, headache, decreased appetite, nausea, pyrexia, and rash. *Renal and/or Hepatic Impairment:* Administer under close medical supervision.

CHANCROID

ANTI-INFECTIVES

▷ *azithromycin* (B)(G) 500 mg x 1 dose on day 1, then 250 mg daily on days 2-5 or 500 mg daily x 3 days or **Zmax** 2 gm in a single dose
Pediatric: 12 mg/kg/day x 5 days; max 500 mg/day; *see* Appendix CC.7.
azithromycin (Zithromax Suspension, Zmax Suspension) *for dose by weight*
    Zithromax *Tab:* 250, 500, 600 mg; *Oral susp:* 100 mg/5 ml (15 ml); 200 mg/5 ml (15, 22.5, 30 ml) (cherry); *Pkt:* 1 gm for reconstitution (cherry-banana)
    Zithromax Tri-pak *Tab:* 3 x 500 mg tabs/pck
    Zithromax Z-pak *Tab:* 6 x 250 mg tabs/pck
    Zmax *Oral susp:* 2 gm ext-rel for reconstitution (cherry-banana) (148 mg Na⁺)

▷ *ceftriaxone* (B)(G) 250 mg IM in a single dose
Pediatric: <45 kg: 125 mg IM in a single dose; ≥45 kg: same as adult
    Rocephin *Vial:* 250, 500 mg; 1, 2 gm

▷ *ciprofloxacin* (C) 500 mg bid x 3 days
Pediatric: <18 years: not recommended; ≥18 years: same as adult
    Cipro *Tab:* 250, 500, 750 mg; *Oral susp:* 250, 500 mg/5 ml (100 ml) (strawberry)
    Cipro XR *Tab:* 500, 1000 mg ext-rel
    ProQuin XR *Tab:* 500 mg ext-rel

▷ *erythromycin base* (B)(G) 500 mg qid x 7 days
Pediatric: 30-50 mg/kg/day divided bid-qid; max 100 mg/kg/day
    Ery-Tab *Tab:* 250, 333, 500 mg ent-coat
    PCE *Tab:* 333, 500 mg

▷ *erythromycin ethylsuccinate* (B)(G) 400 mg qid x 7 days
Pediatric: 30-50 mg/kg/day in 4 divided doses x 7 days; may double dose with severe infection; max 100 mg/kg/day; *see Appendix CC.21. erythromycin ethylsuccinate* (E.E.S. Suspension, Ery-Ped Drops/Suspension) *for dose by weight*
    EryPed *Oral susp:* 200 mg/5 ml (100, 200 ml) (fruit); 400 mg/5 ml (60, 100, 200 ml) (banana); *Oral drops:* 200, 400 mg/5 ml (50 ml) (fruit); *Chew tab:* 200 mg wafer (fruit)
    E.E.S. *Oral susp:* 200, 400 mg/5 ml (100 ml) (fruit)
    E.E.S. Granules *Oral susp:* 200 mg/5 ml (100, 200 ml) (cherry)
    E.E.S. 400 Tablets *Tab:* 400 mg

CHEMOTHERAPY-INDUCED NAUSEA/VOMITING (CINV)

PHENOTHIAZINES

▷ *chlorpromazine* (C)(G) 10-25 mg PO q 4 hours prn or 50-100 mg rectally q 6-8 hours prn
Pediatric: <6 months: not recommended; ≥6 months: 0.25 mg/lb orally q 4-6 hours prn or 0.5 mg/lb rectally q 6-8 hours prn; >12 years: same as adult
Thorazine *Tab:* 10, 25, 50, 100, 200 mg; *Spansule:* 30, 75, 150 mg sust-rel; *Syr:* 10 mg/5 ml (4 oz; orange custard); *Conc:* 30 mg/ml (4 oz); 100 mg/ml (2, 8 oz); *Supp:* 25, 100 mg

▷ *perphenazine* (C) 5 mg IM (may repeat in 6 hours) or 8-16 mg/day PO in divided doses; max 15 mg/day IM; max 24 mg/day PO
Pediatric: <12 years: not recommended; ≥12 years: same as adult
Trilafon *Tab:* 2, 4, 8, 16 mg; *Oral conc:* 16 mg/5 ml (118 ml); *Amp:* 5 mg/ml (1 ml)

▷ *prochlorperazine* (C)(G) 5-10 mg tid-qid prn; usual max 40 mg/day
Compazine
Pediatric: <2 years or <20 lb: not recommended; 20-29 lb: 2.5 mg daily bid prn; max 7.5 mg/day; 30-39 lb: 2.5 mg bid-tid prn; max 10 mg/day; 40-85 lb: 2.5 mg tid or 5 mg bid prn; max 15 mg/day; >85 lb: same as adult
Tab: 5, 10 mg; *Syr:* 5 mg/5 ml (4 oz) (fruit)
Compazine Suppository 25 mg rectally bid prn; usual max 50 mg/day
Pediatric: <2 years or <20 lb: not recommended; 20-29 lb: 2.5 mg daily-bid prn; max 7.5; mg/day; 30-39 lb: 2.5 mg bid-tid prn; max 10 mg/day; 40-85 lb: 2.5 mg tid or 5 mg bid prn; max 15 mg/day; >85 lb: same as adult
Rectal supp: 2.5, 5, 25 mg
Compazine Injectable 5-10 mg tid or qid prn
Pediatric: <2 years or <20 lb: not recommended; ≥2 years or ≥20 lb: 0.06 mg/kg x 1 dose; >12 years: same as adult
Vial: 5 mg/ml (2, 10 ml)
Compazine Spansule 15 mg q AM prn or 10 mg q 12 hours prn usual max 40 mg/day
Pediatric: <12 years: not recommended; ≥12 years: same as adult
Spansule: 10, 15 mg sust-rel

▷ *promethazine* (C)(G) 25 mg PO or rectally q 4-6 hours prn
Pediatric: <2 years: not recommended; ≥2 years: 0.5 mg/lb or 6.25-25 mg every 4-6 hours prn; >12 years: same as adult
Phenergan *Tab:* 12.5*, 25*, 50 mg; *Plain syr:* 6.25 mg/5 ml; *Fortis syr:* 25 mg/5 ml; *Rectal supp:* 12.5, 25, 50 mg
Comment: *Promethazine* is contraindicated in children with uncomplicated nausea, dehydration, Reye's syndrome, history of sleep apnea, asthma, and lower respiratory disorders in children. *Promethazine* lowers the seizure threshold in children and may cause cholestatic jaundice, anticholinergic effects, extrapyramidal effects, and potentially fatal respiratory depression.

SUBSTANCE P/NEUROKININ 1 RECEPTOR ANTAGONIST

▷ *aprepitant* (B)(G) administer with corticosteroid and 5HT-3 receptor antagonist; *Day 1 of chemotherapy cycle:* 125 mg 1 hour prior to chemotherapy *Day 2 and 3:* 80 mg in the morning
Pediatric: <6 months: years: not recommended; ≥6 months-12 years: use oral suspension (see mfr pkg insert for dose by weight); >12 years: same as adult
Emend *Cap:* 40, 80, 125 mg (2 x 80 mg bi-fold pck; 1 x 25 mg/2 x 80 mg tri-fold pck); *Oral susp:* 125 mg pwdr for oral suspension, single-dose pouch w. dispenser; *Vial:* 150 mg pwdr for reconstitution and IV infusion

SUBSTANCE P/NEUROKININ-1 (NK-1) RECEPTOR ANTAGONIST AND SEROTONIN-3 (5-HT3) RECEPTOR ANTAGONIST COMBINATION

▷ *fosnetupitant+palonosetron*

Comment: **Akynzeo** capsules and **Akynzeo for Injection** are indicated in combination with *dexamethasone* for the prevention of acute and delayed nausea and vomiting associated with initial and repeat courses of cancer chemotherapy. The most common adverse reactions (incidence ≥3%) are headache, asthenia, dyspepsia, fatigue, constipation, and erythema. Avoid concomitant CYP3A4 substrates for one week; if not avoidable, consider dose reduction of the CYP3A4 substrate because inhibition of CYP3A4 by *netupitant* can result in increased plasma concentrations of the concomitant drug for 6 days after single dosage administration of **Akynzeo**. CYP3A4 inducers (e.g., *rifampin*) decrease plasma concentrations of *netupitant*.

Pediatric: <18 years: not recommended; ≥18 years: same as adult

Akynzeo administer a single dose approximately 1 hour prior to the start of chemotherapy, with or without food, with concurrent administration of *dexamethasone* 12 mg; on days 2-4, omit *dexamethasone*

Cap: netu 300 mg+palo 0.5 mg

Akynzeo for Injection reconstitute in 50 ml of D$_5$ 0.9% NaCl and administer via IV infusion over 30 minutes starting approximately 30 minutes prior to the start of chemotherapy with concurrent administration of *dexamethasone* 12 mg; on days 2-4, decrease *dexamethasone* to 8 mg each day

Vial: fosn 235 mg+palo 0.25 mg single-dose pwdr for reconstitution and IV infusion

5HT-3 RECEPTOR ANTAGONISTS

Comment: The selective 5HT-3 receptor antagonists indicated for prevention of nausea and vomiting associated with moderately to highly emetogenic chemotherapy.

▷ *dolasetron* (B) administer 100 mg IV over 30 seconds, 30 min prior to administration of chemotherapy or 2 hours before surgery; max 100 mg/dose

Pediatric: <2 years: not recommended; 2-16 years: 1.8 mg/kg; >16 years: same as adult

Anzemet *Tab:* 50, 100 mg; *Amp:* 12.5 mg/0.625 ml; *Prefilled carpuject syringe:* 12.5 mg (0.625 ml); *Vial:* 100 mg/5 ml (single-use); *Vial:* 500 mg/25 ml (multidose)

▷ *granisetron*

Kytril (B) 10 mcg/kg as a single dose; administer IV over 30 seconds, 30 min prior to administration of chemotherapy; max 1 dose/week

Pediatric: <2 years: not recommended; ≥2 years: same as adult

Tab: 1 mg; *Oral soln:* 2 mg/10 ml (30 ml; orange); *Vial:* 1 mg/ml (1 ml single-dose) (preservative-free); 1 mg/ml (4 ml multi-dose) (benzyl alcohol)

Sancuso (B) apply 1 patch 24-48 hours before chemo; remove 24 hours (minimum) to 7 days (maximum) after completion of treatment

Pediatric: <2 years: not recommended; ≥2 years: same as adult

Transdermal patch: 3.1 mg/day

▷ *granisetron extended release injection* administer SC over 20-30 seconds (due to drug viscosity) on Day 1 of chemotherapy and not more frequently than once every 7 days; *CrCl 30-59 mL/min:* repeat dose no more than every 14th day; *CrCl <30 mL/min:* not recommended; for patients receiving MEC, the recommended *dexamethasone* dosage is 8 mg IV on Day 1; for patients receiving AC combination chemotherapy regimens, the recommended *dexamethasone* dosage is 20 mg IV on Day 1, followed by 8 mg PO bid on Days 2, 3 and 4; if **Sustol** is administered with an NK$_1$ receptor antagonist, see that drug's mfr pkg insert for the recommended **dexamethasone** dosing

Pediatric: <18 years: not recommended; ≥18 years: same as adult

> **Sustol** *Syringe:* 10 mg/0.4 ml ext-rel; prefilled single-dose/kit
> Comment: At least 60 minutes prior to administration, remove the **Sustol** kit from refrigeration; activate a warming pouch and wrap the syringe in the warming pouch for 5-6 minutes to warm it to room temperature.

▷ *ondansetron* (C)(G) Oral Forms: *Highly emetogenic chemotherapy:* 24 mg x 1 dose 30 min prior to start of single-day chemotherapy; *Moderately emetogenic chemotherapy:* 8 mg q 8 hours x 2 doses beginning 30 minutes prior to start of chemotherapy; then 8 mg q 12 hours x 1-2 days following

Pediatric: <4 years: not recommended; 4-11 years: *Moderately emetogenic chemotherapy:* 4 mg q 4 hours x 3 doses beginning 30 min prior to start; then 4 mg q 8 hours x 1-2 days following

> **Zofran** *Tab:* 4, 8, 24 mg
> **Zofran ODT** *ODT:* 4, 8 mg (strawberry) (phenylalanine)
> **Zofran Oral Solution** *Oral soln:* 4 mg/5 ml (50 ml) (strawberry) (phenylalanine); *Parenteral form:* see mfr pkg insert
> **Zofran Injection** *Vial:* 2 mg/ml (2 ml single-dose); 2 mg/ml (20 ml multi-dose); 32 mg/50 ml (50 ml multidose); *Prefilled syringe:* 4 mg/2 ml, single-use (24/carton)
> **Zuplenz Oral Soluble Film:** 4, 8 mg oral-dis (10/carton) (peppermint)
> Comment: The FDA has issued a warning against *ondansetron* use in pregnancy *ondansetron* is a 5-HT3 receptor antagonist approved by the FDA for preventing nausea and vomiting related to cancer chemotherapy and surgery. However, it has been used "off label" to treat the nausea and vomiting of pregnancy. The FDA has cautioned against the use of *ondansetron* in pregnancy in light of studies of *ondansetron* in early pregnancy and associated with congenital cardiac malformations and oral clefts (i.e., cleft lip and cleft palate). Further, there are potential maternal risks in pregnancy with electrolyte imbalance caused by severe nausea and vomiting (as with hyperemesis gravidarum). These risks include *serotonin syndrome* (a triad of of cognitive and behavioral changes including confusion, agitation, autonomic instability, and neuromuscular changes). Therefore, *ondansetron* should <u>not</u> be taken during pregnancy.

▷ *palonosetron* (B)(G) *Chemotherapy:* administer 0.25 mg IV over 30 seconds, 30 min prior to administration of chemo; max 1 dose/week <u>or</u> 1 cap 1 hour before chemo; *Post-op:* administer 0.075 mg IV over 10 seconds immediately before induction of anesthesia

Pediatric: <1 month: not recommended; 1 month-17 years: 20 mcg/kg; max 1.5 mg single dose; infuse over 15 minutes beginning 30 minutes prior to administration of chemo

> **Aloxi** *Vial (single-use):* 0.075 mg/1.5 ml; 0.25 mg/5 ml (mannitol)

CANNABINOIDS

▷ *dronabinol* (C)(III) initially 5 mg/m^2 1-3 hours before chemotherapy; then q 2-4 hours prn; max 4-6 doses/day, 15 mg/m^2

Pediatric: <18 years: not recommended; ≥18 years: same as adult

> **Marinol** *Cap:* 2.5, 5, 10 mg (sesame seed oil)

▷ *nabilone* (C)(II) 1-2 mg bid; max 6 mg/day in 3 divided doses; initially 1-3 hours before chemotherapy; may give 1-2 mg the night before chemo; may continue 48 hours after each chemo cycle

Pediatric: <18 years: not recommended; ≥18 years: same as adult

> **Cesamet** *Cap:* 1 mg (sesame seed oil)

CHICKENPOX (VARICELLA)

PROPHYLAXIS

▶ *Varicella virus* vaccine, live, attenuated **(C)**

Varivax 0.5 ml SC; repeat 4-8 weeks later

Pediatric: <12 months: not recommended; 12 months-12 years: 1 dose of
0.5 ml SC; repeat 4-6 weeks later

Vial: 1350 PFU/0.5 ml single-dose w. diluent (preservative-free)

Comment: Administer **Varivax** SC in the deltoid for adults and children.

IMMUNE GLOBULIN

▶ *immune globulin (human)* administer via intramuscular injection <u>only</u> (<u>never</u>
intravenously); ensure adequate hydration prior to administration

Household and Institutional Varicella Case Contacts: promptly administer 0.6-1.2
ml/kg IM as a single dose (if Varicella-Zoster Immune Globulin (Human) is
unavailable

Planned Travel to Varicella Endemic Area: administer 0.6-1.2 ml/kg as a single
dose at least 6 days prior to travel (if Varicella-Zoster Immune Globulin (Human)
is unavailable

Pediatric: 0.25 ml/kg IM (0.5 mg/kg in immunocompromised children)

GamaSTAN S/D *Vial:* 2, 10 ml single-dose

Comment: **GamaSTAN S/D** is the <u>only</u> *gammaglobulin* product FDA-
approved for measles and HAV post-exposure prophylaxis (PEP). **GamaSTAN
S/D** is also FDA-approved for varicella post-exposure prophylaxis (PEP).
Other **GamaSTAN S/D** indications: to prevent <u>or</u> modify measles in a
susceptible person exposed fewer than 6 days previously; to modify varicella;
to modify rubella in exposed women who will <u>not</u> consider a therapeutic
abortion. **GamaSTAN S/D** is <u>not</u> indicated for routine prophylaxis <u>or</u>
treatment of viral hepatitis B, rubella, poliomyelitis, mumps <u>or</u> varicella.
Contraindications to **GamaSTAN S/D** include persons with cancer, chronic
liver disease, and persons allergic to *gammaglobulin*, the HAV vaccine,
<u>or</u> a component of the HAV vaccine. Dosage is higher for HAV PEP than
for measles and varicella PEP based on recently observed decreasing
concentrations of HAV antibodies in **GamaSTAN S/D**, attributed to the
decreasing prevalence of previous HAV infection among plasma donors.

TREATMENT

Antipyretics *see Fever*
Infants and young children: No aspirin

ORAL ANTIPRURITICS

▶ *diphenhydramine* **(B)(OTC)(G)** 25-50 mg q 6-8 hours; max 100 mg/day

Pediatric: <2 years: not recommended; 2-6 years: 6.25 mg q 4-6 hours; max
37.5 mg/day; >6-12 years: 12.5-25 mg q 4-6 hours; max 150 mg/day; >12 years:
same as adult

Benadryl (OTC) *Chew tab:* 12.5 mg (grape; phenylalanine); *Liq:* 12.5
mg/5 ml (4, 8 oz); *Cap:* 25 mg; *Tab:* 25 mg; *dye-free soft gel:* 25 mg; *Dye-free
liq:* 12.5 mg/5 ml (4, 8 oz)

▶ *hydroxyzine* **(C)(G)** 50-100 mg qid; max 600 mg/day

Pediatric: <6 years: 50 mg/day divided qid; ≥6 years: 50-100 mg/day divided qid

AtaraxR *Tab:* 10, 25, 50, 100 mg; *Syr:* 10 mg/5 ml (alcohol 0.5%)

Vistaril *Cap:* 25, 50, 100 mg; *Oral susp:* 25 mg/5 ml (4 oz) (lemon)

ANTIVIRALS

▶ *acyclovir* **(B)(G)** 800 mg qid x 5 days

Pediatric: <2 years: not recommended; ≥2 years, <40 kg: 20 mg/kg qid x 5 days; ≥2 years, >40 kg: 800 mg qid x 5 days; *see* Appendix CC.1. *ayclovir* (Zovirax Suspension) *for dose by weight*

Zovirax *Cap:* 200 mg; *Tab:* 400, 800 mg
Zovirax Oral Suspension *Oral susp:* 200 mg/5 ml (banana)

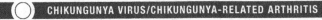

CHIKUNGUNYA VIRUS/CHIKUNGUNYA-RELATED ARTHRITIS

Comment: Chikungunya is a mosquito-borne viral disease first described during an outbreak in southern Tanzania in 1952. It is an RNA virus that belongs to the alphavirus genus of the family *Togaviridae*. The name "chikungunya" derives from a word in the Kimakonde language, meaning "to become contorted," and describes the stooped appearance of sufferers with joint pain (arthralgia). Acute infection with *chikungunya virus* is associated with fever, rash, headache, and muscle and joint pain, with outbreaks having been reported in Africa, Asia, the Indian and Pacific Ocean islands, and Europe. In 2013, for the first time the virus was first detected in the Caribbean region, and more than 1.2 million peoples in the Americas have now been infected. After transmission by an *Aedes aegypti* or *Aedes albopictus* mosquito bite, *chikungunya virus* undergoes local replication and then dissemination to lymphoid tissue," the researchers explained. Viremia is detectable for only 5 to 12 days, but animal studies have indicated that the virus can be found in lymphoid organs, joints, and muscles for several months and that viral RNA can be detected in muscle, liver, and spleen for long periods. But it is not known whether the remnants of the virus actually persist in humans and, if so, whether this can be causatively linked with chronic arthritis, which has implications for treatment. With no evidence of viral persistence, potential mechanisms for arthritis included epigenetic changes to host DNA, as has been observed with *Epstein Barr virus* infection, modification of macrophages, and molecular mimicry. There is currently no cure and no standard treatment for acute *chikungunya virus* infection or chikungunya-related arthritis, but various immunosuppressants such as ***methotrexate*** (**MTX**) and ***hydroxychloroquine*** and biologics such as ***adalimumab*** (**Humira**) and *etanercept* (**Enbrel**) have been tried, despite concerns of renewed viral replication in the synovium and relapse of systemic viral infection. However, no relapses have been reported, and the lack of evidence of viral persistence in the joint seen in this analysis may provide some reassurance that treatment with immunosuppressant anti-rheumatic medications 2 years after infection is a viable option.

CHLAMYDIA TRACHOMATIS

Comment: The following treatment regimens for *C. trachomatis* are published in the **2015 CDC Sexually Transmitted Diseases Treatment Guidelines**. Treatment regimens are presented by generic drug name first, followed by information about brands and dose forms. Treat all sexual contacts. Patients who are HIV-positive should receive the same treatment as those who are HIV-negative. Sexual abuse must be considered a cause of chlamydial infection in preadolescent children, although perinatally transmitted *C. trachomatis* infections of the nasopharynx, urogenital tract, and rectum may persist for >1 year.

RECOMMENDED REGIMENS: ADOLESCENT & >18 YEARS, NON-PREGNANT
Regimen 1
➢ *azithromycin* 1 gm in a single dose

Regimen 2
➢ *doxycycline* 100 mg bid x 7 days

ALTERNATIVE REGIMENS: ADOLESCENT AND ADULT, NON-PREGNANT
Regimen 1
▷ *erythromycin base* 500 mg qid x 7 days

Regimen 2
▷ *erythromycin ethylsuccinate* 800 mg qid x 7 days

Regimen 3
▷ *levofloxacin* 500 mg once daily x 7 days

Regimen 4
▷ *ofloxacin* 300 mg bid x 7 days

RECOMMENDED REGIMENS: PREGNANCY
Regimen 1
▷ *azithromycin* 1 gm in a single dose

Regimen 2
▷ *amoxicillin* 500 mg tid x 7 days

ALTERNATE REGIMENS: PREGNANCY
Regimen 1
▷ *erythromycin base* 500 mg qid x 7 days

Regimen 2
▷ *erythromycin base* 250 mg qid x 14 days

Regimen 3
▷ *erythromycin ethylsuccinate* 800 mg qid x 7 days

Regimen 4
▷ *erythromycin ethylsuccinate* 400 mg qid x 14 days

ALTERNATE REGIMENS: CHILDREN (>8 YEARS)
Regimen 1
▷ *azithromycin* 1 gm in a single dose

Regimen 2
▷ *doxycycline* 100 mg bid x 7 days

ALTERNATE REGIMEN: CHILDREN (>45 KG; <8 YEARS)
Regimen 1
▷ *azithromycin* 1 gm in a single dose

ALTERNATE REGIMENS: INFANTS
Regimen 1
▷ *erythromycin base* 50 mg/kg/day in divided doses qid x 14 days

Regimen 2
▷ *erythromycin ethylsuccinate* 50 mg/kg/day divided qid x 14 days

DRUG BRANDS AND DOSE FORMS
▷ *azithromycin* (B)(G) 500 mg x 1 dose on day 1, then 250 mg daily on days 2-5 or 500 mg daily x 3 days or **Zmax** 2 gm in a single dose

Pediatric: 12 mg/kg/day x 5 days; max 500 mg/day; *see* Appendix CC.7.
azithromycin (Zithromax Suspension, Zmax Suspension) *for dose by weight*
> **Zithromax** *Tab:* 250, 500, 600 mg; *Oral susp:* 100 mg/5 ml (15 ml);
> 200 mg/5 ml (15, 22.5, 30 ml) (cherry); *Pkt:* 1 gm for reconstitution
> (cherry-banana)
> **Zithromax Tri-pak** *Tab:* 3 x 500 mg tabs/pck
> **Zithromax Z-pak** *Tab:* 6 x 250 mg tabs/pck
> **Zmax** *Oral susp:* 2 gm ext-rel for reconstitution (cherry-banana) (148 mg Na⁺)

▷ *doxycycline* (D)(G)
> **Acticlate** *Tab:* 75, 150**mg
> **Adoxa** *Tab:* 50, 75, 100, 150 mg ent-coat
> **Doryx** *Tab:* 50, 75, 100, 150, 200 mg del-rel
> **Doxteric** *Tab:* 50 mg del-rel
> **Monodox** *Cap:* 50, 75, 100 mg
> **Oracea** *Cap:* 40 mg del-rel
> **Vibramycin** *Tab:* 100 mg; *Cap:* 50, 100 mg; *Syr:* 50 mg/5 ml (raspberry-apple)
> (sulfites); *Oral susp:* 25 mg/5 ml (raspberry)
> **Vibra-Tab** *Tab:* 100 mg film-coat

▷ *erythromycin base* (B)(G)
> **Ery-Tab** *Tab:* 250, 333, 500 mg ent-coat
> **PCE** *Tab:* 333, 500 mg

▷ *erythromycin ethylsuccinate* (B)(G)
> **EryPed** *Oral susp:* 200 mg/5 ml (100, 200 ml) (fruit); 400 mg/5 ml (60, 100,
> 200 ml) (banana); *Oral drops:* 200, 400 mg/5 ml (50 ml) (fruit); *Chew tab:* 200
> mg wafer (fruit)
> **E.E.S.** *Oral susp:* 200, 400 mg/5 ml (100 ml) (fruit)
> **E.E.S. Granules** *Oral susp:* 200 mg/5 ml (100, 200 ml) (cherry)
> **E.E.S. 400 Tablets** *Tab:* 400 mg

▷ *levofloxacin* (C)
> **Levaquin** *Tab:* 250, 500, 750 mg

▷ *ofloxacin* (C)(G)
> **Floxin** *Tab:* 200, 300, 400 mg

CHOLANGITIS, PRIMARY BILIARY (PBC)

Comment: Monitor intensity of pruritis and administer antihistamines as
appropriate for dermal pruritis. **Ocaliva** *(obeticholic acid)*, a farnesoid X receptor
(FXR) agonist, is indicated for the treatment of primary biliary cholangitis (PBC),
in combination with ***ursodeoxycholic acid*** (UDCA), in adults with an inadequate
response to UDCA, or as monotherapy in adults unable to tolerate UDCA. This
indication is approved under accelerated approval based on a reduction in alkaline
phosphatase (ALP). An improvement in survival or disease-related symptoms has
not been established. Continued approval for this indication may be contingent
upon verification and description of clinical benefit in confirmatory trials.

FARNESOID X RECEPTOR (FXR) AGONIST

▷ *obeticholic acid* initially 5 mg once daily (this lower starting dose is
recommended to reduce pruritis); then after 3 months of treatment, if an
adequate reduction in ALP and/or total bilirubin is not achieved, and if the
patient is tolerating the drug, increase the dose to 10 mg once daily; take with or
without food
Pediatric: <18 years: not recommended; ≥18 years: same as adult
> **Ocaliva** *Tab:* 5, 10 mg
> **Comment: Ocalvia** is contraindicated in patients with complete biliary
> obstruction. If this complication develops, discontinue **Ocaliva**. Because PBC

management strategies include bile acid binding resin (e.g., *cholestyramine, colestipol, or colesevelam*), concurrent use with *obeticholic acid* should be separated by at least 4 hours. Concurrent use of *obeticholic acid* and *warfarin* may reduce the international normalized ratio (INR), monitor INR and adjust the *warfarin* dose as necessary. Monitor concentrations of CYP1A2 substrates with a narrow therapeutic index (e.g., *theophylline* and *tizanidine*) as *obeticholic acid* a CYP1A2 inhibitor). Reduce the dose of **Ocaliva** in patients with moderate or severe hepatic impairment, and monitor LFTs and lipid levels (especially reduction in HDL).

URSODEOXYCHOLIC ACID (UDCA)

▷ *ursodeoxycholic acid* (UDCA) **(G)** in the first 3 months of treatment, the total daily dose should be divided tid (morning, midday, evening); as liver function values improve, the total daily dose may be taken once a day at bedtime (see mfr pkg insert for dose table based on kilograms weight); monitor hepatic function every 4 weeks for the first 3 months; then, monitor hepatic function once every 3 months
Pediatric: same as adult

Ursofalk *Tab:* 500 mg film-coat; *Cap:* 250 mg, *Oral susp:* 250 mg/5 ml
Comment: *Ursodeoxycholic acid* (UDCA) is indicated for the dissolution of cholesterol gall stones that are radioluscent (not visible on plain x-ray), ≤15 mm, and the gall bladder must still be functioning despite the gall stones.

BILE ACID BINDING RESINS

Comment: This drug class may produce or severely worsen pre-existing constipation. The dosage should be increased gradually in patients to minimize the risk of developing fecal impaction. Increased fluid and fiber intake should be encouraged to alleviate constipation and a stool softener may occasionally be indicated. If the initial dose is well tolerated, the dose may be increased as needed by one dose/day (at monthly intervals) with periodic monitoring of serum lipoproteins. If constipation worsens or the desired therapeutic response is not achieved at one to six doses/day, combination therapy or alternate therapy should be considered. Bile acid sequestrants may decrease absorption of fat-soluble vitamins. Use caution in patients susceptible to fat-soluble vitamin deficiencies.

▷ *cholestyramine* (C)(G) starting dose: 1 packet or 1 scoopful of powder once daily for 5 to 7 days; then, increase to twice daily with monitoring of constipation and of serum lipoproteins, at least twice, 4 to 6 weeks apart; empty one packet into a glass or cup; add 1/2 to 1 cup (4 to 8 ounces) of water, fruit juice, or diet soft drink; stir well and drink immediately; do not swallow dry form; take with meals
Pediatric: 240 mg/kg/day of anhydrous cholestyramine resin in two to three divided doses, normally not to exceed 8 gm/day with dose titration based on response and tolerance.

Prevalite *Pwdr:* 4 gm/pkt, 4 gm/scoopful (1 level tsp) for oral suspension
▷ *colestipol* (C)(G)
Starting dose tabs: 2 gm once or twice daily; then, increases should occur at 1 or 2 month intervals; usual dose is 2 to 16 gm/day given once daily or in divided doses *Starting dose granules:* 1 packet or 1 scoopful (1 level tsp) of granules once daily for 5 to 7 days, increasing to twice daily with monitoring of constipation and of serum lipoproteins, at least twice, 4 to 6 weeks apart; empty one packet or one scoopful (1 level tsp) of granules into a glass or cup; add 1/2 to 1 cup (4 to 8 ounces) of water, fruit juice, or diet soft drink; stir well and drink immediately; do not swallow dry form; take with meals
Pediatric: <12 years: not established; ≥12 years: same as adult

Colestid *Tab:* 1 gm; *Granules:* 5 gm/pkt, 5 gm/scoopful (1 level tsp) for oral suspension
Flavored Colestid *Granules:* 5 gm/pkt, 5 gm/scoopful (1 level tsp) for oral suspension (orange)

▷ **colesevelam** (B)(G)
WelChol recommended dose is 6 tablets once daily or 3 tablets twice daily; take
with a meal and liquid
Pediatric: <10 years: not recommended; ≥10 years: same as adult
  Tab: 625 mg
WelChol for Oral Suspension recommended dose is one 3.75 gm packet once
daily or one 1.875 gm packet twice daily; empty one packet into a glass or cup;
add 1/2 to 1 cup (4 to 8 ounces) of water, fruit juice, or diet soft drink; stir well
and drink immediately; do not swallow dry form; take with meals
Pediatric: <12 years: not established; ≥12 years: same as adult
  Pwdr: 3.75 gm/pkt (30 pkt/carton), 1.875 gm/pkt (60 pkt/carton) for oral
  suspension
Comment: **WelChol** is indicated as adjunctive therapy to improve glycemic
control in adults with type 2 diabetes. It can be added to *metformin*, sulfonylureas,
or insulin alone or in combination with other antidiabetic agents.

CHOLELITHIASIS

▷ **ursodeoxycholic acid** (UDCA) (G) in the first 3 months of treatment, the total daily
dose should be divided tid (morning, midday, evening); as liver function values
improve, the total daily dose may be taken once a day at bedtime; (see mfr pkg
insert for dose table based on kilograms weight); monitor hepatic function every 4
weeks for the first 3 months; then, monitor hepatic function once every 3 months
Pediatric: same as adult
  Ursofalk *Tab:* 500 mg film-coat; *Cap:* 250 mg, *Oral susp:* 250 mg/5 ml
  Comment: *Ursodeoxycholic* (UDCA) is indicated for the dissolution of cholesterol
  gall stones that are radioluscent (not visible on plain x-ray), ≤15 mm, and the gall
  bladder must still be functioning despite the gall stones
▷ **ursodiol** (B) 8-10 mg/kg/day in 2-3 divided doses
Pediatric: <12 years: not recommended; ≥12 years: same as adult
  Actigall *Cap:* 300 mg
  Comment: **Actigall** is indicated for the dissolution of radiolucent,
  noncalciferous, gallstones <20 mm in diameter and for prevention of
  gallstones during rapid weight loss.

BILE ACID BINDING RESINS

Comment: This drug class may produce or severely worsen pre-existing constipation.
The dosage should be increased gradually in patients to minimize the risk of
developing fecal impaction. Increased fluid and fiber intake should be encouraged
to alleviate constipation and a stool softener may occasionally be indicated. If the
initial dose is well tolerated, the dose may be increased as needed by one dose/day (at
monthly intervals) with periodic monitoring of serum lipoproteins. If constipation
worsens or the desired therapeutic response is not achieved at one to six doses/day,
combination therapy or alternate therapy should be considered. Bile acid sequestrants
may decrease absorption of fat-soluble vitamins. Use caution in patients susceptible
to fat-soluble vitamin deficiencies.
▷ **cholestyramine** (C)(G) starting dose: 1 packet or 1 scoopful of powder once daily
for 5 to 7 days; then, increase to twice daily with monitoring of constipation and
of serum lipoproteins, at least twice, 4 to 6 weeks apart; empty one packet into
a glass or cup; add 1/2 to 1 cup (4 to 8 ounces) of water, fruit juice, or diet soft
drink; stir well and drink immediately; do not swallow dry form; take with meals
Pediatric: <12 years: 240 mg/kg/day of anhydrous cholestyramine resin in 2 to
3 divided doses, normally not to exceed 8 gm/day with dose titration based on
response and tolerance.
  Prevalite *Pwdr:* 4 gm/pkt, 4 gm/scoopful (1 level tsp) for oral suspension

▷ *colestipol* (C)(G)

Starting dose tabs: 2 gm once <u>or</u> twice daily; then, increases should occur at one <u>or</u> two month intervals; usual dose is 2 to 16 gm/day given once daily <u>or</u> in divided doses

Starting dose granules: 1 packet <u>or</u> 1 scoopful (1 level tsp) of granules once daily for 5 to 7 days, increasing to twice daily with monitoring of constipation and of serum lipoproteins, at least twice, 4 to 6 weeks apart; empty one packet <u>or</u> one scoopful (1 level tsp) of granules into a glass <u>or</u> cup; add 1/2 to 1 cup (4 to 8 ounces) of water, fruit juice, <u>or</u> diet soft drink; stir well and drink immediately; do <u>not</u> swallow dry form; take with meals

Pediatric: <12 years: not established; ≥12 years: same as adult

  Colestid *Tab:* 1 gm; *Granules:* 5 gm/pkt, 5 gm/scoopful (1 level tsp) for oral suspension

  Flavored Colestid *Granules:* 5 gm/pkt, 5 gm/scoopful (1 level tsp) for oral suspension (orange)

▷ *colesevelam* (B)(G)

WelChol recommended dose is 6 tablets once daily <u>or</u> 3 tablets twice daily; take with a meal and liquid

Pediatric: <10 years: not recommended; ≥10 years: same as adult

  Tab: 625 mg

WelChol for Oral Suspension recommended dose is one 3.75 gm packet once daily <u>or</u> one 1.875 gm packet twice daily; empty one packet into a glass <u>or</u> cup; add 1/2 to 1 cup (4 to 8 ounces) of water, fruit juice, <u>or</u> diet soft drink; stir well and drink immediately; do <u>not</u> swallow dry form; take with meals

Pediatric: <12 years: not established; ≥12 years: same as adult

  Pwdr: 3.75 gm/pkt (30 pkt/carton), 1.875 gm/pkt (60 pkt/carton) for oral suspension

Comment: **WelChol** is indicated as adjunctive therapy to improve glycemic control in adults with type 2 diabetes. It can be added to *metformin*, sulfonylureas, <u>or</u> insulin alone <u>or</u> in combination with other antidiabetic agents.

 CHOLERA (*VIBRIO CHOLERAE*)

Comment: On June 10, 2016, the FDA approved the first vaccine for the prevention of cholera caused by serogroup O1 (the most predominant cause of cholera globally [WHO]) in adults age 18-64 years traveling to cholera-affected areas. https://www.drugs.com/newdrugs/fda-approves-vaxchora-cholera-vaccine-live-oral-prevent-cholera-travelers-4396.html. **Vaxchora** (R) is the <u>only</u> FDA approved vaccine for the prevention of cholera. The bacterium *Vibrio cholerae* is acquired by ingesting contaminated water <u>or</u> food and causes nausea, vomiting, and watery diarrhea that may be mild to severe. Profuse fluid loss may cause life-threatening dehydration if antibiotics and fluid replacement are <u>not</u> initiated promptly.

VACCINE PROPHYLAXIS

▷ *Vibrio cholerae* vaccine

  Vaxchora reconstitute the buffer component in 100 ml purified bottled water; then add the active component (lyophilized V. cholerae CVD 103-HgR); total dose after reconstitution is 100 ml; instruct the patient to avoid eating <u>or</u> drinking fluids for 60 minutes before and after ingestion of the dose

  Comment: **Vaxchora** is a live, attenuated vaccine that is taken as a single oral dose at least 10 days before travel to a cholera-affected area and at least 10 days before starting antimalarial prophylaxis. Diminished immune response when taken concomitantly with *chloroquine*. Avoid concomitant administration with systemic antibiotics since these agents may be active against the vaccine strain. Do <u>not</u> administer to patients who have received an oral <u>or</u> parental antibiotic within 14 days prior to vaccination. **Vaxchora** may be shed in the stool of recipients for at least 7 days. There is potential for transmission of the vaccine strain to non-vaccinated and immunocompromised close contacts. The CDC and several health professional organizations state that vaccines given to a nursing mother do not affect the safety of breastfeeding for mothers or infants and that breastfeeding is not a contraindication to cholera vaccine. **Vaxchora** is not absorbed systemically, and maternal use is not expected to result in fetal exposure to the drug. The **Vaxchora** pregnancy exposure registry for reporting adverse events is 800-533-5899. There are 0 disease interactions, but at least 165 drug-drug interactions with **Vaxchora** (see mfr pkg insert).

TREATMENT

Comment: The first-line treatment for *V. cholerae* is oral rehydration therapy (ORT) and intravenous fluid replacement as indicated. Antibiotic therapy may shorten the duration and severity of symptoms but is optional in other than severe cases. Although *doxycycline* is contraindicated in pregnancy and in children under 7 years-of-age, the benefits may outweigh the risks (WHO, CDC, UNICEF). Although *ciprofloxacin* is contraindicated in children under 18 years-of-age, the benefits may outweigh the risks (WHO, CDC, UNICEF). Cholera is not transmitted from person to person, but rather the fecal-oral route. Therefore, chemoprophylaxis is not usually required with strict hand hygiene and sanitation measures, and avoidance of contaminated food and water. Drugs and dosages for chemoprophylaxis are the same as for treatment.

NON-PREGNANT FEMALES ≥15 YEARS
Regimen 1
▷ *doxycycline* (D)(G) 300 mg in a single dose
    Acticlate *Tab:* 75, 150**mg
    Adoxa *Tab:* 50, 75, 100, 150 mg ent-coat
    Doryx *Tab:* 50, 75, 100, 150, 200 mg del-rel
    Doxteric *Tab:* 50 mg del-rel
    Monodox *Cap:* 50, 75, 100 mg
    Oracea *Cap:* 40 mg del-rel
    Vibramycin *Tab:* 100 mg; *Cap:* 50, 100 mg; *Syr:* 50 mg/ml (raspberry-apple) (sulfites); *Oral susp:* 25 mg/5 ml (raspberry)
    Vibra-Tab *Tab:* 100 mg film-coat

Regimen 2
▷ *azithromycin* (B)(G) 1000 mg in a single dose
    Zithromax *Tab:* 250, 500, 600 mg
    Zmax *Oral susp:* 2 gm ext-rel for reconstitution (cherry-banana) (148 mg Na⁺)
    or
▷ *ciprofloxacin* (C)(G) 1000 mg in a single dose
    Cipro *Tab:* 250, 500, 750 mg;
    Cipro XR *Tab:* 500, 1000 mg ext-rel
    ProQuin XR *Tab:* 500 mg ext-rel

PREGNANT FEMALES ≥15 YEARS
▷ *azithromycin* (B)(G) 1000 mg in a single dose
    Zithromax *Tab:* 250, 500, 600 mg
    Zmax *Oral susp:* 2 gm ext-rel for reconstitution (cherry-banana) (148 mg Na⁺)
    or
▷ *erythromycin* (B)(G) 500 mg q 6 hours x 3 days
    E.E.S. 400 Tablets *Tab:* 400 mg
    Ery-Tab *Tab:* 250, 333, 500 mg ent-coat
    PCE *Tab:* 333, 500 mg

CHILDREN 3-15 YEARS WHO CAN SWALLOW TABLETS
Regimen 1
▷ *erythromycin* (B)(G) 12.5 mg/kg q 6 hours x 3 days
    E.E.S. 400 Tablets *Tab:* 400 mg
    Ery-Tab *Tab:* 250, 333, 500 mg ent-coat
    PCE *Tab:* 333, 500 mg
      or
▷ *azithromycin* (B)(G) 20 mg/kg in a single dose; max 1 gm
    Zithromax *Tab:* 250, 500, 600 mg
    Zmax *Oral susp:* 2 gm ext-rel for reconstitution (cherry-banana) (148 mg Na⁺)

Regimen 2
▷ *ciprofloxacin* (D)(G) <18 years usually not recommended; *erythromycin* or
  azithromycin preferred; consider risk/benefit; 20 mg/kg in a single dose
  Cipro *Tab:* 250, 500, 750 mg;
    Cipro XR *Tab:* 500, 1000 mg ext-rel
    ProQuin XR *Tab:* 500 mg ext-rel
      or
▷ *doxycycline* (D)(G) <8 years usually not recommended; *erythromycin* or
  azithromycin preferred; consider risk benefit; >8 years: 2-4 mg/kg in a single dose
  Acticlate *Tab:* 75, 150**mg
    Adoxa *Tab:* 50, 75, 100, 150 mg ent-coat
    Doryx *Tab:* 50, 75, 100, 150, 200 mg del-rel
    Doxteric *Tab:* 50 mg del-rel
    Monodox *Cap:* 50, 75, 100 mg
    Oracea *Cap:* 40 mg del-rel
    Vibramycin *Tab:* 100 mg; *Cap:* 50, 100 mg; *Syr:* 50 mg/ml (raspberry-apple)
    (sulfites); *Oral susp:* 25 mg/5 ml (raspberry)
    Vibra-Tab *Tab:* 100 mg film-coat

CHILDREN <3 YEARS
Regimen 1
▷ *erythromycin ethylsuccinate* (B)(G) 12.5 mg/kg q 6 hours x 3 days; use suspension
    E.E.S. *Oral susp:* 200, 400 mg/5 ml (100 ml) (fruit)
    E.E.S. Granules *Oral susp:* 200 mg/5 ml (100, 200 ml) (cherry, fruit); *Chew*
    tab: 200 mg wafer (fruit)
    EryPed *Oral susp:* 200 mg/5 ml (100, 200 ml) (fruit); 400 mg/5 ml (60, 100,
    200 ml) (banana); *Oral drops:* 200, 400 mg/5 ml (50 ml) (fruit); *Chew tab:*
    200 mg wafer (fruit)
      or
▷ *azithromycin* (B)(G) 20 mg/kg in a single dose; max 1 gm; use suspension
    Zithromax *Tab:* 250, 500, 600 mg; *Oral susp:* 100 mg/5 ml (15 ml); 200 mg/5 ml
    (15, 22.5, 30 ml) (cherry)
    Zmax *Oral susp:* 2 gm ext-rel for reconstitution (cherry-banana) (148 mg Na⁺)

Regimen 2
▷ *ciprofloxacin* (C)(G) <18 years usually not recommended; *erythromycin* or
  azithromycin preferred; consider risk benefit; 20 mg/kg in a single dose; use
  suspension
    Cipro *Oral susp:* 250, 500 mg/5 ml (100 ml) (strawberry)
      or
▷ *doxycycline* (D)(G) <8 years usually not recommended; *erythromycin* or
  azithromycin preferred; consider risk benefit; 2-4 mg/kg in a single dose; use
  suspension or syrup
    Vibramycin *Syr:* 50 mg/5 ml (raspberry-apple) (sulfites); *Oral susp:* 25 mg/5
    ml (raspberry)

Comment: Acid-suppressing drugs including proton pump inhibitors (PPIs), third- and fourth-generation cephalosporins, carbapenems, and **piperacillin-tazobactam** significantly increase the risk of hospital-onset *Clostridioides difficile* infection (CDI), according to the results of a recent study. Patients who received tetracyclines, macrolides, or **clindamycin** had lower risk of developing hospital-onset CDI.

MACROLIDE ANTIBACTERIAL AGENT

▷ *fidaxomicin* (B) 200 mg bid x 10 days with or without food.
   Pediatric: <18 years: not established; ≥18 years: same as adult
   Dificid *Tab:* 200 mg film-coat
   Comment: Dificid *(fidaxomicin)* is a macrolide antibacterial agent, FDA-approved for treatment of *C. difficile*–associated diarrhea (CDAD). **Dificid** should not be used for treatment of systemic infections. Only use **Dificid** for infection proven or strongly suspected to be caused by *C. difficile*. Prescribing **Dificid** in the absence of a proven or strongly suspected *C. difficile* infection is unlikely to provide benefit to the patient and increases the risk of development of drug-resistant bacteria. Acute hypersensitivity reactions, including dyspnea, rash pruritus, and angioedema of the mouth, throat, and face have been reported with *fidaxomicin*. If a severe hypersensitivity reaction occurs, **Dificid** should be discontinued and appropriate therapy should be instituted. The most common adverse reactions reported in clinical trials are nausea (11%), vomiting (7%), abdominal pain (6%), gastrointestinal hemorrhage (4%), anemia (2%), and neutropenia (2%). Among patients receiving **Dificid**, 5.9% withdrew from trials as a result of adverse reactions. Vomiting was the primary adverse reaction leading to discontinuation of dosing (incidence of 0.5% for both **Dificid** and *vancomycin* patients). No dose adjustment is recommended for patients ≥65 years-of-age. No dose adjustment is recommended for patients with renal impairment. No dosage adjustments are recommended when co-administering *fidaxomicin* with substrates of P-gp or CYP enzymes. The impact of hepatic impairment on the pharmacokinetics of *fidaxomicin* has not been evaluated; however, because *fidaxomicin* and its active metabolite (OP-1118) do not appear to undergo significant hepatic metabolism, elimination of *fidaxomicin* and OP-1118 is not expected to be significantly affected by hepatic impairment. There are no adequate and well-controlled studies in pregnancy; **Dificid** should be used during pregnancy only if clearly needed. It is not known whether fidaxomicin is excreted in human milk.

GLYCOPEPTIDE ANTIBACTERIAL AGENTS

▷ *vancomycin hcl capsule* (B)(G) 500 mg to 2 gm in 3-4 doses x 7-10 days; max 2 gm/day
   Pediatric: 40 mg/kg/day in 3-4 doses x 7-10 days; max 2 gm/day;use caps or oral solution as appropriate
   Vancocin *Cap:* 125, 250 mg
▷ *vancomycin hcl oral solution* see mfr pkg insert for preparation and important administration information; <18 years: *CDAD and Staphylococcal enterocolitis:* 40 mg/kg orally in 3 or 4 divided doses x 7-10 days; total daily dosage max 2 gm; ≥18 years: *CDAD* 125 mg orally 4 x/day x 10 days; *Staphylococcal enterocolitis:* 500 mg to 2 gm orally in 3 or 4 divided doses x 7-10 days
   Firvanq *Kit w. pwdr for oral soln:* 25, 50 mg/ml (150, 300 ml) equivalent to 3.75, 7.5, 10.5, or 15 gm *vancomycin hcl*, plus grape-flavored diluent
   Comment: *Vancomycin hcl,* a glycopeptide antibacterial agent, is FDA approved for treatment of *C. difficile*-associated diarrhea (CDAD) and entercolitis caused by *Staphylococcus aureus,* including methicillin-resistant strains (MRSA). *Vancomycin hcl* should be used only to treat or prevent infections that are proven

or strongly suspected to be caused by susceptible bacteria. Orally administered *vancomycin hcl* is not effective for treatment of other types of infections. Prescribing *vancomycin hcl* in the absence of a proven or strongly suspected bacterial infection is unlikely to provide benefit to the patient and increases the risk of the development of drug-resistant bacteria. Nephrotoxicity has occurred following oral *vancomycin hcl* therapy and can occur either during or after completion of therapy. The risk is increased in geriatric patients. Monitor renal function. Ototoxicity has occurred in patients receiving *vancomycin hcl*. Assessment of auditory function may be appropriate in some instances. The most common adverse reactions ≥10%) have been nausea (17%), abdominal pain (15%) and hypokalemia (13%). There are no available data on **Firvanq** use in the first trimester of pregnancy to inform a drug- associated risk of major birth defects or miscarriage. Available published data on *vancomycin hcl* use in pregnancy during the second and third trimesters have not shown an association with adverse pregnancy-related outcomes. There are insufficient data to inform the levels of *vancomycin hcl* in human milk. However, systemic absorption of *vancomycin hcl* following oral administration is expected to be minimal. There are no data on effects of **Firvanq** on the breastfed infant.

HUMAN IGG1 MONOCLONAL ANTIBODY

Comment: *Bezlotoxumab* is a human IgG1 monoclonal antibody that inhibits the binding of *Clostridioides difficile* toxin B, preventing its effects on mammalian cells. *Bezlotoxumab* does not bind to *C. difficile* toxin A. *Bezlotoxumab* is indicated to reduce the recurrence of CDI in patients who are receiving antibacterial drug treatment of CDI and are at high risk for CDI recurrence. CDI recurrence is defined as a new episode of diarrhea associated with a positive stool test for toxigenic *C. difficile* following a clinical cure of the presenting CDI episode. It is not indicated for the primary treatment of CDI infection. It is to be used only in conjunction with appropriate primary drug treatment of CDI. Patients at high risk for CDI recurrence, studied in clinical trials establishing efficacy, include those ≥65 years-of-age, with a history of CDI in the previous 6 months, immunocompromised state, severe CDI at presentation, and *C. difficile* ribotype 027.

▷ *bezlotoxumab* (C) administer a single dose of 10 mg/kg via IV infusion over 60 minutes
   Pediatric: <18 years: not established; ≥18 years: same as adult
      Zinplava *Vial:* 1,000 mg/40 ml (40 ml, 25 mg/ml) single-use

COLIC: INFANTILE

▷ *hyoscyamine* (C)(G)
   Levsin Drops
      Pediatric: 3-4 kg: 4 drops q 4 hours prn; max 24 drops/day; 5 kg: 5 drops q 4 hours prn; max 30 drops/day; 7 kg: 6 drops q 4 hours prn; max 36 drops/day; 10 kg: 8 drops q 4 hours prn; max 40 drops/day; *Oral drops:* 0.125 mg/ml (15 ml) (orange) (alcohol 5%)
▷ *simethicone* (C) 0.3 ml qid pc and HS
   Mylicon Drops (OTC) *Oral drops:* 40 mg/0.6 ml (30 ml)

COLONOSCOPY PREP/COLON CLEANSE

▷ *polyethylene glycol 3350 with electrolytes* two doses of **Plenvu** are required for a complete preparation for colonoscopy, using a One-Day or Two-Day dosing regimen; reconstitute in water prior to ingestion; additional clear liquids must be consumed after each dose for both dosing regimens; do not take oral medications within 1 hour of starting each dose; for complete information on dosing, preparation, and administration see mfr pkg insert

One-Day Regimen: Dose 1 the morning of the colonoscopy (approximately 3 am to 7 am) and *Dose 2* (Pouch A and B) a minimum of 2 hours after the start of Dose 1
Two-Day Regimen: Dose 1 the evening before the colonoscopy (approximately 4 pm to 8 pm) and *Dose 2* (Pouch A and B) the next morning approximately 12 hours after the start of Dose 1)

Plenvu *Oral soln:* polyethylene glycol 3350 (140 gm), sodium ascorbate (48.11 gm), sodium sulfate (9 gm), ascorbic acid (7.54 gm), sodium chloride (5.2 gm), and potassium chloride (2.2 gm); *Dose 1:* PEG 3350 (100 gm), sodium sulfate (9 gm), sodium chloride (2 gm), potassium chloride (1 gm) ; *Dose 2, Pouch A:* PEG 3350 (40 gm), sodium chloride (3.2 gm), potassium chloride (1.2 gm); *Dose 2, Pouch B:* sodium ascorbate (48.11 gm), ascorbic acid (7.54 gm)
Comment: **Plenvu for Oral Solution** is a lower-volume, polyethylene glycol-based osmotic laxative indicated for cleansing of the colon (bowel prepara- to any ingredient in **Plenvu**. Patients with glucose-6-phosphate dihydrogenase deficiency (G6PD) should use with caution. **Plenvu** contains phenylalanine; there is risk for patients with phenylketonuria (PKA). The most common adverse reactions (incidence ≥2%) are nausea, vomiting, dehydration and abdominal pain/discomfort.

➤ *sodium picosulfate+magnesium oxide+citric acid* reconstitute pwdr with cold water right before use; two dosing regimen options—each requires two separate dosing times; *Split Dose Method* (preferred): 1st dose during evening before the colonoscopy and 2nd dose the next day during the morning prior to the colonoscopy; *Day Before Method* (alternative, if split dose is not appropriate): 1st dose during afternoon or early evening before the colonoscopy and 2nd dose 6 hours later during evening before colonoscopy; additional clear liquids (no solid food or milk) must be consumed after every dose in both dosing regimens
Pediatric: <18 years: not recommended; ≥18 years: same as adult

Prepopik *Pwdr:* sod picos 10 mg+mag oxide 3.5 gm+anhy cit acid 12 gm/pkt pwdr for oral solution (2 pkts)
Comment: **Prepopik** is a combination of sodium picosulfate, a stimulant laxative, and magnesium oxide and anhydrous citric acid which form magnesium citrate, an osmotic laxative, indicated for cleansing of the colon as a preparation for colonoscopy in adults. Rule out diagnosis of suspected GI obstruction or perforation diagnosis before administration. **Prepopik** should be used during pregnancy only if clearly needed. **Prepopik** is contraindicated with severely reduced renal function (CrCl< 30 mL/min), GI obstruction or ileus, bowel perforation, toxic colitis or toxic megacolon, and gastric retention for any reason.

COMMON COLD (VIRAL UPPER RESPIRATORY INFECTION, URI)

Drugs for the Management of Allergy, Cough, and Cold Symptoms *see* Appendix AA. Drugs for the Management of Allergy, Cough, and Cold Symptoms online at https://connect.springerpub.com/content/reference-book/978-0-8261-7935-7/back-matter/part02/back-matter/bmatter27
Oral Decongestants *see* Appendix AA. Drugs for the Management of Allergy, Cough, and Cold Symptoms online at https://connect.springerpub.com/content/reference-book/978-0-8261-7935-7/back-matter/part02/back-matter/bmatter27
Oral Expectorants *see* Appendix AA. Drugs for the Management of Allergy, Cough, and Cold Symptoms online at https://connect.springerpub.com/content/reference-book/978-0-8261-7935-7/back-matter/part02/back-matter/bmatter27
Oral Antitussives *see* Appendix AA. Drugs for the Management of Allergy, Cough, and Cold Symptoms online at https://connect.springerpub.com/content/reference-book/978-0-8261-7935-7/back-matter/part02/back-matter/bmatter27
Oral Antipyretic-Analgesics *see Fever*

NASAL SALINE DROPS & SPRAYS

Comment: Homemade saline nose drops: 1/4 tsp salt added to 8 oz boiled water, then cool water.

▷ *saline* nasal spray (G)

Afrin Saline Mist w. Eucalyptol and Menthol (OTC) 2-6 sprays in each nostril prn
Pediatric: 1 month-2 years: 1-2 sprays in each nostril prn; >2-12 years: 1-4 sprays in each nostril prn; >12 years: same as adult
   Squeeze bottle: 45 ml

Afrin Moisturizing Saline Mist (OTC) 2-6 sprays in each nostril prn
Pediatric: 1 month-2 years: 1-2 sprays in each nostril prn; 2-12 years: 1-4 sprays in each nostril prn; >12 years: same as adult
   Squeeze bottle: 45 ml

Ocean Mist (OTC) 2-6 sprays in each nostril prn
Pediatric: 1 month-2 years: 1-2 sprays in each nostril prn; >2-12 years: 1-4 sprays in each nostril prn; >12 years: same as adult
   Squeeze bottle: saline 0.65% (45 ml) (alcohol-free)

Pediamist (OTC) 2-6 sprays in each nostril prn
Pediatric: 1 month-2 years: 1-2 sprays in each nostril prn; >2-12 years: 1-4 sprays in each nostril prn; >12 years: same as adult
   Squeeze bottle: saline 0.5% (15 ml) (alcohol-free)

NASAL SYMPATHOMIMETICS

▷ *oxymetazoline* (C)(OTC)
4-Hour Formulation: 2-3 drops <u>or</u> sprays in each nostril q 10-12 hours prn; max 2 doses/day; max duration 5 days
Pediatric: <6 years: not recommended; ≥6 years: same as adult
   Afrin 4-Hour:
12-hour Formulation: 2-3 drops <u>or</u> sprays q 4 hours prn; max duration 5 days
Pediatric: <12 years: not recommended; ≥12 years: same as adult
   Afrin 12-Hour Extra Moisturizing Nasal Spray
   Afrin 12-Hour Nasal spray Pump Mist
   Afrin 12-Hour Original Nasal spray
   Afrin 12-Hour Original Nose Drops
   Afrin 12-Hour Severe Congestion Nasal Spray
   Afrin 12-Hour Sinus Nasal Spray
      Nasal spray: 0.05% (45 ml); *Nasal drops:* 0.05% (45 ml)
   Afrin 4-Hour Nasal Spray
   Neo-Synephrine 12 Hour Nasal Spray
   Neo-Synephrine 12 Hour Extra Moisturizing Nasal Spray
      Nasal spray: 0.05% (15 ml)

▷ *phenylephrine* (C)
Afrin Allergy Nasal Spray (OTC) 2-3 sprays in each nostril q 4 hours prn; max duration 5 days
Pediatric: <12 years: not recommended; ≥12 years: same as adult
   Nasal spray: 0.5% (15 ml)

Afrin Nasal Decongestant Children's Pump Mist **(OTC)**
Pediatric: <6 years: not recommended; ≥6 years: 2-3 sprays in each nostril q 4 hours prn; max duration 5 days
   Nasal spray: 0.25% (15 ml)

Neo-Synephrine Extra Strength (OTC) 2-3 sprays <u>or</u> drops in each nostril q 4 hours prn; max duration 5 days
Pediatric: <12 years: not recommended; ≥12 years: same as adult
   Nasal spray: 0.1% (15 ml); *Nasal drops:* 0.1% (15 ml)

Neo-Synephrine Mild Formula (OTC) 2-3 sprays or drops in each nostril q 4 hours prn; max duration 5 days
Pediatric: <6 years: not recommended; ≥6 years: same as adult
Nasal spray: 0.25% (15 ml)

Neo-Synephrine Regular Strength (OTC) 2-3 sprays or drops in each nostril q 4 hours prn; max duration 5 days
Pediatric: <12 years: not recommended; ≥12 years: same as adult
Nasal spray: 0.5% (15 ml); *Nasal drops:* 0.5% (15 ml)

▷ *tetrahydrozoline* (C)
Tyzine 2-4 drops or 3-4 sprays in each nostril q 3-8 hours prn; max duration 5 days
Pediatric: <6 years: not recommended; ≥6 years: same as adult
Nasal spray: 0.1% (15 ml); *Nasal drops:* 0.1% (30 ml)

Tyzine Pediatric Nasal Drops 2-3 sprays or drops in each nostril q 3-6 hours prn
Nasal drops: 0.05% (15 ml)

CONJUNCTIVITIS/BLEPHAROCONJUNCTIVITIS: BACTERIAL

OPHTHALMIC ANTI-INFECTIVES

▷ *azithromycin* (B)(G) ophthalmic solution (B)(G) 1 drop to affected eye(s) bid x 2 days; then 1 drop once daily for the next 5 days
Pediatric: <1 year: not recommended; ≥1 year: same as adult
AzaSite Ophthalmic Solution *Ophth susp:* 1% (2.5 ml) (benzalkonium chloride)

▷ *bacitracin* ophthalmic ointment (C)(G) apply 1/2 inch ribbon to the lower conjunctival sac of affected eye(s) 1-3 x daily x 7 days
Pediatric: same as adult
Bacitracin Ophthalmic Ointment *Ophth oint:* 500 units/gm (3.5 gm)

▷ *besifloxacin* ophthalmic solution (C) 1 drop to affected eye(s) tid x 7 days
Pediatric: <1 year: not recommended; ≥1 year: same as adult
Besivance Ophthalmic Solution *Ophth susp:* 0.6% (5 ml) (benzalkonium chloride)

▷ *ciprofloxacin* ophthalmic ointment (C) apply 1/2 inch ribbon to the lower conjunctival sac of affected eye(s) tid x 2 days; then bid x 5 days
Pediatric: <2 years: not recommended; ≥2 years: same as adult
Ciloxan Ophthalmic Ointment *Ophth oint:* 0.3% (3.5 gm)

▷ *ciprofloxacin* ophthalmic solution (C) 1-2 drops to affected eye(s) q 2 hours while awake x 2 days; then, q 4 hours while awake x 5 days
Pediatric: <1 years: not recommended; ≥1 year: same as adult
Ciloxan Ophthalmic Solution *Ophth soln:* 0.3% (2.5, 5, 10 ml) (benzalkonium chloride)

▷ *erythromycin* ophthalmic ointment (B) apply 1/2 inch ribbon to the lower conjunctival sac of affected eye(s) up to 6 x/day
Pediatric: same as adult
Ilotycin Ophthalmic Ointment *Ophth oint:* 5 mg/gm (1/8 oz)

▷ *gatifloxacin* ophthalmic solution (C)
Pediatric: <1 years: not recommended; ≥1 year: same as adult
Zymar Ophthalmic Solution initially 1 drop to affected eye(s) q 2 hours while awake up to 8 x/day for 2 days; then 1 drop qid while awake x 5 more days
Ophth soln: 0.3% (5 ml) (benzalkonium chloride)

Zymaxid Ophthalmic Solution (G) initially 1 drop to affected eye(s) q 2 hours while awake up to 8 x/day on day 1; then 1 drop bid-qid while awake on days 2-7
Ophth soln: 0.5% (2.5 ml) (benzalkonium chloride)

▷ **gentamicin sulfate** ophthalmic ointment (C)(G) apply 1/2 inch ribbon to the lower conjunctival sac of affected eye(s) bid-tid
Pediatric: same as adult
　　Garamycin Ophthalmic Ointment *Ophth oint:* 3 mg/gm (3.5 gm)
　　(preservative-free formulation available)
　　Genoptic Ophthalmic Ointment *Ophth oint:* 3 mg/gm (3.5 gm)
　　Gentacidin Ophthalmic Ointment *Ophth oint:* 3 mg/gm (3.5 gm)
▷ **gentamicin sulfate** ophthalmic solution (C)(G) 1-2 drops to affected eye(s) q 4 hours x 7-14 days; max 2 drops q 1 h
Pediatric: same as adult
　　Garamycin Ophthalmic Solution *Ophth soln:* 0.3% (5 ml) (benzalkonium chloride)
　　Genoptic Ophthalmic Solution *Ophth soln:* 0.3% (3, 5 ml)
▷ **levofloxacin** ophthalmic solution (C) 1-2 drops to affected eye(s) q 2 hours while awake on days 1 and 2 (max 8 x/day); then 1-2 drops q 4 hours while awake on days 3-7; max 4 x/day
Pediatric: <1 years: not recommended; ≥1 years: same as adult
　　Quixin Ophthalmic Solution *Ophth soln:* 0.5% (2.5, 5 ml) (benzalkonium chloride)
▷ **moxifloxacin** ophthalmic solution (C)(G) 1 drop to affected eye(s) tid x 7 days
Pediatric: <1 years: not recommended; ≥1 year: same as adult
　　Moxeza Ophthalmic Solution (G) *Ophth soln:* 0.5% (3 ml)
　　Vigamox Ophthalmic Solution *Ophth soln:* 0.5% (3 ml)
▷ **ofloxacin** ophthalmic solution (C) 1-2 drops to affected eye(s) q 2-4 hours x 2 days; then qid x 5 days
Pediatric: <1 years: not recommended; ≥1 year: same as adult
　　Ocuflox Ophthalmic Solution *Ophth soln:* 0.3% (5, 10 ml) (benzalkonium chloride)
▷ **sulfacetamide** ophthalmic solution and ointment (C)
　　Bleph-10 Ophthalmic Solution 1-2 drops to affected eye(s) q 2-3 hours x 7-10 days
　　Pediatric: <2 months: not recommended; ≥2 months: 1-2 drops q 2-3 hours during the day x 7-10 days
　　　Ophth soln: 10% (2.5, 5, 15 ml) (benzalkonium chloride)
　　Bleph-10 Ophthalmic Ointment apply 1/2 inch ribbon to the lower conjunctival sac of affected eye(s) q 3-4 hours and HS x 7-10 days
　　Pediatric: <2 years: not recommended; ≥2 years: same as adult
　　　Ophth oint: 10% (3.5 gm) (phenylmercuric acetate)
　　Cetamide Ophthalmic Solution initially 1-2 drops to affected eye(s) q 2-3 hours; then increase dosing interval as condition improves
　　Pediatric: <2 years: not recommended; ≥2 years: same as adult
　　　Ophth soln: 15% (5, 15 ml)
　　Isopto Cetamide Ophthalmic Ointment initially 1/2 inch ribbon in lower conjunctival sac of affected eye(s) q 3-4 hours; then increase dosing interval as condition improves
　　Pediatric: <2 years: not recommended; ≥2 years: same as adult
　　　Ophth oint: 10% (3.5 gm)
　　Isopto Cetamide Ophthalmic Solution initially 1-2 drops to affected eye(s) q 2-3 hours; then increase dosing interval as condition improves
　　Pediatric: <2 years: not recommended; ≥2 years: same as adult
　　　Ophth soln: 15% (5, 15 ml)
▷ **tobramycin** (B)
　　Tobrex Ophthalmic Solution 1-2 drops to affected eye(s) q 4 hours
　　Pediatric: same as adult
　　　Ophth soln: 0.3% (5 ml) (benzalkonium chloride)

Tobrex Ophthalmic Ointment apply 1/2 inch ribbon to the lower conjunctival sac of affected eye(s) bid-tid
Pediatric: same as adult
Ophth oint: 0.3% (3.5 gm) (chlorobutanol)

OPHTHALMIC ANTI-INFECTIVE COMBINATIONS

▷ *polymyxin b sulfate+bacitracin* ophthalmic ointment **(C)** apply 1/2 inch ribbon to the lower conjunctival sac of affected eye(s) q 3-4 hours x 7-10 days
Pediatric: same as adult
  Polysporin Ophthalmic Ointment *Ophth oint:* poly b 10,000 U+bac 500 U (3.75 gm)

▷ *polymyxin b sulfate+bacitracin zinc+neomycin sulfate* ophthalmic ointment **(C)** apply 1/2 inch ribbon to the lower conjunctival sac of affected eye(s) q 3-4 hours x 7-10 days
Pediatric: same as adult
  Neosporin Ophthalmic Ointment *Ophth oint:* poly b 10,000 U+bac 400 U+neo 3.5 mg/gm (3.75 gm)

▷ *polymyxin b sulfate+gramicidin+neomycin* ophthalmic solution **(C)** 1-2 drops to affected eye(s) q 1 hour x 2-3 doses; then 1-2 drops bid-qid x 7-10 days
Pediatric: <12 years: not recommended; ≥12 years: same as adult
  Neosporin Ophthalmic Solution *Ophth soln:* poly b 10,000 U+grami 0.025 mg+neo 1.7 mg/gm (10 ml)

▷ *trimethoprim+polymyxin b sulfate* ophthalmic solution **(C)** 1 drop to affected eye(s) q 3 hours x 7-10 days; max 6 doses/day
Pediatric: <2 years: not recommended; ≥2 years: same as adult
  Polytrim *Ophth soln:* trim 1 mg+poly b 10,000 U/ml (10 ml) (benzalkonium chloride)

OPHTHALMIC ANTI-INFECTIVE+STEROID COMBINATIONS

Comment: Ophthalmic corticosteroids are contraindicated after removal of a corneal foreign body, epithelial herpes simplex keratitis, *varicella*, other viral infections of the cornea or conjunctiva, fungal ocular infections, and mycobacterial ocular infections. Limit ophthalmic steroid use to 2-3 days if possible; usual max 2 weeks. With prolonged or frequent use, there is risk of corneal and scleral thinning and cataract formation.

▷ *gentamicin sulfate+prednisolone acetate* ophthalmic suspension **(C)**
Pediatric: <12 years: not recommended; ≥12 years: same as adult
  Pred-G Ophthalmic Suspension 1 drop to affected eye(s) bid-qid; max 20 ml/therapeutic course
    Ophth susp: gent 0.3%+pred 1%/ml (2, 5, 10 ml) (benzalkonium chloride)
  Pred-G Ophthalmic Ointment apply 1/2 inch ribbon to the lower conjunctival sac of affected eye(s) once daily-tid; max 8 gm/therapeutic course
    Ophth oint: gent 0.3%+pred 0.6%/gm (3.5 gm)

▷ *neomycin sulfate+polymyxin b sulfate+dexamethasone* ophthalmic suspension **(C)**
Pediatric: <12 years: not recommended; ≥12 years: same as adult
  Maxitrol Ophthalmic Suspension 1-2 drops to affected eye(s) q 1 hour (severe infection) or qid (mild to moderate infection)
    Ophth susp: neo 0.35%+poly b 10,000 U+dexa 1%/ml (5 ml) (benzalkonium chloride)
  Maxitrol Ophthalmic Ointment apply 1/2 inch ribbon to the lower conjunctival sac of affected eye(s) q 1 hour (severe infection) or qid (mild to moderate infection)
    Ophth oint: neo 0.35%+poly b 10,000 U+dexa 0.1%/gm (3.5 gm)

▷ **neomycin sulfate+polymyxin b sulfate+prednisolone acetate ophthalmic suspension** (C)

Pediatric: <12 years: not recommended; ≥12 years: same as adult

Poly-Pred Ophthalmic Suspension 1-2 drops to affected eye(s) q 3-4 hours; more often as necessary; max 20 ml/therapeutic course.

Ophth susp: neo 0.35%+poly b 10,000 U+pred 0.5%/ml (10 ml)

▷ **polymyxin b sulfate+neomycin sulfate+hydrocortisone** ophthalmic suspension (C)

Pediatric: <12 years: not recommended; ≥12 years: same as adult

Cortisporin Ophthalmic Suspension 1-2 drops to affected eye(s) tid-qid; more often if necessary; max 20 ml/therapeutic course

Ophth susp: poly b 10,000 U+neo 0.35%+hydro 1%/ml (7.5 ml) (thimerosal)

▷ **polymyxin b sulfate+neomycin sulfate+bacitracin zinc+hydrocortisone** ophthalmic ointment (C)

Pediatric: <12 years: not recommended; ≥12 years: same as adult

Cortisporin Ophthalmic Ointment apply 1/2 inch ribbon to the lower conjunctival sac of affected eye(s) tid-qid; more often if necessary; max 8 gm/therapeutic course

Ophth oint: poly b 10,000 U+neo 0.35%+bac 400 U+hydro 1%/gm (3.5 gm)

▷ **sulfacetamide sodium+fluorometholone** suspension (C) 1 drop to affected eye(s) qid; max 20 ml/therapeutic course

Pediatric: <12 years: not recommended; ≥12 years: same as adult

FML-S *Ophth susp:* sulfa 10%+fluoro 0.1%+ml (5, 10, 15 ml) (benzalkonium chloride)

▷ **sulfacetamide sodium+prednisolone acetate** ophthalmic suspension and ointment (C)

Pediatric: <6 years: not recommended; ≥6 years: same as adult

Blephamide Liquifilm 2 drops to affected eye(s) qid and HS

Ophth susp: sulfa10%+pred 0.2%/ml (5, 10 ml) (benzalkonium chloride)

Blephamide S.O.P. Ophthalmic Ointment apply 1/2 inch ribbon to the lower conjunctival sac of affected eye(s) tid-qid

Ophth oint: sulfa 10%+pred 0.2%/gm (3.5 gm) (benzalkonium chloride)

▷ **sulfacetamide sodium+prednisolone sodium phosphate** ophthalmic solution (C) 2 drops to affected eye(s) every 4 hours

Pediatric: <6 years: not recommended; ≥6 years: same as adult

Vasocidin Ophthalmic Solution *Ophth soln:* sulfa 10%+pred 0.25%/ml (5, 10 ml)

▷ **tobramycin+dexamethasone** ophthalmic solution and ointment (C)

TobraDex Ophthalmic Solution 1-2 drops to affected eye(s) q 2-6 hours x 24-48 hours; then 4-6 hours; reduce frequency of dose as condition improves; max 20 ml per therapeutic course

Pediatric: ≤2 years: not recommended; ≥2 years: 1-2 drops q 4-6 hours; may start with 1-2 drops q 2 hours first 1-2 days

Ophth susp: tobra 0.3%+dexa 0.1%/ml (2.5, 5 ml) (benzalkonium chloride)

TobraDex Ophthalmic Ointment apply 1/2 inch ribbon to the lower conjunctival sac of affected eye(s) tid-qid; may use at bedtime in conjunction with daytime drops; max 8 gm/therapeutic course

Pediatric: <2 years: not recommended; ≥2 years: apply 1/2 inch ribbon to lower conjunctival sac tid-qid

Ophth oint: tobra 0.3%/dexa 0.1%/gm (3.5 gm) (chlorobutanol chloride)

TobraDex ST 1-2 drops to affected eye(s) q 2-6 hours x 24-48 hours; then 4-6 hours; reduce frequency of dose as condition improves; max 20 ml per therapeutic course

Pediatric: <12 years: not recommended; ≥12 years: same as adult
  Ophth susp: tobra 0.3%/dexa 0.5%/ml (2.5, 5, 10 ml) (benzalkonium chloride)
▷ **tobramycin+loteprednol etabonate** ophthalmic suspension **(C)**
  Pediatric: <12 years: not recommended; ≥12 years: same as adult
    Zylet 1-2 drops to affected eye(s) q 1-2 hours first 24-48 hours; reduce
    frequency of dose to q 4-6 hours as condition improves; max 20 ml per
    therapeutic course
      Ophth susp: tobra 0.3%+lote etab 0.5%/ml (2.5, 5, 10 ml) (benzalkonium
      chloride)

CONJUNCTIVITIS: CHLAMYDIAL

Comment: A chlamydial etiology should be considered for all infants aged ≤30 days
that have conjunctivitis, especially if the mother has a history of chlamydia infection.
Topical antibiotic therapy alone is inadequate for treatment for *ophthalmia
neonatorum* caused by chlamydia and is unnecessary when systemic treatment is
administered.

RECOMMENDED FIRST LINE REGIMEN

▷ **erythromycin base (B)(G)** 250 mg qid x 14 days *or* 500 mg qid x 7 days
  Pediatric: <45 kg: 50 mg/kg/day in 4 divided doses x 14 days; ≥45 kg: same as
  adult
    Ery-Tab *Tab:* 250, 333, 500 mg ent-coat
    PCE *Tab:* 333, 500 mg
    OR
▷ **erythromycin ethylsuccinate (B)(G)** 400 mg qid x 14 days *or* 800 mg qid x 7 days
  Pediatric: 50 mg/kg/day in 4 divided doses x 7 days; max 100 mg/kg/day; *see
  Appendix CC.21: erythromycin ethylsuccinate* (E.E.S. Suspension, Ery-Ped Drops/
  Suspension) *for dose by weight*
    EryPed *Oral susp:* 200 mg/5 ml (100, 200 ml) (fruit); 400 mg/5 ml (60, 100,
    200 ml) (banana); Oral drops: 200, 400 mg/5 ml (50 ml) (fruit); *Chew tab:*
    200 mg wafer (fruit)
    E.E.S. *Oral susp:* 200, 400 mg/5 ml (100 ml) (fruit)
    E.E.S. Granules *Oral susp:* 200 mg/5 ml (100, 200 ml) (cherry)
    E.E.S. 400 Tablets *Tab:* 400 mg

ALTERNATE REGIMEN

▷ **azithromycin (B)(G)** 500 mg x 1 dose on day 1; then 250 mg once daily on days;
  2-5 *or* 500 mg daily x 3 days *or* 2 gm in a single dose
  Pediatric: 20 mg/kg in a single dose once daily x 3 days
    Zithromax *Tab:* 250, 500, 600 mg; *Oral susp:* 100 mg/5 ml (15 ml); 200 mg/5
    ml (15, 22.5, 30 ml) (cherry); *Pkt:* 1 gm for reconstitution (cherry-banana)
    Zithromax Tri-pak *Tab:* 3 x 500 mg tabs/pck
    Zithromax Z-pak *Tab:* 6 x 250 mg tabs/pck
    Zmax *Oral susp:* 2 gm ext-rel for reconstitution (cherry-banana) (148 mg Na⁺)

CONJUNCTIVITIS: FUNGAL

▷ **natamycin** ophthalmic suspension **(C)** 1 drop q 1-2 hours x 3-4 days; then 1 drop
  every 6 hours; treat for 14-21 days; withdraw dose gradually at 4- to 7-day intervals
  Pediatric: <1 year: not recommended; ≥1 year: same as adult
    Natacyn Ophthalmic Suspension *Ophth susp:* 0.5% (15 ml) (benzalkonium
    chloride)

CONJUNCTIVITIS: GONOCOCCAL

RECOMMENDED REGIMENS
Regimen 1
➤ *ceftriaxone* **(B)(G)** 250 mg IM x 1 dose
    Pediatric: <45 kg: 50 mg/kg IM x 1 dose; max 125 mg IM
        Rocephin *Vial:* 250, 500 mg; 1, 2 gm

Regimen 2
➤ *erythromycin base* **(B)(G)** 250 mg qid x 10-14 days
    Pediatric: <45 kg: 50 mg/kg/day in 4 divided doses x 10-14 days; ≥45 kg: same as adult
        Ery-Tab *Tab:* 250, 333, 500 mg ent-coat
        PCE *Tab:* 333, 500 mg
➤ *erythromycin ethylsuccinate* **(B)(G)** 400 mg qid x 14 days or 800 mg qid x 7 days
    Pediatric: 50 mg/kg/day in 4 divided doses x 7 days; max 100 mg/kg/day; *see Appendix CC.21: erythromycin ethylsuccinate* (E.E.S. Suspension, Ery-Ped Drops/ Suspension) *for dose by weight*
        EryPed *Oral susp:* 200 mg/5 ml (100, 200 ml) (fruit); 400 mg/5 ml (60, 100, 200 ml) (banana); *Oral drops:* 200, 400 mg/5 ml (50 ml) (fruit); *Chew tab:* 200 mg wafer (fruit)
        E.E.S. *Oral susp:* 200, 400 mg/5 ml (100 ml) (fruit)
        E.E.S. Granules *Oral susp:* 200 mg/5 ml (100, 200 ml) (cherry)
        E.E.S. 400 Tablets *Tab:* 400 mg

ALTERNATE REGIMEN
➤ *azithromycin* **(B)(G)** 500 mg x 1 dose on day 1; then 250 mg once daily on days; 2-5 or 500 mg daily x 3 days or 2 gm in a single dose
    Pediatric: not recommended for bronchitis in children
        Zithromax *Tab:* 250, 500, 600 mg; *Oral susp:* 100 mg/5 ml (15 ml); 200 mg/5 ml (15, 22.5, 30 ml) (cherry); Pkt: 1 gm for reconstitution (cherry-banana)
        Zithromax Tri-pak *Tab:* 3 x 500 mg tabs/pck
        Zithromax Z-pak *Tab:* 6 x 250 mg tabs/pck
        Zmax *Oral susp:* 2 gm ext-rel for reconstitution (cherry-banana) (148 mg Na⁺)

 CONJUNCTIVITIS/KERATITIS/KERATOCONJUNCTIVITIS: ALLERGIC (VERNAL)

Oral Antihistamines *see* Appendix AA. Drugs for the Management of Allergy, Cough, and Cold Symptoms online at https://connect.springerpub.com/content/ reference-book/978-0-8261-7935-7/back-matter/part02/back-matter/bmatter27

OPHTHALMIC CORTICOSTEROIDS
Comment: Concomitant contact lens wear is contraindicated during therapy. Ophthalmic steroids are contraindicated with ocular, fungal, mycobacterial, viral (except herpes zoster), and untreated bacterial infection. Ophthalmic steroids may mask or exacerbate infection, and may increase intraocular pressure, optic nerve damage, cataract formation, or corneal perforation. Limit ophthalmic steroid use to 2-3 days if possible; usual max 2 weeks. With prolonged or frequent use, there is risk of corneal and scleral thinning and cataract formation.
➤ *dexamethasone* **(C)** initially 1-2 drops hourly during the day and q 2 hours at night; then prolong dosing interval to 4-6 hours as condition improves
    Pediatric: <12 years: not recommended; ≥12 years: same as adult
        Maxidex *Ophth susp:* 0.1% (5, 15 ml) (benzalkonium chloride)

▷ *dexamethasone phosphate* (C) initially 1-2 drops hourly during the day and q 2 hours at night; then 1 drop q 4-8 hours or more as condition improves
  Pediatric: <12 years: not recommended; ≥12 years: same as adult
    Decadron *Ophth soln:* 0.1% (5 ml) (sulfites)

▷ *fluorometholone* (C) 1 drop bid-qid or 1/2 inch of ointment 1-3 x/day; may increase dose frequency during initial 24-48 hours
  Pediatric: <2 years: not recommended; ≥2 years: same as adult
    FML *Ophth susp:* 0.1% (5, 10, 15 ml) (benzalkonium chloride)
    FML Forte *Ophth susp:* 0.25% (5, 10, 15 ml) (benzalkonium chloride)
    FML S.O.P. Ointment *Ophth oint:* 0.1% (3.5 gm)

▷ *fluorometholone acetate* (C) initially 2 drops q 2 hours during the first 24-48 hours; then 1-2 drops qid as condition improves
  Pediatric: <12 years: not recommended; ≥12 years: same as adult
    Flarex *Ophth susp:* 0.1% (2.5, 5 10 ml) (benzalkonium chloride)

▷ *loteprednol etabonate* (C)(G)
  Pediatric: <12 years: not recommended; ≥12 years: same as adult
    Alrex 1 drop qid
      Ophth susp: 0.2% (5, 10 ml) (benzalkonium chloride)
    Lotemax 1-2 drops qid
      Ophth susp: 0.5% (5, 10, 15 ml) (benzalkonium chloride)

▷ *medrysone* (C) 1 drop up to q 4 hours
  Pediatric: <12 years: not recommended; ≥12 years: same as adult
    HMS *Ophth susp:* 1% (5, 10 ml) (benzalkonium chloride)

▷ *rimexolone* (C) initially 1-2 drops hourly while awake x 1 week; then 1 drop every 2 hours while awake x 1 week; then taper as condition improves
  Pediatric: <12 years: not recommended; ≥12 years: same as adult
    Vexol *Ophth susp:* 0.1% (5, 10 ml) (benzalkonium chloride)

▷ *prednisolone acetate* (C)(G)
  Pediatric: <12 years: not recommended; ≥12 years: same as adult
    Econopred 2 drops qid
      Ophth susp: 0.125% (5, 10 ml)
    Econopred Plus 2 drops qid
      Ophth susp: 1% (5, 10 ml)
    Pred Forte initially 2 drops hourly x 24-48 hours; then 1-2 drops bid-qid
      Ophth susp: 1% (1, 5, 10, 15 ml) (benzalkonium chloride, sulfites)
    Pred Mild initially 2 drops hourly x 24-48 hours; then 1-2 drops bid-qid
      Ophth susp: 0.12% (5, 10 ml) (benzalkonium chloride)

▷ *prednisolone sodium phosphate* (C) initially 1-2 drops hourly during the day and q 2 hours at night; then 1 drop q 4 hours; then 1 drop tid-qid as condition improves
  Pediatric: <12 years: not recommended; ≥12 years: same as adult
    Inflamase Forte *Ophth soln:* 1% (5, 10, 15 ml) (benzalkonium chloride)
    Inflamase Mild *Ophth soln:* 1/8% (5, 10 ml) (benzalkonium chloride)

OPHTHALMIC H1 ANTAGONISTS (ANTIHISTAMINES)

Comment: May insert contact lens 10 minutes after administration of ophthalmic antihistamine.

▷ *cetirizine* (C) 1 drop bid prn
  Pediatric: <2 years: not established; ≥2 years: same as adult
    Zerviate *Ophth soln:* 0.24%/ml (5 ml [7.5 ml bottle]; 7.5 ml [10 ml bottle])

▷ *emedastine* (C) 1 drop qid prn
  Pediatric: <3 years: not recommended; ≥3 years: same as adult
    Emadine *Ophth soln:* 0.05% (5 ml) (benzalkonium chloride)

▷ *levocabastine* (C) 1 drop qid prn
  Pediatric: <12 years: not recommended; ≥12 years: same as adult
    Livostin *Ophth susp:* 0.05% (2.5, 5, 10 ml) (benzalkonium chloride)

OPHTHALMIC MAST CELL STABILIZERS

Comment: Concomitant contact lens wear is contraindicated during treatment.
▷ *cromolyn sodium* (B) 1-2 drops 4-6 x/day at regular intervals
  Pediatric: <4 years: not recommended; ≥4 years: same as adult
    Crolom *Ophth soln:* 4% (10 ml) (benzalkonium chloride)
▷ *lodoxamide tromethamine* (B) 1-2 drops qid up to 3 months
  Pediatric: <2 years: not recommended; ≥2 years: same as adult
    Alomide *Ophth soln:* 1% (10 ml) (benzalkonium chloride)
▷ *nedocromil* (B) 1-2 drops bid
  Pediatric: <3 years: not recommended; ≥3 years: same as adult
    Alocril *Ophth soln:* 2% (5 ml) (benzalkonium chloride)
▷ *pemirolast potassium* (C) 1-2 drops qid
  Pediatric: <3 years: not recommended; ≥3 years: same as adult
    Alamast *Ophth soln:* 0.1% (10 ml) (lauralkonium chloride)

OPHTHALMIC ANTIHISTAMINE+MAST CELL STABILIZER COMBINATIONS

▷ *alcaftadine* (B) 1 drop each eye daily
  Pediatric: <2 years: not recommended; ≥2 years: same as adult
    Lastacaft *Ophth soln:* 0.25% (6 ml) (benzalkonium chloride)
  Comment: May insert contact lens 10 minutes after ophthalmic administration.
▷ *azelastine* (C) 1 drop each eye bid
  Pediatric: <3 years: not recommended; ≥3 years: same as adult
    Optivar *Ophth soln:* 0.05% (6 ml) (benzalkonium chloride)
  Comment: May insert contact lens 10 minutes after ophthalmic administration.
▷ *bepotastine besilate* (C)(G) 1 drop each eye bid
  Pediatric: <2 years: not recommended; ≥2 years: same as adult
    Bepreve *Ophth soln:* 1.5% (10 ml) (benzalkonium chloride)
  Comment: May insert contact lens 10 minutes after ophthalmic administration.
▷ *epinastine* (C)(G) 1 drop each eye bid
  Pediatric: <3 years: not recommended; ≥3 years: same as adult
    Elestat *Ophth soln:* 0.05% (5 ml) (benzalkonium chloride)
  Comment: May insert contact lens 10 minutes after administration.
▷ *ketotifen fumarate* (C) 1 drop each eye q 8-12 hours
  Pediatric: <3 years: not recommended; ≥3 years: same as adult
    Alaway (OTC) *Ophth soln:* 0.025% (10 ml) (benzalkonium chloride)
    Claritin Eye (OTC) *Ophth soln:* 0.025% (5 ml) (benzalkonium chloride)
    Refresh Eye Itch Relief (OTC) *Ophth soln:* 0.025% (5 ml) (benzalkonium chloride)
    Zaditor (OTC) *Ophth soln:* 0.025% (5 ml) (benzalkonium chloride)
    Zyrtec Itchy Eye (OTC) *Ophth soln:* 0.025% (5 ml) (benzalkonium chloride)
  Comment: May insert contact lens 10 minutes after administration.
▷ *olopatadine* (C)(G) 1 drop each eye bid
  Pediatric: <3 years: not recommended; ≥3 years: same as adult
    Pataday *Ophth soln:* 0.2% (2.5 ml) (benzalkonium chloride)
    Patanol *Ophth soln:* 0.1% (5 ml) (benzalkonium chloride)
    Pazeo *Ophth soln:* 0.7% (2.5 ml) (benzalkonium chloride)
  Comment: May insert contact lens 10 minutes after administration.

OPHTHALMIC VASOCONSTRICTORS

Comment: Concomitant contact lens wear is contraindicated during treatment.

▷ *naphazoline* (C) 1-2 drops each eye qid prn
Pediatric: <12 years: not recommended; ≥12 years: same as adult
  Vasocon-A *Ophth soln:* 0.1% (15 ml) (benzalkonium chloride)
▷ *oxymetazoline* (OTC) 1-2 drops each eye qid prn
Pediatric: <6 years: not recommended; ≥6 years: same as adult
  Visine L-R *Ophth soln:* 0.025% (15, 30 ml)
▷ *tetrahydrozoline* (OTC)(G) 1-2 drops each eye qid prn
Pediatric: <6 years: not recommended; ≥6 years: same as adult
  Visine *Ophth soln:* 0.05% (15, 22.5, 30 ml)

OPHTHALMIC VASOCONSTRICTOR+MOISTURIZER COMBINATION

Comment: Concomitant contact lens wear is contraindicated during treatment.
▷ *tetrahydrozoline+polyethylene glycol 400+povidone+dextran 70* (OTC) 1-2 drops
each eye qid prn
Pediatric: <6 years: not recommended; ≥6 years: same as adult
  Advanced Relief Visine *Ophth soln:* tetra 0.025%+poly 1%+pov 1%+dex
  0.1% (15, 30 ml)

OPHTHALMIC VASOCONSTRICTOR+ASTRINGENT COMBINATION

Comment: Concomitant contact lens wear is contraindicated during treatment.
▷ *tetrahydrozoline+zinc sulfate* (OTC) 1-2 drops each eye qid prn
Pediatric: <6 years: not recommended; ≥6 years: same as adult
  Visine AC *Ophth soln:* tetra 0.025%+zinc 0.05% (15, 30 ml)

OPHTHALMIC VASOCONSTRICTOR+ANTI HISTAMINE COMBINATIONS

Comment: Concomitant contact lens wear is contraindicated during treatment.
▷ *naphazoline+pheniramine* (C) 1-2 drops each eye qid
Pediatric: <6 years: not recommended; ≥6 years: same as adult
  Naphcon-A (OTC) *Ophth soln:* naph 0.025%+phen 0.3% (15 ml)
  (benzalkonium chloride)

OPHTHALMIC NSAIDs

Comment: Concomitant contact lens wear is contraindicated during treatment.

▷ *bromfenac* (C)(G) 1 drop affected eye(s) bid
  Bromday Ophthalmic Solution *Ophth soln:* 0.09% (2.5 ml in 7.5 ml dropper
  bottle; 7.5 ml in 10 ml dropper bottle)
  Xibrom Ophthalmic Solution *Ophth soln:* 0.09% (2.5 ml in 7.5 ml dropper
  bottle; 7.5 ml in 10 ml dropper bottle)
▷ *diclofenac* (B) 1 drop affected eye(s) qid
Pediatric: <12 years: not recommended; ≥12 years: same as adult
  Voltaren Ophthalmic Solution *Ophth soln:* 0.1% (2.5, 5 ml)
▷ *ketorolac tromethamine* (C) 1 drop affected eye(s) qid; max x 4 days
Pediatric: <3 years: not recommended; ≥3 years: same as adult
  Acular *Ophth soln:* 0.5% (3, 5, 10 ml) (benzalkonium chloride)
  Acular LS *Ophth soln:* 0.4% (5 ml) (benzalkonium chloride)
  Acular PF *Ophth soln:* 0.5% (0.4 ml; 12 single-use vials/carton)
  (preservative-free)
▷ *nepafenac* (C) 1 drop affected eye(s) tid
Pediatric: <10 years: not recommended; ≥10 years: same as adult
  Nevanac Ophthalmic Suspension *Ophth susp:* 0.1% (3 ml) (benzalkonium
  chloride)

CONJUNCTIVITIS: VIRAL

Comment: For prevention of secondary bacterial infection, see agents listed under bacterial conjunctivitis. Ophthalmic corticosteroids are contraindicated with herpes simplex, keratitis, *Varicella*, and other viral infections of the cornea.

▷ *trifluridine* ophthalmic suspension **(C)** 1 drop q 2 hours while awake; max 9 drops/day; after re-epithelialization, 1 drop every 4 hours x 7 days (at least 5 drops/day); max 21 days of therapy
  Pediatric: <6 years: not recommended; ≥6 years: same as adult
  Viroptic Ophthalmic Solution *Ophth soln:* 1% (7.5 ml) (thimerosal)

CONSTIPATION: CHRONIC IDIOPATHIC (CIC)

GUANYLATE CYCLASE-C AGONISTS

Comment: Guanylate cyclase-c agonists increase intestinal fluid and intestinal transit time may induce diarrhea and bloating and, therefore, are contraindicated with known *or* suspected mechanical GI obstruction.

▷ *linaclotide* **(C)(G)** 145 mcg orally once daily *or* 72 mcg orally once daily based on individual presentation *or* tolerability; take on an empty stomach at least 30 minutes before the first meal of the day; swallow whole, do *not* crush *or* chew cap *or* cap contents; may open cap and administer with applesauce *or* water (e.g., NGT, PEG tube)
  Pediatric: ≤18 years: not established (<6 years: contraindicated; 6-18 years: avoid); >18 years: same as adult
  Linzess *Cap:* 72, 145, 290 mcg
  Comment: *Linaclotide* and its active metabolite are negligibly absorbed systemically following oral administration and maternal use is *not* expected to result in fetal exposure to the drug. There is no information regarding the presence of *plecanatide* in human milk *or* its effects on the breastfed infant.
▷ *plecanatide* take one tab once daily; if necessary, may crush and administer with applesauce *or* water (e.g., NGT, PEG tube)
  Pediatric: ≤18 years: not established (<6 years: contraindicated; 6-18 years: avoid); >18 years: same as adult
  Trulance *Tab:* 3 mg
  Comment: Suspend *plecanatide* dosing and rehydrate if severe diarrhea occurs. Most common adverse reactions in CIC are sinusitis, URI, diarrhea, abdominal distension and tenderness, flatulence, and increased liver enzymes. *Plecanatide* and its active metabolite are negligibly absorbed systemically following oral administration, and maternal use is *not* expected to result in fetal exposure to the drug. There is no information regarding the presence of *plecanatide* in human milk *or* its effects on the breastfed infant.

CHLORIDE CHANNEL ACTIVATOR

▷ *lubiprostone* **(C)** one 24 mcg cap bid with food and water; swallow whole, do *not* break apart *or* chew
  Pediatric: <18 years: not recommended; ≥18 years: same as adult
  Amitiza *Cap:* 8, 24 mcg
  Comment: **Amitiza** increases intestinal fluid and intestinal transit time. Suspend dosing and rehydrate if severe diarrhea occurs. **Amitiza** is contraindicated with known *or* suspected mechanical GI obstruction. Most common adverse reactions in CIC are nausea, diarrhea, headache, abdominal pain, abdominal distension, and flatulence.

Selective Serotonin Type 4 (5HT4) Receptor Agonist

▷ *prucalopride* 2 mg once daily; *CrCl <30 mL/min:* 1 mg once daily; *ESRD:* avoid
  Pediatric: <18 years: not established; ≥18 years: same as adult
    Motegrity *Tab:* 1, 2 mg film-coat
    Comment: **Motegrity** *(prucalopride)* is a selective serotonin type 4 (5HT4) receptor agonist for the treatment of chronic idiopathic constipation (CIC) in adults. *prucalopride* is a gastrointestinal (GI) prokinetic agent that stimulates colonic peristalsis (high-amplitude propagating contractions [HAPCs]), which increases bowel motility. The most common adverse reactions (incidence ≥2%) have been headache, abdominal pain, nausea, diarrhea, abdominal distension, dizziness, vomiting, flatulence, and fatigue. Contraindications include intestinal perforation or obstruction due to structural or functional disorder of the gut wall, obstructive ileus, severe inflammatory conditions of the intestinal tract such as Crohn's disease, ulcerative colitis, and toxic megacolon/megarectum. Monitor patients for persistent worsening of depression and emergence of suicidal thoughts and behavior. Instruct patients to discontinue **Motegrity** immediately and contact their healthcare provider if their depression is persistently worse, or they experience emerging suicidal thoughts or behaviors. Available data from case reports with *prucalopride* use in pregnancy are insufficient to identify any drug-associated risks of miscarriage, major birth defects, or adverse maternal or fetal outcomes. *prucalopride* is present in breast milk. There are no data on effects of *prucalopride* on the breastfed infant.

CONSTIPATION: OCCASIONAL, INTERMITTENT

BULK-FORMING AGENTS

▷ *calcium polycarbophil* (C) 2 tabs once daily to qid
  Pediatric: <6 years: not recommended; 6-12 years: 1 tab once daily to qid
    FiberCon (OTC) *Cplt:* 625 mg
    Konsyl Fiber Tablets (OTC) *Tab:* 625 mg
▷ *methylcellulose*
    Citrucel 1 heaping tbsp in 8 oz cold water tid
    Pediatric: <6 years: not recommended; 6-12 years: 1/2 adult dose
      Oral pwdr: 16, 24, 30 oz and single-dose pkts (orange)
    Citrucel Sugar-Free 1 heaping tbsp in 8 oz cold water tid
    Pediatric: <6 years: not recommended; 6-12 years: 1/2 adult dose
      Oral pwdr: 16, 24, 30 oz and single-dose pkts (orange) (sugar-free, phenylalanine)
▷ *psyllium husk* (B)
  Pediatric: <6 years: not recommended; 6-12 years: 1/2 adult dose in 8 oz liquid tid
    Metamucil (OTC) wafer or cap or 1 pkt or 1 rounded tsp (1 rounded tbsp for sugar-containing form) in 8 oz liquid tid
      Cap: psyllium husk 5.2 gm (100, 150/carton); Wafer: *psyllium husk* 3.4 gm/ rounded tsp (24/carton) (apple crisp, cinnamon spice); *Plain and flavored pwdr:* 3.4 gm/rounded tsp (15, 20, 24, 29, 30, 36, 44, 48 oz); *Efferv sugar-free flav pkts:* 3.4 gm/pkt (30/carton) (phenylalanine)
▷ *psyllium* hydrophilic mucilloid (B) 2 rounded tsp in 8 oz water qid
  Pediatric: <6 years: not recommended; 6-12 years: 1 rounded tsp in 8 oz liquid tid
    Konsyl (OTC) *Pwdr:* 6 gm/rounded tsp (10.6, 15.9 oz); *Pwdr pkt:* 6 gm/ rounded tsp (30/carton)
    Konsyl-D (OTC) *Pwdr:* 3.4 gm/rounded tsp (11.5, 17.59 oz); *Pwdr pkt:* 3.4 gm/rounded tsp (30/carton)

Konsyl Easy Mix Formula (OTC) *Pwdr:* 3.4 gm/rounded tsp (8 oz)
(sugar-free, low sodium)
Konsyl Orange (OTC) *Pwdr:* 3.4 gm/rounded tsp (19 oz); *Pwdr pkt:* 3.4 gm/
rounded tsp (30/carton)
Konsyl Orange SF (OTC) *Pwdr:* 3.5 gm/rounded tsp (15 oz) (phenylalanine);
Pwdr pkt: 3.5 gm/rounded tsp (30/carton) (phenylalanine)

STOOL SOFTENERS

▷ *docusate sodium* (OTC) 50-200 mg/day
Pediatric: <3 years: 10-40 mg/day; 3-6 years: 20-60 mg/day; >6 years: 40-120 mg/
day
    Cap: 50, 100 mg; *Liq:* 10 mg/ml (30 ml w. dropper); *Syr:* 20 mg/5 ml (8 oz)
    (alcohol ≤1%)
    Dialose 1 tab q HS
    Pediatric: <6 years: not recommended; ≥6 years: same as adult
      Tab: 100 mg
    Surfak (OTC) 240 mg/day
    Pediatric: <12 years: not recommended; ≥12 years: same as adult
      Cap: 240 mg
▷ *docusate* enema
    DocuSol Kids (OTC) <2 years: not established; 2-12 years: 1 x 5 ml mini-enema
      Mini-enema: 100 mg/5 ml (5 ml, 5/box)
    Comment: Results of one mini-enema are usually seen within 5-15 minutes.

OSMOTIC LAXATIVES

▷ *lactulose* (B)(G) take 10-20 gm dissolved in 4 oz water once daily prn; max 40
gm/day
Pediatric: <12 years: not recommended; ≥12 years: same as adult
    Kristalose *Crystals for oral soln:* 10, 20 gm single-dose pkts (30/carton)
▷ *magnesium citrate* (B)(G) 1 full bottle (120-300 ml) once daily prn
Pediatric: <2 years: not recommended; 2-6 years: 4-12 ml once daily prn; ≥6-12
years: 50-100 ml once daily prn
    Citrate of Magnesia (OTC) *Oral soln:* 300 ml
▷ *magnesium hydroxide* (B) 30-60 ml/day in a single or divided doses prn
Pediatric: 2-5 years: 5-15 ml/day in a single or divided doses; 6-11 years: 15-30
ml/day in a single or divided doses; ≥12 years: same as adult
    Milk of Magnesia *Liq:* 390 mg/5 ml (10, 15, 20, 30, 100, 120, 180, 360,
    720 ml)
▷ *polyethylene glycol (PEG)* (C)(OTC)(G) 1 tbsp (17 gm) dissolved in 4-8 oz water
per day for up to max 7 days; may need 2-4 days for results
Pediatric: ≤17: <12 years: not recommended; ≥12 years: same as adult
    GlycoLax Powder for Oral Solution *Oral pwdr:* 7, 14, 30, and 45 dose bottles
    w. 17 gm dosing cup (gluten-free, sugar-free); 17 gm single-dose pkts (20/
    carton)
    MiraLAX Powder for Oral Solution *Oral pwdr:* 7, 14, 30, and 45 dose bottles
    w. 17 gm dosing cup (gluten-free, sugar-free)
    Polyethylene Glycol 3350 Powder for Oral Solution (G) *Oral pwdr:* 3350 gm
    w. dosing cup; 17 gm/scoop
    Comment: *PEG* is an osmotic indicated for occasional constipation without
affecting glucose and electrolyte levels. Contraindicated with suspected or
known bowel obstruction.

STIMULANTS

▷ *bisacodyl* (B) 2-3 tabs or 1 suppository bid prn
    Dulcolax, Gentlax *Tab:* 5 mg; *Rectal supp:* 10 mg

Pediatric: <12 years: 1/2 suppository once daily prn; 6-12 years: 1 tablet or 1/2 suppository once daily prn; >12 years: same as adult

Senokot (OTC) initially 2-4 tabs or 1 level tsp at HS prn; max 4 tabs or 2 tsp bid
Pediatric: <2 years: not recommended; 2-6 years: 1/4 tab or 1/2 tsp once daily prn; max 1 tab or 1/2 tsp bid; 6-12 years: 1 tab or 1/2 tsp once daily prn; max 2 tabs or 1 tsp once daily
  Tab: 8.6*mg; *Granules:* 15 mg/tsp (2, 6, 12 oz) (cocoa)
Senokot Syrup (OTC) initially 10-15 ml at HS prn; max 15 ml bid
Pediatric: use Childrens Syrup
  Syr: 8.8 mg/5 ml (2, 8 oz) (chocolate) (alcohol-free)
Senokot Childrens Syrup (OTC)
Pediatric: <2 years: not recommended; 2-6 years: 2.5-3.75 ml once daily prn; max 3.75 ml bid prn; ≥6-12 years: 5-7.5 ml once daily prn; max 7.5 ml twice daily
  Syr: 8.8 mg/5 ml (2.5 oz) (chocolate) (alcohol-free)
Senokot Xtra (OTC) 1 tab at HS prn; max 2 tabs bid
Pediatric: <2 years: not recommended; 2-6 years: use Childrens Syrup; 6-12 years: 1/2 tab once daily at HS; max 1 tab bid
  Tab: 17*mg

BULK FORMING AGENT+STIMULANT COMBINATIONS

▷ *psyllium+senna* (B)
  Perdiem (OTC) 1-2 rounded tsp swallowed with 8 oz cool liquid once daily to bid
  Pediatric: <7 years: not recommended; 7-11 years: 1 rounded tsp swallowed with 8 oz cool liquid once daily-bid; ≥12 years: same as adult
    Canister: 8.8, 14 oz; *Individual pkt:* 6 gm (6/pck)
  SennaPrompt (OTC) initially 2-5 caps bid
  Pediatric: <12 years: not recommended; ≥12 years: same as adult
    Cap: psyl 500 mg+senna 9 mg

STOOL SOFTENER+STIMULANT COMBINATIONS

▷ *docusate+casanthranol* (C)
    Doxidan (OTC) 1-3 caps/day; max 1 week
    Pediatric: <2 years: not recommended; ≥2 years: 1 cap/day
      Cap: doc 60 mg+cas 30 mg
    Peri-Colace (OTC) 1-2 caps or 15-30 ml q HS; max 2 caps or 30 ml bid or 3 caps q HS
    Pediatric: 5-15 ml q HS
      Cap: doc 100 mg+cas 30 mg; *Syr:* doc 60 mg+cas 30 mg per 15 ml (8, 16 oz)
▷ *docusate+senna* concentrate (C)
    Senokot S (OTC) 2 tabs q HS; max 4 tabs bid
    Pediatric: <2 years: not recommended; 2-6 years: 1/2 tab daily; max 1 tab bid; >6-12 years: 1 tab daily; max 2 tabs bid
      Tab: doc 50 mg+senna 8.6 mg

ENEMAS AND SUPPOSITIRIES

▷ *glycerin* suppository (C)(OTC) 1 adult suppository
  Pediatric: <6 years: 1 pediatric suppository; ≥6 years: 1 adult suppository
▷ *docusate* enema
  Pediatric: <2 years: not established; 2-12 years: 1 x 5 ml mini-enema
    DocuSol Kids (OTC) *Mini-enema:* 100 mg/5 ml (5 ml, 5/box)
    Comment: Results of one mini-enema are usually seen within 5-15 minutes.
▷ *sodium biphosphate+sodium phosphate* enema (C)(OTC)
    Fleets Adult 59-118 ml rectally

Enema: sod biphos 19 gm+sod phos 7 gm (59, 118 ml w. applicator)
Fleets Pediatric 59 ml rectally
Enema: sod biphos 19 gm+sod phos 7 gm (59 ml w. applicator)

CORNEAL EDEMA

▷ *sodium chloride* (G)
Pediatric: same as adult 1-2 drops or 1 inch ribbon q 3-4 hours prn; reduce
frequency as edema subsides
Various (OTC)
Ophth soln: 2, 5% (15, 30 ml); *Ophth oint:* 5% (3.5 gm)

CORNEAL ULCERATION

ANTIBACTERIAL OPHTHALMIC SOLUTION/OINTMENT
see **Conjunctivitis/Blepharoconjunctivitis: Bacterial**

COSTOCHONDRITIS (CHEST WALL SYNDROME)

Acetaminophen for IV Infusion *see Pain*
NSAIDs *see* Appendix J. NSAIDs online at https://connect.springerpub.com/content/
reference-book/978-0-8261-7935-7/back-matter/part02/back-matter/bmatter10
Opioid Analgesics *see Pain*
Topical & Transdermal Analgesics *see Pain*
Parenteral Corticosteroids *see* Appendix M. Parenteral Corticosteroids
Oral Corticosteroids *see* Appendix L. Oral Corticosteroids
Topical Analgesic and Anesthetic Agents *see* Appendix I. Anesthetic Agents for
Local Infiltration and Dermal/Mucosal Membrane Application online at https://
connect.springerpub.com/content/reference-book/978-0-8261-7935-7/back-matter/
part02/back-matter/bmatter9

COVID-19 (*CORONAVIRUS*)

PROPHYLAXIS

▷ **Moderna COVID-19 Vaccine** *(mRNA1237) (100 mcg) vaccine* administer this
2-dose series via IM injection 21 days apart
Pediatric: <16 years: safety and efficacy not established; ≥16 years: same as adult
Moderna COVID-19 Vaccine *(mRNA1237) (100 mcg) Multi-dose Vial:*
contains 10 doses; 100 mcg/dose; frozen suspension requires thawing and
dilution prior to administration; must be used or discarded within 6 hours of
dilution (preservative-free)
Comment: The U.S. Food and Drug Administration (FDA) issued an Emergency
Use Authorization (EUA) to permit the emergency use of the unapproved
product, **Moderna COVID-19 Vaccine,** for active immunization to prevent
COVID-19. Overall, 15,419 participants aged 18 years and older received at least
one dose of **Moderna COVID- 19 Vaccine** in three clinical trials (NCT04283461,
NCT04405076, and NCT04470427). The safety of **Moderna COVID-19
Vaccine** was evaluated in an ongoing Phase 3 randomized, placebo-controlled,
observer-blind clinical trial conducted in the United States involving 30,351
participants 18 years-of-age and older who received at least one dose of **Moderna
COVID-19 Vaccine** (n=15,185) or placebo (n=15,166) (NCT04470427). At the
time of vaccination, the mean age of the population was 52 years (range 18-95);
22,831 (75.2%) of participants were 18 to 64 years-of-age and 7520 (24.8%) of
participants were 65 years-of-age and older. Overall, 52.7% were male, 47.3%
were female, 20.5% were Hispanic or Latino, 79.2% were White, 10.2% were

African American, 4.6% were Asian, 0.8% were American Indian or Alaska Native, 0.2% were Native Hawaiian or Pacific Islander, 2.1% were Other, and 2.1% were Multiracial. Demographic characteristics were similar among participants who received **Moderna COVID-19 Vaccine** and those who received placebo. Vials can be stored refrigerated between 2° to 8°C (36° to 46°F) for up to 30 days prior to first use. Unpunctured vials may be stored between 8° to 25°C (46° to 77°F) for up to 12 hours. Do not refreeze once thawed. Thaw in refrigerated conditions between 2° to 8°C (36° to 46°F) for 2 hours and 30 minutes. After thawing, let vial stand at room temperature for 15 minutes before administering. Alternatively, thaw at room temperature between 15° to 25°C (59° to 77°F) for 1 hour. Swirl vial gently after thawing and between each withdrawal. Do not shake. Do not dilute the vaccine. In clinical studies, the adverse reactions in participants 18 years-of-age and older were pain at the injection site (92.0%), fatigue (70.0%), headache (64.7%), myalgia (61.5%), arthralgia (46.4%), chills (45.4%), nausea/vomiting (23.0%), axillary swelling/tenderness (19.8%), fever (15.5%), swelling at the injection site (14.7%), and erythema at the injection site (10.0%). There is no information on the co-administration of the **Moderna COVID-19 Vaccine** with other vaccines. The **Moderna COVID-19 Vaccine** is a white to off-white suspension. It may contain white or translucent product-related particulates. Visually inspect the **Moderna COVID Vaccine** in the vial and in the syringe. Monitor **Moderna COVID-19 Vaccine** recipients for the occurrence of immediate adverse reactions. Appropriate medical treatment to manage immediate allergic reactions must be immediately available in the event of an acute anaphylactic reaction occurs following administration of the **Moderna COVID-19 Vaccine**. The vaccination provider must communicate to the recipient or their caregiver, information consistent with the "Fact Sheet for Recipients and Caregivers" (and provide a copy or direct the individual to the website www.modernatx.com/covid19vaccine-eua to obtain the Fact Sheet) prior to the individual receiving the **Moderna COVID-19 Vaccine**, including: (1) the FDA has authorized the emergency use of the Moderna **COVID-19 Vaccine**, which is not an FDA-approved vaccine; (2) the recipient or their caregiver has the option to accept or refuse the **Moderna COVID-19 Vaccine**; (3) the significant known and potential risks and benefits of the **Moderna COVID-19 Vaccine**, and the extent to which such risks and benefits are unknown; (4) information about available alternative vaccines and the risks and benefits of those alternatives. The vaccination provider must include vaccination information in the state/local jurisdiction's **Immunization Information System (IIS)** or other designated system. The vaccination provider is responsible for mandatory reporting of the following to the **Vaccine Adverse Event Reporting System (VAERS)**: (1) vaccine administration errors, whether or not associated with an adverse event; (2) serious adverse events (irrespective of attribution to vaccination), (3) cases of **Multisystem Inflammatory Syndrome (MIS)** in adults; (4) cases of COVID-19 that result in hospitalization or death. Complete and submit reports to VAERS online at https://vaers.hhs.gov/reportevent.html. For further assistance with reporting to VAERS, call 1-800-822-7967. The reports should include the words "**Moderna COVID- 19 Vaccine EUA**" in the description section of the report. The vaccination provider is responsible for responding to FDA requests for information about vaccine administration errors, adverse events, cases of MIS in adults and cases of COVID-19 that result in hospitalization or death following administration of the **Moderna COVID-19 Vaccine** to recipients. Available data on **Moderna COVID-19 Vaccine** administered to pregnant women are insufficient to inform vaccine-associated risks in pregnancy. There is a pregnancy exposure registry that monitors pregnancy outcomes in women exposed to **Moderna COVID-19 Vaccine** during pregnancy. Women who are vaccinated with **Moderna COVID-19 Vaccine** during pregnancy are encouraged to enroll in the registry by calling 1-866- MODERNA (1-866-663-3762). Data are <u>not</u> available to assess the effects of **Moderna COVID-19 Vaccine** on the breastfed infant.

▷ **Pfizer COVID-19 Vaccine** *(bnt162b2) (30 mcg) vaccine* administer this 2-dose series via IM injection 21 days apart

Pediatric: <12 years: not established; ≥12 years: same as adult

> **Pfizer COVID-19 Vaccine** *(bnt162b2) (30 mcg) Multi-dose Vial:* contains 5 doses; 30 mcg/dose; frozen requires thawing and diluting prior to administration; must be used <u>or</u> discarded within 6 hours of dilution

Comment: The U.S. Food and Drug Administration (FDA) issued an Emergency Use Authorization (EUA) to permit the emergency use of the unapproved product, **Pfizer COVID-19 Vaccine,** for active immunization for the prevention of *Coronavirus* disease 2019 (COVID-19). The EUA recommendation was based on data from an ongoing phase 3 double-blind, placebo-controlled study in approximately 44,000 participants. Final efficacy data, reported in the *New England Journal of Medicine*, included 36,523 participants, showed that the vaccine was 95% effective (P<.0001) in people without prior severe acute respiratory syndrome coronavirus 2 (SARS-CoV-2), as well as in those with <u>or</u> without evidence of infection before vaccination. Fatigue and headache were noted to be the only grade 3 solicited adverse events (incidence ≥2%). Subgroup analysis of the data has indicated consistent efficacy across age, gender, race, and ethnicity demographics. Among participants over 65 years-of-age, vaccine efficacy was observed to be >94%. At this time, **BNT162b2** is <u>not</u> approved for pregnant <u>or</u> lactating females, persons who are immunocompromised, and children under 16 years-of-age due to insufficient data. More data will be needed to determine duration of protection, effectiveness of the vaccine in certain populations at high risk for severe disease (i.e., those with HIV/AIDS), as well as those with prior SARS-CoV-2 infection.

TREATMENT

▷ *remdesivir Loading Dose on Day 1:* 200 mg via IV infusion; *Maintenance:* 100 mg via IV infusion once daily starting Day 2; administer each infusion over 30 to 120 minutes; *Patients <u>not</u> requiring invasive mechanical ventilation and/or ECMO:* total treatment duration is 5 days; if <u>no</u> clinical improvement, treatment may be extended for up to 5 additional days for total treatment duration up to 10 days; *Patients requiring invasive mechanical ventilation and/or ECMO:* treatment duration is 10 days; *eGFR < 30 mL/min:* not recommended; *Dose Preparation/ Administration:* see mfr pkg insert for full prescribing information

Pediatric: <12 years, <40 kg: not established; ≥12 years, ≥40 kg: same as adult

> **Veklury** *Vial:* 100 mg, single-dose, pwdr, for reconstitution, dilution, and IV infusion; 100 mg/20 ml (5 mg/ml), single-dose, for dilution and IV infusion (preservative-free)

Comment: *Remdesivir* is indicated for patients with COVID-19 requiring hospitalization. **Veklury** should <u>only</u> be administered in a hospital <u>or</u> in a healthcare setting capable of providing acute care comparable to inpatient hospital care. Co-administration of **Veklury** and *chloroquine phosphate* or *hydroxychloroquine sulfate* is <u>not</u> recommended based on cell culture data demonstrating an antagonistic effect of chloroquine on the intracellular metabolic activation and antiviral activity of **Veklury**. In all patients, before initiating **Veklury** and during treatment as clinically appropriate, perform renal and hepatic laboratory testing and assess prothrombin time. The most common adverse reactions (incidence ≥5%, all grades) are nausea and increased ALT and AST. Consider discontinuing **Veklury** if ALT levels increase to >10 times the upper limit of normal (10 x ULN). Discontinue **Veklury** if ALT elevation is accompanied by signs <u>or</u> symptoms of liver inflammation. Hypersensitivity reactions have been observed during and following administration of **Veklury**. Slower infusion rates, with a maximum infusion time of up to 120 minutes, can be considered to potentially prevent signs and symptoms of hypersensitivity. If signs and symptoms of a clinically significant hypersensitivity reaction occur, immediately discontinue administration of **Veklury** and initiate appropriate treatment. Available data from published case reports and compassionate use of *remdesivir* in pregnant females are insufficient to evaluate for a drug-associated risk of major birth defects, miscarriage, or adverse maternal or fetal outcomes. In non-clinical reproductive toxicity studies, *remdesivir* demonstrated no adverse effect on embryo/fetal development when administered to pregnant animals at systemic exposures (AUC) of the predominant circulating metabolite of *remdesivir* (**GS-441524**) that were four times the exposure in humans at the recommended human dose (RHD). There are no available data on the presence of *remdesivir* in human milk or effects on the breastfed infant.

 CRAMPS: ABDOMINAL, INTESTINAL

ANTISPASMODIC-ANTICHOLINERGIC AGENTS

▷ *dicyclomine* (B)(G) initially 20 mg bid-qid; may increase to 40 mg qid PO; usual IM dose 80 mg/day divided qid; do not use IM route for more than 1-2 days
   Pediatric: <12 years: not recommended; ≥12 years: same as adult
      Bentyl *Tab:* 20 mg; *Cap:* 10 mg; *Syr:* 10 mg/5 ml (16 oz); *Vial:* 10 mg/ml (10 ml); *Amp:* 10 mg/ml (2 ml)
▷ *methscopolamine bromide* (B) 1 tab q 6 hours prn
   Pediatric: <12 years: not recommended; ≥12 years: same as adult
      Pamine *Tab:* 2.5 mg
      Pamine Forte *Tab:* 5 mg

ANTICHOLINERGICS

▷ *hyoscyamine* (C)(G)
      Anaspaz 1-2 tabs q 4 hours prn; max 12 tabs/day
      Pediatric: <2 years: not recommended; 2-12 years: 0.0625-0.125 mg q 4 hours prn; max 0.75 mg/day; ≥12 years: same as adult
         Tab: 0.125*mg
      Levbid 1-2 tabs q 12 hours prn; max 4 tabs/day
      Pediatric: <12 years: not recommended; ≥12 years: same as adult
         Tab: 0.375*mg ext-rel
      Levsin 1-2 tabs q 4 hours prn; max 12 tabs/day
      Pediatric: <6 years: not recommended; ≥6-12 years: 1 tab q 4 hours prn
         Tab: 0.125*mg
      Levsinex SL 1-2 tabs q 4 hours SL or PO; max 12 tabs/day
      Pediatric: 2-12 years: 1 tab SL or PO q 4 hours; max 6 tabs/day
         Tab: 0.125 mg sublingual
      Levsinex Timecaps 1-2 caps q 12 hours; may adjust to 1 cap q 8 hours
      Pediatric: 2-12 years: 1 cap q 12 hours; max 2 caps/day
         Cap: 0.375 mg time-rel
      NuLev dissolve 1-2 tabs on tongue, with or without water, q 4 hours prn; max 12 tabs/day
      Pediatric: <2 years: not recommended; 2-12 years: dissolve 1 tab on tongue, with or without water, q 4 hours prn; max 6 tabs/day; >12 years: same as adult
         ODT: 0.125 mg (mint) (phenylalanine)
▷ *simethicone* (C)(G) 0.3 ml qid pc and HS
      Mylicon Drops (OTC) *Oral drops:* 40 mg/0.6 ml (30 ml)
▷ *phenobarbital+hyoscyamine+atropine+scopolamine* (C)(IV)(G)
      Donnatal 1-2 tabs ac and HS
      Pediatric: <12 years: not recommended; ≥12 years: same as adult
         Tab: pheno 16.2 mg+hyo 0.1037 mg+atro 0.0194 mg+scop 0.0065 mg

Donnatal Elixir 1-2 tsp ac and HS
Pediatric: 20 lb: 1 ml q 4 hours <u>or</u> 1.5 ml q 6 hours; 30 lb: 1.5 ml q 4 hours <u>or</u>
2 ml q 6 hours; 50 lb: 1/2 tsp q 4 hours <u>or</u> 3/4 tsp q 6 hours; 75 lb: 3/4 tsp q 4
hours <u>or</u> 1 tsp q 6 hours; 100 lb: 1 tsp q 4 hours <u>or</u> 1 tsp q 6 hours
    Elix: pheno 16.2 mg+hyo 0.1037 mg+atro 0.0194 mg+scop 0.0065 mg per 5 ml
    (4, 16 oz)
Donnatal Extentabs 1 tab q 12 hours
Pediatric: <12 years: not recommended; ≥12 years: same as adult
    Tab: pheno 48.6 mg+hyo 0.3111 mg+atro 0.0582 mg+scop 0.0195 mg ext-
    rel

ANTICHOLINERGIC+SEDATIVE COMBINATION

➤ *chlordiazepoxide+clidinium* (D)(IV) 1-2 caps ac and HS; max 8 caps/day
Pediatric: <12 years: not recommended; ≥12 years: same as adult
    Librax *Cap:* chlor 5 mg+clid 2.5 mg

 CROHN'S DISEASE

Parenteral Corticosteroids *see* Appendix M. Parenteral Corticosteroids
Oral Corticosteroids *see* Appendix L. Oral Corticosteroids

Comment: Standard treatment regimen for active disease (flare) is antibiotic,
antispasmodic, and bowel rest, progress to clear liquids, then progress to high-
fiber diet. Long-term management of chronic disease includes salicylates, immune
modulators, and tumor necrosis factor (TNF) blockers.

ORAL ANTI-INFECTIVES

➤ *metronidazole* (G) 500 mg tid <u>or</u> 750 mg bid; max 8 weeks
Pediatric: 35-50 mg/kg/day in 3 divided doses x 10 days
    Flagyl *Tab:* 250*, 500*mg
    Flagyl 375 *Cap:* 375 mg
    Flagyl ER *Tab:* 750 mg ext-rel

SALICYLATES

➤ *mesalamine* (B)(G)
    Asacol 800 mg tid x 6 weeks; maintenance 1.6 gm/day in divided doses;
    swallow whole, do <u>not</u> crush <u>or</u> chew
    Pediatric: <12 years: not recommended; ≥12 years: same as adult
        Tab: 400 mg del-rel
    Comment: 2 x **Asacol** 400 mg tabs are <u>not</u> bioequivalent to 1 x **Asacol HD** 800 mg
    tab.
    Asacol HD 1600 mg tid x 6 weeks; swallow whole, do <u>not</u> crush <u>or</u> chew
    Pediatric: <12 years: not recommended; ≥12 years: same as adult
        Tab: 800 mg del-rel
    Comment: 1 x **Asacol HD** 800 mg tab is <u>not</u> bioequivalent to 2 x **Asacol** 400 mg
    tabs
    Canasa 1 gm qid for up to 8 weeks
    Pediatric: <12 years: not recommended; ≥12 years: same as adult
        Rectal supp: 1 gm del-rel (30, 42/pck)
    Delzicol *Treatment:* 800 mg tid x 6 weeks; maintenance 1.6 gm/day in 2-4
    divided doses daily; swallow whole; do <u>not</u> crush <u>or</u> chew
    Pediatric: <5 years: not established; ≥5 years: same as adult
        Cap: 400 mg del-rel
    Comment: 2 x **Delzicol** 400 mg caps are <u>not</u> bioequivalent to 1 x *mesalamine*
    800 mg del-rel tab

Lialda 2.4-4.8 gm daily in a single dose for up to 8 weeks; swallow whole, do not crush or chew
Pediatric: <18 years: not recommended; ≥18 years: same as adult
  Tab: 1.2 gm del-rel
Pentasa 1 gm qid for up to 8 weeks; swallow whole, do not crush or chew
Pediatric: <12 years: not recommended; ≥12 years: same as adult
  Cap: 250 mg cont-rel
Rowasa Enema 4 gm rectally by enema q HS; retain for 8 hours x 3-6 weeks
Pediatric: <12 years: not recommended; ≥12 years: same as adult
  Enema: 4 gm/60 ml (7, 14, 28/pck; kit, 7, 14, 28/pck w. wipes)
Rowasa Suppository 1 suppository rectally bid x 3-6 weeks; retain for 1-3 hours or longer
  Rectal supp: 500 mg
Sulfite-Free Rowasa Rectal Suspension 4 gm rectally by enema q HS; retain for 8 hours x 3-6 weeks
  Enema: 4 gm/60 ml (7, 14, 28/pck; kit, 7, 14, 28/pck w. wipes)
▷ *olsalazine* (C)
  Dipentum 1 gm/day in 2 divided doses; max 2 gm/day
  Cap: 250 mg
  Comment: Indicated in persons who cannot tolerate *sulfasalazine*.
▷ *sulfasalazine* (B)(G)
  Azulfidine initially 1-2 gm/day; increase to 3-4 gm/day in divided doses pc until clinical symptoms controlled; maintenance 2 gm/day; max 4 gm/day
  Pediatric: <2 years: not recommended; 2-16 years: initially 40-60 mg/kg/day in 3-6 divided doses; max 2 gm/day
    Tab: 500*mg
  Azulfidine EN initially 500 mg in the PM x 7 days; then 500 mg bid x 7 days; then 500 mg in the AM and 1 gm in the PM x 7 days; then 1 gm bid; max 4 gm/day
  Pediatric: <12 years: not recommended; ≥12 years: same as adult
    Tab: 500 mg ent-coat
▷ *budesonide micronized* (C) (G)
  Pediatric: <12 years: not recommended; ≥12 years: same as adult
  Entocort EC *Treatment* 9 mg once daily in the AM for up to 8 weeks; may repeat an 8-week course; *Maintenance of remission*: 6 mg once daily for up to 3 months
    Cap: 3 mg ent-coat ext-rel granules
  Comment: Taper other systemic steroids when transferring to **Entocort EC**. When corticosteroids are used chronically, systemic effects such as hypercorticism and adrenal suppression may occur. Corticosteroids can reduce the response of the hypothalamus-pituitary-adrenal (HPA) axis to stress. In situations where patients are subject to surgery or other stress situations, supplementation with a systemic corticosteroid is recommended. General precautions concerning corticosteroids should be followed.

PURINE ANTIMETABOLITE IMMUNOSUPPRESSANT
▷ *azathioprine* (D)(G)
  Imuran *Tab:* 50*mg; *Injectable:* 100 mg
  Comment: **Imuran** is usually administered on a daily basis. The initial dose should be approximately 1.0 mg/kg (50 to 100 mg) as a single dose or divided bid. Dose may be increased beginning at 6-8 weeks, and thereafter at 4-week intervals, if there are no serious toxicities and if initial response is unsatisfactory. Dose increments should be 0.5 mg/kg/day, up to max 2.5 mg/kg

per day. Therapeutic response usually occurs after 6-8 weeks of treatment. An adequate trial should be a minimum of 12 weeks. Patients not improved after 12 weeks can be considered refractory. **Imuran** may be continued long-term in patients with clinical response, but patients should be monitored carefully, and gradual dosage reduction should be attempted to reduce risk of toxicities. Maintenance therapy should be at the lowest effective dose, and the dose given can be lowered decrementally with changes of 0.5 mg/kg or approximately 25 mg daily every 4 weeks while other therapy is kept constant. The optimum duration of maintenance **Imuran** has not been determined. **Imuran** can be discontinued abruptly, but delayed effects are possible.

TUMOR NECROSIS FACTOR (TNF) BLOCKERS

▷ *adalimumab* (B) *Day 1:* 160 mg SC (single dose or split over 2 consecutive days); *Day 15:* 80 mg SC; *Starting Day 29:* 40 mg SC every other week; administer SC in the abdomen or thigh; rotate sites administer in abdomen or thigh; rotate sites
Pediatric: <17 kg (37 lb): not recommended; 17 kg (37 lb) to <40 kg (<88 lb): *Day 1:* 80 mg SC; *Day 15:* 40 mg SC; *Starting Day 29:* 20 mg every other week; >40 kg (>88 lb): *Day 1:* 160 mg SC (single dose or split over 2 consecutive days); Day 15: 80 mg SC; Starting Day 29: 40 mg SC every other week
   Humira *Prefilled pen (**Humira Pen**):* 40 mg/0.4 ml, 40 mg/0.8 ml, 80 mg/0.8 ml, single-dose; *Prefilled glass syringe:* 10 mg/0.1 ml, 10 mg/0.2 ml, 20 mg/0.2 ml, 20 mg/0.4 ml, 40 mg/0.4 ml. 40 mg/0.8 ml, 80 mg/0.8 ml, single-dose; *Vial:* 40 mg/0.8 ml, single dose, institutional use only (preservative-free)
   Comment: May use with corticosteroids, salicylates, NSAIDs, or analgesics.
▷ *adalimumab-adaz* (B) *First dose (Day 1):* 160 mg SC (4 x 40 mg injections in 1 day or 2 x 40 mg injections per day x 2 consecutive days); *Second dose 2 weeks later (Day 15):* 80 mg SC; *2 weeks later (Day 29):* begin a maintenance dose of 40 mg SC every other week
Pediatric: <18 years: not recommended; ≥18 years: same as adult
   Hyrimoz *Prefilled syringe:* 40 mg/0.8 ml single-dose (preservative-free)
   Comment: **Hyrimoz** is biosimilar to **Humira** (*adalimumab*).
▷ *adalimumab-adbm* (B) *First dose (Day 1):* 160 mg SC (4 x 40 mg injections in 1 day or 2 x 40 mg injections per day for 2 consecutive days); *Second dose 2 weeks later (Day 15):* 80 mg SC; *2 weeks later (Day 29):* begin a maintenance dose of 40 mg SC every other week
Pediatric: <18 years: not recommended; ≥18 years: same as adult
   Cyltezo *Prefilled syringe:* 40 mg/0.8 ml single-dose (preservative-free)
   Comment: **Cyltezo** is biosimilar to **Humira** (*adalimumab*).
▷ *adalimumab-afzb* 40 mg SC every other week; some patients with RA not receiving *methotrexate* may benefit from increasing the frequency to 40 mg SC every week
   Abrilada *Prefilled pen:* 40 mg/0.8 ml, single-dose; *Prefilled syringe:* 40 mg/0.8 ml, 20 mg/0.4 ml, 10 mg/0.2 ml, single-dose; *Vial:* 40 mg/0.8 ml, single-use (for institutional use only) (preservative-free)
   Comment: **Abrilada** is biosimilar to **Humira** (*adalimumab*).
▷ *adalimumab-bwwd* *Initial Dose (Day 1):* 160 mg SC; *Second Dose: 2 weeks later (Day 15):* 80 mg SC; *2 weeks later (Day 29):* begin maintenance dose of 40 mg every other week
   Hadlima *Prefilled autoinjector:* 40 mg/0.8 ml, single-dose (Hadlima PushTouch); *Prefilled syringe:* 40 mg/0.8 ml, single-dose
   Comment: **Hadlima** is biosimilar to **Humira** (*adalimumab*).
▷ *certolizumab* (B) 400 mg SC (2 x 200 mg inj at two different sites on day 1); then, 400 mg SC at weeks 2 and 4; maintenance 400 mg SC every 4 weeks; administer in abdomen or thigh; rotate sites
Pediatric: <12 years: not recommended; ≥12 years: same as adult

Cimzia *Vial*: 200 mg (2/pck); *Prefilled syringe*: 200 mg/ml single-dose (2/pck; 2, 6/starter pck) (preservative-free)

▷ *infliximab* must be refrigerated at 2°C to 8°C (36°F to 46°F); administer dose intravenously over a period of not less than 2 hours; do not use beyond the expiration date as this product contains no preservative; 5 mg/kg at 0, 2 and 6 weeks, then every 8 weeks.

Pediatric: <6 years: not studied; ≥6-17 years: mg/kg at 0, 2 and 6 weeks, then every 8 weeks; ≥18 years: same as adult

Remicade *Vial*: 100 mg for reconstitution to 10 ml administration volume, single-dose pwdr (presrvative-free)

Comment: **Remicade** is indicated to reduce signs and symptoms, and induce and maintain clinical remission, in adults and children ≥6 years-of-age with moderately to severely active disease who have had an inadequate response to conventional therapy and reduce the number of draining enterocutaneous and rectovaginal fistulas, and maintain fistula closure, in adults with fistulizing disease. Common adverse effects associated with **Remicade** included abdominal pain, headache, pharyngitis, sinusitis, and upper respiratory infections. In addition, **Remicade** might increase the risk for serious infections, including tuberculosis, bacterial sepsis, and invasive fungal infections. Available data from published literature on the use of *infliximab* products during pregnancy have not reported a clear association with *infliximab* products and adverse pregnancy outcomes. *Infliximab* products cross the placenta and infants exposed *in utero* should not be administered live vaccines for at least 6 months after birth. Otherwise, the infant may be at increased risk of infection, including disseminated infection which can become fatal. Available information is insufficient to inform the amount of *infliximab* products present in human milk or effects on the breastfed infant.

▷ *infliximab-abda* (B)
Renflexis *Vial*: 100 mg pwdr for reconstitution to 10 ml administration volume, single-dose
Comment: **Renflexis** is biosimilar to **Remicade**. (*infliximab*).

▷ *infliximab-axxq* *Initially*: 5 mg/kg via IV infusion at 0, 2 and 6 weeks; *Maintenance*: 5 mg/kg via IV infusion every 8 weeks
Pediatric: <6 years: not studied; ≥6 years: same as adult
Avsola *Vial*: 100 mg pwdr in a 20 ml single-dose vial, for reconstitution, dilution, and IV infusion
Comment: **Avsola** is biosimilar to **Remicade** (*infliximab*).

▷ *infliximab-qbtx* (B)
Ixifi *Vial*: 100 pwdr mg for reconstitution to 10 ml administration volume, single-dose
Comment: **Ixifi** is biosimilar to **Remicade**. (*infliximab*).

INTERLEUKIN-12+INTERLEUKIN-23 ANTAGONIST

▷ *ustekinumab* (B) initially a single weight-based IV infusion: <55 *kg*: 260 mg (2 vials); 55-85 *kg*: 390 mg (3 vials)>85 *kg*: 520 mg (4 vials); followed by 90 mg SC every a weeks thereafter
Pediatric: <18 years: not recommended; ≥18 years: same as adult
Stelara *Prefilled sytinge*: 45 mg/0.5 ml, single dose; *Vial*: 45 mg/0.5 ml, 90 mg/ml, single-dose, 130 mg/26 ml, single-dose (preservative-free)

INTEGRIN RECEPTOR ANTAGONIST (IMMUNOMODULATOR)

▷ *natalizumab* (C) administer by IV infusion over 1 hour; monitor during and for 1 hour post-infusion; 300 mg every 4 weeks; discontinue after 12 weeks if no therapeutic response, or if unable to taper off chronic concomitant steroids within 6 months; may continue aminosalicylates
Pediatric: <18 years: not established; ≥18 years: same as adult

Tysabri *Vial:* 300 mg single-dose, soln after dilution for IV infusion (preservative-free)

Stelara *Prefilled syringe:* 45 mg/0.5 ml, single-dose; *Vial:* 45 mg/0.5 ml, 90 mg/ml, single-dose, 130 mg/26 ml, single-dose (preservative-free)

▷ *vedolizumab* (B) administer by IV infusion over 30 minutes; 300 mg at weeks 0, 2, 6; then once every 8 weeks

Pediatric: <18 years: not established; ≥18 years: same as adult

Entyvio *Vial:* 300 mg (20 ml) single-dose, pwdr for IV infusion after reconstitution (preservative-free)

CRYPTOSPORIDIOSIS (*CRYPTOSPORIDIUM PARVUM*)

▷ *nitazoxanide* (B)(G) 500 mg by mouth q 12 hours x 3 days

Pediatric: 12-47 months: 5 ml q 12 hours x 3 days; 4-11 years: 10 ml q 12 hours x 3 days; ≥12 years: same as adult

Alinia *Oral susp:* 100 mg/5 ml (60 ml)

Comment: **Alinia** is an antiprotozoal for the treatment of diarrhea due to *G. lamblia* or *C. parvum.*

CUSHING'S SYNDROME

CORTISOL RECEPTOR BLOCKER

▷ *mifepristone* administer once daily with a meal; initially 300 mg once daily; may increase in 300 mg increments to a maximum of 1200 mg once daily based on clinical response and tolerability; Do not exceed 20 mg/kg per day; *Renal Impairment:* do not exceed 600 mg once daily; *Mild-to-Moderate Hepatic Impairment:* do not exceed 600 mg once daily; *Severe Hepatic Impairment:* do not use

Pediatric: safety and efficacy not established

Korlym *Tab:* 300 mg film-coat

Comment: **Korlym** *(mifepristone)* is a cortisol receptor blocker indicated to control hyperglycemia secondary to hypercortisolism in adult patients with endogenous Cushing's syndrome who have type 2 diabetes mellitus or glucose intolerance and have failed surgery or are not candidates for surgery. The most common adverse reactions in Cushing's syndrome (incidence ≥20%) have been nausea, fatigue, headache, decreased blood potassium, arthralgia, vomiting, peripheral edema, hypertension, dizziness, decreased appetite, and endometrial hypertrophy. Closely monitor patients for signs and symptoms of adrenal insufficiency. Correct hypokalemia prior to treatment and monitor potassium during treatment. Women may experience endometrial thickening or unexpected vaginal bleeding. Use with caution if patient also has a hemorrhagic disorder or is on anticoagulant therapy. Avoid use with QT interval-prolonging drugs and patients with potassium channel variants resulting in a long QT interval. Administer drugs that are metabolized by CYP3A at the lowest dose when used with **Korlym**. Limit *mifepristone* dose to 900 mg per day when used with strong CYP3A inhibitors. Do not use **Korlym** with CYP3A inducers. Use the lowest dose of CYP2C8/2C9 substrates when used with **Korlym**. Use caution when **Korlym** is used concomitantly with *bupropion* and *efavirenz*. Contraindications to **Korlym** include taking drugs metabolized by CYP3A such as *simvastatin*, *lovastatin*, and CYP3A substrates with narrow therapeutic ranges; receiving systemic corticosteroids for lifesaving purposes; history of unexplained vaginal bleeding or endometrial hyperplasia with atypia or endometrial carcinoma. *mifepristone* has potent anti-progestational effects and will result in the termination of pregnancy.

Pregnancy must, therefore, be excluded before the initiation of treatment with
Korlym and if treatment is interrupted for more than 14 days in females of
reproductive potential. **Korlym** interferes with the effectiveness of hormonal
contraceptives; therefore, recommend non-hormonal contraception for
the duration of treatment and for 1 month after the last dose. *mifepristone*
is present in human milk, however, there are no data on the amount of
mifepristone in human milk or effects on the breastfed infant. Developmental
and health benefits of breastfeeding should be considered along with the
mother's clinical need for **Korlym** and any potential adverse effects on the
breastfed infant from **Korlym** or from the underlying maternal condition.
To minimize exposure to a breastfed infant, women who discontinue or
interrupt **Korlym** treatment may consider pumping and discarding milk
during treatment and for 18-21 days (5-6 half-lives) after the last dose, before
breastfeeding.

SOMATASTATIN ANALOG

▷ *pasireotide* initially 0.6 mg or 0.9 mg SC twice daily; recommended dose range
is 0.3 mg to 0.9 mg SC twice daily; titrate dosage based on treatment response
(i.e., clinically meaningful reduction in 24-hour urinary free cortisol [UFC] and/
or improvements in signs and symptoms of disease) and tolerability; *Child-Pugh
Class B:* initially 0.3 mg SC twice daily; max: 0.6 mg twice daily; *Child-Pugh Class
C:* avoid use
Pediatric: safety and efficacy not established

Signifor *Amp:* 0.3 mg/ml (1 ml), 0.6 mg/ml (1ml), 0.9 mg/ml (1ml), single-
dose

Comment: **Signifor** is a somatastatin analog indicated for the treatment
of adult patients with Cushing's disease for whom pituitary surgery is not
an option or has not been curative. *Testing Prior to Dosing:* fasting plasma
glucose (FPG), hemoglobin A1c (HbA1c), liver tests, electrocardiogram
(ECG), gallbladder ultrasound, and serum potassium and magnesium levels.
The most common adverse reactions (incidence ≥20%) of patients have been
diarrhea, nausea, hyperglycemia, cholelithiasis, headache, abdominal pain,
fatigue, and diabetes mellitus. Decreases in circulating levels of cortisol may
occur resulting in biochemical and/or clinical hypocortisolism; **Signifor** dose
reduction or interruption and/or adding a low-dose short-term glucocorticoid
may be necessary. Hyperglycemia and diabetes occurs with initiation of
Signifor; therefore, intensive glucose monitoring is recommended and may
require initiation or adjustment of antidiabetic treatment per standard of care.
Bradycardia and QT prolongation can occur with **Signifor**; use with caution
in at-risk patients; Monitor ECG prior to and during treatment. Evaluate
liver function tests (LFTs) prior to and during treatment. Cholelithiasis
and complications of cholelithiasis may occur; monitor periodically and
discontinue **Signifor** if complications of cholelithiasis are suspected. Use
Signifor with caution in patients who are at significant risk of developing
QTc prolongation. Consider additional monitoring with concomitant use of
cyclosporine. With concomitant *bromocriptine*, consider *bromocriptine* dose
reduction. The limited data with **Signifor** in pregnant females are insufficient
to inform a drug-associated risk for major birth defects and miscarriage. In
embryo/fetal animal development studies, findings indicating developmental
delay were observed with subcutaneous administration of *pasireotide* during
organogenesis at doses less than the exposure in humans at the highest
recommended dose. The reduction or normalization of serum cortisol levels
in female patients with Cushing's disease treated with *pasireotide* may lead
to improved fertility; therefore, females and males of reproductive potential
should be advised of the potential for an unintended pregnancy. There is no

information available on the presence of **Signifor** in human milk or effects of the drug on the breastfed infant. Developmental and health benefits of breastfeeding should be considered along with the mother's clinical need for **Signifor** and any potential adverse effects on the breastfed infant from **Signifor** or from the underlying maternal condition.

CORTISOL SYNTHESIS INHIBITOR

▷ *osilodrostat* initially 2 mg twice daily, with or without food; titrate dose by 1-2 mg twice daily, no more frequently than every 2 weeks based on rate of cortisol changes, individual tolerability and improvement in signs and symptoms; max 30 mg twice daily: *Child-Pugh Class B:* initially 1 mg twice daily; *Child-Pugh Class C:* initially 1 mg once daily in the evening
Pediatric: safety and efficacy not established

    Isturisa *Tab:* 1, 5, 10 mg

    Comment: **Isturisa** is a cortisol synthesis inhibitor indicated for the treatment of adult patients with Cushing's disease. Correct hypokalemia and hypomagnesemia, and obtain baseline electrocardiogram prior to starting **Isturisa**. The most common adverse reactions (incidence >20%) have been adrenal insufficiency, fatigue, nausea, headache, and edema. Monitor patients closely for hypocortisolism and potentially life-threatening adrenal insufficiency. Dosage reduction or interruption may be necessary; ECG is required for all patients; use with caution in patients with risk factors for QTc prolongation. Monitor patients for elevations in adrenal hormone precursors and androgens. Monitor for hypokalemia, worsening of hypertension, edema, and hirsutism. Reduce the dose of **Isturisa** by half with concomitant use of a strong CYP3A4 inhibitor. An increase in **Isturisa** dose may be needed if **Isturisa** is used concomitantly with strong CYP3A4 and CYP2B6 inducers. A reduction in **Isturisa** dosage may be needed if strong CYP3A4 and CYP2B6 inducers are discontinued while using **Isturisa**. There are no available data on *osilodrostat* use in pregnant females to evaluate for a drug-associated risk of major birth defects, miscarriage, or adverse maternal or fetal outcomes. There are risks to the mother and fetus associated with active Cushing's Syndrome during pregnancy. Breastfeeding is not recommended during treatment with **Isturisa** and for at least 1 week after treatment the last dose.

CYCLOSPORIASIS (*CYCLOSPORA CAVETANENSIS*)

Comment: The CDC, state and local health departments, and the US Food and Drug Administration have issued a Health Alert Network advisory after an increase in reported cases of cyclosporiasis, an intestinal illness caused by the parasite *Cyclospora cayetanensis*. Clinicians should consider a diagnosis of cyclosporiasis in patients who experience prolonged or remitting-relapsing diarrhea. Since May 1, 2017, 206 cases have been identified, more than twice the 88 cases reported from May 1 to August 3, 2016. Most laboratories in the United States do not routinely test for *Cyclospora*, even when a stool sample has been tested for parasites, so providers must specifically order the test. Several stool specimens may be required because *Cyclospora* oocysts may be shed intermittently and at low levels, even in persons with profuse diarrhea. Symptoms include watery diarrhea, which can be profuse, anorexia, fatigue, weight loss, nausea, flatulence, stomach cramps, myalgia, vomiting, and low-grade fever. Symptoms begin from 2 days to more than 2 weeks (average 7 days) after ingestion of the parasite. *Cyclospora* is food- and water-borne; it is not transmitted directly from person to person. The recommended treatment is ***trimethoprim-sulfamethoxazole*** (TMP/SMX). There are no effective alternatives for people who are allergic to or who cannot tolerate TMP/SMX; observation and symptomatic care is recommended for those patients. If untreated, illness may last for a few days to a month or longer.

▷ **trimethoprim+sulfamethoxazole (TMP-SMX)(C)(G)** bid x 10 days
Pediatric: <2 months: not recommended; ≥2 months: 40 mg/kg/day of **sulfamethoxazole** in 2 divided doses x 10 days; *see Appendix CC.33: trimethoprim+sulfamethoxazole* (Bactrim Suspension, Septra Suspension) *for dose by weight*

> **Bactrim, Septra** 2 tabs bid x 10 days
> *Tab:* trim 80 mg+sulfa 400 mg*
> **Bactrim DS, Septra DS** 1 tab bid x 10 days
> *Tab:* trim 160 mg+sulfa 800 mg*
> **Bactrim Pediatric Suspension, Septra Pediatric Suspension**
> *Oral susp:* trim 40 mg+sulfa 200 mg per 5 ml (100 ml) (cherry) (alcohol 0.3%)

○ CYSTIC FIBROSIS (CF)

▷ **acetylcysteine (B)(G)** administer via face mask, mouth piece, tracheostomy T-piece, mist tent, or croupette; routine tracheostomy care, 1-2 ml of a 10% to 20% solution may be administered by direct instillation into the tracheostomy every 1-4 hours
Pediatric: same as adult

> **Mucomyst** *Vial:* 10, 20% (4, 10, 30 ml) soln for inhalation
> **Comment:** Mucomyst is a mucolytic. For inhalation, the 10% concentration may be used undiluted; the 20% concentration should be diluted with sterile water or normal saline (either for injection or inhalation).

CYSTIC FIBROSIS TRANSMEMBRANE CONDUCTANCE REGULATOR (CFTR) POTENTIATOR

▷ **ivacaftor (B)** 150 mg every 12 hours; administer with fat-containing food (e.g., eggs, butter, peanut butter, cheese pizza); avoid food and juices containing grapefruit or Seville oranges.
Pediatric: <6 months, <7 kg: not recommended; 6 months-<6 years, 7-<14 kg: 1 x 50 mg pkt oral granules mixed with 1 tsp (5 ml) soft food or liquid every 12 hours with fat-containing food; 6 months-<6 years, ≥14 kg: 1 x 75 mg pkt oral granules mixed with 1 tsp (5 m) soft food or liquid every 12 hours with fat-containing food; ≥6 years: same as adult

> **Kalydeco** *Tab:* 150 mg film-coat; *Oral granules:* 50, 75 mg unit dose pkts (56 pkt/carton)
> **Comment:** Ivacaftor is indicated for the treatment of CF in patients who have a *G551D* co-mutation in the *CFTR* gene. If the patient's genotype is unknown, an FDA-cleared CF mutation test should be used to detect the presence of the *G551D* mutation. **Kalydeco** is not effective in patients with CF who are homozygous for the *F508del* mutation in the *CFTR* gene. Transaminases (ALT and AST) should be assessed prior to initiating **Kalydeco**, every 3 months during the first year of treatment, and annually thereafter. Patients who develop increased transaminase levels should be closely monitored until the abnormalities resolve. Dosing should be interrupted in patients with ALT or AST greater than 5 times the upper limit of normal (ULN). Following resolution of transaminase elevations, consider the benefits and risks of resuming **Kalydeco**. Concomitant use with strong CYP3A inducers (e.g., *rifampin*, St. John's wort) substantially decreases exposure of **Kalydeco** (which may diminish effectiveness); therefore, co-administration is not recommended. Reduce dose to 150 mg twice weekly when co-administered with strong CYP3A inhibitors (e.g., *ketoconazole*). Reduce dose to 150 mg once daily when co-administered with moderate CYP3A inhibitors. Caution

is recommended in patients with severe renal impairment (CrCl ≤30 mL/min) or ESRD. No dose adjustment is necessary for patients with mild hepatic impairment (Child-Pugh Class A). A reduced dose of 150 mg once daily is recommended in patients with moderate hepatic impairment (Child-Pugh Class B). No studies have been conducted in patients with severe hepatic impairment (Child-Pugh Class C). The most commonly reported adverse reactions are headache, sore throat, nasopharyngitis, URI, nasal congestion, abdominal pain, nausea, diarrhea, dizziness, and rash. Excretion of **Kalydeco** into human milk is probable.

(CFTR) POTENTIATOR COMBINATIONS

▷ *lumacaftor+ivacaftor* (B) <6years: not recommended; 6-11 years: 2 x 100/125 tabs q 12 hours; ≥12 years: 2 x 200/125 tabs q 12 hours

Orkambi *Tab*: luma 100 mg+iva 125 mg; luma 200 mg+iva 125 mg film-coat

Comment: **Orkambi** is indicated for the treatment of CF in patients age ≥6 years-of-age who are homozygous for the F508del mutation in the CFTR gene. The efficacy and safety of **Orkambi** have not been established in patients with CF other than those homozygous for the F508del mutation. If the patient's genotype is unknown, an FDA-cleared CF mutation test should be used to detect the presence of the F508del mutation on both alleles of the CFTR gene. Reduce the dose of **Orkambi** in patients with moderate-to severe hepatic impairment. In patients with advanced liver disease, with caution and only if the benefits are expected to outweigh the risks. When initiating **Orkambi** in patients taking strong CYP3A inhibitors, reduce the dose of **Orkambi** for the first week of treatment. There are limited and incomplete human data from clinical trials and postmarketing reports on use of **Orkambi** or its individual components in pregnancy to inform a drug-associated risk. There is no information regarding the presence of *lumacaftor* or *ivacaftor* in human milk or effects on the breastfed infant.

▷ *tezacaftor+ivacaftor plus ivacaftor* (B) <12 years: not established; ≥12 years: 1 x 100/150 fixed dose tab in the morning and 1 x 150 mg *ivacaflor* tab in the evening, approximately 12 hours later. Take with fat-containing food. Avoid grapefruit and Seville oranges.

Symdeko *Tab*: teza 100 mg+iva 150 mg, fixed-dose combination *plus Tab*: iva 150 mg (4-week supply/carton)

Comment: **Symdeko** is indicated for the treatment of the underlying cause of CF in patients ≥12 years-of-age who have two copies of the F508del mutation in the CFTR gene or who have ≥1 mutation that is responsive to *tevacaftor+ivacaftor*. If the patient's genotype is unknown, an FDA-cleared CF mutation test should be used to detect the presence of a CFTR mutation followed by verification with bi-directional sequencing when recommended by the mutation test instructions for use. Reduce dose with moderate-to-severe hepatic impairment. Reduce dose when co-administered with drugs that are moderate or strong CYP3A inhibitors. There are limited and incomplete human data from clinical trials and postmarketing reports on the use of **Symdeko** in pregnancy to inform a drug-associated risk. There is no information regarding the presence of *tezacaftor* or *ivacaftor* in human milk or effects on the breastfed infant.

▷ *elexacaftor+tezacaftor+ivacaftor plus ivacaftor* <12 years: not recommended; ≥12 years: *Morning Dose:* take 2 of the fixed-triple combination tablets; *Evening Dose:* 1 x *ivacaftor* 150 mg tab; morning and evening doses should be taken approximately 12 hours apart with fat-containing food. Avoid food and drink containing grapefruit

Trikafta *Tab*: fixed triple combination (elexa 100 mg+iva 50 mg+teza 75 mg) *plus* iva 150 mg

Comment: Trikafta *(elexacaftor+ivacaftor+tezacaftor)* is a fixed triple combination regimen for the treatment of cystic fibrosis (CF) in patients ages ≥12 years who have at least one copy of the *F508del* mutation in the cystic fibrosis transmembrane conductance regulator *(CFTR)* gene. If the patient's genotype is unknown, an FDA-cleared CF mutation test should be used to confirm the presence of at least one F508del mutation. Liver function should be assessed prior to initiation of **Trikafta**. Monitor LFTs every 3 months during the first year of treatment, and annually thereafter. In patients with a history of hepatobiliary disease or elevated LFTs, more frequent monitoring should be considered. *Moderate Hepatic Impairment:* not recommended unless benefit exceeds risk (if used, reduce dose and monitor liver function tests closely; *Severe Hepatic Impairment:* **Trikafta** should not be used. Dosing should be interrupted in patients with ALT or AST >5 x upper limit of normal (ULN) or ALT or AST >3 x ULN with bilirubin >2 x ULN. Following resolution of transaminase elevations, consider the benefits and risks of resuming treatment. Reduce dose when co-administered with drugs that are moderate or strong CYP3A inducers. Concomitant use with strong CYP3A inducers (e.g., *rifampin*, St. John's wort) significantly decrease *ivacaftor* exposure and are expected to decrease *elexacaftor* and *tezacaftor* exposure, which may reduce **Trikafta** efficacy, and therefore, co-administration is not recommended. Non-congenital lens opacities/cataracts have been reported in pediatric patients treated with *ivacaftor*-containing regimens. Baseline and follow-up examinations are recommended in pediatric patients initiating **Trikafta** treatment. There are limited and incomplete human data from clinical trials on the use of **Trikafta** or its individual components, *elexacaftor*, *tezacaftor,* and *ivacaftor*, in pregnant females to inform a drug-associated risk. There is no information regarding the presence of *elexacaftor*, *tezacaftor*, or *ivacaftor* in human milk or effects on the breastfed infant. The most common adverse drug reactions to **Trikafta** (incidence ≥5% of patients and at a frequency higher than placebo by ≥1%) have been headache, upper respiratory tract infection, abdominal pain, diarrhea, rash, alanine aminotransferase increased, nasal congestion, blood creatine phosphokinase increased, aspartate aminotransferase increased, rhinorrhea, rhinitis, influenza, sinusitis, and blood bilirubin increased.

URSODEOXYCHOLIC ACID (UDCA)

Comment: *Ursodeoxycholic acid (UDCA)* is indicated for liver disease associated with cystic fibrosis in children 6-18 years-of-age.

▷ *ursodeoxycholic acid (UDCA)* (G) in the first 3 months of treatment, the total daily dose should be divided tid (morning, midday, evening); as liver function values improve, the total daily dose may be taken once a day at bedtime; (see mfr pkg insert for dose table based on kilograms weight); monitor hepatic function every 4 weeks for the first 3 months; then, monitor hepatic function once every 3 months

Pediatric: 6-18 years: same as adult

Ursofalk *Tab:* 500 mg film-coat; *Cap:* 250 mg, *Oral susp:* 250 mg/5 ml

Comment: **Ursodeoxycholic (UDCA)** is indicated for the dissolution of cholesterol gall stones that are radioluscent (not visible on plain X-ray), <15 mm, and the gall bladder must still be functioning despite the gall stones.

ANTI-INFECTIVE

▷ *ciprofloxacin* (C)(G) <18 years: 20-40 mg/kg/day divided q 12 hours; ≥18 years: 500 mg bid x 7-10 days; max 1.5 gm/day

Cipro *Tab:* 250, 500, 750 mg; *Oral susp:* 250, 500 mg/5 ml (100 ml) (strawberry)
Cipro XR *Tab:* 500, 1000 mg ext-rel
ProQuin XR *Tab:* 500 mg ext-rel

CYSTINURIA

▷ *tiopronin* recommended initial dosage in adult patients is 800 mg/day (in clinical studies, the average dosage was about 1000 mg/day; avoid doses >50 mg/kg per day; administer in 3 divided doses at the same times each day, at least 1 hour before or 2 hours after meals; measure urinary cystine 1 month after initiation of **Thiola/Thiola EC** and every 3 months thereafter; **Thiola EC** should be swallowed whole (do not break, crush, or chew)
Pediatric: <20 kg: not established; ≥20 kg: recommended initial dosage is 15 mg/kg/day; administer in 3 divided doses at the same times each day, at least 1 hour before or 2 hours after meals; measure urinary cystine 1 month after initiation of **Thiola/Thiola EC** and every 3 months thereafter; **Thiola EC** should be swallowed whole (do not break, crush, or chew)

Thiola *Tab:* 100 mg

Thiola EC *Tab:* 100, 300 mg del-rel

Comment: Oral *tiopronin* undergoes a thiol-disulfide exchange with cystine to form a water-soluble mixed disulfide complex. Thus, the amount of sparingly soluble cystine is reduced. By reducing urinary cystine concentrations below the solubility limit, **tiopronin** helps reduce cystine stone formation. **Thiola, Thiola EC** is a reducing and complexing thiol indicated for the inhibition of cystine stone formation in patients with cystinuria, in combination with high fluid intake, alkali, and diet modification, in adults and pediatric patients weighing ≥20 kg with severe homozygous cystinuria, who are not responsive to these measures alone. Proteinuria, including nephrotic syndrome, and membranous nephropathy, has been reported with *tiopronin* use. Pediatric patients receiving greater than 50 mg/kg of *tiopronin* per day may be at increased risk for proteinuria. Most common adverse reactions (incidence ≥10%) have been nausea, diarrhea or soft stools, oral ulcers, rash, fatigue, fever, arthralgia, proteinuria, and emesis. Choose dose carefully and monitor renal function in the elderly. Available published case report data with *tiopronin* have not identified a drug-associated risk for major birth defects, miscarriage, or adverse maternal or fetal outcomes. Renal stones in pregnancy may result in adverse pregnancy outcomes. Breastfeeding is not recommended.

DEEP VEIN THROMBOSIS (DVT) PROPHYLAXIS

Anticoagulation Therapy *see* Appendix T. Anticoagulants

DEHYDRATION

ORAL REHYDRATION AND ELECTROLYTE REPLACEMENT THERAPY

▷ *oral electrolyte replacement* (OTC)(G)
KaoLectrolyte 1 pkt dissolved in 8 oz water q 3-4 hours
Pediatric: not indicated <2 years
Pkt: sodium 12 mEq+potassium 5 mEq+chloride 10 mEq+citrate 7 mEq+ dextrose 5 gm+calories 22 per 6.2 gm
Pedialyte
Pediatric: <2 years: as desired and as tolerated; ≥2 years: 1-2 liters/day

Oral soln: dextrose 20 gm+fructose 5 gm+sodium 25 mEq+potassium 20 mEq+chloride 35 mEq+citrate 30 mEq+calories 100 per liter (8 oz, 1 L)

Pedialyte Freezer Pops
Pediatric: as desired and as tolerated
Pops: dextrose 1.6 gm+sodium 2.8 mEq+potassium 1.25 mEq+chloride 2.2 mEq+citrate 1.88 mEq+calories 6.25 per 62.5 ml (2.1 fl oz) pop

DELIRIUM: END-OF-LIFE

Comment: "Ultimately ... it is essential for clinicians to focus on the humanness of medicine; to keep dying patients comfortable and as awake as they and their families would like them to be so they can make the last few hours or days of life meaningful; and to make reasonable efforts not to cloud their sensorium unless essential to alleviate patient pain or other severe symptoms" (Pandharipande & Ely, 2017). In a preliminary randomized control study, Hui et al (2017) demonstrated that adding the benzodiazepine *lorazepam* to background *haloperidol* therapy significantly reduced agitated delirium at 8 hours compared with *haloperidol* alone in patients admitted to an acute palliative care unit with advanced cancer and a very short life-expectancy. Moreover, most of the effect the combination had on delirium was achieved in the first 30 minutes following administration (Hui, et al., 2017).

REFERENCES

Hui, D., Frisbee-Hume, S., Wilson, A., Dibaj, S. S., Nguyen, T., De La Cruz, M., ... Bruera, E. (2017). Effect of lorazepam with haloperidol vs haloperidol alone on agitated delirium in patients with advanced cancer receiving palliative care. *Journal of the American Medical Association, 318*(11), 1047–1056. doi:10.1001/jama.2017.11468

Pandharipande, P. P., & Ely, E. W. (2017). Humanizing the treatment of hyperactive delirium in the last days of life. *Journal of the American Medical Association, 318*(11), 1014–1015. doi:10.1001/jama.2017.11466

BENZODIAZEPINE: INTERMEDIATE-ACTING

▷ *lorazepam* (D)(IV)(G) 1-10 mg/day in 2-3 divided doses
Pediatric: <12 years: not recommended; ≥12 years: same as adult
    Ativan *Tab:* 0.5, 1*, 2*mg
    Lorazepam Intensol *Oral conc:* 2 mg/ml (30 ml w. graduated dropper)

ANTIPSYCHOSIS AGENTS

▷ *haloperidol* (C)(G)
Oral route of administration: Moderate Symptomology: 0.5 to 2 mg orally 2 to 3 times a day; *Severe symptomology:* 3 to 5 mg orally 2 to 3 times a day; initial doses of up to 100 mg/day have been necessary in some severely resistant cases; *Maintenance:* after achieving a satisfactory response, the dose should be adjusted as practical to achieve optimum control
Parenteral route of administration: Prompt control of acute agitation: 2 to 5 mg IM every 4 to 8 hours; *Maintenance:* frequency of IM administration should be determined by patient response and may be given as often as every hour; max: 20 mg/day
    Haldol *Tab:* 0.5*, 1*, 2*, 5*, 10*, 20*mg
    Haldol Lactate *Vial:* 5 mg for IM injection, single-dose
▷ *mesoridazine* (C) initially 25 mg tid; max 300 mg/day
    Serentil *Tab:* 10, 25, 50, 100 mg; *Conc:* 25 mg/ml (118 ml)
▷ *olanzapine* (C) initially 2.5-10 mg daily; increase to 10 mg/day within a few days; then by 5 mg/day at weekly intervals; max 20 mg/day
    Zyprexa *Tab:* 2.5, 5, 7.5, 10 mg
    Zyprexa Zydis *ODT:* 5, 10, 15, 20 mg (phenylalanine)

➤ *quetiapine fumarate* (C)(G)

SeroQUEL initially 25 mg bid, titrate q 2nd <u>or</u> 3rd day in increments of 25-50 mg bid-tid; usual maintenance 400-600 mg/day in 2-3 divided doses

Tab: 25, 50, 100, 200, 300, 400 mg

SeroQUEL XR administer once daily in the PM; *Day 1:* 50 mg; *Day 2:* 100 mg; *Day 3:* 200 mg; *Day 4:* 300 mg; usual range 400-600 mg/day

Tab: 50, 150, 200, 300, 400 mg ext-rel

➤ *risperidone* (C) 0.5 mg bid x 1 day; adjust in increments of 0.5 mg bid; usual range 0.5-5 mg/day

Risperdal *Tab:* 1, 2, 3, 4 mg; *Oral soln:* 1 mg/ml (100 ml)

Risperdal M-Tab *Tab:* 0.5, 1, 2 mg

➤ *thioridazine* (C)(G) 10-25 mg bid

Mellaril *Tab:* 10, 15, 25, 50, 100, 150, 200 mg; *Oral susp:* 25 mg/5 ml, 100 mg/5 ml; *Oral conc:* 30 mg/ml, 100 mg/ml (4 oz)

 DEMENTIA

Alzheimer's Disease *see Alzheimer's Disease*
Antidepressants *see Depression*
Hypnotics/Sedatives *see Insomnia*

ANTIPSYCHOTICS

Comment: Underlying cause should be explored, accurately diagnosed, and addressed. All antipsychotic agents are associated with increased risk of mortality in elderly patients with dementia-related psychosis (Black Box Warning.) APA recommends that non-emergency antipsychotic medication should <u>only</u> be used for the treatment of agitation <u>or</u> psychosis in patients with dementia when symptoms are severe, are dangerous <u>and/or</u> cause significant distress to the patient. APA recommends that before non-emergency treatment with an antipsychotic is initiated in patients with dementia, the potential risks and benefits are discussed with the patient and the patient's surrogate decision maker with input from family <u>or</u> others involved with the patient. *haloperidol injection* is <u>not</u> approved for the treatment of patients with dementia-related psychosis.

➤ *haloperidol* (C)(G) 0.5-1 mg q HS

Haldol *Tab:* 0.5, 1, 2, 5, 10, 20 mg

➤ *mesoridazine* (C) initially 25 mg tid; max 300 mg/day

Serentil *Tab:* 10, 25, 50, 100 mg; *Conc:* 25 mg/ml (118 ml)

➤ *olanzapine* (C) initially 2.5-10 mg daily; increase to 10 mg/day within a few days; then by 5 mg/day at weekly intervals; max 20 mg/day

Zyprexa *Tab:* 2.5, 5, 7.5, 10 mg

Zyprexa Zydis *ODT:* 5, 10, 15, 20 mg (phenylalanine)

➤ *quetiapine fumarate* (C)(G)

SeroQUEL initially 25 mg bid, titrate q 2nd <u>or</u> 3rd day in increments of 25-50 mg bid-tid; usual maintenance 400-600 mg/day in 2-3 divided doses

Tab: 25, 50, 100, 200, 300, 400 mg

SeroQUEL XR administer once daily in the PM; *Day 1:* 50 mg; *Day 2:* 100 mg; *Day 3:* 200 mg; *Day 4:* 300 mg; usual range 400-600 mg/day

Tab: 50, 150, 200, 300, 400 mg ext-rel

➤ *risperidone* (C) 0.5 mg bid x 1 day; adjust in increments of 0.5 mg bid; usual range 0.5-5 mg/day

Risperdal *Tab:* 1, 2, 3, 4 mg; *Oral soln:* 1 mg/ml (100 ml)

Risperdal M-Tab *Tab:* 0.5, 1, 2 mg

➤ *thioridazine* (C)(G) 10-25 mg bid

Mellaril *Tab*: 10, 15, 25, 50, 100, 150, 200 mg; *Oral susp*: 25 mg/5 ml,
100 mg/5 ml; *Oral conc*: 30 mg/ml, 100 mg/ml (4 oz)

DENGUE FEVER (*DENGUE VIRUS*)

Dengue is the most common arthropod-borne viral (arboviral) illness in humans.
The CDC reports that cases of dengue in returning US travelers have increased
steadily during the past 20 years, and dengue has become the leading cause of acute
febrile illness in US travelers returning from the Caribbean, South America, and
Asia. Dengue is transmitted by mosquitoes of the genus *Aedes*, which are widely
distributed in subtropical and tropical areas of the world. A small percentage of
persons who have previously been infected by one dengue serotype develop bleeding
and endothelial leak upon infection with another dengue serotype. This syndrome
is termed "dengue hemorrhagic fever." Dengue fever is typically a self-limited
disease, with a mortality rate of less than 1%. When treated, dengue hemorrhagic
fever has a mortality rate of 2%-5%, but when left untreated, the mortality rate
is as high as 50%. Supportive care with analgesics, fluid replacement, and bed
rest is usually sufficient. Acetaminophen may be used to treat fever and relieve
other symptoms. *aspirin*, nonsteroidal anti-inflammatory drugs (NSAIDs), and
corticosteroids should be avoided. Management of severe dengue requires careful
attention to fluid management and proactive treatment of hemorrhage. Single
dose methylprednisolone showed no mortality benefit in the treatment of dengue
shock syndrome in a prospective, randomized, double-blind, placebo-controlled
trial. **There is no specific antiviral treatment currently available for dengue fever.**
Because lack of immunity to a single dengue strain is the major risk factor for
dengue hemorrhagic fever and dengue shock syndrome, a vaccine must provide
high levels of immunity to all four dengue strains to be clinically useful.

A live attenuated tetravalent vaccine against dengue was effective against all four
serotypes of the virus and well-tolerated among children, according to researchers.
Interim results from a phase II study showed that children at four study sites in
dengue-endemic areas of Asia and Latin America who received the vaccine all had
significantly higher levels of antibody titers 18 months later. The vaccine (TAK-003
or TDV) is comprised of a molecularly cloned attenuated strain of dengue serotype
2 (DENV-2), and engineered strains of dengue serotypes 1, 3 and 4 (DENV-1,
DENV-3 and DENV-4). Prior phase I and phase II data found the vaccine was well-
tolerated and immunogenic against all four dengue serotypes. The trial will take 48
months to complete. The trial is ongoing at three sites in the Dominican Republic
(n = 535), Panama (n = 935), and the Philippines (n = 330). Participants are
"healthy" children, ages 2 to 17 years, randomized into three groups plus a placebo
group. A phase III efficacy trial for the vaccine, entitled Tetravalent Immunization
against Dengue Efficacy Study (TIDES) is currently being conducted in eight
dengue-endemic countries.

REFERENCES

Sáez-Llorens, X., Tricou, V., Yu, D., Rivera, L., Jimeno, J., Villarreal, A. C., . . . Wallace, D. (2018). Immunogenicity
and safety of one versus two doses of tetravalent dengue vaccine in healthy children aged 2–17 years in Asia
and Latin America: 18-month interim data from a phase 2, randomised, placebo-controlled study. *The Lancet:
Infectious Diseases, 18*(2), 162–170. doi:10.1016/s1473-3099(17)30632-1

Tricou, V., Sáez-Llorens, X., Yu, D., Rivera, L., Borkowski, A., & Wallace, D. (2017, November 6). *Progress in
development of Takeda's tetravalent dengue vaccine candidate.* Paper presented at the 66th annual meeting
of the American Society of Tropical Medicine & Hygiene, Baltimore, MD. Retrieved from http://www.
abstractsonline.com/pp8/#!/4395/presentation/1438

Yoon, I.-K., & Thomas, S. J. (2018). Encouraging results but questions remain for dengue vaccine. *The Lancet:
Infectious Diseases, 18*(2), 125–126. doi:10.1016/s1473-3099(17)30634-5

▷ **dengue vaccine (CYD-TDV)** >45 years: not recommended
  Pediatric: <9 years: not recommended; ≥9 years: same as adult
    Dengvaxia
Comment: In 2019, **Dengvaxia** was approved external icon by the U.S. Food and Drug Administration (FDA) in the United States for use in children 9 to 16 years old living in an area where dengue is common (the US territories of American Samoa, Puerto Rico and the US Virgin Islands), with laboratory confirmed prior dengue virus infection. *CYD-TDV*, sold under the brand name **Dengvaxia**, is a live attenuated tetravalent chimeric vaccine made using recombinant DNA technology by replacing the PrM (pre-membrane) and E (envelope) structural genes of the yellow fever attenuated 17D strain vaccine with those from the four dengue serotypes. In 2016, a partially effective vaccine for dengue fever (*CYD-TDV*, **Dengvaxia**) became commercially available in 11 countries: Mexico, the Philippines, Indonesia, Brazil, El Salvador, Costa Rica, Paraguay, Guatemala, Peru, Thailand, and Singapore. WHO recommends that countries should consider vaccination with *CYD-TDV* only if the risk of severe dengue in seronegative individuals can be minimized either through pre-vaccination screening or recent documentation of high seroprevalence rates in the area (at least 80% by age 9 years). In 2017 the manufacturer (Sanofi Pasteur) recommended that the vaccine only be used in people who have previously had a dengue infection, as outcomes may be worsened in those who have not been previously infected. WHO updated its recommendations regarding the use of **Dengvaxia** in 2018 based on the evidence that seronegative vaccine recipients have an excess risk of severe dengue compared to unvaccinated seronegative individuals. It is not clear why the vaccinated sereonegative population has more serious adverse outcomes. For the most up-to-date information, guidelines, recommendations, and vaccine availability, contact the CDC at https://www.cdc.gov/dengue or the Vaccine Adverse Events Reporting System (VAERS) at https://wonder.cdc.gov/wonder/help/vaers.html or https://wonder.cdc.gov/wonder/help/vaers.html or VAERS at 1-800-822-7967 or http://vaers.hhs.gov/ or Sanofi Pasteur at 1-800-VACCINE (1-800-822-2463).

⬤ DENTAL ABSCESS

ANTI-INFECTIVES

▷ **amoxicillin+clavulanate** (B)(G)
  Augmentin 500 mg tid or 875 mg bid x 7-10 days
    Pediatric: 40-45 mg/kg/day divided tid x 10 days or 90 mg/kg/day divided bid x 10 days *see* Appendix CC.4. *amoxicillin+clavulanate* (Augmentin Suspension) *for dose by weight*
      Tab: 250, 500, 875 mg; *Chew tab:* 125, 250 mg (lemon-lime); 200, 400 mg (cherry-banana) (phenylalanine); *Oral susp:* 125 mg/5 ml (banana), 250 mg/5 ml (75, 100, 150 ml) (orange); 200, 400 mg/5 ml (50, 75, 100 ml) (orange) (phenylalanine)
  Augmentin ES-600 not recommended for adults
    Pediatric: <3 months: not recommended; ≥3 months, <40 kg: 90 mg/kg/day in 2 divided doses x 7-10 days; ≥40 kg: not recommended
      Oral susp: 42.9 mg/5 ml (50, 75, 100, 125, 150, 200 ml) (strawberry cream) (phenylalanine)
  Augmentin XR 2 tabs q 12 hours x 7-10 days
    Pediatric: <16 years: use other forms; ≥16 years: same as adult
      Tab: 1000*mg ext-rel
▷ **clindamycin** (B) (administer with fluoroquinolone in adults and TMP-SMX in children) 300 mg qid x 10 days
  Pediatric: 8-16 mg/kg/day in 3-4 divided doses x 10 days

Cleocin (G) *Cap:* 75 (tartrazine), 150 (tartrazine), 300 mg
Cleocin Pediatric Granules (G) *Oral susp:* 75 mg/5 ml (100 ml) (cherry)
▷ **erythromycin base (B)(G)** 500 mg q 6 hours x 10 days
Pediatric: 30-40 mg/kg/day in 4 divided doses x 10 days
    Ery-Tab *Tab:* 250, 333, 500 mg ent-coat
    PCE *Tab:* 333, 500 mg
▷ **erythromycin ethylsuccinate (B)(G)** 400 mg qid x 7 days
Pediatric: 30-50 mg/kg/day in 4 divided doses x 7 days; may double dose
with severe infection; max 100 mg/kg/day; *see Appendix CC.21: erythromycin
ethylsuccinate* (E.E.S. Suspension, Ery-Ped Drops/Suspension) *for dose by weight*
    EryPed *Oral susp:* 200 mg/5 ml (100, 200 ml) (fruit); 400 mg/5 ml (60, 100,
    200 ml) (banana); *Oral drops:* 200, 400 mg/5 ml (50 ml) (fruit); *Chew tab:* 200
    mg wafer (fruit)
    E.E.S. *Oral susp:* 200, 400 mg/5 ml (100 ml) (fruit)
    E.E.S. Granules *Oral susp:* 200 mg/5 ml (100, 200 ml) (cherry)
    E.E.S. 400 Tablets *Tab:* 400 mg
▷ **penicillin v potassium (B)** 250-500 mg q 6 hours x 5-7 days
Pediatric: <12 years: 25-50 mg/kg/day divided q 6 hours x 5-7 days; *see* Appendix
CC.29. *penicillin v potassium* (Pen-Vee K Solution, Veetids Solution) *for dose by
weight*; ≥12 years: same as adult
    Pen-Vee K *Tab:* 250, 500 mg; *Oral soln:* 125 mg/5 ml (100, 200 ml);
    250 mg/5 ml (100, 150, 200 ml)

DENTURE IRRITATION

DEBRIDING AGENT/CLEANSER

▷ **carbamide peroxide 10% (OTC)** apply 10 drops to affected area; swish x 2-3
minutes, then spit; do not rinse; repeat treatment qid
Pediatric: with adult supervision only
    Gly-Oxide *Liq:* 10% (15, 60 ml, squeeze bottle w. applicator)

DEPRESSION/MAJOR DEPRESSIVE DISORDER (MDD)

Comment: Antidepressant monotherapy should be avoided until any presence of
(hypo)mania or positive family history for bipolar spectrum disorder has been
ruled out as antidepressant monotherapy can induce mania in the bipolar patient.
Abrupt withdrawal or interruption of treatment with an antidepressant medication
is sometimes associated with an antidepressant discontinuation syndrome which
may be mediated by gradually tapering the drug over a period of 2 weeks or longer,
depending on the dose strength and length of treatment. Common symptoms of
antidepressant withdrawal include flu-like symptoms, insomnia, nausea, imbalance,
sensory disturbances, and hyperarousal. These medications include SSRIs, TCAs,
MAOIs, and atypical agents such as *venlafaxine* (Effexor), *mirtazapine* (Remeron),
trazodone (Desyrel), and *duloxetine* (Cymbalta). Common symptoms of the
serotonin discontinuation syndrome include flu-like symptoms (nausea, vomiting,
diarrhea, headaches, sweating), sleep disturbances (insomnia, nightmares, constant
sleepiness), mood disturbances (dysphoria, anxiety, agitation) cognitive disturbances
(mental confusion, hyperarousal), sensory and movement disturbances (imbalance,
tremors, vertigo, dizziness), and electric-shock-like sensations in the brain, often
described by sufferers as "brain zaps."

SELECTIVE SEROTONIN REUPTAKE INHIBITORS (SSRIs)

Comment: Co-administration of SSRIs with TCAs requires extreme caution.
Concomitant use of MAOIs and SSRIs is absolutely contraindicated. Avoid St. John's
wort and other serotonergic agents. A potentially fatal adverse event is *serotonin*

syndrome, caused by serotonin excess. Milder symptoms require HCP intervention to avert severe symptoms, which can be rapidly fatal without urgent/emergent medical care. Symptoms include restlessness, agitation, confusion, tachycardia, hypertension, dilated pupils, muscle twitching, muscle rigidity, loss of muscle coordination, diaphoresis, diarrhea, headache, shivering, piloerection, hyperpyrexia, cardiac arrhythmias, seizures, loss of consciousness, coma, and death. Common symptoms of the *serotonin discontinuation syndrome* include flu-like symptoms (nausea, vomiting, diarrhea, headaches, sweating), sleep disturbances (insomnia, nightmares, constant sleepiness), mood disturbances (dysphoria, anxiety, agitation), cognitive disturbances (mental confusion, hyperarousal, hallucinations), sensory and movement disturbances (imbalance, tremors, vertigo, dizziness, and electric-shock-like sensations in the brain, often described by sufferers as "brain zaps."

▶ *citalopram* (C)(G) initially 20 mg daily; may increase after one week to 40 mg; max 40 mg
  Pediatric: <12 years: not recommended; ≥12 years: same as adult
    Celexa *Tab:* 10, 20, 40 mg; *Oral soln:* 10 mg/5 ml (120 ml) (peppermint) (sugar-free, alcohol-free, parabens)

▶ *escitalopram* (C)(G) initially 10 mg daily; may increase to 20 mg daily after 1 week; elderly <u>or</u> hepatic impairment, 10 mg once daily
  Pediatric: <12 years: not recommended; 12-17 years: initially 10 mg daily; may increase to 20 mg daily after 3 weeks
    Lexapro *Tab:* 5, 10*, 20*mg
    Lexapro Oral Solution *Oral soln:* 1 mg/ml (240 ml) (peppermint) (parabens)

▶ *fluoxetine* (C)(G)
    Prozac initially 20 mg daily; may increase after 1 week; doses >20 mg/day should be divided into AM and noon doses; max 80 mg/day
    Pediatric: <8 years: not recommended; 8-17 years: initially 10 mg/day; may increase after 1 week to 20 mg/day; range 20-60 mg/day; range for lower weight children, 20-30 mg/day; >17 years: same as adult
      Cap: 10, 20, 40 mg; *Tab:* 30*, 60*mg; *Oral soln:* 20 mg/5 ml (4 oz) (mint)
    Prozac Weekly following daily fluoxetine therapy at 20 mg/day for 13 weeks, may initiate **Prozac Weekly** 7 days after the last 20 mg *fluoxetine* dose
    Pediatric: <12 years: not recommended; ≥12 years: same as adult
      Cap: 90 mg ent-coat del-rel pellets

▶ *levomilnacipran* (C) swallow whole; initially 20 mg once daily for 2 days; then increase to 40 mg once daily; may increase dose in 40 mg increments at intervals of ≥2 days; max 120 mg once daily; *CrCl 30-59 mL/min:* max 80 mg once daily; *CrCl 15-29 mL/min:* max 40 mg once daily
  Pediatric: <12 years: not recommended; ≥12 years: same as adult
    Fetzima *Cap:* 20, 40, 80, 120 mg ext-rel

▶ *paroxetine maleate* (D)(G)
  Pediatric: <12 years: not recommended; ≥12 years: same as adult
    Paxil initially 20 mg daily in AM; may increase by 10 mg/day at weekly intervals as needed; max 60 mg/day
      Tab: 10*, 20*, 30, 40 mg
    Paxil CR initially 25 mg daily in AM; may increase by 12.5 mg at weekly intervals as needed; max 62.5 mg/day
      Tab: 12.5, 25, 37.5 mg cont-rel ent-coat
    Paxil Suspension initially 20 mg daily in AM; may increase by 10 mg/day at weekly intervals as needed; max 60 mg/day
      Oral susp: 10 mg/5 ml (250 ml) (orange)

▶ *paroxetine mesylate* (D)(G) initially 7.5 mg daily in AM; may increase by 10 mg/day at weekly intervals as needed; max 60 mg/day
  Pediatric: <12 years: not established; ≥12 years: same as adult
    Brisdelle *Cap:* 7.5 mg

▷ **sertraline** (C)(G) initially 50 mg daily; increase at 1 week intervals if needed; max 200 mg daily; dilute oral concentrate immediately prior to administration in 4 oz water, ginger ale, lemon-lime soda, lemonade, or orange juice
Pediatric: <6 years: not recommended; 6-12 years: initially 25 mg daily; max 200 mg/day; 13-17 years: initially 50 mg daily; max 200 mg/day; >17 years: same as adult
   Zoloft *Tab:* 25*, 50*, 100*mg; *Oral conc:* 20 mg per ml (60 ml) (alcohol 12%)

SEROTONIN-NOREPINEPHRINE REUPTAKE INHIBITORS (SNRIs)

▷ **desvenlafaxine** (C)(G) swallow whole; initially 50 mg once daily; max 120 mg/day
Pediatric: <12 years: not recommended; ≥12 years: same as adult
   Pristiq *Tab:* 50, 100 mg ext-rel
▷ **duloxetine** (C)(G) swallow whole; initially 30 mg once daily x 1 week; then, increase to 60 mg once daily; max 120 mg/day
Pediatric: <12 years: not recommended; ≥12 years: same as adult
   Cymbalta *Cap:* 20, 30, 40, 60 mg del-rel
▷ **levomilnacipran** (C) swallow whole; initially 20 mg once daily for 2 days; then increase to 40 mg once daily; may increase dose in 40 mg increments at intervals of ≥2 days; max 120 mg once daily; *CrCl 30-59 mL/min:* max 80 mg once daily; *CrCl 15-29 mL/min:* max 40 mg once daily
Pediatric: <12 years: not recommended; ≥12 years: same as adult
   Fetzima *Cap:* 20, 40, 80, 120 mg ext-rel
▷ **venlafaxine** (C)(G)
   Effexor initially 75 mg/day in 2-3 divided doses; may increase at 4 day intervals in 75 mg increments to 150 mg/day; max 225 mg/day
   Pediatric: <18 years: not recommended; ≥18 years: same as adult
      Tab: 37.5, 75, 150, 225 mg
   Effexor XR initially 75 mg q AM; may start at 37.5 mg daily x 4-7 days, then increase by increments of up to 75 mg/day at intervals of at least 4 days; usual max 375 mg/day
   Pediatric: <18 years: not recommended; ≥18 years: same as adult
      Tab/Cap: 37.5, 75, 150 mg ext-rel
▷ **vortioxetine** (C) initially 10 mg once daily; max 30 mg/day
   Pediatric: <18 years: not established; ≥18 years: same as adult
      Brintellix *Tab:* 5, 10, 15, 20 mg

SELECTIVE SEROTONIN REUPTAKE INHIBITOR (SSRI)+5HT-14 RECEPTOR PARTIAL AGONIST COMBINATION

▷ **vilazodone** (C)(G) take with food; initially 10 mg once daily x 7 days; then, 20 mg once daily x 7 days; then, 40 mg once daily
   Pediatric: <18 years: not established; ≥18 years: same as adult
      Viibryd *Tab:* 10, 20, 40 mg

THIENOBENZODIAZEPINE+SSRI COMBINATION

▷ **olanzapine+fluoxetine** (C) initially one 6/25 cap in the PM; titrate; max one 18/75 cap once daily in the PM
   Pediatric: <10 years: not established; ≥10 years: same as adult
      Symbyax
         Cap: Symbyax 3/25 olan 3 mg+fluo 25 mg
            Symbyax 6/25 olan 6 mg+fluo 25 mg
            Symbyax 6/50 olan 6 mg+fluo 50 mg
            Symbyax 12/25 olan 12 mg+fluo 25 mg
            Symbyax 12/50 olan 12 mg+fluo 50 mg
   Comment: Symbyax is a thienobenzodiazepine-SSRI indicated for the treatment of depressive episodes associated with bipolar depression disorder and treatment-resistant depression (TRD).

TRICYCLIC ANTIDEPRESSANTS (TCAs)

Comment: Co-administration of TCAs with SSRIs requires extreme caution.

▶ **amitriptyline** (C)(G) initially 75 mg/day in divided doses or 50-100 mg in a single dose at HS; max 300 mg/day
Pediatric: <12 years: not recommended; ≥12 years: same as adult
   Tab: 10, 25, 50, 75, 100, 150 mg

▶ **amoxapine** (C) initially 50 mg bid-tid; after 1 week may increase to 100 mg bid-tid; usual effective dose 200-300 mg/day; if total dose exceeds 300 mg/day, give in divided doses (max 400 mg/day); may give as a single bedtime dose (max 300 mg q HS)
Pediatric: <12 years: not recommended; ≥12 years: same as adult
   Tab: 25, 50, 100, 150 mg

▶ **desipramine** (C)(G) 100-200 mg/day in single or divided doses; max 300 mg/day
Pediatric: <12 years: not recommended; ≥12 years: same as adult
   Norpramin *Tab:* 10, 25, 50, 75, 100, 150 mg

▶ **doxepin** (C)(G) 75 mg/day; max 150 mg/day
Pediatric: <12 years: not recommended; ≥12 years: same as adult
   Cap: 10, 25, 50, 75, 100, 150 mg; *Oral conc:* 10 mg/ml (4 oz w. dropper)

▶ **imipramine** (C)(G)
Pediatric: <12 years: not recommended; ≥12 years: same as adult
   Tofranil initially 75 mg daily (max 200 mg); adolescents initially 30-40 mg daily (max 100 mg/day); if maintenance dose exceeds 75 mg daily, may switch to **Tofranil PM** for divided or bedtime dose
      Tab: 10, 25, 50 mg
   Tofranil PM initially 75 mg daily 1 hour before HS; max 200 mg
      Cap: 75, 100, 125, 150 mg
   Tofranil Injection 50 mg IM; lower dose for adolescents; switch to oral form as soon as possible
      Amp: 25 mg/2 ml (2 ml)

▶ **nortriptyline** (D)(G) initially 25 mg tid-qid; max 150 mg/day
Pediatric: <12 years: not recommended; ≥12 years: same as adult
   Pamelor *Cap:* 10, 25, 50, 75 mg; *Oral soln:* 10 mg/5 ml (16 oz)

▶ **protriptyline** (C) initially 5 mg tid; usual dose 15-40 mg/day in 3-4 divided doses; max 60 mg/day
Pediatric: <12 years: not recommended; ≥12 years: same as adult
   Vivactil *Tab:* 5, 10 mg

▶ **trimipramine** (C) initially 75 mg/day in divided doses; max 200 mg/day
Pediatric: not recommended
   Surmontil *Cap:* 25, 50, 100 mg

AMINOKETONES

▶ **bupropion HBr** (C)(G)
Pediatric: Safety and effectiveness of **bupropion** in the pediatric population have not been established; when considering the use of **bupropion** in a child or adolescent, balance the potential risks with the clinical need
   Aplenzin initially 100 mg bid for at least 3 days; may increase to 375 or 400 mg/day after several weeks; then after at least 3 more days, 450 mg in 4 divided doses; max 450 mg/day, 174 mg/single dose
      Tab: 174, 348, 522 mg

▶ **bupropion HCl** (C)(G)
Pediatric: Safety and effectiveness of **bupropion** in the pediatric population have not been established; when considering the use of **bupropion** in a child or adolescent, balance the potential risks with the clinical need
   Forfivo XL do not use for initial treatment; use immediate-release **bupropion** forms for initial titration; switch to **Forfivo XL** 450 mg once daily when total dose/day reaches 450 mg; may switch to **Forfivo XL** when total dose/day

reaches 300 mg for 2 weeks and patient needs 450 mg/day to reach therapeutic target; swallow whole, do not crush or chew

    Tab: 450 mg ext-rel

Wellbutrin initially 100 mg bid for at least 3 days; may increase to 375 or 400 mg/day after several weeks; then after at least 3 more days, 450 mg in 4 divided doses; max 450 mg/day, 150 mg/single dose

    Tab: 75, 100 mg

Wellbutrin SR initially 150 mg in AM for at least 3 days; increase to 150 mg bid if well tolerated; usual dose 300 mg/day; max 400 mg/day

    Tab: 100, 150 mg sust-rel

Wellbutrin XL initially 150 mg in AM for at least 3 days; increase to 150 mg bid if well tolerated; usual dose 300 mg/day; max 450 mg/day

    Tab: 150, 300 mg sust-rel

MONOAMINE OXIDASE INHIBITORS (MAOIS)

Comment: Many drug and food interactions with this class of drugs; use cautiously. Should be reserved for refractory depression that has not responded to other classes of antidepressants. Concomitant use of MAOIs and SSRIs is an absolute contraindication. See mfr pkg insert for drug and food interactions.

▷ *isocarboxazid* (C)(G) initially 10 mg bid; increase by 10 mg every 2-4 days up to 40 mg/day; may increase by 20 mg/week to max 60 mg/day divided bid-qid

    Pediatric: <16 years: not recommended; ≥16 years: same as adult

    Marplan *Tab:* 10 mg

▷ *phenelzine* (C)(G) initially 15 mg tid; max 90 mg/day

    Pediatric: <16 years: not recommended; ≥16 years: same as adult

    Nardil *Tab:* 15 mg

▷ *selegiline* (C) initially 10 mg tid; max 60 mg/day

    Emsam *Transdermal patch:* 6 mg/24 Hr, 9 mg/24 Hr, 12 mg/24 Hr

    Comment: With the **Emsam** transdermal patch 6 mg/24 HR dose, the dietary restrictions commonly required when using non-selective MAOIs are not necessary.

▷ *tranylcypromine* (C) initially 10 mg tid; may increase in 10 mg/day every 1-3 weeks; max 60 mg/day

    Parnate *Tab:* 10 mg

TETRACYCLICS

▷ *maprotiline* (B)(G) initially 75 mg/day for 2 weeks then change gradually as needed in 25 mg increments; max 225 mg/day

    Pediatric: <18 years: not recommended; ≥18 years: same as adult

    Ludiomil *Tab:* 25, 50, 75 mg

▷ *mirtazapine* (C) initially 15 mg q HS; increase at intervals of 1-2 weeks; usual range 15-45 mg/day; max 45 mg/day

    Pediatric: <12 years: not recommended; ≥12 years: same as adult

    Remeron *Tab:* 15*, 30*, 45*mg

    Remeron SolTab *ODT:* 15, 30, 45 mg (orange) (phenylalanine)

▷ *chlordiazepoxide+amitriptyline* (C)(IV)

    Pediatric: <12 years: not recommended; ≥12 years: same as adult

    Limbitrol 3-4 tabs in divided doses

        Tab: chlor 5 mg+amit 12.5 mg

    Limbitrol DS 3-4 tabs in divided doses; max 6 tabs/day

        Tab: chlor 10 mg+amit 25 mg

▷ *trazodone* (C)(G) initially 150 mg/day in divided doses with food; increase by 50 mg/day q 3-4 days; max 400 mg/day in divided doses

    Pediatric: <18 years: not recommended; ≥18 years: same as adult

    Oleptro *Tab:* 50, 100*, 150*, 200, 250, 300 mg

ATYPICAL ANTIPSYCHOTICS

▷ *aripiprazole* (C)(G) initially 15 mg daily; may increase to max 30 mg/day
  Pediatric: <10 years: not recommended; 10-17 years: initially 2 mg/day for 2 days;
  then, increase to 5 mg/day for 2 days; then, increase to target dose of 10 mg/day;
  may increase by 5 mg/day at 1 week intervals as needed to max 30 mg/day

  Abilify *Tab:* 2, 5, 10, 15, 20, 30 mg
  Abilify Discmelt *Tab:* 15 mg orally disintegrating (vanilla) (phenylalanine)
  Abilify Maintena *Vial:* 300, 400 mg ext-rel pwdr for IM injection after
  reconstitution; 300, 400 mg single-dose prefilled dual-chamber syringes w.
  supplies
  Comment: **Abilify** is indicated for acute and maintenance treatment of manic
  or mixed episodes in bipolar I disorder, as monotherapy or as an adjunct
  to *lithium* or *valproate*, as adjunct to antidepressants for major depressive
  disorder (MDD), and for irritability associated with autistic disorder.

▷ *brexpiprazole* (C) initially 0.5 or 1 mg once daily; titrate weekly up to target 2 mg/
  day; max 3 mg/day; *Moderate-severe hepatic impairment, renal impairment,* or
  ESRD, max 2 mg/day
  Pediatric: <12 years: not established; ≥12 years: same as adult
  Rexulti *Tab:* 0.25, 0.5, 1, 2, 3, 4 mg

 DEPRESSION: POSTPARTUM

NEUROACTIVE STEROID GAMMA-AMINOBUTYRIC ACID A (GABA_A) RECEPTOR-POSITIVE ALLOSTERIC MODULATOR

▷ *brexanolone* (X) (IV) administer as a continuous intravenous infusion over 60
  hours (2.5 days) by a qualified healthcare provider; patients are at risk for
  excessive sedation or sudden loss of consciousness and must be continuously
  monitored, including continuous pulse oximetry for SpO2 monitoring; the HCP
  must be available on site for the duration of the infusion and intervene as necessary with appropriate supportive care; the diluted product in the infusion bag can
  be used at room temperature for up to 12 hours; if the diluted product is not used
  immediately after dilution, store under refrigerated conditions for up to 96 hours

Infusion Rate	
(0 to 4 hours)	30 mcg/kg/hour
(4 to 24 hours)	60 mcg/kg/hour
(24 to 52 hours)	90 mcg/kg/hour (if not tolerated, reduce rate to 60 mcg/kg/hour)
(52 to 56 hours)	60 mcg/kg/hour
(56 to 60 hours)	30 mcg/kg/hour

Pediatric: safety and effectiveness in children not established
  Zulresso *Vial:* 100 mg/20 ml (5 mg/ml, 20 ml) single-dose for dilution and IV
  infusion (preservative-free)
Comment: **Zulresso** *(brexanolone)* is a GABA_A receptor positive allosteric
modulator indicated for the treatment of postpartum depression (PPD) in adults.
Avoid use in patients with end stage renal disease (ESRD). Most common adverse
reactions (incidence ≥5%) have been sedation/somnolence, dry mouth, loss of
consciousness, and flushing/hot flush. Assess the patient for newly emergent
suicidal thoughts and behaviors. Consider changing the therapeutic regimen,
including discontinuing **Zulresso**, in patients whose PPD becomes worse or
who experience emergent suicidal thoughts and behaviors. Patients must be
accompanied during interactions with their child(ren). May cause fetal harm.
brexanolone is transferred to breastmilk in nursing mothers. Assess risk/benefit of
breastfeeding along with the mother's clinical need for **Zulresso** and any potential
adverse effects on the breastfed infant from **Zulresso** and the underlying maternal
condition. **Zulresso** is available only through a restricted REMS program. The

pregnancy exposure registry monitors pregnancy outcomes in women exposed to antidepressants during pregnancy. Healthcare providers are encouraged to register patients by calling the National Pregnancy Registry for Antidepressants at 1-844-405-6185 or visiting https://womensmentalhealth.org/research/pregnancyregistry/antidepressants/

DEPRESSION: TREATMENT-RESISTANT (TRD)

NON-COMPETITIVE N-METHYL D-ASPARTATE (NMDA) RECEPTOR ANTAGONIST

▷ *esketamine* **nasal spray (III)** administer intra-nasally under the supervision of a qualified healthcare provider in an approved setting; assess BP prior to and after administration; allow each spray to absorb; do not blow nose; during and after **Spravato** administration at each treatment session, observe the patient for at least 2 hours until the patient is safe to leave; evidence of therapeutic benefit should be evaluated at the end of the induction phase to determine need for continued treatment. Administer **Spravato** in conjunction with an oral antidepressant as follows:

Induction Phase	Weeks 1 to 4	Dose
	Administer 2 x/week	Day 1 starting dose: 56 mg
		Subsequent doses:
		56 mg or 84 mg
Maintenance Phase	Weeks 5 to 8	
	Administer once weekly	56 mg or 84 mg
	Week 9 and after	
	Administer every 2 weeks	56 mg or 84 mg
	or once weekly	

Spravato *Nasal spray:* 28 mg/device (one device=2 sprays=total 28 mg; 2 devises=4 sprays=56 mg; 3 devices=6 sprays=84 mg)

Comment: **Spravato** *(esketamine)* is a rapid acting, nasal spray formulation of a non-competitive N-methyl D-aspartate (NMDA) receptor antagonist indicated, in conjunction with an oral antidepressant, for use in adults with treatment-resistant depression (TRD). Contraindications include aneurysm, vascular disease (including thoracic and abdominal aorta, intracranial and peripheral arterial vessels, and arteriovenous malformation), and intracerebral hemorrhage. Patients with cardiovascular and cerebrovascular conditions and risk factors may be at an increased risk of associated adverse effects. Risk factors during a treatment include sedation, dissociation. Risk factors following a treatment are impaired attention, judgment, thinking, reaction speed, and motor skills. The patient should not drive or operate machinery until the next day after a restful sleep. There is potential for abuse/misuse with **Spravato** as a schedule III (CIII) drug. Consider risk v. benefit prior to initiation of treatment in patients at higher risk and monitor for signs and symptoms of abuse/misuse. There is increased risk of suicidal thoughts and behaviors in pediatric and young adult patients taking antidepressants. Therefore, closely monitor all antidepressant-treated patients for clinical worsening and emergence of suicidal thoughts and behaviors. **Spravato** may cause embryo/fetal toxicity. Consider pregnancy planning and prevention in females of reproductive potential. Breastfeeding is not recommended. **Spravato** is only available through the restricted **Spravato** REMS program. Healthcare settings must be certified in the program and ensure that **Spravato** is only dispensed in healthcare settings and administered to patients who are enrolled in the program. Pharmacies must be certified in the REMS program and must only dispense **Spravato** to healthcare settings that are certified in the program. Further information, including a list of certified pharmacies is available at www.SPRAVATOrems.com or 1-855-382-6022.

DERMATITIS: ATOPIC (ECZEMA)

Parenteral Corticosteroids *see* Appendix M. Parenteral Corticosteroids
Oral Corticosteroids *see* Appendix L. Oral Corticosteroids
Topical Corticosteroids *see* Appendix K: Topical Corticosteroids by Potency

PHOSPHODIESTERASE 4 INHIBITOR

▷ *crisaborole 2%* (C) apply sparingly bid; max 4 weeks
   Pediatric: <2 years: not recommended; ≥2 years: same as adult
      Eucrisa *Oint:* 2% (60 gm)

MOISTURIZING AGENTS

   Aquaphor Healing Ointment (OTC) *Oint:* 1.75, 3.5, 14 oz (alcohol)
   Eucerin Daily Sun Defense (OTC) *Lotn:* 6 oz (fragrance-free)
   Comment: **Eucerin Daily Sun Defense** is a moisturizer with SPF-15 sunscreen.
   Eucerin Facial Lotion (OTC) *Lotn:* 4 oz
   Eucerin Light Lotion (OTC) *Lotn:* 8 oz
   Eucerin Lotion (OTC) *Lotn:* 8, 16 oz
   Eucerin Original Creme (OTC) *Crm:* 2, 4, 16 oz (alcohol)
   Eucerin Plus Creme (OTC) *Crm:* 4 oz
   Eucerin Plus Lotion (OTC) *Lotn:* 6, 12 oz
   Eucerin Protective Lotion (OTC) *Lotn:* 4 oz (alcohol)
   Comment: **Eucerin Protective Lotion** is a moisturizer with SPF-25 sunscreen.
   Lac-Hydrin Cream (OTC) *Crm:* 280, 385 gm
   Lac-Hydrin Lotion (OTC) *Lotn:* 25, 400 gm
   Lubriderm Dry Skin Scented (OTC) *Lotn:* 6, 10, 16, 32 oz
   Lubriderm Dry Skin Unscented (OTC) *Lotn:* 3.3, 6, 10, 16 oz (fragrance-free)
   Lubriderm Sensitive Skin Lotion (OTC) *Lotn:* 3.3, 6, 10, 16 oz (lanolin-free)
   Lubriderm Dry Skin (OTC) *Lotn (scented):* 2.5, 6, 10, 16 oz;
         Lotn (fragrance-free): 1, 2.5, 6, 10, 16 oz
   Lubriderm Bath 1-2 capfuls in bath or rub onto wet skin as needed, then rinse
      Oil: 8 oz
   Moisturel (OTC) apply as needed
         Crm: 4, 16 oz; *Lotn:* 8, 12 oz; *Clnsr:* 8.75 oz

OATMEAL COLLOIDS

   Aveeno (OTC) add to bath as needed
         Regular: 1.5 oz (8/pck); *Moisturizing:* 0.75 oz (8/pck)
   Aveeno Oil (OTC) add to bath as needed
         Oil: 8 oz
   Aveeno Moisturizing (OTC) apply as needed
         Lotn: 2.5, 8, 12 oz; *Crm:* 4 oz
   Aveeno Cleansing Bar (OTC) *Bar:* 3 oz
   Aveeno Gentle Skin Cleanser (OTC) *Liq clnsr:* 6 oz

TOPICAL OIL

▷ *fluocinolone acetonide* 0.01% topical oil (C)
   Pediatric: <6 years: not recommended; ≥6 years: apply sparingly bid for up to 4
   weeks
         Derma-Smoothe/FS Topical Oil apply sparingly tid
         Topical oil: 0.01% (4 oz) (peanut oil)

TOPICAL STEROIDS

Comment: Topical steroids should be applied sparingly and for the shortest time
necessary. Do not use in the diaper area. Do not use an occlusive dressing. Systemic

absorption of topical corticosteroids can induce reversible hypothalamic-pituitary-adrenal (HPA) axis suppression with the potential for clinical corticosteroid insufficiency.

▷ *desonide* 0.05% topical gel (C) apply sparingly bid-tid; max 4 weeks
  Pediatric: <3 months: not recommended; ≥3 months: same as adult
    Desonate *Gel:* 0.05% (60 gm) (89% purified water; fragrance-free, surfactant-free, alcohol-free)

SECOND-GENERATION ORAL ANTIHISTAMINES

Comment: The following drugs are second-generation antihistamines. As such they minimally sedating, much less so than the first-generation antihistamines. All antihistamines are excreted into breast milk.

▷ *cetirizine* (C)(OTC)(G) initially 5-10 mg once daily; 5 mg once daily; >65 years: use with caution
  Pediatric: <6 years: not recommended; ≥6 years: same as adult
    cetirizine *Cap:* 10 mg
    Children's Zyrtec Chewable *Chew tab:* 5, 10 mg (grape)
    Children's Zyrtec Allergy Syrup *Syr:* 1 mg/ml (4 oz) (grape, bubble gum) (sugar-free, dye-free)
    Zyrtec *Tab:* 10 mg
    Zyrtec Hives Relief *Tab:* 10 mg
    Zyrtec Liquid Gels *Liq gel:* 10 mg
▷ *desloratadine* (C)
    Clarinex 1/2-1 tab once daily
  Pediatric: <6 years: not recommended; ≥6 years: same as adult
    Tab: 5 mg
    Clarinex RediTabs 5 mg once daily
  Pediatric: <6 years: not recommended; 6-12 years: 2.5 mg once daily; ≥12 years: same as adult
    ODT: 2.5, 5 mg (tutti-frutti) (phenylalanine)
    Clarinex Syrup 5 mg (10 ml) once daily
  Pediatric: <6 months: not recommended; 6-11 months: 1 mg (2 ml) once daily; 1-5 years: 1.25 mg (2.5 ml) once daily; 6-11 years: 2.5 mg (5 ml) once daily; ≥12 years: same as adult
    Syr: 0.5 mg per ml (4 oz) (tutti-frutti) (phenylalanine)
    Desloratadine ODT 1 tab once daily
  Pediatric: <6 years: not recommended; 6-11 years: 1/2 tab once daily; ≥12 years: same as adult
    ODT: 5 mg
▷ *fexofenadine* (C)(OTC)(G) 60 mg once daily-bid <u>or</u> 180 mg once daily; *CrCl <90 mL/min:* 60 mg once daily
  Pediatric: <6 months: not recommended; 6 months-2 years: 15 mg bid; *CrCl ≤90 ml/min:* 15 mg once daily; 2-11 years: 30 mg bid; *CrCl ≤90 ml/min:* 30 mg once daily; ≥12 years: same as adult
    Allegra *Tab:* 30, 60, 180 mg film-coat
    Allegra Allergy *Tab:* 60, 180 mg film-coat
    Allegra ODT *ODT:* 30 mg (phenylalanine)
    Allegra Oral Suspension *Oral susp:* 30 mg/5 ml (6 mg/ml) (4 oz)
▷ *levocetirizine* (B)(OTC)(G) administer dose in the PM; *Seasonal Allergic Rhinitis:* <2 years: not recommended; may start at ≥2 years; *Chronic Idiopathic Urticaria (CIU), Perennial Allergic Rhinitis:* <6 months: not recommended; may start at ≥ 6 months; *Dosing by Age:* 6 months-5 years: max 1.25 mg once daily; 6-11 years: max 2.5 mg once daily; ≥12 years: 2.5-5 mg once daily; *Renal Dysfunction <12 years:* contraindicated; *Renal Dysfunction ≥12 years:* CrCl 50-80 mL/min: 2.5 mg once daily; *CrCl 30-50 mL/min:* 2.5 mg every other day;

CrCl: 10-30 mL/min: 2.5 mg twice weekly (every 3-4 days); CrCl <10 mL/min, ESRD or hemodialysis: contraindicated

>> **Children's Xyzal Allergy 24HR** *Oral Soln:* 0.5 mg/ml (150 ml)
>> **Xyzal Allergy 24HR** *Tab:* 5*mg

▷ *loratadine* (C)(OTC)(G) 5 mg bid or 10 mg once daily; *Hepatic or Renal Insufficiency:* see mfr pkg insert

Pediatric: <2 years: not recommended; 2-5 years: 5 mg once daily; ≥6 years: same as adult

>> **Children's Claritin Chewables** *Chew tab:* 5 mg (grape) (phenylalanine)
>> **Children's Claritin Syrup** 1 mg/ml (4 oz) (fruit) (sugar-free, alcohol-free, dye-free; sodium 6 mg/5 ml)
>> **Claritin** *Tab:* 10 mg
>> **Claritin Hives Relief** *Tab:* 10 mg
>> **Claritin Liqui-Gels** *Liq gel:* 10 mg
>> **Claritin RediTabs 12 Hours** *ODT:* 5 mg (mint)
>> **Claritin RediTabs 24 Hours** *ODT:* 10 mg (mint)

FIRST GENERATION ANTIHISTAMINES

▷ *diphenhydramine* (B)(G) 25-50 mg q 6-8 hours; max 100 mg/day

Pediatric: <2 years: not recommended; 2-6 years: 6.25 mg q 4-6 hours; max 37.5 mg/day; >6-12 years: 12.5-25 mg q 4-6 hours; max 150 mg/day; >12 years: same as adult

>> **Benadryl** (OTC) *Chew tab:* 12.5 mg (grape) (phenylalanine); *Liq:* 12.5 mg/5 ml (4, 8 oz); *Cap:* 25 mg; *Tab:* 25 mg; *Dye-free soft gel:* 25 mg; *Dye-free liq:* 12.5 mg/5 ml (4, 8 oz)

▷ *diphenhydramine injectable* (B)(G) 25-50 mg IM immediately; then q 6 hours prn

Pediatric: <12 years: *See mfr pkg insert:* 1.25 mg/kg up to 25 mg IM x 1 dose; then q 6 hours prn; ≥12 years: same as adult

>> **Benadryl Injectable** *Vial:* 50 mg/ml (1 ml single-use); 50 mg/ml (10 ml multi-dose);
>> *Amp:* 10 mg/ml (1 ml); *Prefilled syringe:* 50 mg/ml (1 ml)

▷ *hydroxyzine* (C)(G) 50 mg/day divided qid prn; 50-100 mg/day divided qid prn

Pediatric: <6 years: 50 mg/day divided qid prn; ≥6 years: same as adult

>> **Atarax** *Tab:* 10, 25, 50, 100 mg; *Syr:* 10 mg/5 ml (alcohol 0.5%)
>> **Vistaril** *Cap:* 25, 50, 100 mg; *Oral susp:* 25 mg/5 ml (4 oz) (lemon)

Comment: *Hydroxyzine* is contraindicated in early pregnancy and in patients with a prolonged QT interval. It is not known whether this drug is excreted in human milk; therefore, **hydroxyzine** should not be given to nursing mothers.

TOPICAL ANALGESICS

▷ *capsaicin* cream (B)(G) apply tid-qid prn

Pediatric: <2 years: not recommended; ≥2 years: apply sparingly tid-qid prn

>> **Axsain** *Crm:* 0.075% (1, 2 oz)
>> **Capsin** (OTC) *Lotn:* 0.025, 0,075% (59 ml)
>> **Capzasin-HP** (OTC) *Crm:* 0.075% (1.5 oz); *Lotn:* 0.075% (2 oz)
>> **Capzasin-P** (OTC) *Crm:* 0.025% (1.5 oz); *Lotn:* 0.025% (2 oz)
>> **Dolorac** *Crm:* 0.025% (28 gm)
>> **Double Cap** (OTC) *Crm:* 0.05% (2 oz)
>> **R-Gel** *Gel:* 0.025% (15, 30 gm)
>> **Zostrix** (OTC) *Crm:* 0.025% (0.7, 1.5, 3 oz)
>> **Zostrix HP** (OTC) *Emol crm:* 0.075% (1, 2 oz)

TOPICAL & TRANSDERMAL ANALGESICS

▷ *capsaicin* 8% patch (B) apply up to 4 patches for one 60-minute application to clean dry skin; may prep area with topical anesthetic; wear non-latex gloves; patches may be cut to size/shape; treatment may be repeated every 3 months
  Pediatric: <18 years: not recommended; ≥18 years: same as adult
    Qutenza *Patch:* 8% 1640 mcg/cm (179 mg) (1 or 2 patches w. 1-50 gm tube cleansing gel/carton)

▷ *diclofenac sodium* (C; D ≥30 wks) apply qid prn to intact skin
  Pediatric: <12 years: not established; ≥12 years: same as adult
    Pennsaid 1.5% in 10 drop increments, dispense and rub into front, side, and back of knee: usually; 40 drops (40 mg) qid
      Topical soln: 1.5% (150 ml)
    Pennsaid 2% apply 2 pump actuations (40 mg) and rub into front, side, and back of knee bid
      Topical soln: 2% (20 mg/pump actuation, 112 gm)
    Solaraze Gel massage in to clean skin bid prn
      Gel: 3% (50 gm) (benzyl alcohol)
    Voltaren Gel (G)(OTC) apply qid prn to intact skin
      Gel: 1% (100 gm)
  Comment: *Diclofenac* is contraindicated with **aspirin** allergy. As with other NSAIDs, should be avoided in late pregnancy (≥30 weeks) because it may cause premature closure of the ductus arteriosus.

▷ *doxepin* (B) cream apply to affected area qid at intervals of at least 3-4 hours; max 8 days
  Pediatric: <12 years: not recommended; >12 years: same as adult
    Prudoxin *Crm:* 5% (45 gm)
    Zonalon *Crm:* 5% (30, 45 gm)

▷ *pimecrolimus* 1% cream (C)(G) <2 years: not recommended; ≥2 years: apply to affected area bid; do not apply an occlusive dressing
    Elidel *Crm:* 1% (30, 60, 100 gm)
  Comment: *Pimecrolimus* is indicated for short-term and intermittent long-term use. Discontinue use when resolution occurs. Contraindicated if the patient is immunosuppressed. Change to the 0.1% preparation or if secondary bacterial infection is present.

▷ *trolamine salicylate* apply tid-qid
  Pediatric: <2 years: not recommended; ≥2 years: same as adult
    Mobisyl Creme *Crm:* 10% (100 gm)

TOPICAL AND TRANSDERMAL ANESTHETICS

Comment: *Lidocaine* should not be applied to non-intact skin.

▷ *lidocaine* cream (B) apply to affected area bid prn
  Pediatric: <12 years: not recommended; ≥12 years: same as adult
    LidaMantle *Crm:* 3% (1, 2 oz)
    Lidoderm *Crm:* 3% (85 gm)
    ZTlido *lidocaine* topical system 1% (30/carton)
      Comment: Compared to **Lidoderm** (*lidocaine* patch 5%), which contains 700 mg/patch, **ZTlido** requires only 35 mg per topical system to achieve the same therapeutic dose.

▷ *lidocaine* lotion (B) apply to affected area bid prn
  Pediatric: <12 years: not recommended; ≥12 years: same as adult
    LidaMantle *Lotn:* 3% (177 ml)

▷ *lidocaine* 5% patch (B)(G) apply up to 3 patches at one time for up to 12 hours/24-hour period (12 hours on/12 hours off); patches may be cut into smaller sizes before removal of the release liner; do not re-use

Pediatric: <12 years: not recommended; ≥12 years: same as adult
  Lidoderm *Patch:* 5% (10x14 cm; 30/carton)
▷ **lidocaine+dexamethasone (B)**
Pediatric: <12 years: not recommended; ≥12 years: same as adult
  Decadron Phosphate with Xylocaine *Lotn:* dexa 4 mg+lido 10 mg per ml (5 ml)
▷ **lidocaine+hydrocortisone (B)(G)** apply to affected area bid prn
Pediatric: <12 years: not recommended; ≥12 years: same as adult
  LidaMantle HC *Crm:* lido 3%+hydro 0.5% (1, 3 oz); *Lotn:* (177 ml)
▷ **lidocaine 2.5%+prilocaine 2.5%** apply sparingly to the burn bid-tid prn
Pediatric: <12 years: not recommended; ≥12 years: same as adult
  Emla Cream (B) 5, 30 gm/tube

INTERLEUKIN-4 RECEPTOR ALPHA ANTAGONIST

▷ **dupilumab** administer SC into the upper arm, abdomen, or thigh; rotate sites; *Initial Dose:* 600 mg (2 x 300 mg SC in different injection sites), then, 300 mg SC once every other week; may use with or without topical corticosteroids; may use with calcineurin inhibitors, but reserve only for problem areas (e.g., face, neck, intertriginous, and genital areas); avoid live vaccines
Pediatric: <12 years: not recommended; ≥12 years: <60 kg: *Initial Dose:* 400 mg (2 x 200 mg SC in different injection sites; then, 200 mg SC once every other week; ≥60 kg: same as adult
  Dupixent *Prefilled syringe:* 200 mg/1.14 ml, 300 mg/2 ml, single-dose (2/pck without needle) (preservative-free)
Comment: *Dupilumab* is a human monoclonal IgG4 antibody that inhibits interleukin-4 (IL-4) and interleukin-13 (IL-13) signaling by specifically binding to the IL4Ra subunit shared by the IL-4 and IL-13 receptor complexes, thereby inhibiting the release of pro-inflammatory cytokines, chemokines, and IgE. **Dupixent** is indicated for the treatment of moderate-to-severe atopic dermatitis when the disease is not adequately controlled with topical prescription therapies or when those therapies are not advisable. **Dupixent** can be used with or without topical corticosteroids. *Dupilumab* is also indicated as an add-on maintenance therapy, at different dosing regimens, for patients ≥12 years-of-age with moderate-to-severe asthma with an eosinophilic subtype or with oral corticosteroid-dependent asthma. Avoid live vaccines.

◯ DERMATITIS: CONTACT

Topical Corticosteroids *see* Appendix K: Topical Corticosteroids by Potency
Parenteral Corticosteroids *see* Appendix M. Parenteral Corticosteroids
Oral Corticosteroids *see* Appendix L. Oral Corticosteroids
OTC diphenhydramine cream

PROPHYLAXIS

▷ **bentoquatam** apply as a wet film to exposed skin at least 15 minutes prior to possible contact; reapply at least q 4 hours; remove with soap and water
Pediatric: <6 years: not recommended; ≥6 years: same as adult
  IvyBlock (OTC) *Soln:* 120 ml
Comment: Provides protection against genus *Rhus* (poison ivy, oak, and sumac).

TREATMENT
Oatmeal Colloids

  Aveeno (OTC) add to bath as needed
    Regular: 1.5 oz (8/pck); *Moisturizing:* 0.75 oz (8/pck)
  Aveeno Oil (OTC) add to bath as needed
    Oil: 8 oz

Aveeno Moisturizing (OTC) apply as needed
   Lotn: 2.5, 8, 12 oz; *Crm:* 4 oz
Aveeno Cleansing Bar (OTC) *Bar:* 3 oz
Aveeno Gentle Skin Cleanser (OTC) *Liq clnsr:* 6 oz

SECOND GENERATION ORAL ANTIHISTAMINES

Comment: The following drugs are second-generation antihistamines. As such they minimally sedating, much less so than the first-generation antihistamines. All antihistamines are excreted into breast milk.

▷ *cetirizine* (C)(OTC)(G) initially 5-10 mg once daily; 5 mg once daily; ≥65 years: use with caution
  Pediatric: <6 years: not recommended; ≥6 years: same as adult
    cetirizine Cap: 10 mg
    Children's Zyrtec Chewable *Chew tab:* 5, 10 mg (grape)
    Children's Zyrtec Allergy Syrup *Syr:* 1 mg/ml (4 oz) (grape, bubble gum) (sugar-free, dye-free)
    Zyrtec *Tab:* 10 mg
    Zyrtec Hives Relief *Tab:* 10 mg
    Zyrtec Liquid Gels *Liq gel:* 10 mg
▷ *desloratadine* (C)
    Clarinex 1/2-1 tab once daily
  Pediatric: <6 years: not recommended; ≥6 years: same as adult
    Tab: 5 mg
    Clarinex RediTabs 5 mg once daily
  Pediatric: <6 years: not recommended; 6-12 years: 2.5 mg once daily; ≥12 years: same as adult
    ODT: 2.5, 5 mg (tutti-frutti) (phenylalanine)
    Clarinex Syrup 5 mg (10 ml) once daily
  Pediatric: <6 months: not recommended; 6-11 months: 1 mg (2 ml) once daily; 1-5 years: 1.25 mg (2.5 ml) once daily; 6-11 years: 2.5 mg (5 ml) once daily; ≥12 years: same as adult
    Syr: 0.5 mg per ml (4 oz) (tutti-frutti) (phenylalanine)
    Desloratadine ODT 1 tab once daily
  Pediatric: <6 years: not recommended; 6-11 years: 1/2 tab once daily; ≥12 years: same as adult
    ODT: 5 mg
▷ *fexofenadine* (C)(OTC)(G) 60 mg once daily-bid <u>or</u> 180 mg once daily; *CrCl <90 mL/min:* 60 mg once daily
  Pediatric: <6 months: not recommended; 6 months-2 years: 15 mg bid; *CrCl ≤90 mL/min:* 15 mg once daily; 2-11 years: 30 mg bid; *CrCl ≤90 mL/min:* 30 mg once daily; ≥12 years: same as adult
    Allegra *Tab:* 30, 60, 180 mg film-coat
    Allegra Allergy *Tab:* 60, 180 mg film-coat
    Allegra ODT *ODT:* 30 mg (phenylalanine)
    Allegra Oral Suspension *Oral susp:* 30 mg/5 ml (6 mg/ml) (4 oz)
▷ *levocetirizine* (B)(OTC)(G) administer dose in the PM; *Seasonal Allergic Rhinitis:* <2 years: not recommended; may start at ≥2 years; *Chronic Idiopathic Urticaria (CIU), Perennial Allergic Rhinitis:* <6 months: not recommended; may start at ≥ 6 months; *Dosing by Age:* 6 months-5 years: max 1.25 mg once daily; 6-11 years: max 2.5 mg once daily; ≥12 years: 2.5-5 mg once daily; *Renal Dysfunction <12 years:* contraindicated; *Renal Dysfunction ≥12 years:* CrCl 50-80 mL/min: 2.5 mg once daily; CrCl 30-50 mL/min: 2.5 mg every other day; CrCl: 10-30 mL/min: 2.5 mg twice weekly (every 3-4 days); CrCl <10 mL/min, ESRD <u>or</u> hemodialysis: contraindicated
    Children's Xyzal Allergy 24HR *Oral Soln:* 0.5 mg/ml (150 ml)
    Xyzal Allergy 24HR *Tab:* 5*mg

➢ **loratadine** (C)(OTC)(G) 5 mg bid or 10 mg once daily; *Hepatic or Renal Insufficiency:* see mfr pkg insert
Pediatric: <2 years: not recommended; 2-5 years: 5 mg once daily; ≥6 years: same as adult

> **Children's Claritin Chewables** *Chew tab:* 5 mg (grape) (phenylalanine)
> **Children's Claritin Syrup** 1 mg/ml (4 oz) (fruit) (sugar-free, alcohol-free, dye-free; sodium 6 mg/5 ml)
> **Claritin** *Tab:* 10 mg
> **Claritin Hives Relief** *Tab:* 10 mg
> **Claritin Liqui-Gels** *Liq gel:* 10 mg
> **Claritin RediTabs 12 Hours** *ODT:* 5 mg (mint)
> **Claritin RediTabs 24 Hours** *ODT:* 10 mg (mint)

FIRST GENERATION ORAL ANTIHISTAMINES

➢ **diphenhydramine** (B)(G) 25-50 mg q 6-8 hours; max 100 mg/day
Pediatric: <2 years: not recommended; 2-6 years: 6.25 mg q 4-6 hours; max 37.5 mg/day; >6-12 years: 12.5-25 mg q 4-6 hours; max 150 mg/day; >12 years: same as adult

> **Benadryl** (OTC) *Chew tab:* 12.5 mg (grape) (phenylalanine); *Liq:* 12.5 mg/5 ml (4, 8 oz); *Cap:* 25 mg; *Tab:* 25 mg; *Dye-free soft gel:* 25 mg; *Dye-free liq:* 12.5 mg/5 ml (4, 8 oz)

➢ **hydroxyzine** (C)(G) 50 mg/day divided qid prn; 50-100 mg/day divided qid prn
Pediatric: <6 years: 50 mg/day divided qid prn; ≥6 years: same as adult

> **Atarax** *Tab:* 10, 25, 50, 100 mg; *Syr:* 10 mg/5 ml (alcohol 0.5%)
> **Vistaril** *Cap:* 25, 50, 100 mg; *Oral susp:* 25 mg/5 ml (4 oz) (lemon)

Comment: *Hydroxyzine* is contraindicated in early pregnancy and in patients with a prolonged QT interval. It is not known whether this drug is excreted in human milk; therefore, *hydroxyzine* should not be given to nursing mothers.

FIRST GENERATION PARENTERAL ANTIHISTAMINE

➢ **diphenhydramine** injectable (B)(G) 25-50 mg IM immediately; then q 6 hours prn
Pediatric: <12 years: See mfr pkg insert: 1.25 mg/kg up to 25 mg IM x 1 dose; then q 6 hours prn; ≥12 years: same as adult

> **Benadryl Injectable** *Vial:* 50 mg/ml (1 ml single-use); 50 mg/ml (10 ml multi-dose); *Amp:* 10 mg/ml (1 ml); *Prefilled syringe:* 50 mg/ml (1 ml)

DERMATITIS: GENUS *RHUS* (POISON OAK, POISON IVY, POISON SUMAC)

Topical Corticosteroids *see* Appendix K: Topical Corticosteroids by Potency
Parenteral Corticosteroids *see* Appendix M. Parenteral Corticosteroids
Oral Corticosteroids *see* Appendix L. Oral Corticosteroids
OTC Calamine Lotion
OTC diphenhydramine cream

PROPHYLAXIS

➢ **bentoquatam** <6 years: not recommended; ≥6 years: apply as a wet film to exposed skin at least 15 minutes prior to possible contact; reapply at least q 4 hours; remove with soap and water

> **IvyBlock** (OTC) *Soln:* 120 ml

Comment: Provides protection against genus *Rhus* (poison oak, poison ivy, and poison sumac).

TREATMENT

Oatmeal Colloids

Aveeno (OTC) add to bath as needed
Regular: 1.5 oz (8/pck); *Moisturizing:* 0.75 oz (8/pck)
Aveeno Oil (OTC) add to bath as needed
Oil: 8 oz
Aveeno Moisturizing (OTC) apply as needed
Lotn: 2.5, 8, 12 oz; *Crm:* 4 oz
Aveeno Cleansing Bar (OTC) *Bar:* 3 oz
Aveeno Gentle Skin Cleanser (OTC) *Liq clnsr:* 6 oz

SECOND-GENERATION ORAL ANTIHISTAMINES

Comment: The following drugs are second-generation antihistamines. As such they are minimally sedating, much less so than the first generation antihistamines. All antihistamines are excreted into breast milk.

▷ *cetirizine* (C)(OTC)(G) initially 5-10 mg once daily; 5 mg once daily; ≥65 years: use with caution
Pediatric: <6 years: not recommended; ≥6 years: same as adult
    cetirizine Cap: 10 mg
    Children's Zyrtec Chewable *Chew tab:* 5, 10 mg (grape)
    Children's Zyrtec Allergy Syrup *Syr:* 1 mg/ml (4 oz) (grape, bubble gum) (sugar-free, dye-free)
    Zyrtec *Tab:* 10 mg
    Zyrtec Hives Relief *Tab:* 10 mg
    Zyrtec Liquid Gels *Liq gel:* 10 mg

▷ *desloratadine* (C)
    Clarinex 1/2-1 tab once daily
    Pediatric: <6 years: not recommended; ≥6 years: same as adult
    Tab: 5 mg
    Clarinex RediTabs 5 mg once daily
    Pediatric: <6 years: not recommended; 6-12 years: 2.5 mg once daily; ≥12 years: same as adult
    ODT: 2.5, 5 mg (tutti-frutti) (phenylalanine)
    Clarinex Syrup 5 mg (10 ml) once daily
    Pediatric: <6 months: not recommended; 6-11 months: 1 mg (2 ml) once daily; 1-5 years: 1.25 mg (2.5 ml) once daily; 6-11 years: 2.5 mg (5 ml) once daily; ≥12 years: same as adult
    Syr: 0.5 mg per ml (4 oz) (tutti-frutti) (phenylalanine)
    Desloratadine ODT 1 tab once daily
    Pediatric: <6 years: not recommended; 6-11 years: 1/2 tab once daily; ≥12 years: same as adult
    ODT: 5 mg

▷ *fexofenadine* (C)(OTC)(G) 60 mg once daily-bid or 180 mg once daily; CrCl <90 mL/min: 60 mg once daily
Pediatric: <6 months: not recommended; 6 months-2 years: 15 mg bid; CrCl ≤90 m/min: 15 mg once daily; 2-11 years: 30 mg bid; CrCl ≤90 m/min: 30 mg once daily; ≥12 years: same as adult
    Allegra *Tab:* 30, 60, 180 mg film-coat
    Allegra Allergy *Tab:* 60, 180 mg film-coat
    Allegra ODT *ODT:* 30 mg (phenylalanine)
    Allegra Oral Suspension *Oral susp:* 30 mg/5 ml (6 mg/ml) (4 oz)

▷ *levocetirizine* (B)(OTC)(G) administer dose in the PM; *Seasonal Allergic Rhinitis:* <2 years: not recommended; may start at ≥2 years; *Chronic Idiopathic Urticaria (CIU), Perennial Allergic Rhinitis:* <6 months: not recommended; may start at ≥ 6 months; *Dosing by Age:* 6 months-5 years: max 1.25 mg once daily; 6-11 years: max 2.5 mg once daily; ≥12 years: 2.5-5 mg once daily; *Renal Dysfunction <12 years:* contraindicated; *Renal Dysfunction ≥12 years:* CrCl 50-80 mL/min: 2.5 mg once daily; *CrCl 30-50 mL/min:* 2.5 mg every other day; CrCl: 10-30 mL/min: 2.5 mg twice weekly (every 3-4 days); CrCl <10 mL/min, ESRD or hemodialysis: contraindicated

> **Children's Xyzal Allergy 24HR** *Oral Soln:* 0.5 mg/ml (150 ml)
> **Xyzal Allergy 24HR** *Tab:* 5*mg

▷ *loratadine* (C)(OTC)(G) 5 mg bid or 10 mg once daily; *Hepatic or Renal Insufficiency:* see mfr pkg insert
Pediatric: <2 years: not recommended; 2-5 years: 5 once daily; ≥6 years: same as adult

> **Children's Claritin Chewables** *Chew tab:* 5 mg (grape) (phenylalanine)
> **Children's Claritin Syrup** 1 mg/ml (4 oz) (fruit) (sugar-free, alcohol-free, dye-free, sodium 6 mg/5 ml)
> **Claritin** *Tab:* 10 mg
> **Claritin Hives Relief** *Tab:* 10 mg
> **Claritin Liqui-Gels** *Lig gel:* 10 mg
> **Claritin RediTabs 12 Hours** *ODT:* 5 mg (mint)
> **Claritin RediTabs 24 Hours** *ODT:* 10 mg (mint)

FIRST GENERATION ANTIHISTAMINES

▷ *diphenhydramine* (B)(G) 25-50 mg q 6-8 hours; max 100 mg/day
Pediatric: <2 years: not recommended; 2-6 years: 6.25 mg q 4-6 hours; max 37.5 mg/day; >6-12 years: 12.5-25 mg q 4-6 hours; max 150 mg/day; >12 years: same as adult

> **Benadryl (OTC)** *Chew tab:* 12.5 mg (grape) (phenylalanine); *Liq:* 12.5 mg/5 ml (4, 8 oz); *Cap:* 25 mg; *Tab:* 25 mg; *Dye-free soft gel:* 25 mg; *Dye-free liq:* 12.5 mg/5 ml (4, 8 oz)

▷ *diphenhydramine injectable* (B)(G) 25-50 mg IM immediately; then q 6 hours prn
Pediatric: <12 years: *See mfr pkg insert:* 1.25 mg/kg up to 25 mg IM x 1 dose; then q 6 hours prn; ≥12 years: same as adult

> **Benadryl Injectable** *Vial:* 50 mg/ml (1 ml single-use); 50 mg/ml (10 ml multi-dose); *Amp:* 10 mg/ml (1 ml); *Prefilled syringe:* 50 mg/ml (1 ml)

▷ *hydroxyzine* (C)(G) 50 mg/day divided qid prn; 50-100 mg/day divided qid prn
Pediatric: <6 years: 50 mg/day divided qid prn; ≥6 years: same as adult

> **Atarax** *Tab:* 10, 25, 50, 100 mg; *Syr:* 10 mg/5 ml (alcohol 0.5%)
> **Vistaril** *Cap:* 25, 50, 100 mg; *Oral susp:* 25 mg/5 ml (4 oz) (lemon)

Comment: *Hydroxyzine* is contraindicated in early pregnancy and in patients with a prolonged QT interval. It is not known whether this drug is excreted in human milk; therefore, *hydroxyzine* should not be given to nursing mothers.

◯ DERMATITIS: SEBORRHEIC

ANTIFUNGAL SHAMPOOS AND TOPICAL AGENTS

▷ *chloroxine* shampoo (C) massage onto wet scalp; wait 3 minutes, rinse, repeat, and rinse thoroughly; use twice weekly
Pediatric: <12 years: not recommended; ≥12 years: same as adult

> **Capitrol Shampoo** *Shampoo:* 2% (4 oz)

▷ *ciclopirox* (B) apply gel once daily or apply cream or lotion twice daily, x 4 weeks or shampoo twice weekly; massage shampoo onto wet scalp; wait 3 minutes, rinse, repeat, and rinse thoroughly; shampoo twice weekly

> **Loprox Cream**
> *Pediatric:* <10 years: not recommended; ≥10 years: same as adult
> *Crm:* 0.77% (15, 30, 90 gm)
> **Loprox Gel**

Pediatric: <16 years: not recommended; ≥16 years: same as adult
  Gel: 0.77% (30, 45 gm)
Loprox Lotion
  Pediatric: <10 years: not recommended; ≥10 years: same as adult
  Lotn: 0.77% (30, 60 ml)
Loprox Shampoo *Shampoo:* 1% (120 ml)
▷ *coal tar* (C)(G)
Pediatric: same as adult
  Scytera (OTC) apply once daily-qid; use lowest effective dose
    Foam: 2%
  T/Gel Shampoo Extra Strength (OTC) use every other day; max 4 x/week;
  massage into wet scalp for 5 minutes; rinse; repeat *Shampoo:* 1%
  T/Gel Shampoo Original Formula (OTC) use every other day; max 7 x/week;
  massage into wet scalp for 5 minutes; rinse; repeat
    Shampoo: 0.5%
  T/Gel Shampoo Stubborn Itch Control (OTC) use every other day; max 7 x/
  week; massage into wet scalp for 5 minutes; rinse; repeat
    Shampoo: 0.5%
▷ *fluocinolone acetonide* (C)
  Derma-Smoothe/FS Shampoo apply up to 1 oz to scalp daily, lather, and leave
  on x 5 minutes, then rinse twice
  Pediatric: <12 years: not recommended; ≥12 years: same as adult
    Shampoo: 0.01% (4 oz)
  Derma-Smoothe/FS Topical Oil *fluocinolone acetonide* 0.01% topical oil (C)
  apply sparingly tid; for scalp psoriasis wet or dampen hair or scalp, then apply
  a thin film, massage well, cover with a shower cap and leave on for at least 4
  hours or overnight, then wash hair with regular shampoo and rinse
  Pediatric: <6 years: not recommended; ≥6 years: apply sparingly bid for up to 4
  weeks
    Topical oil: 0.01% (4 oz) (peanut oil)
▷ *ketoconazole* (C) apply cream or gel once daily x 4 week or apply up to 1 oz
  shampoo to scalp daily, lather, leave on x 5 minutes, then rinse twice
  Pediatric: <12 years: not recommended; ≥12 years: same as adult
  Nizoral Cream *Crm:* 2% (15, 30, 60 gm)
  Nizoral Shampoo *Shampoo:* 2% (4 oz)
  Xolegel *Gel:* 2% (45 gm)
  Xolegel Duo Kit: Xolegel *Gel:* 2% (45 gm) + **Xolex** *Shampoo:* 2% (4 oz)
▷ *selenium sulfide* (C) massage cream into scalp twice weekly x 2 weeks or massage
  into wet scalp, wait 2-3 minutes, rinse; repeat twice weekly x 2 weeks; may
  continue treatment with lotion of shampoo 1-2 x weekly as needed
  Pediatric: <12 years: not recommended; ≥12 years: same as adult
  Exsel Shampoo *Shampoo:* 2.5% (4 oz)
  Selsun Rx *Lotn:* 2.5% (4 oz)
  Selsun Shampoo *Shampoo:* 1% (120, 210, 240, 330 ml); 2.5% (120 ml)
▷ *sodium sulfacetamide+sulfur* (C)
  Clenia Emollient Cream apply daily tid
    Emol crm: sod sulfa 10%+sulfur 5% (10 oz)
  Clenia Foaming Wash wash 1-2 x/day
    Wash: sod sulfa 10%+sulfur 5% (6, 12 oz)
  Rosula Gel apply daily tid
    Gel: sod sulfa 10%+sulfur 5% (45 ml)
  Rosula Lotion apply daily tid
    Lotn: sod sulfa 10%+sulfur 5% (45 ml) (alcohol-free)
  Rosula Wash wash bid
    Clnsr: sod sulfa 10%+sulfur 5% (335 ml)

TOPICAL STEROID

▷ **betamethasone valerate** 0.12% foam **(C)(G)** apply twice daily in AM and PM; invert can and dispense a small amount of foam onto a clean saucer or other cool surface (do not apply directly to hand) and massage a small amount into affected area until foam disappears
Pediatric: <12 years: not recommended; ≥12 years: same as adult
    Luxiq *Foam:* 100 gm

OXIDIZING AGENT

▷ **hydrogen peroxide** 40% apply 4 times to targeted lesion(s) approx 1 min apart during a single session; repeat if lesions have not cleared after 3 weeks; treatments must be applied by a qualified healthcare provider
Pediatric: not applicable
    Eskata *Pen applicator:* 1.5, 2.2 ml/pen (1, 3, 12/carton)
    Comment: Not for oral, ophthalmic, or intravaginal use. Avoid open or infected seborrheic keratoses, lesions within the orbital rim, eyes, and mucous membranes. The most common adverse reactions include erythema (99%), stinging (97%), edema (91%), scaling (90%), crusting (81%), and pruritus (58%).

 DIABETIC MACULAR EDEMA, RETINOPATHY, MACULAR DEGENERATION

VASCULAR ENDOTHELIAL GROWTH FACTOR (VEGF) INHIBITOR

Comment: Diabetic retinopathy is the leading cause of blindness among working-age adults in the US. **Lucentis** *(ranibizumab)* is only one FDA-approved drug for the treatment of diabetic retinopathy. Additional labeled indications include treatment of diabetic macular edema (DME), treatment of neovascular (wet) age-related macular degeneration (AMD), treatment of macular edema following retinal vein occlusion (RVO), and treatment of myopic choroidal neovascularization (mCNV).

▷ **aflibercept** *intravitreal injection* **(C)** 2 mg (0.05 ml) administered by intravitreal injection, with a 30-gauge x ½-inch injection needle, every 4 weeks (monthly) for the first 3 months, followed by 2 mg (0.05 mL) via intravitreal injection once every 8 weeks (2 months); although **Eylea** may be dosed as frequently as 2 mg every 4 weeks (monthly), additional efficacy has not been demonstrated; *Age-related Macular Degeneration (AMD):* although not as effective as the every 8 week dosing regimen, patients with AMD may also be treated with 1 dose every 12 weeks after 1 year of effective therapy; must only be administered by a qualified physician
Pediatric: <18 years: not established; ≥18 years: same as adult
    Eylea *(aflibercept)* **Injection** *Vial:* 2 mg/0.05 ml, single-dose; *Prefilled syringe:* 2 mg/0.05 ml, single-dose
    Comment: **Eylea** *(aflibercept)* is indicated for the treatment of patients with neovascular (wet) age-related macular degeneration, macular edema following retinal vein occlusion, diabetic macular edema, and diabetic retinopathy. It is designed to block the growth of new blood vessels and decrease the ability of fluid to pass through blood vessels (vascular permeability) in the eye by blocking VEGF-A and placental growth factor (PLGF), two growth factors involved in angiogenesis.

▷ **brolucizumab-dbll** administration via intravitreal injection by a qualified healthcare provider; recommended dose is 6 mg (0.05 ml of 120 mg/ml solution) once monthly (approximately every 25-31 days) for the first 3 doses; then, 6 mg (0.05 ml) dose every 8-12 weeks; refrigerate at 2 to 8°C (36 to 46°F). Do not freeze. Prior to use, the unopened glass vial of **Beovu** may be kept at room temperature, 20 to 25°C (68 to 77°F) for up to 24 hours. Store vial in the outer carton to protect from light.

Beovu *Vial:* 6 mg/0.05 ml (120 mg/ml), single-dose, with one sterile 5-micron blunt filter needle (18-gauge x 1½ inch, 1.2 mm x 40 mm)

Comment: **Beovu** *(brolucizumab-dbll)* is a human vascular endothelial growth factor (VEGF) inhibitor indicated for the treatment of neovascular (wet) age-related macular degeneration (AMD). Endophthalmitis and retinal detachments may occur following intravitreal injections. Patients should be instructed to report any symptoms suggestive of endophthalmitis or retinal detachment without delay. Increases in intraocular pressure (IOP) have occurred within 30 minutes of an intravitreal injection. There is a potential risk of an arterial thromboembolic event (ATE) following intravitreal use of VEGF inhibitors. Contraindications include ocular or periocular infection, active intraocular inflammation, and hypersensitivity. The most common adverse reactions (≥5%) reported in patients receiving Beovu have been blurred vision (10%), cataract (7%), conjunctival hemorrhage (6%), eye pain (5%), and vitreous floaters (5%). There are no adequate and well-controlled studies of **Beovu** administration in pregnancy. There is no information regarding the presence of *brolucizumab* in human milk or effects on the breastfed infant.

▷ *ranibizumab* (D)
Pediatric: <18 years: not established; ≥18 years: same as adult

DR: Diabetic retinopathy: Intravitreal: 0.3 mg once a month (approximately every 28 days)

DME: Diabetic macular edema: Intravitreal: 0.3 mg once a month (approximately every 28 days); in clinical trials, monthly doses of 0.5 mg were also studied

AMD: Neovascular (wet) Age-related Macular Degeneration: Intravitreal: 0.5 mg once a month (approximately every 28 days). Frequency may be reduced (e.g., 4 to 5 injections over 9 months) after the first 3 injections or may be reduced after the first 4 injections to once every 3 months if monthly injections are not feasible. *Note:* A regimen averaging 4 to 5 doses over 9 months is expected to maintain visual acuity and an every 3-month dosing regimen has reportedly resulted in a ~5 letter (1 line) loss of visual acuity over 9 months, as compared to monthly dosing which may result in an additional ~1 to 2 letter gain

RVO: macular edema following retinal vein occlusion: Intravitreal: 0.5 mg once a month (approximately every 28 days)

mCNV: myopic choroidal neovascularization: Intravitreal: 0.5 mg once a month (approximately every 28 days) for up to 3 months; may re-treat if necessary

Lucentis *Prefilled Syringe:* 0.3 mg/0.05 ml (0.05 ml); 0.5 mg/0.05 ml (0.05 ml); single-use for intravitreal injection (preservative free); *Vial:* 10 mg/ml (**Lucentis** 0.5 mg); 6 mg/ml solution (**Lucentis** 0.3 mg); single-use; a 5-micron sterile filter needle (19 gauge x 1½ inch) is required for preparation, but not included; keep refrigerated; do not freeze; protect vial from light; see mfr pkg insert for other precautions

Comment: *Ranibizumab* is a recombinant humanized monoclonal antibody fragment that binds to and inhibits human vascular endothelial growth factor A (VEGF-A). **Lucentis** inhibits VEGF from binding to its receptors and thereby suppressing neovascularization and slowing vision loss. Contraindications include ocular or periocular infection, and active intraocular inflammation. For ophthalmic intravitreal injection only. Each vial or prefilled syringe should only be used for the treatment of a single eye. If the contralateral eye requires treatment, a new vial or prefilled syringe should be used and the sterile field, syringe, gloves, drapes, eyelid speculum, filter, and injection needles should be changed before **Lucentis** is administered to the other eye. Adequate anesthesia and a topical broad-spectrum antimicrobial agent should be administered prior to the procedure. Refer to manufacturer labeling for additional detailed information. Based on its mechanism of action, adverse effects on pregnancy would be expected. Information related to use in pregnancy is limited. The intravitreal injection procedure should be carried out under controlled aseptic conditions, which include the use of sterile gloves, a sterile drape, and a sterile eyelid speculum (or equivalent). Adequate anesthesia and a broad-spectrum microbicide should be given prior to the injection. Prior to and 30 minutes following the intravitreal injection, patients should be monitored for elevation in intraocular pressure using tonometry. Each prefilled syringe or vial should only be used for the treatment of a single eye. If the contralateral eye requires treatment, a new prefilled syringe or vial should be used and the sterile field, syringe, gloves, drapes, eyelid speculum, filter needle (vial only), and injection needles should be changed.

REFERENCE

Solomon, S. D., Chew, E., Duh, E. J., Sobrin, L., Sun, J. K., VanderBeek, B. L., . . . Gardner, T. W. (2017). Diabetic retinopathy: A position statement by the American Diabetes Association. *Diabetes Care, 40*(3), 412–418. doi:10.2337/dc16-2641

INTRAVITREAL IMPLANT

▶ *fluocinolone acetonide* surgical intravitreal injection is administered by a qualified healthcare provider under sterile conditions in the office/clinic/hospital setting; the implant is a 36-month sustained-release system

Yutiq 0.18 mg non-bioerodible intravitreal implant, single-dose, preloaded applicator w. 25 g needle, for ophthalmic intravitreal injection

Comment: **Yutiq** is indicated for the treatment of macular edema, diabetic macular edema, and chronic non-infectious posterior uveitis. Placement of a **Yutiq** intravitreal implant is contraindicated with active infection (e.g., ocular herpes simplex, acute blepharoconjunctivitis) or glaucoma. Use of **Yutiq** may increase risk of cataract development and post-procedure blurring of vision, which should clear within 4 weeks. Avoid driving and hazardous activity until vision returns to baseline. If both eyes require treatment, the implants should be placed on separate dates to decrease risk of infection in both eyes.

DIABETIC PERIPHERAL NEUROPATHY (DPN)

Other Oral Analgesics *see Pain*

NUTRITIONAL SUPPLEMENT

▶ *L-methylfolate calcium (as metafolin)+pyridoxyl 5-phosphate+methylcobalamin*
1 cap twice daily or 2 caps once daily
Pediatric: <12 years: not recommended; ≥12 years: same as adult

Metanx *Cap:* meta 3 mg+pyr 35 mg+methyl 2 mg

Comment: **Metanx** is indicated as adjunct treatment for patients with endothelial cell dysfunction, who have loss of protective sensation and neuropathic pain associated with diabetic peripheral neuropathy.

ORAL ANALGESICS

▶ *acetaminophen* (B)(G) *see Fever*
▶ *aspirin* (D)(G) *see Fever*
▶ *tramadol* (C)(IV)(G)

Rybix ODT initially 100 mg once daily; may increase by 100 mg every 5 days; max 300 mg/day; *CrCl <30 mL/min or severe hepatic impairment*: not recommended; *Cirrhosis*: max 50 mg q 12 hours

Pediatric: <18 years: not recommended; ≥18 years: same as adult
> ODT: 50 mg (mint) (phenylalanine)

Ryzolt initially 100 mg once daily; may increase by 100 mg every 5 days; max 300 mg/day; *CrCl <30 mL/min or severe hepatic impairment*: not recommended
Pediatric: <18 years: not recommended; ≥18 years: same as adult
> Tab: 100, 200, 300 mg ext-rel

Ultram 50-100 mg q 4-6 hours prn; max 400 mg/day; *CrCl <30 mL/min*, max 100 mg q 12 hours; cirrhosis, max 50 mg q 12 hours
Pediatric: <18 years: not recommended; ≥18 years: same as adult
> Tab: 50*mg

Ultram ER initially 100 mg once daily; may increase by 100 mg every 5 days; max 300 mg/day; *CrCl <30 mL/min or severe hepatic impairment*: not recommended
Pediatric: <18 years: not recommended; ≥18 years: same as adult
> Tab: 100, 200, 300 mg ext-rel

▷ *tramadol+acetaminophen* **(C)(IV)(G)** 2 tabs q 4-6 hours; max 8 tabs/day x 5 days; *CrCl <30 mL/min:* max 2 tabs q 12 hours; max 4 tabs/day x 5 days
Pediatric: <18 years: not recommended; ≥18 years: same as adult
> **Ultracet** *Tab:* tram 37.5+acet 325 mg

TOPICAL ANALGESICS

▷ *capsaicin* cream **(B)(G)** apply tid-qid after lesions have healed
Pediatric: <2 years: not recommended; ≥2 years: same as adult
> **Axsain** *Crm:* 0.075% (1, 2 oz)
> **Capsin** *Lotn:* 0.025, 0.075% (59 ml)
> **Capzasin-HP (OTC)** *Crm:* 0.075% (1.5 oz); 0.025% (45, 90 gm); *Lotn:* 0.075% (2 oz); 0.025% (45, 90 gm)
> **Capzasin-P (OTC)** *Crm:* 0.025% (1.5 oz); *Lotn:* 0.025% (2 oz)
> **Capsaicin-HP (OTC)** *Crm:* 0.075% (1.5 oz); *Lotn:* 0.075% (2 oz); *Crm:* 0.025%
> **Dolorac** *Crm:* 0.025% (28 gm)
> **Double Cap (OTC)** *Crm:* 0.05% (2 oz)
> **R-Gel** *Gel:* 0.025% (15, 30 gm)
> **Zostrix (OTC)** *Crm:* 0.025% (0.7, 1.5, 3 oz)
> **Zostrix HP** *Emol crm:* 0.075% (1, 2 oz)

▷ *capsaicin* 8% patch **(B)** apply up to 4 patches for one 60-minute application to clean dry skin; may prep area with topical anesthetic; wear non-latex gloves; patches may be cut to size/shape; treatment may be repeated every 3 months
Pediatric: <18 years: not recommended; ≥18 years: same as adult
> **Qutenza** *Patch:* 8% 1640 mcg/cm (179 mg) (1 or 2 patches w. 1-50 gm tube cleansing gel/carton)

▷ *diclofenac sodium* **(C; D ≥30 wks)** apply qid prn to intact skin
Pediatric: <12 years: not established; ≥12 years: same as adult
> **Pennsaid 1.5%** in 10 drop increments, dispense and rub into front, side, and back of knee: usually; 40 drops (40 mg) qid
> > *Topical soln:* 1.5% (150 ml)
> **Pennsaid 2%** apply 2 pump actuations (40 mg) and rub into front, side, and back of knee bid
> > *Topical soln:* 2% (20 mg/pump actuation, 112 gm)
> **Solaraze Gel** massage in to clean skin bid prn
> > *Gel:* 3% (50 gm) (benzyl alcohol)
> **Voltaren Gel (G)(OTC)** apply qid prn to intact skin
> > *Gel:* 1% (100 gm)

Comment: *Diclofenac* is contraindicated with *aspirin* allergy. As with other NSAIDs, should be avoided in late pregnancy (≥30 weeks) because it may cause premature closure of the ductus arteriosus.

▷ *doxepin* (B) cream apply to affected area qid at intervals of at least 3-4 hours; max 8 days
   Pediatric: <12 years: not recommended; ≥12 years: same as adult
     Prudoxin *Crm:* 5% (45 gm)
     Zonalon *Crm:* 5% (30, 45 gm)

▷ *pimecrolimus* 1% cream (C)(G) <2 years: not recommended; ≥2 years: apply to affected area bid; do not apply an occlusive dressing
     Elidel *Crm:* 1% (30, 60, 100 gm)
   Comment: *Pimecrolimus* is indicated for short-term and intermittent long-term use. Discontinue use when resolution occurs. Contraindicated if the patient is immunosuppressed. Change to the 0.1% preparation or if secondary bacterial infection is present.

▷ *trolamine salicylate* apply tid-qid
   Pediatric: <2 years: not recommended; ≥2 years: same as adult
     Mobisyl Creme *Crm:* 10% (100 gm)

TOPICAL AND TRANSDERMAL ANESTHETICS

Comment: *Lidocaine* should not be applied to non-intact skin.

▷ *lidocaine* cream (B) apply to affected area bid prn
   Pediatric: <12 years: not recommended; ≥12 years: same as adult
     LidaMantle *Crm:* 3% (1, 2 oz)
     Lidoderm *Crm:* 3% (85 gm)
     ZTlido *lidocaine* topical system 1% (30/carton)
     Comment: Compared to **Lidoderm** (*lidocaine* patch 5%), which contains 700 mg/patch, **ZTlido** only requires 35 mg per topical system to achieve the same therapeutic dose.

▷ *lidocaine* lotion (B) apply to affected area bid prn
   Pediatric: <12 years: not recommended; ≥12 years: same as adult
     LidaMantle *Lotn:* 3% (177 ml)

▷ *lidocaine* 5% patch (B)(G) apply up to 3 patches at one time for up to 12 hours/24-hour period (12 hours on/12 hours off); patches may be cut into smaller sizes before removal of the release liner; do not re-use
   Pediatric: <12 years: not recommended; ≥12 years: same as adult
     Lidoderm *Patch:* 5% (10x14 cm; 30/carton)

▷ *lidocaine+dexamethasone* (B)
   Pediatric: <12 years: not recommended; ≥12 years: same as adult
     Decadron Phosphate with Xylocaine *Lotn:* dexa 4 mg+lido 10 mg per ml (5 ml)

▷ *lidocaine+hydrocortisone* (B)(G) apply to affected area bid prn
   Pediatric: <12 years: not recommended; ≥12 years: same as adult
     LidaMantle HC *Crm:* lido 3%+hydro 0.5% (1, 3 oz); *Lotn:* (177 ml)

▷ *lidocaine* 2.5%+*prilocaine* 2.5% apply sparingly to the burn bid-tid prn
   Pediatric: <12 years: not recommended; ≥12 years: same as adult
     Emla Cream (B) 5, 30 gm/tube

ANTICONVULSANTS

Gamma Aminobutyric Acid Analog

Comment: The gabapentinoids (*gabapentin* [**Gralise, Neurontin, Horizant**] and *pregabalin* [**Lyrica**]) have respiratory depression risk potential. Therefore, when co-prescribed with other CNS depressant agents, initiate the gabapentinoid at the lowest possible dose and monitor the patient for respiratory depression (especially elders and patients with compromised pulmonary function). Side effects include fatigue, somnolence/sedation, dizziness, vertigo, feeling drunk, headache, nausea, and dry mouth. To discontinue a gabapentinoid, withdraw gradually over 1 week or longer.

▷ *gabapentin* (C)
Pediatric: <3 years: not recommended; 3-12 years: initially 10-15 mg/kg/day in 3 divided doses; max 12 hours between doses; titrate over 3 days; 3-4 years: titrate to 40 mg/kg/day; 5-12 years: titrate to 25-35 mg/kg/day; max 50 mg/kg/day

Gralise initially 300 mg on Day 1; then 600 mg on Day 2; then 900 mg on Days 3-6; then 1200 mg on Days 7-10; then 1500 mg on Days 11-14; titrate up to 1800 mg on Day 15; take entire dose once daily with the evening meal; do not crush, split, or chew
Tab: 300, 600 mg

Neurontin (G) *Tab:* 600*, 800*mg; *Cap:* 100, 300, 400 mg; *Oral soln:* 250 mg/5 ml (480 ml) (strawberry-anise)

▷ *gabapentin enacarbil* (C) 600 mg once daily at about 5:00 PM; if dose is not taken at recommended time, next dose should be taken the following day; swallow whole; take with food; *CrCl 30-59 mL/min:* 600 mg on Day 1, Day 3, and every day thereafter; *CrCl <30 mL/min:* or on hemodialysis: not recommended
Pediatric: <12 years: not recommended; ≥12 years: same as adult

Horizant *Tab:* 300, 600 mg ext-rel

▷ *pregabalin (GABA analog)* (C)(G)(V)
Pediatric: <12 years: not recommended; ≥12 years: same as adult

Lyrica initially 50 mg tid; may titrate to 100 mg tid within 1 week; max 600 mg divided tid; discontinue over 1 week
Cap: 25, 50, 75, 100, 150, 200, 225, 300 mg; *Oral soln:* 20 mg/ml

Lyrica CR usual dose: 165 mg once daily; may increase to 330 mg/day within 1 week; max 660 mg/day
Tab: 82.5, 165, 330 mg ext-rel

TRICYCLIC ANTIDEPRESSANTS (TCAs)

Comment: Co-administration of TCAs with SSRIs requires extreme caution.

▷ *amitriptyline* (C)(G) titrate to achieve pain relief; max 300 mg/day
Pediatric: <12 years: not recommended; ≥12 years: same as adult
Tab: 10, 25, 50, 75, 100, 150 mg

▷ *amoxapine* (C) titrate to achieve pain relief; if total dose exceeds 300 mg/day, give in divided doses; max 400 mg/day
Pediatric: <12 years: not recommended; ≥12 years: same as adult
Tab: 25, 50, 100, 150 mg

▷ *desipramine* (C)(G) titrate to achieve pain relief; max 300 mg/day
Pediatric: <12 years: not recommended; ≥12 years: same as adult
Norpramin *Tab:* 10, 25, 50, 75, 100, 150 mg

▷ *doxepin* (C)(G) titrate to achieve pain relief; max 150 mg/day
Pediatric: <12 years: not recommended; ≥12 years: same as adult
Cap: 10, 25, 50, 75, 100, 150 mg; *Oral conc:* 10 mg/ml (4 oz w. dropper)

▷ *imipramine* (C)(G)
Pediatric: <12 years: not recommended; ≥12 years: same as adult
Tofranil titrate to achieve pain relief; max 200 mg/day; adolescents max 100 mg/day; if maintenance dose exceeds 75 mg/day, may switch to **Tofranil PM** at bedtime
Tab: 10, 25, 50 mg

Tofranil PM titrate to achieve pain relief; initially 75 mg at HS; max 200 mg at HS
Cap: 75, 100, 125, 150 mg

Tofranil Injection 50 mg IM; lower dose for adolescents; switch to oral form as soon as possible
Amp: 25 mg/2 ml (2 ml)

▷ *nortriptyline* (D)(G) titrate to achieve pain relief; initially 10-25 mg tid-qid; max 150 mg/day; lower doses for elderly and adolescents

> *Pediatric:* <12 years: not recommended; ≥12 years: same as adult
>> **Pamelor** titrate to achieve pain relief; max 150 mg/day
>>> *Cap:* 10, 25, 50, 75 mg; *Oral soln:* 10 mg/5 ml (16 oz)
> ▷ *protriptyline* (C) titrate to achieve pain relief; initially 5 mg tid; max 60 mg/day
> *Pediatric:* <12 years: not recommended; ≥12 years: same as adult
>> **Vivactil** *Tab:* 5, 10 mg
> ▷ *trimipramine* (C) titrate to achieve pain relief; max 200 mg/day
> *Pediatric:* <12 years: not recommended; ≥12 years: same as adult
>> **Surmontil** *Cap:* 25, 50, 100 mg

DIAPER RASH

Topical Corticosteroids *see* Appendix K: Topical Corticosteroids by Potency
Comment: Low to intermediate potency topical corticosteroids are indicated if inflammation is present.

BARRIER AGENTS

▷ *aloe+vitamin e+zinc oxide* ointment apply at each diaper change after thoroughly cleansing skin
  Balmex *Oint:* 2, 4 oz tube; 16 oz jar
▷ *vitamin a and e* (G) ointment apply at each diaper change after thoroughly cleansing skin
  A&D Ointment *Oint:* 1.5, 4 oz
▷ *zinc oxide* (G) cream and ointment apply at each diaper change after thoroughly cleansing the skin
  A&D Ointment with Zinc Oxide *Oint:* 10% (1.5, 4 oz)
  Desitin *Oint:* 40% (1, 2, 4, 9 oz)
  Desitin Cream *Crm:* 10% (2, 4 oz)

TOPICAL ANTIFUNGALS

Comment: Use if caused by *Candida albicans*.
▷ *butenafine* (B)(G) apply bid x 1 week or once daily x 4 weeks
  Pediatric: <12 years: not recommended; ≥12 years: same as adult
  Lotrimin Ultra (C)(OTC) *Crm:* 1% (12, 24 gm)
  Mentax *Crm:* 1% (15, 30 gm)
  Comment: *Butenafine* is a benzylamine, not an azole. Fungicidal activity continues for at least 5 weeks after last application.
▷ *clotrimazole* (B) apply to affected area bid x 7 days
  Pediatric: same as adult
  Lotrimin (OTC) *Crm:* 1% (15, 30, 45 gm)
  Lotrimin AF (OTC) *Crm:* 1% (12 gm); *Lotn:* 1% (10 ml); *Soln:* 1% (10 ml)
▷ *econazole* (C) apply bid x 7 days
  Spectazole *Crm:* 1% (15, 30, 85 gm)
▷ *ketoconazole* (C)(G)
  Nizoral Cream *Crm:* 2% (15, 30, 60 gm)
▷ *miconazole* 2% (C)(G) apply bid x 7 days
  Pediatric: same as adult
  Lotrimin AF Spray Liquid (OTC) *Spray liq:* 2% (113 gm) (alcohol 17%)
  Lotrimin AF Spray Powder (OTC) *Spray pwdr:* 2% (90 gm) (alcohol 10%)
  Monistat-Derm *Crm:* 2% (1, 3 oz); *Spray liq:* 2% (3.5 oz); *Spray pwdr:* 2% (3 oz)
▷ *nystatin* (C)(G) apply bid x 7 days
  Mycostatin *Crm:* 100,000 U/gm (15, 30 gm)

COMBINATION AGENT

▷ *clotrimazole+betamethasone* (C)(G) cream apply bid x 7 days
  Lotrisone *Crm:* 15, 45 gm

DIARRHEA: ACUTE

▷ *attapulgite* (C)

Donnagel (OTC) 30 ml after each loose stool; max 7 doses/day x 2 days
Pediatric: <3 years: not recommended; 3-6 years: 7.5 ml; >6-12 years: 15 ml; >12 years: same as adult
Liq: 600 mg/15 ml (120, 240 ml)

Donnagel Chewable Tab (OTC) 2 tabs after each loose stool; max 14 tabs/day
Pediatric: <3 years: not recommended; 3-6 years: 1/2 tab after each loose stool; max 7 doses/day; >6-12 years: 1 tab after each loose stool; max 7 tabs/day
Chew tab: 600 mg

Kaopectate (OTC) 30 ml after each loose stool; max 7 doses/day x 2 days
Pediatric: <3 years: not recommended; 3-6 years: 7.5 ml after each loose stool; >6-12 years: 15 ml after each loose stool; >12 years: same as adult
Liq: 600 mg/15 ml (120, 240 ml)

▷ *bismuth subsalicylate* (C; D in 3rd)(G)

Pepto-Bismol (OTC) 2 tabs or 30 ml q 30-60 minutes as needed; max 8 doses/day
Pediatric: <3 years (14-18 lb): 2.5 ml q 4 hours; max 6 doses/day; <3 years (18-28 lb): 5 ml q 4 hours; max 6 doses/day; 3-6 years: 1/3 tab or 5 ml q 30-60 minutes; max 8 doses/day; >6-9 years: 2/3 tab or 10 ml q 30-60 minutes; max 8 doses/day; >9-12 years: 1 tab or 15 ml q 30-60 minutes; max 8 doses/day
Chew tab: 262 mg; *Liq:* 262 mg/15 ml (4, 8, 12, 16 oz)

Pepto-Bismol Maximum Strength (OTC) 30 ml q 60 minutes; max 4 doses/day
Pediatric: <3 years: not recommended; 3-6 years: 5 ml q 60 minutes; max 4 doses/day; >6-9 years: 10 ml q 60 minutes; max 4 doses/day; >9-12 years: 15 ml q 60 minutes; max 4 doses/day
Liq: 525 mg/15 ml (4, 8, 12, 16 oz)

▷ *calcium polycarbophil* (C)

Pediatric: <6 years: not recommended; 6-12 years: 1 tab daily qid; >12 years: same as adult

Fibercon (OTC) 2 tabs daily qid
Cplt: 625 mg

▷ *crofelemer* (C) 2 tabs once daily; swallow whole with or without food; do not crush or chew

Pediatric: <12 years: not established; ≥12 years: same as adult

Mytesi *Tab:* 125 mg del-rel

Comment: *Crofelemer* is indicated for the symptomatic relief of non-infectious diarrhea in adult patients with HIV/AIDS on antiretroviral therapy.

▷ *difenoxin+atropine* (C)

Pediatric: <2 years: not recommended; ≥2 years: same as adult

Motofen 2 tabs, then 1 tab after each loose stool or 1 tab q 3-4 hours as needed; max 8 tab/day x 2 days
Tab: dif 1 mg+atro 0.025 mg

▷ *diphenoxylate+atropine* (C)(V)(G)

Pediatric: <2 years: not recommended; 2-12 years: initially 0.3-0.4 mg/kg/day in 4 divided doses; >12 years: same as adult

Lomotil 2 tabs or 10 ml qid until diarrhea is controlled
Tab: diphen 2.5 mg+atrop 0.025 mg; *Liq:* diphen 2.5 mg+atrop 0.025 mg per 5 ml (2 oz)

▷ *loperamide* (B)(OTC)(G)

Imodium 4 mg initially, then 2 mg after each loose stool; max 16 mg/day x 2 days
Pediatric: <5 years: not recommended; ≥5 years: same as adult
Cap: 2 mg

Imodium A-D 4 mg initially, then 2 mg after each loose stool; usual max 8 mg/day x 2 days
Pediatric: <2 years: not recommended; 2-5 years (24-47 lb): 1 mg up to tid x 2 days; 6-8 years (48-59 lb): 2 mg initially, then 1 mg after each loose stool; max 4 mg/day x 2 days; 9-11 years (60-95 lb): 2 mg initially, then 1 mg after each loose stool; max 6 mg/day x 2 days
Cplt: 2 mg; *Liq:* 1 mg/5 ml (2, 4 oz) (cherry-mint) (alcohol 0.5%)
▷ *loperamide+simethicone* (B)(OTC)(G)
Imodium Advanced 2 tabs chewed after loose stool, then 1 after the next loose stool; max 4 tabs/day
Pediatric: 6-8 years: chew 1 tab after loose stool, then chew 1/2 tab after next loose stool; 9-11 years: chew 1 tab after loose stool, then chew 1/2 tab after next loose stool; max 3 tabs/day; ≥12 years: same as adult
Chew tab: loper 2 mg+simeth 125 mg (vanilla-mint)

ORAL REHYDRATION AND ELECTROLYTE REPLACEMENT THERAPY
▷ *oral electrolyte replacement* (OTC)
CeraLyte 50 dissolve in 8 oz water
Pediatric: <4 years: not indicated; ≥4 years, same as adult
Pkt: sodium 50 mEq+potassium 20 mEq+chloride 40 mEq+citrate 30 mEq+rice syrup solids 40 gm+calories 190 per liter (mixed berry) (gluten-free)
CeraLyte 70 dissolved in 8 oz water
Pediatric: <4 years: not indicated; ≥4 years: same as adult
Pkt: sodium 70 mEq+potassium 20 mEq+chloride 60 mEq+citrate 30 mEq+rice syrup solids 40 gm+calories 165 per liter (natural, lemon) (gluten-free)
KaoLectrolyte 1 pkt dissolved in 8 oz water q 3-4 hours
Pediatric: <2 years: not indicated; ≥2 years: same as adult
Pkt: sodium 12 mEq+potassium 5 mEq+chloride 10 mEq+citrate 7 mEq+dextrose 5 gm+calories 22 per 6.2 gm
Pedialyte
Pediatric: <2 years: as desired and as tolerated; ≥2 years: 1-2 L/day
Oral soln: dextrose 20 gm+fructose 5 gm+sodium 25 mEq+potassium 20 mEq+chloride 35 mEq+citrate 30 mEq+calories 100 per liter (8 oz, 1 L)
Pedialyte Freezer Pops
Pediatric: as desired and as tolerated
Pops: dextrose 1.6 gm+sodium 2.8 mEq+potassium 1.25 mEq+chloride 2.2 mEq+citrate 1.88 mEq+calories 6.25 per 6.25 ml pop (8 oz, 1 L)

◯ DIARRHEA: CARCINOID SYNDROME (CSD)

TRIPTOPHAN HYDROXYLASE
▷ *telotristat* take with food; 250 mg tid
Pediatric: <18 years: not established; ≥18 years: same as adult
Xermelo *Tab:* 250 mg (4 x 7 daily dose pcks/carton)
Comment: Take **Xermelo,** in combination with somatostatin analog (SSA) therapy, to treat patients inadequately controlled by SSA therapy. Breastfeeding females should monitor the infant for constipation. ESRD requiring dialysis not studied.

◯ DIARRHEA: CHRONIC

▷ *cholestyramine* (C)
Questran Powder for Oral Suspension initially 1 pkt or scoop daily; usual maintenance 2-4 pkts or scoops daily in 2 doses; max 6 pkts or scoops daily

Oral pwdr: 9 gm pkts; 9 gm equal 4 gm anhydrous cholestyramine resin (60/pck); Bulk can: 378 gm w. scoop

Questran Light initially 1 pkt or scoop daily; usual maintenance 2-4 pkts or scoops daily in 2 doses

Light: 5 gm pkts; 5 gm equals 4 gm anhydrous cholestyramine resin (60/pck); Bulk can: 210 gm w. scoop

Comment: Use *cholestyramine* only if diarrhea is due to bile salt malabsorption.

▷ *crofelemer* (C) 2 tabs once daily; swallow whole with or without food; do not crush or chew

Pediatric: <12 years: not established; ≥12 years: same as adult

Mytesi Tab: 125 mg del-rel

Comment: *crofelemer* is indicated for the symptomatic relief of non-infectious diarrhea in adult patients with HIV/AIDS on antiretroviral therapy.

▷ *difenoxin+atropine* (C) 2 tabs, then 1 tab after each loose stool or 1 tab q 3-4 hours prn; max 8 tab/day x 2 days

Pediatric: <2 years: not recommended; ≥2 years: same as adult

Motofen Tab: dif 1 mg+atrop 0.025 mg

▷ *diphenoxylate+atropine* (B)(V)(G)

Pediatric: <2 years: not recommended; 2-12 years: initially 0.3-0.4 mg/kg/day in 4 divided doses; >12 years: same as adult

Lomotil 5-20 mg/day in divided doses

Tab: diphen 2.5 mg+atrop 0.025 mg; Liq: diphen 2.5 mg+atrop 0.025 mg per 5 ml (2 oz w. dropper)

▷ *attapulgite* (C)(G)

Donnagel (OTC) 30 ml after each loose stool; max 7 doses/day

Pediatric: <2 years: not recommended; 2-6 years: 7.5 ml after each loose stool; >6 years: same as adult

Liq: 600 mg/15 ml (120, 240 ml)

Donnagel Chewable Tab 2 tabs after each loose stool; max 14 tabs/day

Pediatric: <3 years: not recommended; 3-6 years: 1/2 tab after each stool; max 7 doses/day; >6-12 years: 1 tab after each loose stool; max 7 tabs/day; >12 years: same as adult

▷ *loperamide* (B)(OTC)(G)

Imodium (OTC) 4-16 mg/day in divided doses

Pediatric: <5 years: not recommended; ≥5 years: same as adult

Cap: 2 mg

Imodium A-D (OTC) 4-16 mg/day in divided doses

Pediatric: <2 years: not recommended; 2-5 years (24-47 lb): 1 mg up to tid x 2 days; 6-8 years (48-59 lb): 2 mg initially, then 1 mg after each loose stool; max 4 mg/day x 2 days; 9-11 years (60-95 lb): 2 mg initially, then 1 mg after each loose stool; max 6 mg/day x 2 days; ≥12 years: same as adult

Cplt: 2 mg; Liq: 1 mg/5 ml (2, 4 oz)

▷ *loperamide+simethicone* (B)(OTC)(G)

Imodium Advanced 2 tabs chewed after loose stool, then 1 after the next loose stool; max 4 tabs/day

Pediatric: 6-8 years: chew 1 tab after loose stool, then chew 1/2 tab after next loose stool; 9-11 years: chew 1 tab after loose stool, then chew 1/2 tab after next loose stool; max 3 tabs/day

Chew tab: loper 2 mg+simeth 125 mg

⊙ DIARRHEA: TRAVELER'S

Comment: Traveler's diarrhea is the most common travel-related illness, affecting an estimated 10-40% of travelers worldwide each year. Traveler's diarrhea is defined by having ≥3 unformed stools in 24 hours, in a person who is traveling. It is caused by a variety of pathogens, but most commonly bacteria found in food and water. The highest-risk destinations are in most of Asia as well as the Middle East, Africa, Mexico, and Central and South America.

ANTI-INFECTIVES

▷ *ciprofloxacin* (C) 500 mg bid x 3 days
  Pediatric: <18 years: not recommended; ≥18 years: same as adult
    Cipro (G) *Tab:* 250, 500, 750 mg; *Oral susp:* 250, 500 mg/5 ml (100 ml) (strawberry)
    Cipro XR *Tab:* 500, 1000 mg ext-rel
    ProQuin XR *Tab:* 500 mg ext-rel

▷ *rifamycin* (C) take 388 mg (2 x 194 mg tabs) bid x 3 days; may be taken with or without food; swallow whole; do not crush, break, or chew; contraindicated with concomitant alcohol; discontinue if diarrhea worsens or persists more than 24 hours; not for use if diarrhea is accompanied by fever or blood in the stool or if causative organism other than *E. coli* is suspected
  Pediatric: <18 years: not recommended; ≥18 years: same as adult
    Aemcolo *Tab:* 194 mg del-rel
    Comment: FDA-approved in November, 2018, **Aemcolo** *(rifamycin)* is an antibacterial drug indicated for the treatment of adult patients with traveler's diarrhea caused by noninvasive strains of *Escherichia coli* (*E. coli*), not complicated by fever or blood in the stool. **Aemcolo** is a broad-spectrum, semi-synthetic, orally administered, minimally absorbed antibiotic. Mechanism of action is inhibition of bacterial DAN-dependent RNA synthesis. **Aemcolo** has the potential to be used for the treatment of other bacterial infections of the colon, such as infectious colitis, *Clostridioides difficile*-associated disease, diverticulitis, and also as supportive treatment of inflammatory bowel diseases and hepatic encephalopathy. **Aemcolo** should not be used in patients with a known hyper-sensitivity to *rifamycin* or any of the other *rifamycin*-class antimicrobial agents (e.g., *rifaximin*). Most common adverse reactions (incidence > 2%) have been headache and constipation. There are no available data on **Aemcolo** use in pregnancy to inform any drug-associated risks for major birth defects, miscarriage, or adverse maternal or fetal outcomes. Systemic absorption of **Aemcolo** in humans is negligible; however, there is no information regarding the presence of **Aemcolo** in human milk, the effects on the breastfed infant.

▷ *rifaximin* (C) 200 mg tid x 3 days; discontinue if diarrhea worsens or persists more than 24 hours; not for use if diarrhea is accompanied by fever or blood in the stool or if causative organism other than *E. coli* is suspected
  Pediatric: <12 years: not recommended; ≥12 years: same as adult
    Xifaxan *Tab:* 200 mg

▷ *trimethoprim+sulfamethoxazole (TMP-SMX)* (C)(G) bid x 10 days
  Pediatric: <2 months: not recommended; ≥2 months: 40 mg/kg/day of *sulfamethoxazole* in 2 divided doses x 10 days; *see Appendix CC.33: trimethoprim+ sulfamethoxazole* (Bactrim Suspension, Septra Suspension) *for dose by weight*
    Bactrim, Septra 2 tabs bid x 10 days
      Tab: trim 80 mg+sulfa 400 mg*
    Bactrim DS, Septra DS 1 tab bid x 10 days
      Tab: trim 160 mg+sulfa 800 mg*
    Bactrim Pediatric Suspension, Septra Pediatric Suspension
      Oral susp: trim 40 mg+sulfa 200 mg per 5 ml (100 ml) (cherry) (alcohol 0.3%)

DIGITALIS TOXICITY

Comment: The digitalis therapeutic index is narrow, 0.8-1.2 ng/mL. Whether acute or chronic toxicity, the patient should be treated in the emergency department and/or admitted to in-patient service for continued monitoring and care. Signs and symptoms of digitalis toxicity include loss of appetite, nausea, vomiting, abdominal pain, diarrhea, visual disturbances (diplopia, blurred, or yellow vision, yellow-green halos around lights and other visual images, spots, blind spots), decreased urine output, generalized edema, orthopnea, confusion, delirium, decreased consciousness, potentially lethal cardiac arrhythmias (ranging from ventricular tachycardia (VT) and ventricular fibrillation (VF) to sino-atrial heart block AVB). Treatment measures include repeated doses of charcoal via NG tube administered after gastric lavage for acute ingestion (methods to induce vomiting are usually discouraged because vomiting can worsen bradyarrhythmias), digitalis binders. Monitoring includes serial ECGs, serum digitalis level, chemistries, potassium (hyperkalemia), magnesium (hypomagnesemia), BUN, and creatinine.

DIGOXIN BINDER

▷ *digoxin (immune fab [ovine]) (B)*
    Digibind contents of 1 vial of **Digibind** neutralizes 0.5 mg digoxin; dose based on amount of *digoxin* or *digitoxin* to be neutralized; see mfr pkg insert
    Pediatric: see mfr pkg insert
      Vial: 38 mg
    Digifab dose is based on amount of digoxin or digitoxin to be neutralized (see mfr pkg insert for dosage; contents of 1 vial neutralizes 0.5 mg digoxin.
    Pediatric: see mfr pkg insert
      Vial: 40 mg for IV injection after reconstitution (preservative-free)

DIPHTHERIA (*CORYNEBACTERIUM DIPHTHERIAE*)

Prophylaxis *see* **Childhood Immunizations**

POST-EXPOSURE PROPHYLAXIS FOR NON-IMMUNIZED PERSONS

▷ *erythromycin base (B)(G)* 500 mg qid x 14 days
    Pediatric: <45 kg: 50 mg/kg/day in 4 divided doses x 14 days; ≥45 kg: same as adult
    Ery-Tab *Tab:* 250, 333, 500 mg ent-coat
    PCE *Tab:* 333, 500 mg
▷ *erythromycin ethylsuccinate (B)(G)* 400 mg qid x 14 days
    Pediatric: 30-50 mg/kg/day in 4 divided doses x 14 days; may double dose with severe infection; max 100 mg/kg/day; *see Appendix CC.21: erythromycin ethylsuccinate* (E.E.S. Suspension, Ery-Ped Drops/Suspension) *for dose by weight*
    EryPed *Oral susp:* 200 mg/5 ml (100, 200 ml) (fruit); 400 mg/5 ml (60, 100, 200 ml) (banana); *Oral drops:* 200, 400 mg/5 ml (50 ml) (fruit); *Chew tab:* 200 mg wafer (fruit)
    E.E.S. *Oral susp:* 200, 400 mg/5 ml (100 ml) (fruit)
    E.E.S. Granules *Oral susp:* 200 mg/5 ml (100, 200 ml) (cherry)
    E.E.S. 400 Tablets *Tab:* 400 mg
▷ *Immunization Series*
    See **Childhood Immunizations**

POST-EXPOSURE PROPHYLAXIS FOR IMMUNIZED PERSONS

▷ *Diphtheria* immunization booster

DIVERTICULITIS

ANTI-INFECTIVES

▷ *amoxicillin* (B)(G) 500 mg q 8 hours or 875 mg q 12 hours x 7 days
    Amoxil *Cap:* 250, 500 mg; *Tab:* 875*mg; *Chew tab:* 125, 200, 250, 400 mg
    (cherry-banana-peppermint) (phenylalanine); *Oral susp:* 125, 250 mg/5 ml
    (80, 100, 150 ml) (strawberry); 200, 400 mg/5 ml (50, 75, 100 ml) (bubble
    gum); *Oral drops:* 50 mg/ml (30 ml) (bubble gum)
    Moxatag *Tab:* 775 mg ext-rel
    Trimox *Tab:* 125, 250 mg; *Cap:* 250, 500 mg; *Oral susp:* 125, 250 mg/5 ml (80,
    100, 150 ml) (raspberry-strawberry)
▷ *amoxicillin+clavulanate* (B)(G)
    Augmentin 500 mg tid or 875 mg bid x 7-10 days
    Pediatric: 40-45 mg/kg/day divided tid x 10 days or 90 mg/kg/day divided
    bid x 10 days *see* Appendix CC.4. *amoxicillin+clavulanate* (Augmentin
    Suspension) *for dose by weight*
        Tab: 250, 500, 875 mg; *Chew tab:* 125, 250 mg (lemon-lime); 200, 400 mg
        (cherry-banana) (phenylalanine); *Oral susp:* 125 mg/5 ml (banana), 250
        mg/5 ml (75, 100, 150 ml) (orange); 200, 400 mg/5 ml (50, 75, 100 ml)
        (orange) (phenylalanine)
    Augmentin ES-600 not recommended for adults
    Pediatric: <3 months: not recommended; ≥3 months, <40 kg: 90 mg/kg/day in
    2 divided doses x 7-10 days; ≥40 kg: not recommended
        Oral susp: 42.9 mg/5 ml (50, 75, 100, 125, 150, 200 ml) (strawberry cream)
        (phenylalanine)
    Augmentin XR 2 tabs q 12 hours x 7-10 days
    Pediatric: <16 years: use other forms; ≥16 years: same as adult
        Tab: 1000*mg ext-rel
▷ *ciprofloxacin* (C) 500 mg bid x 7 days
    Cipro (G) *Tab:* 250, 500, 750 mg; *Oral susp:* 250, 500 mg/5 ml (100 ml)
    (strawberry)
    Cipro XR *Tab:* 500, 1000 mg ext-rel
    ProQuin XR *Tab:* 500 mg ext-rel
▷ *metronidazole* (**not** for use in 1st; B in 2nd, 3rd)(G) 250-500 mg q 8 hours or 750
    mg q 12 hours x 7 days
    Flagyl *Tab:* 250*, 500*mg
    Flagyl 375 *Cap:* 375 mg
    Flagyl ER *Tab:* 750 mg ext-rel
▷ *trimethoprim+sulfamethoxazole* (*TMP-SMX*) (D)(G) bid x 7 days
    Bactrim, Septra 2 tabs bid x 7 days
        Tab: trim 80 mg+sulfa 400 mg*
    Bactrim DS, Septra DS 1 tab bid x 7 days
        Tab: trim 160 mg+sulfa 800 mg*
    Bactrim Pediatric Suspension, Septra Pediatric Suspension 20 ml bid x 7
    days
        Oral susp: trim 40 mg+sulfa 200 mg per 5 ml (100 ml) (cherry) (alcohol
        0.3%)

DIVERTICULOSIS

BULK-PRODUCING AGENTS
See Constipation

DRY EYE SYNDROME (KERATOCONJUNCTIVITIS SICCA)

▷ *lifitegrast* instill 1 drop in each eye twice daily q 12 hours; use 1 single-use container to dose both eyes and discard unused portion; contacts may be reinserted after 15 minutes

Pediatric: <17 years: not recommended; ≥17 years: same as adult

    Xiidra *Ophth soln* 5% (50 mg/ml) (foil pouch containing 5 low density polyethylene 0.2 mL single-use containers, 60 single-use containers/carton) (preservative-free)

Comment: The exact mechanism of action of *lifitegrast* in dry eye disease is <u>not</u> known. However, it is known that *lifitegrast* binds to the integrin lymphocyte function-associated antigen-1 (LFA-1), a cell surface protein found on leukocytes and blocks the interaction of LFA-1 with its cognate ligand intercellular adhesion molecule-1 (ICAM-1). ICAM-1 may be overexpressed in corneal and conjunctival tissues in dry eye disease. LFA-1/ICAM-1 interaction can contribute to the formation of an immunological synapse resulting in T-cell activation and migration to target tissues. *In vitro* studies demonstrated that lifitegrast may inhibit T-cell adhesion to ICAM-1 in a human T-cell line and may inhibit secretion of inflammatory cytokines in human peripheral blood mononuclear cells.

OPHTHALMIC IMMUNOMODULATOR/ANTI-INFLAMMATORY

Comment: Ophthalmic immunomodulators are contraindicated with active ocular infection. Allow at least 15 minutes between doses of artificial tears. May re-insert contact lenses 15 minutes after treatment.

▷ *cyclosporine* (C) using 1 single-use disposable vial, instill 1 drop in each eye twice daily q 12 hours

Pediatric: <16 years: not recommended; ≥16 years: same as adult

    Cequa *Ophth soln:* 0.09% single-use vials (0.25 ml, 6 pouches, 10 vials/pouch per carton) (preservative-free)

    Comment: **Cequa** ophthalmic solution is a calcineurin inhibitor immune-suppressant indicated to increase tear production in patients with kerato-conjunctivitis sicca. It is the first cyclosporine product to utilize nano-micellar technology, facilitating the drug molecule to penetrate the eye's aqueous layer, and preventing the release of active lipophilic molecule prior to penetration.

    Restasis *Ophth emul:* 0.05% (0.4 ml) (preservative-free)

OCULAR LUBRICANTS

Comment: Remove contact lens prior to using an ocular lubricant.

▷ *dextran 70+hypromellose* 1-2 drops prn

Pediatric: same as adult

    Bion Tears (OTC) *Ophth soln:* single-use containers (28/pck) (preservative-free)

▷ *hydroxypropyl cellulose* apply 1/2 inch ribbon <u>or</u> 1 insert in each inferior cul-de-sac 1-2 x/day prn

Pediatric: same as adult

    Lacrisert *Ophth inserts:* 5 mg (60/pck) (preservative-free)

    Hypotears Ophthalmic Ointment (OTC) *Ophth oint:* 1% (3.5 gm) (preservative-free)

Comment: Place insert in the inferior cul-de-sac of the eye, beneath the base of the tarsus, <u>not</u> in apposition to the cornea nor beneath the eyelid at the level of the tarsal plate.

➤ *hydroxypropyl methylcellulose* 1-2 drops prn
  Pediatric: same as adult
> **GenTeal Mild, GenTeal Moderate (OTC)** *Ophth soln:* (15 ml) (perborate)
> **GenTeal Severe (OTC)** *Ophth soln:* (15 ml) (carbopol 980, perborate)

➤ *petrolatum+mineral oil* apply 1/2 inch ribbon prn
  Pediatric: same as adult
> **Hypotears Ophthalmic Ointment (OTC)** *Ophth oint:* 1% (3.5 gm)
> (benzalkonium chloride, alcohol 1%)
> **Hypotears PF Ophthalmic Ointment (OTC)** *Ophth oint:* 1% (3.5 gm)
> (preservative-free, alcohol 1%)
> **Lacri-Lube (OTC)** *Ophth oint:* 1% (3.5, 7 gm)
> **Lacri-Lube NP (OTC)** *Ophth oint:* 1% (0.7 gm, 24/pck) (preservative-free)

➤ *petrolatum+lanolin+mineral oil* apply 1/4 inch ribbon prn
  Pediatric: same as adult
> **Duratears Naturale (OTC)** *Ophth oint:* 3.5 gm (preservative-free)

➤ *polyethylene glycol+glycerin+hydroxypropyl methylcellulose* 1-2 drops prn
  Pediatric: same as adult
> **Visine Tears (OTC)** *Ophth soln:* 1% (15, 30 ml)

➤ *polyethylene glycol* 400 0.4%+*propylene glycol* 0.3% 1-2 drops prn
  Pediatric: same as adult
> **Systane (OTC)** *Ophth soln:* (15, 30, 40 ml) (polyquaternium-1, zinc chloride);
> *Vial:* 0.01 oz (28) (preservative-free)
> **Systane Ultra (OTC)** *Ophth soln:* (10, 20 ml) (aminomethylpropanol,
> polyquaternium-1, sorbitol (zinc chloride); *Vial:* 0.01 oz (24)
> (preservative-free)

➤ *polyvinyl alcohol* 1-2 drops prn
  Pediatric: same as adult
> **Hypotears (OTC)** *Ophth soln:* 1% (15, 30 ml)
> **Hypotears PF (OTC)** 1-2 drops q 3-4 hours prn
>   *Ophth soln:* 1% (0.02 oz single-use containers, 30/pck) (preservative-free)

➤ *propylene glycol* 0.6% 1-2 drops prn
  Pediatric: same as adult
> **Systane Balance (OTC)** *Ophth soln:* (10 ml) (polyquaternium-1)

CORTICOSTEROID

➤ *loteprednol etabonate ophthalmic suspension 0.25%* shake for two to three
  seconds before using; instill 1-2 drops into each eye 4 x/day; max 2 weeks
  Pediatric: safety and efficacy not established
> **Eysuvis** *Ophth susp:* 2.5 mg/ml (8.3 ml) (benzalkonium chloride)
> **Comment:** **Eysuvis** a corticosteroid indicated for the short-term treatment
> of the signs and symptoms of dry eye disease. As with other ophthalmic
> corticosteroids, **Eysuvis** is contraindicated in most viral diseases of the cornea
> and conjunctiva including epithelial herpes simplex keratitis (dendritic
> keratitis), vaccinia, and varicella, and also mycobacterial infection of the eye
> and fungal diseases of ocular structures. The most common adverse reaction
> (incidence 5%) following the use of **Eysuvis** for two weeks has been instillation
> site pain. Potential complications of prolonged ophthalmic corticosteroid
> use include delayed healing, corneal perforation, intraocular pressure (IOP)
> increase, glaucoma with damage to the optic nerve, defects in visual acuity,
> and cataract formation.

◯ DUCHENNE MUSCULAR DYSTROPHY (DMD)

CORTICOSTEROID

➤ *deflazacort* (B) 0.9 mg/kg/day administered once daily; take with or without
  food; may crush and mix with applesauce (then take immediately)

Pediatric: <2 years: not established; ≥ 2 years: same as adult

Emflaza *Tab:* 6, 18, 30, 36 mg; *Oral susp:* 22.75 mg/ml (13 ml)

Comment: **Emflaza** is the first and only FDA-approved corticosteroid indicated for DMD to decrease inflammation and reduce the activity of the immune system. The side effects caused by **Emflaza** are similar to those experienced with other corticosteroids. The most common side effects include facial puffiness (cushingoid appearance), weight gain, increased appetite, upper respiratory tract infection, cough, extraordinary daytime urinary frequency (pollakiuria), hirsutism, and central obesity. Other side effects that are less common include problems with endocrine function increased susceptibility to infection, elevation in blood pressure, risk of gastrointestinal perforation, serious skin rashes, behavioral and mood changes, decrease in the density of the bones, and vision problems such as cataracts. Patients receiving immunosuppressive doses of corticosteroids should not be given live or live attenuated vaccines (LAVs). Moderate or strong CYP3A4 inhibitors, give one-third of the recommended dosage of **Emflaza**. Avoid use of moderate or strong CYP3A4 inducers with **Emflaza**, as they may reduce efficacy. Dosage must be decreased gradually if the drug has been administered for more than a few days. Use only the oral dispenser provided with the product. After withdrawing the appropriate dose into the oral dispenser, slowly add the oral suspension into 3-4 oz of juice or milk and mix well and then the dose should then be administered immediately. Do not administer with grapefruit. Discard any unused **Emflaza** oral suspension remaining after 1 month of first opening the bottle.

ANTISENSE OLIGONUCLEOTIDE

▷ *casimersen* administer 30 mg/kg once weekly as an intravenous (IV) infusion over 35 to 60 minutes via an in-line 0.2 micron filter

Pediatric: same as adult

Amondys 45 *Vial:* 100 mg/2 ml (50 mg/ml), single-dose, soln for dilution in 0.9% NS and IV infusion (preservative-free)

Comment: **Amondys 45** is indicated for patients who have genetic mutations that are amenable to skipping exon 45 of the Duchenne gene

▷ *eteplirsen* 30 mg/kg via IV infusion over 35-60 minutes once weekly

Pediatric: same as adult

Exondys 51 *Vial:* 100 mg/2 ml, 500 mg/10 ml (50 mg/ml), single-dose, for dilution and IV infusion

Comment: **Exondys** is indicated for patients who have a confirmed mutation of the dystrophin gene amenable to exon 51 skipping which affects about 13% of patients with DMD. There are no controlled data to inform safety in human pregnancy, lactation, or effects on the breastfed infant.

▷ *viltolarsen* 80 mg/kg via IV infusion over 60 minutes once weekly; obtain serum cystatin C, urine dipstick, and urine protein-to-creatinine ratio before starting; if the volume of **Viltepso** required is less than 100 ml, dilution in 0.9% NS is required

Viltepso *Vial:* 250 mg/5 ml (50 mg/ml), single-dose (preservative-free)

Comment: **Viltepso** is indicated for the treatment of DMD in patients who have a confirmed mutation of the DMD gene that is amenable to exon 53 skipping. This indication is approved under accelerated approval based on an increase in dystrophin production in skeletal muscle observed in patients treated with **Viltepso**. Continued approval for this indication may be contingent upon verification and description of clinical benefit in a confirmatory trial. Based on animal data, may cause kidney toxicity. Kidney function should be monitored; creatinine may not be a reliable measure of renal function in DMD patients. The most common adverse reactions (incidence ≥15%) have been URI, injection site reaction, cough, and pyrexia. There are no controlled data to inform safety in human pregnancy, lactation, or effects on the breastfed infant.

PHORDIAMIDATE MORPHOLINO OLIGIMER

▷ **golodirsen** 30 mg/kg via IV infusion over 35-60 minutee once weekly; measure GFR prior to initiating treatment

Vyondys 53 *Vial:* 100 mg/2 ml (50 mg/ml), single-dose, for reconstitution, dilution, and IV infusion

Comment: **Vyondys 53** *(golodirsen)* is a phosphordiamidate morpholino oligimer for the treatment of Duchenne muscular dystrophy (DMD) in patients with a confirmed mutation amenable to exon 53 skipping. This indication is approved under accelerated approval based on an increase dystrophin production in skeletal muscle observed in patients treated with **Vyondys 53**. Continued approval for this indication may be contingent upon verification of a clinical benefit in confirmatory trials. Renal function should be monitored. Creatinine may not be a reliable measure of renal function in DMD patients. Measure GFR prior to initiating treatment. The most common adverse reactions (incidence ≥20%) have been pyrexia, fall, abdominal pain, nausea, vomiting, and nasopharyngitis. There are no human or animal data available to assess the use of **Vyondys 53** during pregnancy, presence of *golodirsen* in human milk, or effects on the breastfed infant.

⬤ DUST MITE ALLERGY

ALLERGEN EXTRACT

▷ **dermatophagoides farinae+dermatophagoides pteronyssinus allergen extract** 1 tab SL daily; dissolves in 10 seconds; do not swallow for at least 1 minute; the *First Dose:* should be administered under the supervision of a physician with experience in the diagnosis and treatment of allergic diseases and the patient should be observed in the office for at least 30 minutes; prescribe auto-injectable epinephrine, instruct and train patients on its appropriate use, and instruct patients to seek immediate medical care upon its use

Pediatric: <18 years: not recommended; ≥18 years: same as adult

Odactra *SL tab:* 12 SQ-HDM

Comment: **Odactra** can cause life-threatening allergic reactions, such as anaphylaxis and severe laryngopharyngeal restriction. **Odactra** may not be suitable for patients with certain underlying medical conditions that may reduce their ability to survive a serious allergic reaction. **Odactra** may not be suitable for patients who may be unresponsive to epinephrine or inhaled bronchodilators, such as those taking beta-blockers. Contraindications to **Odactra** include severe, unstable, or uncontrolled asthma; history of any severe systemic allergic reaction or any severe local reaction to sublingual allergen immunotherapy history of eosinophilic esophagitis. The most common solicited adverse reactions reported in ≥10% of subjects treated with **Odactra** were throat irritation/tickle, itching in the mouth, itching in the ear, swelling of the uvula/back of the mouth, swelling of the lips, swelling of the tongue, nausea, tongue pain, throat swelling, tongue ulcer/sore on the tongue, stomach pain, mouth ulcer/sore in the mouth, and taste alteration/food tastes different. Available data on **Odactra** are insufficient to inform associated risks in pregnancy or effects on the breastfed infant.

DYSFUNCTIONAL UTERINE BLEEDING (DUB)

NSAIDs *see* Appendix J. NSAIDs online at https://connect.springerpub.com/content/reference-book/978-0-8261-7935-7/back-matter/part02/back-matter/bmatter10
Opioid Analgesics *see* **Pain**
Oral and Injectable Progesterone-only Contraceptives
Combined Oral Contraceptives

▷ *medroxyprogesterone acetate* **(X)** 10 mg daily x 10-13 days
    Provera *Tab*: 2.5, 5, 10 mg
▷ *combined oral contraceptive* **(X)** with 35 mcg estrogen equivalent

 DYSHIDROSIS (DYSHIDROTIC ECZEMA, POMPHYLOX)

Topical Corticosteroids *see* Appendix K: Topical Corticosteroids by Potency
Comment: Intermediate-to-high potency ophthalmic steroid treatment is indicated for dyshidrosis.

 DYSLIPIDEMIA (HYPERCHOLESTEROLEMIA, HYPERLIPIDEMIA, MIXED DYSLIPIDEMIA)

Comment: As recommended by the American Heart, Lung, and Blood Institute, children and adolescents should be screened for dyslipidemia once between 9 and 11 years and once between 17 and 21 years.

OMEGA 3-FATTY ACID ETHYL ESTERS
Comment: *Vascepa, Lovaza,* and *Epanova* are indicated for the treatment of TG ≥500 mg/dL.

▷ *icosapent ethyl (omega 3-fatty acid ethyl ester of EPA)* **(C)** 2 caps bid with food; max 4 gm/day; swallow whole, do not crush or chew
    Pediatric: <18 years: not recommended; ≥18 years: same as adult
      Vascepa *sgc*: 0.5, 1 gm (α-tocopherol 4 mg/cap)
▷ *omega 3-acid ethyl esters* **(C)(G)** 2 gm bid or 4 gm once daily; swallow whole, do not crush or chew
    Pediatric: <18 years: not recommended; ≥18 years: same as adult
      Lovaza *Soft gel cap*: 1 gm (α-tocopherol 4 mg/cap)
      Epanova *Gelcap*: 1 gm

MICROSOMAL TRIGLYCERIDE-TRANSFER PROTEIN (MTP) INHIBITOR
▷ *lomitapide mesylate* **(X)** 10 mg daily
    Pediatric: <12 years: not established; ≥12 years: same as adult
      Juxtapid *Cap*: 5, 10, 20 mg
      Comment: **Juxtapid** is an adjunct to low-fat diet and other lipid-lowering treatments, including LDL apheresis where available, to reduce LDL-C, total cholesterol, apoB, and non-HDL-C in patients with homozygous familial hypercholesterolemia (HoFH); not for patients with hypercholesterolemia who do not have HoFH.

OLIGONUCLEOTIDE INHIBITOR OF APO B-100 SYNTHESIS
▷ *mipomersen* **(B)** administer 200 mg SC once weekly, on the same day, in the upper arm, abdomen, or thigh; administer 1st injection under appropriate professional supervision
    Pediatric: <12 years: not established; ≥12 years: same as adult

Kynamro *Vial/Prefilled syringe:* 200 mg mg/ml soln for SC inj single-use vial (preservative-free)
Comment: **Kynamro** is an adjunct to low-fat diet and other lipid-lowering treatments, to reduce LDL-C, apo-B, total cholesterol (TC), non-HDL-C in patients with homozygous familial hypercholesterolemia (HoFH).

CHOLESTEROL ABSORPTION INHIBITOR

▷ *ezetimibe* (C)(G) 10 mg daily
   Pediatric: <10 years: not recommended; ≥10 years: same as adult
      Zetia *Tab:* 10 mg
      Comment: *Ezetimibe* is contraindicated with concomitant statins in liver disease, persistent elevations in serum transaminase, pregnancy, and nursing mothers. Concomitant fibrates are not recommended. **Zetia** is potentiated by *fenofibrate*, *gemfibrozil*, and possibly *cyclosporine*. Separate dosing of bile acid sequestrants is required; take *ezetimibe* at least 2 hours before or 4 hours after.

PROPROTEIN CONVERTASE SUBTILISIN KEXIN TYPE 9 (PCSK9) INHIBITOR

Comment: PCSK9 inhibitors are an adjunct to maximally tolerated statin therapy in persons who require additional lowering of LDL-C. There is currently no information regarding the use of PCSK9 inhibitors in pregnancy or the presence of PCSK9 inhibitors in human milk.

▷ *alirocumab* administer SC in the upper outer arm, abdomen, or thigh; initially 75 mg SC once every 2 weeks; measure LDL 4-8 weeks after initiation or titration; if inadequate response, may increase to 150 mg SC every 2 weeks or 300 mg SC once monthly
   Pediatric: <18 years: not established; ≥18 years: same as adult
      Praluent *Soln for SC inj:* 75, 150 mg/ml single-use prefilled syringe (preservative-free)
      Comment: The FDA has approved a new once-monthly 300 mg dosing option for **Praluent** injection, for the treatment of patients with high low-density lipoprotein (LDL) cholesterol. The drug is indicated as an adjunct to diet and other treatments for HoFH for patients with heterozygous familial hypercholesterolemia (HeFH) or clinical atherosclerotic cardiovascular disease (ASCVD) who require additional LDL lowering. The most common side effects of **Praluent** include injection site reactions, symptoms of the common cold, and flu-like symptoms. Each 150 mg pen delivers the dose over 20 seconds. A 300 mg once monthly dose = administration of 2 x 150 mg pens. **Praluent** is contraindicated in the 2nd and 3rd trimester of pregnancy.

▷ *evolocumab* administer SC in the upper outer arm, elbow, or thigh; measure LDL 4-8 weeks after initiation; *HeFH* or *primary hyperlipidemia:* 140 mg SC once every 2 weeks or 420 mg once monthly; *HoFH:* 420 mg once monthly
   Pediatric: HeFH, primary hyperlipidemia: not established; HoFH: <13 years: not established; ≥13 years: same as adult
      Repatha *Soln for SC inj:* single-use prefilled syringe; 140 mg/syringe; single-use prefilled SureClick autoinjector (140 mg/syringe preservative-free)
      Comment: To administer 420 mg of **Repatha**, administer 150 mg SC x 3 within 30 minutes. Although **Repatha**, does not have an assigned pregnancy category, it is contraindicated in pregnancy.

ADENOSINE TRIPHOSPHATE-CITRATE LYASE (ACL) INHIBITOR

▷ *bempedoic acid* take one tablet once daily, with or without food
   Pediatric: safety and efficacy not established
      Nexletol *Tab:* 180mg
      Comment: **Nexletol** (*bempedoic acid*) is a first-in-class, adenosine

triphosphate-citrate lyase (ACL) inhibitor for the treatment of adults with heterozygous familial hypercholesterolemia or established atherosclerotic cardiovascular disease who require additional lowering of LDL-Cholesterol. The most common (incidence ≥2%) adverse reactions have been upper respiratory tract infection, muscle spasms, hyperuricemia, back pain, abdominal pain or discomfort, bronchitis, pain in extremity, anemia, and elevated liver enzymes. Avoid concomitant use of **Nexletol** with *simvastatin* dose greater than 20 mg. Avoid concomitant use of **Nexletol** with *pravastatin* dose greater than 40 mg. Elevations in serum uric acid have occurred. Assess uric acid levels periodically as clinically indicated. Monitor for signs and symptoms of hyperuricemia, and initiate treatment with urate-lowering drugs as appropriate. Tendon rupture has occurred. Discontinue **Nexletol** at the first sign of tendon rupture. Avoid **Nexletol** in patients who have a history of tendon disorders or tendon rupture. Discontinue **Nexletol** when pregnancy is recognized unless the benefits of therapy outweigh the potential risks to the fetus. **Nexletol** decreases cholesterol synthesis and possibly the synthesis of other biologically active substances derived from cholesterol and may cause harm to the breastfed infant; therefore, breastfeeding is not recommended during treatment with **Nexletol**.

HMG-COA REDUCTASE INHIBITORS (STATINS)

Comment: The statins decrease total cholesterol, LDL-C, TG, and apo-B, and increase HDL-C. Before initiating and at 4-6 weeks, 3 months, and 6 months of therapy, check fasting lipid profile and LFTs. Side effects include myopathy and increased liver enzymes. Relative contraindications include concomitant use of cyclosporine, a macrolide antibiotic, various oral antifungal agents, and CYP-450 inhibitors. An absolute contraindication is active or chronic liver disease.

▷ *atorvastatin* (X)(G) initially 10 mg daily; usual range 10-80 mg/day
  Pediatric: <10 years: not recommended; ≥10 years (female post-menarche): same as adult
  Lipitor *Tab:* 10, 20, 40, 80 mg

▷ *fluvastatin* (X)(G) initially 20-40 mg q HS; usual range 20-80 mg/day
  Pediatric: <18 years: not recommended; ≥18 years: same as adult
  Lescol *Cap:* 20, 40 mg
  Lescol XL *Tab:* 80 mg ext-rel

▷ *lovastatin* (X)
  Mevacor initially 20 mg daily at evening meal; may increase at 4-week intervals; max 80 mg/day in single or divided doses; if concomitant fibrates, *niacin,* or *CrCl* <30 *mL/min,* usual max 20 mg/day
  Pediatric: <10 years: not recommended; 10-17 years: initially 10-20 mg daily at evening meal; may increase at 4-week intervals; max 40 mg daily
  Tab: 10, 20, 40 mg
  Altoprev initially 20 mg daily at evening meal; may increase at 4-week intervals; max 60 mg/day; if concomitant fibrates, or *niacin;* >1 gm/day, usual max 40 mg/day; if concomitant *cyclosporine, amiodarone,* or *verapamil,* or *CrCl* <30 *mL/min,* usual max 20 mg/day
  Pediatric: <20 years: not recommended
  Tab: 10, 20, 40, 60 mg ext-rel

▷ *pitavastatin* (X)(G) initially 2 mg q HS; may increase to 4 mg after 4 weeks; max 4 mg/day; if concomitant *erythromycin* or *CrCl* <60 *ml/min;* 1 mg/day with usual max 2 mg/day; if concomitant rifampin, max 2 mg once daily
  Pediatric: <12 years: not established; ≥12 years: same as adult
  Livalo *Tab:* 1, 2, 4 mg
  Nikita *Tab:* 1, 2, 4 mg
  Zypitamag *Tab:* 1, 2, 4 mg

▷ *pravastatin* (**X**) initially 10-20 mg q HS; usual range 10-40 mg/day; may start at 40 mg/day
  Pediatric: <8 years: not recommended; 8-13 years: 20 mg daily; 14-18 years: 40 mg daily
    Pravachol *Tab:* 10, 20, 40, 80 mg

▷ *rosuvastatin* (**X**)(**G**) initially 10-20 mg q HS; usual range 5-40 mg/day; adjust at 4-week intervals
  Pediatric: <10 years: not recommended; 10-17 years: 5-20 mg/day; max 20 mg/day
    Crestor *Tab:* 5, 10, 20, 40 mg

▷ *simvastatin* (**X**) initially 20 mg q PM; usual range 5-80 mg/day; adjust at 4-week intervals
  Pediatric: <10 years: not recommended; ≥10 years (female post-menarche): same as adult
    Zocor *Tab:* 5, 10, 20, 40, 80 mg

CHOLESTEROL ABSORPTION INHIBITOR+HMG-COA REDUCTASE INHIBITOR COMBINATIONS

▷ *ezetimibe+atorvastatin* (**X**)(**G**) Take once daily in the PM; may start at 10/40; swallow whole, do not cut, crush, or chew
  Pediatric: <17 years: not recommended; ≥17 years: same as adult
    Tab: **Liptruzet 10/10** ezet 10 mg+atorva 10 mg
      Liptruzet 10/20 ezet 10 mg+atorva 20 mg
      Liptruzet 10/40 ezet 10 mg+atorva 40 mg
      Liptruzet 10/80 ezet 10 mg+atorva 80 mg

▷ *ezetimibe+rosuvastatin* (**X**) take once daily in the PM; may start at 10/40; swallow whole, do not cut, crush, or chew
  Pediatric: safety and effectiveness not established
    Tab: **Roszet 5/10** rosuva 5 mg+ezet 10 mg
      Roszet 10/10 rosuva10 mg+ezet 10 mg
      Roszet 20/20 rosuva 20 mg+ezet 10 mg
      Roszet 40/40 rosuva 40 mg +ezet 10 mg

▷ *ezetimibe+simvastatin* (**X**)(**G**) Take once daily in the PM; may start at 10/40; swallow whole, do not cut, crush, or chew
  Pediatric: <17 years: not recommended; ≥17 years: same as adult
    Tab: **Vytorin 10/10** ezet 10 mg+simva 10 mg
      Vytorin 10/20 ezet 10 mg+simva 20 mg
      Vytorin 10/40 ezet 10 mg+simva 40 mg
      Vytorin 10/80 ezet 10 mg+simva 80 mg

Comment: These agents decrease total cholesterol, LDL-C, and TG; increase HDL-C. They are indicated when the primary problem is very high TG level. Side effects include epigastric discomfort, dyspepsia, abdominal pain, cholelithiasis, myopathy, and neutropenia. Before initiating, and at 4-6 weeks, 3 months, and 6 months of therapy, check fasting CBC, lipid profile, LFT, and serum creatinine. Absolute contraindications include severe renal disease and severe hepatic disease.

ISOBUTYRIC ACID DERIVATIVES

▷ *gemfibrozil* (**C**)(**G**) 600 mg bid 30 minutes before AM and PM meal
  Pediatric: <12 years: not recommended; ≥12 years: same as adult
    Lopid *Tab:* 600*mg

FIBRATES (FIBRIC ACID DERIVATIVES)

▷ *fenofibrate* (**C**)(**G**) take with meals; adjust at 4- to 8-week intervals; discontinue if inadequate response after 2 months; lowest dose or contraindicated with renal impairment and the elderly

Pediatric: <12 years: not recommended; ≥12 years: same as adult
> **Antara** 43-130 mg daily; max 130 mg/day
>> *Cap:* 43, 87, 130 mg
> **Fenoglide** 40-120 mg daily; max 120 mg/day
>> *Tab:* 40, 120 mg
> **FibriCor** 30-105 mg daily; max 105 mg/day
>> *Tab:* 30, 105 mg
> **TriCor** 48-145 mg daily; max 145 mg/day
>> *Tab:* 48, 145 mg
> **TriLipix** 45-135 mg daily; max 135 mg/day
>> *Cap:* 45, 135 mg del-rel
> **Lipofen** 50-150 mg daily; max 150 mg/day
>> *Cap:* 50, 150 mg
> **Lofibra** 67-200 mg daily; max 200 mg/day
>> *Tab:* 67, 134, 200 mg

NICOTINIC ACID DERIVATIVES

Comment: Nicotinic acid derivatives decrease total cholesterol, LDL-C, and TG; increase HDL-C. Before initiating and at 4-6 weeks, 3 months, and 6 months of therapy, check fasting lipid profile, LFT, glucose, and uric acid. Side effects include hyperglycemia, upper GI distress, hyperuricemia, hepatotoxicity, and significant transient skin flushing. Take with food and take *aspirin* 325 mg 30 minutes before *niacin* dose to decrease flushing. *Relative contraindications:* diabetes, hyperuricemia (gout), and PUD; Absolute contraindications severe gout and chronic liver disease.

▷ *niacin* (C)
> **Niaspan (G)** 375 mg daily for 1st week, then 500 mg daily for 2nd week, then 750 mg daily for 3rd week, then 1 gm daily for weeks 4-7; may increase by 500 mg q 4 weeks; usual range 1-2 gm/day; max 2 gm/day
> *Pediatric:* <21 years: not recommended; ≥21 years: same as adult
>> *Tab:* 500, 750, 1000 mg ext-rel
> **Slo-Niacin** one 250 or 500 mg tab q AM or HS or one-half 750 mg tab q AM or HS
> *Pediatric:* <12 years: not recommended; ≥12 years: same as adult
>> *Tab:* 250, 500, 750 mg cont-rel

BILE ACID SEQUESTRANTS

Comment: Bile acid sequestrants decrease total cholesterol and LDL-C, and increase HDL-C, but have no effect on triglycerides. A relative contraindication is TG ≥200 mg/dL and an absolute contraindication is TG ≥400 mg/dL. Before initiating and at 4-6 weeks, 3 months, and 6 months of therapy, check fasting lipid profile. Side effects include sandy taste in mouth, abdominal gas, abdominal cramping, and constipation. These agents decrease the absorption of many other drugs.

▷ *cholestyramine* (C)
> *Pediatric:* see mfr pkg insert
>> **Questran Powder for Oral Suspension** initially 1 pkt or scoop daily; usual maintenance 2-4 pkts or scoops daily in 2 divided doses; max 6 pkts or scoops daily
>>> *Pwdr:* 9 gm pkts; 9 gm equals 4 gm anhydrous *cholestyramine* resin for reconstitution (60/pck); *Bulk can:* 378 gm w. scoop
>> **Questran Light** initially 1 pkt or scoop daily; usual maintenance 2-4 pkts or scoops daily in 2 doses
>>> *Light:* 5 gm pkts; 5 gm equals 4 gm anhydrous *cholestyramine* resin (60/pck): *Bulk can:* 210 gm w. scoop

▷ *colesevelam* (B)(G)

WelChol recommended dose is 6 tablets once daily or 3 tablets twice daily; take with a meal and liquid

Pediatric: <10 years: not recommended; ≥10 years: same as adult

Tab: 625 mg

WelChol for Oral Suspension recommended dose is one 3.75 gm packet once daily or one 1.875 gm packet twice daily; empty one packet into a glass or cup; add 1/2 to 1 cup (4 to 8 oz) of water, or diet soft drink; stir well and drink immediately; do not swallow dry form; take with meals

Pediatric: <12 years: not established; ≥12 years: same as adult

Pwdr: 3.75 gm/pkt (30 pkt/carton), 1.875 gm/pkt (60 pkt/carton) for oral suspension

Comment: **WelChol** is indicated as adjunctive therapy to improve glycemic control in adults with type 2 diabetes. It can be added to *metformin*, sulfonylureas, or insulin alone or in combination with other antidiabetic agents

▷ *colestipol* (C)

Comment: *Colestipol* lowers LDL and total cholesterol.

Pediatric: <12 years: not recommended; ≥12 years: same as adult

Colestid tabs: 2-16 gm daily in a single or divided doses; granules: 5-30 gm daily in a single or divided dose

Tabs: 1 gm (120); *Granules:* unflavored: 5 gm pkt (30, 90/carton); unflavored bulk: 300, 500 gm w. scoop; orange-flavored: 7.5 gm pkt (60/carton) (aspartame); orange-flavored bulk: 450 gm w. scoop (aspartame) flavored: 7.5 gm pkt; flavored bulk: 450 gm w. scoop

Colestid Tab initially 2 gm bid; increase by 2 gm bid at 1-2-month intervals; usual maintenance 2-16 gm/day

Tab: 1 gm

ANTI-LIPID COMBINATIONS

Zeti Nicotinic Acid Derivative+HMG-CoA Reductase Inhibitors Combinations

Comment: Nicotinic acid derivatives decrease total cholesterol, LDL-C, and TG; increase HDL-C. Before initiating and at 4-6 weeks, 3 months, and 6 months of therapy, check fasting lipid profile, LFT, glucose, and uric acid. Side effects include hyperglycemia, upper GI distress, hyperuricemia, hepatotoxicity, and significant transient skin flushing. Take with food and take *aspirin* 325 mg 30 minutes before *niacin* dose to decrease flushing. Relative contraindications: diabetes, hyperuricemia (gout), and peptic ulcer disease (PUD). *Absolute contraindications:* severe gout and chronic liver disease.

▷ *niacin+lovastatin* (X)

Pediatric: <18 years: not recommended; ≥18 years: same as adult

Advicor swallow whole at bedtime with a low-fat snack; may pretreat with aspirin; start at lowest niacin dose; may titrate niacin by no more than 500 mg/day every 4 weeks; max 2000/40 daily

Tab: **Advicor 500/20** nia 500 mg ext-rel+lova 20 mg

Advicor 750/20 nia 750 mg ext-rel+lova 20 mg

Advicor 1000/20 nia 1000 mg ext-rel+lova 20 mg

Advicor 1000/40 nia 1000 mg ext-rel+lova 40 mg

▷ *niacin+simvastatin* (X)

Pediatric: <18 years: not recommended; ≥18 years: same as adult

Simcor swallow whole at bedtime with a low-fat snack; may pretreat with *aspirin*; to reduce niacin reaction. Start at lowest *niacin* dose; may titrate *niacin* by no more than 500 mg/day every 4 weeks; max 2000/40 daily; take *aspirin* 325 mg 30 minutes before dose to decrease niacin flushing

        Tab: **Simcor 500/20** nia 500 mg ext-rel+simva 20 mg
                Simcor 750/20 nia 750 mg ext-rel+simva 20 mg
                Simcor 1000/20 nia 1000 mg ext-rel+simva 20 mg
                Simcor 500/40 nia 500 mg ext-rel+simva 40 mg
                Simcor 1000/40 nia 1000 mg ext-rel+simva 40 mg

ANTIHYPERTENSIVE+ANTI-LIPID COMBINATIONS
Calcium Channel Blocker+HMG-CoA Reductase Inhibitor (Statin) Combinations
▷ *amlodipine+atorvastatin* (X)(G)
        Caduet select according to blood pressure and lipid values; titrate
        amlodipine over 7-14 days; titrate atorvastatin according to monitored lipid
        values; max amlodipine 10 mg/day and max atorvastatin 80 mg/day; refer to
        contraindications and precautions for CCB and statin therapy
        Pediatric: <10 years: not recommended; ≥10 years (female, post-menarche):
        same as adult
        Tab: **Caduet 5/10** amlo 5 mg+ator 10 mg
                Caduet 5/20 amlo 5 mg+ator 20 mg
                Caduet 5/40 amlo 5 mg+ator 40 mg
                Caduet 5/80 amlo 5 mg+ator 80 mg
                Caduet 10/10 amlo 10 mg+ator 10 mg
                Caduet 10/20 amlo 10 mg+ator 20 mg
                Caduet 10/40 amlo 10 mg+ator 40 mg
                Caduet 10/80 amlo 10 mg+ator 80 mg

DYSMENORRHEA: PRIMARY

NSAIDs *see* Appendix J. NSAIDs online at https://connect.springerpub.com/content/
reference-book/978-0-8261-7935-7/back-matter/part02/back-matter/bmatter10
Opioid Analgesics *see Pain*
Combined Oral Contraceptives *see* Appendix H. Contraceptives

BENZENEACETIC ACID DERIVATIVE
▷ *diclofenac* (C; D ≥30 wks) take on empty stomach; 35 mg tid;
        Hepatic impairment: use lowest dose
        Pediatric: <18 years: not recommended; ≥18 years: same as adult
                Zorvolex *Gelcap:* 18, 35 mg
▷ *diclofenac sodium* (C)
        Pediatric: <18 years: not recommended; ≥18 years: same as adult
                Voltaren 50 mg bid to qid or 75 mg bid or 25 mg qid with an additional 25 mg
                at HS if necessary
                        Tab: 25, 50, 75 mg ent-coat
                Voltaren XR 100 mg once daily; rarely, 100 mg bid may be used
                        Tab: 100 mg ext-rel
Comment: *Diclofenac* is contraindicated with *aspirin* allergy. As with other NSAIDs,
should be avoided in late pregnancy (≥30 weeks) because it may cause premature
closure of the ductus arteriosus.

FENAMATE
Comment: Avoid *aspirin* with a fenamate.
▷ *mefenamic acid* (C) 500 mg once; then 250 mg q 6 hours for up to 2-3 days; take with
food
        Pediatric: <14 years: not recommended; ≥14 years: same as adult
                Ponstel *Cap:* 250 mg

COX-2 INHIBITORS

Comment: Cox-2 inhibitors are contraindicated with history of asthma, urticaria, and allergic-type reactions to *aspirin*, other NSAIDs, and sulfonamides, 3rd trimester of pregnancy, and coronary artery bypass graft (CABG) surgery.

▷ *celecoxib* (C)(G) 400 mg x 1 dose; then 200 mg more on 1st day if needed; then 400 mg daily-bid; max 800 mg/day

  Pediatric: <18 years: not recommended; ≥18 years: same as adult

  Celebrex *Cap:* 50, 100, 200, 400 mg

▷ *meloxicam* (C)(G)

  Mobic <2 years, <60 kg: not recommended; ≥2, >60 kg: 0.125 mg/kg; max 7.5 mg once daily; ≥18 years: initially 7.5 mg once daily; max 15 mg once daily; *Hemodialysis:* max 7.5 mg/day

    Tab: 7.5, 15 mg; *Oral susp:* 7.5 mg/5 ml (100 ml) (raspberry)

  Vivlodex <18 years: not established; ≥18 years: initially 5 mg qd; may increase to max 10 mg/day; *Hemodialysis:* max 5 mg/day

    Cap: 5, 10 mg

▷ *meloxicam injection* administer 30 mg via IV bolus once daily; administer dose over 15 seconds; monitor analgesic response and administer a short-acting, non-NSAID, immediate-release analgesic if response is inadequate; patients must be well hydrated before **Anjeso** administration; use **Anjeso** for the shortest duration consistent with individual patient treatment goals

  Pediatric: safety and efficacy not established

  Anjeso *Vial:* 30 mg/ml (1 ml), single dose

  Comment: **Anjeso** *(meloxicam)* is an NSAID injection indicated for use in adults for the management of moderate-to-severe pain, alone or in combination with non-NSAID analgesics. Because of delayed onset of analgesia, **Anjeso** as monotherapy is not recommended for use when rapid onset of analgesia is required. The most common adverse reactions (incidence ≥2%) in controlled clinical trials have included constipation, GGT increase, and anemia. Use of NSAIDs during the third trimester of pregnancy increases the risk of premature closure of the fetal ductus arteriosus; therefore, avoid **Anjeso** use after 30 weeks gestation. There are no human data available on whether *meloxicam* is present in human milk, or on the effects on breastfed infants NSAIDs are associated with reversible infertility. Consider withdrawal of **Anjeso** in women who have difficulties conceiving. **Anjeso** may also compromise fertility in males of reproductive potential; it is not known if this effect on male fertility is reversible.

 DYSPAREUNIA (POST-MENOPAUSAL PAINFUL INTERCOURSE)

Oral and Transdermal Hormonal Therapy *see Menopause*

NON-HORMONAL THERAPY

▷ *prasterone (dehydroepiandrosterone [DHEA])* (X) insert 1 tab intravaginally daily at bedtime

  Intrarosa *Vaginal inserts:* 6.5 mg (20 tabs+28 applicators/carton)

  Comment: **Intrarosa** is the first local (intravaginal) non-estrogen drug approved for moderate-to-severe dyspareunia. **Prosterone** is an active endogenous steroid converted into active androgens and/or estrogens.

HORMONAL THERAPY

Comment: Estrogen-alone therapy should not be used for the prevention of cardiovascular Disease or dementia. The Women's Health Initiative (WHI) estrogen-alone sub-study reported increased risks of stroke and deep vein thrombosis (DVT). The WHI Memory Study (WHIMS) estrogen-alone ancillary study of WHI reported an increased risk of probable dementia in post-menopausal women 65 years-of-age and older. *Contraindications:* undiagnosed abnormal genital bleeding, known or suspected estrogen-dependent neoplasia (e.g., breast cancer), active DVT, pulmonary embolism (PE), or history of these conditions; active arterial thromoembolic disease (e.g., stroke, myocardial infarction [AMI]), or history of these conditions; known or suspected pregnancy; severe hepatic impairment (Child-Pugh Class C).

▷ *estradiol* (X)(G)

Imvexxy administer 1 vaginal insert once daily x 2 weeks; then 1 vaginal insert twice weekly x 2 weeks (e.g., Mon/Thu); consider the addition of a progestin with intact uterus

Vag inserts: 4, 10 mcg (8, 18/pck) applicator-free

Comment: Imvexxy is the only product in its class that is available in a 4 mcg and 10 mcg dose. The 4-mcg dose is currently the lowest approved dose of vaginal estradiol available. Imvexxy is a bio-identical vaginal estrogen product that offers a fraction of the estrogen contained in the average doses of other products on the market.

Yuvafem Vaginal Tablet insert one 10 mcg or 25 mcg vaginal tablet once daily x 2 weeks; then twice weekly x 2 weeks (e.g., Tues/Fri); consider the addition of a progestin with intact uterus

Vag tab: 10, 25 mcg (8, 18/blister pck with applicator)

ESTROGEN AGONIST-ANTAGONIST

▷ *ospemifene* take 1 tab daily

Osphena *Tab:* 60 mg

Comment: *Ospemifene* is an estrogen agonist-antagonist with tissue selective effects. In the endometrium, OSPHENA has estrogen agonistic effects. There is an increased risk of endometrial cancer in a woman with a uterus who uses unopposed estrogens. Adding a progestin to estrogen therapy reduces the risk of endometrial hyperplasia, which may be a precursor to endometrial cancer. Estrogen-alone therapy has an increased risk of stroke and deep vein thrombosis (DVT). **Osphena** 60 mg had cerebral thromboembolic and hemorrhagic stroke incidence rates of 0.72 and 1.45 per thousand women, respectively v. 1.04 and 0 per thousand women, respectively, in the placebo group. For DVT, the incidence rate for **Osphena** 60 mg is 1.45 per thousand women vs. 1.04 per thousand women in placebo. Do not use estrogen or estrogen agonist/antagonist concomitantly with **Osphena**. *Fluconazole* increases serum concentration of **Osphena**. *Rifampin* decreases serum concentration of **Osphena**.

EBOLA ZAIRE DISEASE (ZAIRE EBOLAVIRUS)

PROPHYLAXIS

Comment: There are six species of Ebolavirus (formerly known as Ebola hemorrhagic fever). *Zaire ebolavirus* is one of four *Ebolavirus* species that can cause a potentially fatal human disease. The most recent outbreaks of Ebola in West Africa (2014–2016) and Democratic Republic of the Congo (2018-2019) were caused by *Zaire ebolavirus*. Until recently, there were no approved vaccines or treatments for *Zaire ebolavirus* infection, with supportive care, and treatment for medical complications the only available options. The first Ebola vaccine was approved by the FDA December 19, 2019. **Ervebo** *(Ebola Zaire Vaccine, Live)* is used for the prevention of disease caused by *Zaire ebolavirus* in adults. **Ervebo** does not protect against other species of Ebolavirus. The first Ebola treatment, **Inmazeb** *(atoltivimab, maftivimab,* and *odesivimab-ebgn)* was approved by the FDA October 14, 2020 for the treatment *Zaire ebolavirus* in adults and children, including newborns of mothers who have tested positive for the virus. A second treatment, **Ebanga** *(ansuvimab-zykl),* was granted orphan drug designation and breakthrough therapy designation December 21, 2020.

▷ *ebola Zaire vaccine, live* administer 1 ml IM once as a single dose
  Pediatric: <18 years: not established; ≥18 years: same as adult
    Ervebo *Vial:* 1 ml, single-dose
    Comment: **Ervebo** *(ebola zaire vaccine, live)* is a vaccine indicated for the prevention of disease caused by *Zaire ebolavirus* in individuals ≥18 years-of-age. The duration of protection conferred by **Ervebo** is unknown. **Ervebo** does not protect against other species of *Ebolavirus* or *Marburgvirus*. Effectiveness of the vaccine when administered concurrently with antiviral medication, immune globulin (IG), and/or blood or plasma transfusions is unknown. Anaphylaxis has been observed following administration of **Ervebo**; appropriate medical treatment and supervision must be available. Vaccinated individuals should continue to adhere to infection control practices to prevent *Zaire ebolavirus* infection and transmission. Vaccine virus RNA has been detected in blood, saliva, urine, and fluid from skin vesicles of vaccinated adults; transmission of vaccine virus is a theoretical possibility. The most common injection-site adverse events have been injection-site pain (70%), swelling (17%), and redness (12%). The most common systemic adverse reactions have been headache (37%), feverishness (34%), muscle pain (33%), fatigue (19%), joint pain (18%), nausea (8%), arthritis (5%), rash (4%) and abnormal sweating (3%). There are no adequate and well-controlled studies of **Ervebo** in pregnancy, and human data available from clinical trials with **Ervebo** are insufficient to establish the presence or absence of vaccine-associated risk during pregnancy. The decision to vaccinate a woman who is pregnant should consider the woman's risk of exposure to *Zaire ebolavirus*. Human data are not available to assess the impact of **Ervebo** on presence in breast milk or effects on the breastfed infant. The developmental and health benefits of breastfeeding should be considered along with the mother's clinical need for **Ervebo** and any potential adverse effects on the breastfed infant from **Ervebo** or from the underlying maternal condition.

TREATMENT

▷ *atoltivimab+maftivimab+odesivimab* recommended dose of INMAZEB is 50 mg of *atoltivimab*, 50 mg of *maftivimab*, and 50 mg of *odesivimab* per kg diluted and administered as a single IV infusion; prior to administration, **Inmazeb** must be further diluted in an IV PVC infusion bag containing 0.9% NS or D5W or Lactated Ringer's; for neonates, **Inmazeb** should be diluted in D5W; total infusion volume is based on the patient's weight; see mfr pkg insert for full prescribing information, and information on preparation (mix by gentle inversion; do not shake), **Inmazeb** volume per kg of body weight (3 ml per kg), total infusion volume (ml) after dilution, and infusion time; the IV infusion must be prepared and administered under the supervision of a qualified healthcare provider
    Inmazeb *Vial:* atolti 241.7 mg + mafti 241.7 mg + odesi 241.7 mg per 14.5 ml (atolti 16.67 mg + mafti 16.67 mg + odesi 16.67 mg per ml), single-dose (preservative-free)
    Comment: **Inmazeb** *(atoltivimab+maftivimab+odesivimab)* is a monoclonal antibody combination indicated for the treatment of *Zaire ebolavirus* infection in adults and children, including newborns of mothers who have tested positive for the virus. Efficacy of **Inmazeb** has not been established for other species of the *Ebolavirus* and *Marburgvirus genera*. *Zaire ebolavirus* can change over time, and factors such as emergence of resistance, or changes in viral virulence, could

diminish the clinical benefit of antiviral drugs. Consider available information on drug susceptibility patterns for circulating *Zaire ebolavirus* strains when deciding whether to use **Inmazeb**. No vaccine interaction studies have been performed. **Inmazeb** may reduce efficacy of the live vaccine. The interval between live vaccination following initiation of **Inmazeb** therapy should be in accordance with current vaccination guidelines. The most common adverse events (incidence ≥20%) have been pyrexia, chills, tachycardia, tachypnea, and vomiting. Hypersensitivity reactions including infusion-associated events have been reported including acute, life-threatening reactions during and after the infusion. In the case of severe or life-threatening hypersensitivity reactions, discontinue the **Inmazeb** immediately and administer appropriate emergency care. Available data are insufficient to evaluate for a drug-associated risk of major birth defects, miscarriage, or adverse maternal/fetal outcome. Maternal, fetal and neonatal outcomes are poor among pregnant women infected with *Zaire ebolavirus* with the majority of pregnancies resulting in maternal death with miscarriage, stillbirth, or neonatal death. Treatment should not be withheld due to pregnancy. There are no data on the presence of *atoltivimab*, *maftivimab*, and *odesivimab-ebgn* in human or animal milk or effects on the breastfed infant. Females infected with *Zaire ebolavirus* should be instructed not to breastfeed due to the potential for *Zaire ebolavirus* transmission.

▷ *ansuvimab-zykl* 50 mg/kg reconstituted, further diluted, and administered as a single IV infusion over 60 minutes; see mfr pkg insert for further instructions on preparation, dilution, and administration

Pediatric: same as adult

    Ebanga *Vial:* 400 mg, single-dose, pwdr for reconstitution, dilution, and IV infusion

    Comment: **Ebanga** *(ansuvimab-zykl)* is a Zaire ebolavirus glycoprotein (EBOV GP)-directed human monoclonal antibody indicated for the treatment of infection caused by Zaire ebolavirus in adult and pediatric patients, including neonates born to a mother who is RT-PCR positive for Zaire ebolavirus infection. The efficacy of **Ebanga** has not been established for other species of the Ebolavirus and Marburgvirus genera. Zaire ebolavirus can change over time, and factors such as emergence of resistance or changes in viral virulence could diminish the clinical benefit of antiviral drugs. Consider available information on drug susceptibility patterns for circulating Zaire ebolavirus strains when deciding whether to use Ebanga. The most frequently reported adverse events (incidence ≥5%) after administration of **Ebanga** have been pyrexia, tachycardia, diarrhea, vomiting, hypotension, tachypnea, and chills. Hypersensitivity reactions including infusion-associated events have been reported with **Ebanga**. These may include acute, life threatening reactions during and after the infusion. Monitor patients and in the case of severe or life-threatening hypersensitivity reactions, discontinue the administration of **Ebanga** immediately and administer appropriate emergency care. No vaccine interaction studies have been performed. **Ebanga** may reduce the efficacy of the live vaccine. The interval between administration of **Ebanga** therapy and live vaccination should be in accordance with current vaccination guidelines. Maternal, fetal and neonatal outcomes are poor among pregnant women infected with Zaire ebolavirus. The majority of such pregnancies result in maternal death with miscarriage, stillbirth, or neonatal death. Treatment should not be withheld due to pregnancy. Monoclonal antibodies, such as Ebanga, are transported across the placenta; therefore, Ebanga has the potential to be transferred from the mother to the developing fetus. Females infected with Zaire ebolavirus should be instructed not to breastfed due to the potential for Zaire ebolavirus transmission.

EDEMA

THIAZIDE DIURETICS

▷ *chlorthalidone* (B)(G) initially 30-60 mg daily or 60 mg on alternate days; max 90-120 mg/day
   Thalitone *Tab:* 15 mg
▷ *chlorothiazide* (B)(G) 0.5-1 gm/day in a single or divided doses; max 2 gm/day
   Pediatric: <6 months: up to 15 mg/lb/day in 2 divided doses; ≥6 months: 10 mg/lb/day in 2 divided doses; max 375 mg/day
   Diuril *Tab:* 250*, 500*mg; *Oral susp:* 250 mg/5 ml (237 ml)
▷ *hydrochlorothiazide* (B)(G)
   Pediatric: <12 years: not recommended; ≥12 years: same as adult
      Esidrix 25-200 mg daily
         Tab: 25, 50, 100 mg
      Microzide 12.5 mg daily; usual max 50 mg/day
         Cap: 12.5 mg
▷ *hydroflumethiazide* (B) 50-200 mg/day in a single or 2 divided doses
   Pediatric: <12 years: not recommended; ≥12 years: same as adult
      Saluron *Tab:* 50 mg
▷ *methyclothiazide+deserpidine* (B) initially 2.5 mg daily; max 5 mg daily
   Pediatric: <12 years: not recommended; ≥12 years: same as adult
      Enduronyl *Tab:* methy 5 mg+deser 0.25 mg*
      Enduronyl Forte *Tab:* methy 5 mg+deser 0.5 mg*
▷ *polythiazide* (C) 1-4 mg daily
   Pediatric: <12 years: not recommended; ≥12 years: same as adult
      Renese *Tab:* 1, 2, 4 mg

POTASSIUM-SPARING DIURETICS

▷ *amiloride* (B)(G) initially 5 mg; may increase to 10 mg; max 20 mg
   Pediatric: <12 years: not recommended; ≥12 years: same as adult
      Tab: 5 mg
▷ *spironolactone* (D) initially 25-200 mg in a single or divided doses; titrate at 2-week intervals
   Pediatric: <12 years: not recommended; ≥12 years: same as adult
      Aldactone (G) *Tab:* 25, 50*, 100*mg
      CaroSpir *Oral susp:* 25 mg/5 ml (118, 473 ml) (banana)
▷ *triamterene* (B) 100 mg bid; max 300 mg
   Pediatric: <12 years: not recommended; ≥12 years: same as adult
      Dyrenium *Cap:* 50, 100 mg

LOOP DIURETICS

▷ *bumetanide* (C)(G) 0.5-2 mg daily; *Tab:* 5 mg; may repeat at 4-5 hour intervals; max 10 mg/day
   Pediatric: <18 years: not recommended; ≥18 years: same as adult
      Tab: 1*mg
   Comment: *Bumetanide* is contraindicated with sulfa drug allergy.
▷ *ethacrynic acid* (B)(G) initially 50-100 mg once daily-bid; max 400 mg/day
   Pediatric: Infants: not recommended; ≥1 month: initially 25 mg/day; then adjust dose in 25 mg increments
      Edecrin *Tab:* 25, 50 mg
▷ *ethacrynate sodium* for IV injection (B)(G) administer smallest dose required to produce gradual weight loss (about 1-2 lb per day); onset of diuresis usually occurs at 50-100 mg in children ≥12 years; after diuresis has been achieved, the minimally effective dose (usually 50-200 mg/day) may be administered on a continuous or intermittent dosage schedule; dose titrations are usually in

25-50 mg increments to avoid derangement electrolyte and water excretion; the patient should be weighed under standard conditions before and during administration of *ethacrynate sodium;* the following schedule may be helpful in determining the lowest effective dose: *Day 1:* 50 mg once daily after a meal; *Day 2:* 50 mg bid after meals, if necessary; *Day 3:* 100 mg in the morning and 50-100 mg following the afternoon or evening meal, depending upon response to the morning dose; a few patients may require initial and maintenance doses as high as 200 mg bid; these higher doses, which should be achieved gradually, are most often required in patients with severe, refractory edema

Pediatric: <1 month: not recommended; ≥1 month-12 years: use the smallest effective dose; initially 25 mg; then careful stepwise increments in dosage of 25 mg to achieve effective maintenance

    Sodium Edecrin *Vial:* 50 mg single-dose

Comment: *Ethacrynate sodium* in is more potent than more commonly used loop and thiazide diuretics. Treatment of the edema associated with congestive heart failure, cirrhosis of the liver, and renal disease, including the nephrotic syndrome, short-term management of ascites due to malignancy, idiopathic edema, and lymphedema, short-term management of hospitalized pediatric patients, other than infants, with congenital heart disease or the nephrotic syndrome. IV **Sodium Edecrin** is indicated when a rapid onset of diuresis is desired, e.g., in acute pulmonary edema or when gastrointestinal absorption is impaired or oral medication is not practical.

▷ *furosemide* (C)(G) initially 20-80 mg as a single dose
    Pediatric: <12 years: not recommended; ≥12 years: same as adult
      Lasix *Tab:* 20, 40*, 80 mg; *Oral soln:* 10 mg/ml (2, 4 oz w. dropper)
    Comment: *Furosemide* is contraindicated with sulfa drug allergy.

▷ *torsemide* (B) 5 mg daily; may increase to 10 mg daily
    Pediatric: <12 years: not recommended; ≥12 years: same as adult
      Demadex *Tab:* 5*, 10*, 20*, 100*mg

OTHER DIURETICS

▷ *indapamide* (B) initially 1.25 mg daily; may titrate every 4 weeks if needed; max 5 mg/day
    Pediatric: <12 years: not recommended; ≥12 years: same as adult
      Lozol *Tab:* 1.25, 2.5 mg
    Comment: *Indapamide* is contraindicated with sulfa drug allergy.

▷ *metolazone* (B)
    Pediatric: <12 years: not recommended; ≥12 years: same as adult
      Mykrox initially 0.5 mg q AM; max 1 mg/day
        Tab: 0.5 mg
      Zaroxolyn 2.5-5 mg once daily
        Tab: 2.5, 5, 10 mg
    Comment: *Metolazone* is contraindicated with sulfa drug allergy.

DIURETIC COMBINATIONS

▷ *amiloride+hydrochlorothiazide* (B)(G) initially 1 tab daily; may increase to 2 tabs/day in a single or divided doses
    Pediatric: <12 years: not recommended; ≥12 years: same as adult
      Moduretic *Tab:* amil 5 mg+hctz 50 mg*

▷ *spironolactone+hydrochlorothiazide* (D)(G) usual maintenance is 100 mg each of *spironolactone* and *hydrochlorothiazide* daily, in a single-dose or in divided doses; range 25-200 mg of each component daily depending on the response to the initial titration
    Pediatric: <12 years: not recommended; ≥12 years: same as adult

Aldactazide
Tab: **Aldactazide 25** spiro 25 mg+hctz 25 mg
  Aldactazide 50 *Tab:* spiro 50 mg+hctz 50 mg
▷ *triamterene+hydrochlorothiazide* (C)(G)
Pediatric: <12 years: not recommended; ≥12 years: same as adult
Dyazide 1-2 caps once daily
  Cap: triam 37.5 mg+hctz 25 mg
Maxzide 1 tab once daily
  Tab: triam 75 mg+hctz 50 mg*
Maxzide-25 1-2 tabs once daily
  Tab: triam 37.5 mg+hctz 25 mg*

 EMPHYSEMA

Inhaled Corticosteroids *see Asthma*
Parenteral Corticosteroids *see* Appendix M. Parenteral Corticosteroids
Oral Corticosteroids *see* Appendix L. Oral Corticosteroids
Inhaled Beta-2 Agonists (Bronchodilators) *see Asthma*
Oral Beta-2 Agonists (Bronchodilators) *see Asthma*

METHYLXANTHINES

see Asthma

LONG-ACTING INHALED BETA-2 AGONIST (LABA)

▷ *indacaterol* (C)
Arcapta Neohaler inhale contents of one 75 mcg cap once daily
  Neohaler Device/Cap: 75 mcg (5 blister cards, 6 caps/card)
Comment: Remove cap from blister cap immediately before use. For oral
inhalation with neohaler device <u>only</u>. **Arcapta Neohaler** is indicated for the
long-term maintenance treatment of bronchoconstriction in persons with
COPD. It is <u>not</u> indicated for treating asthma, for primary treatment of acute
symptoms, <u>or</u> for acute deterioration of COPD.
▷ *olodaterol* (C) 12 mcg q 12 hours
Striverdi Respimat *Inhal soln:* 2.5 mcg/cartridge (metered actuation) (40 gm,
60 metered actuations) (benzalkonium chloride)

CORTICOSTEROID+INHALED LONG-ACTING BETA-2 AGONIST (LABA)

▷ *fluticasone furoate/vilanterol* (C) 1 inhalation 100/25 <u>or</u> 200/25 once daily at the
same time each day
Breo Ellipta 100/25 *Inhal pwdr:* flu 100 mcg+vil 25 mcg dry pwdr per inhal
(30 doses)
Breo Ellipta 200/25 *Inhal pwdr:* flu 200 mcg+vil 25 mcg dry pwdr per inhal
(30 doses)
Comment: **Breo Ellipta** is contraindicated with severe hypersensitivity to milk
proteins.

INHALED ANTICHOLINERGICS (ANTIMUSCARINICS)

▷ *glycopyrrolate inhalation solution* (C) inhale the contents of 1 capsule twice daily
at the same time of day, AM and PM, using the **Neohaler**; do <u>not</u> swallow caps
Pediatric: not indicated
Seebri Neohaler *Inhal cap:* 15.6 mcg (60/blister pck) dry pwdr for inhalation
w. 1 **Neohaler** device (lactose)
▷ *ipratropium* (B)(G)
Atrovent 2 inhalations qid; max 12 inhalations/day
  Inhaler: 14 gm (200 inh)

Atrovent Inhaled Solution 500 mcg by nebulizer tid to qid
Inhal soln: 0.02%; 500 mcg (2.5 ml)

INHALED LONG-ACTING MUSCARINIC-ANTAGONISITS (LAMAs)

Comment: Inhaled LAMAs are indicated for prophylaxis and chronic treatment, only. Not for primary (rescue) treatment of acute attack. Avoid getting powder/ nebulizer solution in the eyes. Caution with narrow-angle glaucoma, BPH, bladder neck obstruction, and pregnancy. Contraindicated with allergy to atropine or its derivatives (e.g., *ipratropium*). Avoid other anticholinergic agents.

▷ *aclidinium bromide* (C) 1 inhalation twice daily using inhaler
 Tudorza Pressair *Inhal device:* 400 mcg/actuation (60 doses per inhalation device)

▷ *glycopyrrolate inhalation solution* (C) administer the contents of one vial twice daily at the same times of day, AM and PM, via the **Magnair** neb inhal device; do not swallow solution; do not use **Magnair** with any other medicine; length of treatment is 2-3 minutes; do not use 2 vials/treatment or more than 2 vials/day
 Pediatric: <18 years: not indicated
 Lonhala Magnair *Vial:* 25 mcg/ml (1 ml) unit dose for use with **Magnair** handset; *Starter Kit:* 60 unit-dose vials w. **Magnair** handset; *Refill Kit:* 60 unit-dose vials (low-density polyethylene [LDPE]) w. **Magnair** handset (preservative-free)
 Comment: **Lonhala Magnair** is the first nebulizing long-acting muscarinic antagonist (LAMA) approved for the treatment of COPD in the United States. Its approval was based on data from clinical trials in the Glycopyrrolate for Obstructive Lung Disease via Electronic Nebulizer (GOLDEN) program, including GOLDEN-3 and GOLDEN-4, 2 phase 3, 12-week, randomized, double-blind, placebo-controlled, parallel-group, multicenter study. Do not initiate **Lonhala Magnair** in acutely deteriorating COPD or to treat acute symptoms. If paradoxical bronchospasm occurs, discontinue **Lonhala Magnair** immediately and institute alternative therapy. Worsening of narrow-angle glaucoma may occur; use with caution in patients with narrow-angle glaucoma and instruct patients to contact a physician immediately if symptoms occur. Worsening of urinary retention may occur. Use with caution in patients with prostatic hyperplasia (BPH) or bladder neck obstruction (BNO) and instruct patients to seek medical care immediately if symptoms occur. Avoid administration with other anticholinergic drugs. Consider risk versus benefit in patients with severe renal impairment. Most common adverse reactions (incidence ≥ 2.0%) have been dyspnea and urinary tract infection. There are no adequate and well-controlled studies in pregnancy. **Lonhala Magnair** should only be used during pregnancy if the expected benefit to the patient outweighs the potential risk to the fetus. There are no data on the presence of *glycopyrrolate* or its metabolites in human milk or effects on the breastfed infant. The developmental and health benefits of breastfeeding should be considered along with the mother's clinical need for **Lonhala Magnair** and any potential adverse effects on the breastfed infant from **Lonhala Magnair** or from the underlying maternal condition.

▷ *revefenacin inhalation solution* administer the contents of one vial via nebulizer once daily at the same times of day; do not swallow solution; do not use more than 1 vial/day; do not use **Yupelri** with any other medicine
 Pediatric: not indicated
 Yupelri *Vial:* 175 mcg/3 ml (3 ml) unit-dose solution for nebulizer
 Comment: **Yupelri** is the first and only long-acting muscarinic antagonist (LAMA) solution for once daily nebulized administration. **Yupelri** is indicated for maintenance treatment of moderate-to-severe. Do not initiate **Yupelri**

in acutely deteriorating COPD or to treat acute symptoms. If paradoxical bronchospasm occurs, discontinue **Yupelri** immediately and institute alternative therapy. Worsening of narrow-angle glaucoma may occur; use with caution in patients with narrow-angle glaucoma and instruct patients to contact a healthcare provider immediately if symptoms occur. Use with caution in patients with prostatic hyperplasia or bladder-neck obstruction and instruct patients to contact a healthcare provider immediately if symptoms occur. May interact additively with other concomitantly used anticholinergic medications; avoid administration of **Yupelri** with other anticholinergic-containing drugs. Co-administration of **Yupelri** with OATP1B1 and OATP1B3 inhibitors (e.g., rifampicin, cyclosporine) may lead to an increase in exposure of the active metabolite; co-administration with **Yupelri** is not recommended. Avoid use of **Yupelri** in patients with hepatic impairment. Most common adverse reactions (incidence ≥2%) include cough, nasopharyngitis, upper respiratory tract infection, headache, and back pain. There are no adequate and well-controlled studies with **Yupelri** in pregnancy and no information regarding the presence of *revefenacin* in human milk or effects on the breastfed infant.

▷ *tiotropium (as bromide monohydrate)* **(C)** 2 inhalations once daily using inhalation device; do not swallow caps
  Spiriva HandiHaler *Inhal device:* 18 mcg/cap pwdr for inhalation (5, 30, 90 caps w. inhalation device)
  Spiriva Respimat *Inhal device:* 1.25, 2.5 mcg/actuation cartridge w. inhalation device (4 gm, 60 metered actuations) (benzylkonian chloride)
  Comment: *Tiotropium* is for prophylaxis and chronic treatment, only. Not for primary (rescue) treatment of acute attack. Avoid getting powder in eyes. Caution with narrow-angle glaucoma, BPH, bladder neck obstruction, and pregnancy. Contraindicated with allergy to *atropine* or its derivatives (e.g., *ipratropium*).

▷ *umeclidinium* **(C)** one inhalation once daily at the same time each day
  Incruse Ellipta *Inhal pwdr:* 62.5 mcg/inhalation (30 doses) (lactose)
  Comment: **Incruse Ellipta** is contraindicated with allergy to atropine or its derivatives.

INHALED BRONCHODILATOR+ANTICHOLINERGIC COMBINATION

▷ *ipratropium/albuterol* **(C)** 2 inhalations qid; max 12 inhalations/day
  Combivent MDI *Inhaler:* 14.7 gm (200 inh)

INHALED ANTICHOLINERGIC+LONG-ACTING BETA-2 AGONIST (LABA) COMBINATIONS

▷ *indacaterol+glycopyrrolate* **(C)**
  Utibron Neohaler inhale the contents of 1 capsule 2 x/day at the same times of day, AM and PM, using the neohaler; do not swallow caps
  Inhal cap: indac 27.5 mcg+glycop 15.6 mcg per cap (60/blister pck) dry pwdr for inhalation w. 1 Neohaler device (lactose)

▷ *ipratropium+albuterol* **(C)** 1 inhalation qid; max 6 inhalations/day
  Combivent Respimat *Inhal soln:* ipra 20 mcg+alb 100 mcg per inhal (4 gm, 120 inhal)
  Comment: When the labeled number of metered actuations (120) has been dispensed from the **Combivent Respimat** inhaler, the locking mechanism engages and no more actuations can be dispensed. **Combivent Respimat** is contraindicated with atropine allergy.

▷ *tiotropium+olodaterol* **(C)** 2 inhalations once daily at the same time each day; max 2 inhalations/day
  Stiolto Respimat *Inhal soln:* tio 2.5 mcg+olo 2.5 mcg per actuation (4 gm, 60 inh) (benzalkonium chloride)
  Comment: **Stiolto Respimat** is not for treating asthma, for relief of acute bronchospasm, or acutely deteriorating COPD.

▷ *umeclidinium+vilanterol* (C) 1 inhalation once daily at the same time each day
   Anoro Ellipta *Inhal soln:* ume 62.5 mcg+vila 25 mcg per inhal (30 doses)
   Comment: **Anoro Ellipta** is contraindicated with severe hypersensitivity to milk proteins.

INHALED CORTICOSTEROID+ANTICHOLINERGIC+ LONG-ACTING BETA AGONIST (LABA) COMBINATION

▷ *fluticasone furoate+umeclidinium+vilanterol* one inhalation once daily
   Trelegy Ellipta flutic furo 100 mcg+umec 62.5 mcg+vilan 25 mcg dry pwdr
   Comment: **Trelegy Ellipta** is maintenance therapy for patients with COPD, including chronic bronchitis and emphysema, who are receiving fixed-dose *furoate* and *vilanterol* for airflow obstruction and to reduce exacerbations, or receiving *umeclidinium* and a fixed-dose combination of *fluticasone furoate* and *vilanterol*. **Trelegy Ellipta** is the first FDA-approved once-daily single-dose inhaler that combines *fluticasone furoate*, a corticosteroid, *umeclidinium*, a long-acting muscarinic antagonist, and *vilantero*, a long-acting beta2-adrenergic agonist. Common adverse reactions reported with **Trelegy Ellipta** included headache, back pain, dysgeusia, diarrhea, cough, oropharyngeal pain, and gastroenteritis. **Trelegy Ellipta** has been found to increase the risk of pneumonia in patients with COPD, and increase the risk of asthma-related death in patients with asthma. **Trelegy Ellipta** is <u>not</u> indicated for the treatment of asthma <u>or</u> acute bronchospasm.

METHYLXANTHINES

see Asthma

METHYLXANTHINE+EXPECTORANT COMBINATION

▷ *dyphylline+guaifenesin* (C)
   Pediatric: <12 years: not recommended; ≥12 years: same as adult
   Lufyllin GG 1 tab qid
      Tab: dyph 200 mg+guaif 200 mg
   Lufyllin GG Elixir 30 ml qid
      Elix: dyph 100 mg+guaif 100 mg per 15 ml (16 oz)

OTHER METHYLXANTHINE COMBINATION

▷ *theophylline+potassium iodide+ephedrine+phenobarbital* (X)(II) 1 tab tid-qid prn;
   add an additional dose q HS as needed
   Pediatric: <6 years: not recommended; ≥6-12 years: 1/2 tab tid
   Quadrinal *Tab:* theo 130 mg+pot iod 320 mg+ephed 24 mg+phenol 24 mg

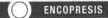 **ENCOPRESIS**

INITIAL BOWEL EVACUATION

▷ *mineral oil* (C) 1 oz x 1 day
   Comment: Mineral oil can inhibit absorption of the fat-soluble vitamins (A, D, E, and K).
▷ *bisacodyl* (B) 1 suppository daily prn
   Pediatric: <12 years: 1/2 suppository daily prn
   Dulcolax *Rectal supp:* 10 mg
▷ *glycerin* suppository (A) 1 adult suppository
   Pediatric: <6 years: 1 pediatric suppository; ≥6 years: same as adult

MAINTENANCE

▷ *mineral oil* (C) 5-15 ml once daily
   Comment: Mineral oil can inhibit absorption of the fat-soluble vitamins (A, D, E, and K).

⊙ ENDOMETRIOSIS

Acetaminophen for IV Infusion *see* **Pain**

NSAIDs *see* Appendix J. NSAIDs online at https://connect.springerpub.com/content/reference-book/978-0-8261-7935-7/back-matter/part02/back-matter/bmatter10

Opioid Analgesics *see* **Pain**

Other Contraceptives *see* Appendix H. Contraceptives

▹ *medroxyprogesterone* (X) 30 mg daily
   Provera *Tab:* 2.5, 5, 10 mg

▹ *medroxyprogesterone acetate* injectable (X) 100-400 mg IM monthly
   Depo-Provera Injectable: 300 mg/ml (2.5, 10 ml)

▹ *norethindrone acetate* (X) initially 5 mg daily x 2 weeks; then increase by 2.5 mg/day every 2 weeks up to 15 mg/day maintenance dose; then continue for 6 to 9 months unless breakthrough bleeding is intolerable
   Aygestin *Tab:* 5*mg

GONADOTROPIN-RELEASING HORMONE (GNRH) RECEPTOR ANTAGONIST

▹ *elagolix* *Normal to mildly impaired hepatic function:* 150 mg once daily for up to 24 months or 200 mg twice daily for up to 6 months; *Moderate hepatic impairment:* 150 mg once daily for up to 6 months
   Pediatric: <18 years: not recommended; ≥18 years: same as adult
      Orlissa *Tab:* 150, 200 mg
      Comment: **Orlissa** *(elagolix)* is an orally administered GnRH receptor antagonist for the managelation of moderate-to-severe pain associated with endometriosis. Contraindications are severe hepatic impairment, pregnancy, concomitant strong organic anion transporting polypeptide (OATP) 1B1 inhibitors, and osteoporosis. Assess BMD in women with additional risk factors for bone loss; dose- and duration-dependent decreases in bone mineral density (BMD) may occur that may not be completely reversible. Due to potential for reduced efficacy with estrogen-containing contraceptives, use non-hormonal contraception during treatment and for 1 week after discontinuing **Orlissa**. **Orlissa** may alter menstrual bleeding, which may reduce the ability to recognize pregnancy. Test if pregnancy is suspected and discontinue if pregnancy is confirmed. Dose-dependent elevations in serum alanine aminotransferase (ALT) may occur; counsel patients on signs and symptoms of liver injury. Counsel patients about potential for suicidal ideation and mood disorders and advise to seek medical attention for suicidal ideation, suicidal behavior, new onset or worsening depression, anxiety, or other mood changes. The most common adverse reactions (incidence >5%) in clinical trials included hot flashes and night sweats, headache, nausea, insomnia, amenorrhea, anxiety, arthralgia, depression-related adverse reactions, and mood changes.

Gonadotropin-Releasing Hormone Analogs (GnRHa)

Comment: These agonists can have unpleasant side effects (e.g., hot flashes, vaginal dryness, bone loss, changes in mood).

▹ *goserelin (GnRH analog)* implant (X) implant SC into upper abdominal wall; 1 SC implant q 28 days for up to 6 months; re-treatment not recommended
   Pediatric: <18 years: not recommended; ≥18 years: same as adult
      Zoladex SC implant in syringe: 3.6 mg

▹ *leuprolide acetate (GnRH analog)* (X)
   Pediatric: <18 years: not recommended; ≥18 years: same as adult
      Lupron Depot 3.75 mg 3.75 mg SC monthly for up to 6 months; may repeat one 6-month cycle
         Syringe: 3.75 mg (single-dose depo susp for SC injection)
      Lupron Depot-3 Month 22.5 mg SC q 3 months (84 days); max 2 injections
         Syringe: 22.5 mg (single-dose depo susp for IM injection)
   Comment: Do not split doses.

▷ *nafarelin acetate* (**X**) 1 spray (200 mcg) into one nostril q AM, then 1 spray (200 mcg) into the other nostril q PM x 6 months; if no response after 2 months, may increase to 2 sprays (400 mcg) bid
Pediatric: <18 years: not recommended; ≥18 years: same as adult
    Synarel *Nasal spray:* 2 mg/ml (10 ml)
Comment: Start *nafarelin acetate* (**Synarel**) on the 3rd or 4th day of the menstrual period or after a negative pregnancy test.

Synthetic Steroid Derived From Ethisterone

▷ *danazol* (**X**) start on 3rd or 4th day of menstrual period or after a negative pregnancy test; initially 400 mg bid; gradual downward titration of dosage may be considered dependent upon patient response; mild cases may respond to 100-200 mg bid
Pediatric: <18 years: not recommended; ≥18 years: same as adult
    Danocrine *Cap:* 50, 100, 200 mg
Comment: *Danazol* is a synthetic steroid derived from ethisterone. It suppresses the pituitary-ovarian axis. This suppression is probably a combination of depressed hypothalamic-pituitary response to lowered *estrogen* production, the alteration of sex steroid metabolism, and interaction of *danazol* with sex hormone receptors. The only other demonstrable hormonal effects are weak androgenic activity and depression of both follicle-stimulating hormone (FSH) and luteinizing hormone (LH) output. Recent evidence suggests a direct inhibitory effect at gonadal sites and a binding of **Danocrine** to receptors of gonadal steroids at target organs. In addition, **Danocrine** has been shown to significantly decrease IgG, IgM and IgA levels, as well as phospholipid and IgG isotope autoantibodies in patients with endometriosis and associated elevations of autoantibodies, suggesting this could be another mechanism by which it facilitates regression of endometrial lesions. **Danocrine** alters the normal and ectopic endometrial tissue so that it becomes inactive and atrophic. Complete resolution of endometrial lesions occurs in the majority of cases. Changes in the menstrual pattern may occur. Generally, the pituitary-suppressive action of **Danocrine** is reversible. Ovulation and cyclic bleeding usually return within 60 to 90 days when therapy with **Danocrine** is discontinued. **Danocrine** is also used to treat fibrocystic breast disease (reduces breast tissue nodularity and breast pain) and hereditary angioedema (to prevent attacks). Contraindications include pregnancy, breastfeeding, active or history of thromboembolic disease/event, porphyria, undiagnosed abnormal genital bleeding, androgen-dependent tumor, and markedly impaired hepatic, renal, or cardiac function.

ENURESIS: PRIMARY, NOCTURNAL

VASOPRESSIN

▷ *desmopressin acetate* (**B**)
    DDAVP usual dosage 0.2 mg before bedtime
    Pediatric: <6 years: not recommended; ≥6 years: same as adult
      Tab: 0.1*, 0.2*mg
    DDAVP Rhinal Tube 10 mcg or 0.1 ml of soln each nostril (20 mcg total dose) before bedtime
    Pediatric: <6 years: not recommended; ≥6 years: same as adult
      Nasal spray: 10 mcg/actuation (5 ml, 50 sprays); *Rhinal tube:* 0.1 mg/ml (2.5 ml)

TRICYCLIC ANTIDEPRESSANTS (TCAs)

Comment: Co-administration of SSRIs and TCAs requires extreme caution.
▷ *amitriptyline* (**C**)(**G**) initially 10 mg before bedtime; use lowest effective dose
Pediatric: <12 years: not recommended; ≥12 years: same as adult
    Tab: 10, 25, 50, 75, 100, 150 mg
Pediatric: <12 years: not recommended; ≥12 years: same as adult

▷ *amoxapine* (C) initially 25 mg before bedtime; use lowest effective dose
  Tab: 25, 50, 100, 150 mg
▷ *clomipramine* (C)(G) initially 25 mg before bedtime; use lowest effective dose
  Pediatric: <10 years: not recommended; ≥10 years: same as adult
    Anafranil *Cap:* 25, 50, 75 mg
▷ *desipramine* (C)(G) initially 25 mg before bedtime; use lowest effective dose
  Pediatric: <12 years: not recommended; ≥12 years: same as adult
    Norpramin *Tab:* 10, 25, 50, 75, 100, 150 mg
▷ *doxepin* (C)(G) initially 10 mg before bedtime; use lowest effective dose
  Pediatric: <12 years: not recommended; ≥12 years: same as adult
    Cap: 10, 25, 50, 75, 100, 150 mg; *Oral conc:* 10 mg/ml (4 oz w. dropper)
▷ *imipramine* (C)(G) initially 10 mg before bedtime; use lowest effective dose
  Pediatric: <12 years: not recommended; ≥12 years: same as adult
    Tofranil initially 10 at bedtime; use lowest effective dose; if bedtime dose
    exceeds 75 mg daily, may switch to **Tofranil PM**
      Tab: 10, 25, 50 mg
    Tofranil PM initially 75 mg before bedtime; use lowest effective dose
      Cap: 75, 100, 125, 150 mg
▷ *nortriptyline* (D)(G)
  Pediatric: <12 years: not recommended; ≥12 years: initially 10 mg before bedtime;
  use lowest effective dose
    Pamelor *Cap:* 10, 25, 50, 75 mg; *Oral soln:* 10 mg/5 ml (16 oz)
▷ *protriptyline* (C) initially 5 mg before bedtime; use lowest effective dose
  Pediatric: <12 years: not recommended; ≥12 years: same as adult
    Vivactil *Tab:* 5, 10 mg
▷ *trimipramine* (C) initially 25 mg before bedtime; use lowest effective dose
  Pediatric: <12 years: not recommended; ≥12 years: same ad adult
    Surmontil *Cap:* 25, 50, 100 mg

EOSINOPHILIC GRANULOMATOSIS WITH POLYANGITIS (FORMERLY CHURG-STRAUSS SYNDROME)

Comment: Eosinophilic granulomatosis with polyangiitis (EGPA) is a rare
autoimmune disease that causes vasculitis, an inflammation in the wall of blood
vessels of the body. EGPA is a characterized by asthma, high levels of eosinophils,
and inflammation of small- to medium-sized blood vessels affecting organ systems,
including the lungs, GI tract, skin, heart, and nervous system. **Nucala** *(mepolizumab)*
is the first FDA-approved therapy specifically to treat EGPA. This expanded indication
of **Nucala** meets a critical, and previously unmet need for EGPA patients. It's notable
that patients taking **Nucala** in clinical trials reported a significant improvement in
their symptoms. The FDA granted this application Priority Review and Orphan Drug
designation.

HUMANIZED INTERLEUKIN-5 ANTAGONIST MONOCLONAL ANTIBODY

▷ *mepolizumab* 100 mg SC once every 4 weeks in upper arm, abdomen, or thigh
  Pediatric: <12 years: not recommended; ≥12 years: same as adult
    Nucala *Vial:* 100 mg pwdr for reconstitution, single-use (preservative-free)
    Comment: **Nucala** is an add-on maintenance treatment for severe asthma.
    There is a pregnancy exposure registry that monitors pregnancy outcomes in
    women exposed to **Nucala** during pregnancy. Healthcare providers can enroll
    patients or encourage patients to enroll themselves by calling 1-877-311-8972
    or visiting www.mothertobaby.org/asthma.

EPICONDYLITIS

NSAIDs *see* Appendix J. NSAIDs online at https://connect.springerpub.com/content/reference-book/978-0-8261-7935-7/back-matter/part02/back-matter/bmatter10
Opioid Analgesics *see Pain*
Topical & Transdermal Analgesics *see Pain*
Parenteral Corticosteroids *see* Appendix M. Parenteral Corticosteroids
Oral Corticosteroids *see* Appendix L. Oral Corticosteroids
Topical Analgesic and Anesthetic Agents *see* Appendix I. Anesthetic Agents for Local Infiltration and Dermal/Mucosal Membrane Application online at https://connect.springerpub.com/content/reference-book/978-0-8261-7935-7/back-matter/part02/back-matter/bmatter9

 EPIDIDYMITIS

Comment: The following treatment regimens for epididymitis are published in the **2015 CDC Transmitted Diseases Treatment Guidelines**. Treatment regimens are presented by generic drug name first, followed by information about brands and dose forms. Empiric treatment requires concomitant treatment of chlamydia. Treat all sexual contacts. Patients who are HIV-positive should receive the same treatment as those who are HIV-negative.

RECOMMENDED REGIMEN
Regimen 1
▷ *ceftriaxone* (B)(G) 250 mg IM in a single dose
  plus
▷ *doxycycline* (D)(G) 100 mg bid x 10 days

RECOMMENDED REGIMENS: LIKELY CAUSED BY ENTERIC ORGANISMS
Regimen 1
▷ *levofloxacin* (C) 500 mg daily x 10 days

Regimen 2
▷ *ofloxacin* (C)(G) 300 mg bid x 10 day

DRUG BRANDS AND DOSE FORMS
▷ *ceftriaxone* (B)(G)
  Rocephin *Vial:* 250, 500 mg; 1, 2 gm
▷ *doxycycline* (D)(G)
  Acticlate *Tab:* 75, 150**mg
  Adoxa *Tab:* 50, 75, 100, 150 mg ent-coat
  Doryx *Tab:* 50, 75, 100, 150, 200 mg del-rel
  Doxteric *Tab:* 50 mg del-rel
  Monodox *Cap:* 50, 75, 100 mg
  Oracea *Cap:* 40 mg del-rel
  Vibramycin *Tab:* 100 mg; *Cap:* 50, 100 mg; *Syr:* 50 mg/5 ml (raspberry-apple) (sulfites); *Oral susp:* 25 mg/5 ml (raspberry)
  Vibra-Tab *Tab:* 100 mg film-coat
▷ *levofloxacin* (C)
  Levaquin *Tab:* 250, 500, 750 mg; *Oral soln:* 25 mg/ml (480 ml) (benzyl alcohol)
▷ *ofloxacin* (C)(G)
  Floxin *Tab:* 200, 300, 400 mg

ERECTILE DYSFUNCTION (ED)

Comment: Due to a degree of cardiac risk with sexual activity, consider cardiovascular status of patient before instituting therapeutic measures for erectile dysfunction.

PHOSPHODIESTERASE TYPE 5 (PDE5) INHIBITORS, CGMP-SPECIFIC

Comment: Oral PDE5 inhibitors (**Cialis**, **Levitra**, **Staxyn**, **Viagra**) are contraindicated in patients taking nitrates. Caution with history of recent MI, stroke, life-threatening arrhythmia, hypotension, hypertension, cardiac failure, unstable angina, retinitis pigmentosa, CYP3A4 inhibitors (e.g., *cimetidine*, the azoles, *erythromycin*, grapefruit juice), protease inhibitors (e.g., *ritonavir*), CYP3A4 inducers (e.g., *rifampin*, *carbamazepine*, *phenytoin*, *phenobarbital*), alcohol, antihypertensive agents. Side effects include headache, flushing, nasal congestion, rhinitis, dyspepsia, and diarrhea. Use with caution in patients with anatomical deformation of the penis (e.g., angulation, cavernosal fibrosis, or Peyronie's disease) or in patients who have conditions, which may predispose them to priapism (e.g., sickle cell anemia, multiple myeloma, or leukemia). In the event of an erection that persists longer than 4 hours, the patient should seek immediate medical assistance. If priapism (painful erection greater than 6 hours in duration) is not treated immediately, penile tissue damage and permanent loss of potency could result.

▷ *avanafil* (B) initially 100 mg taken 30 min prior to sexual activity; may decrease to 50 mg or increase to 200 mg based on response; max 1 administration/day
   Stendra *Tab:* 50, 100, 200 mg
▷ *sildenafil citrate* (B)(G) one dose about 1 hour (range 30 min to 4 hours) before sexual activity; usual initial dose 50 mg; may decrease to 25 mg or increase to max 100 mg/dose based on response; max one administration/day
   Viagra *Tab:* 25, 50, 100 mg
▷ *tadalafil* (B)(G) initially 10 mg prior to sexual activity up to once daily; may decrease to 5 mg or increase to 20 mg based on response; max one administration/day; effect may last 36 hours
   Cialis *Tab:* 2.5, 5, 10, 20 mg
▷ *vardenafil* (B) initially 10 mg taken 60 min prior to sexual activity; may decrease to 5 mg or increase to 20 mg based on response; max one administration/day
   Levitra *Tab:* 2.5, 5, 10, 20 mg film-coat
   Comment: **Levitra** is not interchangeable with **Staxyn**.
▷ *vardenafil (as HCl)* (B)(G) dissolve 1 tab on tongue 60 min prior to sexual activity, max once daily
   Staxyn *Tab:* 10 mg orally disintegrating (peppermint) (phenylalanine)
   Comment: **Staxyn** is not interchangeable with **Levitra**.
▷ *alprostadil* (X) *urethral suppository* initially 125 or 250 mcg inserted in the urethra after urination; adjust dose in stepwise manner on separate occasions; max two administrations/day
   Muse *Urethral supp:* 125, 250, 500, 1000 mcg
   Comment: Contraindicated with urethral stricture, balanitis, severe hypospadias and curvature, urethritis, predisposition to venous thrombosis, and hyperviscosity syndrome. Extreme caution with anticoagulant therapy (e.g., warfarin, heparin). Potential for hypotension and/or syncope.
▷ *alprostadil* (X) *injection* inject over 5-10 seconds into the dorsal lateral aspect of the proximal third of the penis; avoid visible veins; rotate injection sites and sides; if no initial response, may give next higher dose within 1 hour; if partial response, give next higher dose after 24 hours; max 60 mcg and 3 self-injections/week; allow at least 24 hours between doses; reduce dose if erection lasts >1 hour

Caverject *Vial:* 5, 10, 20, 40 mcg/vial (pwdr for reconstitution w. diluent)
Caverject Impulse *Cartridge:* 10, 20 mcg (2 cartridge starter and refill pcks)
Edex *Vial:* 5, 10, 20, 40 mcg (6/pck); *Syringe:* 5, 10, 20, 40 mcg (4/pck);
Cartridge: 10, 20, 40 mcg (2 cartridge starter and refill pcks)
Comment: Determine dose of injectable prostaglandins in the office.
Contraindicated with predisposition to priapism, penile angulation, cavernosal
fibrosis, Peyronies disease, penile implant. Extreme caution with anticoagulant
therapy (e.g., **warfarin, heparin**).

 ERYSIPELAS

Comment: Erysipelas is most commonly due to GABHS (Group A beta-hemolytic
Streptococcus).

TREATMENT OF CHOICE

▷ *penicillin v potassium* (B) 250-500 mg q 6 hours x 10 days
Pediatric: 25-50 mg/kg/day divided q 6 hours x 10 days; *see* Appendix CC.29.
penicillin v potassium (Pen-Vee K Solution, Veetids Solution) *for dose by weight*
Pen-Vee K *Tab:* 250, 500 mg; *Oral soln:* 125 mg/5 ml (100, 200 ml);
250 mg/5 ml (100, 150, 200 ml)

TREATMENT IF PENICILLIN ALLERGIC

▷ *erythromycin base* (B)(G) 250 mg q 6 hours x 10 days
Pediatric: 30-40 mg/kg/day divided q 6 hours x 10 days; >40 kg: same as adult
Ery-Tab *Tab:* 250, 333, 500 mg ent-coat
PCE *Tab:* 333, 500 mg
▷ *erythromycin ethylsuccinate* (B)(G) 400 mg qid x 7 days
Pediatric: 30-50 mg/kg/day in 4 divided doses x 7 days; may double dose
with severe infection; max 100 mg/kg/day; *see Appendix CC.21: erythromycin
ethylsuccinate* (E.E.S. Suspension, Ery-Ped Drops/Suspension) *for dose by weight*
EryPed *Oral susp:* 200 mg/5 ml (100, 200 ml) (fruit); 400 mg/5 ml (60, 100,
200 ml) (banana); *Oral drops:* 200, 400 mg/5 ml (50 ml) (fruit); *Chew tab:*
200 mg wafer (fruit)
E.E.S. *Oral susp:* 200, 400 mg/5 ml (100 ml) (fruit)
E.E.S. Granules *Oral susp:* 200 mg/5 ml (100, 200 ml) (cherry)
E.E.S. 400 Tablets *Tab:* 400 mg

○ **ERYTHROPOIETIC PROTOPORPHYRIA (EPP)**

SELECTIVE AGONIST OF THE MELANOCORTIN 1 RECEPTOR (MC1R)

▷ *afamelanotide* administer a single implant SC, 3-4 cm above the anterior
suprailiac crest, every 2 months using an SFM Implantation Cannula <u>or</u> other
implantation devices that have been determined by the manufacturer to be
suitable for implantation of Scenesse; should be administered by a qualified
healthcare professional who is proficient in the subcutaneous implantation
procedure and has completed training prior to administration; monitor the
patient for 30 minutes following implant administration
Pediatric: safety and efficacy not established
Scenesse *Sub Cu implant:* 16 mg (<u>not</u> supplied with an implant device)
Comment: Scenesse *(afamelanotide)* is a selective agonist of the melanocortin
1 receptor (MC1R) for the prevention of phototoxicity in adult patients with
erythropoietic protoporphyria (EPP). Maintain sun and light protection
measures during treatment with **Scenesse** to prevent phototoxic reactions
related to EPP. The most common adverse reactions (incidence >2%) have
been implant site reaction, nausea, oropharyngeal pain, cough, fatigue,

dizziness, skin hyperpigmentation, somnolence, melanocytic nevus, respiratory tract infection, non-acute porphyria, and skin irritation. **Scenesse** may induce darkening of preexisting nevi and ephelides due to its pharmacological effect. A regular full body skin examination is recommended twice yearly to monitor all nevi and other skin abnormalities. There are no data on **Scenesse** use in pregnancy to evaluate for any drug-associated risk of major birth defects, miscarriage, or adverse maternal or embryo/fetal outcomes. There are no data on the presence of *afamelanotide* or any of its metabolites in human or animal milk or effects on the breastfed infant.

ESOPHAGITIS, EROSIVE

Antacids *see GERD*
H2 Antagonists *see GERD*
Proton Pump Inhibitors *see GERD*
▷ *sucralfate* (B)(G) *Active ulcer:* 1 gm qid; *Maintenance:* 1 gm bid
  Carafate *Tab:* 1*g; *Oral susp:* 1 gm/10 ml (14 oz)

EXOCRINE PANCREAS INSUFFICIENCY (EPI)/ PANCREATIC ENZYME DEFICIENCY

Comment: Seen in chronic pancreatitis, post-pancreatectomy, cystic fibrosis, post-GI tract bypass surgery (Whipple procedure), and ductal obstruction from neoplasia. May sprinkle cap; however, do not crush or chew cap or tab. May mix with applesauce or other acidic food; follow with water or juice. Do not let any drug remain in mouth. Take dose with (not before or after) each meal and snack (half dose with snacks). Base dose on lipase units; adjust per diet and clinical response (i.e., steatorrhea). Pancrelipase products are interchangeable. Contraindicated with pork protein hypersensitivity.

PANCRELIPASE PRODUCTS

▷ *pancreatic enzymes* (C)
  Creon 500 units/kg per meal; max 2,500 units/kg per meal or <10,000 units/kg per day or <4,000 units/gm fat ingested per day
  Pediatric: <12 months: 2,000-4,000 units per 120 ml formula or per breastfeeding (do not mix directly into formula or breast milk; 12 months to 4 years: 1,000 units/kg per meal; max 2,500 units/kg per meal <10,000 units/kg per day; >4 years: same as adult
    Cap: **Creon 3000** lip 3,000 units+pro 9,500 units+amyl 15,000 units del-rel
      Creon 6000 lip 6,000 units+pro 19,000 units+amyl 30,000 units del-rel
      Creon 12000 lip 12,000 units+pro 38,000 units+amyl 60,000 units del-rel
      Creon 24000 lip 24,000 units+pro 76,000 units+amyl 120,000 units del-rel
      Creon 36000 lip 36,000 units+pro 114,000 units+amyl 180,000 units del-rel
  Cotazym 1-3 tabs just prior to each meal or snack
  Pediatric: <12 years: not recommended; ≥12 years: same as adult
    Tab: **Cotazym** lip 1,000 units+pro 12,500 units+amyl 12,500 units del-rel
      Cotazym-S lip 5,000 units+pro 20,000 units+amyl 20,000 units del-rel
  Donnazyme 1-3 caps just prior to each meal or snack
  Pediatric: <12 years: not recommended; ≥12 years: same as adult
    Cap: **Donnazyme** lip 5,000 units+pro 20,000 units+amyl 20,000 units del-rel
  Ku-Zyme 1-2 caps just prior to each meal or snack

Pediatric: <12 years: not recommended; ≥12 years: same as adult

    Cap: **Ku-Zyme:** lip 12,000 units+pro 15,000 units+amyl 15,000 units del-rel

Kutrase 1-2 caps just prior to each meal or snack

Pediatric: <12 years: not recommended; ≥12 years: same as adult

    Cap: **Kutrase:** lip 12,000 units+pro 30,000 units+amyl 30,000 units del-rel

Pancreaze 2,500 lipase units/kg per meal or <10,000 lipase units/kg per day or <4,000 lipase units/gm fat ingested per day

Pediatric: <12 months: 2,000-4,000 lipase units per 120 ml formula or per breastfeeding; >12 months to <4 years 1,000 lipase units/kg per meal; ≥4 years: 500 lipase units/kg per meal; max: adult dose

    Cap: **Pancreaze 4200** lip 4,200 units+pro 10,000 units+amyl 17,500 units ec-microtabs

    Pancreaze 10500 lip 10,500 units+pro 25,000 units+amyl 43,750 units ec-microtabs

    Pancreaze 16800 lip 16,800 units+pro 40,000 units+amyl 70,000 units ec-microtabs

    Pancreaze 21000 lip 21,000 units+pro 37,000 units+amyl 61,000 units ec-microtabs

Pertyze *12 months to 4 years and ≥8 kg:* initially 1,000 lipase units/kg per meal; *≥4 years and ≥16 kg:* initially 500 lipase units/kg per meal; *Both:* 2,500 lipase units/kg per meal or <10,000 units/kg per day or <4,000 lipase units/gm fat ingested per day

    Cap: **Pertyze 8000** lip 8,000 units+pro 28,750 units+amyl 30,250 units del-rel

    Pertyze 16000 lip 16,000 units+pro 57,500 units+amyl 65,000 units del-rel

Ultrase 1-3 tabs just prior to each meal or snack

Pediatric: same as adult

    Cap: **Ultrase** lip 4,500 units+pro 20,000 units+amyl 25,000 units del-rel

    Ultrase MT lip 12,000 units+pro 39,000 units+amyl 39,000 units del-rel

    Ultrase MT 18 lip 18,000 units+pro 58,500 units+amyl 58,500 units del-rel

    Ultrase MT 20 lip 20,000 units+pro 65,000 units+amyl 65,000 units del-rel

Viokace initially 500 lip units/kg per meal; max 2,500 lipase units/kg per meal, or <10,000 lipase units/kg per meal, or <4000 units/gm fat ingested per day

Pediatric: same as adult

    Tab: **Viokace 8000** lip 8,000 units+pro 30,000 units+amyl 30,000 units

    Viokace 16000 lip 16,000 units+pro 60,000 units amyl 60,000 units

    Viokace 10440 lip 10,440 units+pro 39,150 units amyl 39,150 units

    Viokace 20880 lip 20,880 units+pro 78,300 units amyl 78,300 units

Comment: **Viokace 10440** and **Viokase 20880** should be taken with a daily proton pump inhibitor.

Viokace Powder 1/4 tsp (0.7 gm) with meals

Viokace Powder lip 16,800 units+pro 70,000 units+amyl 70,000 units per 1/4 tsp (8 oz)

Zenpep initially 500 lipase units/kg per meal; max 2,500 lipase units/kg per meal or <10,000 lipase units/kg per day or <4,000 units/gm fat ingested per day

Pediatric: Infants-12 months: infants may be given 3,000 lipase units (one capsule) per 120 ml of formula or per breastfeeding; do **not** mix capsule contents directly into formula or breast milk prior to administration; *Children >12 months to <4 Years:* enzyme dosing should begin with 1,000 lipase units/kg of body weight per meal to a maximum of 2,500 lipase units/kg of body weight per meal (or ≤10,000 lipase units/kg/day), or <4,000 lipase units/gm fat ingested per day; *Children >4 Years:* same as adult

Cap: **Zenpep 3000** lip 3000 units+pro 10,000 units+amyl 14,000 units del-rel

Zenpep 5000 lip 5000 units+pro 17,000 units+amyl 24,000 units del-rel

Zenpep 10000 lip 10,000 units+pro 32,000 units+amyl 42,000 units del-rel

Zenpep 15000 lip 15,000 units+pro 47,000 units+amyl 63,000 units del-rel

Zenpep 20000 lip 20,000 units+pro 63,000 units+amyl 84,000 units del-rel

Zenpep 25000 lip 25,000 units+pro 79,000 units+amyl 105,000 units del-rel

Zenpep 40000 lip 40,000 units+pro 126,000 units+amyl 168,000 units del-rel

Comment: **Zenpep** is <u>not</u> interchangeable with any other pancrelipase product. Dosing should <u>not</u> exceed the recommended maximum dosage set forth by the Cystic Fibrosis Foundation Consensus Conferences Guidelines. **Zenpep** should be swallowed whole. For infants <u>or</u> patients unable to swallow intact capsules, the contents may be sprinkled on soft acidic food, e.g., applesauce.

Zymase 1-3 caps just prior to each meal <u>or</u> snack

Pediatric: <12 years: not recommended; ≥12 years: same as adult

Cap: **Zymase** lip 12,000 units+prot 24,000 units+amyl 24,000 units del-rel

EXTRAPYRAMIDAL SIDE EFFECTS (EPS)

▷ *amantadine*

Gocovri *Initially:* 137 mg once daily at bedtime; after 1 week, increase to 274 mg once daily at bedtime; swallow whole; may sprinkle contents on soft food; take with <u>or</u> without food; avoid use with alcohol; a lower dose is recommended for patients with moderate <u>or</u> severe renal impairment; Contraindicated with end-stage renal disease

Cap: 68.5, 137 mg ext-rel

Comment: **Gocovri** is a chrono-synchronous *amantadine* therapy indicated for the treatment of dyskinesia in patients with Parkinson's disease receiving *levodopa*-based therapy, with <u>or</u> without concomitant dopaminergic medications, as adjunctive treatment to *levodopa/carbidopa* in patients with Parkinson's disease experiencing "off" episodes. The most commonly observed adverse reactions (incidence ≥10%) have been hallucination, dizziness, dry mouth, peripheral edema, constipation, fall, and orthostatic hypotension. Advise patients prior to treatment about the potential to fall asleep during activities of daily living; discontinue if this occurs. Monitor patients for depressed mood, depression, <u>or</u> suicidal ideation <u>or</u> behavior. Patients with major psychotic disorder should ordinarily <u>not</u> be treated with **Gocovri**; observe patients for the occurrence of hallucinations throughout treatment, especially at initiation and after dose increases. Monitor patients for dizziness and orthostatic hypotension, especially after starting **Gocovri** and after dose increases. Avoid sudden discontinuation, which can result in withdrawal-emergent hyperpyrexia and confusion. Impulse control and compulsive behaviors may occur, such as gambling urges, sexual urges, uncontrolled spending; consider dose reduction <u>or</u> discontinuation if any occur. Increased risk of anticholinergic effects may require reduction of **Gocovri** <u>or</u> dose of the anticholinergic drug(s). Excretion of *amantadine* increases with acidic urine resulting in possible accumulation with urine change towards alkaline. Live attenuated vaccines (LAVs) are <u>not</u> recommended during treatment with

Gocovri. Concomitant use of alcohol is <u>not</u> recommended due to increased potential for CNS effects. There are <u>no</u> adequate data on embryo/fetal risk associated with use of *amantadine* in pregnant females. Animal studies suggest a potential risk for fetal harm with *amantadine. Amantadine* is excreted in human milk, but amounts have not been quantified. There is <u>no</u> information on the risk to the breastfed infant.

Osmolex ER *Tab:* 129, 193, 258 mg ext-rel

Comment: **Osmolex ER** is <u>not</u> interchangeable with other *amantadine* immediate <u>or</u> extended-release products. Most common adverse reactions (incidence ≥ 5%) are nausea, dizziness/ lightheadedness, and insomnia. **Osmolex ER** is contraindicated in patients with end-stage renal disease (ESRD). Advise patients prior to treatment about potential for falling asleep during activities of daily living (ADLs) and somnolence and discontinue **Osmolex ER** if occurs. Monitor patients for depressed mood, depression, <u>and</u> suicidal ideation <u>or</u> behavior. Patients with major psychotic disorder should ordinarily <u>not</u> be treated with **Osmolex ER**; observe patients throughout treatment for the occurrence of hallucinations, especially at initiation and after dose increases. Monitor patients for dizziness and orthostatic hypotension, especially after starting **Osmolex ER** <u>or</u> increasing the dose. Avoid sudden withdrawal/discontinuation due to risk of Withdrawal-Emergent Hyperpyrexia and confusion: Monitor patient for development of impulse control/compulsive behaviors. Ask patients about increased gambling urges, sexual urges, uncontrolled spending <u>or</u> other urges and consider dose reduction <u>or</u> discontinuation if any occur. Increased risk of anticholinergic effects may require reduction of **Osmolex ER** <u>or</u> dose of the anticholinergic drug(s). Excretion of *amantadine* increases with acidic urine resulting in possible accumulation with urine change towards alkaline. Live Attenuated Influenza Vaccines (LAVs) are <u>not</u> recommended during treatment with **Osmolex ER**. Concomitant use of alcohol is <u>not</u> recommended due to increased potential for CNS effects. There are <u>no</u> adequate data on the developmental risk associated with use of *amantadine* in pregnant females. Animal studies suggest a potential risk for fetal harm with *amantadine. Amantadine* is excreted in human milk, but amounts have <u>not</u> been quantified. There is <u>no</u> information on the risk to the breastfed infant.

 EYE PAIN

OPHTHALMIC NSAIDs

Comment: Concomitant contact lens wear is contraindicated during therapy. Etiology of eye pain must be known prior to use of ophthalmic NSAIDs.

▷ *diclofenac* (B) 1 drop affected eye qid
　Pediatric: <12 years: not recommended; ≥12 years: same as adult
　　Voltaren Ophthalmic Solution *Ophth soln:* 0.1% (2.5, 5 ml)
▷ *ketorolac tromethamine* (C) 1 drop affected eye qid for up to 4 days
　Pediatric: <3 years: not recommended; ≥3 years: same as adult
　　Acular *Ophth soln:* 0.5% (3, 5, 10 ml; benzalkonium chloride)
　　Acular LS *Ophth soln:* 0.4% (5 ml; benzalkonium chloride)
　　Acular PF *Ophth soln:* 0.5% (0.4 ml; 12 single-use vials/carton) (preservative-free)
▷ *nepafenac* (C) 1 drop affected eye tid
　Pediatric: <10 years: not recommended; ≥10 years: same as adult
　　Nevanac Ophthalmic Suspension *Ophth susp:* 0.1% (3 ml) (benzalkonium chloride)

OPHTHALMIC STEROIDS

Comment: Ophthalmic steroids are contraindicated with mycobacterial, fungal, and viral infection. Effectiveness of treatment should be assessed after 2 days. The corticosteroid should be tapered and treatment concluded within 14 days if possible due to risk of corneal and/or scleral thinning with prolonged use.

▸ *difluprednate* (C) 1 drop affected eye qid; *Post-op Pain:* beginning 24 hours after surgery, 1 drop affected eye qid; continue for 2 weeks post-op; then bid x 1 week; then taper until resolved

Pediatric: <12 years: not recommended; ≥12 years: same as adult

Durezol Ophthalmic Solution *Ophth emul:* 0.05% (5 ml)

▸ *etabonate* (C) 1 drop affected eye qid

Pediatric: <12 years: not recommended; ≥12 years: same as adult

Alrex Ophthalmic Solution *Ophth emul:* 0.2% (5 ml) (benzylkonium chloride)

▸ *eoteprednol etabonate 1%* (C) 1-2 drops affected eye bid

Pediatric: <12 years: not established; ≥12 years: same as adult

Inveltys *Ophth soln:* 1% (5 ml) (benzylkonium chloride)

Comment: **Inveltys** is indicated for post-op inflammation and pain following ocular surgery beginning the day after surgery and continuing throughout the first 2 weeks of the post-operative period.

FACIAL HAIR: EXCESSIVE/UNWANTED

TOPICAL HAIR GROWTH RETARDANT

▸ *eflornithine* 13.9% cream (C) apply a thin layer to affected areas of face and under the chin bid at least 8 hours apart; rub in thoroughly; do not wash treated area for at least 4 hours following application

Pediatric: <12 years: not recommended; ≥12 years: same as adult

Vaniqa *Crm:* 13.9% (30, 60 gm)

Comment: After **Vaniqa** dries, may apply cosmetics or sunscreen. Hair removal techniques may be continued as needed.

FECAL ODOR

▸ *bismuth subgallate powder* (B)(OTC) 1-2 tabs tid with meals

Devron *Chew tab:* 200 mg; *Cap:* 200 mg

Comment: **Devron** is an internal (oral) deodorant for control of odors from ileostomy or colostomy drainage or fecal incontinence.

FEVER (PYREXIA)

ACETAMINOPHEN FOR IV INFUSION

▸ *acetaminophen* injectable (B)(G) administer by IV infusion over 15 minutes; 1000 mg q 6 hours prn or 650 mg q 4 hours prn; max 4,000 mg/day

Pediatric: <2 years: not recommended; 2-13 years <50 kg: 15 mg/kg q 6 hours prn or 12.5 mg/kg q 4 hours prn; max 750 mg/single dose; max 75 mg/kg per day

Ofirmev *Vial:* 10 mg/ml (100 ml) (preservative-free)

Comment: The **Ofirmev** vial is intended for single-use. If any portion is withdrawn from the vial, use within 6 hours. Discard the unused portion. For pediatric patients, withdraw the intended dose and administer via syringe pump. Do not ad-mix **Ofirmev** with any other drugs. **Ofirmev** is physically incompatible with diazepam and chlorpromazine hydrochloride.

▸ *acetaminophen* (B)(G)

Children's Tylenol (OTC) 10-20 mg/kg q 4-6 hours prn

Oral susp: 80 mg/tsp

4-11 months (12-17 lb): 1/2 tsp q 4 hours prn; 12-23 months (18-23 lb): 3/4 tsp q 4 hours prn; 2-3 years (24-35 lb): 1 tsp q 4 hours prn; 4-5 years (36-47 lb): 1 tsp q 4 hours prn; 6-8 years (48-59 lb): 2 tsp q 4 hours prn; 9-10 years (60-71 lb): 2 tsp q 4 hours prn; 11 years (72-95 lb): 3 tsp q 4 hours prn; All: max 5 doses/day

Elix: 160 mg/5 ml (2, 4 oz)

Chew tab: 80 mg

2-3 years (24-35 lb): 2 tabs q 4 hours prn; 4-5 years (36-47 lb): 3 tabs q 4 hours prn; 6-8 years (48-59 lb): 4 tabs q 4 hours prn; 9-10 years (60-71 lb): 5 tabs q 4 hours prn; 11 years (72-95 lb): 6 tabs q 4 hours prn; All: max 5 doses/day

Junior Strength:

6-8 years: 2 tabs q 4 hours prn; 9-10 years: 2 tabs q 4 hours prn; 11 years: 3 tabs q 4 hours prn; 12 years: 4 tabs q 4 hours prn; All: max 5 doses/day

Chew tab: 160 mg

Junior cplt: 160 mg

Infant's Drops and Suspension: 80 mg/0.8 ml (1/2, 1 oz)

<3 months: 0.4 ml q 4 hours prn; 4-11 months: 0.8 ml q 4 hours prn; 12-23 months: 1.2 ml q 4 hours prn; 2-3 years (24-35 lb): 1.6 ml q 4 hours prn; 4-5 years (36-47 lb): 2.4 ml q 4 hours prn; All: max 5 doses/day

Extra Strength Tylenol (OTC) 1 gm q 4-6 hours prn; max 4 gm/day

Pediatric: <12 years: not recommended; ≥12 years: same as adult

Tab/Cplt/Gel tab/Gel cap: 500 mg; *Liq*: 500 mg/15 ml (8 oz)

FeverAll Extra Strength Tylenol (OTC)

Pediatric: <3 months: not recommended; 3-36 months: 80 mg q 4 hours prn; 3-6 years: 120 mg q 4 hours prn; ≥6 years: 325 mg q 4 hours prn; *Rectal supp*: 80, 120, 325 mg (6/carton)

Maximum Strength Tylenol Sore Throat (OTC) 500-1000 mg q 4-6 hours prn

Pediatric: <12 years: not recommended; ≥12 years: same as adult

Liq: 1000 mg/30 ml (8 oz)

Tylenol (OTC) 650 mg q 4-6 hours; max 4 gm/day

Pediatric: <6 years: not recommended; 6-11 years: 325 mg q 4-6 hours prn; max 1.625 gm/day; ≥12 years: same as adult

▷ *aspirin* (D)(G)

Bayer (OTC) 325-650 mg q 4 hours prn; max: 5 doses/day

Pediatric: <12 years: not recommended; ≥12 years: same as adult

Tab/Cplt: 325 mg ext-rel

Extra Strength Bayer (OTC) 500 mg-1 gm q 4-6 hours prn; max 4 gm/day

Pediatric: <12 years: not recommended; ≥12 years: same as adult

Cplt: 500 mg

Extended-Release Bayer 8 Hour (OTC) 650-1300 mg q 8 hours prn

Pediatric: <12 years: not recommended; ≥12 years: same as adult

Cplt: 650 mg ext-rel

▷ *aspirin+caffeine* (D)(G)

Anacin (OTC) 800 mg q 4 hours prn; max 4 gm/day

Pediatric: <6 years: not recommended; 6-12 years: 400 mg q 4 hours prn; max 2 gm/day; ≥12 years: same as adult

Tab/Cplt: 400 mg

Anacin Maximum Strength (OTC) 1 gm tid-qid

Pediatric: <12 years: not recommended; ≥12 years: same as adult

Tab: 500 mg

▷ *aspirin+antacid* (D)(G)

Extra Strength Bayer Plus (OTC) 500 mg-1 gm q 4-6 hours prn; usual max 4 gm/day

Pediatric: <12 years: not recommended; ≥12 years: same as adult
> *Cplt:* 500 mg aspirin+calcium carbonate

Bufferin (OTC) 650 mg q 4 hours; max 3.9 mg/day
Pediatric: <12 years: not recommended; ≥12 years: same as adult
> *Tab:* 325 mg aspirin+calcium carbonate+magnesium carbonate+
> magnesium oxide

➤ *ibuprofen* (B; <u>not</u> for use in 3rd)(G)
Comment: *Ibuprofen* is contraindicated in children <6 months-of-age.
**Children's Advil (OTC), ElixSure IB (OTC), Motrin (OTC),
PediaCare (OTC), PediaProfen (OTC)**
Pediatric: 5-10 mg/kg q 6-8 hours; max 40 mg/kg/day; <24 lb (<2 years):
individualize; 24-35 lb (2-3 years): 5 ml q 6-8 hours prn; 36-47 lb (4-5
years): 7.5 ml q 6-8 hours prn; 48-59 lb (6-8 years): 10 ml <u>or</u> 2 tabs q 6-8
hours prn; 60-71 lb (9-10 years): 12.5 ml <u>or</u> 2 tabs q 6-8 hours prn; 72-95 lb
(11 years): 15 ml <u>or</u> 3 tabs q 6-8 hours prn
> *Oral susp:* 100 mg/5 ml (2, 4 oz) (berry); *Junior tabs:* 100 mg

Children's Motrin Drops (OTC), PediaCare Drops (OTC)
Pediatric: <24 lb (<2 years): individualize; 24-35 lb (2-3 years): 2.5 ml q 6-8 hours
prn
> *Oral drops:* 50 mg/1.25 ml (15 ml) (berry)

Children's Motrin Chewables and Caplets (OTC)
Pediatric: 48-59 lb (6-8 years): 200 mg q 6-8 hours prn; 60-71 lb (9-10 years):
250 mg q 6-8 hours prn; 72-95 lb (11 years): 300 mg q 6-8 hours prn; ≥12
years: same as adult
> *Chew tab:* 100*mg (citrus; phenylalanine); *Cplt:* 100 mg

Motrin (OTC) 400 mg q 6 hours prn
Pediatric: <6 months: not recommended; ≥6 months, fever <102.5: 5 mg/kg q
6-8 hours prn; >6 months, fever >102.5: 10 mg/kg q 6-8 hours prn
All: max 40 mg/kg/day
> *Tab:* 400 mg; *Cplt:* 100*mg; *Chew tab:* 50*, 100*mg (citrus; phenylalanine);
> *Oral susp:* 100 mg/5 ml (4, 16 oz) (berry); *Oral drops:* 40 mg/ml (15 ml)
> (berry)

Advil (OTC), Motrin IB (OTC), Nuprin (OTC) 200-400 mg q 4-6 hours; max
1.2 gm/day
Pediatric: <12 years: not recommended; ≥12 years: same as adult
> *Tab/Cplt/Gel cap:* 200 mg

➤ *naproxen* (B)(G)
Pediatric: <2 years: not recommended; ≥2 years: 2.5-5 mg/kg bid-tid; max:
15 mg/kg/day
Aleve (OTC) 400 mg x 1 dose; then 200 mg q 8-12 hours prn; max 10 days
> *Tab/Cplt/Gel cap:* 200 mg

Anaprox 550 mg x 1 dose; then 550 mg q 12 hours <u>or</u> 275 mg q 6-8 hours prn;
max 1.375 gm first day and 1.1 gm/day thereafter
> *Tab:* 275 mg

Anaprox DS 1 tab bid
> *Tab:* 550 mg

EC-Naprosyn 375 <u>or</u> 500 mg bid prn; may increase dose up to max 1500 mg/
day as tolerated
> *Tab:* 375, 500 mg del-rel

Naprelan 1 gm daily <u>or</u> 1.5 gm daily for limited time; max 1 gm/day
thereafter
> *Tab:* 375, 500 mg

Naprosyn initially 500 mg, then 500 mg q 12 hours <u>or</u> 250 mg q 6-8 hours prn;
max 1.25 gm first day and 1 gm/day thereafter
> *Tab:* 250, 375, 500 mg; *Oral susp:* 125 mg/5 ml (473 ml) (pineapple-orange)

FIBROCYSTIC BREAST DISEASE

Contraceptives *see* Appendix H. Contraceptives
▷ *spironolactone* (D) 10 mg bid pre-menstrually
    Aldactone (G) *Tab:* 25, 50*, 100*mg
    CaroSpir *Oral susp:* 25 mg/5 ml (118, 473 ml) (banana)
▷ *vitamin E* (A) 400-600 IU daily
▷ *vitamin B6* (A) 50-100 mg daily

Synthetic Steroid Derived from Ethisterone

▷ *danazol* (X) start on 3rd or 4th day of menstrual period or after a negative
    pregnancy test; 50-200 mg bid x 2-6 months
    Pediatric: <18 years: not recommended; ≥18 years: same as adult
    Danocrine *Cap:* 50, 100, 200 mg
    Comment: *Danazol* is a synthetic steroid derived from ethisterone. It suppresses
    the pituitary-ovarian axis. This suppression is probably a combination of depressed
    hypothalamic-pituitary response to lowered *estrogen* production, the alteration of
    sex steroid metabolism, and interaction of *danazol* with sex hormone receptors.
    The only other demonstrable hormonal effects are weak androgenic activity and
    depression of both follicle-stimulating hormone (FSH) and luteinizing hormone
    (LH) output. Recent evidence suggests a direct inhibitory effect at gonadal sites
    and a binding of **Danocrine** to receptors of gonadal steroids at target organs. In
    addition, **Danocrine** has been shown to significantly decrease IgG, IgM, and IgA
    levels, as well as phospholipid and IgG isotope autoantibodies in patients with
    endometriosis and associated elevations of autoantibodies, suggesting this could be
    another mechanism by which it facilitates regression of fibrocystic breast disease.
    Danocrine usually produces partial-to-complete disappearance of breast tissue
    nodularity and complete relief of pain and tenderness. Changes in the menstrual
    pattern may occur. Generally, the pituitary-suppressive action of **Danocrine** is
    reversible. Ovulation and cyclic bleeding usually return within 60 to 90 days
    when therapy with **Danocrine** is discontinued. **Danocrine** is also used to treat
    endometriosis (to relieve associated abdominal pain) and hereditary angioedema
    (to prevent attacks). Contraindications include pregnancy, breastfeeding, active
    or history of thromboembolic disease/event, porphyria, undiagnosed abnormal
    genital bleeding, androgen-dependent tumor, and markedly impaired hepatic,
    renal, or cardiac function.

FIBROMYALGIA

Acetaminophen for IV Infusion *see Pain*
NSAIDs *see* Appendix J. NSAIDs online at https://connect.springerpub.com/content/
reference-book/978-0-8261-7935-7/back-matter/part02/back-matter/bmatter10
Opioid Analgesics *see Pain*
Topical & Transdermal Analgesics *see Pain*
Parenteral Corticosteroids *see* Appendix M. Parenteral Corticosteroids
Oral Corticosteroids *see* Appendix L. Oral Corticosteroids
Topical Analgesic and Anesthetic Agents *see* Appendix I. Anesthetic Agents for
Local Infiltration and Dermal/Mucosal Membrane Application online at https://
connect.springerpub.com/content/reference-book/978-0-8261-7935-7/back-matter/
part02/back-matter/bmatter9

SEROTONIN-NOREPINEPHRINE REUPTAKE INHIBITORS (SNRIs)

▷ *duloxetine* (C)(G) swallow whole; initially 30 mg once daily x 1 week; then
    increase to 60 mg once daily; max 120 mg/day
    Pediatric: <12 years: not recommended; ≥12 years: same as adult
    Cymbalta *Cap:* 20, 30, 60 mg ent-coat pellets

➤ **milnacipran (C)(G)** *Day 1:* 12.5 mg once; *Days 2-3:* 12.5 mg bid; *Days 4-7:* 25 mg bid; max 100 mg bid
   Pediatric: <17 years: not recommended; ≥17 years: same as adult
     Savella *Tab:* 12.5, 25, 50, 100 mg

GAMMA-AMINOBUTYRIC ACID ANALOGS

Comment: The gabapentinoids (*gabapentin* [**Gralise, Neurontin, Horizant**] and *pregabalin* [**Lyrica**]) have respiratory depression risk potential. Therefore, when co-prescribed with other CNS depressant agents, initiate the gabapentinoid at the lowest possible dose and monitor the patient for respiratory depression (especially elders and patients with compromised pulmonary function). Side effects include fatigue, somnolence/sedation, dizziness, vertigo, feeling drunk, headache, nausea, and dry mouth. To discontinue a gabapentinoid, withdraw gradually over 1 week <u>or</u> longer.

➤ **gabapentin (C)** initially 300 mg on Day 1; then 600 mg on Day 2; then 900 mg on Days 3-6; then 1200 mg on Days 7-10; then 1500 mg on Days 11-14; titrate up to 1800 mg on Day 15; take entire dose once daily with the evening meal; do <u>not</u> crush, split, <u>or</u> chew
   Pediatric: <3 years: not recommended; 3-12 years: initially 10-15 mg/kg/day in 3 divided doses; max 12 hours between doses; titrate over 3 days; 3-4 years: titrate to 40 mg/kg/day; 5-12 years: titrate to 25-35 mg/kg/day; max 50 mg/kg/day; >12 years: same as adult
     Gralise *Tab:* 300, 600 mg
     Neurontin (G) 100 mg daily x 1 day; then 100 mg bid x 1 day; then 100 mg tid continuously <u>or</u> 300 mg bid; max 900 mg tid
       Tab: 600*, 800*mg; *Cap:* 100, 300, 400 mg; *Oral soln:* 250 mg/5 ml (480 ml) (strawberry-anise)
➤ **gabapentin enacarbil (C)** 600 mg once daily at about 5:00 PM; if dose not taken at recommended time, next dose should be taken the following day; swallow whole; take with food; *CrCl 30-59 mL/min:* 600 mg on Day 1, Day 3, and every day thereafter; *CrCl <30 mL/min:* <u>or</u> on hemodialysis: not recommended
   Pediatric: <12 years: not recommended; ≥12 years: same as adult
     Horizant *Tab:* 300, 600 mg ext-rel
➤ **pregabalin (GABA analog) (C)(G)(V)**
   Pediatric: <18 years: not recommended; ≥18 years: same as adult
     Lyrica initially 50 mg tid; may titrate to 100 mg tid within one week; max 600 mg divided tid; discontinue over 1 week
       Cap: 25, 50, 75, 100, 150, 200, 225, 300 mg; *Oral soln:* 20 mg/ml
     Lyrica CR usual dose: 165 mg once daily; may increase to 330 mg/day within 1 week; max 660 mg/day
       Tab: 82.5, 165, 330 mg ext-rel

OTHER AGENTS

➤ **amitriptyline (C)(G)** 20 mg q HS; may increase gradually to max 50 mg q HS
   Pediatric: <12 years: not recommended; ≥12 years: same as adult
     Tab: 10, 25, 50, 75, 100, 150 mg
➤ **cyclobenzaprine (B)(G)** 10 mg tid; usual range 20-40 mg/day in divided doses; max 60 mg/day x 2-3 weeks <u>or</u> 15 mg ext-rel once daily; max 30 mg ext-rel/day x 2-3 weeks
   Pediatric: <15 years: not recommended; ≥15 years: same as adult
     Amrix *Cap:* 15, 30 mg ext-rel
     Fexmid *Tab:* 7.5 mg
     Flexeril *Tab:* 5, 10 mg
➤ **eszopiclone (C)(IV)(G)** (pyrrolopyrazine) 1-3 mg; max 3 mg/day x 1 month; do <u>not</u> take if unable to sleep for at least 8 hours before required to be active again; delayed effect if taken with a meal

Pediatric: <18 years: not recommended; ≥18 years: same as adult
   Lunesta *Tab:* 1, 2, 3 mg

▷ *flurazepam* **(X)(IV)(G)** 15 mg q HS; may increase to 30 mg q HS
  Pediatric: <18 years: not recommended; ≥18 years: same as adult
   Dalmane *Cap:* 15, 30 mg

▷ *trazodone* **(C)(G)** 50 mg q HS
  Pediatric: <18 years: not recommended; ≥18 years: same as adult
   Desyrel *Tab:* 50, 100, 150, 300 mg

▷ *triazolam* **(X)(IV)(G)** 0.125 mg q HS, may increase gradually to 0.5 mg
  Pediatric: <18 years: not recommended; ≥18 years: same as adult
   Halcion *Tab:* 0.125, 0.25*mg

▷ *zaleplon* **(C)(IV)** (imidazopyridine) 5-10 mg at HS <u>or</u> after going to bed if unable
to sleep; do <u>not</u> take if unable to sleep for at least 4 hours before required to be
active again; max 20 mg/day x 1 month; delayed effect if taken with a meal
  Pediatric: <12 years: not recommended; ≥12 years: same as adult
   Sonata *Cap:* 5, 10 mg (tartrazine)
   Comment: **Sonata** is indicated for the treatment of insomnia when a middle-
of-the-night awakening is followed by difficulty returning to sleep.

▷ *zolpidem* oral solution spray **(C)(IV)(G)** (imidazopyridine hypnotic) 2 actuations
(10 mg) immediately before bedtime; *Elderly, debilitated,* <u>or</u> *hepatic impairment:* 2
actuations (5 mg); max 2 actuations (10 mg)
  Pediatric: <18 years: not recommended; ≥18 years: same as adult
   ZolpiMist *Oral soln spray:* 5 mg/actuation (60 metered actuations) (cherry)
   Comment: The lowest dose of *zolpidem* in all forms is recommended for persons
>50 years-of-age and women as drug elimination is slower than in men.

▷ *zolpidem* tabs **(B)(IV)(G)** (pyrazolopyrimidine hypnotic) 5-10 mg <u>or</u> 6.25-12.5
extrel q HS prn; max 12.5 mg/day x 1 month; do <u>not</u> take if unable to sleep for at
least 8 hours before required to be active again; delayed effect if taken with a meal
  Pediatric: <18 years: not recommended; ≥18 years: same as adult
   Ambien *Tab:* 5, 10 mg
   Ambien CR *Tab:* 6.25, 12.5 mg ext-rel
   Comment: The lowest dose of *zolpidem* in all forms is recommended for persons
>50 years-of-age and women as drug elimination is slower than in men.

▷ *zolpidem* sublingual tabs (imidazopyridine hypnotic) **(C)(IV)** dissolve 1 tab under
the tongue; allow to disintegrate completely before swallowing; take <u>only</u> once
per night and <u>only</u> if at least 4 hours of bedtime remain before planned time for
awakening
  Pediatric: <18 years: not recommended; ≥18 years: same as adult
   Edluar *SL Tab:* 5, 10 mg
   Intermezzo *SL Tab:* 1.75, 3.5 mg
   Comment: **Intermezzo** is indicated for the treatment of insomnia when a
middle-of-the-night awakening is followed by difficulty returning to sleep. The
lowest dose of *zolpidem* in all forms is recommended for persons >50 years-
of-age and women as drug elimination is slower than in men.

◯ FIFTH DISEASE (*ERYTHEMA INFECTIOSUM*)

Antipyretics *see* **Fever**

◯ FLATULENCE

▷ *simethicone* **(C)(G)**
   Gas-X (OTC) 2-4 tabs pc and HS prn
    Tab: 40, 80, 125 mg; *Cap:* 125 mg
   Mylicon (OTC) 2-4 tabs pc and HS prn
    Tab: 40, 80, 125 mg; *Cap:* 125 mg

Phazyme-95 1-2 tabs with each meal and HS prn
Tab: 95 mg
Phazyme Infant Oral Drops
Pediatric: <2 years: 0.3 ml qid pc and HS prn; 2-12 years: 0.6 ml qid pc and HS prn; >12 years: 1.2 ml qid pc and HS prn
Oral drops: 40 mg/0.6 ml (15, 30 ml w. calibrated dropper) (orange) (alcohol-free)
Maximum Strength Phazyme 1-2 caps with each meal and HS prn
Cap: 125 mg

FLUORIDATION, WATER, <0.6 PPM

▷ *fluoride* (G)
Luride
Pediatric: Water fluoridation 0.3-0.6 ppm: <3 years: use drops; 3-6 years: 0.25 mg daily; 7-16 years: 0.5 mg daily; *Water fluoridation <0.3 ppm:* <3 years: use drops; 6 months-3 years: 0.25 mg daily; 4-6 years: 0.5 mg daily; 7-16 years: 1 mg daily
Chew tab: 0.25, 0.5, 1 mg (sugar-free)
Luride Drops
Pediatric: Water fluoridation 0.3-0.6 ppm: 6 months-3 years: 0.25 ml once daily; 4-6 years: 0.5 ml once daily; 7-16 years: 1 ml once daily; *Water fluoridation <0.3 ppm:* 6 months-3 years: 0.5 ml once daily; 4-6 years: 1 ml once daily; 7-16 years: 2 ml daily
Oral drops: 0.5 mg/ml (50 ml) (sugar-free)

COMBINATION AGENTS

▷ *fluoride+vitamin a+vitamin d+vitamin c* (G)
Pediatric: Water fluoridation 0.3-0.6 ppm: <3 years: not recommended; 3-6 years: 0.25 mg fluoride/day; 7-16 years: 0.5 mg fluoride/day; *Water fluoridation <0.3 ppm:* <6 months: not recommended; 6 months-3 years: 0.25 mg fluoride/day; 4-6 years: 0.5 mg fluoride/day; 7-16 years: 1 mg fluoride/day
Tri-Vi-Flor Drops
Oral drops: fluoride 0.25 mg+vit a 1500 u+vit d 400 u+vit c 35 mg per ml (50 ml)
Oral drops: fluoride 0.5 mg+vit a 1500 u+vit d 400 u+vit c 35 mg per ml (50 ml)

▷ *fluoride+vitamin a+vitamin d+vitamin c+iron*
Pediatric: Water fluoridation 0.3-0.6 ppm: <3 years: not recommended; 3-6 years: 0.25 mg fluoride/day; 7-16 years: 0.5 mg fluoride/day; *Water fluoridation <0.3 ppm:* <6 months: not recommended; 6 months-3 years: 0.25 mg fluoride/day; 4-6 years: 0.5 mg fluoride/day; 7-16 years: 1 mg fluoride/day
Tri-Vi-Flor w. Iron Drops
Oral drops: fluoride 0.25 mg+vit a 1500 u+vit d 400 u+vit c 35 mg+iron 10 mg per ml (50 ml)

FOLLICULITIS BARBAE

Topical Corticosteroids *see* Appendix K: Topical Corticosteroids by Potency

TOPICAL AGENTS

▷ *benzoyl peroxide* (B) apply after shaving; may discolor clothing and linens.
Benzac-W initially apply to affected area once daily; increase to bid-tid as tolerated
Gel: 2.5, 5, 10% (60 gm)

Benzac-W Wash wash affected area bid
Wash: 5% (4, 8 oz); 10% (8 oz)
Benzagel apply to affected area one or more x/day
Gel: 5, 10% (1.5, 3 oz) (alcohol 14%)
Benzagel Wash wash affected area bid
Gel: 10% (6 oz)
Desquam X₅ wash affected area bid
Wash: 5% (5 oz)
Desquam X₁₀ wash affected area bid
Wash: 10% (5 oz)
Triaz apply to affected area daily bid
Lotn: 3, 6, 9% (bottle), 3% (tube); *Pads:* 3, 6, 9% (jar)
ZoDerm apply once or twice daily
Gel: 4.5, 6.5, 8.5% (125 ml); *Crm:* 4.5, 6.5, 8.5% (125 ml); *Clnsr:* 4.5, 6.5, 8.5% (400 ml)

➤ *clindamycin* topical (B) apply bid
Pediatric: same as adult
Cleocin T *Pad:* 1% (60/pck; alcohol 50%); *Lotn:* 1% (60 ml); *Gel:* 1% (30, 60 gm); *Soln w. applicator:* 1% (30, 60 ml) (alcohol 50%)
Clindagel *Gel:* 1% (42, 77 gm)
Clindets *Pad:* 1% (60/pck)
Evoclin *Foam:* 1% (50, 100 gm) (alcohol)

➤ *clindamycin+benzoyl peroxide* topical (C)
Pediatric: <12 years: not recommended; ≥12 years: same as adult
Acanya (G) apply once daily-bid
Gel: clin 1.2%+*benz* 2.5% (50 gm)
BenzaClin apply bid
Gel: clin 1%+*benz* 5% (25, 50 gm)
Duac apply daily in the evening
Gel: clin 1%+*benz* 5% (45 gm)
Onexton Gel (G) apply once daily
Gel: clin 1.2%+benz 3.75% (50 gm pump) (alcohol-free) (preservative-free)

➤ *dapsone* topical (C)(G) apply bid
Pediatric: <12 years: not recommended; ≥12 years: same as adult
Aczone *Gel:* 5% (30 gm)

➤ *tazarotene* (X)(G) apply daily at HS
Pediatric: <12 years: not recommended; ≥12 years: same as adult
Avage Cream *Crm:* 0.1% (30 gm)
Tazorac Cream *Crm:* 0.05, 0.1% (15, 30, 60 gm)
Tazorac Gel *Gel:* 0.05, 0.1% (30, 100 gm)

➤ *tretinoin* (C) apply q HS
Pediatric: <12 years: not recommended; ≥12 years: same as adult
Atralin Gel *Gel:* 0.05% (45 gm)
Avita *Crm:* 0.025% (20, 45 gm); *Gel:* 0.025% (20, 45 gm)
Renova *Crm:* 0.02% (40 gm); 0.05% (40, 60 gm)
Retin-A Cream *Crm:* 0.025, 0.05, 0.1% (20, 45 gm)
Retin-A Gel *Gel:* 0.01, 0.025% (15, 45 gm; alcohol 90%)
Retin-A Liquid *Soln:* 0.05% (alcohol 55%)
Retin-A Micro Gel *Gel:* 0.04, 0.08, 0.1% (20, 45 gm)
Tretin-X Cream *Crm:* 0.075% (35 gm) (parabens-free, alcohol-free, propylene glycol-free)
Retin-A Micro *Microspheres:* 0.04, 0.1% (20, 45 gm)

FOREIGN BODY: ESOPHAGUS

> *glucagon* (B) 0.02 mg/kg IV *or* IM with serial x-rays; max 1 mg
>> **Glucagon** (rDNA origin *or* beef/pork derived)
>>> *Vial:* 1 mg/ml w. diluent
> Comment: *Glucagon* facilitates passage of foreign body from esophagus into stomach.

FOREIGN BODY: EYE

> *proparacaine* 1-2 drops to anesthetize surface of eye; then flush with normal saline
>> **Ophthaine** *Ophth soln:* 0.5% (15 ml)
> Comment: *Proparacaine* facilitates the search, location, and removal of foreign body and examination of the cornea.

GASTRITIS/DYSPEPSIA

Antacids *see GERD*
H2 Antagonists *see GERD*

GASTRITIS-RELATED NAUSEA/VOMITING

OTC ANTI-EMETIC

> *phosphorylated carbohydrate* solution (C)(G) 1-2 tbsp q 15 minutes until nausea subsides; max 5 doses/day
> *Pediatric:* 1-2 tsp q 15 minutes until nausea subsides; max 5 doses/day
>> **Emetrol** (OTC) *Soln:* dextrose 1.87 gm+fructose 1.87 gm+phosphoric acid 21.5 mg per 5 ml (4, 8, 16 oz)

Rx ANTI-EMETICS

> *ondansetron* (C)(G) 8 mg q 8 hours x 2 doses; then 8 mg q 12 hours
> *Pediatric:* <4 years: not recommended; 4-11 years: 4 mg q 4 hours x 3 doses; then 4 mg q 8 hours
>> **Zofran** *Tab:* 4, 8, 24 mg
>> **Zofran ODT** *ODT:* 4, 8 mg (strawberry) (phenylalanine)
>> **Zofran Oral Solution** *Oral soln:* 4 mg/5 ml (50 ml) (strawberry) (phenylalanine); *Parenteral form:* see mfr pkg insert
>> **Zofran Injection** *Vial:* 2 mg/ml (2 ml single-dose); 2 mg/ml (20 ml multi-dose); 32 mg/50 ml (50 ml multi-dose); *Prefilled syringe:* 4 mg/2 ml, single-use (24/carton)
>> **Zuplenz Oral Soluble Film:** 4, 8 mg oral-dis (10/carton) (peppermint)
> Comment: The FDA has issued an updated warning against *ondansetron* use in pregnancy *ondansetron* is a 5-HT3 receptor antagonist approved by the FDA for preventing nausea and vomiting related to cancer chemotherapy and surgery. However, it has been used "off label" to treat the nausea and vomiting of pregnancy. The FDA has cautioned against the use of *ondansetron* in pregnancy in light of studies of *ondansetron* in early pregnancy and associated with congenital cardiac malformations and oral clefts (i.e., cleft lip and cleft palate). Further, there are potential maternal risks in pregnancy with electrolyte imbalance caused by severe nausea and vomiting (as with hyperemesis gravidarum). These risks include *serotonin syndrome* (a triad of of cognitive and behavioral changes including confusion, agitation, autonomic instability, and neuromuscular changes). Therefore, *ondansetron* should <u>not</u> be taken during pregnancy.

▷ *promethazine* (C)(G) 25 mg PO or rectally q 4-6 hours prn
Pediatric: <2 years: not recommended; ≥2 years: 0.5 mg/lb or 6.25-25 mg q 4-6 hours prn
      Phenergan *Tab:* 12.5*, 25*, 50 mg; *Plain syr:* 6.25 mg/5 ml; *Fortis syr:* 25 mg/5 ml; *Rectal supp:* 12.5, 25, 50 mg
Comment: *Promethazine* is contraindicated in children with uncomplicated nausea, dehydration, Reye's syndrome, history of sleep apnea, asthma, and lower respiratory disorders in children. *Promethazine* lowers the seizure threshold in children, may cause cholestatic jaundice, anticholinergic effects, extrapyramidal effects, and potentially fatal respiratory depression.

GASTROESOPHAGEAL REFLUX (GER), GASTROESOPHAGEAL REFLUX DISEASE (GERD), IDIOPATHIC GASTRIC ACID HYPERSECRETION (IGAH)

Comment: Precipitators of gastric reflux include narcotics, benzodiazepines, calcium antagonists, alcohol, nicotine, chocolate, and peppermint. Issues associated with H2 secretion and gastrointestinal health (e.g., chronic remitting gastritis, Barrett's esophagitis, peptic ulcer disease [PUD)]), other organ system impairments (e.g., CVD, metabolic syndrome, hepatitis, autoimmune and immune-deficiency disorders, renal insufficiency, iatrogenic consequences of treatments (e.g., steroids, NSAIDs, immune modulators), (advanced age), and lifestyle (dietary habits and general nutritional health). Risk/benefit discussions with patients can be challenging, but are necessary for informed decision-making and prudent prescribing.

ANTACIDS

Comment: Antacids with *aluminum hydroxide* may potentiate constipation. Antacids with *magnesium hydroxide* may potentiate diarrhea.

▷ *aluminum hydroxide* (C)
      ALTernaGEL (OTC) 5-10 ml between meals and HS prn; max 90 ml/day
      Pediatric: <12 years: not recommended; ≥12 years: same as adult
        Liq: 500 mg/5 ml (5, 12 oz)
      Amphojel (OTC) 10 ml 5-6 x/day between meals and HS prn; max 60 ml/day
      Pediatric: <12 years: not recommended; ≥12 years: same as adult
        Oral susp: 320 mg/5 ml (12 oz)
      Amphojel Tab (OTC) 600 mg 5-6 x/day between meals and HS prn; max 3.6 gm/day
      Pediatric: <12 years: not recommended; ≥12 years: same as adult
        Tab: 300, 600 mg
▷ *aluminum hydroxide+magnesium hydroxide* (C)(OTC)(G)
      Maalox 10-20 ml qid and HS prn
      Pediatric: <12 years: not recommended; ≥12 years: same as adult
        Oral susp: alum 225 mg+mag 200 mg per 5 ml (5, 12, 26 oz) (mint, lemon, cherry)
      Maalox Therapeutic Concentrate 10-20 ml qid pc and HS prn
      Pediatric: <12 years: not recommended; ≥12 years: same as adult
        Oral susp: alum 600 mg+mag 300 mg per 5 ml (12 oz) (mint)
▷ *aluminum hydroxide+magnesium hydroxide+simethicone* (C)(OTC)(G)
      Maalox Plus 10-20 ml qid pc and HS prn
      Pediatric: <12 years: not recommended; ≥12 years: same as adult
        Tab: alum 200 mg+mag 200 mg+sim 25 mg
      Extra Strength Maalox Plus 10-20 ml qid pc and HS prn

Pediatric: <12 years: not recommended; ≥12 years: same as adult
  Tab: alum 350 mg+mag 350 mg+sim 30 mg
  Oral susp: alum 500 mg+mag 450 mg+sim 40 mg per 5 ml (5, 12, 26 oz)
Extra Strength Maalox Plus Tab 1-3 tabs qid pc and HS prn
Pediatric: <12 years: not recommended; ≥12 years: same as adult
  Tab: alum 350 mg+mag 350 mg+sim 30 mg
Mylanta 10-20 ml between meals and HS prn
Pediatric: <12 years: not recommended; ≥12 years: same as adult
  Liq: alum 200 mg+mag 200 mg+sim 20 mg per 5 ml (5, 12, 24 oz)
Mylanta Double Strength 10-20 ml between meals and HS prn
Pediatric: <12 years: not recommended; ≥12 years: same as adult
  Liq: alum 700 mg+mag 400 mg+sim 40 mg per 5 ml (5, 12, 24 oz)
▷ *aluminum hydroxide+magnesium carbonate* (C)(OTC)(G)
Maalox HRF 10-20 ml qid pc and HS prn
Pediatric: <12 years: not recommended; ≥12 years: same as adults
  Oral susp: alum 280 mg+mag 350 mg per 10 ml (10 oz)
▷ *aluminum hydroxide+magnesium trisilicate* (C)(G)
Gaviscon chew 2-4 tabs qid pc and HS prn
Pediatric: <12 years: not recommended; ≥12 years: same as adult
  Tab: alum 80 mg+mag 20 mg
Gaviscon Liquid 15-30 ml qid pc and HS prn
Pediatric: <12 years: not recommended; ≥12 years: same as adult
  Liq: alum 95 mg+mag 359 mg per 15 ml (6, 12 oz)
Gaviscon Extra Strength 2-4 tabs qid pc and HS prn
Pediatric: <12 years: not recommended; ≥12 years: same as adult
  Tab: alum 160 mg+mag 105 mg
Gaviscon Extra Strength Liquid 10-20 ml qid prn
Pediatric: <12 years: not recommended; ≥12 years: same as adult
  Liq: alum 508 mg+mag 475 mg per 10 ml (12 oz)
▷ *aluminum hydroxide+magnesium hydroxide+simethicone* (C)(OTC)(G)
Maalox Maximum Strength 10-20 ml qid prn; max 60 ml/day
Pediatric: <12 years: not recommended; ≥12 years: same as adult
  Oral susp: alum 500 mg+mag 450 mg+sim 40 mg per 5 ml (5, 12, 26 oz)
  (mint, cherry)
▷ *calcium carbonate* (C)(OTC)(G)
Children's Mylanta Tab
Pediatric: <2 years: not recommended; 2-5 years (24-47 lb): 1 tab as needed up
to tid; 6-11 years (48-95 lb): 2 tabs as needed up to tid
  Tab: 400 mg
Children's Mylanta
Pediatric: <2 years: not recommended; 2-5 years (24-47 lb): 1 tab as needed up
to tid; 6-11 years (48-95 lb): 2 tabs as needed up to tid
  Liq: 400 mg/5 ml (4 oz)
Maalox Tab chew 2-4 tabs prn; max 12 tabs/day
Pediatric: <12 years: not recommended; ≥12 years: same as adult
  Chew tab: 600 mg (wild berry, lemon, wintergreen) (phenylalanine)
Maalox Maximum Strength Tab 1-2 tabs prn; max 8 tabs/day
Pediatric: <12 years: not recommended; ≥12 years: same as adult
  Tab: 1 gm (wild berry, lemon, wintergreen; phenylalanine)
Rolaids Extra Strength 1-2 tabs dissolved in mouth or chewed q 1 hour prn;
max 8 tabs/day
  Tab: 1000 mg
Tums 1-2 tabs dissolved in mouth or chewed q 1 hour prn; max 16 tabs/day
  Tab: 500 mg
Tums E-X 1-2 tabs dissolved in mouth or chewed q 1 hour prn; max 16 tabs/day
  Tab: 750 mg

▷ *calcium carbonate+magnesium hydroxide* (C)
  Mylanta Tab 2-4 tabs between meals and HS prn
  Pediatric: <12 years: not recommended; ≥12 years: same as adult
    Tab: calib 350 mg+mag 150 mg
  Mylanta DS Tab 2-4 tabs between meals and HS prn
  Pediatric: <12 years: not recommended; ≥12 years: same as adult
    Tab: calib 700 mg+mag 300 mg
  Rolaids Sodium-Free 1-2 tabs dissolved in mouth or chewed q 1 hour as needed
    Tab: calib 317 mg+mag 64 mg
▷ *calcium carbonate+magnesium carbonate* (C)
  Mylanta Gel Caps (OTC) 2-4 caps prn
    Gel cap: calib 550 mg+mag 125 mg
▷ *dihydroxyaluminum*
  Rolaids (OTC) 1-2 tabs dissolved in mouth or chewed q 1 hour prn; max 24 tabs/day
    Tab: 334 mg

H2 ANTAGONISTS

▷ *cimetidine* (B)(OTC)(G) 800 mg bid or 400 mg qid; max 12 weeks
  Pediatric: <16 years: not recommended; ≥16 years: same as adult
    Tagamet 800 mg bid or 400 mg qid; max 12 weeks
      Tab: 200, 300, 400*, 800*mg
    Tagamet HB *Prophylaxis:* 1 tab ac; *Treatment:* 1 tab bid
      Tab: 200 mg
    Tagamet HB Oral Suspension *Prophylaxis:* 1-3 tsp ac; *Treatment:* 1 tsp bid
      Oral susp: 200 mg/20 ml (12 oz)
    Tagamet Liquid *Liq:* 300 mg/5 ml (mint-peach) (alcohol 2.8%)
▷ *famotidine* (B)(OTC)(G)
  Pediatric: 0.5 mg/kg/day q HS prn or in 2 divided doses; max 40 mg/day
    Maximum Strength Pepcid AC 1 tab ac
      Tab: 20 mg
    Pepcid 20-40 mg bid; **max 6 weeks**
      Tab: 20 mg; *Tab:* 40 mg; *Oral susp:* 40 mg/5 ml (50 ml)
    Pepcid AC 1 tab ac; max 2 doses/day
      Tab/Rapid dissolving tab: 10 mg
    Pepcid Complete (OTC) 1 tab ac; max 2 doses/day
      Tab: fam 10 mg+CaCO2 800 mg+mag hydroxide 165 mg
    Pepcid RPD *Tab:* 20, 40 mg rapid dissolve
▷ *nizatidine* (B)(OTC)(G) 150 mg bid or 300 mg once daily
  Pediatric: <12 years: not recommended; ≥12 years: same as adult
    Axid *Cap:* 150, 300 mg; *Oral soln:* 15 mg/ml (480 ml) (bubble gum)
▷ *ranitidine* (B)(OTC)(G)
  Pediatric: <1 month: not recommended; 1 month to 16 years: 2-4 mg/kg/day in 2 divided doses; max 300 mg/day; *Duodenal/Gastric Ulcer:* 2-4 mg/kg/day divided bid; max 300 mg/day; *Erosive Esophagitis:* 5-10 mg/kg/day divided bid; max 300 mg/day; 20 lb, 9 kg: 0.6 ml; 30 lb, 13.6 kg: 0.9 ml; 40 lb, 18.2 kg: 1.2 ml; 50 lb, 22.7 kg: 1.5 ml; 60 lb, 27.3 kg: 1.8 ml; 70 lb, 31.8 kg: 2.1 ml
    Zantac 150 mg bid or 300 mg q HS
      Tab: 150, 300 mg
    Zantac 75 1 tab ac
      Tab: 75 mg
    Zantac EFFERdose dissolve 25 mg tab in 5 ml water and dissolve 150 mg tab in 6-8 oz water
      Efferdose: 25, 150 mg effervescent
    Zantac Syrup *Syr:* 15 mg/ml (peppermint) (alcohol 7.5%)

▷ *ranitidine bismuth citrate* (C) 400 mg bid
  Pediatric: <12 years: not recommended; ≥12 years: same as adult
    Tritec *Tab:* 400 mg

PROTON PUMP INHIBITORS (PPIs)

Comment: A study of 144,032 incident users of acid suppression therapy, including 125,596 PPI users and 18,436 histamine H2 receptor antagonist users were followed over 5 years. The researchers reported PPI users had an increased risk of having an eGFR <60 mL/min/1.73m², incident CKD, eGFR decline over 30%, and ESRD or eGFR decline over 50%, as compared to those taking H2 blockers. They concluded, "reliance on antecedent acute kidney injury (AKI) as a warning sign to guard against the risk of chronic kidney disease (CKD) among PPI users is not sufficient as a sole mitigation strategy." Further, timely PPI discontinuation is warranted if there is a first AKI to avoid progression to CKD.

Comment: Practice guidelines from the American Gastroenterological Association (AGA) address risks and recommendations for prescribing PPI therapy based on an extensive review of the literature. PPI use may increase the risk for fracture, vitamin B12 deficiency, hypomagnesemia, iron-deficiency anemia, small intestinal bacterial overgrowth (SIBO), *C. difficile* infection, kidney disease, cardiovascular disease (CVD), pneumonias, and dementia. Healthcare providers are advised to discuss the risks/benefits of PPI therapy with respect to each individual patient's situation.

▷ *dexlansoprazole* (B)(G) 30-60 mg daily for up to 4 weeks
  Pediatric: <18 years: not recommended; ≥18 years: same as adult
    Dexilant *Cap:* 30, 60 mg ent-coat del-rel granules; may open and sprinkle on applesauce; do not crush or chew granules
    Dexilant SoluTab *Tab:* 30 mg del-rel orally disint
▷ *esomeprazole* (B)(OTC)(G) 20-40 mg once daily; max 8 weeks; take 1 hour before food; swallow whole or mix granules with food or juice and take immediately; do not crush or chew granules
  Pediatric: <1 month: not established; 1 month-<1 year, 3-5 kg: 2.5 mg; 5-7.5 kg: 5 mg; 7.5-12 kg: 10 mg; 1-11 years, <20 kg: 10 mg; ≥20 kg: 10-20 mg; 12-17 years: 20 mg; max 8 weeks; >17 years: same as adult
    Nexium *Cap:* 20, 40 mg ent-coat del-rel pellets
    Nexium for Oral Suspension *Oral susp:* 10, 20, 40 mg ent-coat del-rel granules/pkt; mix in 2 tbsp water and drink immediately; 30 pkt/carton
▷ *lansoprazole* (B)(OTC)(G) 15-30 mg daily for up to 8 weeks; may repeat course; take before eating
  Pediatric: <1 year: not recommended; 1-11 years, <30 kg: 15 mg once daily; >11 years: same as adult
    Prevacid *Cap:* 15, 30 mg ent-coat del-rel granules; swallow whole or mix granules with food or juice and take immediately; do not crush or chew granules; follow with water
    Prevacid for Oral Suspension *Oral susp:* 15, 30 mg ent-coat del-rel granules/pkt; mix in 2 tbsp water and drink immediately; 30 pkt/carton (strawberry)
    Prevacid SoluTab *ODT:* 15, 30 mg (strawberry) (phenylalanine)
    Prevacid 24HR 15 mg ent-coat del-rel granules; swallow whole or mix granules with food or juice and take immediately; do not crush or chew granules; follow with water
▷ *omeprazole* (C)(OTC)(G) 20-40 mg daily for 14 days; may repeat course in 4 months; take before eating; swallow whole or mix granules with applesauce and take immediately; do not crush or chew granules; follow with water

Pediatric: <18 years: not recommended; ≥18 years: same as adult
> **Prilosec** *Cap:* 10, 20, 40 mg ent-coat del-rel granules
Pediatric: <1 year: not recommended; ≥1 year: 5-<10 kg: 5 mg daily; 10-<20 kg: 10 mg daily; ≥20 kg: same as adult
> **Prilosec OTC** *Tab:* 20 mg del-rel (regular, wildberry, strawberry)
Pediatric: <18 years: not recommended; ≥18 years: same as adult

▷ *pantoprazole* (B)(G) 40 mg daily
Pediatric: <12 years: not recommended; ≥12 years: same as adult
> **Protonix** *Tab:* 40 mg ent-coat del-rel
> **Protonix for Oral Suspension** *Oral susp:* 40 mg ent-coat del-rel granules/pkt; mix in 1 tsp apple juice for 5 seconds or sprinkle on 1 tsp apple sauce, and swallow immediately; do not mix in water or any other liquid or food; take approximately 30 minutes prior to a meal; 30 pkt/carton

▷ *rabeprazole* (B)(OTC)(G) *Tab:* 20 mg daily after breakfast; do not crush or chew; *Cap:* open cap and sprinkle contents on a small amount of soft food or liquid
Pediatric: <1 year: not recommended; 1-11 years, <15 kg: 5 mg once daily for up to 12 weeks; ≥12 years, ≥15 kg: same as adult
> **AcipHex** *Tab:* 20 mg ent-coat del-rel
> **AcipHex Sprinkle** *Cap:* 5, 10 mg del-rel

PROTON PUMP INHIBITORS+SODIUM BICARBONATE COMBINATION

▷ *omeprazole+sodium bicarbonate* (B)(G) 20 mg daily; do not crush or chew; max 8 weeks
Pediatric: <18 years: not recommended; ≥18 years: same as adult
> **Zegerid** *Cap:* omep 20 mg+sod bicarb 1100 mg; omep 40 mg+sod bicarb 1100 mg
> **Zegerid OTC (OTC)** *Cap:* omep 20 mg+sod bicarb 1100 mg
> **Zegerid for Oral Suspension** *Pwdr for oral susp:* omep 20 mg+sod bicarb 1680 mg; omep 40 mg+sod bicarb 1680 mg (30 pkt/carton)

PROMOTILITY AGENT

▷ *metoclopramide* (B)(G) 10-15 mg qid 30 minutes ac and HS prn; up to 20 mg prior to provoking situation; max 12 weeks per therapeutic course
Pediatric: <18 years: not recommended; ≥18 years: same as adult
> **Metozolv ODT** *ODT:* 5, 10 mg (mint)
> **Reglan** *Tab:* 5*, 10 mg; *Syr:* 5 mg/5 ml
> **Reglan ODT** *ODT:* 5, 10 mg (orange)
Comment: *Metoclopropamide* is contraindicated when stimulation of GI motility may be dangerous. Observe for tardive dyskinesia and Parkinsonism. Avoid concomitant drugs which may cause an extrapyramidal reaction (e.g., phenothiazines, *haloperidol*).

GAUCHER DISEASE, TYPE 1

Comment: Gaucher disease, type 1 (GD1) is the most common form of Gaucher disease. Like other types of Gaucher disease, GD1 is caused when insufficient glucocerebrosidase (GBA), an enzyme that breaks down glucocerebroside, is produced. Fat-filled Gaucher cells build up in areas like the spleen, liver, and bone marrow. Unlike type 2 and 3, GD1 does not usually involve the central nervous system. Symptoms of GD1 include enlarged spleen and liver, low blood cell counts, bleeding problems, and bone disease. Symptoms can range from mild to severe and may appear anytime from childhood to adulthood. Gaucher disease is caused by mutations in the GBA gene and is inherited as an autosomal-recessive gene. Treatments may include enzyme replacement therapy or medications that affect the making of fatty molecules (substrate reduction therapy). Patients with GD1 are usually able to live a normal lifespan. GD2 is universally fatal within 2 years. Patients with GD3 have a 20-40 year life expectancy.

GLUCOSYLCERAMIDE SYNTHASE INHIBITORS

▷ *miglustat* (C)(G) 100 mg 3 x/day at regular intervals; may reduce dose to 100 mg to once daily or twice a day in some patients due to tremor or diarrhea; *CrCl 50-70 mL/min:* start dose at 100 mg bid; *CrCl 30-50 mL/min:* 100 mg once daily; *CrCl <30 mL/min:* not recommended

   Zavesca Cap 100 mg

   Comment: **Zavesca** *(miglustat)* is a glucosylceramide synthase inhibitor indicated as monotherapy for treatment of adult patients with mild/moderate type 1 Gaucher disease for whom enzyme replacement therapy is not a therapeutic option. The most common adverse reactions (incidence ≥5%) diarrhea, weight loss, stomach pain, gas, nausea, and vomiting headache, including migraine, tremor, leg cramps, dizziness, weakness, vision problems, thrombocytopenia, muscle cramps, back pain, constipation, dry mouth, heaviness in arms and legs, memory loss, unsteady walking, anorexia, indigestion, paresthesia, stomach bloating, stomach pain not related to food, and menstrual changes. Based on animal data, may cause fetal harm. Discontinue **Zavesca** or breastfeeding based on importance of drug to mother.

▷ *penicillamine* administer on an empty stomach, at least 1 hour before meals or 2 hours after meals, and at least 1 hour apart from any other drug, food, milk, antacid, zinc or iron-containing preparation; dosage must be individualized, and may require adjustment during the course of treatment; initially, a single daily dose of 125-250 mg; then, increase at 1-3 month intervals by 125-250 mg/day, as patient response and tolerance indicate; if a satisfactory remission of symptoms is achieved, the dose associated with the remission should be continued as the patient's maintenance therapy; if there is no improvement, and there are no signs of potentially serious toxicity after 2-3 months of treatment with doses of 500-750 mg/day, increase by 250 mg/day at 2-3 month intervals until a satisfactory remission occurs or signs of toxicity develop; if there is no discernible improvement after 3-4 months of treatment with 1000-1500 mg/day, discontinue **Cuprimine**; changes in maintenance dosage levels may not be reflected clinically or in the erythrocyte sedimentation rate (ESR) for 2-3 months after each dosage adjustment

   Cuprimine *Cap:* 125, 250 mg
   Depen: 250 mg

Comment: Taking *penicillamine* on an empty stomach permits maximum absorption and reduces the likelihood of inactivation by metal binding in the GI tract. Optimal dosage can be determined by measurement of urinary copper excretion and the determination of free copper in the serum. The urine must be collected in copper-free glassware, and should be quantitatively analyzed for copper before and soon after initiation of therapy with **Cupramine**. Determination of 24-hour urinary copper excretion is of greatest value in the first week of therapy with *penicillamine*. In the absence of any drug reaction, a dose between 0.75 and 1.5 gm that results in an initial 24-hour cupriuresis of over 2 mg should be continued for about 3 months, by which time the most reliable method of monitoring maintenance treatment is the determination of free copper in the serum. This equals the difference between quantitatively determined total copper and ceruloplasmin-copper. Adequately treated patients will usually have less than 10 mcg free copper/dL of serum. It is seldom necessary to exceed a dosage of 2 gm/day. In patients who cannot tolerate as much as 1 gm/day initially, initiating dosage with 250 mg/day, and increasing gradually to the requisite amount, gives closer control of the effects of the drug and may help to reduce the incidence of adverse reactions. If the patient is intolerant to therapy with **Cuprimine**, alternative treatment is *trientine* (**Syprine**).

The use of *penicillamine* has been associated with fatalities due to certain diseases such as aplastic anemia, agranulocytosis, thrombocytopenia, Goodpasture's syndrome, and myasthenia gravis. Because of the potential for serious hematological and renal adverse reactions to occur at any time, routine urinalysis, white and differential blood cell count, hemoglobin, and direct platelet count must be checked twice weekly, together with monitoring of the patient's skin, lymph nodes and body temperature, during the first month of therapy, every 2 weeks for the next 5 months, and monthly thereafter. Patients should be instructed to report promptly the development of signs and symptoms of granulocytopenia and/or thrombocytopenia such as fever, sore throat, chills, bruising or bleeding; the above laboratory studies should then be promptly repeated.

▷ *trientine* (**G**) recommended initial dose is 500-750 mg/day for pediatric patients and 750-1250 mg/day for adults given in divided doses two, three or four x/day; may be increased to max 2000 mg/day for adults or 1500 mg/day for patients ≤12 years-of-age; the daily dose of **Syprine** should be increased only when the clinical response is not adequate or the concentration of free serum copper is persistently above 20 mcg/dL; optimal long-term maintenance dose should be determined at 6-12 month intervals; administer on an empty stomach, at least 1 hour before meals or 2 hours after meals and at least 1 hour apart from any other drug, food, or milk; swallow whole with water; do not open the cap or chew the contents

Syprine Cap 250 mg

Comment: **Syprine** is indicated in the treatment of patients with Wilson's disease who are intolerant of *penicillamine*. Clinical experience with **Syprine** is limited and alternate dosing regimens have not been well-characterized; all endpoints in determining an individual patient's dose have not been well defined. **Syprine** and *penicillamine* cannot be considered interchangeable. **Syprine** should be used when continued treatment with *penicillamine* is no longer possible because of intolerable or life-endangering side effects. Unlike *penicillamine*, **Syprine** is not recommended in cystinuria or rheumatoid arthritis. The absence of a sulfhydryl moiety renders it incapable of binding cystine and, therefore, it is of no use in cystinuria. In 15 patients with rheumatoid arthritis, **Syprine** was reported not to be effective in improving any clinical or biochemical parameter after 12 weeks of treatment. The most reliable index for monitoring treatment is the determination of free copper in the serum, which equals the difference between quantitatively determined total copper and ceruloplasmin-copper. Adequately treated patients will usually have less than 10 mcg free copper/dL of serum. Therapy may be monitored with a 24-hour urinary copper analysis periodically (i.e., every 6-12 months). Urine must be collected in copper-free glassware. Since a low copper diet should keep copper absorption down to <1 mg a day, the patient probably will be in the desired state of negative copper balance if 0.5 to 1.0 mg of copper is present in a 24-hour collection of urine. In general, mineral supplements should not be used since they may block the absorption of **Syprine**. However, iron deficiency may develop, especially in children and menstruating or pregnant females, or as a result of the low copper diet recommended for Wilson's disease. If necessary, iron may be given in short courses, but since iron and **Syprine** each inhibit absorption of the other, 2 hours should elapse between administration of **Syprine** and iron. *trientine* was teratogenic in animals at doses similar to the human dose. The frequencies of both resorptions and fetal abnormalities, including hemorrhage and edema, increased while fetal copper levels decreased when *trientine* was given in the maternal diets. There are no adequate and well-controlled studies in pregnant females. **Syprine** should be used during pregnancy only if the potential benefit justifies the potential risk to the fetus. It is not known whether this drug is excreted in human milk. Caution should be exercised when **Syprine** is administered to a nursing mother. Clinical studies of **Syprine** did not include sufficient numbers of subjects ≥65 years-of-age to determine whether they respond differently from younger subjects. Other reported clinical experience is insufficient to determine differences in responses between the elderly and younger patients. In general, dose selection should be cautious, usually starting at the low end of the dosing range, reflecting the greater frequency of decreased hepatic, renal, or cardiac function, and of concomitant disease or other drug therapy. Clinical experience with **Syprine** has been limited. The following adverse reactions have been reported in a clinical study in patients with Wilson's disease who were on therapy with *trientine:* iron deficiency, systemic lupus erythematosus. In addition, the following adverse reactions have been reported in marketed use: dystonia, muscular spasm, myasthenia gravis.

GIANT CELL ARTERITIS (GCA)/TEMPORAL ARTERITIS

Acetaminophen for IV Infusion *see Pain*
NSAIDs *see* Appendix J. NSAIDs online at https://connect.springerpub.com/content/reference-book/978-0-8261-7935-7/back-matter/part02/back-matter/bmatter10
Opioid Analgesics *see Pain*
Topical & Transdermal Analgesics *see Pain*
Parenteral Corticosteroids *see* Appendix M. Parenteral Corticosteroids
Oral Corticosteroids *see* Appendix L. Oral Corticosteroids

Comment: Giant cell arteritis (GCA), or temporal arteritis, is a systemic inflammatory vasculitis of unknown etiology that occurs in persons ≥50 years-of-age (median age of onset is 75 years) and can result in a wide variety of systemic, neurologic, and ophthalmologic complications. GCA is the most common form of systemic vasculitis in adults. Other names for GCA include arteritis cranialis, Horton disease, granulomatous arteritis, and arteritis of the aged. GCA typically affects the superficial temporal arteries—hence the term temporal arteritis. In addition, GCA most commonly affects the ophthalmic, occipital, vertebral, posterior ciliary, and proximal vertebral arteries. It has also been shown to involve medium- and large-sized vessels, including the aorta and the carotid, subclavian, and iliac arteries. Common early symptoms include headache and visual difficulties. Potential consequences include blindness and aortic aneurysms. Newly recognized GCA should be considered a true neuro-ophthalmic emergency. Prompt initiation of treatment may prevent blindness and other potentially irreversible ischemic sequelae. Corticosteroids are the mainstay of therapy. In steroid-resistant cases, drugs such as *cyclosporine*, *azathioprine*, or *methotrexate* (MTX) may be used as steroid-sparing agents. GCA is the most common systemic vasculitis affecting elderly patients.

INTERLEUKIN-6 RECEPTOR ANTAGONIST

▷ *tocilizumab* (B) *<100 kg:* 162 mg SC every other week on the same day followed by an increase according to clinical response; *≥100 kg:* 162 mg SC once weekly on the same day; SC injections may be self-administered
   Actemra *Vial:* 80 mg/4 ml, 200 mg/10 ml, 400 mg/20 ml, single-use, for IV infusion after dilution; *Prefilled syringe:* 162 mg (0.9 mL, single-dose)

Comment: **Actemra** received FDA approval in May 2017 to treat GCA. This is the first FDA-approved drug specifically for the treatment of this form of vasculitis. *tocilizumab* is an interleukin-6 receptor-α inhibitor also indicated for use in moderate-to-severe rheumatoid arthritis (RA) that has not responded to conventional therapy, and some subtypes of juvenile idiopathic arthritis (JIA). **Actemra** may be used alone or in combination with *methotrexate* (MTX) and in RA, other DMARDs may be used. Monitor patient for dose-related laboratory changes including elevated LFTs, neutropenia, and thrombocytopenia. **Actemra** should not be initiated in patients with an absolute neutrophil count (ANC) <2000/mm³, platelet count <100,000/mm³, or who have ALT or AST above 1.5 times the upper limit of normal (ULN). Registration in the Pregnancy Exposure Registry (1-877-311-8972) is encouraged for monitoring pregnancy outcomes in women exposed to **Atemra** during pregnancy. The limited available data with **Actemra** in pregnant females are not sufficient to determine whether there is a drug-associated risk for major birth defects and miscarriage. Monoclonal antibodies, such as *tocilizumab*, are actively transported across the placenta during the third trimester of pregnancy and may affect immune response in the infant exposed *in utero*. It is not known whether *tocilizumab* passes into breast milk; therefore, breastfeeding is not recommended while using **Actemra**.

GIARDIASIS (*GIARDIA LAMBLIA*)

▷ *metronidazole* (not for use in 1st; B in 2nd, 3rd)(G) 250 mg tid x 5-10 days
Pediatric: 35-50 mg/kg/day in 3 divided doses x 10 days
   Flagyl *Tab:* 250*, 500*mg
   Flagyl 375 *Cap:* 375 mg
   Flagyl ER *Tab:* 750 mg ext-rel
▷ *tinidazole* (C) 2 gm in a single dose; take with food
Pediatric: <3 years: not recommended; ≥3 years: 50 mg/kg daily in a single dose; take with food; max 2 gm
   Tindamax *Tab:* 250*, 500*mg
   Comment: Other than for use in the treatment of *giardiasis* and *amebiasis* in pediatric patients older than 3 years-of-age, safety and effectiveness of *tinidazole* in pediatric patients have not been established. *tinidazole* is excreted in breast milk in concentrations similar to those seen in serum and can be detected in breast milk for up to 72 hours following administration. Interruption of breastfeeding is recommended during *tinidazole* therapy and for 3 days following the last dose.
▷ *nitazoxanide* (B)(G) 500 mg q 12 hours x 3 days; take with food
Pediatric: <1 year: not recommended; 1-3 years; 100 mg q 12 hours x 3 days; 4-11 years: 200 mg q 12 hours x 3 days; ≥12 years: same as adult
   Alinia *Tab:* 500 mg; *Oral susp:* 100 mg/5 ml (60 ml)
   Comment: **Alinia** is an antiprotozoal for the treatment of diarrhea due to *G. lamblia* or *C. parvum*.

GINGIVITIS/PERIODONTITIS

ANTI-INFECTIVE ORAL RINSES
Comment: Oral treatments should be preceded by brushing and flossing the teeth. Avoid foods and liquids for 2-3 hours after a treatment.
▷ *chlorhexidine gluconate* (B)(G) swish 15 ml undiluted for 30 seconds bid; do not swallow; do not rinse mouth after treatment.
   Peridex, PerioGard *Oral soln:* 0.12% (480 ml)

GLAUCOMA: OPEN ANGLE/OCULAR HYPERTENSION

Comment: Other ophthalmic medications should <u>not</u> be administered within 5-10 minutes of administering an ophthalmic antiglaucoma medication. Contact lenses should be removed prior to instillation of antiglaucoma medications and may be replaced 15 minutes later. Interactions with ophthalmic anti-glaucoma agents include MAOIs, CNS depressants, beta-blockers, tricyclic antidepressants, and hypoglycemics. Choices for medical treatment in progressive cases include *betaxolol* eye drops, which have a beneficial effect on optic nerve blood flow in addition to intraocular pressure IOP reduction. Other beta blockers and adrenergic drugs (such as *dipivefrine*) should better be avoided because of the probability of nocturnal systemic hypotension and optic nerve hypoperfusion (e.g., in patients with untreated obstructive sleep apnea). Prostaglandin derivatives tend to have greater IOP-lowering effect which may be of overriding consideration. *dorzolamide-timolol* fixed combination is a safe and effective IOP-lowering agent in patients with normal tension glaucoma (NTG). *Brimonidine* significantly improved retinal vascular autoregulation in NTG patients.

OPHTHALMIC ALPHA-2 ADRENERGIC RECEPTOR AGONISTS

Comment: Ophthalmic alpha-2 agonists are contraindicated with concomitant MAOI use. Cautious use with CNS depressants, beta-blockers (ocular and systemic), antihypertensives, cardiac glycosides, and tricyclic antidepressants.
▸ *apraclonidine* ophthalmic solution (C) 1-2 drops affected eye tid
  Pediatric: <12 years: not recommended; ≥12 years: same as adult
    Iopidine *Ophth soln:* 0.5% (5 ml) (benzalkonium chloride)
▸ *brimonidine tartrate* ophthalmic solution (B) 1 drop affected eye q 8 hours
  Pediatric: <2 years: not recommended; ≥2 years: 1 drop affected eye q 8 hours
    Alphagan P *Ophth soln:* 0.1, 0.15% (5, 10, 15 ml) (purite)

OPHTHALMIC CARBONIC ANHYDRASE INHIBITORS

Comment: Ophthalmic carbonic anhydrase inhibitors are contraindicated in patients with sulfa allergy.
▸ *brinzolamide* (G) ophthalmic suspension (C) 1 drop affected eye tid
  Pediatric: <12 years: not recommended; ≥12 years: same as adult
    Azopt *Ophth susp:* 1% (2.5, 5, 10, 15 ml) (benzalkonium chloride)
▸ *dorzolamide* ophthalmic solution (C)(G) 1 drop affected eye tid
  Pediatric: same as adult
    Trusopt *Ophth soln:* 2% (10 ml) (benzalkonium chloride)

OPHTHALMIC ALPHA-2 ADRENERGIC RECEPTOR AGONIST+CARBONIC ANHYDRASE INHIBITOR

▸ *brimonidine+brinzolamide* (C) 1 drop affected eye tid
  Pediatric: <12 years: not recommended; ≥12 years: same as adult
    Simbrinza *Ophth soln:* brim 1% mg+brinz 0.2% per ml (10 ml)

OPHTHALMIC CHOLINERGICS (MIOTICS)

▸ *carbachol+hydroxypropyl methylcellulose* ophthalmic solution (C) 2 drops affected eye tid
  Pediatric: <12 years: not recommended; ≥12 years: same as adult
    Isopto Carbachol *Ophth soln:* carb 0.75% <u>or</u> 2.25%+hydroxy 1% (15 ml); carb 1.5% <u>or</u> 3%+hydroxy 1% (15, 30 ml) (benzalkonium chloride)
▸ *pilocarpine* (C)(G)
  Pediatric: <12 years: not recommended; ≥12 years: same as adult
    Isopto Carpine 2 drops affected eye tid-qid
      Ophth soln: 1, 2, 4% (15 ml) (benzalkonium chloride)

Ocusert Pilo change ophthalmic insert once weekly
Ophth inserts: 20 mcg/Hr (8/pck)
Pilocar Ophthalmic Solution 1-2 drops affected eye 1-6 x/day
Ophth soln: 0.5, 1, 2, 3, 4, 6, 8% (15 ml)
Pilopine HS apply 1/2 inch ribbon in lower conjunctival sac q HS
Opth gel: 4% (4 gm)

OPHTHALMIC CHOLINESTERASE INHIBITORS

▷ *demecarium bromide* ophthalmic solution (X) 1-2 drops affected eye q 12-48 hours
Pediatric: <12 years: not recommended; ≥12 years: same as adult
Humorsol Ocumeter *Ophth soln:* 0.125, 0.25% (5 ml)
▷ *echothiophate iodide* ophthalmic solution (C) initially 1 drop of 0.03% affected eye bid; then increase strength as needed
Pediatric: <12 years: not recommended; ≥12 years: same as adult
Phospholine Iodide *Ophth soln:* 0.03, 0.06, 0.125, 0.25% (5 ml)

OPHTHALMIC CARDIOSELECTIVE BETA-BLOCKERS

Comment: Ophthalmic beta-blockers are generally contraindicated in severe COPD, history of or current bronchial asthma, sinus bradycardia, 2nd or 3rd degree AV block.
▷ *betaxolol* ophthalmic solution (C)(G) 1-2 drops affected eye bid
Pediatric: <12 years: not recommended; ≥12 years: same as adult
Betoptic *Ophth soln:* 0.5% (5, 10, 15 ml) (benzalkonium chloride)
Betoptic S *Ophth soln:* 0.25% (2.5, 5, 10, 15 ml) (benzalkonium chloride)

OPHTHALMIC BETA-BLOCKERS (NON-CARDIOSELECTIVE)

Comment: Ophthalmic beta-blockers are generally contraindicated in severe COPD, history of or current bronchial asthma, sinus bradycardia, 2nd or 3rd degree AV block.
▷ *carteolol* ophthalmic solution (C)(G) 1 drop affected eye bid
Pediatric: <12 years: not recommended; ≥12 years: same as adult
Ocupress *Ophth soln:* 1% (5, 10, 15 ml) (benzalkonium chloride)
▷ *levobunolol* ophthalmic solution (C) 1-2 drops affected eye bid
Pediatric: <12 years: not recommended; ≥12 years: same as adult
Betagan *Ophth soln:* 0.5% (5, 10, 15 ml) (benzalkonium chloride)
▷ *metipranolol* ophthalmic solution (C)(G) 1 drop affected eye bid
Pediatric: <12 years: not recommended; ≥12 years: same as adult
OptiPranolol *Ophth soln:* 0.3% (5, 10 ml) (benzalkonium chloride)
▷ *timolol* ophthalmic solution and gel (C)(G)
Pediatric: <12 years: not recommended; ≥12 years: same as adult
Betimol 1 drop affected eye bid
Ophth soln: 0.25, 0.5% (5, 10, 15 ml) (benzalkonium chloride)
Istalol 1 drop affected eye daily
Ophth soln: 0.5% (2.5, 5 ml) (preservative-free)
Timoptic 1 drop affected eye bid
Ophth soln: 0.25, 0.5% (5, 10, 15 ml) (benzalkonium chloride)
Timoptic Ocudose 1 drop bid
Ophth soln: 0.25, 0.5% (0.2 ml/dose, 60 dose) (preservative-free)
Timoptic-XE 1 drop affected eye bid
Ophth gel: 0.25, 0.5% (2.5, 5 ml) (preservative-free)

OPHTHALMIC ALPHA-2 ADRENERGIC RECEPTOR AGONIST+ NON-CARDIOSELECTIVE BETA-BLOCKER COMBINATION

Comment: Generally contraindicated in severe COPD, history of or current bronchial asthma, sinus bradycardia, and 2nd or 3rd degree AV block.

▷ *brimonidine tartrate+timolol* ophthalmic solution (C) 1 drop affected eye bid
  Pediatric: <2 years: not recommended; ≥2 years: same as adult
    Combigan *Ophth soln:* brimo 0.2%+timo 0.5% (5, 10, 15 ml)
    (benzalkonium chloride)

OPHTHALMIC PROSTAMIDE ANALOGS

▷ *bimatoprost* ophthalmic solution (C)(G) 1 drop q affected eye HS
  Pediatric: <16 years: not recommended; ≥16 years: same as adult
    Lumigan *Ophth soln:* 0.01, 0.03% (2.5, 5, 7.5 ml) (benzalkonium chloride)
▷ *latanoprost* ophthalmic solution (C) 1 drop affected eye q HS
  Pediatric: <12 years: not recommended; ≥12 years: same as adult
    Xalatan *Ophth soln:* 0.005% (2.5 ml) (benzalkonium chloride)
▷ *tafluprost* ophthalmic solution (C)(G) 1 drop affected eye q HS
  Pediatric: <12 years: not recommended; ≥12 years: same as adult
    Zioptan *Ophth soln:* 0.0015% (0.3 ml single-use, 30-60/carton)
    (preservative-free)
▷ *travoprost* ophthalmic solution (C)(G) 1 drop affected eye q HS
  Pediatric: <16 years: not recommended; ≥16 years: same as adult
    Travatan *Ophth soln:* 0.004% (2.5, 5 ml) (benzalkonium chloride)
    Travatan Z *Ophth soln:* 0.004% (2.5, 5 ml) (boric acid, propylene glycol,
    sorbitol, zinc chloride)

PROSTAGLANDIN F$_{2\alpha}$ ANALOG

▷ *latanoprost* I drop in the affected eye(s) in the evening
    Xelpros *Ophth emul:* 0.005% (2.5 ml) (potassium sorbate 0.47%)
    Comment: *Latanoprost* can cause pigmentation of the iris, periorbital tissue
    (eyelid), and eyelashes (iris pigmentation likely to be permanent) and gradual
    changes to eyelashes including increased length, thickness, and number of lashes
    (usually reversible).

PROSTAGLANDIN ANALOG (WITH NITRIC OXIDE METABOLITE)

▷ *latanoprostene bunod* ophthalmic solution (C) ≤16 years: not recommended
  (because of potential safety concerns related to increased pigmentation following
  long-term chronic use); >16 years: 1 drop affected eye once daily
    Vyzulta *Ophth soln:* 0.024% (5 ml) (benzalkonium chloride)
    Comment: **Vyzulta** is a prostaglandin analog with nitric oxide as one of its
    metabolites. **Vyzulta** exerts a dual mechanism of action through latanoprost
    acid and butanediol mononitrate, working in the uveoscleral pathway and
    Schlemm's canal. Most common ocular adverse reactions with incidence
    ≥ 2% are conjunctival hyperemia (6%), eye irritation (4%), eye pain (3%),
    and instillation site pain (2%). There may be increased pigmentation of
    the iris and periorbital tissue. Iris pigmentation is likely to be permanent.
    There may be gradual changes to eyelashes including increased length,
    increased thickness, and number of eyelashes, that is usually reversible upon
    discontinuation of treatment. There are no available human data for the use
    of **Vyzulta** during pregnancy to inform any drug associated risks. There are
    no data on the presence of **Vyzulta** in human milk or effects on the breastfed
    infant.

OPHTHALMIC RHO KINASE INHIBITOR

▷ *netarsudil* ophthalmic solution (C) 1 drop affected eye once daily in the PM
  Pediatric: <18 years: not established; ≥18 years: same as adult
    Rhopressa *Ophth soln:* 0.02% (0.2 mg/ml, 2.5 ml) (benzalkonium chloride)

OPHTHALMIC RHO KINASE INHIBITOR+PROSTAGLANDIN F2α ANALOGUE COMBINATION

▷ *netarsudil+latanoprost* ophthalmic solution 1 drop in the affected eye(s) once daily in the evening

Pediatric: safety and efficacy not established

Rocklatan *Ophth soln:* netar 0.2 mg (0.02%) + latan 0.05 mg (0.005%) per ml (2.5 ml)

Comment: **Rocklatan** *(netarsudil and latanoprost ophthalmic solution)* is a fixed-dose combination ophthalmic solution of the Rho kinase inhibitor *netarsudil* (**Rhopressa**) and the prostaglandin analog *latanoprost* (**Xalatan**) indicated to reduce elevated intraocular pressure (IOP) in patients with open-angle glaucoma or ocular hypertension. Inform patients that pigmentation of the iris, periorbital tissue (eyelid) and eyelashes can occur. Iris pigmentation likely to be permanent. Gradual change to eyelashes including increased length, thickness and number of lashes can occur, which is usually reversible. *In vitro* studies have shown that precipitation occurs when eye drops containing thimerosal are mixed with *latanoprost* 0.005%. If such drugs are used, they should be administered at least 5 minutes apart. The most common adverse reaction is conjunctival hyperemia (incidence 59%). Other common adverse reactions have been instillation site pain (20%), corneal verticillata (15%), and conjunctival hemorrhage (11%). No overall differences in safety or effectiveness have been observed between elderly and other adult patients.

OPHTHALMIC SYMPATHOMIMETICS

Comment: Contraindicated in narrow-angle glaucoma. Use with caution in cardiovascular disease, hypertension, hyperthyroidism, diabetes, and asthma.

▷ *dipivefrin* ophthalmic solution (**B**) 1 drop affected eye q 12 hours

Propine *Ophth soln:* 0.1% (5, 10, 15 ml) (benzalkonium chloride)

OPHTHALMIC CARBONIC ANHYDRASE INHIBITOR+NON-CARDIOSELECTIVE BETA-BLOCKER

▷ *dorzolamide+timolol* ophthalmic solution (**C**) 1 drop affected eye bid

Pediatric: <12 years: not recommended; ≥12 years: same as adult

Cosopt *Ophth soln:* dorz 2%+tim 0.5% (10 ml) (benzalkonium chloride)

Cosopt PF *Ophth soln:* dorz 2%+tim 0.5% (10 ml) (preservative-free)

OPHTHALMIC SYNTHETIC DOCOSANOID

▷ *unoprostone isopropyl* ophthalmic solution (**C**) 1 drop affected eye bid

Pediatric: <12 years: not recommended; ≥12 years: same as adult

Rescula *Ophth soln:* 0.15% (5 ml) (benzalkonium chloride)

ORAL CARBONIC ANHYDRASE INHIBITORS

▷ *acetazolamide* (**C**) 250-1000 mg/day in divided doses or 500 mg bid sust-rel tabs; max 1 gm/day

Pediatric: <12 years: not recommended; ≥12 years: same as adult

Diamox *Tab:* 125*, 250*mg

Diamox Sequels *Tab:* 500 mg sust-rel

▷ *methazolamide* (**C**)(**G**) 50-100 mg bid-tid times daily

Pediatric: <12 years: not recommended; ≥12 years: same as adult

Neptazane *Tab:* 25, 50 mg

Comment: Administer ophthalmic osmotic and miotic agents concomitantly.

◯ GONORRHEA (*NEISSERIA GONORRHOEAE*)

Comment: The following treatment regimens for *N. gonorrhoeae* are published in the 2015 CDC Transmitted Diseases Treatment Guidelines. Treatment regimens are presented by generic drug name first, followed by information about brands and dose forms. Empiric treatment requires concomitant treatment of chlamydia. Treat all sexual contacts. Patients who are HIV-positive should receive the same treatment as those who are HIV-negative. Sexual abuse must be considered a cause of gonococcal infection in pre-adolescent children.

RECOMMENDED REGIMENS, ≥12 YEARS: UNCOMPLICATED INFECTIONS OF THE CERVIX, URETHRA, AND RECTUM
Regimen 1
▷ *ceftriaxone* 250 mg IM in a single dose
    plus
▷ *azithromycin* 1 gm in a single dose

Regimen 2
▷ *ceftriaxone* 250 mg IM in a single dose
    plus
▷ *doxycycline* 100 mg bid x 7 days

RECOMMENDED REGIMENS, ≥12 YEARS: UNCOMPLICATED INFECTIONS OF THE PHARYNX
Regimen 1
▷ *ceftriaxone* 250 mg IM in a single dose
    plus
▷ *azithromycin* 1 gm in a single dose

Regimen 2
▷ *ceftriaxone* 250 mg IM in a single dose
    plus
▷ *doxycycline* 100 mg bid x 7 days

RECOMMENDED REGIMENS, CHILDREN ≥45 KG, ≥8 YEARS; UNCOMPLICATED INFECTIONS OF THE CERVIX, URETHRA, AND RECTUM
Regimen 1
▷ *ceftriaxone* 250 mg IM in a single dose
    plus
▷ *azithromycin* 1 gm in a single dose

RECOMMENDED REGIMEN: CHILDREN >45 KG
Regimen 1
▷ *ceftriaxone* 250 mg IM in a single dose

RECOMMENDED REGIMEN: CHILDREN >45 KG WHO HAVE GONOCOCCAL BACTEREMIA OR GONOCOCCAL ARTHRITIS
Regimen 1
▷ *ceftriaxone* 50 mg/kg IM or IV in a single dose daily x 7 days

RECOMMENDED REGIMENS, CHILDREN <45 KG, <8 YEARS: UNCOMPLICATED GONOCOCCAL VULVOVAGINITIS, CERVICITIS, URETHRITIS, PHARYNGITIS, OR PROCTITIS
Regimen 1
▷ *ceftriaxone* 250 mg IM in a single dose

RECOMMENDED REGIMEN, CHILDREN <45 KG, <8 YEARS: GONOCOCCAL BACTEREMIA OR ARTHRITIS

Regimen 1

▷ *ceftriaxone* 50 mg/kg (max dose 1 gm) IM or IV in a single dose daily x 7 days

DRUG BRANDS AND DOSE FORMS

▷ *azithromycin* (B)(G)

Zithromax *Tab*: 250, 500, 600 mg; *Oral susp*: 100 mg/5 ml (15 ml); 200 mg/5 ml (15, 22.5, 30 ml) (cherry); *Pkt*: 1 gm for reconstitution (cherry-banana)

Zithromax Tri-pak *Tab*: 3 x 500 mg tabs/pck

Zithromax Z-pak *Tab*: 6 x 250 mg tabs/pck

Zmax *Oral susp*: 2 gm ext-rel for reconstitution (cherry-banana) (148 mg Na$^+$)

▷ *ceftriaxone* (B)(G)

Rocephin *Vial*: 250, 500 mg; 1, 2 gm

▷ *doxycycline* (D)(G)

Acticlate *Tab*: 75, 150**mg

Adoxa *Tab*: 50, 75, 100, 150 mg ent-coat

Doryx *Tab*: 50, 75, 100, 150, 200 mg del-rel

Doxteric *Tab*: 50 mg del-rel

Monodox *Cap*: 50, 75, 100 mg

Oracea *Cap*: 40 mg del-rel

Vibramycin *Tab*: 100 mg; *Cap*: 50, 100 mg; *Syr*: 50 mg/5 ml (raspberry-apple) (sulfites); *Oral susp*: 25 mg/5 ml (raspberry)

Vibra-Tab *Tab*: 100 mg film-coat

ALTERNATE THERAPY

▷ *azithromycin* (B)(G) 2 gm x 1 dose

Pediatric: not recommended for treatment of gonorrhea in children

Zithromax *Tab*: 250, 500, 600 mg; *Oral susp*: 100 mg/5 ml (15 ml); 200 mg/5 ml (15, 22.5, 30 ml) (cherry); *Pkt*: 1 gm for reconstitution (cherry-banana)

Zithromax Tri-pak *Tab*: 3 x 500 mg tabs/pck

Zithromax Z-pak *Tab*: 6 x 250 mg tabs/pck

Zmax *Oral susp*: 2 gm ext-rel for reconstitution (cherry-banana) (148 mg Na$^+$)

▷ *cefotaxime* 500 mg IM x 1 dose

Claforan *Vial*: 500 mg; 1, 2 gm

▷ *cefotetan* 1 gm IM x 1 dose

Pediatric: <12 years: not recommended; ≥12 years: same as adult

Cefotan *Vial*: 1, 2 gm

▷ *cefoxitin* (B) 2 gm IM x 1 dose

Pediatric: <3 months: not recommended; ≥3 months: same as adult

Mefoxin *Vial*: 1, 2 gm

plus

▷ *probenecid* (B)(G)

Benemid 1 gm 30 minutes before *cefoxitin*

Pediatric: <2 years: not recommended; 2-14 years: 25 mg/kg 30 minutes before *cefoxitin*; ≥14 years: same as adult

Tab: 500*mg; *Cap*: 500 mg

▷ *cefpodoxime proxetil* (B) 200 mg x 1 dose

Pediatric: <2 months: not recommended; 2 months-12 years: 10 mg/kg/day (max 400 mg/dose) or 5 mg/kg/day bid (max 200 mg/dose)

Vantin *Tab*: 100, 200 mg; *Oral susp*: 50, 100 mg/5 ml (50, 75, 100 mg) (lemon creme)

▷ *ceftizoxime* (B) 1 gm IM x 1 dose
   Pediatric: <6 months: not recommended; ≥6 months: same as adult
      Cefizox *Vial:* 500 mg; 1, 2, 10 g
▷ *demeclocycline* (X) 600 mg initially, followed by 300 mg q 12 hours x 4 days
   (total 3 gm)
   Pediatric: <8 years: not recommended; ≥8 years: same as adult
      Declomycin *Tab:* 300 mg
▷ *enoxacin* (C) 400 mg x 1 dose
   Pediatric: <18 years: not recommended; ≥18 years: same as adult
      Penetrex *Tab:* 200, 400 mg
▷ *imipramine* (C) 400 mg x 1 dose
   Pediatric: <18 years: not recommended; ≥18 years: same as adult
      Maxaquin *Tab:* 400 mg
▷ *norfloxacin* (C) 800 mg x 1 dose
   Pediatric: <18 years: not recommended; ≥18 years: same as adult
      Noroxin *Tab:* 400 mg
▷ *spectinomycin* (B) 2 gm IM x 1 dose
   Pediatric: 40 mg/kg IM x 1 dose
      Trobicin *Vial:* 2 gm

GOUT (HYPERURICEMIA)

Pseudogout *see* Pseudogout
Acetaminophen for IV Infusion *see* **Pain**
NSAIDs *see* Appendix J. NSAIDs online at https://connect.springerpub.com/content/
reference-book/978-0-8261-7935-7/back-matter/part02/back-matter/bmatter10
Opioid Analgesics *see* **Pain**
Topical & Transdermal Analgesics *see* **Pain**
Parenteral Corticosteroids *see* Appendix M. Parenteral Corticosteroids
Oral Corticosteroids *see* Appendix L. Oral Corticosteroids

XANTHINE OXIDASE INHIBITORS (PROPHYLAXIS)

▷ *allopurinol* (C)(G) initially 100 mg daily; increase by 100 mg weekly; max 800
   mg/day and 300 mg/dose; usual range for mild symptoms 200-300 mg/day; for
   severe symptoms 400-600 mg/day; take with food
   Pediatric: <6 years: max 150 mg/day; 6-10 years: max 400 mg/day; max single
   dose 300 mg; >10 years: same as adult
      Zyloprim *Tab:* 100*, 300*mg
      Comment: Do <u>not</u> take *allopurinol* concurrent with *colchicine*. Gout flares
      may occur after initiation of urate lowering therapy, such as allopurinol, due
      to changing serum uric acid concentrations resulting in mobilization of urate
      from tissue deposits. If a gout flare occurs during treatment, allopurinol does
      <u>not</u> need to be discontinued. Manage the flare concurrently, as appropriate for
      the individual patient. The correct dose and frequency of dosage for maintaining
      the serum uric acid concentration within the normal range are best determined
      by using the serum uric acid concentration as an index. Allopurinol is <u>not</u>
      recommended for the treatment of asymptomatic hyperuricemia. Discontinue
      allopurinol when the potential for overproduction of uric acid is no longer
      present.

ACUTE ATTACK

▷ *colchicine* (C)(G) 0.6-1.2 mg at first sign of attack; then 0.6 mg every hour <u>or</u> 1.2
   mg every 2 hours until pain relief; then consider 0.6 mg/day <u>or</u> every other day
   for maintenance

Pediatric: <12 years: not recommended; ≥12 years: same as adult

    Colcrys *Tab:* 0.6 mg

    Gloperba *Oral soln:* 0.6 mg/5 ml (150 ml) (cherry odor)

    Mitigare *Cap:* 0.6 mg

Comment: Do not take *colchicine* concurrently with *allopurinol*.

▶ *febuxostat* (C)(G) initially 40 mg daily; after 2 weeks, may increase to 80 mg daily.

Pediatric: <18 years: not recommended; ≥18 years: same as adult

    Uloric *Tab:* 40, 80 mg

Comment: Gout flare prophylaxis with *colchicine* or NSAID is recommended on initiation of *febuxostat* (**Uloric**) and up to 6 months. In a recent report of research, gout patients with established cardiovascular (CV) disease treated with **Uloric** had a higher rate of CV death as compared to those treated with *allopurinol*. Therefore, the FDA issued a new BBW (black box warning) to consider the risks and benefits of **Uloric** when deciding to prescribe or continue patients on **Uloric**. Further, **Uloric** should only be used in patients who have an inadequate response to a maximally titrated dose of *allopurinol*, who are intolerant to *allopurinol*, or for whom treatment with *allopurinol* is not advisable.

PEGYLATED URIC ACID SPECIFIC ENZYME

▶ *pegloticase* (C) pre-medicate with antihistamine and corticosteroid; 8 mg once every 2 weeks; administer IV infusion after dilution over at least 2 hours; observe at least 1 hour post-infusion

Pediatric: <18 years: not recommended; ≥18 years: same as adult

    Krystexxa *Vial:* 8 mg/ml (1 ml) single-use pwdr for IV infusion after dilution

    Comment: Slow rate, or stop and restart at lower rate, if infusion reaction occurs (e.g., **Krystexxa** is contraindicated with G6PD deficiency; screen patients of African or Mediterranean descent). **Krystexxa** is not for the treatment of asymptomatic hyperuricemia.

URICOSURIC AGENT

▶ *probenecid* (C)(G) 250 mg bid x 1 week; maintenance 500 mg bid

Pediatric: <18 years: not recommended; ≥18 years: same as adult

    Tab: 500*mg; *Cap:* 500 mg

Comment: Avoid concomitant use of *probenecid* and salicylates.

URICOSURIC+ANTI-INFLAMMATORY COMBINATIONS

▶ *probenecid+colchicine* (G) 1 tab once daily x 1 week; then, 1 tab bid thereafter

Pediatric: <18 years: not recommended; ≥18 years: same as adult

    Tab: prob 500 mg+colch 0.5 mg

Comment: *Probenecid+colchicine* is contraindicated in the treatment of acute gout attack, patients with blood dyscrasias, and patients with uric acid kidney stones. Concomitant salicylates antagonize the uricosuric effects.

▶ *sulfinpyrazone* (C) initially 200-400 mg bid; may gradually increase to 800 mg bid

Pediatric: <18 years: not recommended; ≥18 years: same as adult

    Anturane *Cap:* 100, 200 mg

Comment: Goal is serum uric acid <6.5 mg/dL.

XANTHINE OXIDASE INHIBITOR

▶ *febuxostat* (C) 40 mg once daily x 2 weeks; if serum uric acid is not <6 mg/dL, may increase to 80 mg once daily

Pediatric: <18 years: not established; ≥18 years: same as adult

    Uloric *Tab:* 40, 80 mg

Comment: Gout flare prophylaxis with *colchicine* or NSAID is recommended on initiation of *febuxostat* **Uloric** and up to 6 months. In a recent report of research, gout patients with established cardiovascular (CV) disease treated with *feboxostat* **Uloric** had a higher rate of CV death as compared to those treated with *allopurinol*. Therefore, the FDA issued a new BBW (black box warning) to consider the risks and benefits of **Uloric** when deciding to prescribe or continue patients on **Uloric**. Further, **Uloric** should only be used in patients who have an inadequate response to a maximally titrated dose of *allopurinol*, who are intolerant to *allopurinol*, or for whom treatment with *allopurinol* is not advisable.

XANTHINE OXIDASE INHIBITOR+URATI INHIBITOR COMBINATION

▷ *allopurinol+lesinurad* take 1 tab once daily
 Pediatric: <18 years: not established; ≥18 years: same as adult
   Duzallo *Tab:* 200/200, 300/200 mg
   Comment: The US Food and Drug Administration recently approved **Duzallo** for the treatment of hyperuricemia associated with gout in patients who have not achieved target serum uric acid (sUA) levels with *allopurinol* alone. **Duzallo** is the first drug to combine *allopurinol*, the current standard of care for hyperuricemia associated with gout, and *lesinurad*, the most recent FDA-approved treatment for this condition. The fixed-dose combination addresses the overproduction and underexcretion of serum uric acid. Patients with asymptomatic hyperuricemia are not recommended to receive **Duzallo**. Common adverse reactions associated with **Duzallo** include headache, influenza, higher levels of blood creatinine, and heart burn. In addition, **Duzallo** has a boxed warning for the risk of acute renal failure associated with *lesinurad*. There are no available human data on use of **Duzallo** or *lesinurad* in pregnancy to inform a drug-associated risk of adverse developmental outcomes. Limited published data on *allopurinol* use in pregnancy do not demonstrate a clear pattern or increase in frequency of adverse development outcomes. There is no information regarding the presence of **Duzallo** or *lesinurad* in human milk or the effects on the breastfed infant. Based on information from a single case report, *allopurinol* and its active metabolite, *oxypurinol*, were detected in the milk of a mother at 5 weeks postpartum. The effect of *allopurinol* on the breastfed infant is unknown. CrCl 45-< 60 mL/min: adjust the allopurinol to a medically appropriate dose (200 mg). CrCl <45, *allopurinol* not recommended. Max *lesinurad* 200 mg/day. In clinical trials evaluating the safety and efficacy of this combined therapy among adult patients with gout who failed to achieve target sUA levels on *allopurinol* alone, **Duzallo** was found to nearly double the number of patients who achieved target sUA at 6 months, mean sUA was reduced to less than 6 mg/dL by 1 month, and this level was maintained through 12 months.

SELECTIVE URIC ACID REABSORPTION INHIBITOR (SURI)

▷ *lesinurad* (C) 200 mg once daily in combination with a xanthine oxidase inhibitor (XOI)
 Pediatric: <18 years: not established; ≥18 years: same as adult
   Zurampic *Tab:* 200 mg
   Comment: **Zurampic** inhibits URATI, a urate transporter, which is responsible for the majority of renal absorption of uric acid and (OAT) 4, organic anion transporter, a uric acid transporter involved in diuretic-induced hyperuricemia. Do not use as monotherapy. Use in combination with an XOI, such as *allopurinol* or *febuxostat* to reduce the production of uric acid. Do not initiate if CrCl <45 mL/min, ESRD, dialysis, or kidney transplant.

GOUTY ARTHRITIS

See **Gout (Hyperuricemia)** for gout management drugs
Acetaminophen for IV Infusion *see Pain*
NSAIDs *see* Appendix J. NSAIDs online at https://connect.springerpub.com/content/reference-book/978-0-8261-7935-7/back-matter/part02/back-matter/bmatter10
Opioid Analgesics *see Pain*
Topical & Transdermal Analgesics *see Pain*
Parenteral Corticosteroids *see* Appendix M. Parenteral Corticosteroids
Oral Corticosteroids *see* Appendix L. Oral Corticosteroids
Topical Analgesic and Anesthetic Agents *see* Appendix I. Anesthetic Agents for Local Infiltration and Dermal/Mucosal Membrane Application online at https://connect.springerpub.com/content/reference-book/978-0-8261-7935-7/back-matter/part02/back-matter/bmatter9

TOPICAL AND TRANSDERMAL ANALGESICS

▷ *capsaicin* (B)(G) apply tid-qid prn to intact skin
  Pediatric: <2 years: not recommended; ≥2 years: same as adult
    Axsain *Crm:* 0.075% (1, 2 oz)
    Capsin *Lotn:* 0.025, 0.075% (59 ml)
    Capzasin-HP (OTC) *Crm:* 0.075% (1.5 oz), 0.025% (45, 90 gm); *Lotn:* 0.075% (2 oz); 0.025% (45, 90 gm)
    Capzasin-P (OTC) *Crm:* 0.025% (1.5 oz); *Lotn:* 0.025% (2 oz)
    Dolorac *Crm:* 0.025% (28 gm)
    Double Cap (OTC) *Crm:* 0.05% (2 oz)
    R-Gel *Gel:* 0.025% (15, 30 gm)
    Zostrix (OTC) *Crm:* 0.025% (0.7, 1.5, 3 oz)
    Zostrix HP (OTC) *Emol crm:* 0.075% (1, 2 oz)
▷ *capsaicin* 8% patch (B) apply up to 4 patches for one 60-minute application to clean dry skin; may prep area with topical anesthetic; wear non-latex gloves; patches may be cut to size/shape; treatment may be repeated every 3 months
  Pediatric: <18 years: not recommended; ≥18 years: same as adult
    Qutenza *Patch:* 8% 1640 mcg/cm (179 mg) (1 or 2 patches w. 1-50 gm tube cleansing gel/carton)
▷ *diclofenac sodium* (C; D ≥30 wks) apply qid prn to intact skin
  Pediatric: <12 years: not established; ≥12 years: same as adult
    Pennsaid 1.5% in 10 drop increments, dispense and rub into front, side, and back of knee; usually: 40 drops (40 mg) qid
      Topical soln: 1.5% (150 ml)
    Pennsaid 2% apply 2 pump actuations (40 mg) and rub into front, side, and back of knee bid
      Topical soln: 2% (20 mg/pump actuation, 112 gm)
    Solaraze Gel massage in to clean skin bid prn
      Gel: 3% (50 gm) (benzyl alcohol)
    Voltaren Gel (G)(OTC) apply qid prn to intact skin
      Gel: 1% (100 gm)
  Comment: *Diclofenac* is contraindicated with *aspirin* allergy. As with other NSAIDs, should be avoided in late pregnancy (≥30 weeks) because it may cause premature closure of the ductus arteriosus.
▷ *doxepin* (B) cream apply to affected area qid at intervals of at least 3-4 hours; max 8 days
  Pediatric: <12 years: not recommended; >12 years: same as adult
    Prudoxin *Crm:* 5% (45 gm)
    Zonalon *Crm:* 5% (30, 45 gm)

▷ *pimecrolimus* 1% cream (C)(G) <2 years: not recommended; ≥2 years: apply to affected area bid; do not apply an occlusive dressing

Elidel *Crm:* 1% (30, 60, 100 gm)

Comment: *Pimecrolimus* is indicated for short-term and intermittent long-term use. Discontinue use when resolution occurs. Contraindicated if the patient is immunosuppressed. Change to the 0.1% preparation or if secondary bacterial infection is present.

▷ *trolamine salicylate* apply tid-qid

Pediatric: <2 years: not recommended; ≥2 years: same as adult

Mobisyl Creme *Crm:* 10% (100 gm)

TOPICAL AND TRANSDERMAL ANESTHETICS

Comment: *Lidocaine* should not be applied to non-intact skin.

▷ *lidocaine* cream (B) apply to affected area bid prn

Pediatric: <12 years: not recommended; ≥12 years: same as adult

LidaMantle *Crm:* 3% (1, 2 oz)

Lidoderm *Crm:* 3% (85 gm)

ZTlido *lidocaine* topical system 1% (30/carton)

Comment: Compared to **Lidoderm** (*lidocaine* patch 5%), which contains 700 mg/patch, **ZTlido** requires 35 mg per topical system to achieve the same therapeutic dose.

▷ *lidocaine* lotion (B) apply to affected area bid prn

Pediatric: <12 years: not recommended; ≥12 years: same as adult

LidaMantle *Lotn:* 3% (177 ml)

▷ *lidocaine* 5% patch (B)(G) apply up to 3 patches at one time for up to 12 hours/24-hour period (12 hours on/12 hours off); patches may be cut into smaller sizes before removal of the release liner; do not re-use

Pediatric: <12 years: not recommended; ≥12 years: same as adult

Lidoderm *Patch:* 5% (10x14 cm; 30/carton)

▷ *lidocaine+dexamethasone* (B)

Pediatric: <12 years: not recommended; ≥12 years: same as adult

Decadron Phosphate with Xylocaine *Lotn:* dexa 4 mg+lido 10 mg per ml (5 ml)

▷ *lidocaine+hydrocortisone* (B)(G) apply to affected area bid prn

Pediatric: <12 years: not recommended; ≥12 years: same as adult

LidaMantle HC *Crm:* lido 3%+hydro 0.5% (1, 3 oz); *Lotn:* (177 ml)

▷ *lidocaine* 2.5%+*prilocaine* 2.5% apply sparingly to the burn bid-tid prn

Pediatric: <12 years: not recommended; ≥12 years: same as adult

Emla Cream (B) 5, 30 gm/tube

ORAL SALICYLATE

▷ *indomethacin* (C) initially 25 mg bid-tid; increase as needed at weekly intervals by 25-50 mg/day; max 200 mg/day

Pediatric: <14 years: usually not recommended; ≤2-14 years, if risk warranted: 1-2 mg/kg/day in divided doses; max 3-4 mg/kg/day (or 150-200 mg/day, whichever is less); ≤14 years: ER cap not recommended; >14 years: same as adult

Cap: 25, 50 mg; *Susp:* 25 mg/5 ml (pineapple-coconut, mint; alcohol 1%); *Supp:* 50 mg; *ER Cap:* 75 mg ext-rel

Comment: *Indomethacin* is indicated only for acute painful flares. Administer with food and/or antacids. Use lowest effective dose for shortest duration.

NSAID PLUS PPI

▷ *esomeprazole+naproxen* (C; not for use in 3rd)(G) 1 tab bid; use lowest effective dose for the shortest duration; swallow whole; take at least 30 minutes before a meal

Pediatric: <18 years: not recommended; ≥18 years: same as adult

Vimovo *Tab:* nap 375 mg+eso 20 mg ext-rel; nap 500 mg+eso 20 mg ext-rel

COX-2 INHIBITORS

Comment: Cox-2 inhibitors are contraindicated with history of asthma, urticaria, and allergic-type reactions to *aspirin*, other NSAIDs, and sulfonamides, 3rd trimester of pregnancy, and coronary artery bypass graft (CABG) surgery.

▷ *celecoxib* (C)(G) 100-400 mg bid; max 800 mg/day
  Pediatric: <18 years: not recommended; ≥18 years: same as adult
    Celebrex *Cap:* 50, 100, 200, 400 mg

▷ *meloxicam* (C)(G)
    Mobic initially 7.5 mg once daily; max 15 mg once daily; Hemodialysis: max 7.5 mg/day
    Pediatric: <2 years, <60 kg: not recommended; ≥2 years, >60 kg-12 years: 0.125 mg/kg; max 7.5 mg once daily; ≥12 years: same as adult
      Tab: 7.5, 15 mg; *Oral susp:* 7.5 mg/5 ml (100 ml) (raspberry)
    Vivlodex initially 5 mg qd; may increase to max 10 mg/day; Hemodialysis: max 5 mg/day
      Cap: 5, 10 mg

GRAFT VERSUS HOST DISEASE (GVHD): ACUTE

JANUS ASSOCIATED-ASSOCIATED KINASE (JAK)1/JAK2 INHIBITOR

▷ *ruxolitinib* initially 5 mg twice daily; therapeutic dose should be individualized based on safety and efficacy; *Renal Impairment:* reduce starting dose <u>or</u> avoid use; *Hepatic Impairment:* reduce starting dose <u>or</u> avoid use
  Pediatric: <12 years: not established; ≥12 years: same as adult
    Jakafi *Tab:* 5, 10, 15, 20, 25 mg

Comment: Jakafi *(ruxolitinib)* is approved for the treatment of steroid-refractory acute graft-versus-host disease, myelofibrosis, and polycythemia vera. Manage thrombocytopenia, anemia, and neutropenia with dose reduction, <u>or</u> treatment interruption, <u>or</u> transfusion. Manage thrombocytopenia, anemia, and neutropenia with dose reduction, <u>or</u> treatment interruption, <u>or</u> transfusion. Serious infections should be resolved before starting therapy with **Jakafi**. Assess patients for signs and symptoms of infection during **Jakafi** therapy and initiate appropriate treatment promptly. Manage symptom exacerbation following interruption <u>or</u> discontinuation of **Jakafi** with supportive care and then consider resuming treatment with **Jakafi**. There is risk of non-melanoma skin cancer (NMSC) with **Jakafi** use; perform periodic skin examinations. Assess lipid levels 8-12 weeks from start of **Jakafi** therapy and treat as appropriate. Avoid use of **Jakafi** with *fluconazole* doses greater than 200 mg except in patients with acute graft versus host disease (GVHD). With acute graft versus host disease, the most common hematologic adverse reactions (incidence >50%) are anemia, thrombocytopenia, and neutropenia and the most common nonhematologic adverse reactions (incidence >50%) have been infections and edema. There are <u>no</u> studies with the use of **Jakafi** in pregnant females to inform drug-associated risks. <u>No</u> data are available regarding the presence of *ruxolitinib* in human milk <u>or</u> the effects on the breastfed infant. Patients should be advised to discontinue breastfeeding during treatment with **Jakafi** and for 2 weeks after the final dose.

GRANULOMATOSIS, WEGENER'S GRANULOMATOSIS

Comment: Wegener's granulomatosis is granulomatosis <u>with</u> polyangiitis [GPA].

CD20-DIRECTED CYTOLYTIC ANTIBODY

▷ *rituximab* *Induction:* 375 mg/m² via IV infusion once weekly x 4 weeks, in combination with glucocorticoids; *Follow up, patients who have achieved disease control with induction treatment, in combination with glucocorticoids:* two 500 mg

IV infusions separated by two weeks, followed by one 500 mg IV infusion every 6 months thereafter, based on clinical evaluation; **Rituxan** should only be administered by a qualified healthcare professional with appropriate medical support to manage severe infusion-related reactions that can be fatal if they occur *Pediatric:* <2 years: safety and efficacy not established; ≥2 years: *Induction:* 375 mg/m^2 via IV infusion once weekly x 4 weeks, in combination with glucocorticoids; *Follow up, patients who have achieved disease control with induction treatment, in combination with glucocorticoids:* two 250 mg/m^2 via IV infusions separated by two weeks, followed by one 250 mg/m^2 via IV infusion every 6 months thereafter, based on clinical evaluation; **Rituxan** should only be administered by a qualified healthcare professional with appropriate medical support to manage severe infusion-related reactions that can be fatal if they occur

   Rituxan *Vial:* 100 mg/10 ml (10 mg/ml), 500 mg/50 ml (10 mg/ml), single-dose, soln for dilution and IV infusion (preservative-free)

   Comment: **Rituxan** is indicated for the treatment of Wegener's Granulomatosis, in combination with glucocorticoids, for adults and pediatric patients ≥2 years-of-age. The most adverse common reactions (incidence ≥15%) in clinical trials have been infections, nausea, diarrhea, headache, muscle spasms, anemia, peripheral edema, infusion-related reactions. For tumor lysis syndrome, administer aggressive IV hydration, anti-hyperuricemic agents, and monitor renal function. Monitor for infections; withhold **Rituxan** and institute appropriate anti-infective therapy. For cardiac adverse reactions, discontinue infusions in case of serious or life-threatening events. Discontinue **Rituxan** in patients with rising serum creatinine or oliguria. Bowel obstruction and perforation can occur; consider and evaluate for abdominal pain, vomiting, or related symptoms. Live virus vaccinations prior to or during **Rituxan** treatment is not recommended. **Rituxan** is embryo/fetal toxic. Advise males and females of reproductive potential of the potential risk and to use effective contraception. Advise women not to breastfeed during treatment and for at least 6 months after the last dose.

▷ *rituximab-arrx Induction:* 375 mg/m^2 once weekly x 4 weeks; *then, If Disease Control Achieved:* 500 mg via IV infusion x 2 doses separated by two weeks; then, 500 mg via IV infusion once every 6 months based on clinical evaluation; administer all doses of **Riabni** in combination with glucocorticoids; **Riabni** should only be administered by a qualified healthcare professional with appropriate medical support to manage severe infusion-related reactions that can be fatal

Pediatric: safety and efficacy not established

   Riabni *Vial:* 100 mg/10 ml (10 mg/ml), 500 mg/50 ml (10 mg/ml) soln, single-dose

   Comment: **Riabni** *(rituximab-arrx)* is a biosimilar to **Rituxan** indicated for the treatment of adult patients with granulomatosis with polyangitis (GPA) (Wegener's Granulomatosis) in combination with glucocorticoids. The most common adverse reactions in clinical trials with GPA (incidence ≥15%) have been infections, nausea, diarrhea, headache, muscle spasms, anemia, peripheral edema, and infusion-related reactions. Monitor renal function. Discontinue **Riabni** in patients with rising serum creatinine or oliguria. If tumor lysis syndrome (TLS) is suspected, administer aggressive IV hydration and anti-hyperuricemic agents. If infection occurs, withhold **Riabni** and institute appropriate anti-infective therapy. Bowel obstruction and perforation can occur; evaluate for abdominal pain, vomiting, and related symptoms. Live virus vaccine administration prior to or during treatment with **Riabni** is not recommended. **Riabni** can cause embryo/fetal harm. Advise females of reproductive potential of embryo/fetal risk and to use effective contraception. Advise not to breastfeed.

GRANULOMA INGUINALE (DONOVANOSIS)

Comment: The following treatment regimens are published in the **2015 CDC Sexually Transmitted Diseases Treatment Guidelines**. Treatment regimens are for adults <u>only</u>; consult a specialist for treatment of patients less than 18 years-of-age. Treatment regimens are presented by generic drug name first, followed by information about brands and dose forms. Persons who have sexual contact with a patient who has had granuloma inguinale within the past 60 days before onset of the patient's symptoms should be examined and offered therapy. Patients who are HIV-positive should receive the same treatment as those who are HIV-negative; however, the addition of a parenteral aminoglycoside (e.g., *gentamicin*) can also be considered.

RECOMMENDED REGIMEN

▷ *doxycycline* 100 mg bid x at least 3 weeks and until all lesions have completely healed

ALTERNATE REGIMENS

▷ *azithromycin* 1 gm once weekly for at least 3 weeks and until all lesions have completely healed

▷ *ciprofloxacin* 750 mg bid x at least 3 weeks and until all lesions have completely healed

▷ *erythromycin base* 500 mg qid x 14 days <u>or</u> *erythromycin ethylsuccinate* 400 mg qid x 14 days

▷ *trimethoprim+sulfamethoxazole* take 1 double-strength (160/800) dose bid x at least 3 weeks and until all lesions have completely healed

DRUG BRANDS AND DOSE FORMS

▷ *azithromycin* (B)(G)
  Zithromax *Tab:* 250, 500, 600 mg; *Oral susp:* 100 mg/5 ml (15 ml); 200 mg/5 ml (15, 22.5, 30 ml) (cherry); *Pkt:* 1 gm for reconstitution (cherry-banana)
  Zithromax Tri-pak *Tab:* 3 x 500 mg tabs/pck
  Zithromax Z-pak *Tab:* 6 x 250 mg tabs/pck
  Zmax *Oral susp:* 2 gm ext-rel for reconstitution (cherry-banana) (148 mg Na⁺)
▷ *ciprofloxacin* (C)
  Cipro (G) *Tab:* 250, 500, 750 mg; *Oral susp:* 250, 500 mg/5 ml (100 ml) (strawberry)
  Cipro XR *Tab:* 500, 1000 mg ext-rel
  ProQuin XR *Tab:* 500 mg ext-rel
▷ *doxycycline* (D)(G)
  Acticlate *Tab:* 75, 150** mg
  Adoxa *Tab:* 50, 75, 100, 150 mg ent-coat
  Doryx *Tab:* 50, 75, 100, 150, 200 mg del-rel
  Doxteric *Tab:* 50 mg del-rel
  Monodox *Cap:* 50, 75, 100 mg
  Oracea *Cap:* 40 mg del-rel
  Vibramycin *Tab:* 100 mg; *Cap:* 50, 100 mg; *Syr:* 50 mg/5 ml (raspberry-apple) (sulfites); *Oral susp:* 25 mg/5 ml (raspberry)
  Vibra-Tab *Tab:* 100 mg film-coat
▷ *erythromycin base* (B)(G)
  Ery-Tab *Tab:* 250, 333, 500 mg ent-coat
  PCE *Tab:* 333, 500 mg
▷ *erythromycin ethylsuccinate* (B)(G)
  EryPed *Oral susp:* 200 mg/5 ml (100, 200 ml) (fruit); 400 mg/5 ml (60, 100, 200 ml) (banana); *Oral drops:* 200, 400 mg/5 ml (50 ml) (fruit); *Chew tab:* 200 mg wafer (fruit)

E.E.S. *Oral susp*: 200, 400 mg/5 ml (100 ml) (fruit)
E.E.S. **Granules** *Oral susp*: 200 mg/5 ml (100, 200 ml) (cherry)
E.E.S. **400 Tablets** *Tab*: 400 mg

▷ *trimethoprim+sulfamethoxazole (TMP-SMX)(C)(G)*
Bactrim, Septra
Tab: trim 80 mg+sulfa 400 mg*
Bactrim DS, Septra DS
Tab: trim 160 mg+sulfa 800 mg*
Bactrim Pediatric Suspension, Septra Pediatric Suspension
Oral susp: trim 40 mg+sulfa 200 mg per 5 ml (100 ml) (cherry) (alcohol 0.3%)

GROWTH FAILURE

Comment: Administer growth hormones by SC injection into thigh, buttocks, or abdomen. Rotate sites with each dose. Contraindicated in children with fused epiphyses or evidence of neoplasia.

▷ *mecasermin* (recombinant human insulin-like growth factor-1 [rhIGF-1])
Increlex (B) see mfr pkg insert
Vial: 10 mg/ml (benzyl alcohol)
Comment: **Increlex** is indicated for growth failure in children with severe primary IGF-1 deficiency (primary IGFD) or in those with growth hormone (GH) gene deletion who have developed neutralizing antibodies to GH.

▷ *somatropin* (rDNA origin)
Genotropin (B) initially not more than 0.04 mg/kg/week divided into 6-7 doses; may increase at 4-8 week intervals; max 0.08 mg/kg/week divided into 6-7 doses
Pediatric: usually 0.16-0.024 mg/kg/week divided into 6-7 doses
Intra-Mix Device: 1.5 mg (1.3 mg/ml after reconstitution), 5.8 mg (5 mg/ml after reconstitution) (two-chamber cartridge w. diluent); *Pen* or *Intra-Mix Device*: 5.8 mg (5 mg/ml after reconstitution), 13.8 mg (512 mg/ml after reconstitution) (2-chamber cartridge w. diluent)
Genotropin Miniquick (B) initially not more than 0.04 mg/kg/week divided into 6-7 doses; may increase at 4-8-week intervals; max 0.08 mg/kg/week divided into 6-7 doses
Pediatric: usually 0.16-0.024 mg/kg/week divided into 6-7 doses
MiniQuick: 0.2, 0.4, 0.6, 0.8, 1, 1.2, 1.4, 1.6, 1.8, 2 mg/0.25 ml (pwdr for SC injection after reconstitution) (2-chamber cartridge w. diluent)
Humatrope (C)
Pediatric: initially 0.18 mg/kg/week IM or SC divided into equal doses given either on 3 alternate days or 6 x/week; max 0.3 mg/kg/week
Vial: 5 mg w. 5 ml diluent
Norditropin (C)
Pediatric: 0.024-0.034 mg/kg SC 6-7 x/week
Vial: 4 mg (12 IU), 8 mg (24 IU); *Cartridge for inj*: 5, 10, 15 mg/1.5 ml; *FlexPro prefilled pen*: 5, 10, 15 mg/1.5 ml
NordiFlex prefilled pen: 5, 10, 15 mg/1.5 ml; 30 mg/3 ml
Nutropin (C)
Pediatric: 0.7 mg/kg/week SC in divided daily doses
Vial: 5, 10 mg/vial w. diluent
Nutropin AQ (C)
<35 years: initially not more than 0.006 mg/kg SC daily; may increase to max 0.025 mg/kg SC daily; ≥35 years: initially not more than 0.006 mg/kg SC daily; may increase to max 0.0125 mg/kg SC daily
Pediatric: *Prepubertal*: up to 0.043 mg/kg SC daily; *Pubertal*: up to 0.1 mg/kg SC daily; *Turner Syndrome*: up to 0.0375 mg/kg/week divided into equal doses 3-7 x/week
Vial: 5 mg/ml (2 ml)

Nutropin Depot (C) 1.5 mg/kg SC monthly on same day each month; max 22.5 mg/inj; divide injection if >22.5 mg
Pediatric: same as adult
  Vial: 13.5, 18, 22.5 mg/vial (pwdr for injection after reconstitution; single-use w. diluent and needle)
Omnitrope (B) 0.16-0.24 mg/kg/week SC divided 3-7 x/week
  Vial: 5.8 mg
Omnitrope Pen 5 (B) 0.16-0.24 mg/kg/week SC divided 3-7 x/week
  Cartridge for inj: 5 mg/1.5 ml
Omnitrope Pen 10 (B) 0.16-0.24 mg/kg/week SC divided 3-7 x/week
  Cartridge for inj: 10 mg/1.5 ml
Saizen (B)(G) 0.18 mg/kg/week IM or SC divided 3-7 x/week
  Vial: 5 mg (pwdr for SC injection w. diluent)
Serostim (B) 0.1 mg/kg SC once daily at HS; max 6 mg
  Vial: 5, 4, 6, 8.8 mg (pwdr for SC injection w. diluent) (benzyl alcohol)

GROWTH HORMONE DEFICIENCY, ADULT

HUMAN GROWTH HORMONE ANALOG

▷ *somapacitan-beco* inject SC into the abdomen or thigh with regular rotation of injection sites to avoid lipohypertrophy/Lipoatrophy; *Initially:* 1.5 mg SC once weekly for treatment naïve patients and patients switching from daily growth hormone; *Titration:* increase the weekly dose every 2 to 4 weeks by approximately 0.5 mg to 1.5 mg until the desired response has been achieved based on clinical response and serum insulin-like growth factor 1 (IGF-1) concentrations; max recommended dose is 8 mg SC once weekly. See mfr pkg insert for full prescribing information and for dosage recommendations in patients aged 65 years and older, patients with hepatic impairment, and women receiving oral estrogen
Pediatric: not established
  Sogroya *Prefilled pen:* 10 mg/1.5 ml (6.7 mg/ml)
  Comment: **Sogroya** *(somapacitan-beco)* is a indicated for the replacement of endogenous growth hormone in adults with growth hormone deficiency. Adverse reactions (incidence 2%) have been back pain, arthralgia, dyspepsia, sleep disorder, dizziness, tonsillitis, peripheral edema, vomiting, adrenal insufficiency, hypertension, blood creatine phosphokinase increase, weight increase, and anemia. There are no available data on **Sogroya** use in pregnant females. However, published studies with short-acting recombinant growth hormone (rhGH) use in pregnant females over several decades have not identified any drug-associated risk of major birth defects, miscarriage, or adverse maternal or fetal outcomes. In animal reproduction studies, subcutaneously administered *somapacitan-beco* was not teratogenic during organogenesis at doses approximately 12 times the clinical exposure at the maximum recommended human dose (MRHD) of 8 mg/week. No adverse developmental outcomes were observed in in a pre- and post-natal development study with administration of *somapacitan-beco* to pregnant rats from organogenesis through lactation at approximately 275 times the clinical exposure at the MRHD. Available published data describing administration of short-acting recombinant growth hormone (rhGH) to lactating females for 7 days reported that short-acting rhGH did not increase the normal breastmilk concentration of growth hormone and no adverse effects were reported in breastfed infants. Developmental and health benefits of breastfeeding should be considered along with the mother's clinical need for **Sogroya** and any potential adverse effects on the breastfed infant from **Sogroya** or from the underlying maternal condition. There is no information on with the presence

of *somapacitan-beco* in human milk or effects on the breastfed infant. Risks in pediatric patients associated with growth hormone use include sudden death in pediatric patients with Prader-Willi Syndrome, increased risk of second neoplasm in pediatric cancer survivors treated with radiation to the brain and/or head, slipped capital femoral epiphysis, progression of preexisting scoliosis, pancreatitis.

HAND, FOOT, AND MOUTH DISEASE (*COXSACKIEVIRUS*)

NSAIDs *see* Appendix J. NSAIDs online at https://connect.springerpub.com/content/reference-book/978-0-8261-7935-7/back-matter/part02/back-matter/bmatter10
Opioid Analgesics *see Pain*
OTC Throat Lozenges
OTC Cough Drops and Cough Syrup

Comment: The hand, foot, and mouth disease occurs most commonly in children <10 years-of-age. Although adults are susceptible, most have built up natural immunity. The causative organism, *Coxsackievirus*, is transmitted via droplet spread (coughing and/or sneezing) and contact with contaminated objects and surfaces (same as influenza). Clinical signs and symptoms are typically relatively mild and include fever, sore throat, feeling generally unwell, malaise, headache, and poor appetite. Red spots, some painful blister-like lesions, most often appear on the tongue and roof of the mouth, palms of the hands, and soles of the feet (but not necessarily all three), and are often faint or sparse. Lesions, which are not pruritic, may also be noted on the dorsal surfaces of the hands/fingers and feet/ toes. Medical treatment, per se, is not required. Treatment in the home with age/weight-dosed ibuprofen or acetaminophen for relief of sore throat, lesion pain, and fever. Other comfort measures include salt water gargles, throat lozenges, cough drops or cough syrup, and fluids. The disease typically resolves in 7 to 10 days.

HANSEN'S DISEASE (LEPROMATOUS LEPROSY, *MYCOBACTERIUM LEPRAE*)

Comment: Hansen's disease is treated with a combination of antibiotics. Typically 2 or 3 antibiotics are used at the same time. These are *dapsone* with *rifampicin*, and *clofazimine* is added for some types of the disease. These drugs must never be used alone as monotherapy for leprosy. *Paucibacillary form:* 2 antibiotics are used at the same time, daily *dapsone* and *rifampicin* once per month. *Multibacillary form:* daily *clofazimine* is added to *rifampicin* and *dapsone*. This multi-drug treatment (MDT) strategy helps prevent the development of antibiotic resistance by the bacteria, which may otherwise occur due to length of the treatment. Treatment usually lasts between one to two years. The illness can be cured if treatment is completed as prescribed. A single dose of combination therapy has been used to cure single lesion paucibacillary leprosy: *rifampicin* 600 mg, *ofloxacin* 400 mg, and *minocycline* 100 mg. The child with a single lesion takes half the adult dose of the 3 medications. WHO has designed blister pack medication kits for both paucibacillary leprosy and for multibacillary leprosy. Each kit contains medication for 28 days. The blister pack medication kit for single lesion paucibacillary leprosy contains the necessary medication for the one-time administration of the 3 medications.

ANTIMYCOBACTERIALS

➤ *clofazimine* (G) should be administered with meals or milk
   Dapsone-Sensitive Lepromatous Leprosy: 100 mg daily as a part of a combination regimen for at least 2 years

Dapsone-Resistant Lepromatous Leprosy: 100 mg daily in combination with one or more other agents for 3 years

Leprosy Complicated by Erythema Nodosum Leprosum: 100-200 mg daily for up to 3 months; taper dose to 100 mg as quickly as possible

Pediatric: Safety and effectiveness in pediatric patients have not been established

   Soft gelcap: 50 mg

Comment: *Clofazimine* is sometimes given with other medicines for leprosy. When *clofazimine* is used to treat disease flares, it may be given with a cortisone-like medicine. *Clofazimine* may deposit in intestinal mucosa causing intestinal disturbances, including abdominal obstruction, bleeding, splenic infarction, and death. Reduce dose or discontinue *clofazimine* if patient complains of pain in abdomen or other gastrointestinal symptoms. QT prolongation and Torsade de Pointes may occur with *clofazimine*. Concomitant use with other QT-prolonging drugs or *bedaquiline* may cause additive QT prolongation. Monitor ECGs and discontinue *clofazimine* if significant ventricular arrhythmia or QTcF interval ≥500 ms develop. Advise patients that skin and body fluid discoloration frequently occur. Depression and suicide due to skin discoloration may occur; monitor patients for psychological effects of skin discoloration. The most common adverse reactions reported in 40% to 50% of patients are skin and body fluid discoloration, abdominal and epigastric pain, diarrhea, nausea, vomiting, and gastrointestinal intolerance. No dose adjustment of *clofazimine* is needed for HIV-infected patients. *Severe Renal Impairment:* use with caution. *Hepatic Impairment:* avoid. Monitor for toxicities when used concomitantly with substrates of CYP3A4/5. It may take up to 6 months before the full benefit of *clofazimine* is seen. Sexually active females of reproductive potential should have a pregnancy test prior to starting treatment. There are no studies of *clofazimine* use in pregnant females and few cases of *clofazimine* use during pregnancy have been reported in the literature. These reports indicate that the skin of infants born to women who had received *clofazimine* during pregnancy was deeply pigmented at birth; therefore, *clofazimine* should be used during pregnancy only if the potential benefit justifies the risk to the fetus. *clofazimine* is excreted in human milk. Skin discoloration has been observed in breastfed infants of mothers receiving *clofazimine*. There are no adequate studies in women for determining infant risk when using this medication during breastfeeding; therefore, weigh the potential benefits against the potential risks before taking this medication while breastfeeding. In some areas, *clofazimine* is considered an investigational new drug (IND) that must be prescribed by a registered investigator; providers are encouraged to request investigator status by calling the NDHP at 1-800-642-2477.

SULFONE

▷ *dapsone* topical (C)(G) apply to affected area bid
   Pediatric: <12 years: not recommended; ≥12 years: same as adult
      Aczone Gel: 5, 7.5% (30, 60, 90 gm pump)
▷ *rifampin* (C)(G) 600 mg orally once daily x 12 months
   Pediatric: <12 years: not recommended; ≥12 years: same as adult
      Rifadin, Rimactane Cap: 150, 300 mg

ALTERNATE DRUGS

Comment: *Ofloxacin* may be substituted for *clofazimine*. *Clarithromycin* may be substituted for any of the drugs. *Minocycline* may be substituted for *dapsone* in patients intolerant of *dapsone*, and may also be used to substitute *clofazimine*; however, anti-inflammatory activity is not as substantial as with *clofazimine*.

➤ *clarithromycin* (C)(G) 500 mg/day
    Biaxin *Tab:* 250, 500 mg
    Biaxin Oral Suspension *Oral susp:* 125, 250 mg/5 ml (50, 100 ml) (fruitpunch)
    Biaxin XL *Tab:* 500 mg ext-rel
➤ *ofloxacin* (C)(G) 400 mg/day
    Pediatric: <18 years: not recommended; ≥18 years: same as adult
    Floxin *Tab:* 200, 300, 400 mg
➤ *minocycline* (D)(G) 100 mg/day
    Pediatric: <8 years: not recommended; ≥8 years: same as adult
    Dynacin *Cap:* 50, 100 mg
    Minocin *Cap:* 50, 75, 100 mg; *Oral susp:* 50 mg/5 ml (60 ml) (custard)
    (sulfites, alcohol 5%)

⬤ HEADACHE: MIGRAINE, CLUSTER, VASCULAR

ERGOTAMINE AGENTS

Comment: Do not use an ergotamine-type drug within 24 hours of any triptan or other 5-HT agonist.
➤ *dihydroergotamine mesylate* (X)
    DHE 45 1 mg SC, IM, or IV; may repeat at 1 hour intervals; max 3 mg/day SC or IM/day; max 2 mg IV/day; max 6 mg/week
    Pediatric: <12 years: not recommended; ≥12 years: same as adult
      Amp: 1 mg/ml (1 ml)
    Migranal (G) 1 spray in each nostril; may repeat 15 minutes later; max 6 sprays/day and 8 sprays/week
    Pediatric: <12 years: not recommended; ≥12 years: same as adult
      Nasal spray: 4 mg/ml; 0.5 mg/spray (caffeine)
➤ *ergotamine* (X)(G) 1 tab SL at onset of attack; then q 30 minutes as needed; max 3 tabs/day and 5 tabs/week
    Tab: 2 mg
➤ *ergotamine+caffeine* (X)(G)
    Pediatric: <12 years: not recommended; ≥12 years: same as adult
    Cafergot 2 tabs at onset of attack; then 1 tab every 1/2 hour if needed; max 6 tabs/attack and 10 tabs/week
      Tab: ergot 1 mg+caf 100 mg
    Cafergot Suppository 1 suppository rectally at onset of headache; may repeat x 1 after 1 hour; max 2/attack, 5/week
      Rectal supp: ergot 2 mg+caf 100 mg

5-HT RECEPTOR AGONISTS

Comment: Contraindications to 5-HT receptor agonists include cardiovascular disease, ischemic heart disease, cerebral vascular syndromes, peripheral vascular disease, uncontrolled hypertension, hemiplegic, or basilar migraine. Do not use any triptan within 24 hours of ergot-type drugs or other 5-HT1A agonists, or within 2 weeks of taking an MAOI.
➤ *almotriptan* (C)(G) 6.25 or 12.5 mg; may repeat once after 2 hours; max 2 doses/day
    Pediatric: <12 years: not recommended; ≥12 years: same as adult
    Axert *Tab:* 6.25 mg (6/card), 12.5 mg (12/card)
    Comment: *Almotriptan* is indicated for patients 12-17 years-of-age with PMHx migraine headache lasting ≥4 hours untreated.
➤ *eletriptan* (C)(G) 20 or 40 mg; may repeat once after 2 hours; max 80 mg/day
    Pediatric: <18 years: not recommended; ≥18 years: same as adult
    Relpax *Tab:* 20, 40 mg

▷ *frovatriptan* (C)(G) 2.5 mg with fluids; may repeat once after 2 hours; max 7.5 mg/day

Pediatric: <18 years: not recommended; ≥18 years: same as adult

Frova *Tab:* 2.5 mg

▷ *naratriptan* (C) 1 or 2.5 mg with fluids; may repeat once after 4 hours; max 5 mg/day

Pediatric: <18 years: not recommended; ≥18 years: same as adult

Amerge *Tab:* 1, 2.5 mg

▷ *rizatriptan* (C) initially 5 or 10 mg; may repeat in 2 hours if needed; max 30 mg/day

Pediatric: <18 years: not recommended; ≥18 years: same as adult

Maxalt *Tab:* 5, 10 mg

Maxalt-MLT *ODT:* 5, 10 mg (peppermint) (phenylalanine)

▷ *sumatriptan* (C)(G)

Pediatric: <18 years: not recommended; ≥18 years: same as adult

Alsuma 6 mg SC to the upper arm or lateral thigh only; may repeat after 1 hour if needed; max 2 doses/day

Prefilled syringe: 6 mg/0.5 ml (2/pck with auto injector)

Imitrex Injectable 4-6 mg SC; may repeat after 1 hour if needed; max 2 doses/day

Prefilled syringe: 4, 6 mg/0.5 ml (2/pck with or without autoinjector)

Imitrex Nasal Spray (G) 5-20 mg intranasally; may repeat once after 2 hours if needed; max 40 mg/day

Nasal spray: 5, 20 mg/spray (single-dose)

Imitrex Tab 25-200 mg x 1 dose; may be repeated at intervals of at least 2 hours if needed; max 200 mg/day

Tab: 25, 50, 100 mg rapid-rel

Imitrex STATdose Pen 6 mg/0.5 mg SC; may repeat once after 2 hours if needed; max 2 doses/day

Prefilled needle-free autoinjector delivery system: 6 mg/0.5 ml (6/pck)

Onzetra Xsail each disposable white nosepiece contains half a dose of medication (11 mg of sumatriptan). A full dose is 22 mg. Do not use more than 2 nosepieces per dose; attach the mouthpiece and 1 nasal piece; then press the white button on the delivery device to pierce the capsule in the nasal piece, then insert the nasal piece into one nostril and blow into the mouth piece to deliver the nasal powder in the contents of one capsule (11 mg); repeat in the opposite nostril for a total single 22 mg dose

Cap: 11 mg nasal pwdr; *Kit:* nosepieces (2), capsules (2), reusable breath powered delivery device (1)

Sumavel DosePro 6 mg SC to the upper arm or lateral thigh only; may repeat after 1 hour if needed; max 2 doses/day

Prefilled needle-free delivery system: 6 mg/0.5 ml (6/pck)

Tosymra 10 mg (1 nasal spray); max 3 nasal sprays (30 mg)/24 hours; separate doses by at least one hour

Nasal spray: 10 mg/spray ready-to-use, single-dose, disposable unit (6 units/carton)

Zembrace SymTouch administer 3 mg SC at onset of headache; may repeat hourly; max 12 mg/24 hours

Pediatric: <18 years: not recommended; ≥18 years: same as adult

Autoinjector: 3 mg/0.5 ml (prefilled single-dose disposable autoinjector)

▷ *zolmitriptan* (C)(G) initially 2.5 mg; may repeat after 2 hours if needed; max 10 mg/day

Pediatric: <18 years: not recommended; ≥18 years: same as adult

Zomig *Tab:* 2.5*, 5 mg

Zomig Nasal Spray *Nasal spray:* 5 mg/spray single-dose (6/carton)

Zomig-ZMT *ODT:* 2.5 mg (6 tabs), 5*mg (3 tabs) (orange) (phenylalanine)

Comment: Do not use any *triptan* within 24 hours of ergotamine-type drugs or other 5-HT agonists, or within 2 weeks of taking an MAOI.

SEROTONIN (5-HT) 1F RECEPTOR AGONIST

▷ *lasmiditan* 50 mg, 100 mg, or 200 mg taken orally, as needed; max one dose/24 hours

Pediatric: safety and efficacy not established

Reyvow *Tab:* 50, 100 mg

Comment: **Reyvow** *(lasmiditan)* is the first serotonin (5-HT) 1F receptor agonist indicated for the acute treatment of migraine with or without aura in adults. Advise patients not to drive or operate machinery until at least 8 hours after taking a dose of **Reyvow**. Patients who cannot follow this advice should not take **Reyvow**; these patients may not be able to assess their own driving competence and the degree of impairment caused by **Reyvow**. **Reyvow** has not been studied in patients with severe hepatic impairment (Child-Pugh Class C) and its use in these patients is not recommended. **Reyvow** may further lower heart rate when administered with heart rate lowering drugs. Avoid concomitant use with P-gp and Breast Cancer Resistant Protein (BCRP) substrates. **Reyvow** may cause CNS depression and should be used with caution if used in combination with alcohol or other CNS depressants. A reaction consistent with *serotonin syndrome* has been reported in patients treated with **Reyvow**. Discontinue **Reyvow** if symptoms of serotonin syndrome occur. If medication overuse headache (MOH) develops, detoxification may be necessary. Most common adverse reactions (incidence ≥5% and >placebo) have been dizziness, fatigue, paresthesia, and sedation. In animal studies, adverse effects on development (increased incidences of fetal abnormalities, increased embryo/fetal and offspring mortality, decreased fetal body weight) occurred at maternal exposures less or greater than those observed clinically. There are no adequate data on developmental risk associated with **Reyvow** use in pregnant females. There are no data on the presence of *lasmiditan* in human milk or effects of *lasmiditan* on the breastfed infant. Developmental and health benefits of breastfeeding should be considered along with the mother's clinical need for **Revow** and any potential adverse effects on the breastfed infant from **Revow** or from the underlying maternal condition.

NONSTEROIDAL ANTI-INFLAMMATORY

▷ *celecoxib* 120 mg (4.8 ml) with or without food; max 120 mg/24-hours; limit use to the fewest number of days per month; *Moderate Hepatic Impairment (Child-Pugh Class B):* max 60 mg (2.4 ml); *Poor Metabolizers of CYP2C9 Substrates:* max 60 mg (2.4 ml); *Severe Renal Impairment:* avoid

Pediatric: safety and effectiveness not established; disseminated intravascular coagulation (DIC) has occurred in pediatric patients

Elyxyb *Oral soln:* 120 mg/4.8 ml (25 mg/ml), single-dose glass bottles (9 bottles/carton)

Comment: **Elyxyb** *(celecoxib)* is an oral solution formulation of the nonsteroidal anti-inflammatory drug *celecoxib* (first approved under the brand name **Celebrex**) indicated for the acute treatment of migraine with or without aura in adults. **Elyxyb** is not indicated for the preventive treatment of migraine. Avoid use in pregnancy starting at 30 weeks gestation (due to risk of premature closure of fetal ductus arteriosus). Limited data from 3 published reports that included a total of 12 breastfeeding women showed low levels of *celecoxib* in breast milk.

5-HT IB+ID RECEPTOR AGONIST+NSAID COMBINATION

▷ *sumatriptan+naproxen* (C; D in 3rd)(G)
    Pediatric: <18 years: not recommended; ≥18 years: same as adult
    Treximet initially 1 tab; may repeat after 2 hours; max 2 doses/day
        Tab: suma 85 mg+naprox 500 mg (9/blister card)
    Comment: Do not use *sumatriptan* within 24 hours of ergot-type drugs or other
    5-HT agonists, or within 2 weeks of taking an MAOI.

OTHER ANALGESICS

▷ *acetaminophen+aspirin+caffeine* (D)(G)
    Excedrin Migraine (OTC) 2 tabs q 6 hours prn; max 8 tabs/day x 2 days
        Pediatric: <18 years: not recommended; ≥18 years: same as adult
        Tab: acet 250 mg+asp 250 mg+caf 65 mg
▷ *celecoxib* 120 mg (4.8 ml) with or without food; max 120 mg/24-hours; limit use
    to the fewest number of days per month; *Moderate Hepatic Impairment (Child-
    Pugh Class B):* max 60 mg (2.4 ml); *Poor Metabolizers of CYP2C9 Substrates:* max
    60 mg (2.4 ml); *Severe Renal Impairment:* avoid
    Pediatric: safety and effectiveness not established; disseminated intravascular
    coagulation (DIC) has occurred in pediatric patients
        Elyxyb *Oral soln:* 120 mg/4.8 ml (25 mg/ml), single-dose glass bottles (9
        bottles/carton)
    Comment: **Elyxyb** *(celecoxib)* is an oral solution formulation of the
    nonsteroidal anti-inflammatory drug *celecoxib* (first approved under the
    brand name **Celebrex**) indicated for the acute treatment of migraine with or
    without aura in adults. **Elyxyb** is not indicated for the preventive treatment of
    migraine. Avoid use in pregnancy starting at 30 weeks gestation (due to risk of
    premature closure of fetal ductus arteriosus). Limited data from 3 published
    reports that included a total of 12 breastfeeding women showed low levels of
    celecoxib in breast milk.
▷ *diclofenac potassium powder for oral solution* (C; D ≥30 weeks) empty the
    contents of one pkt into a cup containing 1-2 oz or 2-4 tbsp (30-60 ml) of water,
    mix well, and drink immediately; water only, no other liquids; take on an empty
    stomach; use the closest effective dose for the shortest duration of time; safety and
    effectiveness of a 2nd dose has not been established
    Pediatric: <18 years: not established; ≥18 years: same as adult
        Cambia *Pwdr for oral soln:* 50 mg/pkt (3 pkts/set, conjoined with a perforated
        border
    Comment: **Cambia** is not indicated for migraine prophylaxis. May not be
    bioequivalent with other *diclofenac* forms (e.g., *diclofenac sodium* ent-
    coat tabs, *diclofenac sodium* ext-rel tabs, *diclofenac potassium* immed-rel
    tabs) even of the mg strength is the same, therefore, it is not possible to
    convert dosing from any other *diclofenac* formulation to **Cambia**. **Cambia**
    is contraindicated in the setting of coronary artery bypass graft. Use of
    Cambia should not be considered with hepatic impairment, gastric/duodenal
    ulcer, starting at 30 weeks gestation (risk of premature closure of the ductus
    arteriosus in the fetus), concomitant NSAIDs, SSRIs, anticoagulants/
    antiplatelets, and any risk factor for potential bleeding.
▷ *ibuprofen+acetaminophen*
    Advil Dual Action (OTC) *Cplt:* fixed-dose combination of *ibuprofen* 125
    mg (NSAID, antipyretic, analgesic) and *acetaminophen* 250 mg (antipyretic,
    analgesic)
▷ *isometheptene mucate+dichloralphenazone+acetaminophen* (C)(IV)
    Midrin 2 caps initially; then 1 cap q 1 hour until relieved; max 5 caps/12 hours
        Pediatric: <12 years: not recommended; ≥12 years: same as adult
        Cap: iso 65 mg+dichlor 100 mg+acet 325 mg

CALCITONIN GENE-RELATED PEPTIDE (CGRP) RECEPTOR ANTAGONIST

Comment: The CGRP receptor antagonists are a class of drugs that block the activity of calcitonin gene-related peptide as prophylaxis against migraine attacks.

▷ *erenumab-aooe* administer by SC injection only in the upper arm, abdomen, or thigh; recommended dose is 70 mg SC once monthly; some patients may benefit from a dosage of 140 mg SC once monthly (i.e., two consecutive injections of 70 mg each); the needle shield within the white cap of the prefilled autoinjector and the gray needle cap of the prefilled syringe contain dry natural rubber (a derivative of latex), which may cause allergic reactions in individuals sensitive to latex
  Pediatric: <18 years: not recommended; ≥18 years: same as adult
  Aimovig *Autoinjector:* 70 mg/ml (1 ml), prefilled single-dose, SureClick
  Comment: The most common adverse side effects are injection site reaction and constipation. There are no adequate data on the developmental risk associated with the use of **Aimovig** in pregnant females. There are no data on the presence of *erenumab-aooe* in human milk or effects on the breastfed infant. Safety and effectiveness in pediatric patients have not been established.

▷ *fremanezumab-vfrm* administer by SC injection only in the upper arm, abdomen, or thigh; recommended dose is 225 mg SC once monthly or 675 mg SC once every 3 months (3 x 225 mg SC doses once quarterly)
  Pediatric: <18 years: not recommended; ≥18 years: same as adult
  Ajovy *Prefilled syringe:* 225 mg/1.5 ml (1.5 ml) solution, single-dose;
    Autoinjector: 225 mg/1.5 ml (1.5 ml) solution, single-dose
  Comment: The most common adverse side effects are injection site reaction and constipation. There are no adequate data on the developmental risk associated with the use of **Ajovy** in pregnant females. There are no data on the presence of *erenumab-vfrm* in human milk or effects on the breastfed infant. Safety and effectiveness in pediatric patients have not been established.

▷ *galcanezumab-gnlm* administer by SC injection only in the back of the upper arm, abdomen, thigh, or buttocks; *Loading Dose:* 240 mg (2 x 120 mg) SC; *Maintenance:* 120 mg SC once monthly
  Pediatric: <18 years: not recommended; ≥18 years: same as adult
  Emgality *Prefilled pen/Prefilled syringe:* 120 mg/ml (1 ml) solution single-dose
  Comment: The most common adverse side effect (incidence ≥2%) is injection site reaction. There are no adequate data on the developmental risk associated with the use of **Emgality** in pregnant females. There are no data on the presence of *erenumab-vfrm* in human milk or effects on the breastfed infant. Safety and effectiveness in pediatric patients have not been established.

▷ *rimegepant* 75 mg; max 75 mg/24 hours; safety of treating more than 15 migraines in a 30-day period has not been established
  Pediatric: safety and efficacy not established
  Nurtec ODT *Tab:* 75 mg oral-disint
  Comment: **Nurtec ODT** *(rimegepant)* is a calcitonin gene-related peptide (CGRP) receptor antagonist for the acute treatment of migraine with or without aura. **Nurtec ODT** is not indicated for the preventive treatment of migraine. Avoid use in patients with severe hepatic impairment (Child-Pugh Class C). Avoid concomitant administration of **Nurtec ODT** with strong CYP3A4 inhibitors. When administered with a moderate CYP3A4 inhibitor, avoid another dose of **Nurtec ODT** for the next 48 hours. Avoid concomitant administration of **Nurtec ODT** with strong and moderate CYP3A inducers and inhibitors of P-gp or BCRP. There are no adequate data on embryo/fetal risk associated with the use of **Nurtec ODT** in pregnancy. However, in animal studies, oral administration of *rimegepant* during organogenesis resulted

in decreased fetal body weight and increased incidence of fetal variations at exposures greater than those used clinically and which were associated with maternal toxicity. There are no data on the presence of *rimegepant* or its metabolites in human or animal milk or effects of *rimegepant* on the breastfed infant. The developmental and health benefits of breastfeeding should be considered along with the mother's clinical need for **Nurtec ODT** and any potential adverse effects on the breastfed infant from **Nurtec ODT** or from the underlying maternal condition.

► *ubrogepant* 50 mg or 100 mg; if needed, a second dose may be administered at least 2 hours after the initial dose; max 200 mg/24 hours; *Severe Hepatic or Severe Renal Impairment:* 50 mg; if needed, a second 50 mg dose may be administered at least 2 hours after the initial dose; max 100 mg/24 hours

  Ubrelvy *Tab:* 50, 100 mg

  Comment: **Ubrelvy** *(ubrogepant)* is a potent, orally administered CGRP receptor antagonist for the acute treatment of migraine with or without aura. **Ubrelvy** is not indicated for the preventive treatment of migraine. **Ubrelvy** is contraindicated with concomitant use of strong CYP3A4 inhibitors. Strong CYP3A4 Inducers should be avoided as concomitant use will result in reduction of *ubrogepant* exposure. For additional dose modifications for moderate or weak CYP3A4 inhibitors and inducers or BCRP and/or P-gp only inhibitors, refer to the mfr pkg insert. The most common adverse reactions (incidence ≥2%) have been nausea and somnolence. There are no adequate data on the developmental risks associated with the use of **Ubrelvy** in pregnant females. However, animal studies have demonstrated adverse effects on embryo/fetal development and increased embryo/fetal mortality following administration of *ubrogepant* during pregnancy. There are no data on the presence of *ubrogepant* in human milk or effects on the breastfed infant.

ANTICONVULSANTS

► *divalproex sodium* (D) *Delayed-release:* initially 250 mg bid; titrate weekly to usual max 500 mg bid; *Extended-release:* initially 500 mg once daily; may increase after one week to 1 gm once daily
  Pediatric: <10 years: not recommended; ≥10 years: same as adult
    Depakene *Cap:* 250 mg del-rel; syr: 250 mg/5 ml (16 oz)
    Depakote *Tab:* 125, 250, 500 mg del-rel
    Depakote ER *Tab:* 250, 500 mg ext-rel
    Depakote Sprinkle *Cap:* 125 mg del-rel
► *topiramate* (D)(G) initially 25 mg daily in the PM and titrate up daily as tolerated; then 25 mg bid; then, 25 mg in the AM and 50 mg in the PM; then, 50 mg bid
  Pediatric: <12 years: not recommended; ≥12 years: same as adult
    Topamax *Tab:* 25, 50, 100, 200 mg
    Topamax Sprinkle Caps *Cap:* 15, 25 mg
    Trokendi XR *Cap:* 25, 50, 100, 200 mg ext-rel
    Quedexy XR *Cap:* 25, 50, 100, 150, 200 mg ext-rel

BETA-BLOCKERS

► *atenolol* (D)(G) initially 25 mg bid; max 150 mg/day in divided doses
  Pediatric: <12 years: not recommended; ≥12 years: same as adult
    Tenormin *Tab:* 25, 50, 100 mg
► *metoprolol succinate* (C)
  Pediatric: <12 years: not recommended; ≥12 years: same as adult
    ToprolR-XL initially 25-100 mg in a single dose daily; increase weekly if needed; max 400 mg/day
      Tab: 25*, 50*, 100*, 200*mg ext-rel

▷ **metoprolol tartrate** (C)
    Pediatric: <12 years: not recommended; ≥12 years: same as adult
        Lopressor (G) initially 25-50 mg bid; increase weekly if needed; max 400 mg/day
          Tab: 25, 37.5, 50, 75, 100 mg
▷ **nadolol** (C)(G) initially 20 mg daily; max 240 mg/day in divided doses
    Pediatric: <12 years: not recommended; ≥12 years: same as adult
        Corgard *Tab:* 20*, 40*, 80*, 120*, 160*mg
▷ **propranolol** (C)(G)
    Pediatric: <12 years: not recommended; ≥12 years: same as adult
        Inderal initially 10 mg bid; usual range 160-320 mg/day in divided doses
          Tab: 10*, 20*, 40*, 60*, 80*mg
        Inderal LA initially 80 mg daily in a single dose; increase q 3-7 days; usual range 120-160 mg/day; max 320 mg/day in a single dose
          Cap: 60, 80, 120, 160 mg sust-rel
        InnoPran XL initially 80 mg q HS; max 120 mg/day
          Cap: 80, 120 mg ext-rel
▷ **timolol** (C)(G) initially 5 mg bid; max 60 mg/day in divided doses
    Pediatric: <12 years: not recommended; ≥12 years: same as adult
        Blocadren *Tab:* 5, 10*, 20*mg

CALCIUM ANTAGONISTS

▷ **diltiazem** (C)(G)
    Pediatric: <12 years: not recommended; ≥12 years: same as adult
        Cardizem initially 30 mg qid; may increase gradually every 1-2 days; max 360 mg/day in divided doses
          Tab: 30, 60, 90, 120 mg
        Cardizem CD initially 120-180 mg once daily; adjust at 1- to 2-week intervals; max 480 mg/day
          Cap: 120, 180, 240, 300, 360 mg ext-rel
        Cardizem LA initially 180-240 mg once daily; titrate at 2-week intervals; max 540 mg/day
          Tab: 120, 180, 240, 300, 360, 420 mg ext-rel
        Cardizem SR initially 60-120 mg bid; adjust at 2-week intervals; max 360 mg/day
          Cap: 60, 90, 120 mg sust-rel
▷ **nifedipine** (C)(G)
    Pediatric: <12 years: not recommended; ≥12 years: same as adult
        Adalat initially 10 mg tid; usual range 10-20 mg tid; max 180 mg/day
          Cap: 10, 20 mg
         Procardia initially 10 mg tid; titrate over 7-14 days: max 30 mg/dose and 180 mg/day in divided doses
          Cap: 10, 20 mg
         Procardia XL initially 30-60 mg daily; titrate over 7-14 days; max 90 mg/day in divided doses
▷ **verapamil** (C)(G)
    Pediatric: <12 years: not recommended; ≥12 years: same as adult
        Calan 80-120 mg tid; increase daily <u>or</u> weekly if needed
          Tab: 40, 80*, 120*mg
        Covera HS initially 180 mg q HS; titrate in steps to 240 mg; then to 360 mg; then to 480 mg if needed
          Tab: 180, 240 mg ext-rel
        Isoptin initially 80-120 mg tid
          Tab: 40, 80, 120 mg

Isoptin SR initially 120-180 mg in the AM; may increase to 240 mg in the AM; then, 180 mg q 12 hours or 240 mg in the AM and 120 mg in the PM; then, 240 mg q 12 hours
  Tab: 120, 180*, 240*mg sust-rel

TRICYCLIC ANTIDEPRESSANTS (TCAs)

Comment: Co-administration of TCAs with SSRIs requires extreme caution.
▷ *amitriptyline* (C)(G) 10-20 mg q HS
  Pediatric: <12 years: not recommended; ≥12 years: same as adult
    Tab: 10, 25, 50, 75, 100, 150 mg
▷ *doxepin* (C)(G) 10-200 mg q HS
  Pediatric: <12 years: not recommended; ≥12 years: same as adult
    Cap: 10, 25, 50, 75, 100, 150 mg; *Oral conc:* 10 mg/ml (4 oz w. dropper)
▷ *imipramine* (C)(G) 10-200 mg q HS
    Tofranil 25-50 mg; max 200 mg/day; if maintenance dose exceeds 75 mg daily, may switch to **Tofranil PM**
    Pediatric: <6 years: not recommended; 6-12 years: initially 25 mg; >12 years: 50 mg max 2.5 mg/kg/day
      Tab: 10, 25, 50 mg
    Tofranil PM initially 75 mg once daily 1 hour before HS; max 200 mg
      Cap: 75, 100, 125, 150 mg
▷ *nortriptyline* (D)(G) 10-150 mg q HS
  Pediatric: <12 years: not recommended; ≥12 years: same as adult
    Pamelor *Cap:* 10, 25, 50, 75 mg; *Oral soln:* 10 mg/5 ml (16 oz)

SELECTIVE SEROTONIN REUPTAKE INHIBITORS (SSRIs)

Comment: Co-administration of SSRIs with TCAs requires extreme caution. Concomitant use of MAOIs and SSRIs is absolutely contraindicated. Avoid other serotonergic drugs. A potentially fatal adverse event is *serotonin syndrome,* caused by serotonin excess. Milder symptoms require HCP intervention to avert severe symptoms which can be rapidly fatal without urgent/emergent medical care. Symptoms include restlessness, agitation, confusion, hallucinations, tachycardia, hypertension, dilated pupils, muscle twitching, muscle rigidity, loss of muscle coordination, diaphoresis, diarrhea, headache, shivering, piloerection, hyperpyrexia, cardiac arrhythmias, seizures, loss of consciousness, coma, and death. Abrupt withdrawal or interruption of treatment with an antidepressant medication is sometimes associated with an Antidepressant Discontinuation Syndrome which may be mediated by gradually tapering the drug over a period of 2 weeks or longer, depending on the dose strength and length of treatment. Common symptoms of the *serotonin discontinuation syndrome* include flu-like symptoms (nausea, vomiting, diarrhea, headaches, sweating), sleep disturbances (insomnia, nightmares, constant sleepiness), mood disturbances (dysphoria, anxiety, agitation), cognitive disturbances (mental confusion, hyperarousal), sensory and movement disturbances (imbalance, tremors, vertigo, dizziness), and electric-shock-like sensations in the brain, often described by sufferers as "brain zaps."
▷ *fluoxetine* (C)(G)
    Prozac initially 20 mg daily; may increase after 1 week; doses >20 mg/day may be divided into AM and noon doses; max 80 mg/day
    Pediatric: <8 years: not recommended; 8-17 years: initially 10-20 mg/day; start lower weight children at 10 mg/day; if starting at 10 mg daily, may increase after 1 week to 20 mg once daily
      Cap: 10, 20, 40 mg; *Tab:* 30*, 60*mg; *Oral soln:* 20 mg/5 ml (4 oz) (mint)

Prozac Weekly following daily *fluoxetine* therapy at 20 mg/day for 13 weeks, may initiate **Prozac Weekly** 7 days after the last 20 mg *fluoxetine* dose
Pediatric: <12 years: not recommended; ≥12 years: same as adult
  Cap: 90 mg ent-coat del-rel pellets

OTHER AGENT

▷ *methysergide maleate* (X) 4-8 mg daily in divided doses with food; max 8 mg/day; max 6 month treatment course; wean off over last 2-3 weeks of treatment course; separate treatment courses by 3-4 week drug-free interval
Pediatric: <18 years: not recommended; ≥18 years: same as adult
    Sansert *Tab:* 2 mg
Comment: *Methysergide maleate* is indicated for the prevention or reduction of intensity and frequency of vascular headaches. It is contraindicated in pregnancy due to its oxytocic actions. *Methysergide maleate* is a semi-synthetic compound structurally related to ergotamine, and thus it may appear in breast milk. Ergot alkaloids have been reported to cause nausea, vomiting, diarrhea, and weakness in the nursing infant and suppression of prolactin secretion and lactation in the mother.

MAGNESIUM SUPPLEMENTS

▷ *magnesium* (B)
    Slow-Mag 2 tabs daily
      Tab: 64 mg (as chloride)+110 mg (as carbonate)
▷ *magnesium oxide* (B)
    Mag-Ox 400 1-2 tabs daily
      Tab: 400 mg

◯ HEADACHE: TENSION (MUSCLE CONTRACTION)

Acetaminophen for IV Infusion *see Pain*
NSAIDs *see* Appendix J. NSAIDs online at https://connect.springerpub.com/content/reference-book/978-0-8261-7935-7/back-matter/part02/back-matter/bmatter10
Opioid Analgesics *see Pain*
Topical and Transdermal Analgesics *see Pain*
Parenteral Corticosteroids *see* Appendix M. Parenteral Corticosteroids
Oral Corticosteroids *see* Appendix L. Oral Corticosteroids
Topical Analgesic and Anesthetic Agents *see* Appendix I. Anesthetic Agents for Local Infiltration and Dermal/Mucosal Membrane Application online at https://connect.springerpub.com/content/reference-book/978-0-8261-7935-7/back-matter/part02/back-matter/bmatter9

ORAL ANALGESIC COMBINATIONS

▷ *butalbital+acetaminophen* (C)(G)
Pediatric: <12 years: not recommended; ≥12 years: same as adult
    Phrenilin 1-2 tabs q 4 hours prn; max 6 tabs/day
      Tab: but 50 mg+acet 325 mg
    Phrenilin Forte 1 tab or cap q 4 hours prn; max 6 caps/day
      Cap/Tab: but 50 mg+acet 650 mg
▷ *butalbital+acetaminophen+caffeine* (C)(G)
Pediatric: <12 years: not recommended; ≥12 years: same as adult
    Fioricet 1-2 tabs q 4 hours prn; max 6/day
      Tab: but 50 mg+acet 325 mg+caf 40 mg
    Zebutal 1 cap q 4 hours prn; max 5/day
      Cap: but 50 mg+acet 500 mg+caf 40 mg
▷ *butalbital+acetaminophen+codeine+caffeine* (C)(III)(G)
Pediatric: <18 years: not recommended; ≥18 years: same as adult

Fioricet with Codeine 1-2 tabs at onset q 4 hours prn; max 6 tabs/day
Tab: but 50 mg+acet 325 mg+cod 30 mg+caf 40 mg
▷ *butalbital+aspirin+caffeine* (C)(III)(G)
Pediatric: <12 years: not recommended; ≥12 years: same as adult
Fiorinal 1-2 tabs or caps q 4 hours prn; max 6 caps/tabs/day
Tab/Cap: but 50 mg+asa 325 mg+caf 40 mg
▷ *butalbital+aspirin+codeine+caffeine* (C)(III)(G)
Pediatric: 18 years: not recommended; ≥18 years: same as adult
Fiorinal with Codeine 1-2 caps q 4 hours prn; max 6 caps/day
Cap: but 50 mg+asp 325 mg+cod 30 mg+caf 40 mg
▷ *butorphanol tartrate* (C)(IV)(G) initially 1 spray (1 mg) in one nostril and may
repeat after 60-90 minutes (*Elderly* 90-120 minutes) in opposite nostril if needed
or 1 spray in each nostril and may repeat q 3-4 hours prn
Pediatric: <18 years: not recommended; ≥18 years: same as adult
Butorphanol Nasal Spray *Nasal spray:* 1 mg/actuation (10 mg/ml, 2.5 ml)
Stadol Nasal Spray *Nasal spray:* 10 mg/ml, 1 mg/actuation (10 mg/ml, 2.5
ml)
▷ *tramadol* (C)(IV)(G) initially 100 mg once daily; may increase by 100 mg every
5 days; max 300 mg/day; *CrCl <30 mL/min or severe hepatic impairment:* not
recommended; *Cirrhosis:* max 50 mg q 12 hours
Pediatric: <18 years: not recommended; ≥18 years: same as adult
Rybix ODT *ODT:* 50 mg (mint) (phenylalanine)
Ryzolt *Tab:* 100, 200, 300 mg ext-rel
Ultram *Tab:* 50*mg
Ultram ER *Tab:* 100, 200, 300 mg ext-rel
▷ *tramadol+acetaminophen* (C)(IV)(G) 2 tabs q 4-6 hours prn; max 8 tabs/day; 5
days; *CrCl <30 mL/min:* max 2 tabs q 12 hours; max 4 tabs/day x 5 days; *Cirrhosis
or other liver disease:* contraindicated
Pediatric: <18 years: not recommended; ≥18 years: same as adult
Ultracet *Tab:* tram 37.5+acet 325 mg

TRICYCLIC ANTIDEPRESSANTS (TCAs)

Comment: Co-administration of TCAs with SSRIs requires extreme caution.
▷ *amitriptyline* (C)(G) 50-100 mg/day
Pediatric: <12 years: not recommended; ≥12 years: same as adult
Tab: 10, 25, 50, 75, 100, 150 mg
▷ *desipramine* (C)(G) 50-100 mg bid
Pediatric: <12 years: not recommended; ≥12 years: same as adult
Norpramin *Tab:* 10, 25, 50, 75, 100, 150 mg
▷ *imipramine* (C)(G)
Pediatric: <12 years: not recommended; ≥12 years: same as adult
Tofranil initially 75 mg daily (max 200 mg); adolescents initially 30-40 mg
daily (max 100 mg/day); if maintenance dose exceeds 75 mg daily, may switch
to Tofranil PM for divided or bedtime dosing
Tab: 10, 25, 50 mg
Tofranil PM initially 75 mg once daily 1 hour before HS; max 200 mg
Cap: 75, 100, 125, 150 mg
Tofranil Injection 50 mg IM; lower dose for adolescents; switch to oral form
as soon as possible
Amp: 25 mg/2 ml (2 ml)
▷ *nortriptyline* (D)(G) 25-50 mg/day
Pediatric: <12 years: not recommended; ≥12 years: same as adult
Pamelor *Cap:* 10, 25, 50, 75 mg; *Oral soln:* 10 mg/5 ml (16 oz)

MAGNESIUM SUPPLEMENTS

▷ *magnesium* (B)
> **Slow-Mag** 2 tabs daily
>> *Tab:* 64 mg (as chloride)/110 mg (as carbonate)
▷ *magnesium oxide* (B)
> **Mag-Ox 400** 1-2 tabs daily
>> *Tab:* 400 mg

 HEART FAILURE (HF)

HEART FAILURE AND DIABETES

Comment: Heart failure (HF) in the presence of type 2 diabetes (T2DM) has a 5-year survival rate on par with some of the worst diseases, such as lung cancer, because diabetes makes the pathophysiology of heart failure worse. Diabetes amplifies the neurohormonal response to heart failure, so it drives progressive heart failure and increases the risk for sudden death. **As left ventricular function decreases, patients with diabetes have heightened activation of the renin angiotensin system (RAS).** They have increased left ventricular hypertrophy, and they have increased sympathetic nervous system activation. A "four Ds" framework that clinicians can use to improve prognosis in these patients: (1) *Loop diuretics* to get the patient out of congestive cardiac syndrome as quickly as possible; (2) *Disease modification* with beta-blockers and ACE inhibitors, to the maximal dose tolerated, the mainstays of treatment for patients with heart failure (ACEI's protect these patients against cardiac myocyte cell death and vasoconstriction and beta-blockers protect against the activation of the sympathetic nervous system [SNS]); (3) Consider *device therapy* (including defibrillators and resynchronization therapy); and (4) *Optimize diabetes management*.

ACE INHIBITORS (ACEIs)

▷ *captopril* (C; D in 2nd, 3rd)(G) initially 25 mg tid; after 1-2 weeks may increase to 50 mg tid; max 450 mg/day
> *Pediatric:* <12 years: not recommended; ≥12 years: same as adult
> **Capoten** *Tab:* 12.5*, 25*, 50*, 100*mg
▷ *enalapril* (D) initially 5 mg daily; usual dosage range 10-40 mg/day; max 40 mg/day
> *Pediatric:* <12 years: not recommended; ≥12 years: same as adult
>> **Epaned Oral Solution** *Oral soln:* 1 mg/ml (150 ml) (mixed berry)
>> **Vasotec (G)** *Tab:* 2.5*, 5*, 10, 20 mg
▷ *fosinopril* (C; D in 2nd, 3rd) initially 10 mg daily, usual maintenance 20-40 mg/day in a single or divided doses
> *Pediatric:* <6 years, <50 kg: not recommended; 6-12 years, ≥50 kg: 5-10 mg daily; ≥12 years: same as adult
>> **Monopril** *Tab:* 10*, 20, 40 mg
▷ *lisinopril* (D) initially 5 mg daily
> **Prinivil** initially 10 mg daily; usual range 20-40 mg/day
> *Pediatric:* <12 years: not recommended; ≥12 years: same as adult
>> *Tab:* 5*, 10*, 20*, 40 mg
> **Qbrelis Oral Solution** administer as a single dose once daily
> *Pediatric:* <6 years, GFR <30 mL/min: not recommended; ≥6 years, GFR >30 mL/min: initially 0.07 mg/kg, max 5 mg; adjust according to BP up to a max 0.61 mg/kg (40 mg) once daily
>> *Oral soln:* 1 mg/ml (150 ml)
> **Zestril** initially 10 mg daily; usual range 20-40 mg/day
> *Pediatric:* <12 years: not recommended; ≥12 years: same as adult
>> *Tab:* 2.5, 5*, 10, 20, 30, 40 mg

▷ *quinapril* (C; D in 2nd, 3rd) initially 5 mg bid; increase weekly to 10-20 mg bid
  Pediatric: <12 years: not recommended; ≥12 years: same as adult
    Accupril *Tab:* 5*, 10, 20, 40 mg
▷ *ramipril* (C; D in 2nd, 3rd) initially 2.5 mg bid; usual maintenance 5 mg bid
  Pediatric: <12 years: not recommended; ≥12 years: same as adult
    Altace *Tab/Cap:* 1.25, 2.5, 5, 10 mg
▷ *trandolapril* (C; D in 2nd, 3rd) initially 1 mg daily; titrate to dose of 4 mg daily
  as tolerated
  Pediatric: <12 years: not recommended; ≥12 years: same as adult
    Mavik *Tab:* 1*, 2, 4 mg

BETA-BLOCKERS (CARDIOSELECTIVE)

▷ *carvedilol* (C)(G)
    Coreg initially 3.125 mg bid; may increase at 1-2 week intervals to 12.5 mg
    bid; usual max 50 mg bid
    Pediatric: <18 years: not recommended; ≥18 years: same as adult
      Tab: 3.125, 6.25, 12.5, 25 mg
    Coreg CR initially 10 mg once daily x 2 weeks; may double dose at 2 week
    intervals; max 80 mg once daily; may open caps and sprinkle on food
    Pediatric: <18 years: not recommended; ≥18 years: same as adult
      Cap: 10, 20, 40, 80 mg cont-rel
▷ *metoprolol succinate* (C)
  Pediatric: <12 years: not recommended; ≥12 years: same as adult
    Toprol-XL initially 12.5-25 mg in a single dose daily; increase weekly if
    needed; reduce if symptomatic bradycardia occurs; max 400 mg/day
      Tab: 25*, 50*, 100*, 200*mg ext-rel
▷ *metoprolol tartrate* (C)
  Pediatric: <12 years: not recommended; ≥12 years: same as adult
    Lopressor (G) initially 25-50 mg bid; increase weekly if needed; max 400 mg/day
      Tab: 25, 37.5, 50, 75, 100 mg

ANGIOTENSIN II RECEPTOR BLOCKERS (ARBs)

▷ *valsartan* (C; D in 2nd, 3rd) initially 40 mg bid; increase to 160 mg bid as
  tolerated or 320 mg daily after 2-4 weeks; usual range 80-320 mg/day
  Pediatric: <12 years: not recommended; ≥12 years: same as adult
    Diovan *Tab:* 40*, 80, 160, 320 mg
    Prexxartan Oral Solution *Oral soln:* 20 mg/5 ml, 80 mg/20 ml (120, 473 ml; 20
    ml unit-dose cup)

NEPRILYSIN INHIBITOR+ARB COMBINATION

▷ *sacubitril+valsartan* (D)(G) initially 49/51 bid; double dose after 2-4 weeks;
  maintenance 97/103 bid; *GFR <30 mL/min or moderate hepatic impairment:*
  initially 24/26 bid; double dose every 2-4 weeks to target maintenance 97/103 bid
  Pediatric: <12 years: not established; ≥12 years: same as adult
    Entresto
      Tab: **Entresto 24/26:** sacu 24 mg+val 26 mg
        Entresto 49/51: sacu 49 mg+val 51 mg
        Entresto 97/103: sacu 97 mg+val 103 mg

ALDOSTERONE RECEPTOR BLOCKER

▷ *eplerenone* (B) initially 25 mg once daily; titrate within 4 weeks to 50 mg once
  daily; adjust dose based on serum K^+
  Pediatric: <12 years: not recommended; ≥12 years: same as adult
    Inspra *Tab:* 25, 50 mg

Comment: **Inspra** is contraindicated with concomitant potent CYP3A4 inhibitors. Risk of hyperkalemia with concomitant ACEI or ARB. Monitor serum potassium at baseline, 1 week, and 1 month. Caution with serum Cr >2 mg/dL (male) or >1.8 mg/dL (female) and/or CrCl <50 mL/min, and DM with proteinuria.

THIAZIDE DIURETICS

Comment: Monitor hydration status, blood pressure, urine output, serum K+.
▷ *chlorothiazide* (C)(G) 0.5-1 gm/day in single or divided doses; max 2 gm/day
Pediatric: <6 months: up to 15 mg/lb/day in 2 divided doses; ≥6 months: 10 mg/lb/day in 2 divided doses
 Diuril *Tab:* 250*, 500*mg; *Oral susp:* 250 mg/5 ml (237 ml)
▷ *hydrochlorothiazide* (B)(G)
Pediatric: <12 years: not recommended; ≥12 years: same as adult
 Esidrix 25-100 mg once daily
 Tab: 25, 50, 100 mg
 Microzide 12.5 mg daily; usual max 50 mg/day
 Cap: 12.5 mg
▷ *methyclothiazide+deserpidine* (B) initially 2.5 mg once daily; max 5 mg once daily
Pediatric: <12 years: not recommended; ≥12 years: same as adult
 Enduronyl *Tab:* methy 5 mg+deser 0.25 mg*
 Enduronyl Forte *Tab:* methy 5 mg+deser 0.5 mg*
▷ *polythiazide* (C) 2-4 mg once daily
Pediatric: <12 years: not recommended; ≥12 years: same as adult
 Renese *Tab:* 1, 2, 4 mg

POTASSIUM-SPARING DIURETICS

Comment: Monitor hydration status, blood pressure, urine output, serum K+.
▷ *amiloride* (B) initially 5 mg once daily; may increase to 10 mg; max 20 mg
Pediatric: <12 years: not recommended; ≥12 years: same as adult
 Midamor *Tab:* 5 mg
▷ *spironolactone* (D) initially 50-100 mg in a single or divided doses; titrate at 2 week intervals
Pediatric: <12 years: not established; ≥12 years: same as adult
 Aldactone (G) *Tab:* 25, 50*, 100*mg
 CaroSpir *Oral susp:* 25 mg/5 ml (118, 473 ml) (banana)

LOOP DIURETICS

Comment: Monitor hydration status, blood pressure, urine output, serum K+.
▷ *bumetanide* (C)(G) 0.5-2 mg as a single dose; may repeat at 4-5 hour intervals; max 10 mg/day
Pediatric: <18 years: not recommended; ≥18 years: same as adult
 Bumex *Tab:* 0.5*, 1*, 2*mg
 Comment: **Bumetanide** is contraindicated with sulfa drug allergy.
▷ *ethacrynic acid* (B)(G) initially 50-200 mg once daily
Pediatric: infants: not recommended; >1 month: initially 25 mg/day; then adjust dose in 25 mg increments
 Edecrin *Tab:* 25, 50 mg
▷ *ethacrynate sodium* (B)(G) for IV injection
 Sodium Edecrin *Vial:* 50 mg single-dose
 Comment: **Sodium Edecrin** is more potent than more commonly used loop and thiazide diuretics.
▷ *furosemide* (C)(G) initially 40 mg bid
Pediatric: <12 years: not recommended; ≥12 years: same as adult
 Lasix *Tab:* 20, 40*, 80 mg; *Oral soln:* 10 mg/ml (2, 4 oz w. dropper)

Comment: *Furosemide* is contraindicated with sulfa drug allergy.
▷ *torsemide* (B) 5 mg once daily; may increase to 10 mg daily
  Pediatric: <12 years: not recommended; ≥12 years: same as adult
    Demadex *Tab:* 5*, 10*, 20*, 100*mg

OTHER DIURETICS

Comment: Monitor hydration status, blood pressure, urine output, and serum K⁺.
▷ *indapamide* (B) initially 1.25 mg once daily; may titrate dosage upward every
  4 weeks if needed; max 5 mg/day
    Lozol *Tab:* 1.25, 2.5 mg
  Comment: *Indapamide* is contraindicated with sulfa drug allergy.
▷ *metolazone* (B) 2.5-5 mg once daily
  Pediatric: <12 years: not recommended; ≥12 years: same as adult
    Zaroxolyn *Tab:* 2.5, 5, 10 mg
  Comment: *Metolazone* is contraindicated with sulfa drug allergy.

DIURETIC COMBINATIONS

Comment: Monitor hydration status, blood pressure, urine output, and serum K⁺.
▷ *amiloride+hydrochlorothiazide* (B)(G) initially 1 tab once daily; may increase to
  2 tabs/day in a single or divided doses
  Pediatric: <12 years: not recommended; ≥12 years: same as adult
    Moduretic *Tab:* amil 5 mg+hctz 50 mg*
▷ *spironolactone+hydrochlorothiazide* (D)(G)
  Pediatric: <12 years: not recommended; ≥12 years: same as adult
    Aldactazide 25 usual maintenance 50-100 mg in a single or divided doses
      Tab: spiro 25 mg+hctz 25 mg
    Aldactazide 50 usual maintenance 50-100 mg in a single or divided doses
      Tab: spiro 50 mg+hctz 50 mg
▷ *triamterene+hydrochlorothiazide* (C)(G)
  Pediatric: <12 years: not recommended; ≥12 years: same as adult
    Dyazide 1-2 caps daily
      Cap: triam 37.5 mg+hctz 25 mg
    Maxzide 1 tab once daily
      Tab: triam 75 mg+hctz 50 mg*
    Maxzide-25 1-2 tabs once daily
      Tab: triam 37.5 mg+hctz 25 mg*

NITRATE+PERIPHERAL VASODILATOR COMBINATION

▷ *isosorbide dinitrate+hydralazine* (C) initially 1 tab tid; may reduce to 1/2 tab tid
  if not tolerated; titrate as tolerated after 3-5 days; max 2 tabs tid
  Pediatric: <12 years: not recommended; ≥12 years: same as adult
    BiDil *Tab:* isosor 20 mg+hydral 37.5 mg
    Comment: BiDil is an adjunct to standard therapy in self-identified black
    persons to improve survival, to prolong time to hospitalization for heart
    failure, and to improve patient-reported functional status.

CARDIAC GLYCOSIDES

Comment: In selecting a digoxin dosing regimen, it is important to consider factors
that affect *digoxin* blood levels (e.g., body weight, age, renal function, concomitant
drugs) since *digoxin* has a very narrow therapeutic index (i.e., toxic levels of *digoxin*
are only slightly higher than therapeutic levels). Therapeutic serum level of digoxin
is 0.8-2 mcg/mL. Dosing can be initiated either with a loading dose followed by
maintenance dosing if rapid titration is desired or initiated with maintenance dosing
without a loading dose. Parenteral administration of *digoxin* should be used only
when the need for rapid digitalization is urgent or when the drug cannot be taken
orally. Intramuscular injection can lead to severe pain at the injection site, thus

intravenous administration is preferred. If the drug must be administered by the intramuscular route, it should be injected deep into the muscle followed by massage. For adults, no more than 500 mcg of parenteral *digoxin* (**Lanoxin Injection**) should be injected into a single site. For pediatric patients, no more than 200 mcg of *digoxin* (**Lanoxin Injection Pediatric**) should be injected into a single site. Administer IV *digoxin* dose over a period of 5 minutes or longer and avoid bolus administration to prevent systemic and coronary vasoconstriction. Mixing of **Lanoxin Injection** and **Lanoxin Injection Pediatric** with other drugs in the same container or simultaneous administration in the same intravenous line is not recommended. **Lanoxin Injection** and **Lanoxin Injection Pediatric** can be administered undiluted or diluted with a 4-fold or greater volume of Sterile Water for Injection, 0.9% Sodium Chloride for Injection, or D5W. The use of less than a 4-fold volume of diluent could lead to precipitation of the *digoxin*. Immediate use of the diluted product is recommended. **Lanoxin** (*digoxin*) is a positive inotrope, negative chronotrope, and negative dromatrope. Therefore, monitor the patient for bradycardia and hypotension. The classic features of digitalis toxicity are nausea, vomiting, abdominal pain, headache, dizziness, confusion, delirium, visual disturbance (blurred or yellow vision), and symptomatic/unstable bradycardia and/or hypotension.

For more information on the use of digoxin in pediatric heart failure, see Jain, S & Vaidyanathan, B. Digoxin in management of heart failure in children: Should it be continued or relegated to the history books? *Ann Pediatr Cardiol.* Jul-Dec 2009: 2(2):149–152.

▷ *digoxin* (C)(G) Loading Dose: 1-1.5 mg IM, IV, or PO in divided doses over 1-3 days; Maintenance: 0.125-0.5 mg/day
Pediatric: Total oral pediatric digitalizing dose (in 24 hours): <2 years: 40-50 mcg/kg; 2-10 years: 30-40 mcg/kg; >10 years: 0.75-1.5 mg; Daily oral pediatric maintenance (single dose once daily): <2 years: 10-12 mcg/kg; 2-10 years: 8-10 mcg/kg; >10 years: 0.125–0.5 mg; max: 0.125-0.5 mg; <10 years: use elixir or parenteral form
    Lanoxicap *Cap:* 0.05, 0.1, 0.2 mg soln-filled (alcohol)
    Lanoxin *Tab:* 0.0625, 0.125*, 0.1875, 0.25*mg; *Elix:* 0.05 mg/ml (2 oz w. dropper) (lime) (alcohol 10%)
    Lanoxin Injection *Amp:* 0.25 mg/ml (2 ml)
    Lanoxin Injection Pediatric *Amp:* 0.1 mg/ml (1 ml)

HYPERPOLARIZATION-ACTIVATED CYCLIC NUCLEOTIDE-GATED CHANNEL BLOCKER

▷ *ivabradine* (D) initially 5 mg bid with food; assess after 2 weeks and adjust dose to achieve a resting heart rate of 50-60 bpm; thereafter, adjust dose as needed based on resting heart rate and tolerability; max 7.5 mg bid; in patients with a history of conduction defects, or for whom bradycardia could lead to hemodynamic compromise, initiate at 2.5 mg bid before increasing the dose based on heart rate
Pediatric: <18 years: not established; ≥18 years: same as adult
    Corlanor *Tab:* 5, 7.5 mg
    Comment: **Corlanor** is indicated to reduce the risk of hospitalization for worsening heart failure in patients with stable, symptomatic, chronic heart failure with left ventricular ejection fraction (LVEF) ≤35%, who are in sinus rhythm with resting heart rate ≤70 bpm and either are on maximally tolerated doses of beta-blockers or have a contraindication to beta-blocker use. **Corlanor** is contraindicated with acute decompensated heart failure, BP <90/50, sick sinus syndrome (SSS), sinoatrial block, and 3rd degree AV block (unless patient has a functioning demand pacemaker). **Corlanor** may cause fetal toxicity when administered pregnant females based on embryo-fetal toxicity and cardiac teratogenic to effects observed in animal studies. Therefore, females should be advised to use effective contraception when taking this drug.

SOLUBLE GUANYLATE CYCLASE (SGC) STIMULATOR

▷ *evericiguat* initially 2.5 mg orally once daily with food; then, double the dose approximately every 2 weeks; target maintenance 10 mg once daily; tablets may be crushed and mixed with water for patients who have difficulty swallowing

Verquvo *Tab*: 2.5, 5, 10 mg film-coat

Comment: **Verquvo** indicated to reduce the risk of cardiovascular death and heart failure (HF) hospitalization following a hospitalization for heart failure or need for outpatient IV diuretics, in adults with symptomatic chronic HF and ejection fraction less than 45%. The most common adverse reactions reported (incidence ≥5%) have been hypotension and anemia. **Verquvo** is contraindicated in pregnancy. Exclude pregnancy before the start of treatment. Advise females of reproductive potential to use effective forms of contraception during treatment and for one month after discontinuation. Breastfeeding is not recommended.

 HELICOBACTER PYLORI (*H. PYLORI*) INFECTION

ERADICATION REGIMENS

Comment: There are many H2 receptor blocker-based and PPI-based treatment regimens suggested in the professional literature for the eradication of the *H. pylori* organism and subsequent ulcer healing. Generally, regimens range from 10 to 14 days for eradication and 2-6 more weeks of continued gastric acid suppression. A 3 to 4 antibiotic combination may increase treatment effectiveness and decrease the likelihood of resistant strain emergence. Empirical treatment is not recommended. Diagnosis should be confirmed before treatment is started. Antibiotic choices include *doxycycline, tetracycline, amoxicillin, amoxicillin+clavulanate, clarithromycin, clindamycin,* and *metronidazole*. Follow-up visits are recommended at 2 and 6 weeks to evaluate treatment outcomes.

▷ *Regimen 1:* Helidac Therapy (D)(G) *bismuth subsalicylate* 525 mg qid + *tetracycline* 500 mg qid + *metronidazole* 250 mg qid x 14 days
Pediatric: <12 years: not recommended; ≥12 years: same as adult
Pack: bismuth subsalicylate Chew tab: 262.4 mg (112/pck); *tetracycline cap:* 500 mg (56/pck); *metronidazole Tab:* 250 mg (56/pck)

▷ *Regimen 2:* PrevPac (D)(G) *amoxicillin* 500 mg 2 caps bid + *lansoprazole* 30 mg bid + *clarithromycin* 500 mg bid x 14 days (one card per day)
Pediatric: <12 years: not recommended; ≥12 years: same as adult
Kit: lansoprazole cap: 30 mg (2/card); *amoxicillin cap:* 500 mg (4/card); *clarithromycin Tab:* 500 mg (2/card) (14 daily cards/carton)

▷ *Regimen 3:* Pylera (D) take 3 caps qid after meals and at bedtime x 10 days; take with 8 oz water plus *omeprazole* 20 mg bid, with breakfast and dinner, for 10 days
Pediatric: <12 years: not recommended; ≥12 years: same as adult
Cap: bismuth subsalicylate 140 mg+*tetracycline* 125 mg+*metronidazole* 125 mg (120 caps)
Comment: *Omeprazole* is not included with **Pylera**.

▷ *Regimen 4:* Omeclamox-Pak (C) *omeprazole* 20 mg bid + *amoxicillin* 1000 mg bid + *clarithromycin* 500 mg bid x 10 days
Kit: omeprazole cap: 20 mg (2/pck); *amoxicillin cap:* 500 mg (4/pck); *clarithromycin tab:* 500 mg (2/pck) (10 pcks/carton)

▷ *Regimen 5:* (C) *omeprazole* 40 mg daily + *clarithromycin* 500 mg tid x 2 weeks; then continue *omeprazole* 10-40 mg daily x 6 more weeks

▷ *Regimen 6:* (B) *lansoprazole* 30 mg tid + *amoxicillin* 1 gm tid x 10 days; then continue *lansoprazole* 15-30 mg daily x 6 more weeks

▷ *Regimen 7:* (C) *omeprazole* 40 mg daily + *amoxicillin* 1 gm bid + *clarithromycin* 500 mg bid x 10 days; then continue *omeprazole* 10-40 mg daily x 6 more weeks

▷ *Regimen 8:* (D) *bismuth subsalicylate* 525 mg qid + *metronidazole* 250 mg qid + *tetracycline* 500 mg qid + H₂ receptor agonist x 2 weeks; then continue H₂ receptor agonist x 6 more weeks

▷ *Regimen 9:* (not for use in 1st; B in 2nd, 3rd) *bismuth subsalicylate* 525 mg qid + *metronidazole* 250 mg qid + *amoxicillin* 500 mg qid + H₂ receptor agonist x 2 weeks; then continue H₂ receptor agonist x 6 more weeks

▷ *Regimen 10:* (C) *ranitidine bismuth citrate* 400 mg bid + *clarithromycin* 500 mg bid x 2 weeks; then continue *ranitidine bismuth citrate* 400 mg bid x 2 more weeks

▷ *Regimen 11:* (D) *omeprazole* 20 mg or *lansoprazole* 30 mg q AM + *bismuth subsalicylate* 524 mg qid + *metronidazole* 500 mg tid + *tetracycline* 500 mg qid x 2 weeks; then continue *omeprazole* 20 mg or *lansoprazole* 30 mg q AM for 6 more weeks

▷ *Regimen 12:* **Talicia** administer 4 capsules as a single dose every 8 hours x 14 days; take with food; swallow whole with a full glass of water, do not crush or chew; do not take with alcohol

    Cap: (fixed dose combination) *omeprazole magnesium* 10 mg+*amoxicillin* 250 mg+*rifabutin* 12.5 mg del-rel

HEMOLYTIC UREMIC SYNDROME: ATYPICAL (aHUS)

COMPLEMENT INHIBITORS

▷ *eculizumab* (C) dilute to a final admixture concentration of 5 mg/ml using the following steps: (1) withdraw the required amount of **Soliris** from the vial into a sterile syringe, (2) transfer the dose to an infusion bag, (3) add IV fluid equal to the drug volume (0.9% NaCl or 0.45% NaCl or D5W or Ringer's Lactate); the final admixed **Soliris** 5 mg/ml infusion volume is: 300 mg dose (60 ml), 600 mg dose (120 ml), 900 mg dose (180 ml), 1200 mg dose (240 ml); administer a 900 mg IV infusion once weekly for the first 4 weeks; then, 1200 mg IV infusion for the 5th dose 1 week after the 4th dose; then, 1200 mg IV infusion once every 2 weeks thereafter

Pediatric: <18 years: >40 kg: 900 mg IV infusion once weekly x 4 doses; then, 1200 mg at week 5; then, 1200 mg once every 2 weeks thereafter; 30-<40 kg: 600 mg IV infusion once weekly x 2 doses; then, 900 mg IV infusion at week 3; then, 900 mg IV infusion once every 2 weeks thereafter; 20-<30 kg: 600 mg IV infusion once weekly x 2 doses; then, 600 mg IV infusion at week 3; then, 600 mg IV infusion once every 2 weeks thereafter; 5-<10 kg: 300 mg IV infusion x 1 dose; then, 300 mg IV infusion at week 2; then, 300 mg IV infusion once every 3 weeks thereafter; <5 kg: not established

    Soliris *Vial:* 300 mg (10 mg/ml, 30 ml), single-use, concentrated solution for intravenous infusion (preservative-free)

    Comment: **Soliris** *(eculizumab)* is a complement inhibitor indicated for the treatment of patients with paroxysmal nocturnal hemoglobinuria (PNH) to reduce hemolysis, patients with atypical hemolytic uremic syndrome (aHUS) to inhibit complement-mediated thrombotic acetylcholine receptor (AchR) antibody positive. **Soliris** should be administered at the above recommended dosage regimen time points or within 2 days of each time point. Supplemental dosing of **Soliris** is required in the setting of concomitant support with plasmapheresis (PI) or plasma exchange (PE) or fresh frozen plasma (FFP) infusion (see mfr pkg insert for supplemental dosing). **Soliris** is not indicated for the treatment of patients with Shiga toxin *E. coli*-related hemolytic uremic syndrome (STEC-HUS). **Soliris** is contraindicated in patients with unresolved *Neisseria meningitides* infection and patients who are not currently vaccinated against *Neisseria meningitides,* unless the risks of delaying **Soliris** treatment outweigh the risks of developing meningococcal infection. Prescribers must enroll in the **Soliris** REMS Program (1-888-SOLIRIS, 1-888-765-4747), counsel patients about the risk of meningococcal infection, provide patients with **Soliris** REMS Educational materials, and ensure that patients are vaccinated with meningococcal vaccine. The most frequently reported adverse reactions in the PNH randomized trial (incidence ≥10%) are headache, nasopharyngitis, back pain, and nausea. There are no adequate and well-controlled human studies of **Soliris** in pregnancy or effects on the breastfed infant. Based on animal studies, **Soliris** may cause fetal harm. It is not known whether **Soliris** is excreted in human milk. IgG is excreted in human milk, so it is expected that **Soliris** will be present in human milk. However, published data suggest that antibodies in human milk do not enter the neonatal and infant circulation in substantial amounts. Caution should be exercised when **Soliris** is administered to a breastfeeding patient.

HEMOPHAGOCYTIC LYMPHOHISTIOCYTOSOS (HLH)

INTERFERON GAMMA (IFNγ) BLOCKING ANTIBODY

▶ *emapalumab-lzsg* Starting Dose: 1 mg/kg via IV infusion over 1 hour twice per week; administer concomitant *dexamethasone*

Gamifant *Vial:* 10 mg/2 ml (5 mg/ml), 50 mg/10 ml (5 mg/ml), single dose, for dilution and IV infusion

Comment: Gamifant *(emapalumab-lzsg)* is indicated for the treatment of adult and pediatric (newborn and older) patients with primary hemophagocytic lymphohistiocytosis (HLH) with refractory, recurrent, or progressive disease or intolerance with conventional HLH therapy. The most common adverse reactions (incidence ≥20%) have been infections, hypertension, infusion-related reactions, and pyrexia. Monitor patients for signs and symptoms of infection and treat promptly. Test for latent tuberculosis. Administer prophylactic treatment against Herpes Zoster, Pneumocystis jirovecii and fungal infections. Do not administer live or live attenuated vaccines to patients receiving **Gamifant**. Monitor patients for infusion-related reactions; interrupt infusion for severe reaction and institute appropriate medical management. There are no available data on **Gamifant** use in pregnant females to inform a drug-associated risk of adverse developmental outcomes. In animal studies, no maternal toxicity occurred and there was no evidence of teratogenicity or effects on embryo/fetal survival or growth. There is no information regarding the presence of *emapalumab-lzsg* in human milk of effects on the breastfed infant. Developmental and health benefits of breastfeeding should be considered along with the mother's clinical need for **Gamifant** and any potential adverse effects on the breastfed infant from **Gamifant** or from the underlying maternal condition.

HEMOPHILIA A (CHRISTMAS DISEASE, CONGENITAL FACTOR VIII DEFICIENCY), HEMOPHILIA B (CHRISTMAS DISEASE, FACTOR IX DEFICIENCY), VON WILLEBRAND DISEASE (VWF DEFICIENCY)

BI-SPECIFIC FACTOR IXA- AND FACTOR X-DIRECTED ANTIBODY

▶ *emicizumab-kxwh* initially 3 mg/kg by SC injection once weekly for the first 4 weeks; followed by 1.5 mg/kg once weekly

Pediatric: same as adult

Hemlibra *Vial:* 30 mg/ml (single-dose); 60 mg/0.4 ml (single-dose); 105 mg 0.7 ml (single-dose); 150 mg/ml (single-dose)

Comment: Hemlibra is a bi-specific factor IXa- and factor X-directed antibody indicated for routine prophylaxis to prevent or reduce the frequency of bleeding episodes in adult and pediatric patients with hemophilia A (congenital factor VIII deficiency) with factor VIII inhibitors. *Laboratory Coagulation Test Interference*: **Hemlibra** interferes with activated clotting time (ACT), activated partial thrombo-plastin time (aPTT), and coagulation laboratory tests based on aPTT, including one stage aPTT-based single-factor assays, aPTT-based Activated Protein C Resistance (APC-R), and Bethesda assays (clotting-based) for factor VIII (FVIII) inhibitor titers. Intrinsic pathway clotting-based laboratory tests should <u>not</u> be used. Black Box Warning (BBW): Cases of thrombotic microangiopathy and thrombotic events were reported when on average a cumulative amount of >100 U/kg/24 hours of activated prothrombin complex concentrate (aPCC) was administered for 24 hours <u>or</u> more to patients receiving Hemlibra prophylaxis. Monitor for the development of thrombotic microangiopathy and thrombotic events if aPCC is administered. Discontinue aPCC and suspend dosing of Hemlibra if symptoms occur. The most common adverse reactions (have been injection site reactions, headache, and arthralgia. There are no available data on **Hemlibra** use in pregnant females to inform a drug-associated risk of major birth defects and miscarriage. Women of childbearing potential should use contraception while receiving **Hemlibra** and **Hemlibra** should be used during pregnancy <u>only</u> if the potential benefit for the mother outweighs the risk to the fetus. There is no information regarding the presence of *emicizumab-kxwh* in human milk <u>or</u> effects on the breastfed infant.

COAGULATION FACTOR VIIA [RECOMBINANT]-JNCW

▷ *coagulation factor VIIa [recombinant]-jncw*
Mild/Moderate Bleed: 75 mcg/kg; repeated every 3 hours until hemostasis is achieved <u>or</u> initial dose 225 mcg/kg; if hemostasis is not achieved within 9 hours, additional 75 mcg/kg doses may be administered every 3 hours as needed to achieve hemostasis.
Severe Bleed: 225 mcg/kg, followed if necessary 6 hours later with 75 mcg/kg every 2 hours
Pediatric: <12 years: safety and efficacy not established; ≥12 years: same as adult
  Sevenfact *Vial:* 1, 5 mg, 1 mg/ml (1000 mcg/ml) after reconstitution (see mfr pkg insert), single-use, pwdr for reconstitution and IV infusion w. pre-filled syringe with water for Injection diluent
  Comment: Sevenfact *(coagulation factor VIIa [recombinant]-jncw)* is a recombinant analog of human FVII for the treatment and control of bleeding episodes in patients with hemophilia A or B with inhibitors (neutralizing antibodies). **Sevenfact** is <u>not</u> indicated for treatment of congenital factor VII deficiency. **Sevenfact** is contraindicated in patients with known allergy to rabbits or rabbit proteins. Patients with hemophilia A or B with inhibitors who have other risk factors for thrombosis may be at increased risk of serious arterial and venous thrombotic events. If a hypersensitivity reaction occurs, including anaphylaxis, discontinue **Sevenfact** immediately and institute appropriate medical care. Clinical experience with pharmacologic use of FVIIa-containing products indicates an elevated risk of serious thrombotic events when used simultaneously with activated prothrombin complex concentrates. There are <u>no</u> adequate and well-controlled animal <u>or</u> human studies os Sevenfact use in pregnancy to determine whether there is a drug-associated embryo/fetal risk. There is <u>no</u> information regarding the presence of **Sevenfact** in human milk <u>or</u> effect on the breastfed infant. The developmental and health benefits of breastfeeding should be considered along with the mother's clinical need for **Sevenfact** and any potential adverse effects on the breastfed infant from **Sevenfact** <u>or</u> from the underlying maternal condition. The most common adverse reactions (incidence ≥1%) have been

headache, dizziness, infusion-site discomfort, infusion-site hematoma, infusion-related reaction, and fever.

FACTOR VIII MOLECULE

▷ *turoctocog alfa pegol, N8-GP* dosage must be individualized according to the needs of the patient (weight, severity of hemorrhage, presence of inhibitors); the following general dosages are suggested: Number of AHF I.U. required = (body weight (in kg) x desired Factor VIII increase (% normal)) x 0.5 (see mfr pkg insert)

Minor hemorrhage (superficial, early hemorrhages, hemorrhages into joints): therapeutically necessary plasma level of FVIII activity is 20% to 40% of normal, repeated every 12-24 hours as necessary until resolved (at least 1 day, depending upon the severity of the bleeding episode)

Moderate (bleeding into muscles, mild head trauma, bleeding into the oral cavity): therapeutically necessary plasma level of FVIII activity is 30% to 60% of normal, repeated every 12 to 24 hours for 3-4 days or until adequate local hemostasis is achieved

Major (gastrointestinal bleeding, intracranial, intraabdominal or intrathoracic bleeding, fractures): therapeutically necessary plasma level of FVIII activity is 60% to 100% of normal, repeated every 8 to 24 hours until bleeding is resolved, resolved, or in the case of surgery, until adequate local hemostasis and wound healing are achieved

Esperoct
Pediatric:

Routine prophylaxis to prevent or reduce the frequency of bleeding episodes: <16 years: 20-40 IU/kg every other day (3 to 4 times weekly); alternatively, an every 3rd day dosing regimen targeted to maintain Factor VIII trough levels greater than 1% may be employed

Dosage necessary to maintain the therapeutic plasma level based on an active bleeding episode: although dosage must be individualized according to the needs of the patient (weight, severity of hemorrhage, presence of inhibitors), the following general dosages are suggested: number of Antihemophilic Factor IU required = (body weight (in kg) x desired Factor VIII increase (% normal)) x 0.5

or

Minor hemorrhage (superficial, early hemorrhages, hemorrhages into joints): therapeutically necessary plasma level of Factor VIII activity is 20% to 40% of normal, repeated every 12-24 hours as necessary until resolved (at least 1 day, depending upon the severity of the bleeding episode)

Moderate (bleeding into muscles, mild head trauma, bleeding into the oral cavity): therapeutically necessary plasma level of Antihemophilic Factor VIII activity is 30% to 60% of normal, repeated every 12-24 hours for 3-4 days or until adequate local hemostasis is achieved

Major (gastrointestinal bleeding, intracranial, intra abdominal or intrathoracic bleeding, fractures): therapeutically necessary plasma level of Antihemophilic Factor VIII activity is 60% to 100% of normal, repeated every 8 to 24 hours until bleeding is resolved, resolved, or in the case of surgery, until adequate local hemostasis and wound healing are achieved

Comment: Esperoct (*turoctocog alfa pegol, N8-GP*) is an extended half-life factor VIII molecule for the treatment of adults and children with hemophilia A for routine prophylaxis to reduce the frequency of bleeding episodes, on-demand treatment and control of bleeding episodes, and perioperative management of bleeding. **Esperoct** has been evaluated in 270 people (202 adults/adolescents and 68 children) in five prospective, multicenter clinical trials in previously treated people (PTPs) with severe hemophilia A (<1%

endogenous FVIII activity) and no history of inhibitors. Total exposure to **Esperoct** was 80,425 exposure days corresponding to 889 patient years of treatment. **Esperoct** was well tolerated across all age groups and indications, and no safety concerns were identified after more than 5 years of clinical exposure.

DESMOPRESSIN (DDAVP)

Comment: Desmopressin (DDAVP) acetate 0.3μg/kg administered in 50 mL 0.9% saline solution via IV infusion over 15-30 minutes may enable patients with certain types of hemophilia to undergo minor procedures (e.g., tooth extraction, minor surgery) without needing replacement therapy. If a replacement product is needed, desmopressin may reduce the required dose. One dose of desmopressin is effective for about 8-10 hours. The dose required for hemostasis is approximately 15 times the dose used to treat diabetes insipidus. The regular intranasal preparation (0.1 mg/ml) used to treat diabetes insipidus, is too dilute to elicit a hemostatic response. A high-concentration intranasal preparation (i.e., **Stimate Nasal Spray** (1.5 mg/ml, 150 mcg/actuation, 25 sprays/bottle) has been licensed and has shown a similar response as the intravenous form. **Stimate Nasal Spray** is administered by nasal insufflation, one spray per nostril, to provide a total dose of 300 mcg. In patients weighing less than 50 kg, 150 mcg administered as a single spray provided the expected effect on Factor VIII coagulant activity, Factor VIII ristocetin cofactor activity and skin bleeding time. If **Stimate Nasal Spray** is used pre-operatively, it should be administered 2 hours prior to the scheduled procedure. The necessity for repeat administration of **Stimate Nasal Spray** or use of any blood products for hemostasis should be determined by laboratory response as well as the clinical condition of the patient. Fluid restriction should be observed, and fluid intake should be limited to a minimum, from 1 hour before desmopressin administration, until at least 24 hours after administration. Use of DDAVP in infants and children will require careful fluid intake restriction to prevent possible hyponatremia and water intoxication. **Stimate Nasal Spray** should not be used in infants younger than 11 months in the treatment of hemophilia A or von Willebrand's disease; safety and effectiveness in children between 11 months and 12 years-of-age have been demonstrated.

Treatment of von Willebrand disease involves control of bleeding with replacement therapy (cryoprecipitate or pasteurized intermediate-purity factor VIII concentrate) or desmopressin. Desmopressin (DDAVP) is a synthetic analogue of the antidiuretic hormone vasopressin; it has enhanced antidiuretic activity and no significant pressor activity related to vasopressin. DDAVP controls bleeding by stimulating the body to release more of the von Willebrand factor (VWF) into the plasma, thus increasing levels of factor VIII necessary for normal platelet function. DDAVP causes a 2-fold to 5-fold increase in plasma von Willebrand factor and FVIII concentrations in individuals who are healthy and patients who are responsive. DDAVP is often considered the first treatment for managing von Willebrand disease, type 1 (the most common form of VWD). Some women use the nasal spray at the beginning of their menstrual periods to control excessive bleeding. To ensure adequate response to the drug, a test dose is typically done and the response of VWF antigen is measured. DDAVP will stop bleeding in patients with mild-moderate von Willebrand's disease and Hemophilia A with episodes of spontaneous or trauma-induced injuries, such as hemarthroses, intramuscular hematomas, mucosal bleeding, or menorrhagia. In the outpatient setting during two clinical trials where patients recorded bleeding episodes, desmopression nasal spray (i.e., **Stimate Nasal Spray**) provided effective hemostasis 100% of the time in 75% of the 106 patients (n = 16). For those patients not responding in 100% of bleeding occasions, 78% (64 of 82) of bleeding episodes were effectively controlled with **Stimate Nasal Spray**. In the outpatient setting during two clinical trials where patients recorded bleeding episodes, **Stimate Nasal Spray** provided effective hemostasis 100% of the time in 2 of the 5 patients. For those patients not responding in 100% of bleeding occasions, 45% (14 of 31) of bleeding episodes were effectively controlled with **Stimate Nasal Spray**. **Stimate Nasal Spray** is not indicated for the treatment of severe classic von Willebrand disease (Type I) and when there is evidence of an abnormal molecular form of Factor VIII antigen. **Stimate Nasal Spray** is indicated for patients with hemophilia A with Factor VIII coagulant activity levels greater than 5%. **Stimate Nasal Spray** is not indicated for the treatment of hemophilia A with Factor VIII coagulant activity levels equal to or less than 5%, or for the treatment of hemophilia B, or in patients who have Factor VIII antibodies. **Stimate Nasal Spray** is not appropriate for patients with changes in the nasal mucosa such as scarring, edema, or other disease process which may cause erratic, unreliable absorption.

VON WILLEBRAND FACTOR (RECOMBINANT) (rVWF)

▷ *von Willebrand factor (Recombinant) (rVWF)* physician supervision of the treatment regimen is required; administer via intravenous injection only at max rate 4 ml/min

Pediatric: <18 years: not established; ≥18 years: same as adult *On-Demand Treatment and Control of Bleeding Episode:* for each bleeding episode, administer the first dose of **Vonvendi** with an approved recombinant (non-von Willebrand factor containing) factor VIII, if factor VIII baseline levels are below 40% or are unknown; adjust dose based on the extent and location of bleeding

    Minor: initially 40-50 IU/kg; then, 40-50 IU/kg every 8-24 hours

    Major: initially 50-80 IU/kg; then, 40-60 IU/kg every 8-24 hours for approximately 2 to 3 days

Perioperative Management of Bleeding: continue to monitor the VWF:RCo and FVIII:C plasma levels after any surgical procedure

Elective Surgical Procedure: a single dose of **Vonvendi** may be administered 12-24 hours prior to surgery to allow the endogenous factor VIII levels to increase to at least 30 IU/dL (minor surgery) or 60 IU/dL (major surgery); assess FVIII:C levels within 3 hours prior to surgery; if the FVIII:C levels are at or above the recommended minimum target levels, administer a single dose of **Vonvendi** within 1 hour prior to the procedure; if the FVIII:C levels are below the recommended minimum target levels, administer recombinant factor VIII in addition to **Vonvendi** to raise VWF:RCo and FVIII:C

Emergency Surgery: assess baseline VWF:RCo and FVIII:C levels within 3 hours prior to surgery; if not available, use weight-based dosing calculation; administer **Vonvendi** one hour before surgery with or without recombinant factor VIII and adjust the dose to raise VWF:RCo and FVIII:C to adequate level

Type of Surgery	Target Peak Plasma Level VWF:RCo	FVIII:C	Calculation of rVWF Dose (IU VWF:RCo required)
Minor	50-60 IU/dL	40-50 IU/dL	Δ VWF:RCo x BW (kg)/IR
Major	100 IU/dL	80-100 IU/dL	

Vonvendi Vial: 650, 1300 IU VWF:RCo, single-use, pwdr for reconstitution with diluent supplied, and IV injection (non-pyrogenic)

Comment: Do not use **Vonvendi** in patients who have had life-threatening hypersensitivity reactions to **Vonvendi** or its components (tri-sodium citrate dihydrate, glycine, mannitol, trehalose-dihydrate, polysorbate 80, and hamster or mouse proteins). The most common adverse reactions observed (incidence ≥2%) have been generalized pruritus, vomiting, nausea, dizziness, and vertigo. Thromboembolic reactions can occur, particularly in patients with risk factors for thrombosis. Monitor for early signs of thrombosis and have prophylaxis measures against thromboembolism instituted according to current recommendations. One out of 80 VWD subjects treated with **Vonvendi** in clinical trials developed proximal deep vein thrombosis in the perioperative period after undergoing total hip replacement surgery. In patients requiring frequent doses of **Vonvendi,** in combination with recombinant factor VIII, monitor plasma levels for FVIII:C because sustained excessive factor VIII plasma levels can increase the risk for thromboembolic events. Hypersensitivity reactions, including anaphylaxis, may occur. Discontinue **Vonvendi** if hypersensitivity symptoms occur and administer appropriate emergency treatment. Inhibitors to von Willebrand factor (VWF) and/or factor VIII can occur. If the expected plasma levels of VWF activity (VWF:RCo) are <u>not</u> attained or if bleeding is <u>not</u> controlled with an appropriate dose, perform an appropriate assay to determine if an anti-VWF <u>or</u> anti-factor VIII inhibitors are present.

HEMORRHOIDS

Bulk-Forming Agents, Stool Softeners, and Stimulant Laxatives *see Constipation*

RECTAL PREPARATIONS

▷ *dibucaine* (C)(OTC)(G) 1 applicatorful <u>or</u> suppository bid and after each stool; max 6/day
  Pediatric: <12 years: not recommended; ≥12 years: same as adult
    Nupercainal (OTC) *Rectal oint:* 1% (30, 60 gm); *Rectal supp:* 1% (12, 14/pck)
▷ *hydrocortisone* (C)(OTC)(G)
  Pediatric: <12 years: not recommended; ≥12 years: same as adult
    Anusol-HC 1 suppository rectally bid-tid <u>or</u> 2 suppositories bid x 2 weeks
      Rectal supp: 25 mg (12, 24/pck)
    Anusol-HC Cream 2.5% apply bid-qid prn
      Rectal crm: 2.5% (30 gm)
    Anusol HC-1 apply tid-qid prn; max 7 days
      Rectal crm: 1% (0.7 oz)
    Hydrocortisone Rectal Cream
      Rectal crm: 1, 2.5% (30 gm)
    Nupercainal apply tid-qid prn
      Rectal crm: 1% (30 gm)
    Proctocort 1 suppository rectally bid-tid prn <u>or</u> 2 suppositories bid x 2 weeks
      Rectal supp: 30 mg (12/pck)
    Proctocream HC 2.5% apply rectally bid-qid prn
      Rectal crm: 2.5% (30 gm)
    Proctofoam HC 1% apply rectally tid-qid prn
      Rectal foam: 1% (14 applications/10 gm)
▷ *hydrocortisone+pramoxine* (C) 1 applicatorful tid-qid and after each stool; max 2 weeks
  Pediatric: <12 years: not recommended; ≥12 years: same as adult
    Procort *Rectal crm:* hydrocort 1.85%+pramox 1.15% (30 gm)
▷ *hydrocortisone+lidocaine* (B) apply bid-tid prn
  Pediatric: <12 years: not recommended; ≥12 years: same as adult
    AnaMantle HC, LidaMantle HC *Crm/Lotn:* hydrocort 5%+lido 3% (1 oz)
▷ *petrolatum+mineral oil+shark liver oil+phenylephrine* (C)(OTC)(G)
    Preparation H Ointment apply up to qid prn
      Rectal oint: 1, 2 oz
▷ *petrolatum+glycerin+shark liver oil+phenylephrine* (C)(OTC)(G)
    Preparation H Cream apply up to qid prn
      Rectal crm: 0.9, 1.8 oz

▷ **phenylephrine+cocoa butter+shark liver oil** (C)(OTC)(G)
　　Preparation H Suppositories 1 suppository or 1 application of rectal ointment
　　or cream, up to qid
　　　　Rectal supp: phenyle 0.25%+cocoa 85.5%+shark 3% (12, 24, 45/pck); Rectal
　　　　oint: phenyle 0.25%+petro 1.9%+mineral oil 14%+shark liv 3% (1, 2 oz);
　　　　Rectal crm: *phenyle* 0.25%+petro 18%+gly 12%+shark liv 3% (0.9, 1.8 oz)

TOPICAL AND TRANSDERMAL ANALGESICS

▷ **capsaicin** 8% patch (B) apply up to 4 patches for one 60-minute application to
　　clean dry skin; may prep area with topical anesthetic; wear non-latex gloves;
　　patches may be cut to size/shape; treatment may be repeated every 3 months
　　Pediatric: <18 years: not recommended; ≥18 years: same as adult
　　　　Qutenza *Patch:* 8% 1640 mcg/cm (179 mg) (1 or 2 patches w. 1-50 gm tube
　　　　cleansing gel/carton)
▷ **diclofenac sodium** (C; D ≥30 wks) apply qid prn to intact skin
　　Pediatric: <12 years: not established; ≥12 years: same as adult
　　　　Pennsaid 1.5% in 10 drop increments, dispense and rub into front, side, and
　　　　back of knee: usually; 40 drops (40 mg) qid
　　　　　　Topical soln: 1.5% (150 ml)
　　　　Pennsaid 2% apply 2 pump actuations (40 mg) and rub into front, side, and
　　　　back of knee bid
　　　　　　Topical soln: 2% (20 mg/pump actuation, 112 gm)
　　　　Solaraze Gel massage in to clean skin bid prn
　　　　　　Gel: 3% (50 gm) (benzyl alcohol)
　　　　Voltaren Gel (G)(OTC) apply qid prn to intact skin
　　　　　　Gel: 1% (100 gm)
　　Comment: *Diclofenac* is contraindicated with *aspirin* allergy. As with other
　　NSAIDs, should be avoided in late pregnancy (≥30 weeks) because it may cause
　　premature closure of the ductus arteriosus.
▷ **doxepin** (B) cream apply to affected area qid at intervals of at least 3-4 hours; max
　　8 days
　　Pediatric: <12 years: not recommended; >12 years: same as adult
　　　　Prudoxin *Crm:* 5% (45 gm)
　　　　Zonalon *Crm:* 5% (30, 45 gm)
▷ **pimecrolimus** 1% cream (C)(G) <2 years: not recommended; ≥2 years: apply to
　　affected area bid; do not apply an occlusive dressing
　　　　Elidel *Crm:* 1% (30, 60, 100 gm)
　　Comment: *Pimecrolimus* is indicated for short-term and intermittent long-term
　　use. Discontinue use when resolution occurs. Contraindicated if the patient is
　　immunosuppressed. Change to the 0.1% preparation or if secondary bacterial
　　infection is present.
▷ **trolamine salicylate** apply tid-qid
　　Pediatric: <2 years: not recommended; ≥2 years: same as adult
　　　　Mobisyl Creme *Crm:* 10% (100 gm)
▷ **witch hazel** topical soln/gel (OTC)
　　　　Tucks apply up to 6 x/day; leave on x 5-15 minutes
　　　　　　Pad: 12, 40, 100/pck; *Gel:* 19.8 gm

TOPICAL AND TRANSDERMAL ANESTHETICS

Comment: *Lidocaine* should not be applied to non-intact skin.
▷ **lidocaine** cream (B) apply to affected area bid prn
　　Pediatric: <12 years: not recommended; ≥12 years: same as adult
　　　　LidaMantle *Crm:* 3% (1, 2 oz)
　　　　Lidoderm *Crm:* 3% (85 gm)
　　　　ZTlido *lidocaine* topical system 1% (30/carton)

Comment: Compared to **Lidoderm** (*lidocaine* patch 5%), which contains 700 mg/patch, **ZTlido** requires 35 mg per topical system to achieve the same therapeutic dose.

▷ *lidocaine* lotion (B) apply to affected area bid prn
  Pediatric: <12 years: not recommended; ≥12 years: same as adult
    LidaMantle *Lotn:* 3% (177 ml)
▷ *lidocaine* 5% patch (B)(G) apply up to 3 patches at one time for up to 12 hours/24-hour period (12 hours on/12 hours off); patches may be cut into smaller sizes before removal of the release liner; do not re-use
  Pediatric: <12 years: not recommended; ≥12 years: same as adult
    Lidoderm *Patch:* 5% (10x14 cm; 30/carton)
▷ *lidocaine+dexamethasone* (B)
  Pediatric: <12 years: not recommended; ≥12 years: same as adult
    Decadron Phosphate with Xylocaine *Lotn:* dexa 4 mg+lido 10 mg per ml (5 ml)
▷ *lidocaine+hydrocortisone* (B)(G) apply to affected area bid prn
  Pediatric: <12 years: not recommended; ≥12 years: same as adult
    LidaMantle HC *Crm:* lido 3%+hydro 0.5% (1, 3 oz); *Lotn:* (177 ml)
▷ *lidocaine* 2.5%+*prilocaine* 2.5% apply sparingly to the burn bid-tid prn
  Pediatric: <12 years: not recommended; ≥12 years: same as adult
    Emla Cream (B) 5, 30 gm/tube

HEPATIC PORPHYRIA, ACUTE (AHP)

AMINOLEVULINATE SYNTHASE 1-DIRECTED SMALL INTERFERING RNA

▷ *givosiran* 2.5 mg/kg SC once monthly; administration only by a qualified healthcare provider with access to medical support to appropriately manage anaphylactic reaction; administer injection into the back or side of the upper arm, abdomen, or thigh; rotate injection sites; avoid a 5 cm diameter circle around the navel; if more than one injection is needed for a single dose, separate injection sites at least 2 cm from previous injection sites; divide doses requiring volumes greater than 1.5 ml equally into multiple syringes
    Givlaari *Vial:* 189 mg/m (ml), single-dose
    Comment: **Givlaari** *(givosiran)* is an aminolevulinate synthase 1-directed small interfering RNA indicated for the treatment of adults with acute hepatic porphyria (AHP). Avoid concomitant use of **Givlaari** with CYP1A2 and CYP2D6 substrates for which minimal concentration changes may lead to serious or life-threatening toxicities. The most common adverse reactions (≥20% of patients) included nausea and injection site reactions. If anaphylaxis occurs, discontinue **Givlaari** and administer appropriate medical treatment. Measure liver function at baseline and periodically during the first 6 months of treatment with **Givlaari**. Interrupt or discontinue treatment for severe or clinically significant transaminase elevations. Monitor renal function during treatment with **Givlaari** as clinically indicated. Injection site reaction may occur, including recall reaction; monitor for reactions and manage clinically as needed. Porphyria attacks during pregnancy, often triggered by hormonal changes, occur in 24% to 95% of AHP patients, with maternal mortality ranging from 2% to 42%. Pregnancy in AHP patients is associated with higher rates of spontaneous abortion, hypertension, and low birth weight infants. In animal reproduction studies, subcutaneous administration of *givosiran* during the period of organogenesis resulted in adverse developmental outcomes at doses that produced maternal toxicity. There are no available data with **Givlaari** use in pregnant females to evaluate a drug-associated risk of major birth defects, miscarriage, or adverse maternal

or fetal outcomes. Consider benefits and risks of **Givlaari** for the mother and potential adverse embryo/fetal risk when prescribing **Givlaari** in pregnancy.

 HEPATITIS A (HAV)

Comment: Administer a 2-dose series. Schedule first immunization at least 2 weeks before expected exposure. Booster dose recommended 6-12 months later. Under 1 year-of-age administer in the vastus lateralis; over 1 year-of-age administer in the deltoid.

PROPHYLAXIS (HEPATITIS A)

▷ *hepatitis A vaccine, inactivated* (C)
  Pediatric: <12 years: not approved; ≥12 years: same as adult
   Havrix 1,440 El.U IM; repeat in 6-12 months
   Pediatric: <2 years: not recommended; 2-18 years: 720 El.U IM; repeat in 6-12 months *or* 360 El.U IM; repeat in 1 month
   Vaqta 25 U (1 ml) IM; repeat in 6 months
   Pediatric: <2 years: not recommended; 2-18 years: 0.5 ml IM; repeat in 6-18 months
    Vial: 25 U/ml single-dose (preservative-free); *Prefilled syringe:* 25 U/ml, (0.5, 1 ml, single-dose)

PROPHYLAXIS VACCINE (HAV+HBV COMBINATION)

▷ *hepatitis A inactivated+hepatitis b surface antigen (recombinant vaccine)* (C)
  Pediatric: <18 years: not approved; ≥18 years: same as adult
   Twinrix 1 ml IM in deltoid; repeat in 1 month and 6 months
    Vial (soln): hepatitis a inactivated 720 IU+*hepatitis b* surface antigen (recombinant) 20 mcg/ml (1, 10 ml); *Prefilled syringe: hepatitis a* inactivated 720 IU+*hepatitis b* surface antigen (recombinant) 20 mcg/ml
    Comment: An alternate accelerated 4-dose schedule is approved for **Twinrix** vaccine with doses administered at 0, 7, and 21-30 days, followed by a booster dose at 12 months.

PRE- AND POST-EXPOSURE PROPHYLAXIS

Immune Globulin (Human)

▷ *immune globulin* (human) administer via intramuscular injection *only* (never intravenously); ensure adequate hydration prior to administration; *Household and Institutional HAV Case Contacts:* 0.1 ml/kg IM as a single dose; *Planned Travel to HAV Endemic Area:* administer as a single dose at least 2 weeks prior to travel
  Pediatric: 0.25 ml/kg IM (0.5 mg/kg in immunocompromised children)

Length of Stay	Prior Dose	Dose
Up to 1 month	--------	0.1 ml/kg
Up to 2 months	--------	0.2 ml/kg
More than 2 months	--------	repeat 0.2 ml/kg every 2 months
Less than 3 months	0.02 ml/kg	--------
3 months *or* longer	0.06 ml/kg	repeat every 4-6 months

  GamaSTAN S/D *Vial:* 2, 10 ml single-dose
Comment: **GamaSTAN S/D** is the *only* gammaglobulin product FDA-approved for measles and HAV post-exposure prophylaxis (PEP). **GamaSTAN S/D** is also FDA-approved for varicella post-exposure prophylaxis (PEP). Other **GamaSTAN**

S/D indications: to prevent or modify measles in a susceptible person exposed fewer than 6 days previously; to modify varicella; to modify rubella in exposed women who will not consider a therapeutic abortion. **GamaSTAN S/D** is not indicated for routine prophylaxis or treatment of viral hepatitis B, rubella, poliomyelitis, mumps or varicella. Contraindications to **GamaSTAN S/D** include persons with cancer, chronic liver disease, and persons allergic to gammaglobulin, the HAV vaccine, or a component of the HAV vaccine. Dosage is higher for HAV PEP than for measles and varicella PEP based on recently observed decreasing concentrations of HAV antibodies in **GamaSTAN S/D**, attributed to the decreasing prevalence of previous HAV infection among plasma donors. Defer live vaccines for at least 6 months.

 HEPATITIS B (HBV)

PROPHYLAXIS VACCINE (HBV)

Comment: ACIP 2021 recommends vaccination for the hepatitis B virus (HBV) infection in the setting of adults who have high risk factors for HBV or adults requesting protection against HBV without risk factors. HBV vaccination is recommended by shared clinical decision-making for persons with diabetes age 60 years or older.

Comment: Administer IM; under 1 year-of-age, administer in vastus lateralis. Over 1 year-of-age, administer in the deltoid. Administer a 3-dose series; *First dose:* newborn (or now); *Second dose:* 1-2 months after first dose; *Third dose:* 6 months after first dose.

▷ *hepatitis B recombinant vaccine* (C)

Engerix-B Adult 20 mcg (1 ml) IM; repeat in 1 and 6 months
Pediatric: infant-19 years: 10 mcg (1/2 ml) IM; repeat in 1 and 6 months
Vial: 20 mcg/ml single-dose (preservative-free, thimerosal); *Prefilled syringe:* 20 mcg/ml

Engerix-B Pediatric/Adolescent
Pediatric: infant-19 years: 10 mcg IM; repeat in 1 and 6 months; *Vial:* 10 mcg/0.5 ml single-dose (preservative-free, thimerosal)
Prefilled syringe: 10 mcg/0.5 ml

Recombivax HB Adult 10 mcg (1 ml) IM in deltoid; repeat in 1 and 6 months
Vial: 10 mcg/ml single-dose; *Vial:* 10 mcg/3 ml multi-dose

Recombivax HB Pediatric/Adolescent 5 mcg (0.5 ml) IM; repeat in 1 and 6 months
Pediatric: birth-19 years: 5 mcg (0.5 ml) IM; repeat in 1 and 6 months; >19 years: use adult formulation or 10 mcg (1 ml) pediatric/adolescent formulation
Vial: 5 mcg/0.5 ml single-dose

PROPHYLAXIS VACCINE (HAV+HBV COMBINATION)

Comment: Administer IM; under 1 year-of-age, administer in vastus lateralis. Over 1 year-of-age, administer in the deltoid. Administer a 3-dose series; *First dose:* newborn (or now); *Second dose:* 1-2 months after first dose; *Third dose:* 6 months after first dose.

▷ *hepatitis A inactivated+hepatitis b surface antigen (recombinant) vaccine* (C)
Pediatric: <18 years: not approved; ≥18 years: same as adult
Twinrix 1 ml IM in deltoid; repeat in 1 months and 6 months
Vial (soln): hepatitis A inactivated 720 IU+*hepatitis b* surface antigen (recombinant) 20 mcg/ml (1, 10 ml); *Prefilled syringe: hepatitis A* inactivated 720 IU+*hepatitis b* surface antigen (recombinant) 20 mcg/ml

CHRONIC HBV INFECTION TREATMENT
Nucleoside Analogs (Reverse Transcriptase Inhibitors and HBV Polymerase Inhibitors)
Comment: Nucleoside analogs are indicated for chronic hepatitis infection with viral replication and either elevated ALT/AST or histologically active disease.

▷ *adefovir dipivoxil* (C)(G) 10 mg daily; *CrCl 20-49 mL/min*: 10 mg q 48 hours; *CrCl 10-19 mL/min*: 10 mg q 72 hours
Pediatric: <12 years: not recommended; ≥12 years: same as adult
   Hepsera *Tab*: 10 mg

▷ *entecavir* (C)(G) take on an empty stomach;
Nucleoside naïve: 0.5 mg daily; *Nucleoside naïve, CrCl 30-49 mL/min*: 0.25 mg daily; *Nucleoside naïve, CrCl 10-29 mL/min*: 0.15 mg daily; *Nucleoside naïve, CrCl <10 mL/min*: 0.05 mg daily; *lamivudine-refractory*: 1 mg daily; *lamivudine-refractory, renal impairment*: see mfr pkg insert
Pediatric: <18 years: not recommended; ≥18 years: same as adult
   Baraclude *Tab*: 0.5, 1 mg; *Oral Soln*: 0.05 mg/ml (orange; parabens)

▷ *lamivudine* (C)(G) 100 mg daily; *CrCl <5 mL/min*: 35 mg for 1st dose, then 10 mg once daily; *CrCl 5-14 mL/min*: 35 mg for 1st dose, then 15 mg once daily; *CrCl 15-29 mL/min*: 100 mg for 1st dose, then 25 mg once daily; *CrCl 30-49 mL/min*: 100 mg for 1st dose, then 50 mg once daily
Pediatric: <2 years: not recommended; 2-17 years: 3 mg/kg (max 100 mg) once daily
   Epivir-HBV *Tab*: 100 mg
   Epivir-HBV Oral Solution *Oral Soln*: 5 mg/ml (240 ml) (strawberry-banana)

▷ *telbivudine* (C) 600 mg daily; *CrCl <40 mL/min*: 600 mg q 72 hours; *CrCl 30-49 mL/min*: 600 mg q 48 hours
Pediatric: <16 years: not recommended; ≥16 years: same as adult
   Tyzeka *Tab*: 600 mg

▷ *tenofovir alafenamide (TAF)* (C) take with food; take 1 tab once daily with concomitant carbamazepine 2 tablets
Pediatric: <18 years: not established; ≥18 years: same as adult
   Vemlidy *Tab*: 25 mg
   Comment: No dosage adjustment of **Vemlidy** is required for patients with mild hepatic impairment (Child-Pugh Class A) or compensated liver disease. **Vemlidy** is not recommended in patients with decompensated (Child-Pugh Class B or C) hepatic impairment. No dosage adjustment is required for patients with mild/moderate/severe renal impairment or patients with ESRD who are receiving chronic hemodialysis. Administer **Vemlidy** after the dialysis treatment is completed. **Vemlidy** is contraindicated in patients with ESRD who are not receiving dialysis. Healthcare providers are encouraged to register patients by calling the Antiretroviral Pregnancy Registry (APR) at 1-800-258-4263.

Interferon Alpha

▷ *interferon alfa-2b* (C) 5 million IU SC or IM daily or 10 million IU SC or IM 3 x/week x 16 weeks; reduce dose by half or interrupt dose if WBCs, granulocyte count, or platelet count decreases
Pediatric: <1 year: not recommended; ≥1 year: 3 million IU/m², 3 x/week x 1 week; then increase to 6 million IU/m², 3 x/week to 16-24 weeks; max 10 million IU/dose; reduce dose by half or interrupt dose if WBCs, granulocyte count, or platelet count decreases
   Intron A *Vial (pwdr)*: 5, 10, 18, 25, 50 million IU/vial (pwdr+diluent; single-dose) (benzoyl alcohol); *Vial (soln)*: 3, 5, 10 million IU/vial (single-dose); *Multi-dose vials (soln)*: 18, 25 million IU/vial soln; *Multi-dose pens (soln)*: 3, 5, 10 million IU/0.2 ml (6 doses/pen)

Integrase Strand Transfer Inhibitor (INSTI)

▷ *tenofovir disoproxil fumarate* (C)(G) 300 mg once daily; *CrCl 30-49 mL/min:* 300 mg q 48 hours; *CrCl 10-29 ml/min:* 300 mg q 72-96 hours; *Hemodialysis:* 300 mg once every 7 days or after a total of 12 hours of dialysis; *CrCl <10 mL/min:* not recommended

    Pediatric: <12 years: not recommended; ≥12 years, 35 kg: 300 mg once daily; mix oral pwdr with 2-4 oz soft food

        Viread *Tab:* 150, 200, 250, 300 mg; *Oral pwdr:* 40 mg/gm (60 gm w. dosing scoop)

        Comment: Published studies in HBV-infected subjects do not report an increased risk of adverse pregnancy-related outcomes with the use of **Viread** during the third trimester of pregnancy.

 HEPATITIS C (HCV)

CHRONIC HCV INFECTION TREATMENT

Nucleoside Analogs (Reverse Transcriptase Inhibitors)

Comment: Nucleoside analogs are indicated for patients with compensated liver disease previously untreated with *alpha interferon* or who have relapsed after *alpha interferon* therapy. Primary toxicity is hemolytic anemia. Contraindicated in male partners of pregnant females; use 2 forms of contraception during therapy and for 6 months after discontinuation.

▷ *ribavirin* (X)(G) take with food in 2 divided doses; *Genotype 2, 3:* 800 mg/day x 24 weeks; *Genotype 1, 4, <75 kg:* 1 gm/day x 48 weeks; ≥75 km 1.2 gm/day x 48 weeks; *HIV co-infection:* 800 mg/day x 48 weeks; *CrCl 30-50 mL/min:* alternate 200 mg and 400 mg every other day; *CrCl <30 mL/min or hemodialysis:* reduce dose or discontinue if hematologic abnormalities occur

    Pediatric: <5 years: not established; ≥5–<18 years: 23-33 kg: 400 mg/day; 34-46 kg: 600 mg/day; 47-59 kg: 800 mg/day; 60-75 kg: 1 gm/day; 1.2 gm/day; ≥75 kg: *Genotype 2, 3:* treat for 24 weeks; *Genotype 1, 4:* treat for 48 weeks; reduce dose or discontinue if hematologic abnormalities occur; ≥18 years: same as adult

        Copegus *Tab:* 200 mg

        Rebetol *Cap:* 200 mg

        Rebetol Oral Solution *Oral soln:* 40 mg/ml (120 ml) (bubble gum)

        Ribasphere RibaPak 600 mg *Tab:* 600 mg (14/pck)

        Virazole *Vial:* 6 gm for inhalation

Interferon Alpha

▷ *interferon alfacon-1* (C)

    Pediatric: <18 years: not recommended; ≥18 years: same as adult

        Infergen 9 mcg SC 3 x/week x 24 weeks, then 15 mcg SC 3 x/week x 6 months; allow at least 48 hours between doses

            Vial (soln): 9, 15 mcg/vial soln (6 single-dose/pck) (preservative-free)

▷ *interferon alfa-2b* (C)

        Intron A *Vial (pwdr):* 5, 10, 18, 25, 50 million IU/vial (pwdr w. diluent; single-dose) (benzoyl alcohol); *Vial (soln):* 3, 5, 10 million IU/vial (single-dose); *Multi-dose vials (soln):* 18, 25 million IU/vial; *Multi-dose pens (soln):* 3, 5, 10 million IU/0.2 ml (6 doses/pen)

▷ *peginterferon alfa-2a* (C) administer 180 mcg SC once weekly (on the same day of the week); treat for 48 weeks; consider discontinuing if adequate response after 12-24 weeks

    Pediatric: <18 years: not recommended; ≥18 years: same as adult

        PEGasys *Vial:* 180 mcg/ml (single-dose); *Monthly pck (vials):* 180 mcg/ml (1 ml, 4/pck)

▶ **peginterferon alfa-2b** (C) administer SC once weekly (on the same day of the week); treat for 1 year; consider discontinuing if inadequate response after 24 weeks; 37-45 kg: 40 mcg (100 mg/ml, 0.4 ml); 46-56 kg: 50 mcg (100 mg/ml, 0.5 ml); 57-72 kg: 64 mcg (160 mg/ml, 0.4 ml); 73-88 kg: 80 mcg (160 mg/ml, 0.5 ml); 89-106 kg: 96 mcg (240 mg/ml, 0.4 ml); 107-136 kg: 120 mcg (240 mg/ml, 0.5 ml); 137-160 kg: 150 mcg (300 mg/ml, 0.5 ml)

Pediatric: <18 years: not recommended; ≥18 years: same as adult

  PEG-Intron Vial: 50, 80, 120, 150 mcg/ml (single-dose)
  PEG-Intron Redipen Pen: 50, 80, 120, 150 mcg/ml (disposable pens)

HCV NS5A Inhibitor

▶ **daclatasvir** (X) 60 mg once daily for 12 weeks (with **sofosbuvir**); if **sofosbuvir** is discontinued, **daclatasvir** should also be discontinued; with concomitant CY3P inhibitors, reduce dose to 30 mg once daily; with concomitant CY3P inducers, increase dose to 90 mg once daily

  Daklinza Tab: 30, 60 mg
  Comment: Daklinza is indicated in combination with **sofosbuvir** with or without **ribavirin**, for the treatment of HCV genotypes 1 and 3, and in patients with co-morbid HIV-1 infection, advanced cirrhosis, or post-liver transplant recurrence of HCV.

HCV NS5A Inhibitor+HCV NS3+4A Protease Inhibitor Combinations

▶ **elbasvir+grazoprevir** 1 tab as a single dose once daily; see mfr pkg insert for length of treatment

Pediatric: <18 years: not recommended; ≥18 years: same as adult

  Zepatier Tab: elba 50 mg+grazo 100 mg
  Comment: Zepatier is contraindicated with moderate or severe hepatic impairment, concomitant **atazanavir, carbamazepine, cyclosporine, darunavir, efavirenz, lopinavir, phenytoin, rifampin, saquinavir**, St. John's wort, **tipranavir**. When co-administered with **ribavirin**, pregnancy category (X)

▶ **glecaprevir+pibrentasvir** take 3 tablets (total daily dose: **glecaprevir** 300 mg and **pibrentasvir** 120 mg) once daily with food

Pediatric: <12 years, <45 kg: not established; ≥12 years, ≥45 kg: same as adult

  Mavyret Tab: gleca 100 mg+pibre 40 mg
  Comment: Mavyret is a drug for the treatment of adults who have chronic Hepatitis C virus genotypes 1, 2, 3, 4, 5, or 6 infection and who do not have cirrhosis or who have early stage cirrhosis. Mavyret may cause serious liver problems including liver failure and death in patients who had hepatitis B virus infection. This is because the hepatitis B virus could become active again (i.e., reactivated) during or after treatment with Mavyret. Test all patients for HBV infection by measuring HBsAg and anti-HBc prior to initiating therapy with Mavyret. The most common side effects of Mavyret are headache and tiredness. See mfr insert for table of recommended duration of treatment based on patient characteristics. No adequate human data are available to establish whether or not Mavyret poses a risk to pregnancy outcomes. It is not known whether the components of Mavyret are excreted in human breast milk or have effects on the breastfed infant.

HCV NS5A Inhibitor+HCV NS3/4A Protease Inhibitor+CYP3A Inhibitor Combinations

▶ **ombitasvir+paritaprevir+ritonavir** (B) take 2 tabs once daily in the AM x 12 weeks

Pediatric: <18 years: not established; ≥18 years: same as adult

  Technivie Tab: omvi 25 mg+pari 75 mg+rito 50 mg (4 x 7 daily dose pcks/carton)

Comment: **Technivie** is indicated for use in chronic HCV genotype 4 without cirrhosis. **Technivie** is <u>not</u> for use with moderate hepatic impairment.

HCV NS3/4A Protease Inhibitor

▷ *simeprevir* (C) 150 mg once daily; swallow whole; take with food, <u>not</u> for monotherapy; do <u>not</u> reduce dose <u>or</u> interrupt therapy; if discontinued, do <u>not</u> reinitiate; discontinue if HCV-RNA levels indicate futility; discontinue if *peginterferon, ribavirin,* <u>or</u> *sofosbuvir* is permanently discontinued; *Treatment naïve, treatment relapses, with <u>or</u> without cirrhosis:* treat x 12 weeks (*simeprevir + peginterferon + ribavirin*) followed by additional 12 weeks *peginterferon + ribavirin* (total = 24 weeks). *Partial and non-responders, with <u>or</u> without cirrhosis:* treat x 12 weeks (*simeprevir + peginterferon + ribavirin*) followed by additional 36 weeks *peginterferon + ribavirin* (total = 48 weeks); *Treatment naïve <u>or</u> treatment experienced without cirrhosis:* treat x 12 weeks (*simeprevir + sofosbuvir*); *Treatment naïve <u>or</u> treatment experienced with cirrhosis:* treat x 24 weeks (*simeprevir + sofosbuvir*)

   Olysio *Cap:* 150 mg

HCV NS5A Inhibitor+HCV NS5B Polymerase Inhibitor Combinations

▷ *ledipasvir+sofosbuvir Treatment naïve, without cirrhosis, with pretreatment HCV RNA <6 million IU/ml:* 1 tab daily x 8 weeks; *Treatment naïve with <u>or</u> without cirrhosis <u>or</u> treatment-experienced without cirrhosis:* 1 tab daily x 12 weeks; *Treatment-experienced with cirrhosis:* 1 tab daily x 24 weeks; *In combination with ribavirin:* 1 tab daily x 12 weeks

   Pediatric: <18 years: not established; *≥18 years:* same as adult

   Harvoni *Tab: ledi* 90 mg+*sofo* 400 mg

   Comment: **Harvoni** is indicated for patients with advanced liver disease, genotype 1, 4, 5, <u>or</u> 6 infection: chronic HCV genotype 1- <u>or</u> 4-infected liver transplant recipients with <u>or</u> without cirrhosis <u>or</u> with compensated cirrhosis (Child-Pugh Class A), and for HCV genotype 1-infected patients with decompensated cirrhosis (Child-Pugh Class B <u>or</u> C), including those who have undergone liver transplantation. No adequate human data are available to establish whether <u>or</u> not **Harvoni** poses a risk to pregnancy outcomes; the background risk of major birth defects and miscarriage for the indicated population is unknown. If **Harvoni** is administered with *ribavirin*, the combination regimen is contraindicated (X) in pregnant females <u>and</u> in men whose female partners are pregnant. It is <u>not</u> known whether **Harvoni** and its metabolites are present in human breast milk, affect human milk production, <u>or</u> have effects on the breastfed infant. If **Harvoni** is administered with *ribavirin*, the nursing mother's information for *ribavirin* also applies to this combination regimen.

▷ *sofosbuvir+velpatasvir Without cirrhosis <u>or</u> compensated cirrhosis (Child-Pugh Class A):* 1 tablet daily x 12 weeks; *Decompensated cirrhosis (Child Pugh Class B <u>or</u> C):* 1 tablet daily plus *ribavirin* (RBV)

   Pediatric: <18 years: not established; *≥18 years:* same as adult

   Epclusa *Tab: sofo* 400 mg+*velpa* 100 mg

   Comment: **Epclusa** is indicated for patients with chronic HCV with genotype 1, 2, 3, 4, 5, <u>or</u> 6 infection.

HCV NS5A Inhibitor+HCV NS3/4A Protease Inhibitor+CYP3A Inhibitor Combination

▷ *sofosbuvir+velpatasvir* (B) 1 tab daily

   Pediatric: <12 years: not established; *≥12 years:* same as adult

   Viekira XR *Tab: dasa* 200 mg+*omvi* 8.33 mg+*pari* 50 mg+*rito* 33.33 mg ext-rel (4 weekly cartons, each containing 7 daily dose pcks/carton)

Comment: Viekira XR is indicated for HCV genotype 1 with mild liver dysfunction (Child-Pugh Class A). Viekira XR is contraindicated for moderate (Child-Pugh Class B) to severe (Child-Pugh Class C) liver dysfunction. No adjustment is recommended with mild, moderate, or severe renal dysfunction.

HCV NS5A Inhibitor+HCV NS3/4A Protease Inhibitor+CYP3A Inhibitor PLUS HCV NS5B Polymerase Inhibitor Combination

▷ *ombitasvir+paritaprevir+ritonavir* plus *dasabuvir* (B)
  Pediatric: <12 years: not established; ≥12 years: same as adult
  Viekira Pak *ombitasvir+paritaprevir+ritonavir* fixed-dose combination tablet: 2 tablets orally once a day (in the morning); *dasabuvir*: 250 mg orally twice a day (morning and evening)
    Tab: omvi 12.5 mg+pari 75 mg+rito 50 mg plus *Tab:* dasa 250 mg (28 day supply/pck)
  Comment: Viekira Pak is indicated for mild liver dysfunction (Child-Pugh Class A). Viekira Pak is contraindicated for moderate (Child-Pugh Class B) to severe (Child-Pugh Class C) liver dysfunction. No adjustment is recommended with mild, moderate, or severe renal dysfunction.

HCV NS5B Polymerase Inhibitor+HCV NS5A Inhibitor+HCV NS3/4A Protease Inhibitor Combination

▷ *sofosbuvir+velpatasvir+voxilaprevir* 1 tablet once daily with food x 12 weeks; pre-test for HBV infection by measuring HBsAg and anti-HBc prior to the initiation of therapy
  Pediatric: <12 years: not established; ≥12 years: same as adult
  Vosevi *Tab:* sofo 400 mg+velpa 100 mg+voxil 100 mg fixed-dose combination
  Comment: Vosevi is not recommended in patients with moderate or severe hepatic impairment (Child-Pugh Class B or C). A dosage recommendation cannot be made for patients with severe renal impairment or end stage renal disease. Vosevi is contraindicated while taking any medicines containing *rifampin* (Rifater, Rifamate, Rimactane, Rifadin). Vosevi is indicated for the treatment of adult patients with chronic HCV infection without cirrhosis or with compensated cirrhosis (Child-Pugh Class A) who have: (1) genotype 1, 2, 3, 4, 5, or 6 infection and have previously been treated with an HCV regimen containing an NS5A inhibitor or (2) genotype 1a or 3 infection and have previously been treated with an HCV regimen containing *sofosbuvir* without an NS5A inhibitor. Duration of treatment is 12 weeks. Additional benefit of Vosevi over *sofosbuvir+velpatasvir* has not been demonstrated with genotype 1b, 2, 4, 5, or 6 infection previously treated with *sofosbuvir* without an NS5A inhibitor. Because there is risk of Hepatitis B virus reactivation, test all patients for evidence of current or prior HBV infection before initiation of HCV treatment. Monitor HCV/HBV co-infected patients for HBV reactivation and hepatitis flare during HCV treatment and posttreatment follow-up. Initiate appropriate patient management for HBV infection as clinically indicated. The most common adverse reactions are headache, fatigue, diarrhea, and nausea.

DUAL TREATMENT REGIMEN
Harvoni+Sovaldi

Comment: Patients who are co-infected with hepatitis B are at risk for HBV reactivation during or after treatment with HCV direct-acting retrovirals. Therefore, patients should be screened for current or past HBV infection before starting this treatment protocol.

TRIPLE TREATMENT REGIMEN
Sovaldi+Harvoni+Ribavirin

Comment: For this FDA-approved triple therapy regimen, follow the recommended regimen for each individual drug. Patients who are co-infected with hepatitis B are at risk for HBV reactivation during or after treatment with HCV direct-acting retrovirals. Therefore, patients should be screened for current or past HBV infection before starting this triple therapy regimen.

 HEREDITARY ANGIOEDEMA (HAE)/C1 ESTERASE INHIBITOR DEFICIENCY

Comment: Agents administered for the treatment of hereditary angioedema carry a risk of hypersensitivity reactions, which are similar to HAE attacks, and the patient should be monitored closely for signs and symptoms accordingly (e.g., hives, urticaria, tightness of the chest, wheezing, hypotension and/or anaphylaxis).

HAE PROPHYLAXIS
Synthetic Steroid

▷ *danazol* (X) *Females:* start on 3rd or 4th day of menstrual period or after a negative pregnancy test; *Males/Females:* dosage requirements for continuous treatment of hereditary angioedema should be adjusted based on individual clinical response; initially 200 mg bid-tid; after a favorable initial response is achieved (prevention of episodes of edematous attacks), continuing dosage should be determined by decreasing the dosage by 50% or less at intervals of 1 to 3 months or longer if frequency of attacks prior to treatment dictates; if an attack occurs, daily dosage may be increased by up to 200 mg. During the dose adjusting phase, close monitoring of the patient's response is indicated, particularly if the patient has a history of airway involvement.

Pediatric: <18 years: not recommended; ≥18 years: same as adult

    Danocrine *Cap:* 50, 100, 200 mg

Comment: *Danazol* is a synthetic steroid derived from ethisterone. It suppresses the pituitary-ovarian axis. This suppression is probably a combination of depressed hypothalamic-pituitary response to lowered *estrogen* production, the alteration of sex steroid metabolism, and interaction of *danazol* with sex hormone receptors. The only other demonstrable hormonal effects are weak androgenic activity and depression of both follicle-stimulating hormone (FSH) and luteinizing hormone (LH) output. Recent evidence suggests a direct inhibitory effect at gonadal sites and a binding of **Danocrine** to receptors of gonadal steroids at target organs. In addition, **Danocrine** has been shown to significantly decrease IgG, IgM, and IgA levels, as well as phospholipid and IgG isotope autoantibodies in patients with endometriosis and associated elevations of autoantibodies, suggesting this could be another mechanism by which it facilitates regression of fibrocystic breast disease. Changes in the menstrual pattern may occur. Generally, the pituitary-suppressive action of **Danocrine** is reversible. Ovulation and cyclic bleeding usually return within 60 to 90 days when therapy with **Danocrine** is discontinued. In the treatment of hereditary angioedema, **Danocrine** at effective doses prevents attacks of the disease characterized by episodic edema of the abdominal viscera, extremities, face, and airway, which may be disabling and, if the airway is involved, fatal. In addition, **Danocrine** corrects partially or completely the primary biochemical abnormality of hereditary angioedema by increasing the levels of the deficient C1 esterase inhibitor (C1EI). As a result of this action, the serum levels of the C4 component of the complement system are also increased. **Danocrine** is also used to treat endometriosis (to relieve associated abdominal pain) and fibrocystic breast disease (to reduce breast tissue nodularity and breast pain/tenderness). Contraindications include pregnancy, breastfeeding, active or history of thromboembolic disease/event, porphyria, undiagnosed abnormal genital bleeding, androgen-dependent tumor, and markedly impaired hepatic, renal, or cardiac function.

C1 Esterase Inhibitor [Human]

▷ *C1 esterase inhibitor (human)* administer 60 International Units per kg body weight SC in the abdomen twice weekly (every 3 or 4 days); administer at room temperature within 8 hours after reconstitution; use a silicone-free syringe for reconstitution and administration; use either the Mix2Vial transfer set provided with **Haegarda** or a commercially available 566 double-ended needle and vented filter spike

Pediatric: <12 years: not recommended; ≥12 years: same as adult

Haegarda *Vial:* 2000, 3000 IU C1 INH pwdr for reconstitution, single-use

Comment: **Haegarda** is a plasma-derived concentrate of C1 esterase inhibitor [human], a serine proteinase inhibitor. Indicated for routine prophylaxis to prevent HAE attacks in adults and adolescents. It is not indicated for treating acute attacks of HAE. **Haegarda** is the first C1 esterase inhibitor (human) SC injection approved for self-administration by the patient or caregiver after healthcare provider instruction. An international consensus panel states that human plasma-derived C1 esterase inhibitor is considered to be the therapy of choice for both treatment and prophylaxis of maternal hereditary angioedema during lactation. There are no prospective clinical data from **Haegarda** use in pregnant females. C1-INH is a normal component of human plasma. There is no information regarding the excretion of **Haegarda** in human milk or effect the breastfed infant. The developmental and health benefits of breastfeeding should be considered along with the mother's clinical need for **Haegarda** and any potential adverse effects on the breastfed infant from **Haegarda** or from the underlying maternal condition.

Plasma Kallikrein Inhibitor (Monoclonal Antibody)

▷ *berotralstat* take 1 capsule once daily; take with food; max 150 mg/day

Pediatric: <12 years: not established; ≥12 years: same as adult

Orladeyo *Cap:* 110, 150 mg

Comment: **Orladeyo** *(berotralstat)*, a plasma kallikrein inhibitor, is the first oral, once daily, prophylaxis therapy to prevent attacks of hereditary angioedema (HAE). **Orladeyo** works by binding to plasma kallikrein and inhibiting its proteolytic activity. **Orladeyo** is not used to treat an acute HAE attack. The most common adverse reactions (incidence ≥10%) have been abdominal pain, vomiting, diarrhea, back pain, and gastroesophageal reflux disease. Additionally, an increase in QT prolongation can occur at dosages higher than the recommended 150 mg once daily dosage; additional doses or doses higher than 150 mg once daily are not recommended. Reduce **Orladeyo** dosage when co-administered with P-gp or BCRP inhibitors. Avoid P-gp inducer use with **Orladeyo**. When co-administered with **Orladeyo**, monitor or titrate dose of drugs with a narrow therapeutic index that are predominantly metabolized by CYP2D6, CYP3A4, or are P-gp substrates. There are insufficient data in pregnant females available to inform drug-related risks with **Orladeyo** use in pregnancy. There are no data on the presence of *berotralstat* in human milk or its effects on the breastfed infant.

▷ *lanadelumab-flyo* initially administer 300 mg SC every 2 weeks into the upper arm, abdomen, or thigh; dosing interval of 300 mg every 4 weeks is also effective and may be considered if the patient is well-controlled (i.e., attack free) for more than 6 months; with appropriate healthcare provider instruction, patients may self-administer

Pediatric: <12 years: not established; ≥12 years: same as adult

Takhzyro *Vial:* 300 mg/2 ml (2 ml) soln single-dose (preservative-free)

Comment: Takhzyro *(lanadelumab-flyo)* is a plasma kallikrein inhibitor (monoclonal antibody) indicated for prophylaxis to prevent attacks of hereditary angioedema (HAE). No dedicated drug interaction studies have been conducted. There are no available data on **Takhzyro** use in pregnant females to inform any drug associated risks. Monoclonal antibodies such as *lanadelumab-flyo* are transported across the placenta during the third trimester of pregnancy; therefore, potential effects on a fetus are likely to be greater during the third trimester of pregnancy. Animal studies have revealed no evidence of harm to the developing fetus. There are no data on the presence of *lanadelumab-flyo* in human milk or effects on the breastfed infant.

HAE ACUTE ATTACK

C1 Esterase Inhibitors [Human]

▷ *C1 esterase inhibitor [human]* (C)

Berinert reconstitute pwdr using the sterile water provided; administer 20 IU/kg body weight via IVP injection at approximately 4 ml/min, at room temperature within 8 hours of reconstitution; store the vial at room temperature in the original carton to protect from light; appropriately trained patients may self-administer upon recognition of an HAE attack; hypersensitivity reactions may occur, therefore, have epinephrine immediately available for treatment of acute severe hypersensitivity reaction

Pediatric: <12 years: not established; ≥12 years: same as adult

Vial: 500 Units/10 ml vial, single-use, pwdr for reconstitution with the 10 ml sterile water diluent (provided)

Cinryze administer 1000 Units (2 x 500 U vials) via IVP injection, after reconstitution with 5 ml sterile H2O/vial; reconstitute 1000 U pwdr in a 10 ml syringe with 10 ml sterile water; administer over 10 minutes (1 ml/min) at room temperature within 3 hours of reconstitution; each 1000 Unit treatment is administered every 3-4 days; hypersensitivity reactions may occur, therefore, have epinephrine immediately available for treatment of acute severe hypersensitivity reaction

Pediatric: <16 years: not established; ≥16 years: same as adult

Vial: 500 Units/8 ml vial pwdr for reconstitution (sterile water diluent not provided)

Comment: No adequate and well-controlled studies have been conducted in pregnant women. It is not known whether **Cinryze** can cause fetal harm when administered to a pregnant females or can affect reproduction capacity. **Cinryze** should be administered to a pregnant woman only if clearly needed. It is not known whether **Cinryze** is excreted in human milk.

C1 Esterase Inhibitor [Recombinant]

▷ *C1 esterase inhibitor [recombinant]* (B) reconstitute 2.100 IU pwdr (1 vial) with 14 ml sterile H2O; administer reconstituted solution at room temperature, slow IVP injection over approximately 5 minutes; appropriately trained patients may self-administer upon recognition of HAE attack; Weight-based dose: <84 kg: 50 IU /kg [wt in kg ÷ 3 = vol (ml) reconst soln for administration]; ≥84 kg: 4,200 IU (28 ml, 2 vials); if the attack symptoms persist, an additional (second) dose can be administered at the recommended dose level; do not exceed 4200 IU per dose; max 2 doses within a 24 hour period; hypersensitivity reactions may occur, therefore, have epinephrine immediately available for treatment of acute severe hypersensitivity reaction

Pediatric: <13 years: not established; ≥13 years: same as adult
> **Ruconest** *Vial:* 2100 IU, pwdr, single-use for IVP injection after
> reconstitution (sterile water diluent <u>not</u> provided)

Bradykinen B2 Receptor Antagonist

▷ *icatibant* (C) administer 30 mg SC injection in the abdominal area; if response
is inadequate <u>or</u> symptoms recur, additional injections of 30 mg may be
administered at intervals of at least 6 hours; max 3 injections/24 hours; patients
may self-administer upon recognition of an HAE attack
> *Pediatric:* <18 years: not established; ≥18 years: same as adult
> **Firazyr** *Prefilled syringe:* 10 mg/ml (3 ml) single-dose w. 25 gauge luer lock
> needle (1/carton, 3 cartons/pck)
> **Comment:** **Firazyr**, as a bradykinin B2 receptor antagonist, may attenuate
> the antihypertensive effect of ACE inhibitors. The most commonly reported
> adverse reaction is injection site reaction (97% in clinical trials).

Plasma Kallikrein Inhibitor

▷ *ecallantide* (C) administer 30 mg (3 ml) SC in three 10 mg (I ml) injections; if an
attack persists, an additional dose of 30 mg may be administered within a 24 hour
period; should <u>only</u> be administered by a healthcare professional with appropriate
medical support to manage anaphylaxis and hereditary angioedema
> *Pediatric:* <12 years: not established; ≥12 years: same as adult
> **Kalbitor** *Vial:* 10 mg/ml (1/carton, 3 vials/pkg) single-use
> **Comment:** Anaphylaxis has occurred in 3.9% of patients treated with **Kalbitor**.
> Therefore, **Kalbitor** should <u>only</u> be administered in a setting equipped to
> manage anaphylaxis and hereditary angioedema. Given the similarity in hyper
> sensitivity symptoms and acute HAE symptoms, monitor patients closely for
> hypersensitivity reactions.

  HERPANGINA

Other Oral Analgesics *see* **Pain**

ORAL ANALGESICS

▷ *acetaminophen* (B) *see* **Fever**
▷ *tramadol* (C)(IV)(G)
> **Rybix ODT** initially 100 mg once daily; may increase by 100 mg every 5
> days; max 300 mg/day; *CrCl <30 mL/min* <u>or</u> *severe hepatic impairment:* not
> recommended; *Cirrhosis:* max 50 mg q 12 hours
> *Pediatric:* <18 years: not established; ≥18 years: same as adult
> ODT: 50 mg (mint) (phenylalanine)
> **Ryzolt** initially 100 mg once daily; may increase by 100 mg every 5 days;
> max 300 mg/day; *CrCl <40 mL/min* <u>or</u> *severe hepatic impairment:* not
> recommended
> *Pediatric:* <18 years: not recommended; ≥18 years: same as adult
> Tab: 100, 200, 300 mg ext-rel
> **Ultram** 50-100 mg q 4-6 hours prn; max 400 mg/day; *CrCl <40 mL/min:* max
> 100 mg q 12 hours; *Cirrhosis:* max 50 mg q 12 hours
> *Pediatric:* <18 years: not recommended; ≥18 years: same as adult
> Tab: 50*mg
> **Ultram ER** initially 100 mg once daily; may increase by 100 mg every 5
> days; max 300 mg/day; *CrCl <40 mL/min* <u>or</u> *severe hepatic impairment:* not
> recommended
> *Pediatric:* <18 years: not recommended; ≥18 years: same as adult
> Tab: 100, 200, 300 mg ext-rel

> *tramadol+acetaminophen* (C)(IV)(G) 2 tabs q 4-6 hours; max 8 tabs/day; 5 days;
  CrCl <40 mL/min: max 2 tabs q 12 hours; max 4 tabs/day x 5 days
  Pediatric: <18 years: not recommended; ≥18 years: same as adult
      Ultracet *Tab:* tram 37.5+acet 325 mg

TOPICAL AND TRANSDERMAL ANESTHETICS

Comment: *Lidocaine* should <u>not</u> be applied to non-intact skin.
> *lidocaine* cream (B) apply to affected area bid prn
  Pediatric: <12 years: not recommended; ≥12 years: same as adult
      LidaMantle *Crm:* 3% (1, 2 oz)
      Lidoderm *Crm:* 3% (85 gm)
      ZTlido *lidocaine* topical system 1% (30/carton)
  Comment: Compared to **Lidoderm** (*lidocaine* patch 5%), which contains 700
  mg/patch, **ZTlido** <u>only</u> requires 35 mg per topical system to achieve the same
  therapeutic dose.
> *lidocaine* lotion (B) apply to affected area bid prn
  Pediatric: <12 years: not recommended; ≥12 years: same as adult
      LidaMantle *Lotn:* 3% (177 ml)
> *lidocaine* 5% patch (B)(G) apply up to 3 patches at one time for up to 12
  hours/24-hour period (12 hours on/12 hours off); patches may be cut into smaller
  sizes before removal of the release liner; do <u>not</u> re-use
  Pediatric: <12 years: not recommended; ≥12 years: same as adult
      Lidoderm *Patch:* 5% (10x14 cm; 30/carton)
> *lidocaine+dexamethasone* (B)
  Pediatric: <12 years: not recommended; ≥12 years: same as adult
      Decadron Phosphate with Xylocaine *Lotn:* dexa 4 mg+lido 10 mg per ml
      (5 ml)
> *lidocaine+hydrocortisone* (B)(G) apply to affected area bid prn
  Pediatric: <12 years: not recommended; ≥12 years: same as adult
      LidaMantle HC *Crm:* lido 3%+hydro 0.5% (1, 3 oz); *Lotn:* (177 ml)
> *lidocaine 2.5%+prilocaine 2.5%* apply sparingly to the burn bid-tid prn
  Pediatric: <12 years: not recommended; ≥12 years: same as adult
      Emla Cream (B) 5, 30 gm/tube

  HERPES GENITALIS (HSV TYPE II)

Comment: The following treatment regimens are published in the **2015 CDC
Sexually Transmitted Diseases Treatment Guidelines**. Treatment regimens are for
adults <u>only</u>; consult a specialist for treatment of patients less than 18 years-of-age.
Treatment regimens are presented in alphabetical order by generic drug name,
followed by brands and dose forms.

RECOMMENDED REGIMENS: FIRST CLINICAL EPISODE
Regimen 1
> *acyclovir* 400 mg tid x 7-10 days <u>or</u> 200 mg 5 x/day x 10 days <u>or</u> until clinically
  resolved

Regimen 2
> *acyclovir* cream apply q 3 hours 6 x/day x 7 days

Regimen 3
> *famciclovir* 250 mg tid x 7-10 days <u>or</u> until clinically resolved

Regimen 4
▷ *valacyclovir* 1 gm bid x 10 days <u>or</u> until clinically resolved

RECOMMENDED RECURRENT/EPISODIC REGIMENS

Comment: Initiate treatment of recurrent episodes within 1 day of onset of lesions.

Regimen 1
▷ *acyclovir* 200 mg 5 x/day x 5 days

Regimen 2
▷ *famciclovir* 125 mg bid x 5 days

Regimen 3
▷ *valacyclovir* 500 mg bid x 3-5 days <u>or</u> until clinically resolved

SUPPRESSION THERAPY REGIMENS

Regimen 1
▷ *acyclovir* 400 mg bid x 1 year

Regimen 2
▷ *famciclovir* 250 mg bid x 1 year

Regimen 3
▷ *valacyclovir* 500 mg daily x 1 year (for ≤9 recurrences/year) <u>or</u> 1 gm daily x 1 year (for ≥10 recurrences/year)

DAILY SUPPRESSIVE REGIMENS FOR PERSONS WITH HIV

Regimen 1
▷ *acyclovir* 400-800 mg bid-tid

Regimen 2
▷ *famciclovir* 500 mg bid

Regimen 3
▷ *valacyclovir* 500 mg bid

RECURRENT/EPISODIC REGIMENS FOR PERSONS WITH HIV

Regimen 1
▷ *acyclovir* 400 mg tid x 5-10 days

Regimen 2
▷ *famciclovir* 500 mg bid x 5-10 days

Regimen 3
▷ *valacyclovir* 1 gm bid x 5-10 days

DRUG BRANDS AND DOSE FORMS

▷ *acyclovir* (B)(G)
   Zovirax *Cap:* 200 mg; *Tab:* 400, 800 mg
   Zovirax Oral Suspension *Oral susp:* 200 mg/5 ml (banana)
   Zovirax Cream *Crm:* 5% (3, 15 gm); *Oint:* 5% (3, 15 gm)
▷ *famciclovir* (B)
   Famvir *Tab:* 125, 250, 500 mg
▷ *valacyclovir* (B)
   Valtrex *Cplt:* 500, 1 gm

HERPES LABIALIS/HERPES FACIALIS (HSV TYPE I, COLD SORE, FEVER BLISTER)

PRIMARY INFECTION

▷ *acyclovir* (B)(G) do not chew, crush, or swallow the buccal tab; apply within 1 hour of symptom onset and before appearance of lesion; apply a single buccal tab to the upper gum region on the affected side and hold in place for 30 seconds
Pediatric: see Appendix CC.1. *acyclovir* (Zovirax Suspension) *for dose by weight*
   Sitavig *Buccal tab:* 50 mg
   Comment: **Sitavig** is contraindicated with allergy to milk protein concentrate.
▷ *valacyclovir* (B) 2 gm q 12 hours x 1 day
Pediatric: <12 years: not recommended; ≥12 years: same as adult
   Valtrex *Cplt:* 500, 1000 mg

SUPPRESSION THERAPY (≥6 OUTBREAKS/YEAR)

▷ *acyclovir* (B)(G) 200 mg 2-5 x/day x 1 year
Pediatric: <2 years: not recommended; ≥2 years, <40 kg: 20 mg/kg 2-5 x/day x 1 year; ≥2 years, >40 kg: 200 mg 2-5 x/day x 1 year; *see* Appendix CC.1. *acyclovir* (Zovirax Suspension) *for dose by weight*
   Zovirax *Cap:* 200 mg; *Tab:* 400, 800 mg
   Zovirax Oral Suspension *Oral susp:* 200 mg/5 ml (banana)

TOPICAL ANTIVIRAL THERAPY

▷ *acyclovir* (B)(G) apply q 3 hours 6 x/day x 7 days
Pediatric: <2 years: not recommended; ≥2 years: same as adult
   Zovirax Cream *Crm:* 5% (3, 15 gm); *Oint:* 5% (3, 15 gm)
▷ *docosanol* (B)(G) apply and gently rub in 5 x daily until healed
Pediatric: <12 years: not recommended; ≥12 years: same as adult
   Abreva (OTC) *Crm:* 10% (2 gm)
▷ *penciclovir* (B) apply q 2 hours while awake x 4 days
Pediatric: <12 years: not recommended; ≥12 years: same as adult
   Denavir *Crm:* 1% (2 gm)

TOPICAL ANTIVIRAL+CORTICOSTEROID THERAPY

▷ *acyclovir+hydrocortisone* (B)(G) cream apply to affected area 5 x/day x 5 days
Pediatric: <12 years: not recommended; ≥12 years: same as adult
   Crm: 1% (2, 5 gm)

 HERPES ZOSTER (HZ, SHINGLES)

see **Post-Herpetic Neuralgia**

PROPHYLAXIS VACCINES

Comment: *Herpes zoster* (shingles) vaccine is indicated for adults ≥50 years-of-age (<50 years: not recommended). The vaccine is not for preventing primary infection (chickenpox) or treatment of shingles. Contraindications to *Herpes zoster* vaccine are: history of anaphylactic/anaphylactoid reaction to gelatin, *neomycin*, or any other component of the vaccine, immunosuppression or immunodeficiency, and pregnancy. Pregnancy should be avoided for 3 months following *Varicella zoster* vaccine administration.

▷ *zoster vaccine recombinant, adjuvanted* administer one 0.5 ml dose at month 0 followed by second dose 2 and 6 months later; administer immediately upon reconstitution or store refrigerated and use within 6 hours
Pediatric: <18 years: not established
   Shingrix *Vial:* 0.5 ml single-dose susp for IM injection after reconstitution with diluent (10/carton) (preservative-free)

Comment: Local adverse reactions to **Shringrix** include injection site pain (78%), redness (38.1%), and swelling (25.9%). Generalized adverse reactions include myalgia (44.7%), fatigue (44.5%), headache (37.7%), shivering (26.8%), fever (20.5%), and gastrointestinal symptoms (17.3%). There are no available human data to inform whether there is vaccine-associated risk with **Shingrix** in pregnancy. It is <u>not</u> known whether **Shingrix** is excreted in human milk <u>or</u> effects on the breastfed infant.

ORAL ANTIVIRALS

▷ *acyclovir* (B)(G) 800 mg 5 x/day x 7-10 <u>or</u> 14 days
 Pediatric: <2 years: not recommended; ≥2 years, <40 kg: 20 mg/kg 5 x/day x 7-10 days; *see* Appendix CC.1. *acyclovir* (Zovirax Suspension) *for dose by weight;* >2 years, >40 kg: 800 mg 5 x/day x 7-10 days;
  Zovirax *Cap:* 200 mg; *Tab:* 400, 800 mg
  Zovirax Oral Suspension *Oral susp:* 200 mg/5 ml (banana)
▷ *famciclovir* (B) 500 mg tid x 7-10 days
 Pediatric: <18 years: not recommended; ≥18 years: same as adult
  Famvir *Tab:* 125, 250, 500 mg
▷ *valacyclovir* (B) 1 gm tid x 7-10 days
 Pediatric: <12 years: not recommended; ≥12 years: same as adult
  Valtrex *Cplt:* 500, 1,000 mg

PROPHYLAXIS AGAINST SECONDARY INFECTION

▷ *silver sulfadiazine* (B) apply qid
 Pediatric: <12 years: not recommended; ≥12 years: same as adult
  Silvadene *Crm:* 1% (20, 50, 85, 400, 1,000 gm jar; 20 gm tube)

ORAL ANALGESICS

Other Oral Analgesics *see* **Pain**

▷ *acetaminophen* (B) *see* **Fever**
▷ *aspirin* (D)(G) *see* **Fever**
 Comment: *Aspirin*-containing medications are contraindicated with history of allergic-type reaction to *aspirin*, children and adolescents with *varicella* <u>or</u> other viral illness, and 3rd trimester pregnancy.
▷ *tramadol* (C)(IV)(G)
  Rybix ODT initially 100 mg once daily; may increase by 100 mg every 5 days; max 300 mg/day; *CrCl <30 mL/min* <u>or</u> *severe hepatic impairment:* not recommended; *Cirrhosis:* max 50 mg q 12 hours
  Pediatric: <18 years: not recommended; ≥18 years: same as adult
   ODT: 50 mg (mint) (phenylalanine)
  Ryzolt initially 100 mg once daily; may increase by 100 mg every 5 days; max 300 mg/day; *CrCl <30 mL/min* <u>or</u> *severe hepatic impairment,* not recommended
  Pediatric: <18 years: not recommended; ≥18 years: same as adult
   Tab: 100, 200, 300 mg ext-rel
  Ultram 50-100 mg q 4-6 hours prn; max 400 mg/day; *CrCl <40 mL/min:* max 100 mg q 12 hours; *Cirrhosis:* max 50 mg q 12 hours
  Pediatric: <18 years: not recommended; ≥18 years: same as adult
   Tab: 50*mg
  Ultram ER initially 100 mg once daily; may increase by 100 mg every 5 days; max 300 mg/day; *CrCl <30 mL/min* <u>or</u> *severe hepatic impairment:* not recommended
  Pediatric: <18 years: not recommended; ≥18 years: same as adult
   Tab: 100, 200, 300 mg ext-rel
▷ *tramadol+acetaminophen* (C)(IV)(G) 2 tabs q 4-6 hours; max 8 tabs/day x 5 days; *CrCl <40 mL/min:* max 2 tabs q 12 hours; max 4 tabs/day x 5 days

Pediatric: <18 years: not recommended; ≥18 years: same as adult
    Ultracet *Tab:* tram 37.5+acet 325 mg

TOPICAL AND TRANSDERMAL ANESTHETICS

Comment: *Lidocaine* should <u>not</u> be applied to non-intact skin.

▷ *lidocaine* cream (B) apply to affected area bid prn
    Pediatric: <12 years: not recommended; ≥12 years: same as adult
        LidaMantle *Crm:* 3% (1, 2 oz)
        Lidoderm *Crm:* 3% (85 gm)
        ZTlido *lidocaine* topical system 1% (30/carton)
        Comment: Compared to **Lidoderm** (*lidocaine* patch 5%) which contains 700 mg/patch, **ZTlido** <u>only</u> requires 35 mg per topical system to achieve the same therapeutic dose.

▷ *lidocaine* lotion (B) apply to affected area bid prn
    Pediatric: <12 years: not recommended; ≥12 years: same as adult
        LidaMantle *Lotn:* 3% (177 ml)

▷ *lidocaine* 5% patch (B)(G) apply up to 3 patches at one time for up to 12 hours/24-hour period (12 hours on/12 hours off); patches may be cut into smaller sizes before removal of the release liner; do <u>not</u> re-use
    Pediatric: <12 years: not recommended; ≥12 years: same as adult
        Lidoderm *Patch:* 5% (10x14 cm; 30/carton)

▷ *lidocaine+dexamethasone* (B)
    Pediatric: <12 years: not recommended; ≥12 years: same as adult
        Decadron Phosphate with Xylocaine *Lotn:* dexa 4 mg+lido 10 mg per ml (5 ml)

▷ *lidocaine+hydrocortisone* (B)(G) apply to affected area bid prn
    Pediatric: <12 years: not recommended; ≥12 years: same as adult
        LidaMantle HC *Crm:* lido 3%+hydro 0.5% (1, 3 oz); *Lotn:* (177 ml)

▷ *lidocaine* 2.5%+prilocaine 2.5% apply sparingly to the burn bid-tid prn
    Pediatric: <12 years: not recommended; ≥12 years: same as adult
        Emla Cream (B) 5, 30 gm/tube

SECONDARY INFECTION PROPHYLAXIS

▷ *silver sulfadiazine* (B) apply qid
    Pediatric: <12 years: not recommended; ≥12 years: same as adult
        Silvadene *Crm:* 1% (20, 50, 85, 400, 1,000 gm/jar; 20 gm tube)

◯ HERPES ZOSTER OPHTHALMICUS (HZO, HERPETIC DENDRITIS)

Comment: *Herpes zoster* ophthalmicus (HZO, Herpetic Dendritis) is an ophthalmologic emergency. Standard therapy involves initiating systemic (oral or intravenous) antiviral therapy as soon as possible. Pharmacotherapy options include *acyclovir*, *valacyclovir*, and *famciclovir*. IV acyclovir is recommended for immunocompromised persons. Duration of treatment is 7-10 or 14 days, depending on severity. Ocular complications include conjunctivitis with or without superimposed bacterial infections, episcleritis, scleritis, keratitis, and uveitis, involvement of the 3rd, 4th, and 5th cranial nerves, acute optic neuritis, and necrotizing retinopathy (that often leads to permanent vision loss). Corticosteroids reduce the duration of pain during the acute phase; however, they have <u>not</u> been shown to decrease the incidence of postherpetic neuralgia and can exacerbate some ocular complications. Ophthalmology consultation is mandatory before initiating corticosteroid therapy.

OPHTHALMIC ANTIVIRAL

▷ *acyclovir ophthalmic ointment* apply a 1 cm ribbon in the lower cul-de-sac of the affected eye 5 x/day until healed; then, 3 x/day for 7 more days

Pediatric: <2 years: not established; ≥2years: same as adult

    Avaclyr *Ophth oint:* 3% (3.5 gm) single patient multi-use tube

    Comment: **Avaclyr** *(acyclovir ophthalmic ointment)* is a herpes simplex virus nucleoside analog DNA polymerase inhibitor indicated for the treatment of acute herpetic keratitis (dendritic ulcers) in patients with herpes simplex (HSV-1 and HSV-2) virus. **Avaclyr** is contraindicated in patients with a known hypersensitivity to *acyclovir* or *valacyclovir*. The most common adverse reactions (incidence 2-10%) have been eye pain (stinging), punctate keratitis, and follicular conjunctivitis. There is no information regarding embryo/fetal effects of maternal use of ophthalmic *acyclovir* during pregnancy or presence of ophthalmic *acyclovir* in human milk, or effects on the breastfed infant.

ORAL ANTIVIRALS

▷ *acyclovir* (B)(G) 800 mg 5 x/day x 7-10 days

    Pediatric: <2 years: not recommended; 2 years, ≤40 kg: 20 mg/kg 5 x/day x 7-10 days; 2 years, >40 kg: 800 mg 5 x/day x 7-10 days; *see* Appendix CC.1. *acyclovir (Zovirax Suspension) for dose by weight*

    Zovirax *Cap:* 200 mg; *Tab:* 400, 800 mg; *IVF bag:* 500 mg, 1 gm pre-mixed in 0.9% NS

    Zovirax Oral Suspension *Oral susp:* 200 mg/5 ml (banana)

▷ *famciclovir* (B) 500 mg tid x 7-10 days

    Pediatric: <18 years: not recommended; ≥18 years: same as adult

    Famvir *Tab:* 125, 250, 500 mg

▷ *valacyclovir* (B) 1 gm tid x 7-10 days

    Pediatric: <12 years: not recommended; ≥12 years: same as adult

    Valtrex *Cplt:* 500, 1 gm

HICCUPS: INTRACTABLE

▷ *chlorpromazine* (C) 25-50 mg tid-qid

    Pediatric: <6 months: not recommended; ≥6 months: 0.25 mg/lb orally q 4-6 hours prn or 0.5 mg/lb rectally q 6-8 hours prn

    Thorazine *Tab:* 10, 25, 50, 100, 200 mg; *Spansule:* 30, 75, 150 mg sust-rel; *Syr:* 10 mg/5 ml (4 oz; orange custard); *Oral conc:* 30 mg/ml (4 oz); 100 mg/ml (2, 8 oz); *Supp:* 25, 100 mg

HIDRADENITIS SUPPURATIVA

ORAL ANTI-INFECTIVES

▷ *doxycycline* (D)(G) 100 mg bid x 7-14 days

    Pediatric: <8 years: not recommended; ≥8 years, <100 lb: 2 mg/lb on the first day in 2 divided doses, followed by 1 mg/lb/day in 1-2 divided doses; ≥8 years, ≥100 lb: same as adult; *see Appendix CC.19: doxycycline (Vibramycin Syrup/ Suspension) for dose by weight*

    Acticlate *Tab:* 75, 150******mg

    Adoxa *Tab:* 50, 75, 100, 150 mg ent-coat

    Doryx *Tab:* 50, 75, 100, 150, 200 mg del-rel

    Doxteric *Tab:* 50 mg del-rel

    Monodox *Cap:* 50, 75, 100 mg

    Oracea *Cap:* 40 mg del-rel

    Vibramycin *Tab:* 100 mg; *Cap:* 50, 100 mg; *Syr:* 50 mg/5 ml (raspberry-apple); (sulfites); *Oral susp:* 25 mg/5 ml (raspberry)

    Vibra-Tab *Tab:* 100 mg film-coat

▷ *erythromycin base* (B)(G) 1-1.5 gm divided qid x 7-14 days

    Pediatric: <45 kg: 30-50 mg in 2-4 divided doses x 7-14 days; ≥45 kg: same as adult

        Ery-Tab *Tab*: 250, 333, 500 mg ent-coat
        PCE *Tab*: 333, 500 mg

▷ *erythromycin ethylsuccinate* (B)(G) 1200-1600 mg divided qid x 7-14 days
  Pediatric: 30-50 mg/kg/day in 4 divided doses x 7 days; may double dose
  with severe infection; max 100 mg/kg/day; *see Appendix CC.21: erythromycin*
  ethylsuccinate (E.E.S. Suspension, Ery-Ped Drops/Suspension) *for dose by*
  weight
      EryPed *Oral susp*: 200 mg/5 ml (100, 200 ml) (fruit); 400 mg/5 ml (60, 100,
      200 ml) (banana); *Oral drops*: 200, 400 mg/5 ml (50 ml) (fruit); *Chew tab*: 200
      mg wafer (fruit)
      E.E.S. *Oral susp*: 200, 400 mg/5 ml (100 ml) (fruit)
      E.E.S. Granules *Oral susp*: 200 mg/5 ml (100, 200 ml) (cherry)
      E.E.S. 400 Tablets *Tab*: 400 mg

▷ *minocycline* (D)(G) 100 mg bid x 7-14 days
  Pediatric: <8 years: not recommended, ≥8 years: same as adult
      Dynacin *Cap*: 50, 100 mg
      Minocin *Cap*: 50, 75, 100 mg; *Oral susp*: 50 mg/5 ml (60 ml) (custard)
      (sulfites, alcohol 5%)

▷ *tetracycline* (D)(G) 250 mg qid <u>or</u> 500 mg tid x 7-14 days
  Pediatric: <8 years: not recommended; ≥8 years, <100 lb: 25-50 mg/kg/day in 2-4
  divided doses x 7-14 days; ≥8 years, ≥100 lb: same as adult; *see Appendix CC.31:*
  tetracycline (Sumycin Suspension) *for dose by weight*
      Achromycin V *Cap*: 250, 500 mg
      Sumycin *Tab*: 250, 500 mg; *Cap*: 250, 500 mg; *Oral susp*: 125 mg/5 ml (100,
      200 ml) (fruit) (sulfites)

TOPICAL ANTI-INFECTIVE

▷ *clindamycin* (B) topical apply bid x 7-14 days
      Cleocin T *Pad*: 1% (60/pck; alcohol 50%); *Lotn*: 1% (60 ml); *Gel*: 1% (30, 60
      gm); *Soln w. applicator*: 1% (30, 60 ml) (alcohol 50%)

▷ *adalimumab* (B) 160 mg on Day 1 (administered in one day or split over two
  consecutive days), 80 mg on Day 15, and 40 mg every week <u>or</u> 80 mg every other
  week starting on Day 29. Discontinue in patients without evidence of clinical
  remission by eight weeks (Day 57); administer SC in the abdomen <u>or</u> thigh rotate
  sites
  Pediatric: <12 years: safety and efficacy not established; ≥12 years: <30 kg (<60 lb)
  to 60 kg (132 lb): *Day 1:* 80 mg; *Day 8 and subsequent doses:* 40 mg every other
  week; >60 kg (>132 lb): same as adult; administer SC in the abdomen <u>or</u> thigh;
  rotate sites
      Humira *Prefilled pen* (**Humira Pen**): 40 mg/0.4 ml, 40 mg/0.8 ml, 80 mg/0.8
      ml, single-dose; *Prefilled glass syringe*: 10 mg/0.1 ml, 10 mg/0.2 ml, 20 mg/0.2
      ml, 20 mg/0.4 ml, 40 mg/0.4 ml. 40 mg/0.8 ml, 80 mg/0.8 ml, single-dose;
      Vial: 40 mg/0.8 ml, single dose, institutional use only (preservative-free)

HOOKWORM (UNCINARIASIS, CUTANEOUS LARVAE MIGRANS)

ANTHELMINTICS

▷ *albendazole* (C) 400 mg as a single dose; may repeat in 3 weeks
  Pediatric: <2 years: 200 mg daily x 3 days; may repeat in 3 weeks; ≥2-12 years: 400
  mg daily x 3 days; may repeat in 3 weeks
      Albenza *Tab*: 200 mg

▷ *ivermectin* (C) take with water; chew <u>or</u> crush and mix with food; may repeat in 3
  months if needed; <15 kg: not recommended; ≥15 kg: 200 mcg/kg as a single dose
  Pediatric: <15 kg: not recommended; ≥15 kg: same as adult

Stromectol *Tab:* 3, 6*mg

▷ *mebendazole* (C)(G) chew, swallow, or mix with food; 100 mg bid x 3 days; may repeat in 3 weeks if needed; take with a meal
Pediatric: <2 years: not recommended; ≥2 years: same as adult
  Emverm *Chew tab:* 100 mg
  Vermox *Chew tab:* 100 mg

▷ *pyrantel pamoate* (C) 11 mg/kg x 1 dose; max 1 gm/dose
Pediatric: 25-37 lb: 1/2 tsp x 1 dose; 38-62 lb: 1 tsp x 1 dose; 63-87 lb: 1 tsp x 1 dose; 88-112 lb: 2 tsp x 1 dose; 113-137 lb: 2 tsp x 1 dose; 138-162 lb: 3 tsp x 1 dose; 163-187 lb: 3 tsp x 1 dose; >187 lb: 4 tsp x 1 dose
  Antiminth *Cap:* 180 mg; *Liq:* 50 mg/ml (30 ml); 144 mg/ml (30 ml); *Oral susp:* 50 mg/ml (60 ml)
  Pin-X (OTC) *Cap:* 180 mg; *Liq:* 50 mg/ml (30 ml); 144 mg/ml (30 ml); *Oral susp:* 50 mg/ml (30 ml)

▷ *thiabendazole* (C) take with a meal; may crush and mix with food; treat x 7 days; <30 lb: consult mfr pkg insert; ≥30 lb: 25 mg/kg/dose bid with meals; 30-50 lb: 250 mg bid with meals; >50 lb: 10 mg/lb/dose bid with meals; max 1.5 gm/dose; max 3 gm/day
Pediatric: same as adult
  Mintezol *Chew tab:* 500*mg (orange); *Oral susp:* 500 mg/5 ml (120 ml) (orange)

Comment: *Thiabendazole* is not for prophylaxis. May impair mental alertness. May not be available in the US.

HUMAN IMMUNODEFICIENCY VIRUS (HIV) INFECTION, HIV PRE-EXPOSURE PROPHYLAXIS (PrEP), HIV OCCUPATIONAL POST-EXPOSURE PROPHYLAXIS (oPEP), HIV NON-OCCUPATIONAL POST-EXPOSURE PROPHYLAXIS (nPEP)

ANTIRETROVIRAL HIV PRE-EXPOSURE PROPHYLAXIS (PrEP)

Comment: Descovy and Truvada are each individually used in the treatment of HIV-1 infection and for pre-exposure prophylaxis (PrEP) to reduce the risk of sexually acquired HIV-1 in adults and adolescents weighing ≥35 kg, at high risk for exposure, in combination with safe sex practices. HIV-1 PrEP is contraindicated in individuals with unknown or positive HIV-1 status. HIV-1 PrEP must only be prescribed to individuals confirmed to be HIV-negative immediately prior to initiating and at least every 3 months during use.

▷ **Descovy** (B)(G) *emtricitabine+tenofovir disoproxil fumarate* take1 tablet once daily with or without food
Pediatric: <12 years, <35 kg: not established; ≥12 years, ≥35 kg: same as adult
  Descovy *Tab:* emt 200 mg+teno ala 25 mg

▷ **Truvada** (B)(G) *emtricitabine+tenofovir disoproxil fumarate* <17 kg: not established; 17-<22 kg: 100/150 once daily; 22-<28 kg: 133/200 once daily; 28-35 kg: 167/250 once daily; ≥35 kg: 200/300 once daily
Pediatric: same as adult
  Tab: **Truvada 100/150** emt 100 mg+teno ala 150 mg
  Truvada 133/200 emt 133 mg+teno ala 200 mg
  Truvada 167/250 emt 167 mg+teno 250 mg
  Truvada 200/300 emt 200 mg+teno 300 mg

ANTIRETROVIRAL HIV POST-EXPOSURE PROPHYLAXIS (oPEP and nPEP)

Comment: Antiretroviral prophylactic treatment regimens for occupational HIV post-exposure prophylaxis (oPEP) and non-occupational HIV post-exposure prophylaxis (nPEP) are referenced from the **2015 CDC Sexually Transmitted Diseases Treatment Guidelines, MMWR**, and **NIH,** available at: https://www.cdc.gov/hiv/pdf/programresources/cdc-hiv-npep-guidelines.pdf.

In this section, the 2015 CDC-recommended highly active antiretroviral treatment (HAART) regimens are followed by a listing of the single and combination drugs with dosing regimens and dose forms. Appendix S is an alphabetical listing of the HIV drugs and dose forms. For more information on the management of HIV infection in adults and adolescents, see *Guidelines for the Use of Antiretroviral Agents in HIV-1-Infected Adults and Adolescents:* https://aidsinfo.nih.gov/contentfiles/lvguidelines/adultandadolescentgl.pdf.

For specific dosing information in the management of HIV infection in children, see *Guidelines for Use of Antiretroviral Agents in Pediatric HIV Infection:* www.aidsinfo.nih.gov/contentfiles/lvguidelines/pediatricguidelines.pdf. Providers should consult, and/or refer HIV-infected patients to, a specialist and/or specialty community services for age-appropriate dosing regimens and other patient-specific needs.

Initiation of oPEP/nPEP with ART as soon as possible increases the likelihood of prophylactic benefit. Treatment regimens must be initiated ≥72 hours following exposure. A 28-day course of ART is recommended for persons with *substantial risk for HIV exposure* (i.e., exposure of vagina, rectum, eye, mouth, or other mucous membrane, non-intact skin, or percutaneous contact with blood, semen, vaginal secretions, breast milk, or any body fluid that is visibly contaminated with blood, when the source is known to be infected with HIV). ART is not recommended for persons with *negligible risk for HIV exposure* (i.e., exposure of vagina, rectum, eye, mouth, or other mucus membrane, intact or non-intact skin, or percutaneous contact with urine, nasal secretions, saliva, sweat, or tears, if not visibly contaminated with blood, regardless of the known or suspected HIV status of the source). There is no evidence indicating any specific antiretroviral medication, or combination of medications is optimal for suppressing local viral replication. There is no evidence to indicate that a 3-drug ART regimen is any more beneficial than a 2-drug regimen. When the source person is available for interview and testing, his or her history of retroviral medication use and most recent/current viral load measurement should be considered when selecting an ART treatment regimen (e.g., to help avoid prescribing an antiretroviral medication to which the source virus is likely to be resistant). Register pregnant patients exposed to antiretroviral agents to the Antiretroviral Pregnancy Registry (APR) at 800-258-4263. The CDC recommends that HIV-infected mothers not breastfeed their infants to avoid risking postnatal transmission of HIV infection.

HIV-1 INFECTION ANTIRETROVIRAL TREATMENT REGIMENS

Comment: Immune Reconstitution Syndrome (IRS) has been reported in patients treated with combination antiretroviral therapy. During the initial phase of combination antiretroviral treatment, patients whose immune system responds may develop an inflammatory response to indolent or residual opportunistic infections (such as *Mycobacterium avium* infection, cytomegalovirus, *Pneumocystis jirovecii* pneumonia (PCP), or tuberculosis), which may necessitate further evaluation and treatment. Autoimmune disorders (such as Graves' disease, polymyositis, and Guillain-Barré syndrome) have also been reported to occur in the setting of immune reconstitution; however, the time to onset is more variable and can occur many months after initiation of treatment. Patients with HIV-1 should be tested for the presence of chronic hepatitis B virus (HBV) before initiating antiretroviral therapy.

NONNUCLEOSIDE REVERSE TRANSCRIPTASE INHIBITOR (NNRTI)-BASED REGIMEN

▷ *efavirenz* plus (*lamivudine* or *emtricitabine*) plus (*zidovudine* or *tenofovir*)

PROTEASE INHIBITOR (PI)-BASED REGIMENS

▷ *lopinavir+ritonavir* (co-formulated as **Kaletra**) plus (*lamivudine* or *emtricitabine*) plus *zidovudine*

▷ *darunavir+cobicistat* (co-formulated as **Prezcobix**) plus *other retroviral agents*

ALTERNATIVE REGIMENS

NNRTI-Based Regimen

▷ *efavirenz* plus (*lamivudine* or *emtricitabine*) plus (*abacavir* or *didanosine* or *stavudine*)
   Comment: *Efavirenz* should be avoided in pregnant females and females of child-bearing potential.

Protease Inhibitor-Based Regimens

Regimen 1

▷ *atazanavir* plus (*lamivudine* or *emtricitabine*) plus (*zidovudine* or *stavudine* or *abacavir* or *didanosine*) or (*tenofovir* plus *ritonavir* (100 mg/day)

Regimen 2

▷ *fosamprenavir* plus (*lamivudine* or *emtricitabine*) plus (*zidovudine* or *stavudine*) or (*abacavir* or *tenofovir* or *didanosine*)

Regimen 3

▷ *fosamprenavir+ritonavir* plus (*lamivudine* or *emtricitabine*) plus (*zidovudine* or *stavudine* or *abacavir* or *tenofovir* or *didanosine*)

Regimen 4

▷ *indinavir+ritonavir* plus (*lamivudine* or *emtricitabine*) plus (*zidovudine* or *stavudine* or *abacavir* or *tenofovir* or *didanosine*)
   Comment: Using *ritonavir* with *indinavir* may increase risk for renal adverse events.

Regimen 5

▷ *lopinavir+ritonavir* (co-formulated as **Kaletra**) plus (*lamivudine* or *emtricitabine*) plus (*stavudine* or *abacavir* or *tenofovir* or *didanosine*)

Regimen 6

▷ *nelfinavir* plus (*lamivudine* or *emtricitabine*) plus (*zidovudine* or *stavudine* or *abacavir* or *tenofovir* or *didanosine*)

Regimen 7

▷ *saquinavir+ritonavir* plus (*lamivudine* or *emtricitabine*) plus (*zidovudine* or *stavudine* or *abacavir* or *tenofovir* or *didanosine*)

Triple Nucleoside Reverse Transcriptase Inhibitor (NRTI)-Based Regimen

abacavir plus *lamivudine* plus *zidovudine*
Comment: Triple NRTI therapy should be used <u>only</u> when an NNRTI- <u>or</u> PI-based regimen cannot <u>or</u> should <u>not</u> be used.

BRAND NAMES, DOSING AND DOSE FORMS: SINGLE AGENTS

Integrase Strand Transfer Inhibitors (INSTIs)

▷ *cabotegravir*
   Vocabria *Tab:* 30 mg film-coat

Comment: **Vocabria** *(cabotegravir)* is indicated in combination with **Edurant** *(rilpivirine)* for short-term treatment of HIV-1 infection in adults who are virologically suppressed (HIV-1 RNA less than 50 copies/mL) on a stable antiretroviral regimen with <u>no</u> history of treatment failure and with <u>no</u> known or suspected resistance to either *cabotegravir* <u>or</u> *rilpivirine*, for use as (1) oral lead-in to assess the tolerability of *cabotegravir* prior to administration of **Cabenuva** *(cabotegravir+rilpivirine)* extended-release injectable suspensions and (2) oral therapy for patients who will miss planned injection dosing with **Cabenuva**.

▷ *dolutegravir* (C) *Treatment naïve <u>or</u> treatment experienced but INSTI naïve:* 50 mg once daily; *Treatment experienced <u>or</u> naïve and co-administered with efavirenz, FPV/r, TPV/r, <u>or</u> rifampin:* 50 mg bid; *INSTI experienced with certain INSTI-associated resistance substitutions:* 50 mg bid
  Pediatric: <12 years, <40 kg: not established; ≥12 years, ≥40 kg: same as adult
    Tivicay *Tab:* 10, 25, 50 mg

▷ *raltegravir (as potassium)* (C) 400 mg (one film-coat tab) bid; take with concomitant *rifampin* 800 mg bid; swallow whole; do <u>not</u> crush <u>or</u> chew
  Pediatric: ≥4 weeks, 3-11 kg [oral susp] 3-<4 kg: 20 mg bid; 4-<6 kg: 30 mg bid; 6-<8 kg: 40 mg bid; 8-<11 kg: 60 mg bid; ≥11-<25 kg [oral susp/chew tab]; 6 mg/kg/dose bid; see mfr pkg insert for dose by weight; ≥25 kg and unable to swallow tablet use chewable tab; 25-<28 kg: 150 mg bid; 28-<40 kg: 200 mg bid; ≥40 kg: 300 mg bid; 6 years, ≥25 kg, and able to swallow tablets use film-coat tab; 400 mg bid
    Isentress *Tab:* 400 mg film-coat; *Chew tab:* 25, 100*mg (orange banana) (phenylalanine)
    Isentress HD *Tab:* 600 mg film-coat
    Isentress Oral Suspension *Oral susp:* 100 mg/pkt pwdr for oral susp (banana)
  Comment: Oral suspension, chewable tablets, and film-coat *raltegravir* tablets are <u>not</u> bioequivalent. Maximum dose for chewable tablets is 300 mg twice daily. Previously, the maximum dose for film-coat tablets was 400 mg twice daily. However, the US Food and Drug Administration has recently approved a new 1200 mg daily dosage of **Isentress HD** *(raltegravir)* for the treatment of HIV-1 infection in adults, and pediatric patients who weigh ≥ 40 kg and are treatment-naïve <u>or</u> whose virus has been suppressed on an initial regimen of 400 mg twice-daily dose of **Isentress HD**. **Isentress HD** is administered as two 600 mg film-coat oral tablets, in combination with other antiretroviral agents, and can be taken with <u>or</u> without food. Co-administration of **Isentress HD** can include a wide range of antiretroviral agents and non-antiretroviral agents, however aluminum <u>and/or</u> magnesium-containing antacids, calcium carbonate antacids, *rifampin, tipranavir+ritonavir, etravirine*, and other strong inducers of drug metabolizing enzymes are <u>not</u> recommended to be combined with **Isentress HD**. Healthcare providers should consider the potential for drug-drug interactions prior to and during treatment with **Isentress HD** and any other recommended agents. Adverse effects associated with treatment included abdominal pain, diarrhea, vomiting, and decreased appetite. In addition, severe, potentially life-threatening and fatal skin reactions can occur, including Stevens-Johnson syndrome, hypersensitivity reaction, and toxic epidermal necrolysis. Treatment should be immediately discontinued if severe hypersensitivity, severe rash, <u>or</u> rash with systemic symptoms <u>or</u> liver aminotransferase elevations develop.

Nucleoside Reverse Transcriptase Inhibitors (NRTIs)

▷ *abacavir sulfate* (C)(G) 600 mg once daily <u>or</u> 300 mg bid; *Mild hepatic impairment:* use oral solution for titration
  Pediatric: 3 months-16 years: (tab/oral soln) 16 mg/kg qd <u>or</u> 8 mg/kg bid; max 300 mg bid; >14 kg: see mfr pkg insert for tablet dosing by weight band
    Ziagen (as sulfate) *Tab:* 300*mg

Ziagen Oral Solution *Oral soln:* 20 mg/ml (240 ml) (strawberry-banana) (parabens, propylene glycol)

▷ *didanosine* (C)

Videx EC take once daily on an empty stomach; swallow whole; <20 kg: use oral solution; 20-<25 kg: 200 mg; 25-<60 kg: 250 mg; ≥60 kg: 400 mg; *CrCl 30-59 m/min:* <60 kg: 125 mg; ≥60 kg: 200 mg; *CrCl 10-29 m/min:* 125 mg; *CrCl<10 mL/min or dialysis:*<60 kg: use oral solution ≥60 kg: 125 mg
Pediatric: same as adult

Cap: 125, 200, 250, 400 mg ent-coat del-rel; *Chew tab:* 25, 50, 100, 150, 200 mg (mandarin orange) (buffered with calcium carbonate and magnesium hydroxide, phenylalanine)

Videx Pediatric Pwdr for Solution <60 kg: 125 mg bid; ≥60 kg: 200 mg bid; *If once daily dosing required:* <60 kg: 250 mg once daily; ≥60 kg: 400 mg once daily; *CrCl 30-59 m/min:* <60 kg: 150 mg once daily or 75 mg bid; ≥60 kg: 200 mg once daily or 100 mg bid; *CrCl 10-29 mL/min:* <60 kg: 100 mg once daily; ≥60 kg: 150 mg once daily; *CrCl <10 mL/min or dialysis:* <60 kg: 75 mg once daily; ≥60 kg: 100 mg once daily; take on an empty stomach *Pediatric:* <2 weeks: not recommended; 2 weeks-8 months: 100 mg/m² bid; >8 months: 120 mg/m² bid; *Renal impairment:* consider reducing dose or increasing dosing interval; take on an empty stomach

Pwdr for oral soln: 2, 4 gm (120, 240 ml)

Comment: *Didanosine* is contraindicated with concomitant *allopurinal or ribavirin.*

▷ *emtricitabine* (B)(G) 200 mg once daily; *CrCl 30-49 mL/min:* 200 mg q 48 hours; *CrCl 15-29 mL/min:* 200 mg q 72 hours; *CrCl <15 mL/min or dialysis:* 200 mg q 96 hours
Pediatric: <3 months: 3 mg/kg oral soln once daily; 3 months-17 years, 6 mg/kg once daily; ≤33 kg: use oral soln, max 240 mg (24 ml); >33 kg: 200 mg cap once daily; max 240 mg/day; ≥18 years: same as adult

Emtriva Cap: 200 mg

Emtriva Oral Solution *Oral soln:* 10 mg/ml (170 ml) (cotton candy)

▷ *lamivudine* (C)(G) *CrCl ≥50 mL/min:* 300 mg qd or 150 mg bid; *CrCl >30-50 mL/min:* 150 mg qd; *CrCl 15-29:* first dose 150 mg, then 100 mg once daily; *CrCl 5-14 mL/min:* first dose 150 mg, then 50 mg qd; *CrCl <5 mL/min:* first dose 50 mg, the 25 mg once daily; max 8 mg/kg once daily or 150 mg bid
Pediatric: <3 months: not established; 3 months-16 years: 4 mg/kg oral soln or tab bid; [tab] 14-<20 kg: 150 mg once daily or 75 mg bid; ≥20-<25 kg: 225 mg once daily or 75 mg in the AM and 150 mg in the PM; ≥25 kg: 300 mg once daily or 150 mg bid; max 8 mg/kg once daily or 150 mg bid or 300 mg once daily

Epivir *Tab:* 150*, 300 mg

Epivir Oral Solution *Oral soln:* 10 mg/ml (240 ml) (strawberry-banana) (sucrose 3 gm/15 ml)

Comment: With renal impairment reduce *lamivudine* dose or extend dosing interval.

▷ *stavudine* (C)(G) ≥60 kg: 40 mg q 12 hours; ≤60 kg: 30 mg q 12 hours; *If peripheral neuropathy develops:* discontinue; *After resolution, ≥60 kg:* may re-start at 20 mg q 12 hours; *After resolution, ≤60 kg:* may restart at 15 mg q 12 hours; *if neuropathy returns:* consider permanent discontinuation; *CrCl 10-50 mL/min, ≥60 kg:* 20 mg q 12 hours; *CrCl 10-50 mL/min, ≥60 kg:* 15 mg q 12 hours; *Hemodialysis, ≥60 kg:* 20 mg q 24 hours; *Hemodialysis, ≤60 kg:* 15 mg q 24 hours; administer at the same time of day; *Hemodialysis:* administer at the end of dialysis
Pediatric: birth-13 days: [tab/oral soln] 0.5 mg/kg q 12 hours; >14 days, <30 kg: [tab/oral soln] 1 mg/kg q 12 hours; ≥30-<60 kg: 30 mg q 12 hours; ≥60 kg: 40 mg q 12 hours

Zerit *Cap:* 15, 20, 30, 40 mg
Zerit for Oral Solution *Oral soln:* 1 mg/ml pwdr for reconstitution (fruit) (dye-free)

Comment: Withdraw *stavudine* if peripheral neuropathy occurs. After complete resolution, may restart at half the recommended dose. If peripheral neuropathy recurs, consider permanent discontinuation.

▷ *tenofovir disoproxil fumarate* (C)(G) 300 mg once daily; *CrCl 30-49 mL/min:* 300 mg q 48 hours; *CrCl 10-29:* 300 mg q 72-96 hours; *Hemodialysis:* 300 mg once every 7 days or after a total of 12 hours of dialysis; *CrCl <10 mL/min:* not recommended
Pediatric: <2 years: not established; 2-12 years: 8 mg/kg once daily; >12 years, 35 kg: 300 mg once daily; mix oral pwdr with 2-4 oz soft food
Viread *Tab:* 150, 200, 250, 300 mg; *Oral pwdr:* 40 mg/gm (60 gm w. dosing scoop)

Comment: Published studies in HBV-infected subjects do not report an increased risk of adverse pregnancy-related outcomes with the use of **Viread** during the third trimester of pregnancy.

▷ *zidovudine* (C)(G) 600 mg daily divided bid-tid; *ESRD/dialysis:* 100 mg q 6-8 hours; *Vertical transmission, severe anemia, or neutropenia:* see mfr pkg insert
Pediatric: Treatment of HIV-1 infection: 4-<9 kg: 24 mg/kg/day divided bid or tid; ≥9-<30 kg: 18 mg/kg/day divided bid or tid; ≥30 kg: 600 mg/day divided bid or tid; *Prevention of maternal-fetal neonatal transmission: <12 hours after birth until 6 weeks of age:* [Soln] 2 mg/kg q 6 hours until 6 weeks-of-age; [IV] 1.5 mg/kg infused over 30 minutes q 6 hours until 6 weeks-of-age; max 200 mg q 8 hours
Retrovir Tablets *Tab:* 300 mg
Retrovir Capsules *Cap:* 100 mg
Retrovir Syrup *Syrup:* 50 mg/5 ml (strawberry)
Retrovir IV *Vial:* 10 mg/ml after dilution (20 ml) (preservative-free)

Nonnucleoside Reverse Transcriptase Inhibitors (NNRTIs)

▷ *delavirdine mesylate* (C) 400 mg (4 x 100-mg or 2 x 200 mg) tablets tid in combination with other antiretroviral agents
Pediatric: <16 years: not established; ≥16 years: same as adult
Rescriptor *Tab:* 100, 200 mg

Comment: The 100 mg **Rescriptor** tablets may be dispersed in water prior to consumption. To prepare a dispersion, add four 100 mg **Rescriptor** tablets to at least 3 oz of water, allow to stand for a few minutes, and then stir until a uniform dispersion occurs. The dispersion should be consumed promptly. The glass should be rinsed with water and the rinse swallowed to insure the entire dose is consumed. The 200 mg tablets should be taken as intact tablets, because they are not readily dispersed in water.

▷ *doravirine* 100 mg once daily in combination with other antiretroviral agents; as a dosage adjustment when taking *rifabutin* with **Delstrigo**, administer 100 mg of *doravirine* (**Pifeltro**) approximately 12 hours after the dose of **Delstrigo**
Pediatric: <18 years: not established; ≥18 years: same as adult
Pifeltro *Tab:* 100 mg

▷ *efavirenz* (D)(G) 600 mg once daily
Pediatric: >3 months, 3.5 kg: [tab/cap] 3.5 to < 5 kg: 100 mg once daily 5 to <7.5 kg: 150 mg once daily; 7.5 to <15 kg: 200 mg once daily; 15 to <20 kg: 250 mg once daily; 20 to <25 kg: 300 mg once daily; 25 to <32.5 kg: 350 once daily; 32.5 to <40 kg: 400 mg once daily; >40 kg: 600 mg once daily; max 600 mg once daily

Comment: For children who cannot swallow capsules, the capsule contents can be administered with a small amount of food or infant formula using the capsule sprinkle method of administration. See mfr pkg insert for instructions. Tablets should not be crushed or chewed. Administer at bedtime to limit CNS effects.
Sustiva *Tab:* 75, 150, 600, 800 mg; *Cap:* 50, 200 mg

▷ **etravirine (B)** 200 mg (1 x 200 mg tablet or 2 x 100 mg tablets) bid following a meal

Pediatric: <3 year: not recommended; ≥3 years, >16 kg: 16-< 20 kg: 100 mg bid; 20-<25 kg: 125 mg bid; 25-<30 kg: 150 mg bid; ≥30 kg: 200 mg bid; max 200 mg bid; take following a mail

   Intelence *Tab:* 25*, 100, 200 mg

▷ **nevirapine (B)(G)** initially one 200 mg tablet of immediate-release **Viramune** once daily for the first 14 days, in combination with other antiretroviral agents; then, one 400 mg tablet of **Viramune XR** once daily

Comment: The 14-day lead-in period has been found to lessen the frequency of rash.

Pediatric: <6 years: not recommended; 6-<18 years: BSA 0.58-0.83 kg/m²: 200 mg once daily; BSA 0.84-1.16 kg/m²: 300 mg once daily; BSA ≥1.17 kg/m²: 400 mg; once daily; max 400 mg once daily

Comment: Children must initiate therapy with immediate-release **Viramune** for the first 14 days; ≥15 days: [oral susp/tab]: 150 mg/m² once daily for 14 days, then 150 mg/m² bid

   Viramune *Tab:* 200*mg
   Viramune Oral Suspension *Oral susp:* 50 mg/5 ml (240 ml)
   Viramune XR *Tab:* 100, 400 mg ext-rel

▷ **rilpivirine (D)** 25 mg once daily; *If concomitant* **rifabutin**: 50 mg once daily: *If concomitant* **rifabutin** *stopped:* 25 mg once daily

Pediatric: <12 years: not recommended; ≥12 years, >35 kg: same adult

   Edurant *Tab:* 25 mg

Protease Inhibitors (PIs)

▷ **atazanavir (B)(G)** *Treatment naive: Recommended regimen:* 300 mg plus **ritonavir** 100 mg once daily; *Unable to tolerate* **ritonavir**: 400 mg once daily; *In combination with efavirenz:* 400 mg plus **ritonavir** 100 mg once daily; *Treatment experienced: Recommended regimen:* 300 mg plus **ritonavir** 100 mg once daily; *In combination with both an H2-blocker or PPI and tenofovir:* 400 mg plus **ritonavir** 100 mg once daily; take with food

Pediatric: <3 months: not recommended; ≥3 months, 5 kg: [oral pwdr] 5-<15 kg: 200 mg (4 packets) plus **ritonavir** 80 mg once daily; 15-<25 kg: 250 mg (5 packets) plus **ritonavir** 80 mg once daily; ≥25 kg, unable to swallow capsules: 300 mg (6 packets) plus **ritonavir** once daily; 6 years, <15 kg: [cap] 15-<20 kg: 150 mg plus **ritonavir** 100 mg once daily; 20-<40 kg: 200 mg plus **ritonavir** 100 mg once daily; ≥40 kg: 300 mg plus **ritonavir** 100 mg once daily; [capsule]15-<20 kg: 150 mg plus **ritonavir** 100 mg once daily; 20-<40 kg: 200 mg plus **ritonavir** 100 mg once daily; ≥40 kg: 300 mg plus **ritonavir** 100 mg once daily; max dose 400 mg once daily; take with food

   Reyataz *Cap:* 100, 150, 200, 300 mg; *Oral pwdr:* 50 mg/pkt (30/carton) (phenylalanine)

Comment: Administration of **atazanavir** with **ritonavir** is preferred. Dose for treatment-naïve children ≥13 years of age and ≥40 kg unable to tolerate **ritonavir**, administer 400 mg once daily. See mfr pkg insert for special dosing considerations when combining **atazanavir** with other retrovirals.

▷ **darunavir (C)(G)** *Treatment naïve and treatment experienced with no darunavir resistance associated substitutions:* 800 mg once daily with **ritonavir** 100 mg once daily; *Treatment-experienced with at least one darunavir resistance associated substitution:* 600 mg bid with ritonavir 100 mg bid; *Severe hepatic impairment:* not recommended

Pediatric: ≥3 years, 10 kg [oral soln/tab/cap] *Treatment naïve or experienced without darunavir-associated substitutions:* 10-<15 kg: 35 mg/kg once daily plus **ritonavir** 7 mg/kg once daily; 15-<30 kg: 600 mg plus **ritonavir** 100 mg once daily; 30-<40 kg: 675 mg plus **ritonavir** 100 mg once daily; >40 kg: 800 mg plus *ritonavir* 100 mg once daily; *Treatment experienced with ≥1* ***darunavir****-associated substitution(s):* 10-15 kg: 20 mg/kg bid <u>plus</u> ***ritonavir*** 3 mg/kg bid; 15-<30 kg: 375 mg <u>plus</u> ***ritonavir*** 48 mg bid; 30-<40 kg: 450 mg <u>plus</u> ***ritonavir*** 60 mg bid; >40 kg: 600 mg <u>plus</u> ***ritonavir*** 100 mg bid

    Prezista *Tab:* 75, 150, 600, 800 mg film-coat

    Prezista Oral Suspension *Susp:* 100 mg/ml (strawberry cream)

    Comment: **Prezista** is FDA approved for treatment of HIV-1-infected pregnant females and for the treatment of children >3 years-of-age in combination with ***ritonavir*** and other antiretrovirals.

▷ ***fosamprenavir*** **(C)(G)** *Treatment-naïve:* 1,400 mg bid <u>or</u> 1400 mg once daily <u>plus</u> ***ritonavir*** 200 mg once daily <u>or</u> 1400 mg once daily <u>plus</u> ***ritonavir*** 100 mg once daily <u>or</u> 700 mg bid <u>plus</u> ***ritonavir*** 100 mg bid; *Protease inhibitor-experienced:* 700 mg bid <u>plus</u> ***ritonavir*** 100 mg bid

Pediatric: <4 weeks: not recommended; *Protease inhibitor-naïve, ≥4 weeks* <u>or</u> *protease inhibitor-experienced:* ≥6 Months, <11 kg: 45 mg/kg <u>plus</u> ***ritonavir*** 7 mg/kg bid; 11-<15 kg: 30 mg/kg <u>plus</u> ***ritonavir*** 3 mg/kg bid; 15 kg-<20 kg: 23 mg/kg <u>plus</u> ***ritonavir*** 3 mg/kg bid; ≥20 kg: 18 mg/kg <u>plus</u> ***ritonavir*** 3 mg/kg bid; *Protease-inhibitor naïve, ≥2 years:* 30 mg/kg bid <u>without</u> ***ritonavir***: max dose 700 mg <u>plus</u> ***ritonavir*** 100 mg bid

    Lexiva: *Tab:* 700 mg film-coat

    Lexiva Oral Suspension *Oral susp:* 50 mg/ml (225 ml) (grape-bubble gum-peppermint)

    Comment: *Fosamprenavir* 1 ml is equivalent to approximately 43 mg of ***amprenavir*** 1 ml.

▷ ***indinavir sulfate*** **(C)** 800 mg q 8 hours; *Concomitant* ***rifabutin***: 1 gm q 8 hours and reduce ***rifabutin*** dose by half; *Hepatic insufficiency* <u>or</u> *concomitant* ***ketoconazole, itraconazole,*** <u>or</u> ***delavirdine***: 600 mg q 8 hours; take with water on an empty stomach <u>or</u> with a light meal

Pediatric: <3 years: not established ≥3-18 years, doses of 500 mg/m² every 8 hours have been used; see mfr pkg insert)

    Crixivan *Cap:* 100, 200, 333, 400 mg

▷ ***nelfinavir mesylate*** **(B)** 1250 mg (5 x 250 mg tablets <u>or</u> 2 x 625 mg tablets) bid <u>or</u> 750 mg (3 x 250 mg tablets) tid; take with a meal; may dissolve tablets in a small amount of water; max 2500 mg/day

Pediatric: <2 years: not established; 2-13 years: 45-55 mg/kg bid <u>or</u> 25-35 mg/kg tid; take with a meal; max 2500 mg/day; ≥13 years: same as adult

    Viracept *Tab:* 250, 625 mg

    Viracept Oral Powder *Oral pwdr:* 50 mg/gm (144 gm) (phenylalanine)

    Comment: The 250 mg **Viracept** tabs are interchangeable with oral powder, the 625 mg tabs are <u>not</u>.

▷ ***raltegravir (as potassium)*** **(C)** 400 mg bid

Pediatric: ≥4 weeks, 3-11 kg: [oral susp] 3-<4 kg: 20 mg bid; 4-<6 kg: 30 mg bid; 6-<8 kg: 40 mg bid; 8-<11 kg: 60 mg bid; ≥11-<25 kg: [oral susp/chew tab] 6 mg/kg/dose bid; see mfr pkg insert for dosage by weight; ≥25 kg and unable to swallow tablet: [chew tab] 25-<28 kg: 150 mg bid; 28-<40 kg: 200 mg bid; ≥40 kg: 300 mg bid; ≥6 years, ≥25 kg, able to swallow tablets: 400 mg film-coat tablet bid

Comment: Oral suspension, chewable tablets, and film-coat tablets are <u>not</u> bioequivalent. Chewable tablet max dose 300 mg bid. Film-coat tablets max dose 400 mg bid. Oral suspension max dose 100 mg bid

    Isentress *Tab:* 400 mg film-coat; *Chew tab:* 25, 100*mg (orange-banana) (phenylalanine)

    Isentress Oral Suspension *Oral susp:* 100 mg/pkt pwdr for oral susp (banana)

▷ ***ritonavir*** **(B)(G)** initially 300 mg bid; increase at 2-3 day intervals by 100 mg bid; max 600 mg bid

Pediatric: <1 month: not recommended; ≥1 month: 350-400 mg/m² bid; initiate at 250 mg/m² bid and titrate upward every 2-3 days by 50 mg/m² bid; max dose 600 mg bid

Comment: Lower doses of *ritonavir* have been used to boost other protease inhibitors but the *ritonavir* doses used for boosting have not been specifically approved in children.

> **Norvir** *Tab:* 100 mg film-coat; *Gel cap:* 100 mg (alcohol)
> **Norvir Oral Solution** *Oral soln:* 80 mg/ml, 600 mg/7.5 ml (8 oz) (peppermint-caramel) (alcohol)
> Comment: **Norvir** tablets should be swallowed whole. Take **Norvir** with meals. Patients may improve the taste of **Norvir Oral Solution** by mixing with chocolate milk, **Ensure**, or **Advera** within 1 hour of dosing. Dose reduction of **Norvir** is necessary when used with other protease inhibitors (*atazanavir, darunavir, fosamprenavir, saquinavir,* and *tipranavir.* Patients who take the 600 mg gel cap bid may experience more gastrointestinal side effects such as nausea, vomiting, abdominal pain, or diarrhea when switching from the gel cap to the tablet because of greater maximum plasma concentration (Cmax) achieved with the tablet. These adverse events (gastrointestinal or paresthesias) may diminish as treatment is continued.

▷ *saquinavir mesylate* (B)
Pediatric: <16 years: not established; ≥16 years: same as adult
> **Fortovase** *Tab/Cap:* 200 mg
> **Invirase** *Tab:* 500 mg; *Cap:* 200 mg

▷ *tipranavir* (C) 500 mg bid plus ritonavir 200 mg bid
Pediatric: <2 years: not recommended; 2-18 years: [cap/oral soln] 14 mg/kg plus ritonavir 6 mg/kg bid or 375 mg/m² plus *ritonavir* 150 mg/m² bid; max 500 mg plus *ritonavir* 200 mg bid
> **Aptivus** *Gel cap:* 250 mg (alcohol)
> **Aptivus Oral Solution** *Oral soln:* 100 mg/ml (buttermint-butter toffee) (Vit E 116 IU/ml)

FUSION INHIBITORS—CCR5 CO-RECEPTOR ANTAGONISTS

▷ *enfuvirtide* (B) 90 mg (1 ml) SC bid; administer in upper arm, abdomen, or anterior thigh; rotate injection sites
Pediatric: <6 years: not established; 6-16 years: administer 2 mg/kg SC bid; max 90 mg SC bid; >16 years: same as adult; rotate injection sites
> **Fuzeon** *Vial:* 90 mg/ml pwdr for SC inj after reconstitution (1 ml, 60 vials/kit) (preservative-free)

▷ *maraviroc* (B) must be administered concomitant with other retrovirals; *Concomitant potent CYP3A inhibitors (with or without a potent CYP3A inducer) including protease inhibitors (except tipranavir+ritonavir), delavirdine, ketoconazole, itraconazole, clarithromycin, other potent CYP3A inhibitors (e.g., nefazodone, telithromycin):* CrCl ≥30 mL/min: 150 mg bid; <30 mL/min, dialysis: not recommended; *Potent CYP3A inducers (without a potent CYP3A inhibitor) including efavirenz, rifampin, etravirine, carbamazepine, phenobarbital, and phenytoin:* 300 mg bid; *CrCl ≥30 mL/min:* 600 mg bid; <30 mL/min: not recommended; *Other concomitant agents, including tipranavir+ritonavir, nevirapine, raltegravir, all NRTIs, and enfuvirtide:* 300 mg bid
Pediatric: <16 years: not established; ≥16 years: same as adult
> **Selzentry** *Tab:* 150, 300 mg film-coat

CD4-DIRECTED POST-ATTACHMENT HIV-1 INHIBITOR

▷ *ibalizumab-uiyk* administer as an IV injection once every 14 days
Pediatric: <18 years: not established; ≥18 years: same as adult
> **Trogarzo** *Vial:* 200 mg/1.33 ml (1.33 ml) single-dose

Comment: **Trogarzo** *(ibalizumab)* is indicated for the treatment of patients with HIV infection who are heavily treatment-experienced and multi-drug resistant infection. It is intended for use in combination with other anti-retroviral medications.

GP120-DIRECTED ATTACHMENT INHIBITOR

➤ *fostemsavir* take one tablet twice daily, with or without food
 Pediatric: not established
  Rokubia *Tab:* 600 mg, film-coat, ext-rel
  Comment: Rokubia *(fostemsavir)*, a human immunodeficiency virus type 1 (HIV-1) gp120-directed attachment inhibitor, in combination with other antiretroviral(s), is indicated for the treatment of HIV-1 infection in heavily treatment-experienced adults with multidrug-resistant HIV-1 infection failing their current antiretroviral regimen due to resistance, intolerance, or safety considerations. The most common adverse reaction (incidence 5%) has been nausea. See mfr pkg insert for complete list of significant drug interactions. Co-administration of **Rokubia** with strong cytochrome P450 (CYP)3A inducers is contraindicated as significant decreases in *temsavir* plasma concentrations may occur, which may result in loss of virologic response. Immune reconstitution syndrome has been reported in patients treated with combination antiretroviral therapies. Concomitant oral contraceptive should not contain more than 30 mcg of *ethinyl estradiol* per day. Use **Rukobia** with caution in patients with a history of QTc prolongation or with relevant pre-existing cardiac disease or who are taking drugs with a known risk of Torsade de Pointes. Elevations in hepatic transaminases have been observed in a greater proportion of subjects with HBV and/or HCV co-infection, compared with those with HIV mono-infection. There are insufficient human data on the use of **Rukobia** during pregnancy to adequately assess a drug-associated risk of birth defects and miscarriage. In animal reproduction studies, oral administration of *fostemsavir* during organogenesis resulted in no adverse developmental effects at clinically relevant *temsavir* exposures. There is a pregnancy exposure registry that monitors pregnancy outcomes in individuals exposed to **Rokubia** during pregnancy. Healthcare providers are encouraged to register patients by calling the Antiretroviral Pregnancy Registry (APR) at 1-800-258-4263. Breastfeeding is not recommended due to the potential for HIV-1 transmission.

CYP3A INHIBITOR

➤ *cobicistat* 150 mg once daily; must be co-administer with *atazanavir* 300 mg once daily or *darunavir* 800 mg once daily, at the same time, with food, and in combination with other HIV-1 antiretroviral agents
 Pediatric: <35 kg: not established; ≥35 kg: 150 mg once daily, co-administered with *atazanavir* or ≥40 kg: 150 mg once daily, co-administered with *darunavir*; at the same time, with food, and in combination with other HIV-1 antiretroviral agents; For dosage recommendations of the co-administered protease inhibitor *atazanavir* or darunavir, refer to Table 2 of the **Tybost** pkg insert
  Tybost *Tab:* 150 mg
  Comment: Tybost *(cobicistat)* is a CYP3A inhibitor indicated to increase systemic exposure of *atazanavir* or *darunavir* in combination with other antiretroviral agents in the treatment of HIV-1 infection. **Tybost**, in combination with *atazanavir* or *darunavir*, can alter the concentration of drugs metabolized by CYP3A or CYP2D6. Drugs that induce CYP3A can alter the concentrations of **Tybost**, *atazanavir* and *darunavir*. Consult the mfr pkg insert prior to and during treatment for potential drug interactions. Assess CrCl before initiating treatment. When **Tybost** is used

in combination with a TDF-containing regimen, cases of acute renal failure (ARF) and Fanconi syndrome have been reported. Assess urine glucose and urine protein at baseline and monitor CrCl, urine glucose, and urine protein. Monitor serum phosphorus in patients with or at risk for renal impairment. **Tybost** in combination with more than one antiretroviral agent that requires pharmacokinetic enhancement (i.e., two protease inhibitors or *elvitegravir* in combination with a protease inhibitor) is not recommended. Use with HIV-1 protease inhibitors other than *atazanavir* or *darunavir* administered once daily is not recommended. Co-administration with drugs or regimens containing *ritonavir* is not recommended. **Tybost** co-administered with *atazanavir* or *darunavir* is not recommended during pregnancy or lactation.

BRAND NAMES, DOSING, AND DOSE FORMS: COMBINATION AGENTS

▷ **Atripla (B)(G)** *efavirenz+emtricitabine+tenofovir disoproxil fumarate* 1 tablet once daily on an empty stomach; bedtime dosing may improve the tolerability of nervous system symptoms; *CrCl <50 mL/min:* not recommended
Pediatric: <12 years, <40 kg: not established; ≥12 years, ≥40 kg: same as adult
   Tab: efa 600 mg+emtri 200 mg+teno dis fum 300 mg film-coat

▷ **Biktarvy** *bictegravir+emtricitabine+tenofovir alafenamide* take 1 tablet once daily with or without food
Pediatric: <18 years: not established; ≥18 years: same as adult
   Tab: bict 50 mg+emtri 200 mg+teno alaf 25 mg
Comment: Biktarvy is a 3-drug fixed-dose combination of *bictegravir*, a human immunodeficiency virus type 1 (HIV-1) integrase strand transfer inhibitor (INSTI), and *emtricitabine* and *tenofovir alafenamide*, both HIV-1 nucleoside analog reverse transcriptase inhibitors (NRTIs) indicated as a complete regimen for the treatment of HIV-1 infection in adults who have no antiretroviral treatment history or to replace the current antiretroviral regimen in those who are virologically suppressed (HIV-1 RNA less than 50 copies per mL) on a stable antiretroviral regimen for at least 3 months with no history of treatment failure and no known substitutions associated with resistance to the individual components of **Biktarvy**. **Biktarvy** is not recommended in patients with estimated CrCl <30 mL/min and/or with severe hepatic impairment.

▷ **Cabenuva** *cabotegravir* and *rilpivirine*
   2 Vial Kit: **cabo** 400 mg single-dose and rilpiv 600 mg single-dose; *2 Vial Kit:* **cabo** 400 mg single-dose and **rilpiv** 900 mg single-dose
Comment: Cabenuva *(cabotegravir* and *rilpivirine)* is a 2-drug co-packaged product containing a single-dose vial of **cabotegravir** (HIV-1 integrase the strand transfer inhibitor [NSTI]) and a single-dose vial of *rilpivirine* (HIV-1 non-nucleoside reverse transcriptase inhibitor [NNRTI]). This combination provides a complete long-acting once-monthly injectable regimen (depot) option for treatment of HIV-1 infection in adults. Prior to initiation with **Cabenuva**, an oral lead-in should be used for approximately 1 month (at least 28 days) to assess the tolerability of *cabotegravir* and *rilpivirine*.

▷ **Cimduo** *lamivudine+tenofovir disoproxil fumarate* 1 tablet once daily with or without food
Pediatric: <35 kg: not recommended; ≥35 kg: same as adult
   Tab: lami 300 mg+teno teno diso 300 mg
Comment: Cimduo is a two-drug fixed-dose combination of *lamivudine* and *tenofovir disoproxil fumarate*, both nucleoside reverse transcriptase inhibitors (NRTIs) and is indicated for the treatment of HIV-1 infection in combination with other antiretroviral agents. Prior to initiation and during treatment with **Cimduo**, patients should be tested for hepatitis B virus (HBV) infection, and estimated CrCl, serum phosphorus, urine glucose, and urine protein should be

obtained. **Cimduo** is not recommended in patients with CrCL < 50 ml/min or patients with end-stage renal disease (ESRD) requiring hemodialysis. Discontinue treatment in patients who develop symptoms or laboratory findings suggestive of lactic acidosis or pronounced hepatotoxicity.

▷ **Combivir (C)(G)** *lamivudine+zidovudine*
  Pediatric: <12 years: not recommended; ≥12 years, ≥30 kg: 1 tablet bid with food
   Tab: lami 150 mg+zido 300 mg

▷ **Complera (B)** *emtricitabine+tenofovir disoproxil fumarate+rilpivirine* 1 tablet once daily; *CrCl <50 mL/min:* not recommended
  Pediatric: <12 years, <40 kg: not recommended; ≥12 years, ≥40 kg: same as adult
   Tab: emtri 200 mg+teno dis 300 mg+rilpiv 25 mg

▷ **Delstrigo** *doravirine+lamivudine+tenofovir disoproxil fumarate* 1 tablet once daily with or without food; *CrCl <50 mL/min:* not recommended
  Pediatric: <18 years: not established; ≥18 years: same as adult
   Tab: dora 100 mg+lami ala 300 mg+teno dis 300 mg

Comment: **Delstrigo** is approved as a complete 3-drug fixed-dose once daily regimen for patients with no prior antiretroviral treatment experience. Monitor for new onset or worsening renal impairment. Prior to or when initiating **Delstrigo**, and during treatment on a clinically appropriate schedule, assess serum creatinine, estimated creatinine clearance, urine glucose, and urine protein in all patients. Avoid administering **Delstrigo** with concurrent or recent use of nephrotoxic drugs. In patients with chronic kidney disease (CKD), also assess serum phosphorus. Severe acute exacerbations of hepatitis B (HBV) have been reported in patients co-infected with HIV-1 and HBV who have discontinued *lamivudine* or *tenofovir disoproxil fumarate* (TDF), two of the components of **Delstrigo**. Closely monitor hepatic function in these patients. If appropriate, initiation of anti-hepatitis B therapy may be warranted. Dosage adjustment with *rifabutin:* Take one tablet of **Delstrigo** once daily, followed by one tablet of *doravirine* 100 mg (**Pifeltro**) approximately 12 hours after the dose of **Delstrigo**. There is a pregnancy exposure registry that monitors pregnancy outcomes in individuals exposed to **Delstrigo** during pregnancy. Healthcare providers are encouraged to register patients by calling the Antiretroviral Pregnancy Registry (APR) at 1-800-258-4263.

▷ **Descovy (D)** *emtricitabine+tenofovir alafenamide* 1 tablet once daily with or without food; *CrCl <30 mL/min:* not recommended
  Pediatric: <12 years, <35 kg: not recommended; ≥12 years, ≥35 kg: same as adult
   Tab: emtri 200 mg+teno ala 25 mg

Comment: Patients with HIV-1 should be tested for the presence of chronic hepatitis B virus (HBV) before initiating antiretroviral therapy. **Descovy** is not approved for the treatment of chronic HBV infection, and the safety and efficacy of **Descovy** have not been established in patients co-infected with HIV-1 and HBV.

▷ **Dovato** *dolutegravir+lamivudine* one tab daily
  Pediatric: safety and efficacy not established
   Tab: dolu 50 mg+lami 300 mg film-coat

Comment: **Dovato** (*dolutegravir+lamivudine*) is a once-daily, single-tablet, two-drug fixed-dose combination of *dolutegravir* (**Tivicay**, an integrase strand transfer inhibitor (INSTI) and *lamivudine* (**Epivir**, a nucleoside analogue reverse transcriptase inhibitor [NRTI]) indicated for the treatment of HIV-1 infection in adults with no antiretroviral (ARV) treatment history and with no known resistance to either *dolutegravir* or *lamivudine*.

▷ **Epzicom (B)(G)** *abacavir sulfate+lamivudine* 1 tab daily; *Mild hepatic impairment* or *CrCl<50 mL/min:* not recommended
  Pediatric: <25 kg: use individual components; ≥25 kg: one tablet once daily; *Mild hepatic impairment* or *CrCl<50 mL/min:* not recommended
   Tab: aba 600 mg/lami 300 mg

▷ **Evotaz (B)** *atazanavir+cobicistat* 1 tab once daily
Pediatric: <12 years, <35 kg: not established; ≥12 years, ≥35 kg: same as adult
   Tab: ataz 600 mg+cobi 300 mg

▷ **Genvoya (B)** *elvitegravir+cobicistat+emtricitabine+tenofovir alafenamide* 1 tab once daily; *Severe hepatic impairment or CrCl <30 mL/min:* not recommended; take with food
Pediatric: <12 years, <35 kg: not established; ≥12 years, ≥35 kg: same as adult
   Tab: elvi 150 mg+cobi 150 mg+emtri 200 mg+teno 10 mg

▷ **Juluca** *dolutegravir+rilpivirine* take one tablet once daily with or without food
Pediatric: <18 years: not established; ≥18 years: same as adult
   Tab: dolu 50 mg+rilp 25 mg film-coat
Comment: **Juluca** is a complete two-drug fixed-dose combination of *dolutegravir*, a human immunodeficiency virus type 1 (HIV-1) integrase strand transfer inhibitor (INSTI) and *rilpivirine*, a HIV-1 non-nucleoside reverse transcriptase inhibitor (NNRTI), indicated for treatment of HIV infection to replace the current antiretroviral regimen in those who are virologically suppressed (HIV-1 RNA <50 copies per mL) on a stable antiretroviral regimen for at least 6 months, with no history of treatment failure, and no known substitutions associated with resistance to the individual components of **Juluca.** Pregnancy testing and contraception are recommended before initiation of **Juluca** in females of childbearing potential. Avoid use of **Juluca** at the time of conception through the first trimester due to the risk of neural tube defects.

▷ **Kaletra, Kaletra Oral Solution (C)(G)** *lopinavir+ritonavir* 800+200 mg (4 tablets or 10 ml) once daily or 400/100 (2 tablets or 5 ml) bid; *May administer once daily or bid:* patients with <3 *lopinavir* resistance-associated substitutions; *May dose bid only:* patients with ≥3 resistance-associated substitutions; *Dose must be increased:* when administered in combination with *efavirenz, nevirapine,* or *nelfinavir* (500 mg/125 mg (2 x 200/50 tab plus 1 x 100/25 tab) bid or 520/130 (6.5 ml) bid; *Once daily dosing regimen not recommended:* in combination with ≥3 *lopinavir* resistance-associated substitutions or in combination with: *carbamazepine, phenobarbital,* or *phenytoin*; Patients receiving *nevirapine* or *efavirenz* with **Kaletra** should have their **Kaletra** dose increased; swallow whole with or without food
Pediatric: dose calculation is based on the *lopinavir* component; 14 days-6 months: 16 mg/kg bid; 6 months-12 years: [tab/cap/soln] 7-<15 kg: 12 mg/kg bid (13 mg/kg plus *nevirapine*); 15-40 kg: 10 mg/kg bid (11 mg/kg plus *nevirapine*), ≥40 kg, >12 years: *lopinavir* 400 mg bid (533 mg plus *nevirapine*); max *lopinavir* 400 mg bid for patients who are not receiving *nevirapine* or *efavirenz*; **Kaletra** should not be used in combination with NNRTIs in children <6 months-of-age; see mfr pkg insert for BSA-based dosing
   Tab: **Kaletra 100/25** lopin 100 mg+riton 25 mg
      Kaletra 200/50 lopin 200 mg+riton 50 mg
   Oral Soln: lopin 80 mg+riton 20 mg per ml, lopin 400 mg+riton 500 mg per 5 ml (160 ml) (cotton candy) (alcohol 42.4%)

▷ **Odefsey (D)** *emtricitabine+rilpivirine+tenofovir alafenamide* 1 tab once daily with food; *CrCl <30 mL/min:* not recommended
Pediatric: <12 years, <35 kg: not established; ≥12 years, >35 kg: same as adult
   Tab: emtri 200 mg+rilpi 25 mg+teno alafen 25 mg

▷ **Prezcobix (C)** *darunavir+cobicistat* 1 tab once daily; *Treatment naïve and treatment experienced with no darunavir resistance-associated substitution:* 800 mg once daily plus *ritonavir* 100 mg once daily; *Treatment experienced with at least one darunavir resistance associated substitution:* 600 mg bid plus *ritonavir* 100 mg bid; take with food; *CrCl <70 mL/min:* not recommended
Pediatric: not recommended
   Tab: darun 800 mg+cobi 150 mg

▷ **Stribild (B)(G)** *elvitegravir+cobicistat+emtricitabine+tenofovir disoproxil fumarate* 1 tab once daily; *CrCl <70 mL/min*: <u>not</u> recommended; *if CrCl declines to <50 mL/min during treatment*: discontinue; *Severe hepatic impairment*: <u>not</u> recommended
Pediatric: <12 years: not recommended; ≥12 years: same as adult
  Tab: elvi 150 mg+cobi 150 mg+emtri 200 mg+teno dis fum 300 mg

▷ **Symfi** *efavirenz+lamivudine+tenofovir disoproxil fumarate* take 1 tablet once daily with <u>or</u> without food
Pediatric: <40 kg: not studied; ≥40 kg: same as adult
  Tab: efav 600 mg+lami 300 mg+teno diso fum 300 mg
Comment: **Symfi** is a complete 3-drug fixed-dose regimen for the treatment of HIV-1 infection in adults and children weighing >40 kg. It contains the same triple-combination ingredients found in **Symfi** Lo but with a 600 mg dose of *efavirenzvs* v. the 400 mg in **Symfi** Lo. Safety and effectiveness of **Symfi** as a fixed-dose tablet in pediatric patients weighing ≥40 kg have been established based on clinical studies using the individual components.

▷ **Symfi Lo** *efavirenz+lamivudine+tenofovir disoproxil fumarate* 1 tablet once daily with <u>or</u> without food
Pediatric: <35 kg: not studied; ≥35 kg: same as adult
  Tab: efav 400 mg+lami 300 mg+teno diso fum 300 mg
Comment: **Symfi Lo** is a complete three-drug fixed-dose regimen for the treatment HIV-1 infection in adults and children weighing ≥45 kg. It contains the same triple combination ingredients found in **Symfi** but with a 400 mg dose of *efavirenz* vs the 600 mg in **Symfi** Lo. Safety and effectiveness of **Symfi** as a fixed-dose tablet in pediatric patients weighing ≥40 kg have been established based on clinical studies using the individual components.

▷ **Symtuza** *darunavir+cobicistat+emtricitabine+tenofovir alafenamide* 1 tablet once daily with food
Pediatric: <18 years: not recommended; ≥18 years: same as adult
  Tab: daru 800 mg+cobic 150 mg+emtri 200 mg+tenofo alafen 10 mg
Comment: **Symtuza** is indicated as a complete regimen for the treatment of HIV infection in adults who have no prior antiretroviral treatment history <u>or</u> who are virologically suppressed (HIV-1 RNA less than 50 copies per ml) on a stable antiretroviral regimen for at least 6 months and have no known substitutions associated with resistance to *darunavir* <u>or</u> *tenofovir*. Assess serum creatinine, estimated creatinine clearance, urine glucose, and urine protein on a clinically appropriate schedule. In patients with chronic kidney disease, also assess serum phosphorus. **Symtuza** is <u>not</u> recommended in patients with estimated CrCl <30 mL/min and patients with severe hepatic impairment. **Symtuza** is <u>not</u> recommended during pregnancy due to substantially lower exposures of *darunavir* and *cobicistat* during pregnancy. Breastfeeding is <u>not</u> recommended. Co-administration of **Symtuza** with other drugs can alter the concentration of other drugs and other drugs may alter the concentrations of **Symtuza** components. Consult the mfr pkg insert prior to and during treatment for potential drug interactions.

▷ **Temixys** *lamivudine+tenofovir disoproxil fumarate* 1 tab once daily with <u>or</u> without food
Pediatric: <35 kg: not recommended; ≥35 kg: same as adult
  Tab: lami 300 mg+teno diso fum 300mg
Comment: **Temixys**, a fixed-dose combination of two nucleoside reverse transcriptase inhibitors, is indicated in combination with other antiretroviral agents. Discontinue treatment in patients who develop symptoms <u>or</u> laboratory findings suggestive of lactic acidosis <u>or</u> pronounced hepatotoxicity including severe hepatomegaly with steatosis. In patients at risk for renal dysfunction, assess estimated creatinine clearance, serum phosphorus, urine

glucose, and urine protein before initiating treatment with **Temixys** and periodically during treatment. Avoid administering **Temixys** with concurrent or recent use of nephrotoxic drugs. Healthcare providers are encouraged to register patients exposed to **Temexis** by calling the Antiretroviral Pregnancy Registry (APR) at 1-800-258-4263. Instruct mothers not to breastfeed if they are receiving **Temixys**.

▷ **Triumeq (C)(G)** *abacavir sulfate+dolutegravir+lamivudine* 1 tab once daily
   Pediatric: <12 years: not recommended; ≥12 years: same as adult
      Tab: aba 600 mg+dolu 50 mg+lami 300 mg

▷ **Trizivir (C)(G)** *abacavir sulfate+lamivudine+zidovudine* 1 tab bid
   Pediatric: <40 kg: not recommended; ≥40 kg: same as adult
      Tab: aba 300 mg+lami 150 mg+zido 300 mg

▷ **Truvada (B)(G)** *emtricitabine+tenofovir disoproxil fumarate* <17 kg: not established; *17-<22 kg:* 100/150 once daily; *22-<28 kg:* 133/200 once daily; *28-35 kg:* 167/250 once daily; *≥35 kg:* 200/300 once daily
   Pediatric: same as adult
      Tab: **Truvada 100/150** emt 100 mg+teno ala 150 mg
         Truvada 133/200 emt 133 mg+teno ala 200 mg
         Truvada 167/250 emt 167 mg+teno 250 mg
         Truvada 200/300 emt 200 mg+teno 300 mg

HUMAN PAPILLOMAVIRUS (HPV, VENEREAL WART)

Comment: Vaccination for HPV is recommended at 11-12 years-of-age, but can also be started at age 9 years. Catch-up is recommended through age 26 years. Although public health benefit is generally minimal for adults aged 27 through 45 years, shared clinical decision-making is recommended because some may benefit from the HPV vaccine Additional doses of HPV are not recommended after completing a series at the recommended dosing intervals using any HPV vaccine. The 3-dose series is recommended regardless of age of initial vaccination in immunocompromising conditions. The dose series does not need to be restarted if the vaccination schedule is interrupted. (ACIP 2021)

TREATMENT
see Wart: Venereal

PROPHYLAXIS

▷ *human papillomavirus 9-valent (types 6, 11, 16, 18, 31, 33, 45, 52, and 58) vaccine, recombinant, aluminum adsorbed* **(B)**
   Males and Females 9 to 45 Years-of-Age: administer IM in the deltoid or thigh *9-14 years (2-dose regimen):* 0.5 ml IM at 0 and 6-12 months (if the second dose is administered earlier than 5 months after the first dose, administer a third dose at least 4 months after the second dose) *9-14 years: (3-dose regimen):* administer 0.5 ml IM at 0, 2, and 6 months *15-45 years (3-dose regimen):* administer 0.5 ml IM at 0, 2, and 6 months
      Gardasil 9 *Vial:* 0.5 ml (single-dose); *Prefilled syringe w. needles or tip caps:* 0.5 ml (single-dose) (preservative-free)
   Comment: Gardasil 9 is indicated for prevention of genital warts (*condyloma acuminata*) caused by HPV types 6 and11 and prevention of cervical, vulvar, vaginal, and anal cancer caused by HPV types 16, 18, 31, 33, 45, 52, and 58. There are no adequate and well-controlled studies of **Gardasil 9** in pregnancy. Available human data do not demonstrate vaccine-associated increase in risk of major birth defects and miscarriages when **Gardasil 9** is administered during pregnancy. Register pregnant patients exposed to **Gardasil 9** by calling 1-800-986-8999. Available data are not sufficient to assess the effects of **Gardasil 9** on the breastfed infant.

HUNTINGTON DISEASE-ASSOCIATED CHOREA

VESICULAR MONOAMINE TRANSPORTER 2 (VMAT2) INHIBITOR

▷ *deutetrabenazine* take with food; initially 6 mg once daily; titrate up at weekly intervals by 6 mg per day to a tolerated dose that reduces chorea; administer total daily dosages ≥12 mg in two divided doses; max recommended daily dose 36 mg/day divided bid (18 mg twice daily); swallow whole; do not chew, crush, or break; if switching from *tetrabenazine,* discontinue *tetrabenazine* and initiate *Austedo* the following day; see mfr pkg insert for full prescribing information and for a recommended conversion table

Pediatric: <12 years: not established; ≥12 years: same as adult

    Austedo Tab: 6, 9, 12 mg

Comment: The most common adverse effects of *deutetrabenazine* are somnolence, diarrhea, dry mouth, fatigue, and sedation, as well as an increased risk of depression and suicidal thoughts and behaviors. **Austedo** is contraindicated for patients with untreated or inadequately treated depression, who are suicidal, have hepatic impairment, are taking MAOIs, *reserpine,* or *tetrabenazine.* **Austedo** may increase the risk of akathisia, agitation, and restlessness, and may cause parkinsonism in patients with Huntington disease. There are no adequate data on the developmental risk associated with the use of **Austedo** in pregnant females or lactation.

▷ *trabenazine* individualization of dose with careful weekly titration is required. *Week 1:* starting dose is 12.5 mg daily; *Week 2:* 25 mg (12.5 mg twice daily); then slowly titrate dose by 12.5 mg/day at weekly intervals as tolerated to a dose that reduces chorea; doses of 37.5 mg and up to 50 mg per day should be administered in three divided doses per day with a maximum recommended single dose not to exceed 25 mg; patients requiring doses above 50 mg per day should be genotyped for the drug metabolizing enzyme CYP2D6 to determine if the patient is a poor metabolizer (PM) or an extensive metabolizer (EM); max daily dose in PMs is 50 mg with a max single dose of 25 mg

Pediatric: <12 years: not established; ≥12 years: same as adult

    Xenazine *Tab:* 12.5, 25*mg

Comment: Most common adverse reactions are sedation/somnolence, fatigue, insomnia, depression, akathisia, anxiety/anxiety aggravated, and nausea.

BBW: **Xenazine** increases the risk of depression and suicidal thoughts and behavior (suicidality) in patients with Huntington's disease. Balance risks of depression and suicidality with the clinical need for control of chorea when considering the use of **Xenazine**. Monitor patients for the emergence or worsening of depression, suicidality, or unusual changes in behavior. Inform patients, caregivers and families of the risk of depression and suicidality and instruct to report behaviors of concern promptly to the treating healthcare provider. Exercise caution when treating patients with a history of depression or prior suicide attempts or ideation.

Xenazine is contraindicated in patients who are actively suicidal, and in patients with untreated or inadequately treated depression, hepatic impairment, concomitant an MAOI or reserpine, taking *deutetrabenazine* or *valbenazine.*

▷ *valbenazine* initially 40 mg once daily; after 1 week, increase to the recommended 80 mg once daily; take with or without food; recommended dose for patients with moderate or severe hepatic impairment is 40 mg once daily; consider dose reduction based on tolerability in known CYP2D6 poor metabolizers; concomitant use of strong CYP3A4 inducers is not recommended; avoid concomitant use of MAOIs

Pediatric: <18 years: not established; ≥18 years: same as adult

    Ingrezza *Cap:* 40 mg

Comment: Safety and effectiveness of **Ingrezza** have <u>not</u> been established in pediatric patients. No dose adjustment is required for elderly patients. The limited available data on **Ingrezza** use in pregnant females are insufficient to inform a drug-associated risk. There is no information regarding the presence of **Ingrezza** <u>or</u> its metabolites in human milk, the effects on the breastfed infant, <u>or</u> the effects on milk production. However, women are advised <u>not</u> to breastfeed during treatment and for 5 days after the final dose.

HYPERCALCEMIA

CALCIUM-SENSING RECEPTOR AGONIST

See *Hyperparathyroidism (HPT)* for *cinacalcet* dosing in adult patients with secondary hyperparathyroidism (HPT) due to chronic kidney disease CKD.

▷ *cinacalcet* (C)(G) take tabs whole; with food <u>or</u> shortly after a meal;
Hypercalcemia, including hypercalcemia in patients with primary HPT: initially 30 mg 2 x/day; titrate dose every 2 to 4 weeks through sequential doses of 30 mg 2 x/day, 60 mg 2 x/day, 90 mg 2 x/day, and 90 mg 3 <u>or</u> 4 x/day as necessary to normalize serum calcium levels; once the maintenance dose has been established, monitor serum calcium approximately every 2 months; iPTH levels should be measured no earlier than 12 hours after most recent dose
Pediatric: <18 years: not indicated; ≥18 years: same as adult
　Sensipar *Tab*: 30, 60, 90 mg
　Comment: **Sensipar** is indicated for the treatment of hypercalcemia in adult patients with parathyroid carcinoma and patients with primary HPT for whom parathyroidectomy would be indicated on the basis of serum calcium levels, but who are unable to undergo parathyroidectomy. Co-administration with a strong CYP3A4 inhibitor may increase serum levels of *cinacalcet*; dose adjustment and monitoring of iPTH serum phosphorus and serum calcium may be required. *cinacalcet* is a strong inhibitor of CYP2D6. Dose adjustments may be required for concomitant medications that are predominantly metabolized by CYP2D6. **Sensipar** has been shown to cross the placental barrier in animal studies. There are no adequate and well-controlled studies of **Sensipar** in pregnancy. **Sensipar** should be used during pregnancy only if the potential benefit justifies the potential risk to the fetus. Animal studies have shown that **Sensipar** is excreted in milk with a high milk-to-plasma ratio. It is <u>not</u> known whether **Sensipar** is excreted in human milk. Because of the potential for clinically significant adverse reactions in infants from **Sensipar**, risk/benefit should be discussed and a decision should be made whether to discontinue breastfeeding <u>or</u> to discontinue the drug. No differences in the safety and efficacy of **Sensipar** were observed in patients > <u>or</u> < than 65 years-of-age.

HYPEREMESIS GRAVIDARUM/NAUSEA AND VOMITING OF PREGNANCY

ANTIHISTAMINE+VITAMIN B ANALOG

Comment: **Bonjesta** and **Diclegis** are indicated for nausea/vomiting of pregnancy in women who do <u>not</u> respond to conservative management. Somnolence (severe drowsiness) can occur when used in combination with alcohol <u>or</u> other sedating medications. Use with caution in patients with asthma, increased intraocular pressure, narrow angle glaucoma, stenosing peptic ulcer, pyloroduodenal obstruction, and urinary bladder-neck obstruction. Concomitant monoamine oxidase inhibitors (MAOIs) are contraindicated because MAOIs prolong and intensify the anticholinergic effects of antihistamines, especially long-acting formulations. *doxylamine* is secreted in breast milk; therefore, breastfeeding is not recommended.

▷ *doxylamine* succinate+*pyridoxine* **hydrochloride** take 1 tab at HS prn; if symptoms are not adequately controlled, the dose can be increased to max 1 tablet in the AM and 1 tablet at HS
  Pediatric: <18 years: not established; ≥18 years: same as adult
    Bonjesta *Tab:* doxy 20 mg+pyri 20 mg ext-rel
    Diclegis *Tab:* doxy 10 mg+pyri 10 mg ext-rel

HYPERHIDROSIS (PERSPIRATION, EXCESSIVE)

Comment: Hyperhidrosis is a common, self-limiting problem that affects 2% to3% of the US population. Patients may complain of localized sweating of the hands, feet, face, or underarms, or more systemic, generalized sweating in multiple locations and report a significant impact on their quality of life.

REFERENCE
Varella, A. Y., Fukuda, J. M., Telvelis, M. P., Campos, J. R., Kauffman, P., Cucato, G. G., . . . Wolosker, N. (2016). Translation and validation of hyperhidrosis disease severity scale. *Revista da Associação Médica Brasileira*, 62(9), 843–847. doi:10.1590/1806-9282.62.09.843

▷ *aluminum chloride* 20% solution apply q HS; wash treated area the following morning; after 1-2 treatments, may reduce frequency to 1-2 x/week
    Drysol *Soln:* 35, 60 ml (alcohol 93%) cont-rel
  Comment: Apply to clean dry skin (e.g., underarms). Do not apply to broken, irritated, or recently shaved skin.

TOPICAL ANTICHOLINERGIC

▷ *glycopyrronium* unfold one **Qbrexza** cloth and apply by wiping across one entire underarm one time; using the same cloth, wipe across the other under arm one time; discard used cloth; wash hands immediately; repeat once every 24 hours
  Pediatric: <9 years: not recommended; ≥9 years:
    Qbrexza Pre-moistened cloth (single-use pouche)
    Comment: **Qbrexza** (*glycopyrronium*) is the first FDA-approved, once-daily, topical treatment indicated for patients ≥9 years-of-age with primary axillary hyperhidrosis. *glycopyrronium* is anticholinergic; it is important to wash hands after **Qbrexza** cloths are used because it can cause blurred vision if the eyes are touched. Do not re-use **Qbrexza** cloths. **Qbrexza** is flammable. Avoid heat and flame while applying **Qbrexza**. **Qbrexza** is contraindicated in patients with medical conditions that can be exacerbated by the anticholinergic effect of *glycopyrronium* (e.g., glaucoma, paralytic ileus, unstable cardiovascular status in acute hemorrhage, severe ulcerative colitis, toxic megacolon complicating ulcerative colitis, myasthenia gravis, and Sjogren's syndrome). The most common adverse reactions (incidence ≥2%) have been dry mouth (24.2%), mydriasis (6.8%), oropharyngeal pain (5.7%), headache (5.0%), urinary hesitation (3.5%), vision blurred (3.5%), nasal dryness (2.6%), dry throat (2.6%), dry eye (2.4%), dry skin (2.2%) and constipation (2.0%). Local skin reactions, including erythema (17.0%), burning/stinging (14.1%), and pruritus (8.1%). Co-administration of Qbrexza with anticholinergic medications may result in additive interaction; therefore, avoid co-administration of **Qbrexza** with other anticholinergic drugs. There are no available data on Qbrexza use in pregnancy to inform a drug-associated risk for adverse developmental outcomes. There are no data on the presence of *glycopyrrolate* or its metabolites in human milk or effects on the breastfed infant.

ORAL ANTICHOLINERGIC

Comment: *Oxybutynin*, a cholinergic antagonist commonly prescribed for overactive bladder, is the first oral agent to emerge as a treatment option for hyperhidrosis.

▷ *oxybutynin chloride* (B)(G)

Ditropan 5 mg bid-tid; max 20 mg/day
Pediatric: <5 years: not recommended; 5-12 years: 5 mg bid; max 15 mg/day; ≥16 years: same as adult
   Tab: 5*mg; *Syr:* 5 mg/5 ml
Ditropan XL initially 5 mg daily; may increase weekly in 5-mg increments as needed; max 30 mg/day
Pediatric: <6 years: not recommended; ≥6 years: initially 5 mg once daily; may increase weekly in 5-mg increments as needed; max 20 mg/day
   Tab: 5, 10, 15 mg ext-rel
GelniQUE 3 mg Pump: apply 3 pumps (84 mg) once daily to clean dry intact skin on the abdomen, upper arm, shoulders, or thighs; rotate sites; wash hands; avoid washing application site for 1 hour after application
Pediatric: <12 years: not recommended; ≥12 years: same as adult
   Gel: 3% (92 gm, metered pump dispenser) (alcohol)
GelniQUE 1 gm Sachet: apply 1 gm gel (1 sachet) once daily to dry intact skin on abdomen, upper arms/shoulders, or thighs; rotate sites; wash hands; avoid washing application site for 1 hour after application
Pediatric: <12 years: not recommended; ≥12 years: same as adult
   Gel: 10%, 1 gm/sachet (30/carton) (alcohol)
Oxytrol Transdermal Patch (OTC): apply patch to clean dry area of the abdomen, hip, or buttock; one patch twice weekly; rotate sites
Pediatric: <12 years: not recommended; ≥12 years: same as adult
   Transdermal patch: 3.9 mg/day

▷ *etelcalcetide Starting Dose:* 5 mg via IV bolus 3 x/week at the end of hemodialysis treatment; *Maintenance Dose:* individualized, determined by titration, based on parathyroid hormone (PTH) and corrected serum calcium response; *Dose Range:* is 2.5 to 15 mg 3 x/week; dose may be increased in 2.5 mg or 5 mg increments no more frequently than every 4 weeks; ensure corrected serum calcium is at or above the lower limit of normal prior to initiation, dose increase, or re-initiation; do not mix or dilute prior to administration; administer via IV bolus injection into the venous line of the dialysis circuit after hemodialysis, during rinse back or after rinse back; administer a sufficient volume of saline (e.g., 150 ml of rinse back) after injection into the dialysis tubing; if administered after rinse back, administer intravenously followed by at least 10 ml of saline flush
Parsabiv *Vial:* 2.5 mg/0.5 ml, 5 mg/ml, 10 mg/2 ml soln, single-dose
Comment: **Parsabiv** *(etelcalcetide)* is indicated for secondary hyperparathyroidism (HPT) in adult patients with chronic kidney disease (CKD) on hemodialysis. Parsabiv has not been studied in adult patients with parathyroid carcinoma, primary hyperparathyroidism, or with CKD who are not on hemodialysis and is not recommended for use in these populations. Measure serum calcium within 1 week after initiation or dose adjustment and every 4 weeks for maintenance. Measure PTH after 4 weeks from initiation or dose adjustment. Decrease or temporarily discontinue **Parsabiv** in individuals with PTH levels below the target range. Consider decreasing or temporarily discontinuing **Parsabiv** or use concomitant therapies to increase corrected serum calcium in patients with a corrected serum calcium below the lower limit of normal but at or above 7.5 mg/dL without symptoms of hypocalcemia. Stop **Parsabiv** and treat hypocalcemia if the corrected serum calcium falls below 7.5 mg/dL or patients report symptoms of hypocalcemia. The most common

adverse reactions (incidence ≥ 5%) have been decreased serum calcium, muscle spasms, diarrhea, nausea, vomiting, headache, hypocalcemia, and paresthesia. Hypocalcemia may sometimes be severe and severe hypocalcemia can cause paresthesias, myalgias, muscle spasms, seizures, QT prolongation, and ventricular arrhythmias. Patients predisposed to QT interval prolongation, ventricular arrhythmias, and seizures may be at increased risk and require close monitoring. Educate patients on the symptoms of hypocalcemia and advise them to contact an HCP if they occur. Reductions in corrected serum calcium may be associated with CHF; however, a causal relationship to **Parsabiv** could not be completely excluded. Closely monitor patients for worsening signs and symptoms of HF. Patients with risk factors for upper GI bleeding may be at increased risk. Monitor patients and promptly evaluate and treat any suspected GI bleeding. Adynamic bone may develop if PTH levels are chronically suppressed. If PTH levels decrease below the recommended target range, the dose of **Parsabiv** should be reduced or discontinued. **Parsabiv** is not recommended when breastfeeding.

HYPERHOMOCYSTEINEMIA

Comment: Elevated homocysteine is associated with cognitive impairment, vascular dementia, and dementia of the Alzheimer's type.

HOMOCYSTEINE-LOWERING NUTRITIONAL SUPPLEMENTS

▷ *L-methylfolate calcium (as metafolin)+pyridoxyl 5-phosphate+methylcobalamin* take 1 cap daily
   Pediatric: <12 years: not recommended; ≥12 years: same as adult
   Metanx *Cap:* metafo 3 mg+pyrid 35 mg+methyl 2 mg (gluten-free, yeast-free, lactose-free)
   Comment: **Metanx** is indicated as adjunct treatment of endothelial dysfunction and/or hyperhomocysteinemia in patients who have lower extremity ulceration.

▷ *L-methylfolate calcium (as metafolin)+methylcobalamin+n-acetylcysteine* take 1 cap daily
   Pediatric: <12 years: not recommended; ≥12 years: same as adult
   Cerefolin *Cap:* metafo 5.6 mg+methyl 2 mg+N-ace 600 mg (gluten-free, yeast-free, lactose-free)
   Comment: **Cerefolin** is indicated in the dietary management of patients treated for early memory loss, with emphasis on those at risk for neurovascular oxidative stress, hyperhomocysteinemia, mild-to-moderate cognitive impairment with or without vitamin B12 deficiency, vascular dementia, or Alzheimer's disease.

HYPERKALEMIA

POTASSIUM BINDERS

Comment: Normal serum K+ range is approximately 3.5-5.5 mEq/L. Hyperkalemia is associated with cardiac dysrhythmias and metabolic acidosis. Risk factors include kidney disease, heart failure, and drugs that inhibit the renin-angiotensin-aldosterone system (RAAS), including ACEIs, ARBs, direct renin inhibitors, and aldosterone antagonists. Cation exchange resins are not for emergency treatment of life-threatening hyperkalemia, severe constipation, and bowel obstruction or impaction. May cause GI irritability, ulceration, necrosis, sodium retention, hypocalcemia, hypomagnesemia, fecal impaction, and ischemic colitis. Avoid non-absorbable cation-donating antacids and laxatives (e.g., *magnesium hydroxide, aluminum hydroxide*). Concomitant sorbitol should be avoided because it may cause intestinal necrosis.

▷ *patiromer sorbitex calcium* (B) initially 8.4 gm once daily; adjust dosage as prescribed based on potassium concentration and target range; may increase dosage at 1-week (or longer) intervals in increments of 8.4 gm; max dose 25.2 gm once daily; prepare immediately prior to administration; do not take in dry form; administer with food; measure 1/3 cup of water and pour half into a glass; then add **Veltassa** and stir; add the remaining water and stir well; the powder will not dissolve and the mixture will look cloudy; add more water as needed for desired consistency; take with or without food; do not heat or mix with heated food or fluids; take other oral drugs at least 6 hours before or 6 hours after taking **Veltassa**
Pediatric: <18 years: not recommended; ≥18 years: same as adult

Veltassa *Pkt:* 8, 4, 16.8, 25.2 gm pwdr for oral susp, 30 single-use pkts/carton
Comment: Store packets in the refrigerator. If stored at room temperature, product must be used within 3 months.

▷ *sodium polystyrene sulfonate* (C)(G) *Oral:* average total daily adult dose is 15-60 gm, administered as a 15 gm dose (4 level teaspoons), 1-4 x/day; *Rectal:* average adult dose is 30-50 gm every 6 hours
Pediatrics: Use 1 gm/1 mEq of K+ as basis of calculation; in pediatric patients, as in adults, **Kayexalate** is expected to bind potassium at the practical exchange ratio of 1mEq potassium per 1 gm of resin; in neonates, **Kayexalate** should not be given by the oral route; in both children and neonates, excessive dosage or inadequate dilution could result in impaction of the resin; premature infants or low birth weight infants may have an increased risk for gastrointestinal adverse effects

Kayexalate *Jar:* 1 lb (453.6 gm) pwdr for dilution
Comment: **Kayexalate** should not be used an emergency treatment for life-threatening hyperkalemia because of its delayed onset of action. Contraindications are hypersensitivity to polystyrene sulfonate resins, obstructive bowel disease, and neonates with reduced gut motility. Take other orally administered drugs at least 3 hours before or 3 hours after **Kayexalate**. Cation-donating antacids may reduce the resin's potassium exchange capability and increase risk of systemic alkalosis. Concomitant use of sorbitol may contribute to the risk of intestinal necrosis and is not recommended. **Kayexalate** is not absorbed systemically so breastfeeding is not expected to result in risk to the infant.

▷ *sodium zirconium cyclosilicate* *Starting dose:* 10 gm administered 3 x/day for up to 48 hours; *Maintenance treatment:* 10 gm once daily; adjust dose at 1-week intervals by 5 gm daily, as needed, to obtain desired serum potassium target range; in general, other oral medications should be administered at least 2 hours before or 2 hours after a **Lokelma** dose
Pediatric: <18 years: not established; >18 years: same as adult

Lokelma for Oral Suspension *Pwdr for oral susp:* 5, 10 gm/pkt (30 pkts/box)
Comment: **Lokelma** (*sodium zirconium cyclosilicate*) is a potassium binder. ≥18 years-of-age. *In vitro*, **Lokelma** has a high affinity for potassium ions, even in the presence of other cations such as calcium and magnesium. **Lokelma** increases fecal potassium excretion through binding of potassium in the lumen of the GI tract. **Lokelma** should not be used as an emergency treatment for life-threatening hyperkalemia because of its delayed onset of action. The most common adverse reaction with **Lokelma** is mild-to-moderate edema. Patients with motility disorders may experience gastrointestinal adverse reactions. As **Lokelma** is not absorbed systemically, maternal use is not expected to result in fetal exposure and breastfeeding is not expected to result in infant exposure.

HYPERPARATHYROIDISM (HPT)

▷ *calcifediol* (C)(G) 1 cap daily
    Pediatric: <18 years: not established; ≥18 years: same as adult
        Rayaldee *Cap:* 30 mcg ext-rel
        Comment: **Rayaldee** is indicated for the prevention and treatment of
        secondary hyperparathyroidism associated with chronic kidney disease
        (CKD), stage 3 or 4 and serum total 25-hydroxyvitamin D levels <30 mg/mL.
▷ *paricalcitol* (C)(G) administer 0.04-1 mcg/kg (2.8-7 mcg) IV bolus, during
    dialysis, no more than every other day; may be increased by 2-4 mcg every
    2-4 weeks; monitor serum calcium and phosphorus during dose adjustment
    periods; if Ca x P ≥75, immediately reduce dose or discontinue until these levels
    normalize; discard unused portion of single-use vials immediately
    Pediatric: <18 years: not established; ≥18 years: same as adult
        Zemplar *Vial:* 2, 5 mcg/ml soln for inj
        Comment: **Zemplar** is indicated for the prevention and treatment of
        secondary hyperparathyroidism associated with chronic kidney disease
        (CKD), stage 5.

CALCIUM-SENSING RECEPTOR AGONIST

▷ *cinacalcet* (C) *Initial Dose:* 30 mg bid; titrate every 2 to 4 weeks through
    sequential doses of 30 mg bid, then 60 mg bid, then 90 mg bid, then 90 mg tid-
    qid as needed to normalize serum calcium levels; swallow whole, do not break;
    take with food or shortly after a meal; *Maintenance:* serum calcium and serum
    phosphorus should be measured approximately monthly, and PTH every 1 to 3
    months
        Sensipar Tab 30, 60, 90 mg
        Comment: **Sensipar** (*cinacalet*) is indicated (1) for the treatment of
        hypercalcemia in adult patients with primary hyperparathyroidism (pHPT)
        for whom parathyroidectomy would be indicated on the basis of serum
        calcium levels, but who are unable to undergo parathyroidectomy, (2) for
        the treatment of secondary hyperparathyroidism in patients with Chronic
        Kidney Disease (CKD) on dialysis (see *Hypercalcemia*), and (3) for the
        treatment of hypercalcemia in patients with parathyroid carcinoma. **Sensipar**
        can be used as monotherapy or in combination with vitamin D sterols and/
        or phosphate binders. Secondary hyperparathyroidism (sHPT) in patients
        with chronic kidney disease (CKD) is a progressive disease, associated
        with increases in parathyroid hormone (PTH) levels and derangements in
        calcium and phosphorus metabolism. Increased PTH stimulates osteoclastic
        activity resulting in cortical bone resorption and marrow fibrosis. The goals
        of treatment of secondary hyperparathyroidism are to lower levels of PTH,
        calcium, and phosphorus in the blood, in order to prevent progressive bone
        disease and the systemic consequences of disordered mineral metabolism.
        In CKD patients on dialysis with uncontrolled secondary HPT, reductions
        in PTH are associated with a favorable impact on bone-specific alkaline
        phosphatase (BALP), bone turnover and bone fibrosis. The calcium-sensing
        receptor on the surface of the chief cell of the parathyroid gland is the
        principal regulator of PTH secretion. **Sensipar** directly lowers PTH levels
        by increasing the sensitivity of the calcium-sensing receptor to extracellular
        calcium. The reduction in PTH is associated with a concomitant decrease in
        serum calcium levels. Patients should be aware of potential manifestations
        of hypocalcemia, including paresthesias, myalgias, cramping, tetany, and
        convulsions. **Sensipar** treatment should not be initiated if serum calcium is
        less than the lower limit of the normal range (8.4 mg/dL). Serum calcium
        should be measured within 1 week after any **Sensipar** dose adjustment. If

serum calcium falls below 8.4 mg/dL but remains above 7.5 mg/dL, or if symptoms of hypocalcemia occur, calcium-containing phosphate binders and/or vitamin D sterols can be used to raise serum calcium. If serum calcium falls below 7.5 mg/dL, or if symptoms of hypocalcemia persist and the dose of vitamin D cannot be increased, withhold administration of **Sensipar** until serum calcium levels reach 8.0 mg/dL, and/or symptoms of hypocalcemia have resolved. Treatment should be re-initiated using the next lowest dose of **Sensipar**. Adynamic bone disease may develop if iPTH levels are suppressed below 100 pg/mL. **Sensipar** is metabolized in part by the enzyme CYP3A4. Co-administration of *ketoconazole*, a strong inhibitor of CYP3A4, can cause an approximate 2-fold increase in *cinacalcet* exposure. Dose adjustment of **Sensipar** may be required and PTH and serum calcium concentrations should be closely monitored if a patient initiates or discontinues therapy with a strong CYP3A4 inhibitor (e.g., *ketoconazole, erythromycin, itraconazole*). Patients with congenital long QT syndrome, history of QT interval prolongation, family history of long QT syndrome or sudden cardiac death, and other conditions that predispose to QT interval prolongation and ventricular arrhythmia may be at increased risk for QT interval prolongation and ventricular arrhythmias if they develop hypocalcemia due to **Sensipar**. Closely monitor corrected serum calcium and QT interval in patients at risk receiving **Sensipar**. Seizure threshold is lowered by significant reductions in serum calcium levels. Monitor patients with seizure disorders receiving **Sensipar**. Patients with risk factors for upper GI bleeding (e.g., known gastritis, esophagitis, ulcers, or severe vomiting) may be at increased risk for GI bleeding when receiving **Sensipar** treatment. In postmarketing safety surveillance, isolated, idiosyncratic cases of hypotension, worsening heart failure, and/or arrhythmia have been reported in patients with impaired cardiac function.

▷ *etelcalcetide* Starting Dose: 5 mg via IV bolus 3 x/week at the end of hemodialysis treatment; *Maintenance Dose:* individualized, determined by titration, based on parathyroid hormone (PTH) and corrected serum calcium response; *Dose Range:* is 2.5 to 15 mg 3 x/week; dose may be increased in 2.5 mg or 5 mg increments no more frequently than every 4 weeks; ensure corrected serum calcium is at or above the lower limit of normal prior to initiation, dose increase, or re-initiation; do not mix or dilute prior to administration; administer via IV bolus injection into the venous line of the dialysis circuit after hemodialysis, during rinse back or after rinse back; administer a sufficient volume of saline (e.g., 150 ml of rinse back) after injection into the dialysis tubing; if administered after rinse back, administer intravenously followed by atleast 10 ml of saline flush

Parsabiv *Vial:* 2.5 mg/0.5 ml, 5 mg/ml, 10 mg/2 ml soln, single-dose

Comment: **Parsabiv** *(etelcalcetide)* is indicated for secondary hyperparathyroidism (HPT) in adult patients with chronic kidney disease (CKD) on hemodialysis. **Parsabiv** has not been studied in adult patients with parathyroid carcinoma, primary hyperparathyroidism, or with CKD who are not on hemodialysis and is not recommended for use in these populations. Measure serum calcium within 1 week after initiation or dose adjustment and every 4 weeks for maintenance. Measure PTH after 4 weeks from initiation or dose adjustment. Decrease or temporarily discontinue **Parsabiv** in individuals with PTH levels below the target range. Consider decreasing or temporarily discontinuing **Parsabiv** or use concomitant therapies to increase corrected serum calcium in patients with a corrected serum calcium below the lower limit of normal but at or above 7.5 mg/dL without symptoms of hypocalcemia. Stop **Parsabiv** and treat hypocalcemia if the corrected serum calcium falls below 7.5 mg/dL or patients report symptoms of hypocalcemia. The most common adverse reactions (incidence ≥ 5%) have been decreased serum calcium, muscle spasms, diarrhea, nausea, vomiting, headache, hypocalcemia, and paresthesia. Hypocalcemia may sometimes be severe and severe hypocalcemia can cause paresthesias, myalgias, muscle spasms, seizures, QT prolongation, and ventricular arrhythmias. Patients predisposed to QT interval prolongation, ventricular arrhythmias, and seizures may be at increased risk and require close monitoring. Educate patients on the symptoms of hypocalcemia and advise them to contact an HCP if they occur. Reductions in corrected serum calcium may be associated with CHF; however, a causal relationship to **Parsabiv** could not be completely excluded. Closely monitor patients for worsening signs and symptoms of HF. Patients with risk factors for upper GI bleeding may be at increased risk. Monitor patients and promptly evaluate and treat any suspected GI bleeding. Adynamic bone may develop if PTH levels are chronically suppressed. If PTH levels decrease below the recommended target range, the dose of **Parsabiv** should be reduced or discontinued. **Parsabiv** is <u>not</u> recommended when breastfeeding.

HYPERPHOSPHATEMIA

FERRIC CITRATE

▶ **ferric citrate** *Hyperphosphatemia in Chronic Kidney Disease on Dialysis:* starting dose is 2 tabs orally 3 x/day with meals; adjust dose by 1 to 2 tabs as needed to maintain serum phosphorus at target levels, up to max 12 tabs/day; dose can be titrated at 1 week <u>or</u> longer intervals; *Iron Deficiency Anemia in Chronic Kidney Disease <u>Not</u> on Dialysis:* starting dose is 1 tablet 3 x/day with meals; adjust dose as needed to achieve and maintain hemoglobin goal, up to max 12 tabs/day *Pediatric:* <18 years: not recommended; ≥18 years: same as adult

Aurexia *Tab:* 210 mg *ferric iron* (equivalent to 1 gm *ferric citrate*)
Comment: Auryxia is a phosphate binder indicated for the control of serum phosphorus levels in patients ≥18 years-of-age with chronic kidney disease (CKD) on dialysis. Ferric iron binds dietary phosphate in the GI tract and precipitates as ferric phosphate. This compound is insoluble and is excreted in the stool. **Auryxia** is also an iron replacement product indicated for the treatment of iron deficiency anemia in patients >18 years-of-age with chronic kidney (CKD) <u>not</u> on dialysis. Ferric iron is reduced from the ferric to the ferrous form by ferric reductase in the GI tract. After transport through the enterocytes into the blood, oxidized ferric iron circulates bound to the plasma protein transferrin, for incorporation into hemoglobin. **Auryxia** is contraindicated in iron overload syndromes (e.g., hemochromatosis). Monitor ferritin and TSAT. When clinically significant drug interactions are expected, consider separation of the timing of administration. Consider monitoring clinical responses <u>or</u> blood levels of the concomitant medication. The most common adverse reactions (incidence ≥5%) are discolored feces, diarrhea, constipation, nausea, vomiting, cough, abdominal pain, and hyperkalemia. There are no available data on **Auryxia** use in pregnancy to inform a drug-associated risk of major birth defects and miscarriage; however, an overdose of iron may carry a risk for spontaneous abortion, gestational diabetes and fetal malformation. There are no human data regarding effects of **Auryxia** on the breastfed infant. Accidental overdose of iron-containing products is a leading cause of fatal poisoning in children under 6 years-of-age. Keep this product out of reach of children. In case of accidental overdose, contact poison control center immediately and transfer to emergency care.

PHOSPHATE BINDERS

Comment: Monitor for development of hypercalcemia. Normal serum PO4⁻ is 2.5 to 4.5 mg/dL and normal serum calcium is 8.5-10.5 mg/dL.

▷ *calcium acetate* (C)(G) initially 2 tabs or caps with each meal; then titrate gradually to keep serum phosphate at <6 mg/dL; usual maintenance is 3-4 tabs or caps with each meal

Pediatric: <12 years: not recommended; ≥12 years: same as adult

PhosLo *Tab:* 667 mg; *Cap:* 667 mg

▷ *lanthanum carbonate* (C)(G) initially 750 mg to 1.5 gm per day in divided doses; take with meals; titrate at 2-3-week intervals in increments of 750 mg/day based on serum phosphate; usual range 1.5-3 gm/day; usual max 3750 mg/day

Pediatric: <12 years: not recommended; ≥12 years: same as adult

Fosrenol *Chew tab:* 250, 500, 750 mg; 1 gm

▷ *sevelamer* (C)(G) for patients not taking a phosphate binder, take tid with meals; swallow whole; titrate by 1 tab per meal at 1-week intervals to keep serum phosphorus 3.5-5.5 mg/dL; switching from calcium acetate to *sevelamer*, see mfr pkg insert. *Serum phosphorus* ≥5.5 to ≤7.5 mg/dL: 800 mg tid; *Serum phosphorus* 7.5 to 9: 1.2 to 1.6 gm tid

Pediatric: <12 years: not recommended; ≥12 years: same as adult

Renagel *Tab:* 400, 800 mg

Renvela *Tab:* 800 mg

HYPERPIGMENTATION

Comment: Depigmenting agents may be used for hyperpigmented skin conditions, including chloasma, melasma, freckles, and senile lentigines. Limit treatments to small areas at one time. Sunscreen ≥30 SPF recommended.

▷ *hydroquinone* (C)(G) apply sparingly to affected area and rub in bid

Lustra *Crm:* 4% (1, 2 oz) (sulfites)

Lustra AF *Crm:* 4% (1, 2 oz) (sunscreen, sulfites)

▷ *monobenzone* (C) apply sparingly to affected area and rub in bid-tid; depigmentation occurs in 1-4 months

Benoquin *Crm:* 20% (1.25 oz)

▷ *tazarotene* (X)(G) apply daily at HS

Pediatric: <12 years: not recommended; ≥12 years: same as adult

Avage Cream *Crm:* 0.1% (30 gm)

Tazorac Cream *Crm:* 0.05, 0.1% (15, 30, 60 gm)

Tazorac Gel *Gel:* 0.05, 0.1% (30, 100 gm)

▷ *tretinoin* (C) apply daily at HS

Pediatric: <12 years: not recommended; ≥12 years: same as adult

Avita *Crm/Gel:* 0.025% (20, 45 gm)

Renova *Crm:* 0.02% (40 gm); 0.05% (40, 60 gm)

Retin-A Cream *Crm:* 0.025, 0.05, 0.1% (20, 45 gm)

Retin-A Gel *Gel:* 0.01, 0.025% (15, 45 gm) (alcohol 90%)

Retin-A Liquid *Liq:* 0.05% (28 ml) (alcohol 55%)

Retin-A Micro *Microspheres:* 0.04, 0.1% (20, 45 gm)

COMBINATION AGENTS

▷ *hydroquinone+fluocinolone+tretinoin* (C) apply sparingly to affected area and rub in daily at HS

Pediatric: <12 years: not recommended; ≥12 years: same as adult

Tri-Luma *Crm:* hydroquin 4%+fluo 0.01%+tretin 0.05% (30 gm) (parabens, sulfites)

▷ *hydroquinone+padimate o+oxybenzone+octyl methoxcinnamate* (C) apply
sparingly to affected area and rub in bid
Pediatric: <12 years: not recommended; ≥16 years: same as adult
   Glyquin *Crm:* 4% (1 oz jar)
▷ *hydroquinone+ethyl dihydroxypropyl PABA+dioxybenzone+oxybenzone* (C) apply
sparingly to affected area and rub in bid; max 2 months
Pediatric: <12 years: not recommended; ≥12 years: same as adult
   Solaquin *Crm:* hydroquin 2%+PABA 5%+dioxy 3%+oxy 2% (1 oz) (sulfites)
▷ *hydroquinone+padimate+dioxybenzone+oxybenzone* (C) apply sparingly to
affected area and rub in bid; max 2 months
Pediatric: <12 years: not recommended; ≥12 years: same as adult
   Solaquin Forte *Crm:* hydroquin 4%+pad 0.5%+dioxy 3%+oxy 2% (1oz) (sunscreen,
   sulfites)
▷ *hydroquinone+padimate+dioxybenzone* (C) apply sparingly to affected area and
rub in bid; max 2 months
Pediatric: <12 years: not recommended; ≥12 years: same as adult
   Solaquin Forte Gel: hydroquin 4%+pad 0.5%+dioxy 3% (1 oz) (alcohol,
   sulfites)

 HYPERPROLACTINEMIA

DOPAMINE RECEPTOR AGONIST

▷ *dostinex* (B)(G) initial therapy is 0.25 mg twice a week; may increase by 0.25 mg
twice weekly up to 1 mg twice a week according to the patient's serum prolactin
level; dose increases should <u>not</u> occur more than every 4 weeks; after a normal
serum prolactin level has been maintained for 6 months, may be discontinued,
with periodic monitoring of serum prolactin level to determine if/when
treatment should be reinstituted
Pediatric: <12 years: not established; ≥12 years: same as adult
   Cabergoline *Tab:* 0.5 mg
   Comment: **Cabergoline** is indicated to treat hyperprolactinemia disorders due
   to idiopathic <u>or</u> pituitary adenoma.

 HYPERTENSION: PRIMARY, ESSENTIAL

see JNC-8 Recommendations

BETA-BLOCKERS (CARDIOSELECTIVE)

Comment: Cardioselective beta-blockers are less likely to cause bronchospasm,
peripheral vasoconstriction, <u>or</u> hypoglycemia than non-cardioselective beta-blockers.
▷ *acebutolol* (B)(G) initially 400 mg in 1-2 divided doses; usual range 200-800 mg/
day; max 1.2 gm/day in 2 divided doses
Pediatric: <12 years: not recommended; ≥12 years: same as adult
   Sectral *Cap:* 200, 400 mg
▷ *atenolol* (D)(G) initially 50 mg daily; may increase after 1-2 weeks to 100 mg
daily; max 100 mg/day
Pediatric: <12 years: not recommended; ≥12 years: same as adult
   Tenormin *Tab:* 25, 50, 100 mg
▷ *betaxolol* (C) initially 10 mg daily; may increase to 20 mg/day after 7-14 days;
usual max 20 mg/day
Pediatric: <12 years: not recommended; ≥12 years: same as adult
   Kerlone *Tab:* 10*, 20 mg
▷ *bisoprolol* (C) 5 mg daily; max 20 mg daily
Pediatric: <12 years: not recommended; ≥12 years: same as adult
   Zebeta *Tab:* 5*, 10 mg

▷ *metoprolol succinate* (C)
    Pediatric: <12 years: not recommended; ≥12 years: same as adult
        Toprol-XL initially 25-100 mg in a single dose once daily; increase weekly if needed; max 400 mg/day; as monotherapy or with a diuretic
            Tab: 25*, 50*, 100*, 200*mg ext-rel
▷ *metoprolol tartrate* (C) initially 25-50 mg bid; increase weekly if needed; max 400 mg/day; as monotherapy or with a diuretic
    Pediatric: <12 years: not recommended; ≥12 years: same as adult
        Lopressor (G) *Tab:* 25, 37.5, 50, 75, 100 mg
▷ *nebivolol* (C)(G) initially 5 mg once daily; may increase at 2 week intervals; max 40 mg/day
    Pediatric: <12 years: not recommended; ≥12 years: same as adult
        Bystolic *Tab:* 2.5, 5, 10, 20 mg

BETA-BLOCKERS (NON-CARDIOSELECTIVE)

Comment: Non-cardioselective beta-blockers are more likely to cause bronchospasm, peripheral vasoconstriction, and/or hypoglycemia than cardioselective beta-blockers.
▷ *nadolol* (C)(G) initially 40 mg daily; usual maintenance 40-80 mg daily; max 320 mg/day
    Pediatric: <12 years: not recommended; ≥12 years: same as adult
        Corgard *Tab:* 20*, 40*, 80*, 120*, 160*mg
▷ *penbutolol* (C) 10-20 mg once daily
    Pediatric: <12 years: not recommended; ≥12 years: same as adult
        Levatol *Tab:* 20*mg
▷ *pindolol* (B)(G) initially 5 mg bid; may increase after 3-4 weeks in 10 mg increments; max 60 mg/day
    Pediatric: <12 years: not recommended; ≥12 years: same as adult
        Pindolol *Tab:* 5, 10 mg
        Visken *Tab:* 5, 10 mg
▷ *propranolol* (C)(G)
        Inderal initially 40 mg bid; usual maintenance 120-240 mg/day; max 640 mg/day
    Pediatric: initially 1 mg/kg/day; usual range 2-4 mg/kg/day in 2 divided doses; max 16 mg/kg/day
            Tab: 10*, 20*, 40*, 60*, 80*mg
        Inderal LA initially 80 mg daily in a single dose; increase q 3-7 days; usual range 120-160 mg/day; max 320 mg/day in a single dose
    Pediatric: <12 years: not recommended; ≥12 years: same as adult
        Cap: 60, 80, 120, 160 mg sust-rel
        InnoPran XL initially 80 mg q HS; max 120 mg/day
    Pediatric: <12 years: not recommended; ≥12 years: same as adult
        Cap: 80, 120 mg ext-rel
▷ *timolol* (C)(G) initially 10 mg bid, increase weekly if needed; usual maintenance 20-40 mg/day; max 60 mg/day in 2 divided doses
    Pediatric: <12 years: not recommended; ≥12 years: same as adult
        Blocadren *Tab:* 5, 10*, 20*mg

BETA-BLOCKER (NON-CARDIOSELECTIVE)+ALPHA-1 BLOCKER COMBINATIONS

▷ *carvedilol* (C)(G)
    Pediatric: <12 years: not recommended; ≥12 years: same as adult
        Coreg initially 6.25 mg bid; may increase at 1-2-week intervals to 12.5 mg bid; max 25 mg bid
            Tab: 3.125, 6.25, 12.5, 25 mg

Coreg CR initially 20 mg once daily for 2 weeks; may increase at 1-2-week intervals; max 80 mg once daily
Tab: 10, 20, 40, 80 mg cont-rel

▷ *carteolol* (C) initially 2.5 mg daily, gradually increase to 5 or 10 mg once daily; usual maintenance 2.5-5 mg once daily
Pediatric: <12 years: not recommended; ≥12 years: same as adult
Cartrol *Tab:* 2.5, 5 mg

▷ *labetalol* (C)(G) initially 100 mg bid; increase after 2-3 days if needed; usual maintenance 200-400 mg bid; max 2.4 gm/day
Pediatric: <12 years: not recommended; ≥12 years: same as adult
Normodyne *Tab:* 100*, 200*, 300 mg
Trandate *Tab:* 100*, 200*, 300*mg

DIURETICS

Thiazide Diuretics

▷ *chlorthalidone* (B)(G) initially 15 mg daily; may increase to 30 mg once daily based on clinical response; max 45-60 mg/day
Pediatric: <12 years: not established; ≥12 years: same as adult
Chlorthalidone *Tab:* 25, 50 mg
Thalitone *Tab:* 15 mg

▷ *chlorothiazide* (B)(G) 0.5-1 gm/day in a single or divided doses; max 2 gm/day
Pediatric: <6 months: up to 15 mg/lb/day in 2 divided doses; ≥6 months: 10 mg/lb/day in 2 divided doses
Diuril *Tab:* 250*, 500*mg; *Oral susp:* 250 mg/5 ml (237 ml)

▷ *hydrochlorothiazide* (B)(G)
Pediatric: <12 years: not recommended; ≥12 years: same as adult
Esidrix 25-100 mg once daily
Tab: 25, 50, 100 mg
Hydrochlorothiazide 12.5 mg once daily; usual max 50 mg/day
Tab: 25*, 50*mg
Microzide 12.5 mg once daily; usual max 50 mg/day
Cap: 12.5 mg

▷ *methyclothiazide+deserpidine* (B) initially 5/0.25 mg once daily; titrate individual components
Pediatric: <12 years: not recommended; ≥12 years: same as adult
Enduronyl *Tab:* methy 5 mg+deser 0.25 mg*
Enduronyl Forte *Tab:* methy 5 mg+deser 0.5 mg*

▷ *polythiazide* (C) 2-4 mg once daily
Pediatric: <12 years: not recommended; ≥12 years: same as adult
Renese *Tab:* 1, 2, 4 mg

Potassium-Sparing Diuretics

▷ *amiloride* (B)(C) initially 5 mg; may increase to 10 mg; max 20 mg
Pediatric: <12 years: not recommended; ≥12 years: same as adult
Midamor *Tab:* 5 mg

▷ *spironolactone* (D)(G) initially 50-100 mg in a single or divided doses; titrate at 2-week intervals
Pediatric: <12 years: not established; ≥12 years: same as adult
Aldactone *Tab:* 25, 50*, 100*mg
CaroSpir *Oral susp:* 25 mg/5 ml (118, 473 ml) (banana)

▷ *triamterene* (B) 100 mg bid; max 300 mg
Pediatric: <12 years: not recommended; ≥12 years: same as adult
Dyrenium *Cap:* 50, 100 mg

Loop Diuretics

▷ *bumetanide* (C)(G) 0.5-2 mg daily; may repeat at 4-5-hour intervals; max 10 mg/day
   Pediatric: <18 years: not recommended; ≥18 years: same as adult
   Tab: 1*mg
   Comment: *Bumetanide* is contraindicated with sulfa drug allergy.

▷ *ethacrynic acid* (B)(G) initially 50-200 mg/day
   Pediatric: <1 month: not recommended; ≥1 month: initially 25 mg/day; then adjust dose in 25-mg increments
      Edecrin *Tab:* 25, 50 mg

▷ *ethacrynate sodium* (B)(G) <1 month: not recommended; ≥1 month-12 years: use the smallest effective dose; initially 25 mg; then careful stepwise increments in dosage of 25 mg to achieve effective maintenance; ≥12 years: administer smallest dose required to produce gradual weight loss (about 1-2 pounds per day); onset of diuresis usually occurs at 50-100 mg in children ≥12 years; after diuresis has been achieved, the minimally effective dose (usually 50-200 mg/day) may be administered on a continuous or intermittent dosage schedule; dose titrations are usually in 25-50 mg increments to avoid derangement electrolyte and water excretion; the patient should be weighed under standard conditions before and during administration of *ethacrynate sodium;* the following schedule may be helpful in determining the lowest effective dose; *Day 1:* 50 mg once daily after a meal; *Day 2:* 50 mg bid after meals, if necessary; *Day 3:* 100 mg in the morning and 50-100 mg following the afternoon or evening meal, depending upon response to the morning dose; a few patients may require initial and maintenance doses as high as 200 mg bid; these higher doses, which should be achieved gradually, are most often required in patients with severe, refractory edema
      Sodium Edecrin *Vial:* 50 mg single-dose
      Comment: Sodium Edecrin is more potent than more commonly used loop and thiazide diuretics. Treatment of the edema associated with congestive heart failure, cirrhosis of the liver, and renal disease, including the nephrotic syndrome, short-term management of ascites due to malignancy, idiopathic edema, and lymphedema, short-term management of hospitalized pediatric patients, other than infants, with congenital heart disease or the nephrotic syndrome. IV Sodium Edecrin is indicated when a rapid onset of diuresis is desired, for example, in acute pulmonary edema or when gastrointestinal absorption is impaired or oral medication is not practical.

▷ *furosemide* (C)(G) initially 40 mg bid
   Pediatric: <12 years: not recommended; ≥12 years: same as adult
      Lasix *Tab:* 20, 40*, 80 mg; *Oral Soln:* 10 mg/ml (2, 4 oz w. dropper)
   Comment: *Furosemide* is contraindicated with sulfa drug allergy.

▷ *torsemide* (B) 5 mg once daily; may increase to 10 mg once daily
   Pediatric: <12 years: not recommended; ≥12 years: same as adult
      Demadex *Tab:* 5*, 10*, 20*, 100*mg

Indoline Diuretic

▷ *indapamide* (B) initially 1.25 mg daily; may titrate dosage upward every 4 weeks if needed; max 5 mg/day
   Pediatric: <12 years: not recommended; ≥12 years: same as adult
      Lozol *Tab:* 1.25, 2.5 mg
   Comment: *Indapamide* is contraindicated with sulfa drug allergy.

Quinazoline Diuretic

▷ *metolazone* (B) 2.5-5 mg daily
　Pediatric: <12 years: not recommended; ≥12 years: same as adult
　　Zaroxolyn 2.5-5 mg daily
　　Tab: 2.5, 5, 10 mg
　Comment: *Metolazone* is contraindicated with sulfa drug allergy.

DIURETIC COMBINATIONS

▷ *amiloride+hydrochlorothiazide* (B)(G) initially 1 tab daily; may increase to 2
tabs/day in a single or divided doses
　Pediatric: <12 years: not recommended; ≥12 years: same as adult
　　Moduretic *Tab:* amil 5 mg+hctz 50 mg*
▷ *methyclothiazide+deserpidine* (C) initially 5/0.25 mg once daily; titrate individual
components
　Pediatric: Safety and effectiveness in children have not been established; therefore,
age at which this drug may be initially prescribed is not specified
　　Enduronyl *Tab:* methyl 5 mg+deser 0.25 mg*
　　Enduronyl Forte *Tab:* methyl 5 mg+deser 0.5 mg*
　Comment: **Enduronyl** (*methyclothiazide* and *deserpidine*) is indicated in
the treatment of mild-to-moderately severe hypertension. The combined
antihypertensive actions of *methyclothiazide* and *deserpidine* result in a
total clinical antihypertensive effect, which is greater than can ordinarily be
achieved by either drug, given individually and more potent agents can be
administered at reduced dosage. *methylchlorothiazide* (**Enduron**) is a thiazide
(benzothiadiazine) diuretic-antihypertensive. *deserpidine* is a purified
rauwolfia alkaloid. The pharmacologic actions of *deserpidine* are essentially
the same as those of other active rauwolfia alkaloids. *deserpidine* probably
produces its antihypertensive effects through depletion of tissue stores of
catecholamines (epinephrine and norepinephrine) from peripheral sites. By
contrast, its sedative and tranquilizing properties are thought to be related
to depletion of 5-hydroxytryptamine from the brain. The antihypertensive
effect is often accompanied by bradycardia. There is no significant alteration
in cardiac output or renal blood flow. The carotid sinus reflex is inhibited,
but postural hypotension is rarely seen with the use of conventional doses of
deserpidine alone. *Methyclothiazide* is contraindicated in patients with anuria
and in patients with a history of hypersensitivity to this or other sulfonamide-
derived drugs. *deserpidine* is contraindicated in patients with known
hypersensitivity, active peptic ulcer, history of mental depression, especially
with suicidal tendencies and patients receiving electroconvulsive therapy.
Animal reproduction studies have not been conducted with methyclothiazide
or deserpidine. It is also not known whether *methyclothiazide* or
deserpidine can cause fetal harm when administered to a pregnant woman.
methyclothiazide and *deserpidine* should be given to a pregnant woman only
if clearly needed. *methyclothiazide* and *deserpidine* are excreted in human
milk. Effects on the breastfed infant are unknown; therefore, assess maternal
need/benefit as against potential fetal risk.
▷ *spironolactone+hydrochlorothiazide* (D)(G)
　Pediatric: <12 years: not recommended; ≥12 years: same as adult
　　Aldactazide 25 usual maintenance 1-4 tabs in a single or divided doses
　　　Tab: spiro 25 mg+hctz 25 mg
　　Aldactazide 50 usual maintenance 1-2 tabs in a single or divided doses
　　　Tab: spiro 50 mg+hctz 50 mg
▷ *triamterene+hydrochlorothiazide* (C)(G)
　Pediatric: <12 years: not recommended; ≥12 years: same as adult
　　Dyazide 1-2 caps once daily
　　　Cap: triam 37.5 mg/hctz 25 mg

Maxzide 1 tab once daily
  Tab: triam 75 mg/hctz 50 mg*
Maxzide-25 1-2 tabs once daily
  Tab: triam 37.5 mg/hctz 25 mg*

ANGIOTENSIN CONVERTING ENZYME INHIBITORS (ACEIS)

Comment: Black patients receiving ACEI monotherapy have been reported to have a higher incidence of angioedema as compared to non-Blacks. Non-Blacks have a greater decrease in BP when ACEIs are used as compared to Black patients.

▷ *benazepril* (D)(G) initially 10 mg daily; usual maintenance 20-40 mg/day in 1-2 divided doses; usual max 80 mg/day
  Pediatric: <12 years: not recommended; ≥12 years: same as adult
    Lotensin *Tab:* 5, 10, 20, 40 mg
▷ *captopril* (D)(G) initially 25 mg bid-tid; after 1-2 weeks increase to 50 mg bid-tid
  Pediatric: <12 years: not recommended; ≥12 years: same as adult
    Capoten *Tab:* 12.5*, 25*, 50*, 100*mg
▷ *enalapril* (D) initially 5 mg daily; usual dosage range 10-40 mg/day; max 40 mg/day
  Pediatric: <12 years: not recommended; ≥12 years: same as adult
    Epaned Oral Solution *Oral soln:* 1 mg/ml (150 ml) (mixed berry)
    Vasotec (G) *Tab:* 2.5*, 5*, 10, 20 mg
▷ *fosinopril* (D) initially 10 mg daily; usual maintenance 20-40 mg/day in a single or divided doses; max 80 mg/day
  Pediatric: <6 years, <50 kg: not recommended; ≥6-12 years, ≥50 kg: 5-10 mg once daily
    Monopril *Tab:* 10*, 20, 40 mg
▷ *lisinopril* (D)
    Prinivil initially 10 mg daily; usual range 20-40 mg/day
    Pediatric: <12 years: not recommended; ≥12 years: same as adult
      Tab: 5*, 10*, 20*, 40 mg
    Qbrelis Oral Solution administer as a single dose once daily
    Pediatric: <6 years, GFR <30 mL/min: not recommended; ≥6 years, GFR >30 mL/min: initially 0.07 mg/kg, max 5 mg; adjust according to BP up to a max 0.61 mg/kg (40 mg) once daily
      Oral soln: 1 mg/ml (150 ml)
    Zestril initially 10 mg daily; usual range 20-40 mg/day
    Pediatric: <12 years: not recommended; ≥12 years: same as adult
      Tab: 2.5, 5*, 10, 20, 30, 40 mg
▷ *moexipril* (D) initially 7.5 mg daily; usual range 15-30 mg/day in 1-2 divided doses; max 30 mg/day
  Pediatric: <12 years: not recommended; ≥12 years: same as adult
    Univasc *Tab:* 7.5*, 15*mg
▷ *perindopril* (D) initially 2-8 mg daily-bid; max 16 mg/day
  Pediatric: <12 years: not recommended; ≥12 years: same as adult
    Aceon *Tab:* 2*, 4*, 8*mg
▷ *quinapril* (D) initially 10 mg once daily; usual maintenance 20-80 mg daily in 1-2 divided doses
  Pediatric: <12 years: not recommended; ≥12 years: same as adult
    Accupril *Tab:* 5*, 10, 20, 40 mg
▷ *ramipril* (D)(G) initially 2.5 mg bid; usual maintenance 2.5-20 mg in 1-2 divided doses
  Pediatric: <12 years: not established; ≥12 years: same as adult
    Altace *Tab/Cap:* 1.25, 2.5, 5, 10 mg
▷ *trandolapril* (C; D in 2nd, 3rd) initially 1-2 mg once daily; adjust at 1-week intervals; usual range 2-4 mg in 1-2 divided doses; max 8 mg/day
  Pediatric: <12 years: not recommended; ≥12 years: same as adult
    Mavik *Tab:* 1*, 2, 4 mg

ANGIOTENSIN II RECEPTOR BLOCKERS (ARBs)

▷ *azilsartan medoxomil* (D) *Monotherapy, <u>not</u> volume depleted*: 80 mg once daily;
Volume-depleted (concomitant high-dose diuretic): initially 40 mg once daily
Pediatric: <12 years: not recommended; ≥12 years: same as adult
   Edarbi *Tab*: 40, 80 mg

▷ *candesartan* (D)(G) initially 16 mg daily; range 8-32 mg in 1-2 divided doses
Pediatric: <12 years: not recommended; ≥12 years: same as adult
   Atacand *Tab*: 4, 8, 16, 32 mg

▷ *eprosartan* (D)(G) initially 400 mg bid <u>or</u> 600 mg once daily; max 800 mg/day
Pediatric: <12 years: not established; ≥12 years: same as adult
   Teveten *Tab*: 400, 600 mg

▷ *irbesartan* (D)(G) initially 150 mg daily; titrate up to 300 mg
Pediatric: <12 years: not recommended; ≥12 years: same as adult
   Avapro *Tab*: 75, 150, 300 mg

▷ *losartan* (D)(G) initially 50 mg daily; max 100 mg/day
Pediatric: <12 years: not recommended; ≥12 years: same as adult
   Cozaar *Tab*: 25, 50, 100 mg

▷ *olmesartan medoxomil* (D)(G) initially 20 mg once daily; after 2 weeks, may
increase to 40 mg daily
Pediatric: <6 years: not recommended; ≥6-16 years: 20-35 kg: initially 10 mg once
daily; after 2 weeks, may increase to max 20 mg once daily; ≥6-16 years: >35 kg:
initially 20 mg once daily; after 2 weeks, may increase to max 40 mg once daily
   Benicar *Tab*: 5, 20, 40 mg

▷ *valsartan* (D)(G) initially 80 mg once daily; may increase to 160 <u>or</u> 320 mg once
daily after 2-4 weeks; usual range 80-320 mg/day
Pediatric: <12 years: not recommended; ≥12 years: same as adult
   Diovan *Tab*: 40*, 80, 160, 320 mg
   Prexxartan Oral Solution *Oral soln*: 20 mg/5 ml, 80 mg/20 ml (120, 473 ml; 20
   ml unit dose cup)

CALCIUM CHANNEL BLOCKERS (CCBs)
Benzothiazepines

▷ *diltiazem* (C)(G)
Pediatric: <12 years: not established; ≥12 years: same as adult
   Cardizem initially 30 mg qid; may increase gradually every 1-2 days; max 360
   mg/day in divided doses
      Tab: 30, 60, 90, 120 mg
   Cardizem CD initially 120-180 mg daily; adjust at 1-2-week intervals; max
   480 mg/day
      Cap: 120, 180, 240, 300, 360 mg ext-rel
   Cardizem LA initially 180-240 mg daily; titrate at 2-week intervals; max 540
   mg/day
      Tab: 120, 180, 240, 300, 360, 420 mg ext-rel
   Cardizem SR initially 60-120 mg bid; adjust at 2-week intervals; max 360 mg/
   day
      Cap: 60, 90, 120 mg sust-rel
   Cartia XT initially 180 <u>or</u> 240 mg once daily; max 540 mg once daily
      Cap: 120, 180, 240, 300 mg ext-rel
   Dilacor XR initially 180 <u>or</u> 240 mg in AM; usual range 180-480 mg/day; max
   540 mg/day
      Cap: 120, 180, 240 mg ext-rel
   Tiazac (G) initially 120-240 mg daily; adjust at 2-week intervals; usual max
   540 mg/day
      Cap: 120, 180, 240, 300, 360, 420 mg ext-rel

▷ *diltiazem maleate* (C) initially 120-180 mg daily; adjust at 2-week intervals; usual range 120-480 mg daily

Pediatric: <12 years: not recommended; ≥12 years: same as adult

Tiamate *Cap:* 120, 180, 240 mg ext-rel

Dihydropyridines

▷ *amlodipine* (C) initially 5 mg once daily; max 10 mg/day

Pediatric: <12 years: not recommended; ≥12 years: same as adult

Norvasc *Tab:* 2.5, 5, 10 mg

▷ *amlodipine benzoate* recommended starting dose 5 mg orally once daily; max 10 mg once daily; small stature, fragile, or elderly patients, or patients with hepatic insufficiency may be started on 2.5 mg once daily

Pediatric: <6 years: not studied; ≥6 years: starting dose: 2.5-5 mg once daily

Katerzia *Oral susp:* 1 mg/ml (150 ml), keep refrigerated

Comment: **Katerzia** *(amlodipine benzoate)* is a calcium channel blocker in an oral suspension formulation indicated for the treatment of hypertension in adults and children ≥6 years-of-age, to lower blood pressure. Lowering blood pressure reduces the risk of fatal and nonfatal cardiovascular events, primarily strokes and myocardial infarctions. **Katerzia** is also indicated for adult patients with Coronary Artery Disease (CAD), Chronic Stable Angina (CSA), Vasospastic Angina (Prinzmetal's or Variant Angina), Angiographically Documented Coronary Artery Disease in patients without heart failure or an ejection fraction <40%, at the same dose as for blood pressure management (2.5-10 mg once daily).

▷ *clevidipine butyrate* (C) administer by IV infusion; initially 1-2 mg/hour; double dose at 90-second intervals until BP approaches goal; then titrate slower; adjust at 5-10-minute intervals; maintenance 4-6 mg/hour; usual max, 16-32 mg/hour; do not exceed 1,000 ml (21 mg/hour for 24 hours) due to lipid load

Pediatric: <18 years: not recommended; ≥18 years: same as adult

Cleviprex *Vial:* 0.5 mg/ml soln for IV infusion (single-use, 50, 100 ml) (lipids)

Comment: **Cleviprex** is indicated to reduce blood pressure when oral therapy is not feasible or desirable. **Cleviprex** is contraindicated with egg or soy allergy.

▷ *felodipine* (C)(G) initially 5 mg daily; usual range 2.5 mg to 10 mg daily; adjust at 2-week intervals; max 10 mg/day

Pediatric: <12 years: not recommended; ≥12 years: same as adult

Plendil *Tab:* 2.5, 5, 10 mg ext-rel

▷ *isradipine* (C)

Pediatric: <12 years: not recommended; ≥12 years: same as adult

DynaCirc initially 2.5 mg bid; adjust in increments of 5 mg/day at 2 to 4 week intervals; max 20 mg/day

Cap: 2.5, 5 mg

DynaCirc CR initially 5 mg daily; adjust in increments of 5 mg/day at 2-4-week intervals; max 20 mg/day

Tab: 5, 10 mg cont-rel

▷ *levamlodipine maleate* initially 2.5 mg once daily; max 5 mg/day; small, fragile, or elderly patients, or patients with hepatic insufficiency may be started on 1.25 mg once daily

Pediatric: <6 years: not established; ≥6 years: initially 1.25 mg to 2.5 mg once daily

Conjupri *Tab:* 1.25*, 2.5*, 5*mg

▷ *nicardipine* (C)(G)

Pediatric: <18 years: not recommended; ≥18 years: same as adult

Cardene initially 10-20 mg tid; adjust at intervals of at least 3 days; max 120 mg/day

Cap: 20, 30 mg

Cardene SR 30-60 mg bid

Cap: 30, 45, 60 mg sust-rel

▷ *nifedipine* (C)(G)

Pediatric: <12 years: not recommended; ≥12 years: same as adult

Adalat initially 10 mg tid; usual range 10-20 mg tid; max 180 mg/day
Cap: 10, 20 mg

Adalat CC initially 10 mg tid; usual range 10-20 mg tid; max 180 mg/day
Cap: 30, 60, 90 mg ext-rel

Afeditab CR initially 30 mg once daily; titrate over 7-14 days; max 90 mg/day
Cap: 30, 60 mg ext-rel

Procardia initially 10 mg tid; titrate over 7-14 days: max 30 mg/dose and 180 mg/day in divided doses
Cap: 10, 20 mg

Procardia XL initially 30-60 mg daily; titrate over 7-14 days; max dose 90 mg/day
Tab: 30, 60, 90 mg ext-rel

▷ *nisoldipine* (C) initially 20 mg daily; may increase by 10 mg weekly; usual maintenance 20-40 mg/day; max 60 mg/day

Pediatric: <12 years: not recommended; ≥12 years: same as adult

Sular Tab: 10, 20, 30, 40 mg ext-rel

Diphenylalkylamines

▷ *verapamil* (C)(G)

Pediatric: <12 years: not recommended; ≥12 years: same as adult

Calan 80-120 mg tid; may titrate up; usual max 360 mg in divided doses
Tab: 40, 80*, 120*mg

Calan SR initially 120 mg in the AM; may titrate up; max 480 mg/day in divided doses
Cplt: 120, 180*, 240*mg sust-rel

Covera HS initially 180 mg q HS; titrate to 240 mg; then to 360 mg; then to 480 mg if needed
Tab: 180, 240 mg ext-rel

Isoptin initially 80-120 mg tid
Tab: 40, 80, 120 mg

Isoptin SR initially 120-180 mg in the AM; may increase to 240 mg in the AM; then 180 mg q 12 hours or 240 mg in the AM and 120 mg in the PM; then 240 mg q 12 hours
Tab: 120, 180*, 240*mg sust-rel

Verelan initially 240 mg once daily; adjust in 120 mg increments; max 480 mg/day
Cap: 120, 180, 240, 360 mg sust-rel

Verelan PM initially 200 mg q HS; may titrate upward to 300 mg; then 400 mg if needed
Cap: 100, 200, 300 mg ext-rel

ALPHA-1 ANTAGONISTS

Comment: Educate the patient regarding potential side effects of hypotension when taking an alpha-1 antagonist, especially with first dose ("first dose effect"). Start at lowest dose and titrate upward.

▷ *doxazosin* (C)(G) initially 1 mg once daily at HS; increase dose slowly every 2 weeks if needed; max 16 mg/day

Pediatric: <12 years: not recommended; ≥12 years: same as adult

Cardura Tab: 1*, 2*, 4*, 8*mg

Cardura XL Tab: 4, 8 mg

▷ *prazosin* (C)(G) first dose at HS, 1 mg bid-tid; increase dose slowly; usual range 6-15 mg/day in divided doses; max 20-40 mg/day

Pediatric: <12 years: not recommended; ≥12 years: same as adult

Minipress Cap: 1, 2, 5 mg

▷ *terazosin* (C) 1 mg at bedtime, then increase dose slowly; usual range 1-5 mg at bedtime; max 20 mg/day
  Pediatric: <12 years: not recommended; ≥12 years: same as adult
    Hytrin *Cap:* 1, 2, 5, 10 mg

CENTRAL ALPHA-AGONISTS

▷ *clonidine* (C)
  Pediatric: <12 years: not recommended; ≥12 years: same as adult
    Catapres initially 0.1 mg bid; usual range 0.2-0.6 mg/day in divided doses; max 2.4 mg/day
      Tab: 0.1*, 0.2*, 0.3*mg
    Catapres-TTS initially 0.1 mg patch weekly; increase after 1-2 weeks if needed; max 0.6 mg/day
      Patch: 0.1, 0.2 mg/day (12/carton); 0.3 mg/day (4/carton)
    Kapvay (G) initially 0.1 mg bid; usual range 0.2-0.6 mg/day in divided doses; max 2.4 mg/day
      Tab: 0.1, 0.2 mg
    Nexiclon XR initially 0.18 mg (2 ml) suspension or 0.17 mg tab once daily; usual max 0.52 mg (6 ml suspension) once daily
      Tab: 0.17, 0.26 mg ext-rel; *Oral susp:* 0.09 mg/ml ext-rel (4 oz)
▷ *guanabenz* (C)(G) initially 4 mg bid; may increase by 4-8 mg/day every 1-2 weeks; max 32 mg/day
  Pediatric: <12 years: not recommended; ≥12 years: same as adult
    Tab: 4, 8 mg
▷ *guanfacine* (B)(G) initially 1 mg/day q HS; may increase to 2 mg/day q HS; usual max 3 mg/day
  Pediatric: <12 years: not recommended; ≥12 years: same as adult
    Tenex *Tab:* 1, 2 mg
▷ *methyldopa* (B)(G) initially 250 mg bid-tid; titrate at 2-day intervals; usual maintenance 500 mg/day to 2 gm/day; max 3 gm/day
  Pediatric: initially 10 mg/kg/day in 2-4 divided doses; max 65 mg/kg/day or 3 gm/day, whichever is less
    Aldomet *Tab:* 125, 250, 500 mg; *Oral susp:* 250 mg/5 ml (473 ml)

ALDOSTERONE RECEPTOR BLOCKER

▷ *eplerenone* (B) initially 25-50 mg daily; may increase to 50 mg bid; max 100 mg/day
  Pediatric: <12 years: not recommended; ≥12 years: same as adult
    Inspra *Tab:* 25, 50 mg
  Comment: Contraindicated with concomitant potent CYP3A4 inhibitors. Risk of hyperkalemia with concomitant ACE-I or ARB. Monitor serum potassium at baseline, 1 week, and 1 month. Caution with serum Cr >2 mg/dL (male) or >1.8 mg/dL (female) and/or CrCl <50 mL/min, and DM with proteinuria.

PERIPHERAL ADRENERGIC BLOCKER

▷ *guanethidine* (C) initially 10 mg daily; may adjust dose at 5-7 day intervals; usual range 25-50 mg/day
  Pediatric: <12 years: not recommended; ≥12 years: same as adult
    Ismelin *Tab:* 10, 25 mg

DIRECT RENIN INHIBITOR

▷ *aliskiren* (D)(G) initially 150 mg once daily; max 300 mg/day
  Pediatric: <18 years: not recommended; ≥18 years: same as adult
    Tekturna *Tab:* 150, 300 mg

PERIPHERAL VASODILATORS

▷ *hydralazine* (C)(G) initially 10 mg qid x 2-4 days; then increase to 25 mg 4 x/day
for remainder of 1st week; then increase to 50 mg qid; max 300 mg/day
Pediatric: initially 0.75 mg/kg/day in 4 divided doses; increase gradually over 3-4
weeks; max 7.5 mg/kg/day or 2,000 mg/day
    Tab: 10, 25, 50, 100 mg

▷ *minoxidil* (C) initially 5 mg daily; may increase at 3-day intervals to 10 mg/day,
then 20 mg/day, then 40 mg/day; usual range 10-40 mg/day; max 100 mg/day
Pediatric: initially 0.2 mg/kg daily; may increase in 50%-100% increments every 3
days; usual range 0.25-1 gm/kg/day; max 50 mg/day
    Loniten *Tab:* 2.5*, 10*mg

ACEI+DIURETIC COMBINATIONS

▷ *benazepril+hydrochlorothiazide* (D)
Pediatric: <12 years: not recommended; ≥12 years: same as adult
    Lotensin HCT
      Tab: **Lotensin HCT 5/6.25** benaz 5 mg+hctz 6.25 mg*
        Lotensin HCT 10/12.5 benaz 10 mg+hctz 12.5 mg*
        Lotensin HCT 20/12.5 benaz 20 mg+hctz 12.5 mg*
        Lotensin HCT 20/25 benaz 20 mg+hctz 25 mg*

▷ *captopril+hydrochlorothiazide* (D)(G)
Pediatric: <12 years: not recommended; ≥12 years: same as adult
    Capozide 1 tab once daily; titrate individual components
      Tab: **Capozide 25/15** capt 25 mg+hctz 15 mg*
        Capozide 25/25 capt 25 mg+hctz 25 mg*
        Capozide 50/15 capt 50 mg+hctz 15 mg*
        Capozide 50/25 capt 50 mg+hctz 25 mg*

▷ *enalapril+hydrochlorothiazide* (D)
Pediatric: <12 years: not recommended; ≥12 years: same as adult
    Vaseretic 1 tab once daily; titrate individual components
      Tab: **Vaseretic 5/12.5** enal 5 mg+hctz 12.5 mg
        Vaseretic 10/25 enal 10 mg+hctz 25 mg

▷ *lisinopril+hydrochlorothiazide* (D)
Pediatric: <12 years: not recommended; ≥12 years: same as adult
    Prinzide 1 tab once daily; titrate individual components
      Tab: **Prinzide 10/12.5** lis 10 mg+hctz 12.5 mg
        Prinzide 20/12.5 lis 20 mg+hctz 12.5 mg
        Prinzide 20/25 lis 20 mg+hctz 25 mg
    Zestoretic 1 tab once daily; titrate individual components; *CrCl <40 mL/min:*
<u>not</u> recommended
      Tab: **Zestoretic 10/12.5** lis 10 mg+hctz 12.5 mg
        Zestoretic 20/12.5 lis 20 mg+hctz 12.5 mg*
        Zestoretic 20/25 lis 20 mg+hctz 25 mg

▷ *moexipril+hydrochlorothiazide* (D)
Pediatric: <12 years: not recommended; ≥12 years: same as adult
    Uniretic 1 tab once daily; titrate individual components
      Tab: **Uniretic 7.5/12.5** moex 7.5 mg+hctz 12.5 mg*
        Uniretic 15/12.5 moex 15 mg+hctz 12.5 mg*
        Uniretic 15/25 moex 15 mg+hctz 25 mg*

▷ *quinapril+hydrochlorothiazide* (D)
Pediatric: <12 years: not recommended; ≥12 years: same as adult
    Accuretic 1 tab once daily; titrate individual components
      Tab: **Accuretic 10/12.5** quin 10 mg+hctz 12.5 mg*
        Accuretic 20/12.5 quin 20 mg+hctz 12.5 mg*
        Accuretic 20/25 quin 20 mg+hctz 25 mg*

ARB+DIURETIC COMBINATIONS

▷ *azilsartan+chlorthalidone* (D)
  Pediatric: <18 years: not recommended; ≥18 years: same as adult
    Edarbyclor 1 tab once daily; titrate individual components
      Tab: **Edarbyclor 40/12.5** azil 40 mg+chlor 12.5 mg
        Edarbyclor 40/25 azil 40 mg+chlor 25 mg

▷ *candesartan+hydrochlorothiazide* (D)
  Pediatric: <12 years: not recommended; ≥12 years: same as adult
    Atacand HCT
      Tab: **Atacand HCT 16/12.5** cande 16 mg+hctz 12.5 mg
        Atacand HCT 32/12.5 cande 32 mg+hctz 12.5 mg

▷ *eprosartan+hydrochlorothiazide* (D)
  Pediatric: <12 years: not recommended; ≥12 years: same as adult
    Teveten HCT 1 tab once daily; titrate individual components
      Tab: **Teveten HCT 600/12.5** epro 600 mg+hctz 12.5 mg
        Teveten HCT 600/25 epro 600 mg+hctz 25 mg

▷ *irbesartan+hydrochlorothiazide* (D)
  Pediatric: <12 years: not recommended; ≥12 years: same as adult
    Avalide 1 tab once daily; titrate individual components
      Tab: **Avalide 150/12.5** irbes 150 mg+hctz 12.5 mg
        Avalide 300/12.5 irbes 300 mg+hctz 12.5 mg

▷ *losartan+hydrochlorothiazide* (D)(G)
  Pediatric: <12 years: not recommended; ≥12 years: same as adult
    Hyzaar 1 tab once daily; titrate individual components
      Tab: **Hyzaar 50/12.5** losar 50 mg+hctz 12.5 mg
        Hyzaar 100/12.5 losar 100 mg+hctz 12.5 mg
        Hyzaar 100/25 losar 100 mg+hctz 25 mg

▷ *olmesartan medoxomil+hydrochlorothiazide* (D)(G)
  Pediatric: <12 years: not recommended; ≥12 years: same as adult
    Benicar HCT 1 tab once daily; titrate individual components
      Tab: **Benicar HCT 20/12.5** olmi 20 mg+hctz 12.5 mg
        Benicar HCT 40/12.5 olmi 40 mg+hctz 12.5 mg
        Benicar HCT 40/25 olmi 40 mg+hctz 25 mg

▷ *telmisartan+hydrochlorothiazide* (D)(G)
  Pediatric: <12 years: not recommended; ≥12 years: same as adult
    Micardis HCT 1 tab once daily; titrate individual components
      Tab: **Micardis HCT 40/12.5** telmi 40 mg+hctz 12.5 mg
        Micardis HCT 80/12.5 telmi 80 mg+hctz 12.5 mg
        Micardis HCT 80/25 telmi 80 mg+hctz 25 mg

▷ *valsartan+hydrochlorothiazide* (D)
  Pediatric: <12 years: not recommended; ≥12 years: same as adult
    Diovan HCT 1 tab once daily; titrate individual components
      Tab: **Diovan HCT 80/12.5** vals 80 mg+hctz 12.5 mg
        Diovan HCT 160/12.5 vals 160 mg+hctz 12.5 mg
        Diovan HCT 160/25 vals 160 mg+hctz 25 mg
        Diovan HCT 320/12.5 vals 320 mg+hctz 12.5 mg
        Diovan HCT 320/25 vals 320 mg+hctz 25 mg

CENTRAL ALPHA-AGONIST+DIURETIC COMBINATIONS

▷ *clonidine+chlorthalidone* (C)
  Pediatric: <12 years: not recommended; ≥12 years: same as adult
    Combipres 1 tab daily-bid
      Tab: **Combipres 0.1** clon 0.1 mg+chlor 15 mg*
        Combipres 0.2 clon 0.2 mg+chlor 15 mg*
        Combipres 0.3 clon 0.3 mg+chlor 15 mg*

▷ *methyldopa+hydrochlorothiazide* (C)(G)
  Pediatric: <12 years: not recommended; ≥12 years: same as adult
    Aldoril initially **Aldoril 15** bid-tid or **Aldoril 25** bid; titrate individual components
      Tab: **Aldoril 15** meth 250 mg+hctz 15 mg
        Aldoril 25 meth 250 mg+hctz 25 mg
        Aldoril D30 meth 500 mg+hctz 30 mg
        Aldoril D50 meth 500 mg+hctz 50 mg

BETA-BLOCKER (CARDIOSELECTIVE)+DIURETIC COMBINATIONS

▷ *atenolol+chlorthalidone* (D)(G)
  Pediatric: <12 years: not recommended; ≥12 years: same as adult
    Tenoretic initially *tenoretic* 50 mg once daily; may increase to *tenoretic* 100 mg once daily
      Tab: **Tenoretic 50/25** aten 50 mg+chlor 25 mg*
        Tenoretic 100/25 aten 100 mg+chlor 25 mg
▷ *bisoprolol+hydrochlorothiazide* (C)
  Pediatric: <12 years: not recommended; ≥12 years: same as adult
    Ziac initially one 2.5/6.25 mg tab daily; adjust at 2 week intervals; max two 10/6.25 mg tabs daily
      Tab: **Ziac 2.5** biso 2.5 mg+hctz 6.25 mg
        Ziac 5 biso 5 mg+hctz 6.25 mg
        Ziac 10 biso 10 mg+hctz 6.25 mg
▷ *metoprolol succinate+hydrochlorothiazide* (C)
  Pediatric: <12 years: not recommended; ≥12 years: same as adult
    Lopressor HCT titrate individual components
      Tab: **Lopressor HCT 50/25** meto succ 50 mg+hctz 25 mg*
        Lopressor HCT 100/25 meto succ 100 mg+hctz 25 mg*
        Lopressor HCT 100/50 meto succ 100 mg+hctz 50 mg*
▷ *metoprolol succinate+ext-rel hydrochlorothiazide* (C)
  Pediatric: <12 years: not established; ≥12 years: same as adult
    Dutoprol titrate individual components; may titrate to max 200/25 mg once daily
      Tab: **Dutoprol 25/12.5** meto succ 25 mg+hctz 12.5 mg *ext-rel*
        Dutoprol 50/12.5 meto succ 50 mg+hctz 12.5 mg *ext-rel*
        Dutoprol 100/12.5 meto succ 100 mg+hctz 12.5 mg *ext-rel*

BETA-BLOCKER (NON-CARDIOSELECTIVE)+DIURETIC COMBINATIONS

▷ *nadolol+bendroflumethiazide* (C)
  Pediatric: <12 years: not recommended; ≥12 years: same as adult
    Corzide titrate individual components
      Tab: **Corzide 40/5** nado 40 mg+bend 5 mg*
        Corzide 80/5 nado 80 mg+bend 5 mg*
▷ *propranolol+hydrochlorothiazide* (C)(G)
  Pediatric: <12 years: not recommended; ≥12 years: same as adult
    Inderide titrate individual components
      Tab: **Inderide 40/25** prop 40 mg+hctz 25 mg*
        Inderide 80/25 prop 80 mg+hctz 25 mg*
    Inderide LA titrate individual components
      Cap: **Inderide LA 80/50** prop 80 mg+hctz 50 mg *sust-rel*
        Inderide LA 120/50 prop 120 mg+hctz 50 mg *sust-rel*
        Inderide LA 160/50 prop 160 mg+hctz 50 mg *sust-rel*
▷ *timolol+hydrochlorothiazide* (C)
  Pediatric: <12 years: not recommended; ≥12 years: same as adult
    Timolide usual maintenance 2 tabs/day in a single or 2 divided doses
      Tab: timo 10 mg+hctz 25 mg

BETA-BLOCKER (CARDIOSELECTIVE)+ARB COMBINATION

▷ *nebivolol+valsartan* (X)(G) 1 tab daily; may initiate when inadequately controlled on *nebivolol* 10 mg or *valsartan* 80 mg
    Pediatric: <12 years: not established; ≥12 years: same as adult
      Byvalson *Tab:* nebi 5 mg+val 80 mg

ALPHA-1 ANTAGONIST+DIURETIC COMBINATIONS

▷ *prazosin+polythiazide* (C)
    Pediatric: <12 years: not recommended; ≥12 years: same as adult
      Minizide titrate individual components
        Cap: Minizide 1 praz 1 mg+poly 0.5 mg
           Minizide 2 praz 2 mg+poly 0.5 mg
           Minizide 5 praz 5 mg+poly 0.5 mg

PERIPHERAL ADRENERGIC BLOCKER+HCTZ COMBINATION

▷ *guanethidine+hydrochlorothiazide* (C)
    Pediatric: <12 years: not recommended; ≥12 years: same as adult
      Esimil titrate individual components
        Tab: Esimil 10/25 guan 10 mg+hctz 25 mg

ACEI+CCB COMBINATIONS

▷ *amlodipine+benazepril* (D)
    Pediatric: <12 years: not recommended; ≥12 years: same as adult
      Lotrel titrate individual components
        Cap: Lotrel 2.5/10 amlo 2.5 mg+benaz 10 mg
           Lotrel 5/10 amlo 5 mg+benaz 10 mg
           Lotrel 5/20 amlo 5 mg+benaz 20 mg
           Lotrel 10/20 amlo 10 mg+benaz 20 mg
           Lotrel 5/40 amlo 5 mg+benaz 40 mg
           Lotrel 10/40 amlo 10 mg+benaz 40 mg
▷ *amlodipine+perindopril* (D)
    Pediatric: <12 years: not recommended; ≥12 years: same as adult
      Prestalia titrate individual components
        Cap: Prestalia 2.5/3.5 amlo 2.5 mg+peri 3.5 mg
           Prestalia 5/7 amlo 5 mg+peri 7 mg
           Prestalia 5/14 amlo 5 mg+peri 14 mg
▷ *enalapril+diltiazem* (D)
    Pediatric: <12 years: not recommended; ≥12 years: same as adult
      Teczem titrate individual components
        Tab: enal 5 mg+dil 180 mg ext-rel
▷ *enalapril+felodipine* (D)
    Pediatric: <18 years: not recommended; ≥18 years: same as adult
      Lexxel titrate individual components
        Tab: Lexxel 5/2.5 enal 5 mg+felo 2.5 mg ext-rel
           Lexxel 5/5 enal 5 mg+felo 5 mg ext-rel
▷ *perindopril+amlodipine* (D)
    Pediatric: <12 years: not established; ≥12 years: same as adult
      Prestalia titrate individual components; max 14/10 once daily
        Tab: Prestalia 3.5/2.5 peri 3.5 mg+amlo 2.5 mg
           Prestalia 7/5 peri 7 mg+amlo 5 mg
           Prestalia 14/10 peri 14 mg+amlo 10 mg
▷ *trandolapril+verapamil* (D)
    Pediatric: <12 years: not established; ≥12 years: same as adult
      Tarka titrate individual components

Tab: **Tarka 1/240** tran 1 mg+ver 240 mg ext-rel
Tarka 2/180 tran 2 mg+ver 180 mg ext-rel
Tarka 2/240 tran 2 mg+ver 240 mg ext-rel
Tarka 4/240 tran 4 mg+ver 240 mg ext-rel

DRI+HCTZ COMBINATIONS

▷ *aliskiren+hydrochlorothiazide* (D) initially *aliskiren* 150 mg once daily; max *aliskiren* 300 mg/day
Pediatric: <18 years: not recommended; ≥18 years: same as adult
Tekturna HCT
Tab: **Tekturna HCT 150/12.5** alisk 150 mg+hctz 12.5 mg
Tekturna HCT 150/25 alisk 150 mg+hctz 25 mg
Tekturna HCT 300/12.5 alisk 300 mg+hctz 12.5 mg
Tekturna HCT 300/25 alisk 300 mg+hctz 25 mg

DRI+ARB COMBINATION

▷ *aliskiren+valsartan* (D)
Pediatric: <12 years: not recommended; ≥12 years: same as adult
Valturna initially 150/160 once daily; may increase to max 300/320 once daily
Tab: **Valturna 150/160** alisk 150 mg+vals 160 mg
Valturna 300/320 alisk 300 mg+vals 320 mg

DRI+CCB COMBINATION

▷ *aliskiren+amlodipine* (D)
Pediatric: <12 years: not recommended; ≥12 years: same as adult
Tekamlo initially 150/5 once daily; may increase to max 300/10 once daily
Tab: **Tekamlo 150/5** alisk 150 mg+amlo 5 mg
Tekamlo 150/10 alisk 150 mg+amlo 10 mg
Tekamlo 300/5 alisk 300 mg+amlo 5 mg
Tekamlo 300/10 alisk 300 mg+amlo 10 mg

DRI+CCB+HCTZ COMBINATIONS

▷ *aliskiren+amlodipine+hydrochlorothiazide* (D)
Pediatric: <12 years: not established; ≥12 years: same as adult
Amturnide initially 150/5/12.5 once daily; may increase to max 300/10/25 once daily
Tab: **Amturnide 150/5/12.5** alisk 150 mg+amlo 5 mg+hctz 12.5 mg
Amturnide 300/5/12.5 alisk 300 mg+amlo 5 mg+hctz 12.5 mg
Amturnide 300/5/25 alisk 300 mg+amlo 5 mg+hctz 25 mg

ARB+CCB COMBINATIONS

▷ *amlodipine+valsartan medoxomil* (D)(G)
Pediatric: <12 years: not recommended; ≥12 years: same as adult
Exforge 1 tab daily; titrate individual components at 1-week intervals; max 10/320 once daily
Tab: **Exforge 5/160** amlo 5 mg+vals 160 mg
Exforge 5/320 amlo 5 mg+vals 320 mg
Exforge 10/160 amlo 10 mg+vals 160 mg
Exforge 10/320 amlo 10 mg+vals 320 mg
▷ *amlodipine+olmesartan medoxomil* (D)(G)
Pediatric: <12 years: not established; ≥12 years: same as adult
Azor titrate individual components
Tab: **Azor 5/20** amlo 5 mg+olme 20 mg
Azor 10/20 amlo 10 mg+olme 20 mg
Azor 5/40 amlo 5 mg+olme 40 mg
Azor 10/40 amlo 10 mg+olme 40 mg

▷ *telmisartan+amlodipine* (D)(G)
  Pediatric: <12 years: not established; ≥12 years: same as adult
    Twynsta initially 40/5 once daily; titrate at 1 week intervals; max 80/10 once daily
      Tab: **Twynsta 40/5** telmi 40 mg+amlo 5 mg
             Twynsta 40/10 telmi 40 mg+amlo 10 mg
             Twynsta 80/5 telmi 80 mg+amlo 5 mg
             Twynsta 80/10 telmi 80 mg+amlo 10 mg

ARB+CCB+HCTZ COMBINATIONS

▷ *amlodipine+valsartan medoxomil+hydrochlorothiazide* (D)(G)
  Pediatric: <12 years: not recommended; ≥12 years: same as adult
    Exforge HCT: initially 5/160/12.5 once daily; may titrate at 1-week intervals to max 10/320/25 once daily
      Tab: **Exforge HCT 5/160/12.5** amlo 5 mg+vals 160 mg+hctz 12.5 mg
             Exforge HCT 5/160/25 amlo 5 mg+vals 160 mg+hctz 25 mg
             Exforge HCT 10/160/12.5 amlo 10 mg+vals 160 mg+hctz 12.5 mg
             Exforge HCT 10/160/25 amlo 10 mg+vals 160 mg+hctz 25 mg
             Exforge HCT 10/320/25 amlo 10 mg+vals 320 mg+hctz 25 mg
▷ *olmesartan medoxomil+amlodipine+hydrochlorothiazide* (D)(G)
  Pediatric: <12 years: not recommended; ≥12 years: same as adult
    Tribenzor: initially 20/5/12.5 once daily; may titrate at 1-week intervals to max 40/10/25 daily
      Tab: **Tribenzor 20/5/12.5** olme 20 mg+amlo 5 mg+hctz 12.5 mg
             Tribenzor 40/5/12.5 olme 40 mg+amlo 5 mg+hctz 12.5 mg
             Tribenzor 40/5/25 olme 40 mg+amlo 5 mg+hctz 25 mg
             Tribenzor 40/10/12.5 olme 40 mg+amlo 10 mg+hctz 12.5 mg
             Tribenzor 40/10/25 olme 40 mg+amlo 10 mg+hctz 25 mg

OTHER COMBINATION AGENTS

▷ *clonidine+chlorthalidone* (C)
  Pediatric: <12 years: not recommended; ≥12 years: same as adult
    Clorpres initially 0.1/15 once daily; may titrate to max 0.3/15 bid
      Tab: **Clorpres 0.1/15** clon 0.1 mg+chlor 15 mg
             Clorpres 0.2/15 clon 0.2 mg+chlor 15 mg
             Clorpres 0.3/15 clon 0.3 mg+chlor 15 mg
▷ *reserpine+hydroflumethiazide* (C)
  Pediatric: <12 years: not recommended; ≥12 years: same as adult
    Salutensin initially 1.25/25 once daily; may titrate to 1.25/25 bid or 1.25/50 once daily
      Tab: **Salutensin 1.25/25** enal 1.25 mg+hydro 25 mg
             Salutensin 1.25/50: enal 1.25 mg+hydro 50 mg

ANTIHYPERTENSION+ANTILIPID COMBINATIONS
CCB+Statin Combinations

▷ *amlodipine+atorvastatin* (X)
  Pediatric: <10 years: not established; ≥10 years (female postmenarche): same as adult
    Caduet select according to blood pressure and lipid values; titrate *amlodipine* over 7-14 days; titrate *atorvastatin* according to monitored lipid values; max *amlodipine* 10 mg/day and max *atorvastatin* 80 mg/day; refer to contraindications and precautions for CCB and statin therapy
      Tab: **Caduet 2.5/10** amlo 2.5 mg+ator 10 mg
             Caduet 2.5/20 amlo 2.5 mg+ator 20 mg
             Caduet 5/10 amlo 5 mg+ator 10 mg
             Caduet 5/20 amlo 5 mg+ator 20 mg

Caduet 5/40 amlo 5 mg+ator 40 mg
Caduet 5/80 amlo 5 mg+ator 80 mg
Caduet 10/10 amlo 10 mg+ator 10 mg
Caduet 10/20 amlo 10 mg+ator 20 mg
Caduet 10/40 amlo 10 mg+ator 40 mg
Caduet 10/80 amlo 10 mg+ator 80 mg

ANTIHYPERTENSION+ANTI-OSTEOARTHRITIS COMBINATION

CCB + Cox-2 Inhibitor

▷ *amlodipine+celecoxib*
Pediatric: safety and efficacy not established
Cosensi take as a single dose once daily; max *amlodipine* 10 mg and max *celecoxib* 200 mg per day
Tab: Consensi 2.5/200 *Tab:* amlo 2.5 mg + celecox 200 mg
Consensi 5/200 *Tab:* amlo 5 mg + celecox 200 mg
Consensi 10/200 *Tab:* amlo 10 mg + celecox 200 mg
Comment: Consensi is a combination of *amlodipine besylate* (calcium channel blocker) and *celecoxib* (Cox-2 inhibitor) indicated for patients for whom treatment with are appropriate. Lowering blood pressure reduces the risk of fatal and nonfatal CV events, primarily stroke, and myocardial infarction.

HYPERTHYROIDISM

▷ *methimazole* (D) initially 15-60 mg/day in 3 divided doses; maintenance 5-15 mg/day
Pediatric: initially 0.4 mg/kg/day in 3 divided doses; maintenance 0.2 mg/kg/day or 1/2 initial dose
Tapazole *Tab:* 5*, 10*mg
Comment: *Methimazole* potentiates anticoagulants. Contraindicated in nursing mothers.

▷ *propylthiouracil (ptu)* (D)(G)
Propyl-Thyracil initially 100-900 mg/day in 3 divided doses; maintenance usually 50-600 mg/day in 2 divided doses
Pediatric: <6 years: not recommended; ≥6-10 years: initially 50-150 mg/day or 5-7 mg/kg/day in 3 divided doses; ≥10 years: initially 150-300 mg/day or 5-7 mg/kg/day in 3 divided doses; *maintenance:* 0.2 mg/kg/day or 1/2 to 2/3 of initial dose
Tab: 50*mg
Comment: Preferred agent in pregnancy. Side effects include dermatitis, nausea, agranulocytosis, and hypothyroidism. Should be taken regularly for 2 years. Do not discontinue abruptly.

BETA-ADRENERGIC BLOCKER

▷ *propranolol* (C)(G) 40-240 mg daily
Pediatric: <12 years: not recommended; ≥12 years: same as adult
Inderal *Tab:* 10*, 20*, 40*, 60*, 80*mg
Inderal LA initially 80 mg daily in a single dose; increase q 3-7 days; usual range 120-160 mg/day; max 320 mg/day in a single dose
Cap: 60, 80, 120, 160 mg sust-rel
InnoPran XL initially 80 mg q HS; max 120 mg/day
Cap: 80, 120 mg ext-rel

HYPERTRIGLYCERIDEMIA

OMEGA 3-FATTY ACID ETHYL ESTERS

Comment: Vascepa, Lovaza, and Epanova are indicated for the treatment of TG ≥500 mg/dl.

▷ *icosapent ethyl (omega 3-fatty acid ethyl ester of EPA)* (C) 2 caps bid with food; max 4 gm/day; swallow whole, do not crush or chew
Pediatric: <18 years: not recommended; ≥18 years: same as adult
Vascepa *sgc:* 0.5, 1 gm (α-tocopherol 4 mg/cap)

▷ *omega 3-fatty acid ethyl esters* (C)(G) 2 gm bid or 4 gm daily; swallow whole, do not crush or chew
Pediatric: <18 years: not recommended; ≥18 years: same as adult
Lovaza *Gelcap:* 1 gm (α-tocopherol 4 mg/cap) *omega 3-carcartonyl acids* (C) take 2-4 gel caps (2-4 gm) daily without regard to meals
Epanova *Gelcap:* 1 gm

ISOBUTYRIC ACID DERIVATIVE

▷ *gemfibrozil* (C)(G)
Pediatric: <12 years: not recommended; ≥12 years: same as adult
Lopid 600 mg bid 30 minutes before AM and PM meals
Tab: 600*mg

FIBRATES (FIBRIC ACID DERIVATIVES)

▷ *fenofibrate* (C) take with meals; adjust at 4-8-week intervals; discontinue if inadequate response after 2 months; lowest dose or contraindicated with renal impairment and the elderly
Pediatric: <12 years: not recommended; ≥12 years: same as adult
Antara 43-130 mg once daily; max 130 mg/day
Cap: 43, 87, 130 mg
FibriCor 30-105 mg once daily; max 105 mg/day
Tab: 30, 105 mg
TriCor (G) 48-145 mg once daily; max 145 mg/day
Tab: 48, 145 mg
TriLipix (G) 45-135 mg once daily; max 135 mg/day
Cap: 45, 135 mg del-rel
Lipofen (G) 50-150 mg once daily; max 150 mg/day
Cap: 50, 150 mg
Lofibra 67-200 mg daily; max 200 mg/day
Tab: 67, 134, 200 mg

NICOTINIC ACID DERIVATIVES

Comment: Contraindicated in liver disease. Decrease total cholesterol, LDL-C, and TG; increase HDL-C. Before initiating and at 4-6 weeks, 3 months, and 6 months of therapy, check fasting lipid profile or as indicated by manufacturer, LFT, glucose, and uric acid. Significant side effect of transient skin flushing. Take with food and take *aspirin* 325 mg 30 minutes before *niacin* dose to decrease flushing.

▷ *niacin* (C)
Niaspan 375 mg daily for 1st week, then 500 mg daily for 2nd week, then 750 mg daily for 3rd week, then 1 gm daily for weeks 4-7; may increase by 500 mg q 4 weeks; usual range 1-3 gm/day
Pediatric: <12 years: not recommended; ≥12 years: same as adult
Tab: 500, 750, 1000 mg ext-rel
Slo-Niacin 250 mg or 500 mg or 750 mg q AM or HS
Pediatric: <12 years: not recommended; ≥12 years: same as adult
Tab: 250, 500, 750 mg cont-rel

HMG-COA REDUCTASE INHIBITORS (STATINS)

▷ *atorvastatin* (X)(G) initially 10 mg daily; usual range 10-80 mg daily
Pediatric: <10 years: not recommended; ≥10 years (female post-menarche): same as adult
Lipitor *Tab:* 10, 20, 40, 80 mg

▷ *fluvastatin* (X)(G) initially 20-40 mg q HS; usual range 20-80 mg/day
  Pediatric: <18 years: not established; ≥18 years: same as adult
    Lescol *Cap*: 20, 40 mg
    Lescol XL *Tab*: 80 mg ext-rel

▷ *lovastatin* (X) initially 20 mg daily at evening meal; may increase at 4 week intervals; max 80 mg/day in a single or divided doses; *Concomitant fibrates, niacin,* or *CrCl <40 mL/min*: usual max 20 mg/day
  Pediatric: <10 years: not recommended; 10-17 years: initially 10-20 mg daily at evening meal; may increase at 4 week intervals; max 40 mg daily; *Concomitant fibrates, niacin,* or *CrCl <40 mL/min*: usual max 20 mg/day
    Mevacor *Tab*: 10, 20, 40 mg

▷ *pravastatin* (X)(G) initially 10-20 mg q HS; usual range 10-80 mg/day; may start at 40 mg/day
  Pediatric: <8 years: not recommended; 8-13 years: 20 mg q HS; 14-17 years: 40 mg q HS; >17 years: same as adult
    Pravachol *Tab*: 10, 20, 40, 80 mg

▷ *rosuvastatin* (X) initially 20 mg q HS; usual range 5-40 mg/day; adjust at 4 week intervals
  Pediatric: <10 years: not recommended; 10-17 years: 5-20 mg q HS; max 20 mg q HS; >17 years: same as adult
    Crestor *Tab*: 5, 10, 20, 40 mg

▷ *simvastatin* (X)(G) initially 20 mg q HS; usual range 5-80 mg/day; adjust at 4 week intervals
  Pediatric: <10 years: not recommended; 10-17 years: initially 10 mg q HS; may increase at 4 week intervals; max 40 mg q HS; >17 years: same as adult
    Zocor *Tab*: 5, 10, 20, 40, 80 mg

NICOTINIC ACID DERIVATIVE+HMG-COA REDUCTASE INHIBITOR COMBINATION

Comment: Nicotinic acid derivatives decrease total cholesterol, LDL-C, and TG; increase HDL-C. Before initiating and at 4-6 weeks, 3 months, and 6 months of therapy, check fasting lipid profile, LFT, glucose, and uric acid. Side effects include hyperglycemia, upper GI distress, hyperuricemia, hepatotoxicity, and significant transient skin flushing. Take with food and take **aspirin** 325 mg 30 minutes before **niacin** dose to decrease flushing. *Relative contraindications:* diabetes, hyperuricemia (gout), and PUD. *Absolute contraindications:* severe gout and chronic liver disease.

▷ *niacin+lovastatin* (X)
  Pediatric: <18 years: not recommended; ≥18 years: same as adult
    Advicor monitor lab values; may titrate up to max 1,000/20 once daily
    Tab: **Advicor 500/20** niac 500 mg ext-rel+lova 20 mg
      Advicor 750/20 niac 750 mg ext-rel+lova 20 mg
      Advicor 1000/20 niac 1000 mg ext-rel+lova 20 mg

◯ HYPOCALCEMIA

Comment: Hypocalcemia resulting in metabolic bone disease may be secondary to hyperparathyroidism, pseudoparathyroidism, and chronic renal disease. Normal serum Ca^{++} range is approximately 8.5-12 mg/dL. Signs and symptoms of hypocalcemia include confusion, increased neuromuscular excitability, muscle spasms, paresthesias, hyperphosphatemia, positive Chvostek's sign, and positive Trousseau's sign. Signs and symptoms of hypercalcemia include fatigue, lethargy, decreased concentration and attention span, frank psychosis, anorexia, nausea, vomiting, constipation, bradycardia, heart block, and shortened QT interval. Foods high in calcium include almonds, broccoli, baked beans, salmon, sardines, buttermilk, turnip greens, collard greens, spinach, pumpkin, rhubarb, and bran. Recommended daily calcium intake: 1-3 years: 700 mg; 4-8 years: 1000 mg; 9-18 years: 1300 mg; 19-50 years: 1000 mg: 51-70 years (males): 1000 mg; ≥51 years (females): 1200 mg; pregnancy or nursing: 1000-1300 mg. Recommended daily vitamin D intake: >1 year: 600 IU; 50+ years: 800-1000 IU. The American Academy of Rheumatology (AAR) recommends the following daily doses for anyone on a chronic oral corticosteroid regimen: Calcium 1200-1500 mg/day and vitamin D 800-1000 IU/day.

CALCIUM SUPPLEMENTS

Comment: Take *calcium* supplements after meals to avoid gastric upset. Dosages of *calcium* over 2000 mg/day have not been shown to have any additional benefit. *Calcium* decreases *tetracycline* absorption. *Calcium* absorption is decreased by corticosteroids.

▶ *calcitonin-salmon* (C)

    Miacalcin 200 units (1 spray intranasally) once daily; alternate nostrils each day

      Nasal spray: 14 dose (2 ml)

    Miacalcin injection 100 units/day SC or IM

      Vial: 2 ml

▶ *calcium carbonate* (C)(OTC)(G)

    Rolaids chew 2 tabs bid; max 14 tabs/day

      Tab: calcium carbonate: 550 mg

    Rolaids Extra Strength chew 2 tabs bid; max 8 tabs/day

      Tab: 1000 mg

    Tums chew 2 tabs bid; max 16 tabs/day

      Tab: 500 mg

    Tums Extra Strength chew 2 tabs bid; max 10 tabs/day

      Tab: 750 mg

    Tums Ultra chew 2 tabs bid; max 8 tabs/day

      Tab: 1000 mg

    Os-Cal 500 (OTC) 1-2 tab bid-tid

      Tab: elemental calcium carbonate 500 mg

▶ *calcium carbonate+vitamin D* (C)(G)

    Os-Cal 250+D (OTC) 1-2 tabs tid

      Tab: elemental calcium carbonate 250 mg+vit d 125 IU

    Os-Cal 500+D (OTC) 1-2 tabs bid-tid

      Tab: elemental calcium carbonate 500 mg+vit d 125 IU

    Viactiv (OTC) 1 tab tid

      Chew tab: elemental calcium 500 mg+vit d and vit a100 IU+Vit k 40 mEq

▶ *calcium citrate*

    Citracal (OTC) 1-2 tabs bid

      Tab: elemental calcium citrate 200 mg

▶ *calcium citrate+vitamin D* (C)(G)

    Citracal+D (OTC) 1-2 cplts bid

      Cplt: elemental calcium citrate 315 mg+vit d 200 IU

    Citracal 250+D (OTC) 1-2 tabs bid

      Tab: elemental calcium citrate 250 mg+vit d 62.3 IU

VITAMIN D ANALOGS

Comment: Concurrent *vitamin D* supplementation is contraindicated for patients taking *calcitriol* or *doxercalciferol* due to the risk of *vitamin D* toxicity. Symptoms of hypervitaminosis D: hypercalcemia, hypercalciuria, elevated creatinine, erythema multiforme, and hyperphosphatemia. Maintain adequate daily calcium and fluid intake. Keep serum calcium times phosphate (Ca x P) product below 70. Monitor serum calcium (esp. during dose titration), phosphorus, and other lab values (see literature for frequency).

▷ **calcitriol** (C)(G) *Predialysis:* initially 0.25 mcg daily; may increase to 0.5 mcg daily; *Dialysis:* initially 0.25 mcg daily; may increase by 0.25 mcg/day at 4-8-week intervals; usual maintenance 0.5-1 mcg/day; *Hypoparathyroidism:* initially 0.25 mcg q AM; may increase by 0.25 mcg/day at 4-8 week intervals; usual maintenance 0.5-2 mcg/day
Pediatric: <12 years: *Predialysis:* <3 years: 10-15 ng/kg per day; ≥3 years: initially 0.25 mcg daily; may increase to 0.5 mcg daily; *Dialysis:* not recommended; *Hypoparathyroidism:* initially 0.25 mcg daily in the AM; may increase by 0.25 mcg/day at 2-4 week intervals; usual maintenance: (1-5 years): 0.25-0.75 mcg daily; (≥6 years): 0.5-2 mcg daily; *Pseudohypoparathyroidism:* (<6 years): insufficient data, see mfr pkg insert; ≥12 years: *Predialysis:* initially 0.25 mcg daily; may increase to 0.5 mcg daily *Dialysis:* initially 0.25 mcg daily; may increase by 0.25 mcg daily at 4-8 week intervals; usual maintenance: 0.5-1 mcg daily.
    Rocaltrol *Cap:* 0.25, 0.5 mcg
    Rocaltrol Solution *Soln:* 1 mcg/ml (15 ml, single-use dispensers)
    Comment: *Calcitriol* is indicated for the treatment of secondary hyperparathyroidism and resultant metabolic bone disease in predialysis patients (CrCl 15-55 mL/min), hypocalcemia and resultant metabolic bone disease in patients on chronic renal dialysis, hypocalcemia in hypoparathyroidism, and pseudohypoparathyroidism.

▷ **doxecalciferol** (C)(G) *Dialysis:* initially 10 mcg 3 x/week at dialysis; adjust to maintain intact parathyroid hormone (iPTH) 150-300 pg/mL; if iPTH is not lowered by 50% and fails to reach target range, may increase by 2.5 mcg at 8-week intervals; max 20 mcg 3 x/week; if iPTH <100 pg/mL, suspend for 1 week, then resume at a dose that is at least 2.5 mcg lower; *Predialysis:* initially 1 mcg once daily; may increase by 0.5 mcg at 2 week intervals to target iPTH levels; max 3.5 mcg/day
Pediatric: <12 years: not established; ≥12 years: same as adult
    Hectorol *Cap:* 0.25, 0.5, 1, 2.5 mcg
    Comment: Oral **Hectorol** is indicated for the treatment of secondary hyperparathyroidism in patients with chronic kidney disease (CKD) on dialysis; Predialysis stage 3 or 4 CKD: use oral form only.
    Hectoral Injection <12 years: not recommended; ≥12 years: 4 mcg 3 x weekly after dialysis; adjust dose to maintain intact parathyroid hormone (iPTH) 150-300 pg/mL; if iPTH is not lowered by 50% and fails to reach target range, may increase by 1-2 mcg at 8 week intervals; max 18 mcg/week; if iPTH <100 pg/mL, suspend for 1 week, then resume at a dose that is at least 1 mcg lower
    Vial: 2 mcg/ml (1, 2 ml single-dose; 2 ml multi-dose)
    Comment: **Hectorol Injection** is indicated for the treatment of secondary hyperparathyroidism in patients with chronic kidney disease (CKD) on dialysis.

▷ **paricalcitol** (C)(G) administer 0.04-1 mcg/kg (2.8-7 mcg) IV bolus, during dialysis, no more than every other day; may be increased by 2-4 mcg/dose every 2-4 weeks; monitor serum calcium and phosphorus during dose adjustment periods; if Ca x P >75, immediately reduce dose or discontinue until these levels normalize; discard unused portion of single-use vials immediately
Pediatric: <18 years: not established; ≥18 years: same as adult
    Zemplar *Vial:* 2, 5 mcg/ml soln for inj
    Comment: *Paricalcitol* is indicated for the prevention and treatment of secondary hyperparathyroidism associated with chronic kidney disease (CKD) stage 5.

BIOENGINEERED REPLICA OF HUMAN PARATHYROID HORMONE

▷ **bioengineered replica of human parathyroid hormone** (C) before starting, confirm 25-hydroxyvitamin D stores are sufficient; if insufficient, replace to sufficient levels per standard of care; confirm serum calcium is above 7.5 mg/dL; the goal of treatment is to achieve serum calcium within the lower half of the normal range; administer SC into the thigh once daily; alternate thighs; initially, 50 mcg/day; when initiating, decrease dose of active vitamin D by 50%, if serum calcium is above 7.5 mg/dL; monitor serum calcium levels every 3 to 7 days after starting or adjusting dose and when adjusting either active vitamin D or calcium supplements dose. Abrupt interruption or discontinuation of **Natpara** can result in severe hypocalcemia. Resume treatment with, or increase the dose of, an active form of vitamin D and calcium supplements. Monitor for signs and symptoms of hypocalcemia and monitor serum calcium levels, In the case of a missed dose, the next **Natpara** dose should be administered as soon as reasonably feasible and additional exogenous calcium should be taken in the event of hypocalcemia.

Natpara *Soln for inj:* 25, 50, 75, 100 mcg (2/pkg) multiple dose, dual-chamber glass cartridge containing a sterile powder and diluent

Comment: **Natpara** is indicated as an adjunct to calcium and vitamin D in patients with hypoparathyroidism. Because of a potential risk of osteosarcoma, use **Natpara** only in patients who cannot be well-controlled on calcium and active forms of vitamin D alone and for whom the potential benefits are considered to outweigh the potential risk. Avoid use of **Natpara** in patients who are at increased baseline risk for osteosarcoma, such as patients with Paget's disease of bone or unexplained elevations of alkaline phosphatase, pediatric and young adult patients with open epiphyses, patients with hereditary disorders predisposing to osteosarcoma or patients with a prior history of external beam or implant radiation therapy involving the skeleton. Because of the risk of osteosarcoma, **Natpara** is available only through a restricted program under a Risk Evaluation and Mitigation Strategy (REMS) (www.natparaREMS.com).

HYPOGLYCEMIA: ACUTE

GLUCAGON/GLUCAGON ANALOG

Comment: Necrolytic Migratory Erythema (NME), a skin rash, has been reported postmarketing following continuous *glucagon* infusion and resolved with discontinuation of the *glucagon*. The following are alternative treatments for the treatment of acute hypoglycemia: *glucagon* (**Gvoke**) injection for SC administration; *glucagon* nasal powder (**Basqimi**) for nasal administration; *glucagon analog (desglucagon,* **Zegalogue***)* for SC administration; orally administered glucose or a parenteral form of glucose for IV administration; orally administered non-diuretic benzothiadiazine derivative *diazoxide* (**Proglycem**) for patients with pheochromocytoma or insulinoma.

▷ *glucagon injection*

Gvoke 1 mg SC; administer via SC injection only in the upper outer arm, lower abdomen, or outer thigh; call for emergency assistance immediately after administration of the dose; if there has been no response after 15 minutes, an additional weight-appropriate dose may be administered while waiting for emergency assistance; do not re-use an injection device when the patient has responded to treatment, administer oral carbohydrates

Pediatric: <2 years: not established; 2-12 years: <45 kg: 0.5 mg SC; ≥45 kg: same as adult; administer via SC injection only in the upper outer arm, lower abdomen, or outer thigh; call for emergency assistance immediately after administering the dose; if there has been no response after 15 minutes, an additional weight-appropriate dose may be administered while waiting for emergency assistance; do not re-use an injection device; when the patient has responded to treatment, administer oral carbohydrates

HypoPen auto-injector: 0.5 mg/0.1 ml, 1 mg/0.2 ml, single-use; *Pre-filled syringe:* 0.5 mg/0.1 ml, 1 mg/0.2 ml, single-use

Comment: **Gvoke** *(glucagon injection)* is a ready-to-use, room-temperature stable, liquid *glucagon* for the treatment of severe hypoglycemia in adult and pediatric patients ≥2 years-of-age with diabetes. Patients taking a beta-blocker may have a transient increase in pulse and blood pressure. In patients taking *indomethacin*, **Gvoke** may lose its ability to raise glucose or may produce hypoglycemia. **Gvoke** may increase the anticoagulant effect of *warfarin*. **Gvoke** is contraindicated in patients with pheochromocytoma because **Gvoke** may stimulate the release of catecholamines from the tumor. In patients with insulinoma, **Gvoke** administration may produce an initial increase in blood glucose; however, **Gvoke** may stimulate exaggerated insulin release from an insulinoma and cause hypoglycemia; if a patient develops symptoms of hypoglycemia after a dose of **Gvoke**, administer glucose orally or intravenously. Allergic reactions have been reported and include generalized rash, anaphylactic shock with breathing difficulties, and hypotension. **Gvoke** is effective in treating hypoglycemia only if sufficient hepatic glycogen is present; patients in states of starvation, with adrenal insufficiency or chronic hypoglycemia may not have adequate levels of hepatic glycogen for **Gvoke** to be effective (use glucose instead). *glucagon* administered to patients with glucagonoma may cause secondary hypoglycemia. Test patients suspected of having glucagonoma for blood levels of glucagon prior to treatment, and monitor blood glucose levels during treatment; if hypoglycemia develops, administer glucose orally or intravenously. Most common adverse reactions to **Gvoke** (incidence ≥2%) reported have been: *Adult*—nausea, vomiting, injection site edema raised ≥1 mm, and headache; *Pediatric*—nausea, hypoglycemia, vomiting, headache, abdominal pain, hyperglycemia, injection site discomfort and reaction, and urticaria. Available data from case reports and a small number of observational studies with *glucagon* use in pregnant females over decades of use have not identified a drug-associated risk of major birth defects, miscarriage or adverse maternal or embryo/fetal outcomes. There is no information available on the presence of *glucagon* in human or animal milk or effects on the breastfed infant. However, *glucagon* is a peptide and would be expected to be broken down to its constituent amino acids in the infant's digestive tract and is, therefore, unlikely to cause harm to an exposed infant.

▷ *glucagon nasal powder* 3 mg administered as one actuation of the intranasal device into one nostril; administer the dose by inserting the tip into one nostril and pressing the device plunger all the way in until the green line is no longer showing; the dose does not need to be inhaled; call for emergency assistance immediately after administering the dose; when the patient responds to treatment, administer oral carbohydrates; do not attempt to re-use the device (each device contains only one dose of *glucagon*); if there has been no response after 15 minutes, administer an additional 3 mg using an unused device
Pediatric: <4 years: not approved: ≥4 years: same as adult

  Basqimi *Intranasal device:* 3 mg pwdr, single-dose
  Comment: Baqsimi is a nasally administered antihypoglycemic agent indicated for the treatment of severe hypoglycemia in diabetes patients ≥4 years-of-age. Pheochromocytoma (**Baqsimi** may stimulate the release of catecholamines from the tumor) and insulinoma (**Baqsimi** may stimulate exaggerated insulin release from an insulinoma) are contraindications to **Baqsimi** use. Patients taking a beta-blocker may experience a transient increase in HR and BP. For patients taking *indomethacin*, **Baqsimi** may lose its ability to raise glucose or may produce hypoglycemia. **Baqsimi** may increase the anticoagulant effect of *warfarin*. **Baqsimi** is effective in treating hypoglycemia only if sufficient hepatic glycogen is present. Patients in states of starvation, with adrenal insufficiency, or chronic hypoglycemia may not have adequate levels of hepatic glycogen for **Baqsimi** to be effective; therefore, patients with any of these conditions should be treated with glucose. The most common (incidence ≥10%) adverse reactions associated with **Baqsimi** are

nausea, vomiting, headache, upper respiratory tract irritation (i.e., rhinorrhea, nasal discomfort, nasal congestion, cough, and epistaxis), watery eyes, redness of eyes, itchy nose, throat, and eyes.

GLUCAGON ANALOG

▷ *dasiglucagon* 0.6 mg SC into the outer upper arm, lower abdomen, thigh, or buttocks; if there has been no response after 15 minutes, an additional dose from a new device may be administered while waiting for emergency assistance; when the patient has responded to treatment, give oral carbohydrates
Pediatric: <6 years: safety and efficacy not established; ≥6 years: same as adult
Zegalogue *Prefilled syringe:* 0.6 mg/0.6 ml, single-dose; *Autoinjector:* 0.6 mg/0.6 ml, single-dose
Comment: Zegalogue is a glucagon analog for the treatment of severe hypoglycemia in patients with diabetes. Contraindications to Zegalogue include pheochromocytoma and insulinoma. In patients with pheochromocytoma, Zegalogue may stimulate the release of catecholamines from the tumor. In patients with insulinoma, Zegalogue may produce an initial increase in blood glucose, but then stimulate exaggerated insulin release from an insulinoma, causing subsequent hypoglycemia. If the patient develops symptoms of hypoglycemia after a dose of Zegaloque, administer glucose orally or intravenously. Zegalogue is effective in treating hypoglycemia only if sufficient hepatic glycogen is present. Patients in states of starvation, with adrenal insufficiency, or chronic hypoglycemia may not have adequate levels of hepatic glycogen for Zegalogue to be effective and patients with these conditions should be treated with glucose. Drug interactions with Zegalogue include beta blockers, *indomethacin*, and *warfarin*. Patients taking a beta-blocker may have a transient increase in HR and BP. With patients taking *indomethacin*, Zegalogue may lose its ability to raise serum glucose or may produce hypoglycemia. Co-administration of Zegalogue with *warfarin* may increase *warfarin*'s anticoagulant effect. The most common adverse reactions (incidence ≥2%) associated with Zegalogue have been: *Adult:* nausea, vomiting, headache, diarrhea, and injection site pain; *Pediatric:* nausea, vomiting, headache, and injection site pain. Allergic reactions have been reported with glucagon products. These reactions may include generalized rash, and in some cases anaphylactic shock with breathing difficulties and hypotension. There are no available data on *dasiglucagon* use in pregnant women to evaluate for a drug-associated risk of major birth defects, miscarriage or adverse maternal or embryo/fetal outcomes. In animal reproduction studies, daily subcutaneous administration of *dasiglucagon* to during the period of organogenesis did not cause adverse developmental effects at exposures 7 and 709 times the human dose of 0.6 mg based on AUC, respectively. There is no information on the presence of *dasiglucagon* in either human or animal milk or effects on the breastfed infant. *Dasiglucagon* is a peptide and would be expected to be broken down to its constituent amino acids in the infant's digestive tract and is, therefore, unlikely to cause harm to the exposed infant.

NONDIURETIC BENZOTHIADIAZINE DERIVATIVE

▷ *diazoxide* (C)(G)
Proglycem *Cap:* 50 mg, *Oral Suspension:* 50 mg/ml (chocolate mint) (sodium benzoate) (alcohol 7.25%)
Comment: Proglycem is useful in the management of hypoglycemia due to hyperinsulinism associated with the following conditions: *Adults:* inoperable islet cell adenoma or carcinoma, or extrapancreatic malignancy. *Infants and Children:* Leucine sensitivity, islet cell hyperplasia, nesidioblastosis,

extrapancreatic malignancy, islet cell adenoma, or adenomatosis. **Proglycem** may be used preoperatively as a temporary measure, and postoperatively, if hypoglycemia persists. Treatment with **Proglycem** should be initiated under close clinical supervision, with careful monitoring of blood glucose and clinical response until the patient's condition has stabilized. This usually requires several days. If not effective in 2 to 3 weeks, **Proglycem** should be discontinued. **Proglycem**-induced hyperglycemia is reversed by the administration of insulin or *tolbutamide*. The inhibition of insulin release by **Proglycem** is antagonized by alpha-adrenergic blocking agents. The antidiuretic property of *diazoxide* may lead to significant fluid retention, which in patients with compromised cardiac reserve, may precipitate CHF. The fluid retention will respond to conventional therapy with diuretics. There have been postmarketing reports of pulmonary hypertension occurring in infants and neonates treated with *diazoxide*. The cases were reversible upon discontinuation of the drug. Monitor patients, especially those with risk factors for pulmonary hypertension, for respiratory distress and discontinue *diazoxide* if pulmonary hypertension is suspected. Development of abnormal facial features in four children treated chronically (>4 years) with **Proglycem** for hypoglycemia hyperinsulinism has been reported. *diazoxide* is highly bound to serum proteins (>90%) and, therefore, may displace other substances which are also protein bound—such as bilirubin or *coumarin* and its derivatives, resulting in higher blood levels of these substances. Concomitant administration of oral *diazoxide* and *diphenylhydantoin* may result in a loss of seizure control. IV administration of **Proglycem** during labor may cause cessation of uterine contractions, and administration of oxytocic agents may be required to reinstate labor; caution is advised in administering **Proglycem** at that time. *diazoxide* crosses the placental barrier and appears in cord blood. When given to the mother prior to delivery of the infant, the drug may produce fetal or neonatal hyperbilirubinemia, thrombocytopenia, altered carbohydrate metabolism, and possibly other side effects that have occurred in adults. Alopecia and hypertrichosis lanuginosa have occurred in infants whose mothers received oral *diazoxide* during the last 19 to 60 days of pregnancy. Reproduction animal studies using the oral preparation have revealed increased fetal resorptions and delayed parturition, as well as fetal skeletal anomalies; evidence of skeletal and cardiac teratogenic effects have also been noted with IV administration. **Proglycem** has also been demonstrated to cross the placental barrier in animals and to cause degeneration of the fetal pancreatic beta cells. When use of **Proglycem** is considered, potential benefits to the mother must be weighed against possible harmful effects to the fetus. Information is not available concerning the passage of diazoxide in breast milk. Because many drugs are excreted in human milk and because of the potential for adverse reactions from *diazoxide* in nursing infants, a decision should be made whether to discontinue nursing or to discontinue the drug, taking into account the importance of the drug to the mother.

HYPOKALEMIA

Comment: Normal serum K+ range is approximately 3.5-5.5 mEq/L. Signs and symptoms of hypokalemia include neuromuscular weakness, muscle twitching and cramping, hyporeflexia, postural hypotension, anorexia, nausea and vomiting, depressed ST segments, flattened T waves, and cardiac tachyarrhythmias. Signs and symptoms of hyperkalemia include peaked T waves, elevated ST segment, and widened QRS complexes.

PROPHYLAXIS

Comment: Usual dose range is 8-10 mEq/day.

TREATMENT OF HYPOKALEMIA: NON-EMERGENCY (K⁺ <3.5 mEq/L)

Comment: Usual dose range 40-120 mEq/day in divided doses. Solutions are preferred; potentially serious GI side effects may occur with tablet formulations or when taken on an empty stomach.

POTASSIUM SUPPLEMENTS

Comment: Potassium supplements should be taken with food. Solutions are the preferred form. Extended-release and sustained-release forms should be swallowed whole; do not crush or chew. Potassium supplementation is indicated for hypokalemia including that caused by diuretic use, and digitalis intoxication without atrioventricular (AV) block.

▷ *potassium* (C)(G)

    Pediatric: <12 years: not established; ≥12 years: same as adult

      KCL Solution *Oral soln:* 10% (30 ml unit dose, 50/case)

      K-Dur (as chloride) *Tab:* 10, 20* mEq sust-rel

      K-Lor for Oral Solution (as chloride) *Pkts* for reconstitution: 20 mEq/pkt (fruit)

      Klor-Con/25 (as chloride) *Pkts* for reconstitution: 25 mEq/pkt

      Klor-Con/EF 25 (as bicarbonate) *Pkts* for reconstitution: 25 mEq/pkt (effervescent) (fruit)

      Klor-Con Extended-Release (as chloride) *Tab:* 8, 10 mEq ext-rel

      Klor-Con M (as chloride) *Tab:* 10, 15*, 20* mEq ext-rel

      Klor-Con Powder (as chloride) 20, 25 mEq *Pkts* for reconstitution: (30/carton) (fruit)

      Klorvess (as bicarbonate and citrate) *Tab:* 20 mEq effervescent for solution; *Granules:* 20 mEq/pkt effervescent for solution; *Oral liq:* 20 mEq/15 ml (16 oz)

      Klotrix (as chloride) *Tab:* 10 mEq sust-rel

      K-Lyte (as bicarbonate and citrate) *Tab:* 25 mEq effervescent for solution (lime, orange)

      K-Lyte/CL (as chloride) *Tab:* 25 mEq effervescent for solution (citrus, fruit)

      K-Lyte/CL 50 (as chloride) *Tab:* 50 mEq effervescent for solution (citrus, fruit)

      K-Lyte/DS (as bicarbonate and citrate) *Tab:* 50 mEq effervescent for solution (lime, orange)

      K-Tab (as chloride) *Tab:* 10 mEq sust-rel

      Micro-K (as chloride) *Cap:* 8, 10 mEq sust-rel

      Potassium Chloride Extended Release Caps *Cap:* 8, 10 mEq ext-rel

      Potassium Chloride Sust-Rel Tabs *Tab/Cap:* 10 mEq sust-rel

      Potassium Chloride ER *Tab:* 8 mEq (600 mg), 10 mEq (750 mg)

HYPOMAGNESEMIA

Comment: Normal serum Mg⁺⁺ range is approximately 1.2-2.6 mEq/L. Signs and symptoms of hypomagnesemia include confusion, disorientation, hallucinations, hyperreflexia, tetany, convulsions, tachyarrhythmia, positive Chvostek's sign, and positive Trousseau's sign. Signs and symptoms of hypermagnesemia include drowsiness, lethargy, muscle weakness, hypoactive reflexes, slurred speech, bradycardia, hypotension, convulsions, and cardiac arrhythmias.

MAGNESIUM SUPPLEMENTS

▷ *magnesium* (B) 2 tabs daily

    Slow-Mag

      Tab: 64 mg (as chloride)+110 mg (as carbonate)

▷ *magnesium oxide* (B) 1-2 tabs daily
>   **Mag-Ox 400**
>   *Tab:* 400 mg

⬤ HYPOPARATHYROIDISM

VITAMIN D ANALOGS

Comment: Concurrent vitamin D supplementation is contraindicated for patients taking *calcitriol* or *doxecalciferol* owing to the risk of vitamin D toxicity.

▷ *calcitriol* (C) initially 0.25 mcg q AM; may increase by 0.25 mcg/day at 4-8-week intervals; usual maintenance 0.5-2 mcg/day
Pediatric: initially 0.25 mcg daily; may increase by 0.25 mcg/day at 2-4-week intervals; usual maintenance (1-5 years) 0.25-0.75 mcg/day, (≥6 years) 0.5-2 mcg/day
>   **Rocaltrol** *Cap:* 0.25, 0.5 mcg
>   **Rocaltrol Solution** *Soln:* 1 mcg/ml (15 ml, single-use dispensers)

▷ *doxecalciferol* (C) initially 0.25 mcg q AM; may increase by 0.25 mcg/day at 4 to 8 week intervals; usual maintenance 0.5-2 mcg/day
Pediatric: initially 0.25 mcg daily; may increase by 0.25 mcg/day at 2-4-week intervals; usual maintenance (1-5 years) 0.25-0.75 mcg/day, (≥6 years) 0.5-2 mcg/day
>   **Hectorol** *Cap:* 0.25, 0.5 mcg

HUMAN PARATHYROID HORMONE

▷ *teriparatide* (C) 20 mcg SC daily in the thigh or abdomen; may treat for up to 2 years
>   **Forteo** *Multi-dose pen:* 250 mcg/ml (3 ml)
>   Comment: **Forteo** is indicated for the treatment of postmenopausal osteoporosis in women who are at high risk for fracture and to increase bone mass in men with primary or hypogonadal osteoporosis who are at high risk for fracture.

HUMAN PARATHYROID HORMONE-RELATED PEPTIDE (PTHrP) ANALOG

▷ *abaloparatide* (C) Administer 80 mcg SC once daily into the periumbilical region of the abdomen; sit or lie down in case of orthostatic hypotension, especially for first dose; patients should receive supplemental calcium and vitamin D if dietary intake is inadequate
>   **Tymlos** *Multi-dose pen:* 3120 mcg/1.56 ml (2000 mcg/ml, 30 daily doses) disposable
>   Comment: **Tymlos** is indicated for the treatment of post-menopausal osteoporosis in women who are at high risk for fracture (defined as a history of osteoporotic fracture, or multiple risk factors for fracture, or patients who have failed or are intolerant to other available osteoporosis therapy. **Tymlos** is not recommended in patients who are at risk for osteosarcoma (boxed warning). Cumulative use of **Tymlos** or other parathyroid analogs (e.g., *teriparatide*) for >2 years during a patient's lifetime is not recommended (boxed warning). Avoid use in patients with preexisting hypercalcemia and those known to have an underlying hypercalcemic disorder, such as primary hyperparathyroidism. Monitor urine calcium if preexisting hypercalciuria or active urolithiasis are suspected.

BIOENGINEERED REPLICA OF HUMAN PARATHYROID HORMONE

▷ *bioengineered replica of human parathyroid hormone* (C) initially inject mg IM into the thigh once daily; when initiating, decrease dose of active vitamin D by 50% if serum calcium is above 7.5 mg/d; monitor serum calcium levels every 3-7 days after starting or adjusting dose and when adjusting either active vitamin D or calcium supplements dose

Natpara *Soln for inj:* 25, 50, 75, 100 mcg (2/pkg) multiple dose, dual-chamber glass cartridge containing a sterile powder and diluent

Comment: **Natpara** is indicated as an adjunct to calcium and vitamin D in patients with parathyroidism.

HYPOPHOSPHATASIA (OSTEOMALACIA, RICKETS)

Comment: Hypophosphatasia (HPP) is an inborn error of metabolism marked by abnormally low serum alkaline phosphatase activity and phosphoethanolamine in the urine. It is manifested by osteomalacia in adults and rickets in infants and children. It is most severe in infants under 6 months-of-age. With congenital absence of alkaline phosphatase, an enzyme essential to the calcification of bone tissue, complications include vomiting, growth retardation, and often death in infancy. Surviving children have numerous skeletal abnormalities and dwarfism.

▷ *asfotase alfa* 6 mg/kg/week SC, administered as 2 mg/kg or 1 mg/kg 6 x/week; max 9 mg/kg/week SC administered as 3 mg/kg 3 x/week
Pediatric: same as adult
Strensiq *Vial:* 18 mg/0.45 ml, 28 mg/0.7 ml, 40 mg/ml, 80 mg/0.8 ml for SC inj, single-use (1, 12/carton) (preservative-free)
Comment: **Strensiq** is the first FDA-approved (2015) treatment for perinatal, infantile, and juvenile onset HPP. Prior to the availability of **Strensiq**, there was no effective treatment and patient prognosis was very poor.

HYPOPHOSPHATEMIA, X-LINKED (XLH)

FIBROBLAST GROWTH FACTOR (FGF23) BLOCKING ANTIBODY

▷ *burosumab-twza* (C) 1 mg/kg body weight rounded to the nearest 10 mg up to max dose of 90 mg administered every 4 weeks
Pediatric: <1 year: not recommended; ≥1-17 years: starting dose 0.8 mg/kg rounded to the nearest 10 mg; min starting dose 10 mg; max dose 90 mg; administer SC every 2 weeks; dose may be increased up to approximately 2 mg/kg (max 90 mg), administered every 2 weeks to achieve normal serum phosphorus; ≥18 years: same as adult
Crysvita *Vial:* 10, 20, 30 mg/ml (1 ml) single-dose
Comment: The most common adverse side effects associated with **Crysvita** in pediatric XLH patients are headache, injection site reaction, vomiting, pyrexia, pain in extremity, and decreased serum vitamin D. The most common adverse side effects associated with **Crysvita** in patients with XLH ≥18 years-of-age are back pain, headache, tooth infection, restless leg syndrome, dizziness, constipation, decreased serum vitamin D, and increased serum phosphorus. There are no available data on *burosumab-twza* use to inform a drug-associated risk of adverse developmental outcomes in pregnancy. There are no data to inform the presence of *burosumab-twza* in human milk or effects on the breastfed infant.

HYPOTENSION: NEUROGENIC, ORTHOSTATIC

ALPHA-1 AGONIST

▷ *midodrine* (C)(G) 10 mg tid at 3-4-hour intervals; take while upright; take last dose at least 4 hours before bedtime
Pediatric: <12 years: not recommended; ≥12 years: same as adult
ProAmatine *Tab:* 2.5*, 5*, 10*mg

SYNTHETIC AMINO ACID PRECURSOR OF NOREPINEPHRINE

▷ *droxidopa* (C)(G) initially 100 mg, taken 3 x/day (upon arising in the morning, at midday, and in the late afternoon at least 3 hours prior to bedtime (to reduce the potential for supine hypertension during sleep); administer with or without; swallow whole; titrate to symptomatic response, in increments of 100 mg tid every 24-48 hours; max 600 mg tid (max total 1800 mg/day)
Pediatric: <12 years: not recommended; ≥12 years: same as adult
  Northera *Cap:* 100, 200, 300 mg
  Comment: **Northera** is indicated for the treatment of orthostatic dizziness, lightheadedness, or feeling about to black out in adult patients with symptomatic neurogenic orthostatic hypotension (NOH) caused by primary autonomic failure (Parkinson's disease [PD], multiple system atrophy [MSA], and pure autonomic failure), dopamine beta-hydroxylase deficiency, and non-diabetic autonomic neuropathy. Effectiveness beyond 2 weeks of treatment has not been established. The continued effectiveness of **Northera** should be assessed. Administering **Northera** in combination with other agents that increase blood pressure (e.g., norepinephrine, ephedrine, midodrine, triptans) would be expected to increase the risk for supine hypertension.

 HYPOTHYROIDISM

Comment: Take thyroid replacement hormone in the morning on an empty stomach. For the elderly, start thyroid hormone replacement at 25 mcg/day. Target TSH is 0.4-5.5 mIU/L; target T4 is 4.5-12.5 ng/L. Signs and symptoms of thyroid toxicity include tachycardia, palpitations, nervousness, chest pain, heat intolerance, and weight loss.

ORAL THYROID HORMONE SUPPLEMENTS
T3

▷ *liothyronine* (A) initially 25 mcg daily; may increase by 25 mcg every 1-2 weeks as needed; usual maintenance 25-75 mcg/day
Pediatric: initially 5 mcg/day; may increase by 5 mcg/day every 3-4 days;
Cretinism: maintenance dose: <1 year: 20 mcg/day; 1-3 years: 50 mcg/day; >3 years: same as adult
  Cytomel *Tab:* 5, 25, 50 mcg

T4

▷ *levothyroxine* (A)(G)
  Levoxyl initially 25-100 mcg/day; increase by 25 mcg/day q 2-3 weeks as needed; maintenance 100-200 mcg/day
  Pediatric: <6 months: 8-10 mcg/kg/day; 6-12 months: 6-8 mcg/kg/day; >1-5 years: 5-6 mcg/kg/day; 6-12 years: 4-5 mcg/kg/day; >12 years: same as adult
    Tab: 25*, 50* (dye-free), 75*, 88*, 100*, 112*, 125*, 137*, 150*, 175*, 200*, 300*mcg
  Synthroid initially 50 mcg/day; increase by 25 mcg/day q 2-3 weeks as needed; max 300 mcg/day
  Pediatric: <6 months: 8-10 mcg/kg/day; 6-12 months: 6-8 mcg/kg/day; >1-5 years: 5-6 mcg/kg/day; 6-12 years: 4-5 mcg/kg/day; >12 years: same as adult
    Tab: 25*, 50* (dye-free), 75*, 88*, 100*, 112*, 125*, 137*, 150*, 175*, 200*, 300*mcg
  Unithroid initially 50 mcg/day; increase by 25 mcg/day every 2-3 weeks as needed; max 300 mcg/day
  Pediatric: 0-3 months: 10-15 mcg/kg/day; 3-6 months: 8-10 mcg/kg/day; 6-12 months: 6-8 mcg/kg/day; 1-5 years: 5-6 mcg/kg/day; 6-12 years: 4-5 mcg/kg/day; >12 years: 2-3 mcg/kg/day; *Growth and puberty complete:* same as adult

Tab: 25*, 50* (dye-free), 75*, 88*, 100*, 112*, 125*, 150*, 175*, 200*, 300*mcg

T3+T4 Combination

▷ *liothyronine+levothyroxine* (A) initially 15-30 mg/day; increase by 15 mg/day q 2-3 weeks to target goal; usual maintenance 60-120 mg/day
Pediatric: <6 months: 4.6-6 mcg/kg/day; 6-12 months: 3.6-4.8 mcg/kg/day; >1-5 years: 3-3.6 mcg/kg/day; 6-12 years: 2.4-3 mcg/kg/day; >12 years: 1.2-1.8 mcg/kg/day; *Growth and puberty complete:* same as adult
  Armour Thyroid Tab *Tab:* per grain: T3 9 mcg+T4 38 mcg: 1/4, 1/2, 1, 1, 2, 3*, 4*, 5* gr; 15, 30, 60, 90, 120, 180*, 240*, 300*mg
  Thyrolar *Tab: per grain:* T3 12.5 mcg+T4 50 mcg: 1/4, 1/5, 1, 2, 3 gr

PARENTERAL THYROID HORMONE SUPPLEMENT

▷ *levothyroxine sodium* (A)(G) 1/2 oral dose by IV or IM and titrate; *Myxedema Coma:* 200-500 mcg IV x 1 dose; may administer 100-300 mcg (or more) IV on second day if needed; then 50-100 mcg IV daily; switch to oral form as soon as possible
Pediatric: <12 years: not recommended; ≥12 years: same as adult
  T4 *Vial:* 100, 200, 500 mcg (pwdr for IM or IV administration after reconstitution)

 HYPOTRICHOSIS (THIN/SPARSE EYELASHES)

PROSTAGLANDIN ANALOG

▷ *bimatoprost* ophthalmic solution (C)(G) apply one drop nightly directly to the skin of the upper eyelid margin at the base of the eyelashes using the accompanying applicators; blot any excess solution beyond the eyelid margin; dispose of the applicator after one use; repeat for the opposite eyelid margin using a new sterile applicator. Repeat treatment of the opposite eye using a new applicator
Pediatric: <16 years: not recommended; ≥16 years: same as adult
  Latisse *Ophth soln:* 0.03% (3 ml in 5 ml bottle w. 70 disposable sterile applicators; 5 ml in 5 ml bottle w. 140 disposable sterile applicators)
  Comment: **Latisse** is indicated to treat hypotrichosis of the eyelashes by increasing their growth including length, thickness, and darkness. Ensure the face is clean, all makeup is removed, and contact lenses removed. Place one drop of **Latisse** on the disposable sterile applicator and brush cautiously along the skin of the upper eyelid margin at the base of the eyelashes. Do not to apply to the lower eyelash line. If eyelid skin darkening occurs, it may be reversible after discontinuation of **Latisse**. If any **Latisse** solution gets into the eye proper, it will not cause harm; the eye should not be rinsed. Any excess solution outside the upper eyelid margin should be blotted with a tissue or other absorbent material. Onset of effect is gradual but is not significant in the majority of patients until 2 months. The effect is not permanent and can be expected to gradually return to previous. Additional applications of **Latisse** will not increase the growth of eyelashes.

IDIOPATHIC (IMMUNE) THROMBOCYTOPENIA PURPURA (ITP)

SPLEEN TYROSINEKINASE (SYK) INHIBITOR

▷ *fostamatinib disodium hexahydrate* initially 100 mg twice daily; increase to 150 mg twice daily if platelet count not at ≥50x10⁹/L after 4 weeks; discontinue if insufficient increase in platelet count after 12 weeks; for dose modifications, see mfr pkg insert

Pediatric: <18 years: not recommended; ≥18 years: same as adult

Tavalisse *Tab:* 100, 150 mg

Comment: **Tavalisse** *(fostamatinib)* is an oral spleen tyrosine kinase (SYK) inhibitor for the treatment of patients with chronic immune thrombocytopenia (ITP). Monitor CBCs, including platelets, monthly until stable count (≥50 x 10⁹/L) achieved, then periodically thereafter. Monitor LFTs monthly. Discontinue if AST/ALT >5XULN for ≥2 weeks or ≥3XULN and total bilirubin >2XULN. Monitor blood pressure every 2 weeks until stable dose established, then monthly thereafter. Interrupt or discontinue dose if hypertensive crisis (>180/120 mm Hg) occurs; discontinue if repeat BP >160/100 mmHg for >4 weeks. Temporarily interrupt if severe diarrhea (Grade ≥3) occurs; resume at next lower daily dose if improved to Grade 1. Monitor ANC monthly and for infection. Temporarily interrupt if ANC <1 x 10⁹/L occurs and remains low after 72 hours until resolved; resume at next lower daily dose. Use lowest effective dose. Due to potential for embryo/fetal toxicity, use effective contraception during and for ≥1 month after last dose. Confirm negative pregnancy status prior to initiation. Breastfeeding not recommended (during and for ≥1 month after last dose). Concomitant strong CYP3A4 inducers not recommended. Concomitant strong CYP3A4 inhibitors or substrates; monitor for toxicity. May potentiate concomitant BCRP (eg, *rosuvastatin*) or P-gp (e.g., *digoxin*) substrates; monitor for toxicity. Adverse reactions include diarrhea, hypertension, nausea, respiratory infection, dizziness, ALT/AST increase, rash, abdominal pain, fatigue, chest pain, and neutropenia.

IMMUNODEFICIENCY: PRIMARY HUMORAL (PHI)

Comment: Primary Humoral Immunodeficiency (PHI) includes, but is not limited to, Congenital or X-linked Agammaglobulinemia, Common Variable Immunodeficiency, Wiskott-Aldrich Syndrome, and Severe Combined Immunodeficiencies.

IMMUNE GLOBULIN, HUMAN

▶ *immune globulin intravenous, human–slra* 300-800 mg/kg via IV infusion every 3-4 weeks; rate 0.5 mg/kg/min (0.005 ml/kg/min) for the first 15 minutes; then, increase rate gradually every 5 minutes as tolerated; max 8 mg/kg/min (0.08 ml/kg/min); ≥65 years-of-age: infuse **Asceniv** at the minimum infusion rate practicable. monitor renal function, including blood urea nitrogen (BUN), serum creatinine (sCr), and urine output; ensure that patients with pre-existing renal insufficiency are not volume depleted; discontinue **Asceniv** if renal function deteriorates; for patients at risk of renal dysfunction or thrombotic events, administer **Asceniv** at the minimum infusion rate practicable; IgA-deficient patients with antibodies against IgA are at greater risk of developing severe hypersensitivity and anaphylactic reactions; have epinephrine available to treat any acute severe hypersensitivity reaction.

Pediatric: **Asceniv** was evaluated in 11 pediatric subjects (6 children [age 12 years] and 5 adolescents [ages 12-16 years]) with primary humoral immunodeficiency (PHI). The pharmacokinetic (PK), safety, and effectiveness profile of **Asceniv** in adolescent subjects appeared to be comparable to that demonstrated in adult subjects. There are insufficient PK, safety, and effectiveness data from pediatric subjects <12 years-of-age and safety and effectiveness have not been studied in pediatric patients with PHI who are <3 years-of-age.

Asceniv *Vial:* 5 gm/50 ml (100 mg/ml), single use, liquid solution containing 10% IgG for intravenous infusion (preservative-free)

Comment: **Asceniv** *(immune globulin intravenous, human–slra)* is a 10% immune globulin liquid for intravenous infusion, indicated for the treatment of primary humoral immunodeficiency (PHI) in adults and adolescents (12 to 17 years-of-age). Clinical studies of **Asceniv** have not included sufficient numbers of subjects ≥65 years-of-age to determine whether they respond differently from younger subjects. Hyperproteinemia, increased serum viscosity, and hyponatremia or pseudohyponatremia can occur in patients receiving IGIV treatment. Aseptic meningitis syndrome (AMS) has been reported with IGIV treatment, especially with high doses or rapid infusion. Hemolytic anemia can develop subsequent to IGIV treatment; monitor patients for hemolysis and hemolytic anemia. Monitor patients for pulmonary adverse reactions (Transfusion-related acute lung injury [TRALI]). If transfusion-related acute lung injury is suspected, test the product and patient for antineutrophil antibodies. Because this product is made from human blood, it may carry a risk of transmitting infectious agents, e.g., viruses, and theoretically, the Creutzfeldt-Jakob disease (CJD) agent. There are no controlled data in human pregnancy. Intact immune globulins cross the placenta increasingly after 30 weeks gestation. Clinical experience with immunoglobulins does not suggest a harmful effect on pregnancy or the fetus. When administered prior to delivery in mothers with immune thrombocytopenic purpura, the platelet response and clinical effect were similar in the mother and the neonate.

▷ *immune globulin subcutaneous [human] 20% liquid* administer via SC Infusion only; up to 8 infusion sites are allowed simultaneously, with at least 2 inches between sites; *Infusion volume:* for the first infusion, up to 15 ml per injection site; may increase to 20 ml per site after the fourth infusion; max 25 ml per site as tolerated; *Infusion rate:* first infusion, up to 15 ml/hr per site; may increase, to max 25 ml/hr per site as tolerated; however, maximum flow rate is not to exceed a total of 50 ml/hr for all sites combined before switching to **Hizentra**, obtain the patient's serum IgG trough level to guide subsequent dose adjustments; adjust the dose based on clinical response and serum IgG trough levels; administer at regular intervals from daily up to every 2 week. *Weekly dosing:* start **Hizentra** 1 week after last Immune Globulin Intravenous, Human (IGIV) infusion; initial weekly dose: (previous IGIV dose [in grams] x 1.37) divided by # of weeks between IGIV doses *Biweekly dosing (every 2 weeks):* start **Hizentra** 1 or 2 weeks after the last IGIV infusion or 1 week after the last weekly IGSC infusion; administer twice the calculated weekly dose *Frequent dosing (2 to 7 times per week):* start **Hizentra** 1 week after the last IGIV or IGSC infusion; divide the calculated weekly dose by the desired number of times per week *Pediatric:* <12 years: not established; ≥12 years: same as adult

Hizentra *Vial:* 0.2 mg/ml (20%; 5, 10, 20, 50 ml)

Comment: IgA-deficient patients with anti-IgA antibodies are at greater risk of severe hypersensitivity and anaphylactic reactions. Thrombosis may occur following treatment with immune globulin products, including **Hizentra**. Aseptic meningitis syndrome has been reported with IGIV and IGSC, including **Hizentra**. Monitor renal function in patients at risk of acute renal failure (ARF). Monitor for clinical signs and symptoms of hemolysis. Monitor for pulmonary adverse reactions (transfusion-related acute lung injury [TRALI]). **Hizentra** is made from human blood and may contain infectious agents (e.g., viruses, the variant Creutzfeldt-Jakob disease [vCJD] agent and, theoretically, the Creutzfeldt-Jakob disease [CJD] agent). Monitor for clinical signs and symptoms of hemolysis. The most common adverse reactions observed in ≥5% of study subjects were local infusion site reactions, headache, diarrhea, fatigue, back pain, nausea, pain in extremity, cough, upper respiratory tract infection, rash, pruritus, vomiting, abdominal pain (upper), migraine, arthralgia, pain, fall, and nasopharyngitis. No human or animal reproduction studies have not been conducted with **Hizentra**. It is not known whether **Hizentra** can cause fetal harm when administered during pregnancy. No human data are available to inform maternal use of **Hizentra** on the breastfed infant. Safety and effectiveness of weekly **Hizentra** administration have <u>not</u> been established in children <2 years-of-age.

Hizentra *Vial:* 0.2 mg/ml (20%; 5, 10, 20, 50 ml)

Comment: IgA-deficient patients with anti-IgA antibodies are at greater risk of severe hypersensitivity and anaphylactic reactions. Thrombosis may occur following treatment with immune globulin products, including **Hizentra**. Aseptic meningitis syndrome has been reported with IGIV and IGSC, including **Hizentra**. Monitor renal function in patients at risk of acute renal failure ARF). Monitor for clinical signs and symptoms of hemolysis. Monitor for pulmonary adverse reactions (transfusion-related acute lung injury [TRALI]). **Hizentra** is made from human blood and may contain infectious agents (e.g., viruses, the variant Creutzfeldt-Jakob disease (vCJD) agent and, theoretically, the Creutzfeldt-Jakob disease (CJD) agent). Monitor for clinical signs and symptoms of hemolysis. The most common adverse reactions observed in ≥5% of study subjects were local infusion site reactions, headache, diarrhea, fatigue, back pain, nausea, pain in extremity, cough, upper respiratory tract infection, rash, pruritus, vomiting, abdominal pain (upper), migraine, arthralgia, pain, fall, and nasopharyngitis. No human <u>or</u> animal reproduction studies have <u>not</u> been conducted with **Hizentra**. It is <u>not</u> known whether **Hizentra** can cause fetal harm when administered during pregnancy. No human data are available to inform maternal use of **Hizentra** on the breastfed infant. Safety and effectiveness of weekly **Hizentra** administration have <u>not</u> been established in children <2 years of age.

 IMPETIGO CONTAGIOSA (INDIAN FIRE)

Comment: The most common infectious organisms are *Staphylococcus aureus* and *Streptococcus pyogenes*.

TOPICAL ANTI-INFECTIVES

▷ *mupirocin* (B)(G) apply to lesions bid; apply to walls of nares bid
   Pediatric: same as adult
      Bactroban *Oint:* 2% (22 gm); *Crm:* 2% (15, 30 gm)
      Centany *Oint:* 2% (15, 30 gm)

ORAL ANTI-INFECTIVES

▷ *amoxicillin* (B)(G) 500-875 mg bid <u>or</u> 250-500 mg tid x 10 days
   Pediatric: <40 kg (88 lb): 20-40 mg/kg/day in 3 divided doses x 10 days <u>or</u> 25-45 mg/kg/day in 2 divided doses x 10 days; ≥40 kg: same as adult; *see* Appendix CC.3. *amoxicillin* (Amoxil Suspension, Trimox Suspension) *for dose by weight*
      Amoxil *Cap:* 250, 500 mg; *Tab:* 875*mg; *Chew tab:* 125, 200, 250, 400 mg (cherry-banana-peppermint) (phenylalanine); *Oral susp:* 125, 250 mg/5 ml (80, 100, 150 ml) (strawberry); 200, 400 mg/5 ml (50, 75, 100 ml) (bubble gum); Oral drops: 50 mg/ml (30 ml) (bubble gum)
      Moxatag *Tab:* 775 mg ext-rel
      Trimox *Tab:* 125, 250 mg; *Cap:* 250, 500 mg; *Oral susp:* 125, 250 mg/5 ml (80, 100, 150 ml) (raspberry-strawberry)

▷ *amoxicillin+clavulanate* (B)(G)
      Augmentin 500 mg tid <u>or</u> 875 mg bid x 7-10 days
      Pediatric: 40-45 mg/kg/day divided tid x 10 days <u>or</u> 90 mg/kg/day divided bid x 10 days *see* Appendix CC.4. *amoxicillin+clavulanate* (Augmentin Suspension) *for dose by weight*
         Tab: 250, 500, 875 mg; *Chew tab:* 125, 250 mg (lemon-lime); 200, 400 mg (cherry-banana) (phenylalanine); *Oral susp:* 125 mg/5 ml (banana), 250

mg/5 ml (75, 100, 150 ml) (orange); 200, 400 mg/5 ml (50, 75, 100 ml) (orange) (phenylalanine)

Augmentin ES-600 not recommended for adults
Pediatric: <3 months: not recommended; ≥3 months, <40 kg: 90 mg/kg/day in 2 divided doses x 7-10 days; ≥40 kg: not recommended
   Oral susp: 42.9 mg/5 ml (50, 75, 100, 125, 150, 200 ml) (strawberry cream) (phenylalanine)

Augmentin XR 2 tabs q 12 hours x 7-10 days
Pediatric: <16 years: use other forms; ≥16 years: same as adult
   Tab: 1000*mg ext-rel

▷ *azithromycin* **(B)(G)** 500 mg x 1 dose on day 1, then 250 mg daily on days 2-5 or 500 mg daily x 3 days or 2 gm in a single dose
   Zithromax *Tab:* 250, 500, 600 mg; *Oral susp:* 100 mg/5 ml (15 ml); 200 mg/5 ml (15, 22.5, 30 ml) (cherry); *Pkt:* 1 gm for reconstitution (cherry-banana)
   Zithromax Tri-pak *Tab:* 3 x 500 mg tabs/pck
   Zithromax Z-pak *Tab:* 6 x 250 mg tabs/pck
   Zmax *Oral susp:* 2 gm ext-rel for reconstitution (cherry-banana) (148 mg Na+)

▷ *cefaclor* **(B)(G)**
   Ceclor 250 mg tid or 375 mg bid 3-10 days
   Pediatric: <1 month: not recommended; 1 month-12 years: 20-40 mg/kg divided bid or q 12 hours x 3-10 days; max 1 gm/day; see Appendix CC.8.
   cefaclor (Ceclor Suspension) for *dose by weight*; >12 years: same as adult
      Tab: 500 mg; *Cap:* 250, 500 mg; *Susp:* 125 mg/5 ml (75, 150 ml) (strawberry); 187 mg/5 ml (50, 100 ml) (strawberry); 250 mg/5 ml (75, 150 ml) (strawberry); 375 mg/5 ml (50, 100 ml) (strawberry)
   Ceclor Extended Release 375-500 mg bid x 3-10 days
   Pediatric: <16 years: ext-rel not recommended; ≥16 years: same as adult
      Tab: 375, 500 mg ext-rel

▷ *cefadroxil* **(B)** 1-2 gm in 1-2 divided doses x 10 days
   Pediatric: 30 mg/kg/day in 2 divided doses x 10 days; *see* Appendix CC.9.
   cefadroxil (Duricef Suspension) for *dose by weight*
      Duricef *Cap:* 500 mg; *Tab:* 1 gm; *Oral susp:* 250 mg/5 ml (100 ml); 500 mg/5 ml (75, 100 ml) (orange-pineapple)

▷ *cefpodoxime proxetil* **(B)** 200 mg bid x 10 days
   Pediatric: <2 months: not recommended; 2 months-12 years: 10 mg/kg/day (max 400 mg/dose) or 5 mg/kg/day bid (max 200 mg/dose) x 10 days; *see* Appendix CC.12. *cefpodoxime proxetil* (Vantin Suspension) for *dose by weight*
      Vantin *Tab:* 100, 200 mg; *Oral susp:* 50, 100 mg/5 ml (50, 75, 100 mg) (lemon creme)

▷ *cefprozil* **(B)** 500 mg bid x 10 days
   Pediatric: ≤6 months: not recommended; 6 months-12 years: *see* Appendix CC.13. *cefprozil* (Cefzil Suspension) for *dose by weight*
      Cefzil *Tab:* 250, 500 mg; *Oral susp:* 125, 250 mg/5 ml (50, 75, 100 ml) (bubble gum) (phenylalanine)

▷ *ceftaroline fosamil* **(B)** administer by IV infusion after reconstitution every 12 hours x 5-14 days; *CrCl >50 mL/min:* 600 mg; *CrCl >30-<50 mL/min:* 400 mg; *CrCl >1 5-<30 mL/min:* 300 mg; *ESRD:* 200 mg
   Teflaro *Vial:* 400, 600 mg

▷ *cephalexin* **(B) (G)** 250-500 mg qid or 500 mg bid x 10 days
   Pediatric: 25-50 mg/kg/day in 4 divided doses x 10 days; *see* Appendix CC.15.
   cephalexin (Keflex Suspension) for *dose by weight*
      Keflex *Cap:* 250, 333, 500, 750 mg; *Oral susp:* 125, 250 mg/5 ml (100, 200 ml) (strawberry)

▷ *clarithromycin* (C)(G) 500 mg bid or 500 mg ext-rel once daily x 7 days
  Pediatric: <6 months: not recommended; ≥6 months: 7.5 mg/kg bid x 7 days; *see*
  Appendix CC.16. *clarithromycin* (Biaxin Suspension) *for dose by weight*
    Biaxin *Tab:* 250, 500 mg
    Biaxin Oral Suspension *Oral susp:* 125, 250 mg/5 ml (50, 100 ml) (fruit
    punch)
    Biaxin XL *Tab:* 500 mg ext-rel
▷ *dicloxacillin* (B) (G) 500 mg q 6 hours x 10 days
  Pediatric: 12.5-25 mg/kg/day in 4 divided doses x 10 days; *see* Appendix CC.18.
  dicloxacillin (Dynapen Suspension) *for dose by weight*
    Dynapen *Cap:* 125, 250, 500 mg; *Oral susp:* 62.5 mg/5 ml (80, 100, 200 ml)
▷ *erythromycin base* (B)(G) 250 mg qid, or 333 mg tid, or 500 mg bid x 7-10 days
  Pediatric: ≤45 kg: 30-50 mg in 2-4 divided doses x 7-10 days; ≥45 kg: same as
  adult
    Ery-Tab *Tab:* 250, 333, 500 mg ent-coat
    PCE *Tab:* 333, 500 mg
▷ *erythromycin ethylsuccinate* (B)(G) 400 mg tid x 7-10 days
  Pediatric: 30-50 mg/kg/day in 4 divided doses x 7-10 days; may double dose
  with severe infection; max 100 mg/kg/day; *see Appendix CC.21: erythromycin
  ethylsuccinate* (E.E.S. Suspension, Ery-Ped Drops/Suspension) for dose by weight
    EryPed *Oral susp:* 200 mg/5 ml (100, 200 ml) (fruit); 400 mg/5 ml (60, 100,
    200 ml) (banana); *Oral drops:* 200, 400 mg/5 ml (50 ml) (fruit); *Chew tab:*
    200 mg wafer (fruit)
    E.E.S. *Oral susp:* 200, 400 mg/5 ml (100 ml) (fruit)
    E.E.S. Granules *Oral susp:* 200 mg/5 ml (100, 200 ml) (cherry)
    E.E.S. 400 Tablets *Tab:* 400 mg
▷ *loracarbef* (B) 200 mg bid x 10 days
  Pediatric: 15 mg/kg/day in 2 divided doses x 10 days; *see* Appendix CC.27.
  loracarbef (Lorabid Suspension) *for dose by weight*
  Pediatric: 30 mg/kg/day in 2 divided doses x 7 days
    Lorabid *Pulvule:* 200, 400 mg; *Oral susp:* 100 mg/5 ml (50, 100 ml); 200 mg/5
    ml (50, 75, 100 ml) (strawberry bubble gum)
▷ *ozenoxacin* <2 months: not recommended; ≥2 months: apply a thin layer topically
  to the affected area bid x 5 days; affected area may be up to 100 cm² in patients
  ≥12 years-of-age or 2% of the total BSA and not exceeding 100 cm² in patients
  <12 years-of-age
    Xepi *Crm:* 1% 10 mg/gm (45 gm)
    Comment: Xepi (azenoxacin) is indicated for the topical treatment of impetigo
    due *to Staphylococcus aureus* or *Streptococcus pyogenes*. There are no available
    data on the use of **Xepi** in pregnancy to inform a drug associated risk; however,
    systemic absorption of *ozenoxacin* in humans is negligible following topical
    administration. No data are available regarding the presence of *ozenoxacin* in
    human milk or effects on the breastfed infant; however, breastfeeding is not
    expected to result in infant exposure due to the negligible systemic absorption.
    There are no available data on the use of **Xepi** in pregnancy to inform a drug
    associated risk; however, systemic absorption of *ozenoxacin* in humans is
    negligible following topical administration. No data are available regarding the
    presence of *ozenoxacin* in human milk or effects on the breastfed infant; however,
    breastfeeding is not expected to result in infant exposure due to the negligible
    systemic absorption.
▷ *penicillin g (benzathine)* (B)(G) 1.2 million units IM x 1 dose
  Pediatric: <60 lb: 300,000-600,000 units IM x 1 dose; ≥60 lb: 900,000 units x 1 dose
    Bicillin L-A *Cartridge-needle unit:* 600,000 units (1 ml); 1.2 million units (2 ml)
▷ *penicillin g (benzathine procaine)* (B)(G) 2.4 million units IM x 1 dose
  Pediatric: <30 lb: 600,000 units IM x 1 dose; 30-60 lb: 900,000-1.2 million units
  IM x 1 dose

Bicillin C-R *Cartridge-needle unit:* 600,000 units (1 ml); 1.2 million units (2 ml); 2.4 million units (4 ml)

▷ *penicillin v potassium* (B) 250-500 mg q 6 hours x 10 days
Pediatric: 50 mg/kg/day in 4 divided doses x 3 days; ≥12 years: same as adult; *see* Appendix CC.29. *penicillin v potassium (Pen-Vee K Solution, Veetids Solution) for dose by weight*
Pen-Vee K *Tab:* 250, 500 mg; *Oral soln:* 125 mg/5 ml (100, 200 ml); 250 mg/ 5 ml (100, 150, 200 ml)

INCONTINENCE: FECAL

Comment: Treatment of fecal incontinence in patients who have failed conservative therapy (e.g., diet, fiber therapy, antimotility agents).

▷ *dextranomer microspheres+sodium hyaluronate*
Pediatric: <18 years: not recommended; ≥18 years: same as adult
Pre-treatment: bowel preparation using enema (required) and prophylactic antibiotics (recommended) prior to injection
Treatment: inject slowly into the deep submucosal layer in the proximal part of the high pressure zone of the anal canal about 5 mm above the dentate line; four 1-ml injections in the following order: posterior, left lateral, anterior, right lateral; keep needle in place 15-30 seconds to minimize leakage; use a new needle for each syringe and injection site
Post-treatment: avoid hot baths and physical activity during first 24 hours; avoid antidiarrheal drugs, sexual intercourse, and strenuous activity for 1 week; avoid anal manipulation for 1 month
Re-treatment: may repeat if needed with max 4 ml, no sooner than 4 weeks after the first injection; point of injection should be made in between initial injection sites (i.e., shifted 1/8 of a turn)
Solesta dex micro 50 mg+sod hyal 15 mg per ml
Syringe: 1 ml (4 w. needles)

INCONTINENCE: URINARY OVERACTIVE BLADDER, STRESS INCONTINENCE, URGE INCONTINENCE

See **Enuresis**
▷ *estrogen* replacement (X) *see Menopause*
▷ *pseudoephedrine* (C)(G) 30-60 mg tid
Sudafed (OTC) *Tab:* 30 mg; *Liq:* 15 mg/5 ml (1, 4 oz)

VASOPRESSIN

▷ *desmopressin acetate (DDAVP)* (B)(G)
DDAVP usual dosage 0.1-1.2 mg/day in 2-3 divided doses; 0.2 mg q HS prn for nocturnal enuresis
Pediatric: <6 years: not recommended; ≥6 years: 0.5 mg daily or q HS prn
Tab: 0.1*, 0.2*mg
DDAVP Rhinal Tube
Pediatric: <6 years: not recommended; ≥6 years: 10 mcg or 0.1 ml of soln each nostril (20 mcg total dose) q HS prn; max 40 mcg total dose
Rhinal tube: 0.1 mg/ml (2.5 ml)

BETA-3 ADRENERGIC AGONIST

▷ *mirabegron* (C) initially 25 mg once daily; max 50 mg once daily; severe renal impairment, 25 mg once daily
Myrbetriq *Tab:* 25, 50 mg ext-rel

Comment: **Myrbetriq** *(mirabegron)* is FDA-approved to be taken in combination with **VESIcare** *(solifenacin succinate)* for the treatment of overactive bladder (OAB) with symptoms of frequency, urgency, and urge urinary incontinence.

MUSCARINIC RECEPTOR ANTAGONISTS

▷ *vibegron* take one 75 mg tablet once daily; swallow tablet whole with water; may be crushed and mixed with applesauce
  Pediatric: safety and effectiveness not established
      Gemtesa *Tab:* 75 mg
      Comment: **Gemtesa** is indicated for the treatment of overactive bladder (OAB) with symptoms of urge urinary incontinence, urgency, and urinary frequency in adults. The most common adverse reactions (incidence ≥2%) have been headache, UTI, nasopharyngitis, diarrhea, nausea, and URI. Measure serum *digoxin* concentrations before initiating **Gemtesa**; monitor serum *digoxin* concentrations to titrate *digoxin* dose to desired clinical effect. Monitor for urinary retention, especially in patients with bladder outlet obstruction and patients taking muscarinic antagonist medications for OAB, in whom the risk of urinary retention may be greater. If urinary retention develops, discontinue **Gemtesa**. *ESRD with or without Hemodialysis:* not recommended. *Severe Hepatic Impairment:* not recommended. There are no available data on **Gemtesa** use in pregnant females to evaluate for a drug-associated risk of major birth defects, miscarriage, or adverse maternal or fetal outcomes. In animal studies, no effects on embryo/fetal development were observed following administration of *vibegron* during organogenesis at exposures approximately 275-fold and 285-fold greater than clinical exposure at the recommended daily dose. There are no data on the presence of *vibegron* in human milk or effects on the breastfed infant. Developmental and health benefits of breastfeeding should be considered along with the mother's clinical need for **Gemtesa** and any potential adverse effects on the breastfed infant from **Gemtesa** or from the underlying maternal condition.

▷ *fesoterodine* (C)(G) 4 mg daily; max 8 mg/day
  Pediatric: <12 years: not recommended; ≥12 years: same as adult
      Toviaz *Tab:* 4, 8 mg ext-rel

▷ *tolterodine tartrate* (C)(G) **Detrol** 1-2 mg bid or **Detrol LA** 2-4 mg once daily or **Detrol XL** one tab daily
  Pediatric: <12 years: not recommended; ≥12 years: same as adult
      Detrol *Tab:* 1, 2 mg
      Detrol *Cap:* 2, 4 mg ext-rel
      Detrol XL *Tab:* 5, 10, 15 mg ext-rel

ANTISPASMODIC/ANTICHOLINERGICS AGENTS

▷ *darifenacin* (C) 7.5-15 mg daily with liquid; max 15 mg/day
  Pediatric: <12 years: not recommended; ≥12 years: same as adult
      Enablex 7.5-15 mg daily with liquid; max 15 mg/day
          Tab: 7.5, 15 mg ext-rel

▷ *dicyclomine* (B)(G) 10-20 mg qid
  Pediatric: <12 years: not recommended; ≥12 years: same as adult
      Bentyl *Tab:* 20 mg; *Cap:* 10 mg; *Syr:* 10 mg/5 ml (16 oz)

▷ *flavoxate* (B) 100-200 mg tid-qid
  Pediatric: <12 years: not recommended; ≥12 years: same as adult
      Urispas *Tab:* 100 mg

▷ *hyoscyamine* (C)(G)
      Anaspaz 1-2 tabs q 4 hours prn; max 12 tabs/day
      Pediatric: <2 years: not recommended; 2-12 years: 0.0625-0.125 mg q 4 hours prn; max 0.75 mg/day

Tab: 0.125*mg

Levbid 1-2 tabs q 12 hours prn; max 4 tabs/day

Pediatric: <12 years: not recommended; ≥12 years: same as adult

Tab: 0.375*mg ext-rel

Levsin 1-2 tabs q 4 hours prn; max 12 tabs/day

Pediatric: <6 years: not recommended; 6-12 years: 1 tab q 4 hours prn

Tab: 0.125*mg

Levsin Drops 1-2 ml q 4 hours prn; max 60 ml/day

Pediatric: 3.4 kg: 4 drops q 4 hours prn; max 24 drops/day; 5 kg: 5 drops q 4 hours prn; max 30 drops/day; 7 kg: 6 drops q 4 hours prn; max 36 drops/day; 10 kg: 8 drops q 4 hours prn; max 40 drops/day; 2-12 years: 0.25-1 ml; max 6 ml/day

Oral drops: 0.125 mg/ml (15 ml) (orange) (alcohol 5%)

Levsin Elixir 5-10 ml q 4 hours prn

Pediatric: <10 kg: use drops; 10-19 kg: 1.25 ml q 4 hours prn; 20-39 kg: 2.5 ml q 4 hours prn; 40-49 kg: 3.75 ml q 4 hours prn; ≥50 kg: 5 ml q 4 hours prn

Elix: 0.125 mg/5 ml (16 oz) (orange) (alcohol 20%)

Levsinex SL 1-2 tabs q 4 hours SL or PO; max 12 tabs/day

Pediatric: <2 years: not recommended; 2-12 years: 1 tab q 4 hours; max 6 tabs/day; >12 years: same as adult

Tab: 0.125 mg sublingual

Levsinex Timecaps 1-2 caps q 12 hours; may adjust to 1 cap q 8 hours

Pediatric: 2-12 years: 1 cap q 12 hours; max 2 caps/day; >12 years: same as adult

Cap: 0.375 mg time-rel

NuLev dissolve 1-2 tabs on tongue, with or without water, q 4 hours prn; max 12 tabs/day

Pediatric: <2 years: not recommended; 2-12 years: dissolve 1 tab on tongue, with or without water, q 4 hours prn; max 6 tabs/day; ≥12 years: same as adult

ODT: 0.125 mg (mint) (phenylalanine)

▷ *oxybutynin chloride* (B)

Ditropan 5 mg bid-tid; max 20 mg/day

Pediatric: <5 years: not recommended; 5-12 years: 5 mg bid; max 15 mg/day; ≥16 years: same as adult

Tab: 5*mg; *Syr:* 5 mg/5 ml

Ditropan XL initially 5 mg daily; may increase weekly in 5-mg increments as needed; max 30 mg/day

Pediatric: <6 years: not recommended; ≥6 years: initially 5 mg once daily; may increase weekly in 5-mg increments as needed; max 20 mg/day

Tab: 5, 10, 15 mg ext-rel

GelniQUE 3 mg Pump: apply 3 pumps (84 mg) once daily to clean dry intact skin on the abdomen, upper arm, shoulders, or thighs; rotate sites; wash hands; avoid washing application site for 1 hour after application

Pediatric: <12 years: not recommended; ≥12 years: same as adult

Gel: 3% (92 gm, metered pump dispenser) (alcohol)

GelniQUE 1 gm Sachet: apply 1 gm gel (1 sachet) once daily to dry intact skin on abdomen, upper arms/shoulders, or thighs; rotate sites; wash hands; avoid washing application site for 1 hour after application

Pediatric: <12 years: not recommended; ≥12 years: same as adult

Gel: 10%, 1 gm/sachet (30/carton) (alcohol)

Oxytrol Transdermal Patch (OTC): apply patch to clean dry area of the abdomen, hip, or buttock; one patch twice weekly; rotate sites

Pediatric: <12 years: not recommended; ≥12 years: same as adult

Transdermal patch: 3.9 mg/day

▷ *propantheline* (C) 15-30 mg tid

Pediatric: <12 years: not recommended; ≥12 years: same as adult

Pro-Banthine *Tab:* 7.5, 15 mg

▷ **solifenacin** (C)(G) 5-10 mg daily
    Pediatric: <12 years: not recommended; ≥12 years: same as adult
        VESIcare *Tab:* 5, 10 mg
        Comment: **VESIcare** *(solifenacin succinate)* is FDA-approved to be taken in combination with **Myrbetriq** *(mirabegron)* for the treatment of overactive bladder (OAB) with symptoms of frequency, urgency, and urge urinary incontinence.
▷ **trospium chloride** (C)(G)
    Pediatric: <12 years: not recommended; ≥12 years: same as adult
        Sanctura 20 mg twice daily; ≥75 years: *CrCl ≤30 mL/min:* 20 mg once daily
            Tab: 20 mg
        Sanctura XR 60 mg daily in the morning
            Cap: 60 mg ext-rel
    Comment: Take *trospium chloride* on an empty stomach.

OVERFLOW INCONTINENCE: ATONIC BLADDER

▷ **bethanechol** (C) 10-30 mg tid
    Urecholine *Tab:* 5, 10, 25, 50 mg

OVERFLOW INCONTINENCE: PROSTATIC ENLARGEMENT
Alpha-1 Blockers

Comment: Educate the patient regarding the potential side effect of hypotension when taking an alpha-1 blocker, especially with first dose. Start at lowest dose and titrate upward.
▷ **terazosin** (C) initially 1 mg q HS; titrate to 10 mg q HS; max 20 mg/day
    Hytrin *Cap:* 1, 2, 5, 10 mg
▷ **doxazosin** (C) initially 1 mg q HS; may double dose every 1-2 weeks; max 8 mg/day
    Cardura *Tab:* 1*, 2*, 4*, 8*mg
    Cardura XL *Tab:* 4, 8 mg
▷ **prazosin** (C)(G) 1-15 mg q HS; max 15 mg/day
    Minipress *Tab:* 1, 2, 5 mg
▷ **tamsulosin** (C) initially 0.4 mg daily; may increase to 0.8 mg daily after 2-4 weeks if needed
    Flomax *Cap:* 0.4 mg

5-ALPHA REDUCTASE INHIBITOR

▷ **finasteride** (X)(G) 5 mg daily
    Proscar *Tab:* 5 mg

ALPHA 1A-BLOCKER

▷ **silodosin** (B)(G) take 8 mg with food once daily; *CrCl 30-50 mL/min:* take 4 mg
    Rapaflo *Cap:* 4, 8 mg

INFLUENZA, SEASONAL (FLU)

Comment: Routine annual influenza vaccination is recommended for all persons aged 6 months and older without contraindications for the 2020-2021 flu season. ACIP does not prefer one vaccine over another for persons in which more than one influenza vaccine product is applicable based on age and health status.

The live attenuated influenza vaccine (LAIV4) is an option for adults through age 49 years, except with immunocompromising conditions. According to the LAIV4 mfr pkg insert, antiviral agents may reduce the effectiveness of LAIV4 if it is given within the interval from 48 hours before to 14 days after vaccination. Considering the longer half-lives of newer antiviral agents, ACIP recommends that LAIV4 should not be used if a person received either *oseltamivir* or *zanamivir* within the previous 48 hours, *peramivir* within the previous 5 days, or *baloxavir* within the previous 17 days.

Regarding persons with egg allergy with symptoms other than hives, if an influenza vaccine other than **Flublok** or **Flucelvax** is used, the vaccine should be administered in a medical setting under supervision of a health care provider who can recognize and manage severe allergic reactions.

The influenza vaccine is contraindicated in persons with a previous severe allergic reaction to the vaccine. Adults who have received a previous influenza dose and developed Guillain-Barre syndrome within 6 weeks of vaccination should not be vaccinated again unless benefits outweigh the risks.

PROPHYLAXIS (NASAL SPRAY)

▷ *trivalent, live attenuated influenza* vaccine, types A and B (C) 1 spray each nostril; ≥50 years not recommended
  Pediatric: ≤5 years: not recommended; ≥5 years: same as adult
    Never vaccinated with FluMist: 5-8 years: 2 divided doses 46-74 days apart.
    Previously vaccinated with FluMist: 5-8 years: same as adult
    FluMist Nasal Spray 0.5 ml spray annually
      Nasal spray: 0.5 ml (0.25 ml/spray) (10/carton) (preservative-free)

PROPHYLAXIS (INJECTABLE)

▷ *quadrivalent inactivated influenza subvirion vaccine, types a and b* (C)
  Afluria Quadrivalent (B) <6 months: not recommended; 6 months-18 years: 1-2 doses/season at least 4 weeks apart; >9 years: 1 dose/season
  Vial/Prefilled Pen/PharmaJet Stratis Needle-Free Injection System: 0.5 ml single-dose (preservative-free); Vial: 5 ml multi-dose (thimerosol)
  Comment: Contraindicated with allergy to egg or chicken protein, neoeomycin, polymyxin, or history of life-threatening reaction to any previous flu vaccine. PharmaJet Stratis Needle-Free Injection System is only approved as a method of administration for patients 18-64 years-of-age.
    Fluad 0.5 ml IM annually
    Comment: **Fluad** is the first seasonal influenza vaccine with adjuvant, indicated for persona ≥65 years-of-age. Adjuvants are incorporated into some vaccine formulations to enhance or direct the immune response.
    Fluarix Quadrivalent 0.5 ml IM annually
    Pediatric: <3 years: not recommended; ≥3 years: same as adult
      Prefilled syringe: 0.5 ml (10/carton) (preservative-free, latex-free)
▷ *trivalent inactivated influenza subvirion vaccine, types a and b*
    Fluarix (B) 0.5 ml IM annually
    Pediatric: <3 years: not recommended; 3-9 years (previously unvaccinated or vaccinated for the first time last season with one dose of flu vaccine): 2 doses per season at least 1 month apart; 3-9 years (previously vaccinated with two doses of flu vaccine); and >9 years: 1 dose per season
      Prefilled syringe: 0.5 ml single-dose (5/carton) (may contain trace amounts of hydrocortisone, gentamicin; preservative-free)
    Flublok 0.5 ml IM annually; ≥49 years, not recommended
    Pediatric: <18 years: not recommended; ≥18 years: same as adult
      Vial: 0.5 ml single-dose (10/carton) (preservative-free, egg protein-free, antibiotic-free, latex-free)

Comment: Flublok is a cell culture-derived vaccine and, therefore, is an alternative to the traditional egg-based vaccines. Contains 3 times the amount of active ingredient in traditional flu vaccines Flucelvax 0.5 ml IM annually
Pediatric: <18 years: not recommended; ≥18 years: same as adult
   Prefilled syringes: 0.5 ml (10/carton; preservative-free, latex-free)
Comment: Flucelvax is a cell culture-derived vaccine and, therefore, is an alternative to the traditional egg-based vaccines.
FluLaval (C) 0.5 ml IM annually
Pediatric: <6 months: not recommended; ≥6 years: same as adult
   Vial: (5 ml)
FluShield 0.5 ml IM annually
Pediatric: <6 months: not recommended; *Never vaccinated:* <9 years: 2 doses at least 4 weeks apart; 9-12 years: same as adult; *Previously vaccinated:* 6-35 months: 0.25 ml IM x 1 dose; 3-8 years: same as adult
Fluzone 0.5 ml IM annually
   Vial: 5 ml (thimerosal)
Fluzone High-Dose Quadrivalent 0.5 ml IM annually
   Vial: 5 ml (thimerosal)
Fluzone Preservative-Free: Adult Dose 0.5 ml IM annually
Pediatric: <6 months: not recommended; *Not previously vaccinated:* 6 months-8 years: 0.25 ml IM; repeat in 1 month; *Previously vaccinated:* 6-35 months: 0.25 ml IM x 1 dose; >3sss years: same as adult
   Prefilled syringe: 0.5 ml (10/carton) (preservative-free, trace thimerosal)
Fluzone Preservative-Free: Pediatric Dose
Pediatric: <6 months: not recommended; *Not previously vaccinated:* 6 months-8 years: 0.25 ml IM; repeat in 1 month; *Previously vaccinated:* 6-35 months: 0.25 ml IM x 1 dose; ≥3 years: 0.5 ml IM (use Fluzone for Adult)
   Prefilled syringe: 0.5 ml (10/carton; preservative-free; trace thimerosal)
Comment: Contraindicated with allergy to egg protein, or history of life-threatening reaction to any previous flu vaccine.

PROPHYLAXIS AND TREATMENTS
Neuraminidase Inhibitors
Comment: Effective for influenza type A and B. Indicated for treatment of uncomplicated acute illness in patients who have been symptomatic for no more than 2 days; therefore, start within 2 days of symptom onset or exposure. Indicated for influenza prophylaxis in patients ≥3 months of age.
▷ *oseltamivir* phosphate (C)(G)
   Prophylaxis: 75 mg daily for at least 7 days and up to 6 weeks for community outbreak
      Pediatric: <1 year: not recommended; 1-12 years: <15 kg: 30 mg once daily x 10 days; 16-23 kg: 45 mg once daily x 10 days; 24-40 kg: 60 mg once daily x 10 days; >40 kg: same as adult
   Treatment: 75 mg bid x 5 days; initiate treatment only if symptomatic <2 days
      Pediatric: <1 year: not recommended; 1-12 years: <15 kg: 30 mg bid x 5 days; 16-23 kg: 45 mg bid x 5 days; 24-40 kg: 60 mg bid x 5 days; >40 kg: same as adult
      Tamiflu *Cap:* 30, 45, 75 mg; *Oral susp:* 6 mg/ml pwdr for reconstitution (60 ml w. oral dispenser) (tutti-frutti)
      Comment: Tamiflu is effective for influenza type A and B.
▷ *peramivir* start within 2 days of symptom onset; administer via IV infusion over 15-30 minutes; 600 mg as a single dose; *CrCl 30-49 mL/min:* 200 mg; *CrCl 10-29 mL/min:* 100 mg; *Hemodialysis:* administer after dialysis

Pediatric: start within 2 days of symptom onset; administer via IV infusion over 15-30 minutes;<2 years: <u>not</u> established; 2-12 years: 12 mg/kg as a single dose; max 600 mg; ≥13 years: same as adult; *CrCl 30-49 mL/min*: 4 mg/kg; *CrCl 10-29 mL/min*: 2 mg/kg; *Hemodialysis*: administer after dialysis

Rapivab *Vial*: 10 mg/ml (20 ml) single-use soln for IV administration after dilution (preservative-free)

Comment: Avoid live attenuated influenza vaccine 2 weeks prior and 48 hours after treatment with **Rapivab** (*peramivir*).

▷ *zanamivir* (C) 2 inhalations (10 mg) bid x 5 days

Pediatric: <7 years: not recommended; ≥7 years: same as adult

Relenza Inhaler *Inhaler*: 5 mg/inh blister; 4 blisters/Rotadisk (5 Rotadisks/ carton w. 1 inhaler)

Comment: **Relenza Inhaler** is effective for influenza type A and B. Use caution with asthma and COPD.

Polymerase Acidic (PA) Endonuclease Inhibitor

▷ *baloxavir marboxil* take as a single dose within 48 hours of symptom onset; *40-<80 kg*: 40 mg; *≥80 kg*: 80 mg; take with <u>or</u> without food; do <u>not</u> take with dairy products, calcium-fortified beverages, laxatives, antacids <u>or</u> oral supplements containing iron, zinc, selenium, calcium <u>or</u> magnesium (polyvalent cations)

Pediatric: <12 years, <88 lb (40 kg): not established; ≥12 years, ≥88 lb (40 kg): same as adult

Xofluza *Tab*: 20, 40 mg

Comment: **Xofluza** (*baloxavir marboxil*) is a first-in-class, single-dose, oral antiviral drug with a novel mechanism of action designed to target the influenza A and B viruses, including *oseltamivir*-resistant strains and avian strains (e.g., H7N9, H5N1). Unlike other currently available antiviral treatments, *baloxavir marboxil* is the first polymerase acidic [PA] endonuclease inhibitor designed to inhibit the cap-dependent endonuclease protein within the flu virus, which is essential for viral replication, thereby reducing symptoms and duration of the illness. This is the first new antiviral flu treatment with a novel mechanism of action approved by the FDA in nearly 20 years. Safety and efficacy of **Xofluza** was demonstrated in two randomized controlled clinical trials of 1832 patients, where participants were randomly assigned to receive a single dose of 40 mg <u>or</u> 80 mg of *baloxavir marboxil* (according to body weight), placebo, <u>or</u> 75 mg of *oseltamivir* twice a day for five days, within 48 hours of experiencing flu symptoms. **Xofluza** was granted priority review (FDA action on an application within an expedited time frame where the agency determines that the drug, if approved, would significantly improve the safety <u>or</u> effectiveness of treating, diagnosing, <u>or</u> preventing a serious condition). Co-administration with polyvalent cation-containing products may decrease plasma concentrations of *baloxavir,* which may reduce **Xofluza** efficacy. Therefore, avoid co-administration of **Xofluza** with polyvalent cation-containing laxatives, antacids, <u>or</u> oral supplements (e.g., calcium, iron, magnesium, selenium, <u>or</u> zinc). The concurrent use of **Xofluza** with intranasal live attenuated influenza vaccine (LAIV) has <u>not</u> been evaluated. Concurrent administration of antiviral drugs may inhibit viral replication of LAIV and thereby decrease the effectiveness of LAIV vaccination. Interactions between inactivated influenza vaccines and **Xofluza** have <u>not</u> been evaluated. It is <u>not</u> known if **Xofluza** is safe and effective in children younger than 12 years-of-age <u>or</u> weighing less than 88 pounds (40 kg). Safety in pregnancy is unknown. It is <u>not</u> known whether **Xofluza** is present in breastmilk <u>or</u> effects on the breastfed infant.

INSECT BITE/STING

Topical Corticosteroids *see* Appendix K: Topical Corticosteroids by Potency
Parenteral Corticosteroids *see* Appendix M. Parenteral Corticosteroids
Oral Corticosteroids *see* Appendix L. Oral Corticosteroids

TOPICAL AND TRANSDERMAL ANESTHETICS

Comment: *lidocaine* should <u>not</u> be applied to non-intact skin.

▷ *lidocaine* cream (B) apply to affected area bid prn
   Pediatric: <12 years: not recommended; ≥12 years: same as adult
      LidaMantle *Crm:* 3% (1, 2 oz)
      Lidoderm *Crm:* 3% (85 gm)
      ZTlido *lidocaine* topical system 1% (30/carton)
      Comment: Compared to **Lidoderm** (*lidocaine* patch 5%), which contains 700 mg/patch, **ZTlido** <u>only</u> requires 35 mg per topical system to achieve the same therapeutic dose.

▷ *lidocaine* lotion (B) apply to affected area bid prn
   Pediatric: <12 years: not recommended; ≥12 years: same as adult
      LidaMantle *Lotn:* 3% (177 ml)

▷ *lidocaine* 5% patch (B)(G) apply up to 3 patches at one time for up to 12 hours/24-hour period (12 hours on/12 hours off); patches may be cut into smaller sizes before removal of the release liner; do <u>not</u> re-use
   Pediatric: <12 years: not recommended; ≥12 years: same as adult
      Lidoderm *Patch:* 5% (10x14 cm; 30/carton)

▷ *lidocaine+dexamethasone* (B)
   Pediatric: <12 years: not recommended; ≥12 years: same as adult
      Decadron Phosphate with Xylocaine *Lotn:* dexa 4 mg+lido 10 mg per ml (5 ml)

▷ *lidocaine+hydrocortisone* (B)(G) apply to affected area bid prn
   Pediatric: <12 years: not recommended; ≥12 years: same as adult
      LidaMantle HC *Crm:* lido 3%+hydro 0.5% (1, 3 oz); *Lotn:* (177 ml)

▷ *lidocaine 2.5%+prilocaine 2.5%* apply sparingly to the burn bid-tid prn
   Pediatric: <12 years: not recommended; ≥12 years: same as adult
      Emla Cream (B) 5, 30 gm/tube

EPINEPHRINE

▷ *epinephrine* (C)(G) 1:1,000 0.3-0.5 ml SC
   Pediatric: 0.01 ml/kg SC

TETANUS PROPHYLAXIS

▷ *tetanus toxoid* vaccine (C)(G) 0.5 ml IM x 1 dose if previously immunized
   Vial: 5 Lf units/0.5 ml (0.5, 5 ml); *Prefilled syringe:* 5 Lf units/0.5 ml (0.5 ml) (For patients <u>not</u> previously immunized *see Tetanus*)

○ **INSOMNIA**

Tricyclic Antidepressants *see Depression*

MELATONIN RECEPTOR AGONIST

▷ *ramelteon* (C)(IV) 8 mg within 30 minutes of bedtime; delayed effect if taken with a meal
   Pediatric: <12 years: not recommended; ≥12 years: same as adult
      Rozerem *Tab:* 8 mg

NON-BENZODIAZEPINES

▷ *eszopiclone* (C)(IV)(G) (pyrrolopyrazine) 1-3 mg; max 3 mg/day x 1 month; do <u>not</u> take if unable to sleep for at least 8 hours before required to be active again; delayed effect if taken with a meal

Pediatric: <18 years: not recommended; ≥18 years: same as adult
> **Lunesta** *Tab:* 1, 2, 3 mg

▷ *zaleplon* (C)(IV) (imidazopyridine) 5-10 mg at HS or after going to bed if unable to sleep; do not take if unable to sleep for at least 4 hours before required to be active again; max 20 mg/day x 1 month; delayed effect if taken with a meal
Pediatric: <12 years: not recommended; ≥12 years: same as adult
> **Sonata** *Cap:* 5, 10 mg (tartrazine)
> Comment: **Sonata** is indicated for the treatment of insomnia when a middle-of-the-night awakening is followed by difficulty returning to sleep.

▷ *zolpidem* oral solution spray (C)(IV) (imidazopyridine hypnotic) 2 actuations (10 mg) immediately before bedtime; *Elderly, debilitated, or hepatic impairment:* 2 actuations (5 mg); max 2 actuations (10 mg)
Pediatric: <18 years: not recommended; ≥18 years: same as adult
> **ZolpiMist** *Oral soln spray:* 5 mg/actuation (60 metered actuations) (cherry)
> Comment: The lowest dose of *zolpidem* in all forms is recommended for persons >50 years-of-age and women as drug elimination is slower than in men.

▷ *zolpidem* tabs (B)(IV)(G) (pyrazolopyrimidine hypnotic) 5-10 mg or 6.25-12.5 ext-rel q HS prn; max 12.5 mg/day x 1 month; do not take if unable to sleep for at least 8 hours before required to be active again; delayed effect if taken with a meal
Pediatric: <18 years: not recommended; ≥18 years: same as adult
> **Ambien** *Tab:* 5, 10 mg
> **Ambien CR** *Tab:* 6.25, 12.5 mg ext-rel
> Comment: The lowest dose of *zolpidem* in all forms is recommended for persons >50 years-of-age and women as drug elimination is slower than in men.

▷ *zolpidem* sublingual tabs (C)(IV)(G) (imidazopyridine hypnotic) dissolve 1 tab under the tongue; allow to disintegrate completely before swallowing; take only once per night and only if at least 4 hours of bedtime remain before planned time for awakening
Pediatric: <18 years: not recommended; ≥18 years: same as adult
> **Edluar** *SL Tab:* 5, 10 mg
> **Intermezzo** *SL Tab:* 1.75, 3.5 mg
> Comment: **Intermezzo** is indicated for the treatment of insomnia when a middle-of-the-night awakening is followed by difficulty returning to sleep. The lowest dose of *zolpidem* in all forms is recommended for persons >50 years-of-age and women as drug elimination is slower than in men.

OREXIN RECEPTOR ANTAGONIST

▷ *suvorexant* (C)(IV) use lowest effective dose; take 30 minutes before bedtime; do not take if unable to sleep for ≥7 hours, max 20 mg
Pediatric: <12 years: not recommended; ≥12 years: same as adult
> **Belsomra** *Tab:* 5, 10, 15, 20 mg (30/blister pck)

BENZODIAZEPINES

▷ *estazolam* (X)(IV)(G) initially 1 mg q HS prn; may increase to 2 mg q HS
Pediatric: <18 years: not recommended; ≥18 years: same as adult
> **ProSom** *Tab:* 1*, 2*mg

▷ *flurazepam* (X)(IV)(G) 30 mg q HS prn; elderly or debilitated, 15 mg
Pediatric: <15 years: not recommended; ≥15 years: same as adult
> **Dalmane** *Cap:* 15, 30 mg

▷ *temazepam* (X)(IV)(G) 7.5-30 mg q HS prn; short term, 7-10 days; max 30 mg; max 1 month
Pediatric: <18 years: not recommended; ≥18 years: same as adult
> **Restoril** *Cap:* 7.5, 15, 22.5, 30 mg

▷ *triazolam* (X)(IV) 0.125-0.25 mg q HS prn; short term, 7-10 days; max 0.5 mg; max 1 month
  Pediatric: <18 years: not recommended; ≥18 years: same as adult
    Halcion *Tab:* 0.125, 0.25*mg
    Barbiturates
▷ *pentobarbital* (D)(II)(G)
    Nembutal 100 mg q HS prn
      Cap: 50, 100 mg
    Nembutal Suppository 120 or 200 mg suppository rectally q HS prn
    Pediatric: 2-12 months (10-20 lb): 30 mg supp; 1-4 years (21-40 lb): 30 or 60 mg supp; 5-12 years (41-80 lb): 60 mg supp; 12-14 years (81-110 lb): 60 or 120 mg sup
      Rectal supp: 30, 60, 120, 200 mg

ORAL H1 RECEPTOR AGONIST (FIRST GENERATION ANTIHISTAMINE)

▷ *doxepin* (C)
    Silenor 3-6 mg q HS prn; *Elderly, hepatic impairment, tendency to urinary retention:* initially 3 mg
      Tab: 3, 6 mg

Other Oral 1st Generation Antihistamines *see* Appendix AA. Drugs for the Management of Allergy, Cough, and Cold Symptoms online at https://connect. springerpub.com/content/reference-book/978-0-8261-7935-7/back-matter/part02/back-matter/bmatter27

DUAL OREXIN RECEPTOR ANTAGONIST (DORA)

▷ *lemborexant* (controlled substance schedule pending) *Recommended Dose:* 5 mg once nightly, immediately before going to bed, with at least 7 hours remaining before the planned time of awakening; time to sleep onset may be delayed if taken with or soon after a meal; may increase to max 10 mg based on clinical response and tolerability; *Moderate Hepatic Impairment:* max 5 mg once nightly; *Severe Hepatic Impairment:* not recommended
  Pediatric: safety and efficacy not established
    Dayvigo *Tab:* 5, 10 mg
    Comment: Dayvigo *(lemborexant)* is dual orexin receptor antagonist (DORA) for the treatment of adult patients with insomnia, characterized by difficulties with sleep onset and/or sleep maintenance. The CNS depressant effects of **Dayvigo** impair alertness and motor coordination, including morning impairment. Risk increases with dose and concomitant use with other CNS depressants. **Dayvigo** is contraindicated in patients with narcolepsy. Sleep Paralysis, hypnogogic/hypnopompic hallucinations, and cataplexy-like symptoms may be experienced. Complex sleep behaviors (CSB) including sleep-walking, sleep-driving, and engaging in other activities while not fully awake may occur; if this happens, discontinue **Dayvigo** immediately. Patients should be cauthioned regarding potential worsening of depression or suicidal ideation. The most common adverse reaction reported (incidence ≥5% and at least twice the rate of placebo) has been somnolence. Avoid concomitant use of strong or moderate CYP3A inhibitors, weak CYP3A inhibitors, and strong or moderate CYP3A inducers. There are no available data on **Dayvigo** use in pregnant women to assess drug-associated risk of major birth defects, miscarriage, or adverse maternal or fetal outcomes. There are no data on the presence of *lemborexant* in human milk or effects on the breastfed infant. There is a pregnancy exposure registry that monitors pregnancy outcomes in women who are exposed to **Dayvigo** during pregnancy. Healthcare providers are encouraged to register patients in the **Dayvigo** pregnancy registry by calling 1-888-274-2378.

ANALGESIC+FIRST GENERATION ANTIHISTAMINE COMBINATIONS

▷ *acetaminophen+diphenhydramine* (B)

    Excedrin PM (OTC) 2 tabs q HS prn
      Pediatric: <12 years: not recommended; ≥12 years: same as adult
      Tab/Geltab: acet 500 mg+diphen 38 mg

    Tylenol PM (OTC) 2 caps q HS prn
      Pediatric: <12 years: not recommended; ≥12 years: same as adult
      Tab/Cap/Gel cap: acet 500 mg+diphen 25 mg

 INTERSTITIAL CYSTITIS

Acetaminophen for IV Infusion *see* **Pain**
Oral Prescription NSAIDs *see* Appendix J. NSAIDs online at https://connect.
springerpub.com/content/reference-book/978-0-8261-7935-7/back-matter/part02/
back-matter/bmatter10
Comment: Avoid peppers and spicy food, citrus, vinegar, caffeine (e.g., coffee, tea,
colas), alcohol, carbonated beverages, and other GU tract irritants.

MANAGEMENT OF PAIN AND URINARY URGENCY

▷ *phenazopyridine* (B)(G) 95-200 mg q 6 hours prn; max 2 days
    Pediatric: <12 years: not recommended; ≥12 years: same as adult
      AZO Standard, Prodium, Uristat (OTC) *Tab:* 95 mg
      AZO Standard Maximum Strength (OTC) *Tab:* 97.5 mg
      Pyridium, Urogesic *Tab:* 100, 200 mg *phenazopyridine* (B)(G) 190-200 mg
      tid; max 2 days
      Azo Standard (OTC) *Tab:* 95 mg
      Azo Standard Maximum Strength (OTC) *Tab:* 97.5 mg
      Pyridium *Tab:* 100, 200 mg ent-coat
      Uristat (OTC) *Tab:* 95 mg
      Urogesic *Tab:* 100, 200 mg

▷ *hyoscyamine* (C)(G)
      Anaspaz 1-2 tabs q 4 hours prn; max 12 tabs/day
      Pediatric: <2 years: not recommended; 2-12 years: 0.0625-0.125 mg q 4 hours
      prn; max 0.75 mg/day; ≥12 years: same as adult
        Tab: 0.125*mg
      Levbid 1-2 tabs q 12 hours prn; max 4 tabs/day
      Pediatric: <12 years: not recommended; ≥12 years: same as adult
        Tab: 0.375*mg ext-rel
      Levsin 1-2 tabs q 4 hours prn; max 12 tabs/day
      Pediatric: <6 years: not recommended; 6-12 years: 1 tab q 4 hours prn; ≥12
      years: same as adult
        Tab: 0.125*mg
      Levsin Drops 1-2 ml q 4 hours prn; max 60 ml/day
      Pediatric: 3.4 kg: 4 drops q 4 hours prn; max 24 drops/day; 5 kg: 5 drops q 4
      hours prn; max 30 drops/day; 7 kg: 6 drops q 4 hours prn; max 36 drops/day;
      10 kg: 8 drops q 4 hours prn; max 40 drops/day
        Oral drops: 0.125 mg/ml (15 ml) (orange) (alcohol 5%)
      Levsin Elixir 5-10 ml q 4 hours prn
      Pediatric: <10 kg: use drops; 10-19 kg: 1.25 ml q 4 hours prn; 20-39 kg: 2.5 ml
      q 4 hours prn; 40-49 kg: 3.75 ml q 4 hours prn; ≥50 kg: 5 ml q 4 hours prn;
        Elix: 0.125 mg/5 ml (16 oz) (orange) (alcohol 20%)
      Levsinex SL 1-2 tabs q 4 hours SL <u>or</u> PO; max 12 tabs/day
      Pediatric: <2 years: not recommended; 2-12 years: 1 tab q 4 hours; max 6 tabs/
      day; ≥12 years: same as adult
        SL tab: 0.125 mg

Levsinex Timecaps 1-2 caps q 12 hours; may adjust to 1 cap q 8 hours
Pediatric: <2 years: not recommended; 2-12 years: 1 cap q 12 hours; max 2 caps/day; ≥12 years: same as adult
   Cap: 0.375 mg time-rel

NuLev dissolve 1-2 tabs on tongue, with or without water, q 4 hours prn; max 12 tabs/day
Pediatric: <2 years: not recommended; 2-12 years: dissolve 1 tab on tongue, with or without water, q 4 hours prn; max 6 tabs/day; ≥12 years: same as adult
   ODT: 0.125 mg (mint) (phenylalanine)

▷ *methenamine+sod phosphate monobasic+phenyl salicylate+methylene blue+hyoscyamine sulfate* (C) 1 cap qid
Pediatric: <6 years: not recommended; ≥6 years: individualize dose
   Uribel *Cap:* meth 118 mg+sod phos 40.8 mg+phenyl sal 36 mg+meth blue 10 mg+hyoscy 0.12 mg

▷ *methenamine+phenyl salicylate+methylene blue+benzoic acid+atropine sulfate+hyoscyamine sulfate* (C)(G) 2 tabs qid
Pediatric: <6 years: not recommended; ≥6 years: same as adult
   Urised *Tab:* meth 40.8 mg+phenyl sal 18.1 mg+meth blue 5.4 mg+benz acid 4.5 mg+atro sul 0.03 mg+hyoscy 0.03 mg
   Comment: **Urised** imparts a blue-green color to urine which may stain fabrics.

▷ *oxybutynin chloride* (B)
   Ditropan 5 mg bid-tid; max 20 mg/day
Pediatric: <5 years: not recommended; 5-12 years: 5 mg bid; max 15 mg/day; ≥12 years: same as adult
   Tab: 5*mg; *Syr:* 5 mg/5 ml
   Ditropan XL initially 5 mg daily; may increase weekly in 5-mg increments as needed; max 30 mg/day
Pediatric: <5 years: not recommended; ≥5 years: same as adult
   Tab: 5, 10, 15 mg ext-rel

▷ *pentosan* (B) 100 mg tid; reevaluate at 3 and 6 months
Pediatric: <16 years: not recommended; ≥16 years: same as adult
   Elmiron *Cap:* 100 mg

URINARY TRACT ANALGESIA

▷ *phenazopyridine* (B)(G) 95-200 mg q 6 hours prn; max 2 days
Pediatric: <12 years: not recommended; ≥12 years: same as adult
   AZO Standard, Prodium, Uristat (OTC) *Tab:* 95 mg
   AZO Standard Maximum Strength (OTC) *Tab:* 97.5 mg
   Pyridium, Urogesic *Tab:* 100, 200 mg
   Azo Standard (OTC) *Tab:* 95 mg
   Azo Standard Maximum Strength (OTC) *Tab:* 97.5 mg
   Pyridium *Tab:* 100, 200 mg ent-coat
   Uristat (OTC) *Tab:* 95 mg
   Urogesic *Tab:* 100, 200 mg
   Comment: *Phenazopyridine* imparts an orange-red color to urine which may stain fabrics.

▷ *propantheline* (C) 15-30 mg tid
   Pro-Banthine *Tab:* 7.5, 15 mg

▷ *tolterodine tartrate* (C)(G) **Detrol** 1-2 mg bid or **Detrol LA** 2-4 mg once daily or **Detrol XL** one tab daily
Pediatric: <12 years: not recommended; ≥12 years: same as adult
   Detrol *Tab:* 1, 2 mg
   Detrol *Cap:* 2, 4 mg ext-rel
   Detrol XL *Tab:* 5, 10, 15 mg ext-rel

ANTICHOLINERGIC+SEDATIVE COMBINATION

▷ *chlordiazepoxide+clidinium* (D)(IV) 1-2 caps ac and HS; max 8 caps/day
  Pediatric: <12 years: not recommended; ≥12 years: same as adult
    Librax *Cap:* chlor 5 mg+clid 2.5 mg

TRICYCLIC ANTIDEPRESSANTS (TCAs)

▷ *amitriptyline* (C)(G) 25-50 mg q HS
  Pediatric: <12 years: not recommended; ≥12 years: same as adult
    Tab: 10, 25, 50, 75, 100, 150 mg
▷ *imipramine* (C)(G)
  Pediatric: <12 years: not recommended; ≥12 years: same as adult
    Tofranil initially 75 mg daily (max 200 mg); adolescents initially 30-40 mg
    daily (max 100 mg/day); if maintenance dose exceeds 75 mg daily, may switch
    to **Tofranil PM** for divided or bedtime dose
    Tab: 10, 25, 50 mg
    Tofranil PM initially 75 mg daily 1 hour before HS; max 200 mg
    Cap: 75, 100, 125, 150

◯ INTERTRIGO

See **Candidiasis: Skin**
Topical Antifungals *see Tinea Corporis*
Topical Anti-infectives *see Skin Infection: Bacterial*
Topical Corticosteroids *see* Appendix K: Topical Corticosteroids by Potency
OTC hydrocortisone 1% paste or ointment
OTC Zinc Oxide paste or ointment
OTC A&D Ointment

Comment: Intertrigo is an irritant dermatitis in the intertriginous zones (skin
creases and folds) characterized by inflammation and excoriation caused by
skin-to-skin friction, moisture, and heat and may be itching, stinging, burning
with a musty odor. Common areas at risk include breast folds, axillae, groin folds,
buttocks folds, and the abdominal panniculus in obese persons, finger, and toe
webs. Treatment includes keeping the areas clean, moisture-free, application of a
steroid cream, and a protective lubricant barrier. Intertrigo may be complicated by
a superimposed infection such as yeast (*Candida albicans*), dermatophytic fungi, or
bacteria. Oral agents may be required based on severity of the skin breakdown and
invasive infectious process. Apply appropriate topical anti-infective first and barrier
product last. Non-medicated powders (e.g., corn starch) are contraindicated in the
affected areas as they trap moisture. Exposure to light and air when possible and as
appropriate facilitates integumentary healing.

◯ INTRA-ABDOMINAL INFECTION: COMPLICATED (cIAI)

PARENTERAL CEPHALOSPORIN ANTIBACTERIAL+BETA-LACTAMASE INHIBITOR

▷ *ceftazidime+avibactam* (B) infuse dose over 2 hours; recommended duration of
  treatment: 5 to 4 days; *CrCl 31-50 mL/min:* 1.25 gm every 8 hours; *CrCl 16-30
  mL/min:* 0.94 gm every 12 hours; *CrCl 6-15 mL/min:* 0.94 gm every 24 hours;
  CrCl ≤5 mL/min: 0.94 gm every 48 hours; both *ceftazidime* and *avibactam* are
  hemodialyzable; thus, administer **Avycaz** after hemodialysis on hemodialysis days
  Pediatric: <18 years: not recommended; ≥18 years: same as adult
    Avycaz *Vial:* 2.5 gm, single-dose, pwdr for reconstitution and IV infusion
    Comment: **Avycaz** 2.5 gm contains *ceftazidime* (a cephalosporin) 2 gm
    (equivalent to 2.635 gm of *ceftazidime pentahydrate/sodium carbonate*

powder) and *avibactam* (a beta lactam inhibitor) 0.5 gm (equivalent to 0.551 gm of *avibactam sodium*). As only limited clinical safety and efficacy data for **Avycaz** are currently available, reserve **Avycaz** for use in patients who have limited or no alternative treatment options. To reduce the development of drug-resistant bacteria and maintain the effectiveness of **Avycaz** and other antibacterial drugs, **Avycaz** should be used only to treat infections that are proven or strongly suspected to be caused by susceptible bacteria. Seizures and other neurologic events may occur, especially in patients with renal impairment. Adjust dose in patients with renal impairment. Decreased efficacy in patients with baseline CrCl 30--≤50 mL/min. Monitor CrCl at least daily in patients with changing renal function and adjust the dose of **Avycaz** accordingly. Monitor for hypersensitivity reactions, including anaphylaxis and serious skin reactions. Cross-hypersensitivity may occur in patients with a history of penicillin allergy. If an allergic reaction occurs, discontinue **Avycaz**. *Clostridioides difficile*-associated diarrhea CDAD) has been reported with nearly all systemic antibacterial agents, including **Avycaz**. There are no adequate and well-controlled studies of **Avycaz**, *ceftazidime*, or *avibactam* in pregnant females. *ceftazidime* is excreted in human milk in low concentrations. It is not known whether *avibactam* is excreted into human milk. There are no studies to inform effects on the breastfed infant.

▷ *ceftolozane+tazobactam* administer 1.5 gm every 8 hours via IV infusion over 1 hour x 4-14 days; *CrCl 30-50 ml/min:* 750 mg via IV infusion every 8 hours; *CrCl 15-29 ml/min:* 375 mg via IV infusion every 8 hours; *ESRD:* a single loading dose of 750 mg via IV infusion, followed by 150 mg via IV infusion every 8 hours for the remainder of the treatment period (on hemodialysis days, administer the dose at the earliest possible time following completion of dialysis)

Pediatric: <18: not established; ≥18 years: same as adult

Zerbaxa *Vial:* 1.5 gm (*ceftolozane* 1 gm+*tazobactam* 0.5 gm), single-dose, pwdr for reconstitution and IV infusion

Comment: For doses >1.5 gm, reconstitute a second vial in the same manner as the first one, withdraw an appropriate volume (see Table 3 in the mfr pkg insert) and add to the same infusion bag. The most common adverse reactions in patients with cIAI (incidence ≥5%) have been nausea, diarrhea, headache, and pyrexia.

PARENTERAL PENEM ANTIBACTERIAL+RENAL DEHYDROPEPTIDASE INHIBITOR+ BETA-LACTAMASE INHIBITOR

▷ *imipenem+cilastatin+relebactam* administer dose via IV infusion over 30 minutes every 6 hours; *CrCL ≥90 mL/min:* 1.25 gm/dose (*imipenem* 500 mg, *cilastatin* 500 mg, *relebactam* 250 mg); *CrCL 60-89 mL/min:* 1 gm/dose (*imipenem* 400 mg, *cilastatin* 400 mg, *relebactam* 200 mg) *CrCL 30-59 mL/min:* 0.75 gm/dose (*imipenem* 300 mg, *cilastatin* 300 mg, *relebactam* 150 mg); *CrCL 15-29 mL/min:* 0.5 gm/dose (*imipenem* 200 mg, *cilastatin* 200 mg, *relebactam* 100 mg); *ESRD/Dialysis:* 0.5 gm/dose (*imipenem* 200 mg, *cilastatin* 200 mg, *relebactam* 100 mg)

Pediatric: <18 years: not established; ≥18 years: same as adult

Recarbrio *Vial:* impen 500 mg+cilast 500 mg+relebac 250 mg, single-dose, pwdr for reconstitution, dilution, and IV infusion

Comment: **Recarbrio** (*imipenem+cilastatin+relebactam)* is a fixed-dose triple combination of *imipenem* (a penem antibacterial), *cilastatin* (a renal dehydropeptidase inhibitor), and *relebactam* (a beta-lactamase inhibitor) indicated for the treatment of complicated urinary tract infection (cUTI), including pyelonephritis, and complicated intra-abdominal infection (cIAI) caused by susceptible gram-negative bacteria in patients who have limited or no alternative treatment options, hospital-acquired bacterial pneumonia

(HABP), and ventilator-associated bacterial pneumonia (VABP) in adults. Avoid concomitant use of **Recarbrio** with *ganciclovir*, *valproic acid*, or *divalproex sodium*. Based on clinical reports on patients treated with imipenem/cilastatin plus relebactam 250 mg, the most frequent adverse reactions (incidence ≥2 %) have been diarrhea, nausea, headache, vomiting, alanine aminotransferase increased, aspartate aminotransferase increased, phlebitis/infusion site reactions, pyrexia, and hypertension. There are insufficient human data to establish whether there is a drug-associated risk for major birth defects, miscarriage, or adverse maternal or fetal outcomes with *imipenem*, *cilastatin*, or *relebactam* in prenanancy. However, embryonic loss has been observed in monkeys treated with *imipenem/cilastatin*, and fetal abnormalities have been observed in *relebactam*-treated mice; therefore, advise pregnant females of the potential risks to pregnancy and the fetus. There are insufficient data on the presence of *imipenem/cilastatin* and *relebactam* in human milk, and no data on the effects on the breastfed infant; However, *relebactam* is present in the milk of lactating rats and, therefore, developmental and health benefits of breastfeeding should be considered along with the mother's clinical need for **Recarbrio** and any potential adverse effects on the breastfed child from **Recarbrio** or from the underlying maternal condition.

PARENTERAL TETRACYCLINE-CLASS (FLUOROCYCLINE) ANTIBACTERIAL

▶ *eravacycline* 1 mg/kg by intravenous infusion over approximately 60 minutes every 12 hours x 4-14 days; *Severe Hepatic Impairment (Child Pugh Class C)*: 1 mg/kg every 12 hours on Day 1, then 1 mg/kg every 24 hours starting on Day 2 for a total duration of 4-14 days; *Concomitant Use of a Strong Cytochrome P450 Isoenzymes (CYP)3A Inducer*: 1.5 mg/kg every 12 hours x 4-14 days
Pediatric: <18 years: not established; ≥18 years: same as adult

Xerava *Vial*: 50 mg pwdr for IV reconstitution and further dilution for IV infusion, single use

Comment: **Xerava** *(eravacycline)* is a tetracycline-class (fluorocycline) antibacterial indicated for the treatment of complicated intra-abdominal infections in patients ≥18 years-of-age. **Xerava** is not indicated for the treatment of complicated urinary tract infections (cUTI). Patients who are on anticoagulant therapy may require downward adjustment of their anticoagulant dosage. Most common adverse reactions (incidence ≥3%) have been infusion site reactions, nausea, and vomiting. The use of **Xerava** during tooth development (last half of pregnancy, infancy and childhood up to 8 years-of-age) may cause permanent discoloration of the teeth (yellow-gray-brown) and enamel hypoplasia. The use of **Xerava** during the second and third trimester of pregnancy, infancy and childhood up to 8 years-of-age may cause reversible inhibition of bone growth. *erevacycline* and its metabolites are excreted in breast milk. Breastfeeding is not recommended; consider fetal risk and maternal benefit.

IRITIS: ACUTE

▶ *loteprednol etabonate* (C)(G) 1-2 drops qid; may increase to 1 drop hourly as needed
Pediatric: <12 years: not recommended; ≥12 years: same as adult

Lotemax Ophthalmic Gel *Ophth gel*: 0.5% (5 gm)
Lotemax Ophthalmic Ointment *oint*: 0.5% (3.5 gm)
Lotemax Ophthalmic Solution *Ophth soln*: 0.3% (2.5, 5, 10, 15 ml)
Lotemax SM *Ophth gel*: 0.38% (5 gm)

▷ *prednisone acetate* (C)(G) 1 drop q 1 hour x 24-48 hours, then 1 drop q 2 hours while awake x 24-48 hours, then 1 drop bid-qid until resolved
Pediatric: <12 years: not recommended; ≥12 years: same as adult
  Pred Forte Ophth soln: 1% (1, 5, 10, 15 ml)

⊙ IRON OVERLOAD

IRON CHELATING AGENTS

▷ *deferiprone* 25 mg/kg to 33 mg/kg 3 x/day (total daily dose 75 mg/kg to 99 mg/)
Pediatric: <3 years: safety and efficacy not established; ≥3-8 years: same as adult (use oral soln); ≥8 years: same as adult (use tablet form)
  Ferriprox Tab: 500, 1000 mg film-coat (5 x 10-count blister packs/carton), adults and patients ≥8 years-of-age; *Oral soln:* 80, 100 mg/ml (20 gm/250 ml, 40 gm/500 ml w. graduated measuring cup)
  Comment: **Ferriprox** is an iron chelator agent indicated for the treatment of transfusional iron overload in patients with thalassemia syndromes and patients with sickle cell disease or other anemias. Safety and efficacy have not been established for the treatment of transfusional iron overload in patients with myelodysplastic syndrome or in patients with Diamond Blackfan anemia. The most common adverse reactions in patients with thalassemia (incidence ≥6%) have been nausea, vomiting, abdominal pain, arthralgia, increased ALT, and neutropenia. The most common adverse reactions in patients with sickle cell disease or other anemias (incidence ≥6%) have been pyrexia, abdominal pain, bone pain, headache, vomiting, pain in extremity, sickle cell anemia with crisis, back pain, increased ALT, increased AST, arthralgia, oropharyngeal pain, nasopharyngitis, decreased neutrophil count, cough, and nausea. Monitor liver enzymes monthly and discontinue for persistent elevations. Monitor for zinc deficiency and supplement as indicated. *BBW:* **Ferriprox** can cause agranulocytosis that can lead to serious infections and death. Neutropenia may precede the development of agranulocytosis; Measure the absolute neutrophil count (ANC) before starting **Ferriprox** and monitor weekly while on therapy. Interrupt **Ferriprox** if infection develops and monitor the ANC more frequently. Advise patients to immediately report any symptoms indicative of infection. Avoid co-administration of drugs associated with neutropenia or agranulocytosis. If co-administration is unavoidable, closely monitor the absolute neutrophil count. Avoid co-administration with UGT1A6 inhibitors. Allow at least a 4-hour interval between administration of **Ferriprox** and drugs or supplements containing polyvalent cations (e.g., iron, aluminum, or zinc). Limited available data from *deferiprone* use in pregnant females are insufficient to inform a drug-associated risk of major birth defects and miscarriage. Based on animal studies, **Ferriprox** can cause embryo/fetal harm. Advise pregnant females and males and females of reproductive potential of the potential risk and advise to use effective contraception. Advise not to breastfeed.

▷ *deferasirox* (*tridentate ligand*) (C)(G) initially 20 mg/kg/day; titrate; may increase 5-10 mg/kg q 3-6 months based on serum ferritin trends; max 30 mg/kg/day
Pediatric: <2 years: not recommended; ≥2 years: same as adult
  Exjade Tab for oral soln: 125, 250, 500 mg
  Jadenu Tab: 90, 180, 360 mg film-coat
  Jadenu Sprinkle Sachet: 90, 180, 360 mg (30/carton)
  Comment: *Deferasirox* is an orally active chelator selective for iron. It is indicated for the treatment of chronic iron overload due to blood transfusions (transfusional hemosiderosis). Monitor serum ferritin monthly. Consider interrupting therapy if serum ferritin falls below 500 mcg/L. Take *deferasirox* (**Exjade, Jadenu, Jadenu**

Sprinkle) on an empty stomach. Completely disperse tablet(s) or granules in 3.5 oz liquid if dose is ≤1 gm or 7 oz liquid if dose is ≥1 gm.

▷ *Succimer* (C) initially 10 mg/kg q 8 hours x 5 days; then, reduce frequency to every 12 hours x 14 more days; allow at least 14 days between courses unless blood lead levels indicate need for prompt treatment

Pediatric: <12 months: not recommended; ≥12 months: same as adult

Chemet Cap: 100 mg

Comment: **Chemet** is indicated for the treatment of lead poisoning when blood lead level 45 mcg/dL. Treatment for more than 3 consecutive weeks is not recommended. Monitor hydration, renal, and hepatic function.

IRRITABLE BOWEL SYNDROME WITH CONSTIPATION (IBS-C)

Bulk-Producing Agents, Laxatives, Stool Softeners *see Constipation*

GUANYLATE CYCLASE-C AGONIST

Comment: Guanylate cyclase-c agonists increase intestinal fluid and intestinal transit time may induce diarrhea and bloating and, therefore, are contraindicated with known or suspected mechanical GI obstruction.

▷ *linaclotide* (C)(G) 290 mcg once daily; take on an empty stomach at least 30 minutes before the first meal of the day; swallow whole or may open cap and sprinkle on applesauce or in water for administration

Pediatric: <6 years: not recommended; 6-17 years: avoid; >17 years: same as adult

Linzess Cap: 145, 290 mcg

Comment: *Linaclotide* and its active metabolite are negligibly absorbed systemically following oral administration and maternal use is not expected to result in fetal exposure to the drug. There is no information regarding the presence of *plecanatide* in human milk or its effects on the breastfed infant.

CHLORIDE CHANNEL ACTIVATOR

▷ *lubiprostone* (C) 8 mcg bid; *Severe hepatic impairment (Child-Pugh Class C):* 8 mcg once daily; take with food and water; do not break apart or chew

Pediatric: <18 years: not recommended; ≥18 years: same as adult

Amitiza Cap: 8, 24 mcg

Comment: **Amitiza** increases intestinal fluid and intestinal transit time. Suspend dosing and rehydrate if severe diarrhea occurs. **Amitiza** is contraindicated with known or suspected mechanical GI obstruction. Most common adverse reactions in CIC are nausea, diarrhea, headache, abdominal pain, abdominal distension, and flatulence.

SODIUM/HYDROGEN EXCHANGER 3 (NHE3) INHIBITOR

▷ *tenapanor* 50 mg twice daily; administer immediately prior to breakfast or the first meal of the day and immediately prior to dinner; if a dose is missed, skip the missed dose and take the next dose at the regular time; do not take 2 doses at the same time

Pediatric: <6 years: contraindicated; 6-<12 years: avoid use; <18 years: safety not established; ≥18 years: same as adult

Ibsrela Tab: 50 mg

Comment: **Ibsrela** *(tenapanor)* is a first-in-class, sodium/hydrogen exchanger 3 (NHE3) inhibitor indicated for the treatment of adults with irritable bowel syndrome with constipation (IBS-C). **Ibsrela** is contraindicated in pediatric patients <6 years-of-age and patients with known or suspected mechanical gastrointestinal obstruction. Most common adverse reactions (incidence

≥2%) have been diarrhea, abdominal distension, flatulence, and dizziness. If severe diarrhea occurs, suspend dosing and rehydrate the patient. *tenapanor* is minimally absorbed systemically, with plasma concentrations below the limit of quantification (<0.5 ng/mL) following oral administration. Therefore, maternal use is not expected to result in embryo/fetal exposure to the drug. Animal studies, and available data on **Ibsrela** exposure from a small number of pregnant females, have not identified any drug associated risk for major birth defects, miscarriage, or adverse maternal or embryo/fetal outcomes. The minimal systemic absorption of *tenapanor* will not result in a clinically relevant exposure to breastfed infants.

GUANYLATE CYCLASE-C AGONIST

▷ *plecanatide* 3 mg once daily; take with or without food; swallow whole; for patients who have difficulty swallowing tablets whole or those with a nasogastric or gastric feeding tube, see full prescribing information with instructions for crushing the tablet and administering with applesauce or water; if serious dehydration occurs, suspend dosing and institute rehydration measures
Pediatric: <6 years: contraindicated; 6-<18 years: avoid use, safety and efficacy not established; ≥18 years: same as adult
    Trulance Tab: 3 mg
    Comment: **Trulance** *(plecanatide)* is a guanylate cyclase-C agonist indicated for adults for treatment of chronic idiopathic constipation (CIC) and irritable bowel syndrome with constipation (IBS-C). **Trulance** is contraindicated children <6 years-of-age (due to risk of serious dehydration) and patients with known or suspected gastrointestinal obstruction *plecanatide* and its active metabolite are negligibly absorbed systemically following oral administration and maternal use is not expected to result in fetal exposure. No lactation studies in animals have been conducted and there is no information regarding the presence of *plecanatide* in human milk or effects on the breastfed infant.

IRRITABLE BOWEL SYNDROME WITH DIARRHEA (IBS-D)

Bulk-Producing Agents *see Constipation*

CONSTIPATING AGENTS

▷ *difenoxin+atropine* (C) 2 tabs, then 1 tab after each loose stool or 1 tab q 3-4 hours as needed; max 8 tab/day x 2 days
Pediatric: <12 years: not recommended; ≥12 years: same as adult
    Motofen *Tab:* difen 1 mg+atro 0.025 mg
▷ *diphenoxylate+atropine* (C)(G) 2 tabs or 10 ml qid
Pediatric: <2 years: not recommended; 2-12 years: initially 0.3-0.4 mg/kg/day in 4 divided doses; ≥12 years: same as adult
    Lomotil *Tab:* difen 2.5 mg+atro 0.025 mg; *Liq:* difen 2.5 mg+atro 0.025 mg per 5 ml (2 oz)
▷ *eluxadoline* (NA)(IV) 100 mg bid; 75 mg bid if unable to tolerate 100 mg, or without a gall bladder, or mild-to-moderate hepatic impairment, or receiving concomitant OATP1B1 inhibitors
Pediatric: <12 years: not established; ≥12 years: same as adult
    Viberzi 4 mg initially, then 2 mg after each loose stool; max 16 mg/day
      Tab: 75, 100 mg film-coat
Comment: *Eluxadoline* is a mu-opioid receptor agonist. It is contraindicated with biliary obstruction, Sphincter of Oddi disease or dysfunction, alcohol abuse or addiction, pancreatitis, pancreatic duct obstruction, severe hepatic impairment, and mechanical GI obstruction.

▷ *loperamide* (B)(G)

Imodium (OTC) 4 mg initially, then 2 mg after each loose stool; max 16 mg/day

Pediatric: <5 years: not recommended; ≥5 years: same as adult

Cap: 2 mg

Imodium A-D (OTC) 4 mg initially, then 2 mg after each loose stool; usual max 8 mg/day x 2 days

Pediatric: <2 years: not recommended; 2-5 years (24-47 lb): 1 mg up to tid x 2 days; 6-8 years (48-59 lb): 2 mg initially, then 1 mg after each loose stool; max 4 mg/day x 2 days; 9-11 years (60-95 lb): 2 mg initially, then 1 mg after each loose stool; max 6 mg/day x 2 days; ≥12 years: same as adult

Cplt: 2 mg; *Liq:* 1 mg/5 ml (2, 4 oz)

▷ *loperamide+simethicone* (B)(G)

Imodium Advanced (OTC) 2 tabs chewed after loose stool, then 1 after the next loose stool; max 4 tabs/day

Pediatric: <6 years: not recommended; 6-8 years: 1 tab chewed after loose stool, then 1/2 after next loose stool; max 2 tabs/day; 9-11 years: 1 tab chewed after loose stool, then 1/2 after next loose stool; max 3 tabs/day; ≥12 years: same as adult

Chew tab: lop 2 mg+sim 125 mg

SEROTONIN (5-HT3) RECEPTOR ANTAGONIST

▷ *alosetron* (B)(G) initially 0.5 mg bid; may increase to 1 mg bid after 4 weeks if starting dose is tolerated but inadequate

Pediatric: <12 years: not recommended; ≥12 years: same as adult

Lotronex *Tab:* 0.5, 1 mg

ANTISPASMODIC+ANTICHOLINERGIC COMBINATIONS

▷ *dicyclomine* (B)(G) initially 20 mg bid-qid; may increase to 40 mg qid PO; usual IM dose 80 mg/day divided qid; do not use IM route for more than 1-2 days

Pediatric: <12 years: not recommended; ≥12 years: same as adult

Bentyl *Tab:* 20 mg; *Cap:* 10 mg; *Syr:* 10 mg/5 ml (16 oz); *Vial:* 10 mg/ml (10 ml); *Amp:* 10 mg/ml (2 ml)

▷ *methscopolamine bromide* (B) 1 tab q 6 hours prn

Pediatric: <12 years: not recommended; ≥12 years: same as adult

Pamine *Tab:* 2.5 mg

Pamine Forte *Tab:* 5 mg

ANTICHOLINERGICS

▷ *hyoscyamine* (C)(G)

Anaspaz 1-2 tabs q 4 hours prn; max 12 tabs/day

Pediatric: <2 years: not recommended; 2-12 years: 0.0625-0.125 mg q 4 hours prn; max 0.75 mg/day; ≥12 years: same as adult

Tab: 0.125*mg

Levbid 1-2 tabs q 12 hours prn; max 4 tabs/day

Pediatric: <12 years: not recommended; ≥12 years: same as adult

Tab: 0.375*mg ext-rel

Levsin 1-2 tabs q 4 hours prn; max 12 tabs/day

Pediatric: <6 years: not recommended; 6-12 years: 1 tab q 4 hours prn; >12 years: same as adult

Tab: 0.125*mg

Levsinex SL 1-2 tabs q 4 hours SL or PO; max 12 tabs/day

Pediatric: <2 years: not recommended; 2-12 years: 1 tab q 4 hours; max 6 tabs/day; >12 years: same as adult

Tab: 0.125 mg sublingual

Levsinex Timecaps 1-2 caps q 12 hours; may adjust to 1 cap q 8 hours
Pediatric: <2 years: not recommended; 2-12 years: 1 cap q 12 hours; max 2 caps/day; >12 years: same as adult
   Cap: 0.375 mg time-rel
NuLev dissolve 1-2 tabs on tongue, with or without water, q 4 hours prn; max 12 tabs/day
Pediatric: <2 years: not recommended; 2-12 years: dissolve 1 tab on tongue, with or without water, q 4 hours prn; max 6 tabs/day; >12 years: same as adult
   ODT: 0.125 mg (mint; phenylalanine)
▷ *simethicone* (C)(G) 0.3 ml qid pc and HS
   Mylicon Drops (OTC) *Oral drops:* 40 mg/0.6 ml (30 ml)
▷ *phenobarbital+hyoscyamine+atropine+scopolamine* (C)(IV)(G)
   Donnatal 1-2 tabs ac and HS
   Pediatric: <12 years: not recommended; ≥12 years: same as adult
     Tab: pheno 16.2 mg+hyo 0.1037 mg+atro 0.0194 mg+scop 0.0065 mg
   Donnatal Elixir 1-2 tsp ac and HS
   Pediatric: 20 lb: 1 ml q 4 hours or 1.5 ml q 6 hours; 30 lb: 1.5 ml q 4 hours or 2 ml q 6 hours; 50 lb: 1/2 tsp q 4 hours or 3/4 tsp q 6 hours; 75 lb: 3/4 tsp q 4 hours or 1 tsp q 6 hours; 100 lb: 1 tsp q 4 hours or 1 tsp q 6 hours
     Elix: pheno 16.2 mg+hyo 0.1037 mg+atro 0.0194 mg+scop 0.0065 mg per 5 ml (4, 16 oz)
   Donnatal Extentabs 1 tab q 12 hours
   Pediatric: <12 years: not recommended; ≥12 years: same as adult
     Tab: pheno 48.6 mg+hyo 0.3111 mg+atro 0.0582 mg+scop 0.0195 mg ext-rel

ANTICHOLINERGIC+SEDATIVE COMBINATION

▷ *chlordiazepoxide+clidinium* (D)(IV) 1-2 caps ac and HS: max 8 caps/day
   Pediatric: <12 years: not recommended; ≥12 years: same as adult
   Librax *Cap:* chlor 5 mg+clid 2.5 mg

TRICYCLIC ANTIDEPRESSANTS (TCAs)

▷ *amitriptyline* (C)(G) 25-50 mg q HS
   Pediatric: <12 years: not recommended; ≥12 years: same as adult
   Tab: 10, 25, 50, 75, 100, 150 mg
▷ *imipramine* (C)(G) 25-50 mg tid
   Pediatric: <12 years: not recommended; ≥12 years: same as adult
   Tofranil initially 75 mg daily (max 200 mg); adolescents initially 30-40 mg daily (max 100 mg/day); if maintenance dose exceeds 75 mg daily, may switch to **Tofranil PM** for divided or bedtime dose
     Tab: 10, 25, 50 mg
   Tofranil PM initially 75 mg daily 1 hour before HS; max 200 mg
     Cap: 75, 100, 125, 150
   Tofranil Injection 50 mg IM; lower dose for adolescents; switch to oral form as soon as possible
     Amp: 25 mg/2 ml (2 ml)
▷ *nortriptyline* (D)(G) initially 25 mg tid-qid; max 150 mg/day
   Pediatric: <12 years: not recommended; ≥12 years: same as adult
   Pamelor *Cap:* 10, 25, 50, 75 mg; *Oral soln:* 10 mg/5 ml (16 oz)
▷ *protriptyline* (C) initially 5 mg tid; usual dose 15-40 mg/day in 3-4 divided doses; max 60 mg/day
   Pediatric: <12 years: not recommended; ≥12 years: same as adult
   Vivactil *Tab:* 5, 10 mg
▷ *trimipramine* (C) initially 75 mg/day in divided doses; max 200 mg/day
   Pediatric: <12 years: not recommended; ≥12 years: same as adult
   Surmontil *Cap:* 25, 50, 100 mg

JAPANESE ENCEPHALITIS VIRUS (JEV)

Comment: Japanese encephalitis is a viral disease spread by the bite of an infected mosquito. It is not spread from person-to-person. Currently there is no cure. A person with encephalitis can experience fever, neck stiffness, seizures, and coma. About 1 person in 4 with encephalitis dies. Up to half of those who don't die have permanent disability. There is one vaccine for Japanese encephalitis, currently licensed in the UK, for use in adults and children >2 months-of-age. The **live** attenuated vaccine is administered in two doses for full protection, with the second dose administered 28 days after the first. The second dose should be given at least a week before travel. Children younger than 3 years of age get a smaller dose than patients who are 3 or older. A booster dose might be recommended for anyone 17 or older who was vaccinated more than a year ago and is still at risk of exposure. There is no information yet on the need for a booster dose for children. The (JEV) vaccine is usually available through the local health department.

▷ *Japanese encephalitis vaccine (JEV), inactivated, adsorbed* (B) shake the prefilled syringe containing 0.5 ml to obtain a homogeneous suspension; *18-65 years:* 0.5 ml IM x 2 doses 7-28 days apart; *>65 years:* 0.5 ml IM x 2 doses 28 days apart
Pediatric: shake the prefilled syringe containing 0.5 ml to obtain a homogeneous suspension; <2 months: not recommended; 2 months to <3 years: 0.25 ml IM x 2 doses 28 days apart; 3 to <18 years: 0.5 ml IM x 2 doses 28 days apart

   Ixiaro *Prefilled syringe:* 0.5 ml (protamine sulfate)
   Comment: Administer **Ixiaro** intramuscularly only. Preferred injection sites are the anterolateral aspect of the thigh (LAT) in infants 2 to 11 months-of-age, the anterolateral aspect of the thigh (LAT) or the deltoid muscle if muscle mass is adequate) in children 1 to <3 years-of-age, and the deltoid muscle in patients ≥3 years-of-age. To administer a 0.25 ml JEV dose, expel and discard half of the volume from the 0.5 ml prefilled syringe by pushing the plunger stopper up to the edge of the red line on the syringe barrel prior to injection. Complete the primary immunization series at least 1 week prior to potential exposure to JEV. A booster dose (third dose) may be administered at least 11 months after completion of the primary immunization series if ongoing exposure or re-exposure to JEV is expected. Embryo/fetal effects of JEV exposure in pregnancy and effects on the breastfed infant have not been studied.

JUVENILE IDIOPATHIC ARTHRITIS (JIA), POLYARTICULAR JUVENILE IDIOPATHIC ARTHRITIS (PJIA), SYSTEMIC JUVENILE IDIOPATHIC ARTHRITIS (SJIA)

Acetaminophen for IV Infusion *see Pain*
NSAIDs *see* Appendix J. NSAIDs online at https://connect.springerpub.com/content/reference-book/978-0-8261-7935-7/back-matter/part02/back-matter/bmatter10
Opioid Analgesics *see Pain*
Topical & Transdermal Analgesics *see Pain*
Parenteral Corticosteroids *see* Appendix M. Parenteral Corticosteroids
Oral Corticosteroids *see* Appendix L. Oral Corticosteroids
Topical Analgesic and Anesthetic Agents *see* Appendix I. Anesthetic Agents for Local Infiltration and Dermal/Mucosal Membrane Application online at https://connect.springerpub.com/content/reference-book/978-0-8261-7935-7/back-matter/part02/back-matter/bmatter9

TOPICAL & TRANSDERMAL ANALGESICS

▷ *capsaicin* (B)(G) apply tid or qid prn to intact skin
   Pediatric: <2 years: not recommended; ≥2 years: same as adult
      Axsain *Crm:* 0.075% (1, 2 oz)

Capsin *Lotn:* 0.025, 0.075% (59 ml)
Capzasin-HP (OTC) *Crm:* 0.075% (1.5 oz), 0.025% (45, 90 gm); *Lotn:* 0.075% (2 oz); 0.025% (45, 90 gm)
Capzasin-P (OTC) *Crm:* 0.025% (1.5 oz); *Lotn:* 0.025% (2 oz)
Dolorac *Crm:* 0.025% (28 gm)
Double Cap (OTC) *Crm:* 0.05% (2 oz)
R-Gel *Gel:* 0.025% (15, 30 gm)
Zostrix (OTC) *Crm:* 0.025% (0.7, 1.5, 3 oz)
Zostrix HP (OTC) *Emol crm:* 0.075% (1, 2 oz)

▶ *capsaicin* 8% patch (B) apply up to 4 patches for one 60-minute application to clean dry skin; may prep area with topical anesthetic; wear non-latex gloves; patches may be cut to size/shape; treatment may be repeated every 3 months
Pediatric: <18 years: not recommended; ≥18 years: same as adult
Qutenza *Patch:* 8% 1640 mcg/cm (179 mg) (1 or 2 patches w. 1-50 gm tube cleansing gel/carton)

▶ *diclofenac sodium* (C; D ≥30 wks) apply qid prn to intact skin
Pediatric: <12 years: not established; ≥12 years: same as adult
Pennsaid 1.5% in 10 drop increments, dispense and rub into front, side, and back of knee: usually; 40 drops (40 mg) qid
Topical soln: 1.5% (150 ml)
Pennsaid 2% apply 2 pump actuations (40 mg) and rub into front, side, and back of knee bid
Topical soln: 2% (20 mg/pump actuation, 112 gm)
Solaraze Gel massage in to clean skin bid prn
Gel: 3% (50 gm) (benzyl alcohol)
Voltaren Gel (G)(OTC) apply qid prn to intact skin
Gel: 1% (100 gm)

Comment: *Diclofenac* is contraindicated with *aspirin* allergy. As with other NSAIDs, should be avoided in late pregnancy (≥30 weeks) because it may cause premature closure of the ductus arteriosus.

▶ *doxepin* (B) cream apply to affected area qid at intervals of at least 3-4 hours; max 8 days
Pediatric: <12 years: not recommended; >12 years: same as adult
Prudoxin *Crm:* 5% (45 gm)
Zonalon *Crm:* 5% (30, 45 gm)

▶ *pimecrolimus* 1% cream (C)(G) <2 years: not recommended; ≥2 years: apply to affected area bid; do not apply an occlusive dressing
Elidel *Crm:* 1% (30, 60, 100 gm)

Comment: *Pimecrolimus* is indicated for short-term and intermittent long-term use. Discontinue use when resolution occurs. Contraindicated if the patient is immunosuppressed. Change to the 0.1% preparation or if secondary bacterial infection is present.

▶ *trolamine salicylate* apply tid-qid
Pediatric: <2 years: not recommended; ≥2 years: same as adult
Mobisyl Creme *Crm:* 10% (100 gm)

TOPICAL AND TRANSDERMAL ANESTHETICS

Comment: *Lidocaine* should not be applied to non-intact skin.
▶ *lidocaine* cream (B) apply to affected area bid prn
Pediatric: <12 years: not recommended; ≥12 years: same as adult
LidaMantle *Crm:* 3% (1, 2 oz)
Lidoderm *Crm:* 3% (85 gm)
ZTlido *lidocaine* topical system 1% (30/carton)
Comment: Compared to Lidoderm (*lidocaine* patch 5%), which contains 700 mg/patch, ZTlido requires 35 mg per topical system to achieve the same therapeutic dose.

▷ *lidocaine* lotion (B) apply to affected area bid prn
  Pediatric: <12 years: not recommended; ≥12 years: same as adult
    LidaMantle *Lotn:* 3% (177 ml)

▷ *lidocaine* 5% patch (B)(G) apply up to 3 patches at one time for up to 12 hours/24-hour period (12 hours on/12 hours off); patches may be cut into smaller sizes before removal of the release liner; do <u>not</u> re-use
  Pediatric: <12 years: not recommended; ≥12 years: same as adult
    Lidoderm *Patch:* 5% (10x14 cm; 30/carton)

▷ *lidocaine+dexamethasone* (B)
  Pediatric: <12 years: not recommended; ≥12 years: same as adult
    Decadron Phosphate with Xylocaine *Lotn:* dexa 4 mg+lido 10 mg per ml (5 ml)

▷ *lidocaine+hydrocortisone* (B)(G) apply to affected area bid prn
  Pediatric: <12 years: not recommended; ≥12 years: same as adult
    LidaMantle HC *Crm:* lido 3%+hydro 0.5% (1, 3 oz); *Lotn:* (177 ml)

▷ *lidocaine 2.5%+prilocaine 2.5%* apply sparingly to the burn bid-tid prn
  Pediatric: <12 years: not recommended; ≥12 years: same as adult
    Emla Cream (B) 5, 30 gm/tube

ORAL SALICYLATES

▷ *indomethacin* (C) initially 25 mg bid <u>or</u> tid, increase as needed at weekly intervals by 25-50 mg/day; max 200 mg/day
  Pediatric: <14 years: usually not recommended; >2 years, if risk warranted: 1-2 mg/kg/day in divided doses; max 3-4 mg/kg/day (<u>or</u> 150-200 mg/day, whichever is less; <14 years: ER cap not recommended
  Cap: 25, 50 mg; *Susp:* 25 mg/5 ml (pineapple-coconut, mint) (alcohol 1%); *Supp:* 50 mg; *ER Cap:* 75 mg ext-rel
  Comment: *Indomethacin* is indicated <u>only</u> for acute painful flares. Administer with food <u>and/or</u> antacids. Use lowest effective dose for shortest duration.

METHOTREXATE (MTX)

▷ *methotrexate* (MTX)(X) 7.5 mg x 1 dose per week <u>or</u> 2.5 mg x 3 at 12 hour intervals once a week; max 20 mg/week; therapeutic response begins in 3-6 weeks; administer *methotrexate* injection SC <u>only</u> into the abdomen <u>or</u> thigh
  Pediatric: <2 years: not recommended; ≥2 years: 10 mg/m² once weekly; max 20 mg/m²
    Rasuvo *Autoinjector:* 7.5 mg/0.15 ml, 10 mg/0.20 ml, 12.5 mg/0.25 ml, 15 mg/0.30 ml, 17.5 mg/0.35 ml, 20 mg/0.40 ml, 22.5 mg/0.45 ml, 25 mg/0.50 ml, 27.5 mg/0.55 ml, 30 mg/0.60 ml (solution concentration for SC injection is 50 mg/ml)
    Redi-Trex *Prefilled syringe (in needle safety device):* 7.5, 10, 12.5, 15, 17.5, 20, 22.5, 25 mg, single-dose
    Rheumatrex *Tab:* 2.5*mg (5, 7.5, 10, 12.5, 15 mg/week, 4/card unit dose pack)
    Trexall *Tab:* 5*, 7.5*, 10*, 15*mg (5, 7.5, 10, 12.5, 15 mg/week, 4/card unit dose pack)
  Comment: *Methotrexate* (MTX) is contraindicated with immunodeficiency, blood dyscrasias, alcoholism, and chronic liver disease.

INTERLEUKIN-6 RECEPTOR ANTAGONIST

▷ *tocilizumab* (B) *IV Infusion:* administer over 1 hour; do <u>not</u> administer as bolus <u>or</u> IV push; *Adults, PJIA, and SJIA,* ≥30 kg: dilute to 100 mL in 0.9% <u>or</u> 0.45% NaCl. *PJIA and SJIA,* <30 kg: dilute to 50 mL in 0.9% <u>or</u> 0.45% NaCl.
  Pediatric: <2 years: not recommended; ≥2 years: same as adult
    Adults: IV Infusion: Whether used in combination with DMARDs <u>or</u> as monotherapy, the recommended IV infusion starting dose is 4 mg/kg IV every 4 weeks followed by an increase to 8 mg/kg IV every 4 weeks based on clinical

response; Max 800 mg per infusion in RA patients; *SC Administration:* ≥100 kg: 162 mg SC once weekly on the same day; <100 kg: 162 mg SC every other week on the same day followed by an increase according to clinical response *Pediatric:* <2 years: not recommended; ≥2 years: weight-based dosing according to diagnosis: *PJIA:* ≥30 kg: 8 mg/kg SC every 4 weeks; <30 kg: 10 mg/kg SC every 4 weeks; *SJIA:* ≥30 kg: 8 mg/kg SC every 2 weeks; <30 kg: 12 mg/kg SC every 2 weeks

> **Actemra** *Vial:* 80 mg/4 ml, 200 mg/10 ml, 400 mg/20 ml, single-use, for IV infusion after dilution; *Prefilled syringe:* 162 mg (0.9 ml, single-dose)

Comment: *Tocilizumab* is an interleukin-6 receptor-α inhibitor indicated for use in moderate-to-severe rheumatoid arthritis (RA) that has not responded to conventional therapy, and also for some subtypes of juvenile idiopathic arthritis (JIA). **Actemra** may be used alone or in combination with *methotrexate* (MTX) and in RA, other DMARDs may be used. Monitor patient for dose-related laboratory changes, including elevated LFTs, neutropenia, and thrombocytopenia. **Actemra** should not be initiated in patients with an absolute neutrophil count (ANC) below 2000 per mm^3, platelet count below 100,000 per mm^3, or who have ALT or AST above 1.5 times the upper limit of normal (ULN). Registration in the Pregnancy Exposure Registry (1-877-311-8972) is encouraged for monitoring pregnancy outcomes in women exposed to **Actemra** during pregnancy. The limited available data with **Actemra** in pregnant females are not sufficient to determine whether there is a drug-associated risk for major birth defects and miscarriage. Monoclonal antibodies, such as *tocilizumab*, are actively transported across the placenta during the third trimester of pregnancy and may affect immune response in the infant exposed in *utero*. It is not known whether *tocilizumab* passes into breast milk; therefore, breastfeeding is not recommended while using **Actemra**.

Selective Co-stimulation Modulator

▶ *abatacept* (C) <2 years: not recommended; 2- 17 years: administer as an IV Infusion over 30 minutes at weeks 0, 2, and 4; then every 4 weeks thereafter; <75 kg, administer 10 mg/kg; same as adult (max 1 gm); administer as an IV infusion over 30 minutes at weeks 0, 2, and 4; then every 4 weeks thereafter; <60 kg, administer 500 mg/dose; 60-100 kg, administer 750 mg/dose; >100 kg, administer 1 gm/dose

> **Orencia** *Vial:* 250 mg pwdr for IV infusion after reconstitution (silicone-free) (preservative-free); *Prefilled syringe:* 125 mg/ml soln for SC injection (preservative-free); *ClickJect Autoinjector:* 125 mg/ml soln for SC injection

Comment: **Orencia** is indicated to reduce signs/symptoms of moderate-to-severe active polyarticular juvenile idiopathic arthritis (PJIA) in patients >2 years-of-age as monotherapy or with *methotrexate* (MTX). **Orencia** is also indicated to reduce signs/symptoms, induce major clinical response, inhibit progression of structural damage, and improve physical function in adult patients with moderate-to-severe active RA. **Orencia** may be used as monotherapy or with DMARDs other than TNF antagonists.

TUMOR NECROSIS FACTOR (TNF) BLOCKER

▶ *adalimumab* (B) <10 kg (<22 lb): safety and efficacy not established; 10 kg (22 lb) to <15 kg (<33 lb): 10 mg every other week; 15 kg (33 lb) to <30 kg (<66 lb): 20 mg every other week; ≥30 kg (66 lb) 40 mg every other week; administer SC in the abdomen or thigh; rotate sites

> **Humira** *Prefilled pen (Humira Pen):* 40 mg/0.4 ml, 40 mg/0.8 ml, 80 mg/0.8 ml, single-dose; *Prefilled glass syringe:* 10 mg/0.1 ml, 10 mg/0.2 ml, 20 mg/0.2 ml, 20 mg/0.4 ml, 40 mg/0.4 ml. 40 mg/0.8 ml, 80 mg/0.8 ml, single-dose; *Vial:* 40 mg/0.8 ml, single dose, institutional use only (preservative-free)

Comment: May use with *methotrexate* (MTX), DMARDs, corticosteroids, salicylates, NSAIDs, or analgesics.

▷ *adalimumab-adaz* (B) <4 years, <30 kg (<66 lbs): not recommended; ≥4 years, ≥30 kg (≥66 lbs): 40 mg every other week; inject into thigh or abdomen; rotate sites

Hyrimoz *Prefilled syringe:* 40 mg/0.8 ml single-dose (preservative-free)
Comment: **Hyrimox** is biosimilar to **Humira** (*adalimumab*).

▷ *adalimumab-adbm* (B) <30 kg, <66 lbs: not recommended; ≥30 kg, ≥66 lbs: 40 mg every other week; inject into thigh or abdomen; rotate sites

Cyltezo *Prefilled syringe:* 40 mg/0.8 ml single-dose (preservative-free)
Comment: **Cyltezo** is biosimilar to **Humira** (*adalimumab*).

▷ *adalimumab-afzb* 40 mg SC every other week; some patients with RA not receiving *methotrexate* (MTX) may benefit from increasing the frequency to 40 mg SC every week

Abrilada *Prefilled pen:* 40 mg/0.8 ml, single-dose; *Prefilled syringe:* 40 mg/0.8 ml, 20 mg/0.4 ml, 10 mg/0.2 ml, single-dose; *Vial:* 40 mg/0.8 ml, single-use (for institutional use only) (preservative-free)
Comment: **Abrilada** is biosimilar to **Humira** (*adalimumab*).

▷ *adalimumab-bwwd* Initial Dose (Day 1): 160 mg SC; *Second Dose: two weeks later (Day 15):* 80 mg SC; *Two weeks later (Day 29):* begin maintenance dose of 40 mg every other week

Hadlima *Prefilled autoinjector:* 40 mg/0.8 ml, single-dose (Hadlima PushTouch); *Prefilled syringe:* 40 mg/0.8 ml, single-dose
Comment: **Hadlima** is biosimilar to **Humira** (*adalimumab*).

▷ *etanercept* (B) inject SC into thigh, abdomen, or upper arm; rotate sites; initially 50 mg twice weekly (3-4 days apart) for 3 months; then 50 mg/week maintenance or 25 mg or 50 mg per week for 3 months; then 50 mg/week maintenance
Pediatric: <4 years: not recommended; 4-17 years: Chronic moderate-to-severe plaque psoriasis; >17 years: same as adult

Enbrel *Vial:* 25 mg pwdr for SC injection after reconstitution (4/carton w. supplies) (preservative-free, diluent contains benzyl alcohol); *Prefilled syringe:* 25, 50 mg/ml (preservative-free); *SureClick autoinjector:* 50 mg/ml (preservative-free)

▷ *etanercept-ykro* 50 mg SC once weekly
Pediatric: <4 years: not established; ≥4 years, ≥63 kg, 138 lbs: same as adult

Eticovo *Prefilled syringe:* 25 mg/0.5 ml, 50 mg/ml solution, single-dose
Comment: **Eticovo** (*etanercept-ykro*) is a tumor necrosis factor (TNF) blocker biosimilar to **Enbrel** *etanercept*.

▷ *golimumab* (B) administer SC or IV infusion
Simponi 50 mg SC once monthly; rotate sites
Pediatric: <18 years: not recommended; ≥18 years
Prefilled syringe, SmartJect autoinjector: 50 mg/0.5 ml, single-use (preservative-free)
Simponi Aria 2 mg/kg IV infusion week 0 and week 4; then every 8 weeks thereafter
Pediatric: <2 years: not recommended; ≥2 years, with active (pJIA): 80 mg/m^2 via IV infusion over 30 minutes at weeks 0 and 4, and every 8 weeks thereafter
Vial: 50 mg/4 ml, single-use, soln for IV infusion after dilution (latex-free, preservative-free)

JUVENILE RHEUMATOID ARTHRITIS (JRA)

See Juvenile Idiopathic Arthritis (JIA), Polyarticular Juvenile Idiopathic Arthritis (PJIA), Systemic Juvenile Idiopathic Arthritis (SJIA)

Acetaminophen for IV Infusion *see Pain*

NSAIDs *see* Appendix J. NSAIDs online at https://connect.springerpub.com/content/reference-book/978-0-8261-7935-7/back-matter/part02/back-matter/bmatter10

Opioid Analgesics *see Pain*

Topical & Transdermal Analgesics *see Pain*

Parenteral Corticosteroids *see* Appendix M. Parenteral Corticosteroids

Oral Corticosteroids *see* Appendix L. Oral Corticosteroids

TOPICAL & TRANSDERMAL ANALGESICS

➤ *capsaicin* **(B)(G)** apply tid-qid prn to intact skin
  Pediatric: <2 years: not recommended; ≥2 years: same as adult
      Axsain *Crm:* 0.075% (1, 2 oz)
      Capsin *Lotn:* 0.025, 0.075% (59 ml)
      Capzasin-HP (OTC) *Crm:* 0.075% (1.5 oz), 0.025% (45, 90 gm); *Lotn:* 0.075% (2 oz); 0.025% (45, 90 gm)
      Capzasin-P (OTC) *Crm:* 0.025% (1.5 oz); *Lotn:* 0.025% (2 oz)
      Dolorac *Crm:* 0.025% (28 gm)
      Double Cap (OTC) *Crm:* 0.05% (2 oz)
      R-Gel *Gel:* 0.025% (15, 30 gm)
      Zostrix (OTC) *Crm:* 0.025% (0.7, 1.5, 3 oz)
      Zostrix HP (OTC) *Emol crm:* 0.075% (1, 2 oz)
➤ *capsaicin* 8% patch **(B)** apply up to 4 patches for one 60-minute application to clean dry skin; may prep area with topical anesthetic; wear non-latex gloves; patches may be cut to size/shape; treatment may be repeated every 3 months
  Pediatric: <18 years: not recommended; ≥18 years: same as adult
      Qutenza *Patch:* 8% 1640 mcg/cm (179 mg) (1 or 2 patches w. 1-50 gm tube cleansing gel/carton)
➤ *diclofenac sodium* **(C; D ≥30 wks)** apply qid prn to intact skin
  Pediatric: <12 years: not established; ≥12 years: same as adult
      Pennsaid 1.5% in 10 drop increments, dispense and rub into front, side, and back of knee: usually; 40 drops (40 mg) qid
        Topical soln: 1.5% (150 ml)
      Pennsaid 2% apply 2 pump actuations (40 mg) and rub into front, side, and back of knee bid
        Topical soln: 2% (20 mg/pump actuation, 112 gm)
      Solaraze Gel massage in to clean skin bid prn
        Gel: 3% (50 gm) (benzyl alcohol)
      Voltaren Gel (G)(OTC) apply qid prn to intact skin
        Gel: 1% (100 gm)
  Comment: *Diclofenac* is contraindicated with *aspirin* allergy. As with other NSAIDs, should be avoided in late pregnancy (≥30 weeks) because it may cause premature closure of the ductus arteriosus.
➤ *doxepin* **(B)** cream apply to affected area qid at intervals of at least 3-4 hours; max 8 days
  Pediatric: <12 years: not recommended; >12 years: same as adult
      Prudoxin *Crm:* 5% (45 gm)
      Zonalon *Crm:* 5% (30, 45 gm)
➤ *pimecrolimus* 1% cream **(C)(G)** <2 years: not recommended; ≥2 years: apply to affected area bid; do not apply an occlusive dressing
      Elidel *Crm:* 1% (30, 60, 100 gm)
  Comment: *Pimecrolimus* is indicated for short-term and intermittent long-term use. Discontinue use when resolution occurs. Contraindicated if the patient is immunosuppressed. Change to the 0.1% preparation or if secondary bacterial infection is present.

▷ *trolamine salicylate* apply tid-qid
  Pediatric: <2 years: not recommended; ≥2 years: same as adult
    Mobisyl Creme *Crm:* 10% (100 gm)

TOPICAL & TRANSDERMAL ANESTHETICS

Comment: *Lidocaine* should <u>not</u> be applied to non-intact skin.
▷ *lidocaine* cream (B) apply to affected area bid prn
  Pediatric: <12 years: not recommended; ≥12 years: same as adult
    LidaMantle *Crm:* 3% (1, 2 oz)
    Lidoderm *Crm:* 3% (85 gm)
    ZTlido *lidocaine* topical system 1% (30/carton)
    Comment: Compared to **Lidoderm** (*lidocaine* patch 5%), which contains
    700 mg/patch, **ZTlido** requires 35 mg per topical system to achieve the same
    therapeutic dose.
▷ *lidocaine* lotion (B) apply to affected area bid prn
  Pediatric: <12 years: not recommended; ≥12 years: same as adult
    LidaMantle *Lotn:* 3% (177 ml)
▷ *lidocaine* 5% patch (B)(G) apply up to 3 patches at one time for up to 12
  hours/24-hour period (12 hours on/12 hours off); patches may be cut into smaller
  sizes before removal of the release liner; do <u>not</u> re-use
  Pediatric: <12 years: not recommended; ≥12 years: same as adult
    Lidoderm *Patch:* 5% (10x14 cm; 30/carton)
▷ *lidocaine+dexamethasone* (B)
  Pediatric: <12 years: not recommended; ≥12 years: same as adult
    Decadron Phosphate with Xylocaine *Lotn:* dexa 4 mg+lido 10 mg per ml
    (5 ml)
▷ *lidocaine+hydrocortisone* (B)(G) apply to affected area bid prn
  Pediatric: <12 years: not recommended; ≥12 years: same as adult
    LidaMantle HC *Crm:* lido 3%+hydro 0.5% (1, 3 oz); *Lotn:* (177 ml)
  lidocaine 2.5%+*prilocaine* 2.5% apply sparingly to the burn bid-tid prn
  Pediatric: <12 years: not recommended; ≥12 years: same as adult
    Emla Cream (B) 5, 30 gm/tube

ORAL SALICYLATE

▷ *indomethacin* (C) initially 25 mg bid-tid, increase as needed at weekly intervals
  by 25-50 mg/day; max 200 mg/day
  Pediatric: <14 years: usually not recommended; ≥2 years, if risk warranted:
  1-2 mg/kg/day in divided doses; max 3-4 mg/kg/day (<u>or</u> total 150-200 mg/day,
  whichever is less); ≤14 years: ER cap not recommended
  Cap: 25, 50 mg; *Susp:* 25 mg/5 ml (pineapple-coconut, mint; alcohol 1%); *Supp:* 50
  mg; ER Cap: 75 mg ext-rel
  Comment: *Indomethacin* is indicated <u>only</u> for acute painful flares. Administer
  with food <u>and/or</u> antacids. Use lowest effective dose for shortest duration.

METHOTREXATE (MTX)

▷ *methotrexate* (MTX)(X) 7.5 mg x 1 dose per week <u>or</u> 2.5 mg x 3 at 12-hour
  intervals once a week; max 20 mg/week; therapeutic response begins in 3-6
  weeks; administer *methotrexate* (MTX) injection SC <u>only</u> into the abdomen <u>or</u>
  thigh
  Pediatric: <2 years: not recommended; ≥2 years: 10 mg/m² once weekly; max 20
  mg/m²
    Rasuvo *Autoinjector:* 7.5 mg/0.15 ml, 10 mg/0.20 ml, 12.5 mg/0.25 ml, 15
    mg/0.30 ml, 17.5 mg/0.35 ml, 20 mg/0.40 ml, 22.5 mg/0.45 ml, 25 mg/0.50
    ml, 27.5 mg/0.55 ml, 30 mg/0.60 ml (solution concentration for SC injection is
    50 mg/ml)

Rheumatrex *Tab:* 2.5*mg (5, 7.5, 10, 12.5, 15 mg/week, 4/card unit-of-use dose pack)

Trexall *Tab:* 5*, 7.5*, 10*, 15*mg (5, 7.5, 10, 12.5, 15 mg/week, 4/card unit-of-use dose pack)

Comment: *Methotrexate* (MTX) is contraindicated with immunodeficiency, blood dyscrasias, alcoholism, and chronic liver disease.

INTERLEUKIN-6 RECEPTOR ANTAGONIST

▷ *tocilizumab* (B) <2 years: not recommended; ≥2 years: weight-based dosing ≥30 kg: 8 mg/kg SC every 2 weeks; <30 kg: 12 mg/kg SC every 2 weeks; *IV Infusion:* administer over 1 hour; do not administer as bolus or IV push; ≥30 kg: dilute to 100 mL in 0.9% or 0.45% NaCl. <30 kg: dilute to 50 mL in 0.9% or 0.45% NaCl; ≥18 years: whether used in combination with DMARDs or as monotherapy, the recommended IV infusion starting dose is 4 mg/kg IV every 4 weeks followed by an increase to 8 mg/kg IV every 4 weeks based on clinical response; Max 800 mg per infusion in RA patients; *SC Administration:* ≥100 kg: 162 mg SC once weekly on the same day; <100 kg: 162 mg SC every other week on the same day followed by an increase according to clinical response

Actemra *Vial:* 80 mg/4 ml, 200 mg/10 ml, 400 mg/20 ml, single-use, for IV Infusion after dilution; *Prefilled syringe:* 162 mg (0.9 ml, single-dose)

Comment: *Tocilizumab* is an interleukin-6 receptor-α inhibitor indicated for use in moderate-to-severe rheumatoid arthritis (RA) that has not responded to conventional therapy, and also for some subtypes of JRA. **Actemra** may be used alone or in combination with *methotrexate* (MTX) and in RA, other DMARDs may be used. Monitor patient for dose-related laboratory changes, including elevated LFTs, neutropenia, and thrombocytopenia. **Actemra** should not be initiated in patients with an absolute neutrophil count (ANC) below 2000 per mm3, platelet count below 100,000 per mm3, or who have ALT or AST above 1.5 times the upper limit of normal (ULN). Registration in the Pregnancy Exposure Registry (1-877-311-8972) is encouraged for monitoring pregnancy outcomes in women exposed to **Actemra** during pregnancy. The limited available data-associated risk for major birth defects and miscarriage. Monoclonal antibodies, such as *tocilizumab*, are actively transported across the placenta during the third trimester of pregnancy and may affect immune response in the infant exposed *in utero*. It is not known whether *tocilizumab* passes into breast milk; therefore, breastfeeding is not recommended while using **Actemra**.

Selective Co-stimulation Modulator

▷ *abatacept* (C) <2 years: not recommended; 2-17 years: administer as an IV infusion over 30 minutes at weeks 0, 2, and 4; then every 4 weeks thereafter; <75 kg, administer 10 mg/kg; same as adult (max 1 gm); administer as an IV infusion over 30 minutes at weeks 0, 2, and 4; then every 4 weeks thereafter; <60 kg, administer 500 mg/dose; 60-100 kg, administer 750 mg/dose; >100 kg, administer 1 gm/dose

Orencia *Vial:* 250 mg pwdr for IV infusion after reconstitution (silicone-free) (preservative-free); *Prefilled syringe:* 125 mg/ml soln for SC injection (preservative-free); *ClickJect Autoinjector:* 125 mg/ml soln for SC injection

Comment: **Orencia** is also indicated to reduce signs/symptoms, induce major clinical response, inhibit progression of structural damage, and improve physical function in adult patients with moderate-to-severe active RA. **Orencia** may be used as monotherapy or with DMARDs other than TNF antagonists. **Orencia** is also indicated to reduce signs/symptoms of moderate-to-severe active polyarticular juvenile idiopathic arthritis (PJIA) in patients >2 years-of-age as monotherapy or with *methotrexate* (MTX).

KERATITIS/KERATOCONJUNCTIVITIS SICCA/DRY EYE SYNDROME

▷ *cyclosporine* (C) using 1 single-use disposable vial, instill 1 drop in each eye twice daily q 12 hours

Pediatric: <16 years: not recommended; ≥16 years: same as adult

Cequa *Ophth soln:* 0.09% single-use vials (0.25 ml, 6 pouches, 10 vials/pouch per carton) (preservative-free)

Comment: Cequa ophthalmic solution is a calcineurin inhibitor immune-suppressant indicated to increase tear production in patients with keratoconjunctivitis sicca. It is the first cyclosporine product to utilize nanomicellar technology, facilitating the drug molecule to penetrate the eye's aqueous layer, and preventing the release of active lipophilic molecule prior to penetration.

Restasis *Ophth emul:* 0.05% (0.4 ml) (preservative-free)

KERATITIS/KERATOCONJUNCTIVITIS: HERPES SIMPLEX

▷ *acyclovir ophthalmic ointment* apply a 1 cm ribbon in the lower cul-de-sac of the affected eye 5 x/day until healed; then, 3 x/day for 7 more days

Pediatric: <2 years: not established; ≥2 years: same as adult

Avaclyr *Ophth oint:* 3% (3.5 gm) single patient multi-use tube

Comment: Avaclyr *(acyclovir ophthalmic ointment)* is a herpes simplex virus nucleoside analog DNA polymerase inhibitor indicated for the treatment of acute herpetic keratitis (dendritic ulcers) in patients with herpes simplex (HSV-1 and HSV-2) virus. Avaclyr is contraindicated in patients with a known hypersensitivity to *acyclovir* or *valacyclovir*. The most common adverse reactions (incidence 2-10%) have been eye pain (stinging), punctate keratitis, and follicular conjunctivitis. There is no information regarding embryo/fetal effects of maternal use of ophthalmic *acyclovir* during pregnancy or presence of ophthalmic *acyclovir* in human milk, or effects on the breastfed infant.

▷ *ganciclovir* (C) instill 1 drop 5 x/day (every 3 hours) while awake until corneal ulcer heals; then 1 drop tid x 7 days

Pediatric: <2 years: not recommended; ≥2 years: same as adult

Zirgan *Ophth gel:* 0.15% (5 gm) (benzalkonium chloride)

▷ *idoxuridine* (C) instill 1 drop q 1 hour during day and every other hour at night or 1 drop every minute for 5 minutes and repeat q 4 hours during day and night

Herplex *Ophth soln:* 0.1% (15 ml)

▷ *trifluridine* (C) instill 1 drop q 2 hours while awake (max 9 drops/day until re-epithelialization; then 1 drop q 4 hours x 7 more days (at least 5 drops/day); max 21 days

Pediatric: <6 years: not recommended; ≥6 years: same as adult

Viroptic *Ophth soln:* 1% (7.5 ml) (thimerosal)

▷ *vidarabine* (C) apply 1/2 inch in lower conjunctival sac 5 x/day q 3 hours until re-epithelialization occurs, then bid x 7 more days

Pediatric: <2 years: not recommended; ≥2 years: same as adult

Vira-A *Ophth oint:* 3% (3.5 gm)

KERATITIS: NEUROTROPHIC

Comment: Oxervate is a recombinant form of human nerve growth factor (hNGF) structurally similar to endogenous NGF protein. NGF is an endogenous protein involved in the differentiation and maintenance of neurons, which acts through specific high-affinity (i.e., TrkA) and low-affinity (i.e., p75NTR) nerve growth factor receptors in the anterior segment of the eye to support corneal innervation and integrity. Prior to FDA- approval of **Oxervate**, treatment was limited to symptomatic relief such as artificial tears, antibiotics, autologous serum-derived eye drops, tarsorrhaphy, and botulinum-induced ptosis, or surgical intervention.

▷ *cenegermin-bkbj* 1 drop in affected eye(s) 6 x/ day at 2-hour intervals x 8 weeks; pharmacy storage of the weekly carton in the freezer at or below -4°F (-20°C) until dispensed in the insulated pack in the Delivery System Kit; within 5 hours of leaving the pharmacy, store the weekly carton in the refrigerator between 36°F to 46°F (2°C to 8°C) for up to 14 days; opened vials may be stored in the original weekly carton in the refrigerator between 36°F to 46°F (2°C to 8°C) or at room temperature up to 77°F (25°C) for up to 12 hours; do not re-freeze; do not shake the vial; discard any unused portion after 12 hours

Pediatric: <2 years: not recommended; ≥2 years: same as adult

Oxervate *Vial:* 0.002% multi-dose (7/carton; Delivery System Kit contains, insulated pack, 8 vial adapters, 45 pipettes, 45 sterile disinfectant wipes, dose card) (preservative-free)

KERATITIS/KERATOCONJUNCTIVITIS: VERNAL

OPHTHALMIC MAST CELL STABILIZERS

Comment: Contact lens wear is contraindicated
▷ *cromolyn sodium* (B) 1-2 drops 4-6 x/day
Pediatric: <4 years: not recommended; ≥4 years: same as adult
Crolom, Opticrom *Ophth soln:* 4% (10 ml) (benzalkonium chloride)
▷ *lodoxamide tromethamine* (B) 1-2 drops qid; max 3 months
Pediatric: <2 years: not recommended; ≥2 years: same as adult
Alomide *Ophth susp:* 0.1% (10 ml)

LABYRINTHITIS

▷ *meclizine* (B) 25 mg tid
Pediatric: <12 years: not recommended; ≥12 years: same as adult
Antivert *Tab:* 12.5, 25, 50*mg
Bonine (OTC) *Cap:* 15, 25, 30 mg; *Tab:* 12.5, 25, 50 mg; *Chew tab/Film-coat tab:* 25 mg
Dramamine II (OTC) *Tab:* 25*mg
Zentrip *Strip:* 25 mg orally disintegrating
▷ *promethazine* (C)(G) 25 mg tid
Pediatric: <2 years: not recommended; ≥2 years: 0.5 mg/lb or 6.25-25 mg tid
Phenergan *Tab:* 12.5*, 25*, 50 mg; *Plain syr:* 6.25 mg/5 ml; *Fortis syr:* 25 mg/5 ml; *Rectal supp:* 12.5, 25, 50 mg
Comment: *Promethazine* is contraindicated in children with uncomplicated nausea, dehydration, Reye's syndrome, history of sleep apnea, asthma, and lower respiratory disorders in children. *Promethazine* lowers the seizure threshold in children, may cause cholestatic jaundice, anticholinergic effects, extrapyramidal effects, and potentially fatal respiratory depression.
▷ *scopolamine* (C)
Transderm Scop 1 patch behind ear at least 4 hours before travel; each patch is effective for 3 days
Transdermal patch: 1.5 mg (4/carton)

LACTOSE INTOLERANCE

▷ *lactase* enzyme 9000 FCC units taken with dairy food; adjust based on abatement of symptoms; usual max 18,000 units/dose

Pediatric: same as adult

Lactaid Drops (OTC) 5-7 drops to each quart of milk and shake gently; may increase to 10-15 drops if needed; hydrolyzes 70%-99% of lactose at refrigerator temperature in 24 hours

  Oral drops: 1250 units/5 gtts (7 ml w. dropper)

Lactaid Extra (OTC) *Cplt:* 4500 FCC units

Lactaid Fast ACT (OTC) *Cplt:* 9000 FCC units; *Chew tab:* 9000 FCC units (vanilla twist)

Lactaid Original (OTC) *Cplt:* 3000 FCC units

Lactaid Ultra (OTC) *Cplt:* 9000 FCC units; *Chew tab:* 9000 FCC units (vanilla twist)

LAMBERT-EATON MYASTHENIC SYNDROME (LEMS)

BROAD SPECTRUM POTASSIUM CHANNEL BLOCKER

▷ *amifampridine*

Pediatric: <6 years: not established; *6-<17 years, <45 kg:* initially 7.5-15 mg daily in divided doses; then, increase daily in 2.5 mg to 5 mg increments, divided in up to 5 doses daily; max single dose is 15 mg; max total 50 mg/day; *6 -<17 years, ≥45 kg :* initially 15-30 mg daily in individed doses; then, increase daily in 5 mg to 10 mg increments, divided in up to 5 doses daily; max single dose is 30 mg; max total 100 mg/day; if the patient requires doses in less than 5 mg increments, has difficulty swallowing, or requires a feeding tube, a 1 mg/ml suspension can be prepared; for patients with renal or hepatic impairment, or are poor N-acetyltransferase 2 metabolizers, use the lowest recommended initial dose of **Rusurgi.**

  Rusurgi *Tab:* 10*mg

  Comment: **Rusurgi** *(amifampridine)* is a broad spectrum potassium channel blocker. **Rusurgi** is contraindicated for patients with a history of seizures or hypersensitivity to *amifampridine* or other *aminopyridine*. **Rusurgi** can cause seizures. Consider discontinuation or dose-reduction of **Rusurgi** in patients who have a seizure while on treatment. If a hypersensitivity reaction such as anaphylaxis occurs, **Rusurgi** should be discontinued and appropriate therapy initiated. Concomitant use of **Rusurgi** and drugs known to lower seizure threshold may lead to an increased risk of seizures. Concomitant use of **Rusurgi** and drugs with cholinergic effects (e.g., direct or indirect cholinesterase inhibitors) may increase the cholinergic effects of **Rusurgi** and of those drugs, and increase the risk of adverse reaction. The most common adverse reactions (incidence 10% and 2% greater than placebo) are paresthesia/dysesthesia, abdominal pain, dyspepsia, dizziness, and nausea. There are no human or animal data on the developmental risk associated with the use of **Rusurgi** in pregnancy. There are no data on the presence of *amifampridine* or the 3-N-acetyl-amifampridine metabolite in human milk or effects on the breastfed infant.

LARVA MIGRANS: CUTANEOUS, VISCERAL

▷ *thiabendazole* (C) adult and pediatric dosing schedules are the same; dosing is bid, is based on weight in pounds, and must be taken with meals

  Cutaneous Larva Migrans: treat bid x 2 days

  Visceral Larva Migrans: treat bid x 7 days

    <30 lbs: consult mfr pkg insert; 30 lbs: 250 mg bid; 50 lbs: 500 mg bid; 75 lbs: 750 mg bid; 100 lbs: 1000 mg bid; 125 lbs: 1250 mg bid: ≥150 lbs: 1500 mg bid; max 3000 mg/day.

  Mintezol *Chew tab:* 500*mg (orange); *Oral susp:* 500 mg/5 ml (120 ml) (orange)

Comment: *Thiabendazole* is not for prophylaxis. May impair mental alertness. May not be available in the US.

LEAD POISONING

Comment: Chelation therapy for lead poisoning requires maintenance of adequate hydration, close monitoring of renal and hepatic function, and monitoring for neutropenia; discontinue therapy at first sign of toxicity. Contraindicated with severe renal disease or anuria.

CHELATING AGENTS

▷ *deferoxamine mesylate* (C) initially 1 gm IM, followed by 500 mg IM every 4 hours x 2 doses; then repeat every 4-12 hours if needed; max 6 gm/day
   Pediatric: <3 months: not recommended; ≥3 months: same as adult
      Desferal *Vial:* 250 mg/ml after reconstitution (500 mg)

▷ *edetate calcium disodium (EDTA)* (B) administer IM or IV; use IM route of administration for children and overt lead encephalopathy
   Pediatric: same as adult; *Serum lead level: 20-70 mcg/dL:* 1 gm/m² per day; *IV:* infuse over 8-12 hours; *IM:* divided doses q 8-12 hours; Treat for 5 days; then stop for 2-4 days; may repeat if serum lead level is ≥70 mcg/dL
      Calcium Disodium Versenate *Amp:* 200 mg/ml (5 ml)

▷ *succimer* (C) may swallow caps whole or put contents onto a small amount of soft food or a spoon and swallow, followed by a fruit drink
   Pediatric: <12 months: not recommended; ≥12 months: same as adult; *Serum lead level: >45 mcg/dL:* initially 10 mg/kg (or 350 mg/m²) every 8 hours for 5 days; then reduce frequency to every 12 hours for 14 more days; allow at least 14 days between courses unless serum lead levels indicate a need for more prompt treatment; for more than 3 consecutive weeks not recommended
      Chemet *Cap:* 100 mg

 LEG CRAMPS: NOCTURNAL, RECUMBENCY

▷ *quinine sulfate* (C)(G) 1 tab or cap q HS
   Pediatric: <16 years: not recommended; ≥16 years: same as adult
      Qualaquin *Tab:* 260 mg; *Cap:* 260, 300, 325 mg
   Comment: If **hypokalemia** is the cause of leg cramps, treat with potassium supplementation (*see* **hypokalemia**).

 LEISHMANIASIS: CUTANEOUS, MUCOSAL, VISCERAL

Comment: The leishmanial parasite species addressed in this section are: **cutaneous leishmaniasis** (due to *Leishmania braziliensis*, *Leishmania guyanensis*, *Leishmania panamensis*), **mucosal leishmaniasis** (due to *Leishmania braziliensis*), and **visceral leishmaniasis** (due to *Leishmania donovani*). The weight-based treatment for adults and adolescents is the same for each of the species, the anti-leishmanial drug *miltefosone* (**Impavido**). Contraindications to this drug include pregnancy, lactation, and Sjogren-Larsson-Syndrome. The contraindication in pregnancy is due to embryo/fetal toxicity, teratogenicity, and fetal death. Obtain a serum or urine pregnancy test for females of reproductive potential and advise females to use effective contraception during therapy and for 5 months following treatment. Breastfeeding is contraindicated while taking this drug and for 5 months following termination of breastfeeding. Potential ASEs include loss of appetite, abdominal pain, nausea, vomiting, diarrhea, headache, dizziness, pruritis, somnolence, elevated liver transaminases, bilirubin, and serum creatinine and thrombocytopenia. *miltefosine* is associated with impaired fertility in females and males in animal studies.

▷ *miltefosine* (D)(G) 30-44 kg: one cap bid x 28 consecutive days; ≥45 kg: one cap tid x 28 consecutive days; take with a full meal
   Pediatric: <12 years, <30 kg (60 lbs): not established; ≥12 years, ≥30 kg (≥60 lbs): same as adult
      Impavido *Cap:* 50 mg

LENNOX-GASTAUT SYNDROME (LGS)/DRAVET SYNDROME

CANNABINOID-DERIVED TREATMENT

Comment: The FDA Peripheral and Central Nervous System Drugs Advisory Committee's **Epidiolex** (*cannabidiol*) recommendation was based on three randomized, double-blind, placebo-controlled clinical trials. These trials showed a 50% reduction of drop seizure frequency in 40%-44% of patients with Lennox-Gastaut syndrome, and a 39% decrease in convulsive seizure frequency for trial participants with Dravet Syndrome. A total of 516 patients with one of the two seizure disorders participated in the clinical trials. The FDA Advisory Committee judged that CBD-OS, derived from a non-psychoactive chemical found in marijuana, was very unlikely to have potential for abuse.

▷ *cannabidiol* initially 2.5mg/kg 2 x/day (5mg/kg/day); after one week, may be increased to a maintenance dose of 5 mg/kg 2 x/day (10 mg/kg/day); max 10 mg/kg 2 x/day (20 mg/kg/day); titration based on effectiveness and tolerability; dose adjustment is recommended for patients with moderate or severe hepatic impairment.

Pediatric: <1 years: not established; ≥1 year: weight-based dosing as above
  Epidiolex *Oral soln*: 100 mg/ml (100 ml) (strawberry)
  Comment: **Epidiolex** (*cannabidiol*) is a prescription pharmaceutical formulation of highly-purified, marijuana plant-derived cannabidiol (CBD) indicated for the treatment of seizures associated with Lennox-Gastaut syndrome, Dravet syndrome, and tuberous sclerosis complex in patients ≥2 years-of-age. Obtain serum transaminases (ALT and AST) and total bilirubin levels in all patients prior to starting treatment. Concomitant use of *valproate* and higher doses of **Epidiolex** increase the risk of transaminase elevations. Consider dose reduction of **Epidiolex** with concomitant moderate or strong inhibitors of CYP3A4 or CYP2C19. Consider dose increase of **Epidiolex** with strong inducers of CYP3A4 or CYP2C19. Consider dose reduction of substrates of UGT1A9, UGT2B7, CYP2C8, CYP2C9, and CYP2C19 (e.g., *clobazam*). Substrates of CYP1A2 and CYP2B6 may also require dose adjustment. Monitor for somnolence and sedation and advise patients not to drive or operate machinery until they have gained sufficient experience on **Epidiolex**. Monitor patients for suicidal behavior and thoughts. Advise patients to seek immediate medical care for any hypersensitivity reaction. Discontinue and do not restart **Epidiolex** if hypersensitivity occurs. **Epidiolex** should be gradually withdrawn to minimize the risk of increased seizure frequency and status epilepticus. The most common adverse reactions (incidence ≥10%) include somnolence, decreased appetite, diarrhea, transaminase elevations, fatigue, malaise, and asthenia, rash, insomnia, sleep disorder, and poor quality sleep, and infections. There are no adequate data on the developmental risks associated with the use of **Epidiolex** in pregnant females. However, animal studies have demonstrated **Epidiolex** may cause fetal harm. There are no data on the presence of *cannabidiol* or its metabolites in human milk or effects on the breastfed infant. Encourage females who take **Epidiolex** during pregnancy to enroll in the North American Antiepileptic Drug (NAAED) Pregnancy Registry by calling 1-888-233-2334 or visiting www.aedpregnancyregistry.org/.

OTHER ANTICONVULSANTS

▷ *clobazam* (C)(IV)(G) take with or without food; for doses above 5 mg/day, administer in two divided doses; ≤*30 kg body weight*: initiate at 5 mg daily and titrate as tolerated up to 20 mg daily; >*30 kg body weight*: initiate at 10 mg daily and titrate as tolerated up to 40 mg daily; *Tablets*: administer whole, broken in half along the score line, or crushed and mixed in applesauce; *Suspension:* measure prescribed amount using provided adapter and dosing syringe; *Mild-to-Moderate Hepatic Impairment:* reduce dose or discontinue gradually; *Severe Hepatic Impairment:* no information; *Geriatric Patients and CYP2C19 poor metabolizers:* adjust dose

Pediatric: <2 years: not recommended; ≥2 years: same as adult

Onfi *Tab:* 10*, 20*mg

Onfi Oral Suspension *Oral susp:* 2.5 mg/ml (120 ml w. adapter and 2 dosing syringes) (berry)

Sympazan Oral Film *Oral film:* 5, 10, 20 mg, single-dose (60/pkg) (berry)

Comment: **Clobazam** is a benzodiazepine indicated for adjunctive treatment of seizures associated with Lennox-Gastaut syndrome (LGS) in patients ≥2 years-of-age. Monitor for central nervous system (CNS) depression (somnolence, sedation), caution with concomitant CNS depressants, avoid rapid dose reduction or discontinuation. Monitor for potential Stevens-Johnson syndrome and toxic epidermal necrolysis. Discontinue *clobazam* at first sign of rash unless the rash is clearly not drug-related. Monitor patients with a history of substance abuse for signs of habituation and dependence. Monitor for suicidal thoughts or behaviors. Adverse reactions which have occurred (incidence ≥ 10%) with any *clobazam* dose included constipation, somnolence or sedation, pyrexia, lethargy, and drooling. *clobazam* is excreted in human milk. Breastfed infants of mothers taking benzodiazepines, such as *clobazam*, may have effects of lethargy, somnolence, and poor sucking. *clobazam* is excreted in human milk. Breastfed infants of mothers taking benzodiazepines, such as *clobazam*, may have effects of lethargy, somnolence and poor sucking. There is insufficient evidence to assess the effect of benzodiazepine pregnancy exposure on neurodevelopment. Prescribers are advised to recommend pregnant patients taking **Onfi** or **Sympazan** self-enroll in the North American Antiepileptic Drug (NAAED) Pregnancy Registry by calling 1-888-233-2334 or visiting www.aedpregnancyregistry.org

▶ *stiripentol* 50 mg/kg/day in 2 or 3 divided doses; reduce dose or discontinue dose gradually; capsules must be swallowed whole with a glass of water during a meal; do not break or open capsules; mix contents of one packet in a glass of water and take immediately after mixing during a meal

Pediatric: <2 years: not recommended; ≥2 years: same as adult

Diacomit *Cap:* 250, 500 mg; *Pwdr for Oral Susp:* 250, 500 mg (60 pkts/carton) (fruit)

Comment: **Diacomit** is indicated for the treatment of seizures associated with Dravet syndrome in patients ≥2 years-of-age taking *clobazam*. There are no clinical data to support the use of **Diacomit** as monotherapy in Dravet syndrome.

LENTIGINES: BENIGN, SENILE

Comment: Wash affected area with a soap-free cleanser; pat dry and wait 20-30 minutes; then apply agent sparingly to affected area; use only once daily in PM. Avoid eyes, ears, nostrils, mouth, and healthy skin. Avoid sun exposure. Cautious use of concomitant astringents, alcohol-based products, sulfur-containing products, salicylic acid-containing products, soap, and other topical agents.

TOPICAL RETINOIDS

▶ *tazarotene* (X)(G) apply daily at HS

Pediatric: <12 years: not recommended; ≥12 years: same as adult

Avage Cream *Crm:* 0.1% (30 gm)

Tazorac Cream *Crm:* 0.05, 0.1% (15, 30, 60 gm)

Tazorac Gel *Gel:* 0.05, 0.1% (30, 100 gm)

▷ *tretinoin* (C)(G) apply daily at HS
  Pediatric: <12 years: not recommended; ≥12 years: same as adult
    Avita *Crm:* 0.025% (20, 45 gm); *Gel:* 0.025% (20, 45 gm)
    Renova *Crm:* 0.02% (40 gm); 0.05% (40, 60 gm)
    Retin-A Cream *Crm:* 0.025, 0.05, 0.1% (20, 45 gm)
    Retin-A Gel *Gel:* 0.01, 0.025% (15, 45 gm) (alcohol 90%)
    Retin-A Liquid *Liq:* 0.05% (28 ml; alcohol 55%)
    Retin-A Micro *Microspheres:* 0.04, 0.1% (20, 45 gm)
    Retin-A Micro Gel *Gel:* 0.04, 0.1% (20, 45 gm)

LISTERIOSIS (*LISTERIA MONOCYTOGENES*)

Comment: *L. monocytogenes* is a potentially lethal foodborne pathogen that is a common contaminant of food and food preparation equipment, and has been isolated in soil, farm environments, produce, raw foods, dairy products, and the feces of asymptomatic people. IV *ampicillin* is the mainstay of treatment, but penicillin may be as effective. Some experts recommend combination antibiotic therapy for neuro-invasive *L. monocytogenes*. The most common antimicrobial combination is IV *ampicillin* and IV *gentamycin* (which is usually discontinued when the patient shows signs of improvement to limit the potential for toxicity). If the patient is penicillin-allergic, IV *trimethoprim-sulfamethoxazole* (TMP-SMX) as mono therapy x 28 days. Patients with bacteremia but without CNS involvement may be treated with combination (*ampicillin+gentamycin*) therapy for 14 days, but patients with meningitis require a full 21 day combination course of antibiotics. Endocarditis, encephalitis, and brain abscesses may require a longer duration of high dose antimicrobials. Cephalosporins are ineffective. Supportive care and standard isolation precautions are required.

▷ *ampicillin* (B)(G) 2 gm IV infusion every 4 hours (in combination with IV gentamycin every 8 hours)
  Pediatric: 50-100 mg/kg (max 3 gm) IV infusion q 6 hours
    Unasyn *Vial:* 1.5, 3 gm
▷ *gentamicin* (C)(G) 1-2 mg/kg q 8 hours (in combination with IV ampicillin every 4 hours; monitor plasma levels; dilution not less than 1 mg/ml in D5W or NS; administer dose over 30 minutes-2 hours
  Pediatric: 2 mg/kg/dose q 8 hours; monitor plasma levels; dilution not less than 1 mg/ml in D5W or NS; administer dose over 30 minutes-2 hours
    Geramycin *Vial:* 20, 80 mg/2 ml (2 ml) for dilution (not less than 1 mg/ml) and IV infusion (over 30 minutes-2 hours
▷ *penicillin g potassium (B)(G)* 4 million units via IV infusion q 4 hours
  Pediatric: 65,000 units/kg/dose via IV infusion q 4 hours; max 4 million units/dose; infuse dose over 1-2 hours
    Vial: 5, 20 MU pwdr for reconstitution (in D5W or NS) and IV infusion; *Pre-mixed bag:* 1, 2, 3 MU (50 ml); infuse dose over 1-2 hours
▷ *trimethoprim-sulfamethoxazole (TMP-SMX)* (C)(G) TMP 5 mg/kg IV infusion q 6 hours; max TMP 160 mg/dose
  Pediatric: <2 months: contraindicated: ≥2 months: 2-5 mg/kg/dose q 8 hours; max TMP 160 mg/dose

LIVER FLUKES: FASCIOLIASIS (*FASCIOLA GIGANTICA, FASCIOLA HEPATICA*)

BENZIMIDAZOLE ANTHELMINTIC

▷ *triclabendazole* recommended dose is 2 doses of 10 mg/kg administered 12 hours apart; take with food; swallow dose with waters; swallow whole or divide tablet in half; may crush and administer with applesauce; if the dose cannot be adjusted exactly, round dose upwards

Pediatric: <6 years: not established; ≥6 years: same as adult

Egaten *Tab:* 250*mg

Comment: *Triclabendazole* is indicated for the treatment of fascioliasis, a neglected tropical disease (NTD) caused by liver flukes *Fasciola hepatica* and *Fasciola gigantica*. It is contraindicated in patients with known hypersensitivity to *triclabendazole* or other *benzimidazole* derivatives. *triclabendazole* may prolong QT interval; therefore, monitor ECG in patients with a history of QTprolongation or who are taking medications which prolong the QT interval. The most common adverse reactions (incidence >2%) with *triclabendazole* ≥20 mg/kg dose are abdominal pain, hyperhidrosis, nausea, decreased appetite, headache, urticaria, diarrhea, vomiting, musculoskeletal chest pain, and pruritus. There are no available data on **Egaten** use in pregnant females to inform a drug associated risk of major birth defects, miscarriage or adverse maternal or fetal outcomes. There are no data on the presence of *triclabendazole* in human milk or effects on the breastfed infant. Clinical studies of **Egaten** have not included sufficient numbers of patients ≥65 to inform whether the elderly respond differently from younger patients.

TREMATODICIDE

Comment: *Praziquantel* is a trematodicide indicated for the treatment of infections due to all species of Schistosoma (e.g., *Schistosoma mekongi, Schistosoma japonicum, Schistosoma mansoni,* and *Schistosoma hematobium*) and infections due to liver flukes (i.e., *Clonorchis sinensis, Opisthorchis viverrini*). *Praziquantel* induces a rapid contraction of schistosomes by a specific effect on the permeability of the cell membrane. The drug further causes vacuolization and disintegration of the schistosome tegument.

▶ *praziquantel* (B) 25 mg/kg tid as a one-day treatment; take the 3 doses at intervals of not less than 4 hours and not more than 6 hours; swallow whole with water during meals; holding the tablets in the mouth leaves a bitter taste which can trigger gagging or vomiting.

Pediatric: <4 years: not established; >4 years: same as adult

Biltricide *Tab:* 600mg*** film-coat (3 scores, 4 segments, 150 mg/segment)

Comment: Concomitant administration with strong Cytochrome P450 (P450) inducers, such as *rifampin*, is contraindicated since therapeutically effective blood levels of *praziquantel* may not be achieved. In patients receiving *rifampin* who need immediate treatment for schistosomiasis, alternative agents for schistosomiasis should be considered. However, if treatment with *praziquantel* is necessary, *rifampin* should be discontinued 4 weeks before administration of *praziquantel*. Treatment with *rifampin* can then be restarted one day after completion of *praziquantel* treatment. Concomitant administration of other P450 inducers (e.g., antiepileptic drugs such as *phenytoin, phenobarbital, carbamazepine*) and *dexamethasone*, may also reduce plasma levels of *praziquantel*. Concomitant administration of P450 inhibitors (e.g., *cimetidine, ketoconazole, itraconazole, erythromycin*) may increase plasma levels of *praziquantel*. Patients should be warned not to drive a car or operate machinery on the day of **Biltricide** treatment and the following day. There are no adequate or well-controlled studies in pregnant females. This drug should be used during pregnancy only if clearly needed. *praziquantel* appears in the milk of nursing women at a concentration of about 1/4 that of maternal serum. It is not known whether a pharmacological effect is likely to occur in children. Women should not nurse on the day of **Biltricide** treatment and during the subsequent 72 hours.

LOW BACK STRAIN (LBS)

Acetaminophen for IV Infusion *see **Pain***
NSAIDs *see* Appendix J. NSAIDs online at https://connect.springerpub.com/content/reference-book/978-0-8261-7935-7/back-matter/part02/back-matter/bmatter10
Opioid Analgesics *see **Pain***
Topical & Transdermal Analgesics *see **Pain***
Muscle Relaxants *see* Muscle Strain
Parenteral Corticosteroids *see* Appendix M. Parenteral Corticosteroids
Oral Corticosteroids *see* Appendix L. Oral Corticosteroids
Topical Analgesic and Anesthetic Agents *see* Appendix I. Anesthetic Agents for Local Infiltration and Dermal/Mucosal Membrane Application online at https://connect.springerpub.com/content/reference-book/978-0-8261-7935-7/back-matter/part02/back-matter/bmatter9

 LOW LIBIDO, HYPOACTIVE SEXUAL DESIRE DISORDER (HSDD)

5-HT1A AGONIST/5-HT2A

▷ *flibanserin* 1 tab once daily at bedtime; discontinue if no improvement in 8 weeks
Pediatric: <18 years: not recommended; ≥18 years: same as adult
    Addyi *Tab:* 100 mg
    Comment: **Addyi** is for use in pre-menopausal women. **Addyi** is not for use in men, postmenopausal women, and is not recommended in pregnancy, or lactation. Potential ASEs include dry mouth, nausea, hypotension, dizziness, syncope, fatigue, somnolence, and insomnia.

MELANOCORTIN RECEPTOR AGONIST (MRA)

▷ *bremelanotide* inject 1.75 mg SC via the autoinjector to the abdomen or thigh, as needed, at least 45 minutes before anticipated sexual activity; do not administer more than one dose within 24 hours; more than 8 doses per month is not recommended
Pediatric: <18 years: not established; ≥18 years: same as adult
    Vyleesi *Prefilled autoinjector:* 1.75 mg (0.3 ml) solution, single-dose (4/carton)
    Comment: **Vyleesi** *(bremelanotide)* is a melanocortin receptor agonist for the treatment of acquired, generalized, and hypoactive sexual desire disorder (HSDD) in pre-menopausal women as characterized by low sexual desire that causes marked distress or interpersonal difficulty and is not due to a co-existing medical or psychiatric condition, problems with the relationship, or effects of a medication or drug. **Vyleesi** is not indicated for treatment of HSDD in postmenopausal women or in men, and **Vyleesi** is not indicated to enhance sexual performance. **Vyleesi** is contraindicated in patients with uncontrolled hypertension or known cardiovascular disease. Transient increase in blood pressure and decrease in heart rate occurs after each dose and usually resolves within 12 hours. Consider the patient's cardiovascular risk before initiating **Vyleesi** and periodically. Focal hyperpigmentation has been eported by 1% of patients who received up to 8 doses per month, including involvement of the face, gingiva, and breasts with higher risk in patients with darker skin and with daily dosing. Resolution was not confirmed in some patients. Consider discontinuing **Vyleesi** if hyperpigmentation develops. Nausea has been reported by 40% of patients receiving up to 8 monthly doses, requiring anti-emetic therapy in 13% of patients and leading to premature discontinuation for 8% of patients. Improvement has been reported for most patients with the second dose. Consider discontinuing **Vyleesi** or initiating anti-emetic therapy for persistent or severe nausea. **Vyleesi** may slow gastric emptying and impact absorption of concomitantly administered oral medications. Avoid use of

Vyleesi with orally administered *naltrexone*-containing products intended to treat alcohol or opioid addiction as **Vyleesi** may significantly decrease the systemic exposure of orally-administered *naltrexone*. Use of **Vyleesi** during pregnancy is not recommended. Advise females of reproductive potential to use effective contraception while taking **Vyleesi**, and to discontinue **Vyleesi** if pregnancy is suspected. Pregnant females exposed to **Vyleesi** and healthcare providers are encouraged to call the Vyleesi Pregnancy Exposure Registry at (877) 411-2510. There is no information on the presence of *bremelanotide* or its metabolites in human milk or effects on the breastfed infant.

▷ *selpercatinib* < 50 kg: 120 mg twice daily; >50 kg: 160 mg twice daily; reduce dose in patients with severe hepatic impairment

Pediatric: <12 years: not established; ≥12 years: same as adult

Retevmo *Cap:* 40, 80 mg

Comment: Retevmo *(selpercatinib)* is a kinase inhibitor indicated for adult patients with metastatic RET fusion-positive non-small cell lung cancer, adult and pediatric patients ≥12 years-of-age with advanced or metastatic RET-mutant medullary thyroid cancer (MTC) who require systemic therapy; adult and pediatric patients ≥12 years-of-age with advanced or metastatic RET fusion-positive thyroid cancer who require systemic therapy and who are radioactive iodine-refractory (if radioactive iodine is appropriate). The most common adverse reactions, including laboratory abnormalities, (incidence ≥ 25%) have been increased aspartate aminotransferase (AST), increased alanine aminotransferase (ALT), increased glucose, decreased leukocytes, decreased albumin, decreased calcium, dry mouth, diarrhea, increased creatinine, increased alkaline phosphatase, hypertension, fatigue, edema, decreased platelets, increased total cholesterol, rash, decreased sodium, and constipation. Monitor ALT and AST prior to initiating **Retevmo**, every 2 weeks during the first 3 months, then monthly thereafter and as clinically indicated. Do not initiate **Retevmo** in patients with uncontrolled hypertension; optimize BP prior to initiating **Retevmo** and monitor BP after 1 week, at least monthly thereafter and as clinically indicated. Monitor patients who are at significant risk of developing QTc prolongation. Assess QT interval, electrolytes and TSH at baseline and periodically during treatment. Monitor QT interval more frequently when **Retevmo** is concomitantly administered with strong and moderate CYP3A inhibitors or drugs known to prolong QTc interval. Permanently discontinue **Retevmo** in patients with severe or life-threatening hemorrhage. Withhold **Retevmo** and initiate corticosteroids in the occurrence of any hypersensitivity reaction and, upon resolution, resume at a reduced dose and increase dose by 1 dose level each week until reaching the dose taken prior to onset of hypersensitivity. Continue steroids until the patient reaches target dose of **Retevmo** and then taper. Withhold **Retevmo** for at least 7 days prior to elective surgery. Do not administer for at least 2 weeks following major surgery and until adequate wound healing. The safety of resumption of **Retevmo** after resolution of wound healing complications has not been established. Avoid co-administration with PPIs; if co-administration cannot be avoided, take **Retevmo** with food (with PPI) or modify its administration time (with H2 receptor antagonist or locally-acting antacid). Avoid co-administration strong and moderate CYP3A inhibitors; if co-administration cannot be avoided, reduce the **Retevmo** dose. Avoid co-administration with strong and moderate CYP3A inducers. Avoid co-administration with CYP2C8 and CYP3A substrates; if co-administration cannot be avoided, modify the substrate dosage as recommended in its product labeling. Based on findings from animal studies, and its mechanism of action, **Retevmo** can cause fetal harm. There are no available data on **Retevmo** use in pregnant females to inform drug-associated risk. Therefore, verify pregnancy status in females of reproductive potential prior to initiating **Retevmo** and advise females of reproductive potential of the possible risk to the fetus and to use effective contraception. There are no data on the presence of *selpercatinib* or its metabolites in human milk or effects on the breastfed infant. Because of the potential for serious adverse embryo/fetal effects, advise women not to breastfeed during treatment with **Retevmo** and for 1 week after the final dose.

○ LUPUS NEPHRITIS

CALCINEURIN-INHIBITOR IMMUNOSUPPRESSANT

▷ *voclosporin Recommended Starting Dose*: 23.7 mg twice daily; *Severe Renal Impairment*: 15.8 mg twice daily; *Mild/Moderate Hepatic Impairment*: 15.8 mg twice daily; *Severe Hepatic Impairment*: avoid use with administer consistently as close to a 12-hour schedule as possible, and with at least 8 hours between doses; if a dose is missed, take it as soon as possible within 4 hours after the missed the dose; beyond the 4-hour time frame, wait until the usual scheduled time to take the next regular dose; do not to double the next dose; must be swallowed whole on an empty stomach; avoid eating grapefruit or drinking grapefruit juice while taking **Lupkynis**

Lupkynis *Cap*: 7.9 mg

Comment: **Lupkynis** *(voclosporin)* is indicated in combination with a background immunosuppressive therapy regimen. Use **Lupkynis** in combination with *mycophenolate mofetil* (**MMF**) and corticosteroids. Before initiating **Lupkynis**, establish an accurate baseline estimated glomerular filtration rate (eGFR) and blood pressure.

Baseline eGFR ≤45 mL/min: not recommended unless the benefit exceeds the risk (these patients may be at increased risk for acute and/or chronic nephrotoxicity). Assess eGFR every two weeks for the first month, and every four weeks thereafter. If eGFR <60 mL/min and reduced from baseline by >20% and <30%, reduce the dose by 7.9 mg twice daily; then re-assess within 2 weeks; if eGFR is still reduced from baseline by >20%, reduce the dose again by 7.9 mg twice daily.

If eGFR <60 mL/min and reduced from baseline by ≥30%, discontinue **Lupkynis**; then, re-assess eGFR within two weeks; consider re-initiating **Lupkynis** at a lower dose (7.9 mg twice daily) only if eGFR has returned to ≥80% of baseline.

For patients who had a decrease in dose due to eGFR, consider increasing the dose by 7.9 mg twice a day for each eGFR measurement that is ≥80% of baseline; do not exceed the starting dose. Do not initiate **Lupkynis** in patients with baseline BP >165/105 or with hypertensive emergency. Monitor BP every two weeks for the first month and as clinically indicated thereafter. For patients with If BP >165/105 or with hypertensive emergency, discontinue **Lupkynis** and initiate antihypertensive therapy. Concomitant use of strong CYP3A4 inhibitors (e.g., ketoconazole, itraconazole, clarithromycin) with **Lupkynis** is contraindicated. The most commonly reported adverse reactions (incidence ≥3%) have been decreased eGFR, hypertension, diarrhea, headache, anemia, cough, urinary tract infection, abdominal pain upper, dyspepsia, alopecia, renal impairment, abdominal pain, mouth ulceration, fatigue, tremor, acute kidney injury, and decreased appetite. When **Lupkynis** is co-administered with moderate CYP3A4 inhibitors, reduce the **Lupkynis** daily dose to 15.8 mg in the morning and 7.9 mg in the evening. Avoid co-administration of **Lupkynis** with strong and moderate CYP3A4 inducers. Reduce dosage of certain P-gp substrates with a narrow therapeutic window when co-administered with **Lupkynis**. Avoid live vaccines. **Lupkynis** may cause embryo/fetal harm. Advise not to breastfeed.

LYME DISEASE (*ERYTHEMA CHRONICUM MIGRANS*)

Comment: The bite of the deer tick (*Ioxodes scapularis*) carries the *Borrelia burgdorferi* organism causing Lyme disease. Proper removal of the tick, and early diagnosis and treatment are essential to effective management of this disease.

STAGE 1

▶ *amoxicillin* (B)(G) 500-875 mg bid or 250-500 mg tid x 10 days
  Pediatric: <40 kg (88 lb): 20-40 mg/kg/day in 3 divided doses x 10 days or 25-45 mg/kg/day in 2 divided doses x 10 days; ≥40 kg: same as adult; *see* Appendix CC.3. *amoxicillin* (Amoxil Suspension, Trimox Suspension) *for dose by weight*
    Amoxil *Cap:* 250, 500 mg; *Tab:* 875*mg; *Chew tab:* 125, 200, 250, 400 mg (cherry-banana-peppermint) (phenylalanine); *Oral susp:* 125, 250 mg/5 ml (80, 100, 150 ml) (strawberry); 200, 400 mg/5 ml (50, 75, 100 ml) (bubble gum); *Oral drops:* 50 mg/ml (30 ml) (bubble gum)
    Moxatag *Tab:* 775 mg ext-rel
    Trimox *Tab:* 125, 250 mg; *Cap:* 250, 500 mg; *Oral susp:* 125, 250 mg/5 ml (80, 100, 150 ml) (raspberry-strawberry)
▶ *clarithromycin* (C)(G) 500 mg bid or 500 mg ext-rel once daily x 14-21 days
  Pediatric: <6 months: not recommended; ≥6 months: 7.5 mg/kg bid x 7 days; *see* Appendix CC.16. *clarithromycin* (Biaxin Suspension) *for dose by weight*
    Biaxin *Tab:* 250, 500 mg
    Biaxin Oral Suspension *Oral susp:* 125, 250 mg/5 ml (50, 100 ml)
    Biaxin XL *Tab:* 500 mg ext-rel
▶ *doxycycline* (D)(G) 100 mg bid x 14-21 days
  Pediatric: <8 years: not recommended; ≥8 years, ≤100 lb: 2 mg/lb on first day in 2 divided doses, followed by 1 mg/lb/day in 1-2 divided doses; ≥8 years, >100 lb: same as adult; *see Appendix CC.19: doxycycline* (Vibramycin Syrup/Suspension) *for dose by weight*
    Acticlate *Tab:* 75, 150**mg
    Adoxa *Tab:* 50, 75, 100, 150 mg ent-coat
    Doryx *Tab:* 50, 75, 100, 150, 200 mg del-rel
    Doxteric *Tab:* 50 mg del-rel
    Monodox *Cap:* 50, 75, 100 mg
    Oracea *Cap:* 40 mg del-rel
    Vibramycin *Tab:* 100 mg; *Cap:* 50, 100 mg; *Syr:* 50 mg/5 ml (raspberry-apple) (sulfites); *Oral susp:* 25 mg/5 ml (raspberry)
    Vibra-Tab *Tab:* 100 mg film-coat
▶ *minocycline* (D)(G) 200 mg on first day; then 100 mg q 12 hours x 9 more days
  Pediatric: ≤8 years: not recommended; ≥8 years, <100 lb: 2 mg/lb on first day in 2 divided doses, followed by 1 mg/lb q 12 hours x 9 more days; ≥8 years, >100 lb: same as adult
    Dynacin *Cap:* 50, 100 mg
    Minocin *Cap:* 50, 75, 100 mg; *Oral susp:* 50 mg/5 ml (60 ml) (custard) (sulfites, alcohol 5%)
▶ *tetracycline* (D)(G) 250-500 mg qid ac x 21 days
  Pediatric: <8 years: not recommended; ≥8 years, ≤100 lb: 25-50 mg/kg/day in 2-4 divided doses x 7 days; ≥8 years, >100 lb: same as adult; *see Appendix CC.31: tetracycline* (Sumycin Suspension) *for dose by weight*
    Achromycin V *Cap:* 250, 500 mg
    Sumycin *Tab:* 250, 500 mg; *Cap:* 250, 500 mg; *Oral susp:* 125 mg/5 ml (100, 200 ml) (fruit) (sulfites)

 LYMPHADENITIS

Comment: Therapy should continue for no less than 5 days after resolution of symptoms.

▷ *amoxicillin+clavulanate* (B)(G)
  Augmentin 500 mg tid *or* 875 mg bid x 7-10 days
  Pediatric: 40-45 mg/kg/day divided tid x 10 days *or* 90 mg/kg/day divided
  bid x 10 days *see* Appendix CC.4. *amoxicillin+clavulanate* (Augmentin
  Suspension) *for dose by weight*
    Tab: 250, 500, 875 mg; *Chew tab:* 125, 250 mg (lemon-lime); 200, 400
    mg (cherry-banana) (phenylalanine); *Oral susp:* 125 mg/5 ml (banana),
    250 mg/5 ml (75, 100, 150 ml) (orange); 200, 400 mg/5 ml (50, 75, 100 ml)
    (orange) (phenylalanine)
  Augmentin ES-600 not recommended for adults
  Pediatric: <3 months: not recommended; ≥3 months, <40 kg: 90 mg/kg/day in
  2 divided doses x 7-10 days; ≥40 kg: not recommended
    Oral susp: 42.9 mg/5 ml (50, 75, 100, 125, 150, 200 ml) (strawberry cream)
    (phenylalanine)
  Augmentin XR 2 tabs q 12 hours x 7-10 days
  Pediatric: <16 years: use other forms; ≥16 years: same as adult
    Tab: 1000*mg ext-rel
▷ *cephalexin* (B)(G) 500 mg bid x 10 days
  Pediatric: 25-50 mg/kg/day in 4 divided doses x 10 days; *see* Appendix CC.15.
  cephalexin (Keflex Suspension) *for dose by weight*
    Keflex *Cap:* 250, 333, 500, 750 mg; *Oral susp:* 125, 250 mg/5 ml (100, 200 ml)
    (strawberry)
▷ *dicloxacillin* (B) 500 mg qid x 10 days
  Pediatric: 12.5-25 mg/kg/day in 4 divided doses x 10 days; *see* Appendix CC.18.
  dicloxacillin (Dynapen Suspension) *for dose by weight*
    Dynapen *Cap:* 125, 250, 500 mg; *Oral susp:* 62.5 mg/5 ml (80, 100, 200 ml)

 LYMPHOGRANULOMA VENEREUM

Comment: The following treatment regimens are published in the **2015 CDC Sexually
Transmitted Diseases Treatment Guidelines.** This section contains treatment regimens
for adults <u>only</u>; consult a specialist for treatment of patients less than 18 years of age.
Treatment regimens are presented in alphabetical order by generic drug name, followed
by brands and dose forms. Treat all sexual contacts. Persons with both LGV and HIV
infection should receive the same treatment regimens as those who are HIV-negative;
however, prolonged treatment may be required and delay in resolution of symptoms
may occur.

RECOMMENDED REGIMEN
Regimen 1
▷ *doxycycline* 100 mg bid x 21 days

ALTERNATIVE REGIMEN
Regimen 1
▷ *erythromycin base* 500 mg qid x 21 days *or* *erythromycin ethylsuccinate* 400 mg
  qid x 21 days

RECOMMENDED REGIMENS FOR THE MANAGEMENT OF SEXUAL CONTACTS
Comment: LGV is caused by *C. trachomatis* serovars L1, L2, *or* L3. Persons who
have had sexual contact with a patient who has LGV within 60 days before onset
of the patient's symptoms should be examined, tested for urethral *or* cervical
chlamydial infection, and treated with a chlamydia regimen.

Regimen 1
▷ *azithromycin* 1 gm in a single dose

Regimen 2

▷ *doxycycline* 100 mg bid x 7 days

DRUG BRANDS AND DOSE FORMS

▷ *azithromycin* (B)(G)
Zithromax *Tab:* 250, 500, 600 mg; *Oral susp:* 100 mg/5 ml (15 ml); 200 mg/5 ml
(15, 22.5, 30 ml) (cherry); *Pkt:* 1 gm for reconstitution (cherry-banana)
Zithromax Tri-pak *Tab:* 3 x 500 mg tabs/pck
Zithromax Z-pak *Tab:* 6 x 250 mg tabs/pck
Zmax *Oral susp:* 2 gm ext-rel for reconstitution (cherry-banana) (148 mg Na$^+$)

▷ *doxycycline* (D)(G)
Acticlate *Tab:* 75, 150**mg
Adoxa *Tab:* 50, 75, 100, 150 mg ent-coat
Doryx *Tab:* 50, 75, 100, 150, 200 mg del-rel
Doxteric *Tab:* 50 mg del-rel
Monodox *Cap:* 50, 75, 100 mg
Oracea *Cap:* 40 mg del-rel
Vibramycin *Tab:* 100 mg; *Cap:* 50, 100 mg; *Syr:* 50 mg/5 ml (raspberry-apple)
(sulfites); *Oral susp:* 25 mg/5 ml (raspberry)
Vibra-Tab *Tab:* 100 mg film-coat

▷ *erythromycin base* (B)(G)
Ery-Tab *Tab:* 250, 333, 500 mg ent-coat
PCE *Tab:* 333, 500 mg

▷ *erythromycin ethylsuccinate* (B)(G)
EryPed *Oral susp:* 200 mg/5 ml (100, 200 ml) (fruit); 400 mg/5 ml (60, 100,
200 ml) (banana); *Oral drops:* 200, 400 mg/5 ml (50 ml) (fruit); *Chew tab:*
200 mg wafer (fruit)
E.E.S. *Oral susp:* 200, 400 mg/5 ml (100 ml) (fruit)
E.E.S. Granules *Oral susp:* 200 mg/5 ml (100, 200 ml) (cherry)
E.E.S. 400 Tablets *Tab:* 400 mg

MALARIA (*PLASMODIUM FALCIPARUM, PLASMODIUM VIVAX*)

▷ *doxycycline* (D)(G) 100 mg daily; initiate 1-2 days prior to travel; take during
travel; continue for 4 weeks after leaving the endemic area
Pediatric: ≤8 years: not recommended; ≥8 years, ≤100 lb: 1 mg/lb/day prior to
travel; take during travel; continue for 4 weeks after leaving the endemic area;
≥8 years, ≥100 lb: same as adult; *see Appendix CC.19: doxycycline* (Vibramycin
Syrup/Suspension) *for dose by weight*
Acticlate *Tab:* 75, 150**mg
Adoxa *Tab:* 50, 75, 100, 150 mg ent-coat
Doryx *Tab:* 50, 75, 100, 150, 200 mg del-rel
Doxteric *Tab:* 50 mg del-rel
Monodox *Cap:* 50, 75, 100 mg
Oracea *Cap:* 40 mg del-rel
Vibramycin *Tab:* 100 mg; *Cap:* 50, 100 mg; *Syr:* 50 mg/5 ml (raspberry-apple)
(sulfites); *Oral susp:* 25 mg/5 ml (raspberry)
Vibra-Tab *Tab:* 100 mg film-coat

▷ *minocycline* (D)(G) 100 mg daily; initiate 1-2 days prior to travel; take during
travel; continue for 4 weeks after leaving the endemic area
Pediatric: <8 years: not recommended; ≥8 years, ≤100 lb: 2 mg/lb on first day in
2 divided doses, followed by 1 mg/lb q 12 hours x 9 more days; ≥8 years, >100 lb:
same as adult
Dynacin *Cap:* 50, 100 mg
Minocin *Cap:* 50, 75, 100 mg; *Oral susp:* 50 mg/5 ml (60 ml) (custard) (sulfites,
alcohol 5%)

▷ *tetracycline* (D) 250 mg daily; initiate 1-2 days prior to travel; take during travel; continue for 4 weeks after leaving the endemic area
Pediatric: <8 years: not recommended; ≥8 years, ≤100 lb: 25-50 mg/kg/day in 4 divided doses x 10 days; ≥8 years, >100 lb: same as adult; *see Appendix CC.31: tetracycline* (Sumycin Suspension) *for dose by weight*
   Achromycin V *Cap:* 250, 500 mg
   Sumycin *Tab:* 250, 500 mg; *Cap:* 250, 500 mg; *Oral susp:* 125 mg/5 ml (100, 200 ml) (fruit) (sulfites)

INITIAL BOLUS TREATMENT FOR SEVERE MALARIA

▷ *artesunate for injection* 2.4 mg/kg administered intravenously at 0 hours, 12 hours, and 24 hours; thereafter, administer once daily until the patient is able to tolerate oral antimalarial therapy; using only the sterile diluent supplied, swirl gently (do not shake) for up to 5-6 minutes until the powder is fully dissolved; administer as a slow IV bolus over 1-2 minutes within 1.5 hours after reconstitution; do not administer via continuous IV infusion; see mfr pkg insert for instructions on preparation
Pediatric: for patients <6 months, a pharmacokinetic (PK) extrapolation approach using modeling and simulation indicated comparable or higher predicted PK steady-state AUC of DHA between this age group and older children or adults at the recommended 2.4 mg/kg dose regimen; no notable safety issues have been identified in limited published safety and outcome data in patients <6 months with severe malaria; no dose adjustment is necessary for pediatric patients regardless of age or bodyweight
   Artesunate for Injection *Vial:* 110 mg, single-dose, pwdr for reconstitution w. supplied sterile diluent (12 ml) (natural rubber latex-free)
   Comment: **Artesunate** for Injection is an antimalarial indicated for the initial treatment of severe malaria in adult and pediatric patients. Treatment of severe malaria with **Artesunate** for Injection should always be followed by a complete treatment course of an appropriate oral antimalarial regimen. **Artesunate for Injection** does not treat the hypnozoite liver stage forms of *Plasmodium* and will, therefore, not prevent relapses of malaria due to *Plasmodium vivax* or *Plasmodium ovale*. Concomitant therapy with an antimalarial agent, such as an 8-aminoquinoline drug, is necessary for the treatment of severe malaria due to *P. vivax* or *P. ovale*. Cases of posttreatment hemolytic anemia severe enough to require transfusion have been reported; monitor patients for 4 weeks after treatment for evidence of hemolytic anemia. Serious hypersensitivity reactions including anaphylaxis have been reported; discontinue if signs of serious hypersensitivity occur. The most common adverse reactions (incidence ≥2%) reported in clinical trials of severe malaria include acute renal failure requiring dialysis, hemoglobinuria, and jaundice. Monitor for possible reduced antimalarial efficacy if **Artesunate for Injection** is used concomitantly with *nevirapine* or *ritonavir* antiretrovirals or strong UGT inducers (e.g., *rifampin, carbamazepine, phenytoin*). Delaying treatment of severe malaria in pregnancy may result in serious morbidity and mortality to the mother and fetus. Based on animal data, **Artesunate for Injection** may cause fetal harm. However, administration for the treatment of severe malaria may be lifesaving for the pregnant female and fetus; therefore, treatment should not be delayed due to pregnancy.

ANTIMALARIALS

▷ *atovaquone* (C)(G) take as a single dose with food or a milky drink at the same time each day; repeat dose if vomited within 1 hour; *Prophylaxis:* 1500 mg once daily; *Treatment:* 750 mg bid x 21 days
   Mepron *Susp:* 750 mg/5 ml

▷ *atovaquone+proguanil* (C)(G) take as a single dose with food or a milky drink at the same time each day; repeat dose if vomited within 1 hour; *Prophylaxis:* 1 tab daily starting 1-2 days before entering endemic area, during stay, and for 7 days after return; *Treatment (acute, uncomplicated):* 4 tabs daily x 3 days
Pediatric: <5 kg: not recommended; 5-40 kg:
Prophylaxis: daily dose starting 1-2 days before entering endemic area, during stay, and for 7 days after return; 5-20 kg: 1 ped tab; 21-30 kg: 2 ped tabs; 31-40 kg: 3 ped tabs; ≥40 kg: same as adult; *Treatment (acute, uncomplicated):* daily dose x 3 days; 5-8 kg: 2 ped tabs; 9-10 kg: 3 ped tabs; 11-20 kg: 1 adult tab; 21-30 kg: 2 adult tabs; 31-40 kg: 3 adult tabs; >40 kg: same as adult

   Malarone *Tab:* atov 250 mg+prog 100 mg

   Malarone Pediatric *Tab:* atov 62.5 mg+prog 25 mg

Comment: *Atovaquone* is antagonized by **tetracycline** and **metoclopramide**. Concomitant **rifampin** is not recommended (may elevate LFTs).

▷ *chloroquine* (C)(G) *Prophylaxis:* 500 mg once weekly (on the same day of each week); start 2 weeks prior to exposure, continue while in the endemic area, and continue 4 weeks after departure; *Treatment:* initially 1 gm; then 500 mg 6 hours, 24 hours, and 48 hours after initial dose or initially 200-250 mg IM; may repeat in 6 hours; max 1 gm in first 24 hours; continue to 1.875 gm in 3 days
Pediatric: Suppression: 8.35 mg/kg (max 500 mg) weekly (on the same day of each week); *Treatment:* initially 16.7 mg/kg (max 1 gm); then 8.35 mg/kg (max 500 mg) 6 hours, 24 hours, and 48 hours after initial dose, or initially 6.25 mg/kg IM; may repeat in 6 hours; max 12.5 mg/kg/day

   Aralen *Tab:* 500 mg; *Amp:* 50 mg/ml (5 ml)

▷ *hydroxychloroquine* (C)(G) *Prophylaxis:* 400 mg once weekly (on the same day of each week); start 2 weeks prior to exposure, continue while in the endemic area, and continue 8 weeks after departure; *Treatment:* initially 800 mg; then 400 mg 6 hours, 24 hours, and 48 hours after initial dose
Pediatric: Suppression: 6.45 mg/kg (max 400 mg) weekly (on the same day of each week) beginning 2 weeks prior to arrival, continuing while in endemic area, and continuing 4 weeks after departure; *Treatment:* initially 12.9 mg/kg (max 800 mg); then 6.45 mg/kg (max 400 mg) 6 hours, 24 hours, and 48 hours after initial dose hours after initial dose

   Plaquenil *Tab:* 200 mg

▷ *mefloquine* (C) *Prophylaxis:* 250 mg once weekly (on the same day of each week); start 1 week prior to exposure, continue while in the endemic area, and continue for 4 weeks after departure; *Treatment:* 1,250 mg as a single dose
Pediatric: <6 months: not recommended; *Prophylaxis:* ≥6 months: 3-5 mg/kg (max 250 mg) weekly (on the same day of each week); start 1 week prior to exposure, continue while in the endemic area, and continue for 4 weeks after departure; *Treatment:* ≥6 months: 25-50 mg/kg as a single dose; max 250 mg

   Lariam *Tab:* 250*mg

Comment: **Mefloquine** is contraindicated with active or recent history of depression, generalized anxiety disorder, psychosis, schizophrenia or any other psychiatric disorder or history of convulsions.

▷ *quinine sulfate* (C)(G) 1 tab or cap every 8 hours x 7 days
Pediatric: <16 years: not recommended; ≥16 years: same as adult

   Tab: 260 mg; *Cap:* 260, 300, 325 mg

   Qualaquin *Cap:* 324 mg

   Comment: **Qualaquin** is indicated in the treatment of uncomplicated *P. falciparum* malaria (including **chloroquine**-resistant strains).

▷ *tafenoquine* (C)(G) *Loading Regimen:* take 200 mg (2 x 100 mg tabs) once daily x 3 days before travel to endemic area; *Maintenance:* take 200 mg (2 x 100 mg tabs) once weekly beginning 7 days after the last loading regimen dose; maintenance dose may be continued for up to 6 months; take with food

Pediatric: <18 years: not recommended; ≥18 years: same as adult

Arakoda *Tab:* 100 mg

Comment: **Arakoda** *(tafenoquine)* is an 8-aminoquinoline antimalarial drug indicated for the prophylaxis of malaria. **Arakoda** provides effective protection against both of the major types of malaria (*P. vivax* and *P. falciparum*), killing the parasites in both the blood and liver. **Arakoda** is not recommended for with a history of psychosis or current psychotic symptoms. **Arakoda** is not recommended for patients with G6PD deficiency or unknown G6PD status. Because **Arakoda** may cause fetal harm when administered to a pregnant female with a G6PD-deficient fetus, **Arakoda** is not recommended during pregnancy, breastfeeding when the infant is found to be G6PD deficient or if G6PD status is unknown and during treatment and for 3 months after the last dose of **Arakoda**. All patients must be tested for glucose-6-phosphate dehydrogenase (G6PD) deficiency prior to prescribing **Arakoda** and pregnancy testing is recommended for females of reproductive potential prior to initiating treatment. Due to the long half-life of **Arakoda** (approximately 17 days), psychiatric effects, hemolytic anemia, methemoglobinemia, and hypersensitivity reactions may be delayed in onset and/or duration. Avoid co-administration with drugs that are substrates of organic cation transporter-2 (OCT2) or multidrug and toxin extrusion (MATE) transporters. The most common adverse reactions (incidence ≥1%) have been headache, dizziness, back pain, diarrhea, nausea, vomiting, increased alanine, aminotransferase (ALT), motion sickness, insomnia, depression, abnormal dreams, and anxiety.

RADICAL CURE (PREVENTION OF RELAPSE)
8-AMINOQUINOLINE DERIVATIVE

▷ *tafenoquine* take 300 mg (2 x 150 mg tabs) as a single dose with food; co-administer on the first or second day of the appropriate antimalarial therapy for acute *P. vivax* malaria

Pediatric: <16 years: not recommended; ≥16 years: same as adult

Krintafel *Tab:* 150 mg

Comment: **Krintafel** *(tafenoquine)* is an 8-aminoquinoline derivative antimalarial for the radical cure (prevention of relapse) of *Plasmodium vivax* malaria in patients who are receiving appropriate antimalarial therapy for acute *P. vivax* infection. **Krintafel** is not indicated for the treatment of acute *P. vivax* malaria. Contraindications are glucose-6-phosphate dehydrogenase (G6PD) deficiency or unknown G6PD status and breastfeeding by a lactating woman when the infant is found to be G6PD deficient or if G6PD status is unknown (due to the risk of hemolytic anemia in patients with G6PD deficiency). All patients must be tested for G6PD deficiency prior to prescribing **Krintafel** and pregnancy testing is recommended for females of reproductive potential prior to initiating treatment with **Krintafel**. Also, the G6PD-deficient infant may be at risk for hemolytic anemia from exposure to **Krintafel** through breast milk; check infant's G6PD status before breastfeeding begins. Asymptomatic elevations in blood methemoglobin have been observed; initiate appropriate therapy if signs or symptoms of methemoglobinemia occur. Serious psychiatric adverse reactions have been observed in patients with a previous history of psychiatric conditions at doses higher than the approved dose. Therefore, benefit of treatment with **Krintafel** must be weighed against the potential risk for psychiatric adverse reactions in patients with a history of psychiatric illness. Due to the long half-life of **Krintafel** (15 days), psychiatric effects and hypersensitivity reactions may be delayed in onset and/or duration. Common adverse reactions (incidence ≥5%) have been dizziness, nausea, vomiting, headache, and decreased hemoglobin.

MASTITIS (BREAST ABSCESS)

ANTI-INFECTIVES

▷ *amoxicillin+clavulanate* (B)(G)

Augmentin 500 mg tid <u>or</u> 875 mg bid x 7-10 days
Pediatric: 40-45 mg/kg/day divided tid x 10 days <u>or</u> 90 mg/kg/day divided bid x 10 days *see* Appendix CC.4. *amoxicillin+clavulanate* (Augmentin Suspension) *for dose by weight*
  Tab: 250, 500, 875 mg; *Chew tab:* 125, 250 mg (lemon-lime); 200, 400 mg (cherry-banana) (phenylalanine); *Oral susp:* 125 mg/5 ml (banana), 250 mg/5 ml (75, 100, 150 ml) (orange); 200, 400 mg/5 ml (50, 75, 100 ml) (orange) (phenylalanine)

Augmentin ES-600 not recommended for adults
Pediatric: <3 months: not recommended; ≥3 months, <40 kg: 90 mg/kg/day in 2 divided doses x 7-10 days; ≥40 kg: not recommended
  Oral susp: 42.9 mg/5 ml (50, 75, 100, 125, 150, 200 ml) (strawberry cream) (phenylalanine)

Augmentin XR 2 tabs q 12 hours x 7-10 days
Pediatric: <16 years: use other forms; ≥16 years: same as adult
  Tab: 1000*mg ext-rel

▷ *cefaclor* (B)(G)

Ceclor 250 mg tid <u>or</u> 375 mg bid 3-10 days
Pediatric: <1 month: not recommended; 1 month-12 years: 20-40 mg/kg divided bid or q 12 hours x 3-10 days; max 1 gm/day; see Appendix CC.8. *cefaclor* (Ceclor Suspension) for *dose by weight*; >12 years: same as adult
  Tab: 500 mg; *Cap:* 250, 500 mg; *Susp:* 125 mg/5 ml (75, 150 ml) (strawberry); 187 mg/5 ml (50, 100 ml) (strawberry); 250 mg/5 ml (75, 150 ml) (strawberry); 375 mg/5 ml (50, 100 ml) (strawberry)

Ceclor Extended Release 375-500 mg bid x 3-10 days
Pediatric: <16 years: ext-rel not recommended; ≥16 years: same as adult
  Tab: 375, 500 mg ext-rel

▷ *ceftriaxone* (B)(G) 1-2 gm IM daily continued 2 days after signs of infection have disappeared; max 4 gm/day
Pediatric: 50 mg/kg IM daily continued 2 days after signs of infection have disappeared
  Rocephin *Vial:* 250, 500 mg; 1, 2 gm

▷ *cephalexin* (B)(G) 500 mg bid x 10 days
Pediatric: 25-50 mg/kg/day in 4 divided doses x 10 days; *see* Appendix CC.15. *cephalexin* (Keflex Suspension) *for dose by weight*
  Keflex *Cap:* 250, 333, 500, 750 mg; *Oral susp:* 125, 250 mg/5 ml (100, 200 ml) (strawberry)

▷ *clindamycin* (B)(G) 300 mg tid x 10 days
Pediatric: <12 years: not recommended; ≥12 years: same as adult
  Cleocin *Cap:* 75 (tartrazine), 150 (tartrazine), 300 mg
  Cleocin Pediatric Granules *Oral susp:* 75 mg/5 ml (100 ml) (cherry)

▷ *erythromycin base* (B)(G) 250-500 mg qid x 10 days
Pediatric: <45 kg: 30-40 mg/kg/day in 4 divided doses x 10 days; ≥45 kg: same as adult
  Ery-Tab *Tab:* 250, 333, 500 mg ent-coat
  PCE *Tab:* 333, 500 mg

MELASMA/CHLOASMA

SKIN DEPIGMENTING AGENTS

▷ *hydroquinone* (C) apply a thin film to clean dry affected areas bid; discontinue if lightening does <u>not</u> occur after 2 months

Pediatric: <12 years: not recommended; ≥12 years: same as adult
> **Lustra** *Crm:* hydro 4% (1, 2 oz) (sulfites)
> **Lustra AF** *Crm:* hydro 4% (1, 2 oz) (sunscreens, sulfites)

▶ ***hydroquinone+fluocinolone acetonide+tretinoin*** (C) apply a thin film to clean dry affected areas once daily at least 30 minutes before bedtime
Pediatric: <12 years: not recommended; ≥12 years: same as adult
> **Tri-Luma** *Crm:* hydro 4%+fluo acet 0.01%+tret 0.05% (30 gm) (sulfites, parabens)

MÉNIÈRE'S DISEASE

▶ ***diazepam*** (D)(IV)(G) initially 1-2.5 mg tid-qid; may increase gradually
Pediatric: <6 months: not recommended; ≥6 months: same as adult
> **Diastat** *Rectal gel delivery system:* 2.5 mg
> **Diastat AcuDial** *Rectal gel delivery system:* 10, 20 mg
> **Valium** *Tab:* 2*, 5*, 10*mg
> **Valium Intensol Oral Solution** *Conc oral soln:* 5 mg/ml (30 ml w. dropper) (alcohol 19%)
> **Valium Oral Solution** *Oral soln:* 5 mg/5 ml (500 ml) (wintergreen-spice)

▶ ***dimenhydrinate*** (B) 50 mg q 4-6 hours
Pediatric: <2 years: not recommended; 2-6 years: 12.5-25 mg q 6-8 hours; max 75 mg/day; >6-11 years: 25-50 mg q 6-8 hours; max 150 mg/day; >11 years: same as adult
> **Dramamine (OTC)** *Tab:* 50*mg; *Chew tab:* 50 mg (phenylalanine, tartrazine); *Liq:* 12.5 mg/5 ml (4 oz)

▶ ***diphenhydramine*** (B)(OTC)(G) 25-50 mg q 6-8 hours; max 100 mg/day
Pediatric: <2 years: not recommended; 2-6 years: 6.25 mg q 4-6 hours; max 37.5 mg/day; >6-12 years: 12.5-25 mg q 4-6 hours; max 150 mg/day; >12 years: same as adult
> **Benadryl (OTC)** *Chew tab:* 12.5 mg (grape; phenylalanine); *Liq:* 12.5 mg/5 ml (4, 8 oz); *Cap:* 25 mg; *Tab:* 25 mg; *dye-free softgel:* 25 mg; Dye-free liq: 12.5 mg/5 ml (4, 8 oz)

▶ ***meclizine*** (B)(G) 25-100/day in divided doses
Pediatric: <12 years: not recommended; ≥12 years: same as adult
> **Antivert** *Tab:* 12.5, 25, 50*mg; *Amp:* 50 mg/ml (1 ml); *Vial:* 50 mg/ml (1 ml single-use); 50 mg/ml (10 ml multi-dose)
> **Bonine (OTC)** *Cap:* 15, 25, 30 mg; *Tab:* 12.5, 25, 50 mg; *Chew tab/Film-coat tab:* 25 mg
> **Dramamine II** 25 mg bid; max 50 mg/day
> *Tab:* 25*mg
> **Zentrip** *Strip:* 25 mg orally disintegrating

▶ ***promethazine*** (C) 12.5-25 q 4-6 hours PO or rectally
Pediatric: <2 years: not recommended; ≥2 years: 0.5 mg/lb or 6.25-25 mg q 4-6 hours PO or rectally
> **Phenergan** *Tab:* 12.5*, 25*, 50 mg; *Plain syr:* 6.25 mg/5 ml; *Fortis syr:* 25 mg/5 ml; *Rectal supp:* 12.5, 25, 50 mg

Comment: *Promethazine* is contraindicated in children with uncomplicated nausea, dehydration, Reye's syndrome, history of sleep apnea, asthma, and lower respiratory disorders in children. *Promethazine* lowers the seizure threshold in children, may cause cholestatic jaundice, anticholinergic effects, extrapyramidal effects, and potentially fatal respiratory depression.

▶ ***scopolamine*** transdermal patch (C) 1 patch behind ear; each patch is effective for 3 days; change patch every 4th day; alternate sites
Pediatric: <12 years: not recommended; ≥12 years: same as adult
> **Transderm Scop** *Patch:* 1.5 mg (4/carton)

MENINGITIS (*NEISSERIA MENINGITIDIS*)

PROPHYLAXIS

Comment: Meningitis vaccine is a 3-dose series (0, 2, 6 month schedule) indicated for persons age ≥10-25 years. Have epinephrine 1:1000 readily available and monitor for 15 minutes post-dose of meningitis vaccine.

Meningococcal A, C, W, Y Vaccination

ACIP recommends routine vaccination with a quadrivalent meningococcal conjugate vaccine (**MenACWY**) for persons at risk for meningococcal disease caused by serogroups A, C, W, or Y and booster doses for those who were previously vaccinated who become or remain at risk. **MenACWY-TT** was first licensed in 2020 for the prevention of meningococcal disease caused by serogroups A, C, W, Y in persons age ≥2 years.

Meningococcal B Vaccination

ACIP recommends routine vaccination with serogroup B meningococcal (**MenB**) vaccine in persons age >10 years who are at risk for serogroup B meningococcal disease and **MenB** boosters are recommended for those who were previously vaccinated who become or remain at risk. ACIP recommends a **MenB** series for adolescents and young adults age 16-23 years by shared clinical decision-making to provide short-term protection against most strains of the serogroup B meningococcal disease.

▷ *Meningococcal group b vaccine (recombinant, absorbed)* administer first dose IM in the deltoid; administer second dose 2 months later; administer the third dose 6 months from the first dose;
Pediatric: <10 years: not established; ≥10 years: same as adult
  Bexsero *Susp for IM inj:* 0.5 ml single-dose prefilled syringes (1, 10/carton)
  Trumenba *Susp for IM inj:* 0.5 ml single-dose prefilled syringes (5, 10/carton)

▷ *Neisseria meningitides oligosaccharide conjugate* quadrivalent meningococcal vaccine (**B**) contains *Corynebacterium diphtheria* CRM197 protein; 10 mcg of Group A + 5 mcg each of Group C, Y, and W-135 + 32.7-64.1 mcg of diphtheria CRM 197 protein per 0.5 m.
Pediatric: <11 years: not recommended; ≥11-55 years: 0.5 ml IM x 1 dose in the deltoid
  Menveo *Vial multi-dose:* 5 doses/vial (MenA conjugate component pwdr for reconstitution + 1 vial liquid MenCWY conjugate component for reconstitution) (preservative-free)

▷ *Neisseria meningitidis polysaccharides* vaccine (**C**) 0.5 ml SC x 1 dose; if at high risk, may revaccinate after 3-5 years; age ≥55 years contact mfr
  Menactra (A/C/Y/W-135)
  Pediatric: <2 years: see mfr pkg insert; ≥2 years: same as adult; if at high risk, may revaccinate children first vaccinated ≤4 years-of-age after 2-3 years
    Vial (single-dose): 4 mcg each of group A, C, Y, and W-135 per 0.5 ml (pwdr for SC inj after reconstitution) (preservative-free diluent); *Vial (multi-dose):* 4 mcg each of group A, C, Y, and W-130 per 0.5 ml pwdr for SC inj after reconstitution (5 doses/vial) (preservative-free)
  Comment: Latex allergy is a contraindication to **Menactra**.
  Menomune-A/C/Y/W-135
  Pediatric: <2 years: not recommended (except ≥3 months of age as short-term protection against group A); ≥2 years: same as adult; if at high risk, may revaccinate children first vaccinated ≤4 years of age after 2-3 years (older children after 3-5 years)
    Vial (single-dose): 50 mcg each of group A, C, Y, and W-135 per 0.5 ml (pwdr for SC inj after reconstitution; preservative-free diluent); *Vial (multi-*

dose): 50 mcg each of group A, C, Y, and W-130 per 0.5 ml [pwdr for SC inj after reconstitution (10 doses/vial) (thimerosal-preserved diluent)]

Comment: Use precaution with latex allergy.

▷ *meningococcal (groups A, C, W, Y) conjugate vaccine Primary Vaccination:* 0.5 ml IM as a single one-time dose; *Booster Vaccination:* a single 0.5 ml IM dose may be administered to individuals ≥15 years-of-age and older who are at continued risk for meningococcal disease if at least 4 years have elapsed since a prior dose of meningococcal (Groups A, C, W, Y) conjugate vaccine
Pediatric: <2 years: not established; ≥2 years: same as adult

MenQuadfi *Vial:* 0.5 ml, single-dose

Comment: MenQuadfi is a quadrivalent (MenACWY) vaccine indicated for active immunization for the prevention of Invasive meningococcal disease caused by *Neisseria meningitidis* serogroups A, C, W, and Y. MenQuadfi is contraindicated with patient history of severe allergic reaction to any component of the vaccine, or after a previous dose of MenQuadfi or any other tetanus toxoid-containing vaccine. The most commonly reported adverse reactions (incidence ≥10%) following a primary dose have been as follows: *2-9 Years:* pain (38.6%), erythema (22.6%), swelling at the injection site (13.8%), malaise (21.1%), (13.8%) myalgia (20.1%), and headache (12.5%); *10-17 Years:* injection site pain (34.8%–45.2%), myalgia (27.4%–35.3%), headache (26.5%–30.2%), and malaise (19.4%–26.0%); *18-55 Years:* injection site pain (41.9%), myalgia (35.6%), headache (29.0%), and malaise (22.9%). *≥56 Years:* pain at the injection site.

MENOMETRORRHAGIA: IRREGULAR HEAVY MENSTRUAL BLEEDING, MENORRHAGIA: HEAVY CYCLICAL MENSTRUAL BLEEDING

ANTIFIBROLYTIC AGENT

▷ *tranexamic acid* (B)(G) 1,300 mg tid; treat for up to 5 days during menses; *Normal renal function (SCr ≤1.4 mg/dL):* 1,300 mg tid; *SCr ≥1.4-2.8 mg/dL:* 1,300 mg bid; *SCr ≥2.8-5.7 mg/dL:* 1,300 mg once daily; *SCr ≥5.7 mg/dL:* 650 mg once daily
Pediatric: <18 years: not recommended; ≥18 years: same as adult

Lysteda *Tab:* 650 mg

Injectible Progesterone Only Contraceptives

▷ *medroxyprogesterone* (X)(G)

Depo-Provera 150 mg deep IM q 3 months
Vial: 150 mg/ml (1 ml)
Prefilled syringe: 150 mg/ml
Depo-SubQ 104 mg SC q 3 months
Prefilled syringe: 104 mg/ml (0.65 ml) (parabens)

Comment: Administer first dose within 5 days of onset of normal menses, within 5 days postpartum if not breastfeeding, or at 6 weeks postpartum if breastfeeding exclusively. Do not use for >2 years unless other methods are inadequate.

Combined Oral Contraceptives *see* Appendix H.2. 28-Day Oral Contraceptives with Estrogen and Progesterone Content

Intrauterine Contraceptives *see* Appendix H.9. Intrauterine Contraceptives

MENOPAUSE

Comment:

Adverse Side Effects of Estrogen Supplementation: Inform patients of possible less serious but common adverse reactions that may occur with estrogen-alone therapy: headaches, breast/nipple tenderness/pain, and nausea/vomiting. Estrogen-alone therapy increases the risk of gallbladder disease; discontinue estrogen if severe hypercalcemia, loss of vision, severe hypertriglyceridemia, or cholestatic jaundice occurs.

Estrogen Therapy: should be used with caution in women with hypoparathyroidism as estrogen-induced hypocalcemia may occur. Monitor thyroid function in women on thyroid replacement therapy. Retinal vascular thrombosis has been reported in women receiving estrogen; discontinue medication pending examination if there is sudden partial or complete loss of vision, or a sudden onset of proptosis, diplopia, or migraine. If examination reveals papilledema or retinal vascular lesions, estrogens should be permanently discontinued. In a small number of case reports, substantial increases in blood pressure have been attributed to idiosyncratic reactions to estrogens. In a large, randomized, placebo-controlled clinical trial, a generalized effect of estrogens on blood pressure was not seen. Exogenous estrogen may exacerbate symptoms of angioedema in women with hereditary angioedema. Estrogen therapy may cause exacerbation of asthma, diabetes mellitus, epilepsy, migraine, porphyria, systemic lupus erythematosus and hepatic hemangiomas; use with caution in women with any of these conditions.

Inducers and inhibitors of CYP3A4 may alter estrogen drug metabolism and decrease or increase the estrogen plasma concentration.

Contraindications to Estrogen-Replacement Therapy (ERT): known or suspected pregnancy. undiagnosed abnormal genital bleeding, breast cancer or a history of breast cancer, estrogen-dependent neoplasia, active DVT, PE, or history of these conditions, active arterial thromboembolic disease (e.g., stroke, MI), or history of these conditions, known anaphylactic reaction, angioedema, or hypersensitivity to exogenous estrogen, hepatic impairment/disease, protein C, protein S, or antithrombin deficiency, or other known thrombophilic disorder. A woman who takes estrogen but does not have a uterus, generally does not need a progestin. In some cases, however, hysterectomized women who have a history of endometriosis may need a progestin. Use estrogen-alone, or in combination with a progestin, at the lowest effective dose and for the shortest duration consistent with treatment goals and risks for the individual woman. Re-evaluate post-menopausal women periodically as clinically appropriate to determine if treatment is still necessary.

Estrogen-Alone Therapy: There is increased risk of endometrial cancer in a woman with a uterus who uses unopposed estrogens. Estrogen-alone therapy should not be used for the prevention of cardiovascular disease or dementia. The Women's Health Initiative (WHI) estrogen-alone substudy reported increased risks of stroke and deep vein thrombosis (DVT). The WHI Memory Study (WHIMS), estrogen-alone ancillary study of WHI, reported an increased risk of probable dementia in post-menopausal women ≥65 years-of-age.

Estrogen plus Progestin Therapy: Estrogen plus progestin therapy should not be used for the prevention of cardiovascular disease or dementia. The WHI estrogen plus progestin substudy reported increased risks of stroke, DVT, pulmonary embolism (PE), and myocardial infarction (MI) (5.1). The WHI estrogen plus progestin study reported increased risks of invasive breast cancer. The WHIMS estrogen plus progestin ancillary study of WHI reported an increased risk of probable dementia in post-menopausal women ≥65 years-of-age.

VAGINAL RINGS

▷ *estradiol, acetate* (X)
    Femring Vaginal Ring insert high into vagina; replace every 90 days
▷ *estradiol, micronized* (X)
    Estring Vaginal Ring insert high into vagina; replace every 90 days
      Vag ring: 7.5 mcg/24 hours (1/pck)

REGIMENS FOR PATIENTS WITH INTACT UTERUS

Vaginal Preparations (With Uterus)

Comment: Vaginal preparations provide relief from vaginal and urinary symptoms only (i.e., atrophic vaginitis, dyspareunia, dysuria, and urinary frequency).

▷ *estradiol* (X)(G)

Vagifem Tabs insert one 10 mcg or 25 mcg vaginal tablet once daily x 2 weeks; then twice weekly for 2 weeks (e.g., tues/fri); consider the addition of a progestin
Vag tab: 10, 25 mcg (8, 18/blister pck with applicator)

Yuvafem Vaginal Tablet 1 tab intravaginally daily x 2 weeks; then 1 tab intravaginally twice weekly
Vag tab: 10 mcg (15 tabs w. applicators)

▷ *estradiol, micronized* (X)(G)

Estrace Vaginal Cream 2-4 gm daily x 1-2 weeks, then gradually reduced to 1/2 initial dose x 1-2 weeks, then maintenance dose of 1 gm 1-3 x/week
Vag crm: 0.01% (12, 42.5 gm w. calib applicator)

▷ *estrogen, conjugated equine* (X)

Premarin Vaginal Cream 0.5-2 gm/day intravaginally; cyclically (3 weeks on, 1 week off)
Vag crm: 1.5 oz w. applicator marked in 1/2 gm increments to max of 2 gm

Transdermal Systems (With Uterus)

Comment: Alternate sites. Do not apply patches on or near breasts.

▷ *estradiol* (X)(G)

Climara initially 0.025 mg/day patch once/week to trunk (3 weeks on and 1 week off)
Transdermal patch: 0.025, 0.0375, 0.05, 0.075, 0.1 mg/day (4/pck)

Esclim apply twice weekly x 3 weeks, then 1 week off; use with an oral progestin to prevent endometrial hyperplasia
Transdermal patch: 0.025, 0.0375, 0.05, 0.075, 0.1 mg/day (8, 48/pck)

Vivelle initially one 0.0375 mg/day patch twice weekly to trunk area; use with an oral progestin to prevent endometrial hyperplasia
Transdermal patch: 0.025, 0.0375, 0.05, 0.075, 0.1 mg/day (8, 48/pck)

Vivelle-Dot initially one 0.05 mg/day patch twice weekly to lower-abdomen, below the waist; use with an oral progestin to prevent endometrial-hyperplasia
Transdermal patch: 0.025, 0.0375, 0.05, 0.075, 0.1 mg/day (8, 24/pck)

▷ *estradiol+levonorgestrel* (X) apply 1 patch weekly to lower abdomen; avoid waistline; alternate sites

Climara Pro *Transdermal patch*: estra 0.045 mg+levo 0.015 mg per day (4/pck)

▷ *estradiol+norethindrone* (X)

CombiPatch apply twice weekly or q 3-4 days
Transdermal patch: 9 cm^2: estra 0.05 mg+noreth 0.14 mg; 16 cm^2: estra 0.05 mg+*noreth* 0.25 mg

Comment: May cause irregular bleeding in first 6 months of therapy, but usually decreases over time (often to amenorrhea).

ORAL AGENTS (WITH UTERUS)

▷ *estradiol* (X)(G)

Estrace 1-2 mg daily cyclically (3 weeks on and 1 week off)
Tab: 0.5, 1, 2*mg (tartrazine)

▷ *estradiol+drospirenone* (X)

Angeliq 1 tab daily
Tab: **Angeliq 0.5/0.25** estra 0.5 mg+dros 0.25 mg
Angeliq 1/0.5 estra 1 mg+dros 0.5 mg

➢ *estradiol+norethindrone* (X) 1 tab daily
    Activella (G) *Tab:* estra 1 mg+noreth 0.5 mg
    FemHRT (G) **1/5** *Tab:* estra 5 mcg+noreth 1 mg
    Fyavolv (G) *Tab:* estra 0.25 mg+noreth 1 mg; *Tab:* estra 0.5 mg+noreth 1 mg
    Mimvey LO *Tab:* estra 0.5 mg+noreth 0.1 mg
➢ *estradiol+norgestimate* (X) 1 x estradiol 1 mg tab once daily x 3 days, then 1
  x estradiol 1 mg+norgestimate 0.09 mg tab daily x 3 days; repeat this pattern
  continuously
    Ortho-Prefest *Tab:* estra 1 mg+norgest 0.09 mg (30/blister pck)
➢ *estradiol+progesterone* (X) 1 cap each evening with food
    Bijuva *Cap:* estradiol 1 mg+progesterone 100 mg
➢ *estrogen, conjugated+medroxyprogesterone* (X)
    Prempro 1 tab daily
        Tab: **Prempro 0.3/1.5** estro, conj 0.3 mg+medroxy 1.5 mg
            Prempro 0.45/1.5 estro, conj 0.45 mg+medroxy 1.5 mg
            Prempro 0.625/2.5 estro, conj 0.625 mg+medroxy 2.5 mg
            Prempro 0.625/5 estro, conj 0.625 mg+medroxy 5 mg
    Premphase 0.625 *estrogen* on days 1-14, then 0.625 mg *estrogen*+5 mg
    medroxyprogesterone on days 15-28
        Tab (in dial dispenser): estro, conj 0.625 mg (14 maroon tabs) + medroxy 5
        mg (14 blue tabs)
➢ *estrogen, esterified (plant derived)* (X)
    Menest 0.3-2.5 mg daily cyclically, 3 weeks on and 1 week off (with progestins
    in the latter part of the cycle to prevent endometrial hyperplasia)
        Tab: 0.3, 0.625, 1.25, 2.5 mg
➢ *estrogen, esterified+methyltestosterone* (X)
    Estratest 1 tab daily cyclically, 3 weeks on and 1 week off
        Tab: estro ester 1.25 mg+meth 2.5 mg
    Estratest HS 1-2 tabs daily cyclically, 3 weeks on and 1 week off
        Tab: estro ester 0.625 mg+meth 1.25 mg
➢ *ethinyl estradiol* (X) 0.02-0.05 mg q 1-2 days cyclically, 3 weeks on and
  1 week off (with progestins in the latter part of the cycle to prevent
  endometrial hyperplasia)
    Estinyl *Tab:* 0.02 (tartrazine), 0.05 mg
➢ *estropipate, piperazine estrone sulfate* (X)(G)
    Ogen 0.625-1.25 mg daily cyclically (3 weeks on and 1 week off)
        Tab: 0.625, 1.25, 2.5 mg
    Ortho-Est 0.75-6 mg daily cyclically (3 weeks on and 1 week off)
        Tab: 0.625, 1.25 mg
➢ *medroxyprogesterone* (X) 5-10 mg daily for 12 sequential days of each 28-day
  cycle to prevent endometrial hyperplasia in the post-menopausal women with an
  intact uterus receiving conjugated estrogens
    Provera *Tab:* 2.5, 5, 10 mg
➢ *norethindrone acetate* (X) 2.5-10 mg daily x 5-10 days during second half of
  menstrual cycle
    Aygestin *Tab:* 5*mg
➢ *progesterone, micronized* (X)(G)
    Prometrium 200 mg daily in the PM for 12 sequential days of each 28-day
    cycle to prevent endometrial hyperplasia in the post-menopausal woman with
    an intact uterus receiving conjugated estrogens
        Cap: 100, 200 mg (peanut oil)

BIO-IDENTICAL ESTRADIOL+PROGESTERONE

➢ *estradiol+projesterone (bio-identical)* take 1 gelcap once daily
    Bijuvia *Gelap:* estro 1 mg+progest 100 mg

Comment: **Bijuva** is the first and <u>only</u> bio-identical estradiol and bio-identical progesterone product offering women an alternative to the available FDA-approved synthetic (non-bio-identical) hormones, the separate FDA-approved bio-identical estrogen and progesterone products that are used together but are <u>not</u> approved for combination use, and the unapproved compounded bio-identical hormone products.

ESTROGENS, CONJUGATED+ESTROGEN AGONIST-ANTAGONIST

▷ *estrogen, conjugated+bazedoxifene* (X)
    Duavee 1 tab daily
        Tab: conj estra 0.45 mg+baze 20 mg

REGIMENS FOR PATIENTS WITHOUT UTERUS
Oral Agents (Without Uterus)

▷ *estradiol* (X)(G)
    Estrace 1-2 mg daily
        Tab: 0.5*, 1*, 2*mg (tartrazine)
▷ *estrogen, conjugated (equine)* (X)
    Premarin 1 tab daily
        Tab: 0.3, 0.45, 0.625, 0.9, 1.25, 2.5 mg
▷ *estrogen, conjugated (synthetic)* (X) 1 tab daily; may titrate up to max 1.25 mg/day
    Cenestin *Tab:* 0.3, 0.625, 0.9, 1.25 mg
    Enjuvia *Tab:* 0.3, 0.45, 0.625 mg
▷ *estrogen, esterified (plant derived)* (X) 1 tab daily
    Estratab *Tab:* 0.3, 0.625, 2.5 mg
    Menest *Tab:* 0.3, 0.625, 1.25, 2.5 mg
▷ *ethinyl estradiol* (X) 0.02-0.05 mg q 1-2 days
    Estinyl *Tab:* 0.02 (tartrazine), 0.05 mg

Vaginal Preparations (Without Uterus)

Comment: Vaginal preparations provide relief from vaginal and urinary symptoms <u>only</u> (i.e., atrophic vaginitis, dyspareunia, dysuria, and urinary frequency).
▷ *estradiol* (X)(G)
    Vagifem Tabs insert one 10 mcg <u>or</u> 25 mcg vaginal tablet once daily x 2 weeks; then twice weekly for 2 weeks (e.g., tues/fri); consider the addition of a progestin
        Vag tab: 10, 25 mcg (8, 18/blister pck with applicator)
    Yuvafem Vaginal Tablet 1 tab intravaginally daily x 2 weeks; then 1 tab intravaginally twice weekly
        Vag tab: 10 mcg (15 tabs w. applicators)

Topical Agents (Without Uterus)

▷ *estradiol* (X)
    Divigel apply 0.25 to 1.25 gm of **Divigel** to the right <u>or</u> left upper thigh once daily; alternate thighs every other day; start with the lowest effective dose and re-evaluate periodically; max 1.25 mg (1.25 gm/pkt) once daily
        Gel: 0.25 mg (0.25 gm/pkt), 0.5 mg (0.5 gm/pkt), 0.75 mg (0.75 gm/pkt), 1.0 mg (1.0 gm/pkt), 1.25 mg (1.25 gm/pkt), single-dose, foil packets (30 pkts/carton) (alcohol)
    Elestrin once daily, apply one pump actuation (0.87 gm of gel, 0.52 mg *estradiol*) <u>or</u> two pump actuations (1.7 gm of gel, 1.04 *mg estradiol*) to the upper arm; alternate arms every other day
        Metered Dose Pump: 0.52 mg of *estradiol* in 0.87 gm of gel per non-aerosol pump actuation (30 metered doses/container) (hydroalcohol)

Estrasorb apply 3.48 gm (2 pouches) every morning; apply one pouch to each leg from the upper thigh to the calf; rub in for 3 minutes; rub excess on hands onto buttocks

Emul: 0.025 mg/day/pouch (2.5 mg/gm; 1.74 gm/pouch) (56 pouches/carton)
EstroGel apply 1.25 gm (one compression) to one arm from wrist to shoulder once daily at the same time each day

Gel: (32 metered 1.25 gm doses/pump container) (50 gm)
Evamist apply one spray once daily each morning to forearm; may increase to two or three sprays once daily to forearm based upon clinical response

Spray: 1.53 mg (90 mcl) per metered spray actuation (56 sprays) (alcohol)

Transdermal Systems (Without Uterus)

Comment: Do not apply patches on or near breasts. Alternate sites.
▷ *estradiol* (X)

Alora initially 0.05 mg/day apply patch twice weekly to lower abdomen, upper quadrant of buttocks or outer aspect of hip

Transdermal patch: 0.025, 0.05, 0.075, 0.1 mg/day (8, 24/pck)
Climara initially 0.025 mg/day patch once/week to trunk

Transdermal patch: 0.025, 0.0375, 0.05, 0.075, 0.1 mg/day (4, 8, 24/pck)
Esclim initially 0.025 mg/day apply patch twice weekly to buttocks, femoral triangle, or upper arm

Transdermal patch: 0.025, 0.0375, 0.05, 0.075, 0.1 mg/day (8/pck)
Estraderm initially apply one 0.05 mg/day patch twice weekly to trunk

Transdermal patch: 0.05, 0.1 mg/day (8, 24/pck)
Menostar apply one patch weekly to lower abdomen, below the waist; avoid the breasts; alternate sites

Transdermal patch: 14 mcg/day (4/pck)
Minivelle initially one 0.0375 mg/day patch twice weekly to trunk area; adjust after one month of therapy

Transdermal patch: 0.025, 0.0375, 0.05, 0.075, 0.1 mg/day (8/pck)
Vivelle initially one 0.0375 mg/day patch twice weekly to trunk area; adjust after one month of therapy

Transdermal patch: 0.025, 0.0375, 0.05, 0.075, 0.1 mg/day (8, 48/pck)
Vivelle-Dot initially apply one 0.05 mg/day patch twice weekly to lower abdomen, below the waist; adjust after one month of therapy

Transdermal patch: 0.025, 0.0375, 0.05, 0.075, 0.1 mg/day (8, 24/pck)
Comment: The estrogens in **Alora**, **Climara**, **Estraderm**, and **Vivelle-Dot** are plant derived.

MESOTHELIOMA

KINASE INHIBITOR

▷ *capmatinib* 400 mg twice daily with or without food
Tabrecta *Tab:* 150, 200 mg
Comment: **Tabrecta** *(capmatinib)* is a kinase inhibitor indicated for the treatment of adult patients with metastatic non-small cell lung cancer (NSCLC) whose tumors have a mutation that leads to mesenchymal-epithelial transition (MET) exon 14 skipping as detected by an FDA-approved test. The most common adverse reactions (incidence ≥ 20%) have been peripheral edema, nausea, fatigue, vomiting, dyspnea, and decreased appetite. Monitor for new or worsening pulmonary symptoms indicative of interstitial lung disease ILD/pneumonitis. Permanently discontinue **Tabrecta** in patients with ILD/pneumonitis. Monitor liver function tests. In the event of hepatotoxicity, withhold, reduce dose, or permanently discontinue **Tabrecta** based on severity.

Tabrecta may cause photosensitivity reactions. Advise patients to limit direct ultraviolet exposure. Tabrecta can cause embryo/fetal harm. Advise patients of reproductive potential to use effective contraception. Advise not to breastfeed.

FOLATE ANALOG METABOLIC INHIBITOR

▷ *pemetrexed* for injection *Recommended dose, administered as a single agent or with cisplatin, in patients with CrCl ≥45 mL/min:* 500 mg/m2 via IV infusion over 10 minutes on Day 1 of each 21-day cycle; *Initiate Folic Acid:* 400 mcg to 1000 mcg orally once daily beginning 7 days prior to the first dose and continue until 21 days after the last dose; *Administer vitamin B12:* 1 mg IM 1 week prior to the first dose and every 3 cycles thereafter; *Administer dexamethasone:* 4 mg orally twice daily the day before, the day of, and the day after Pemfexy administration
Pediatric: safety and efficacy not established

Pemfexy *Vial:* 500 mg/20 ml (25 mg/ml), single dose, for dilution and IV infusion

Comment: Pemfexy is a branded alternative to Alimta for the treatment of nonsquamous non-small cell lung cancer (NSCLC) and malignant pleural mesothelioma. Pemfexy is indicated: (1) in combination with *cisplatin* for the initial treatment of patients with locally advanced or metastatic non-squamous, non-small cell lung cancer (NSCLC), (2) as a single agent for the maintenance treatment of patients with locally advanced or metastatic non-squamous NSCLC whose disease has not progressed after 4 cycles of *platinum-based first-line chemotherapy*, and (3) as a single agent for the treatment of patients with recurrent, metastatic non-squamous NSCLC after prior chemotherapy. Pemfexy is not indicated for the treatment of patients with squamous cell non-small cell lung cancer SCLC. Pemfexy can cause severe bone marrow suppression resulting in cytopenia and an increased risk of infection. Do not administer Pemfexy when the absolute neutrophil count is less than 1500 cells/mm^3 and platelets are <100,000 cells/mm^3. Initiate supplementation with oral folic acid and vitamin B12 IM to reduce the severity of hematologic and gastrointestinal toxicity. Pemfexy can cause severe, and sometimes fatal, renal failure. Do not administer when CrCl <45 mL/min. Permanently discontinue for severe and life-threatening bullous, blistering or exfoliating skin toxicity. Withhold for acute onset of new or progressive unexplained pulmonary symptoms and permanently discontinue if interstitial pneumonitis is confirmed. Radiation recall can occur in patients who received radiation weeks to years previously; permanently discontinue for signs of radiation recall. The most common adverse reactions (incidence ≥20%) of *pemetrexed*, when administered as a single agent have been fatigue, nausea, and anorexia. The most common adverse reactions (incidence ≥20%) of *pemetrexed* when administered with *cisplatin* have been vomiting, neutropenia, anemia, stomatitis/pharyngitis, thrombocytopenia, and constipation. Pemfexy is embryo/fetal toxic. Advise males and females of reproductive potential of the potential risk and to use effective contraception. Advise not to breastfeed.

 METHAMPHETAMINE-INDUCED PSYCHOSIS

ANTIPSYCHOSIS AGENTS

For more antipsychotics, see Appendix Q. Antipsychosis Drugs
see Tardive Dyskinesia

Comment: First-generation antipsychotics (e,g., *haloperidol or fluphenazine*) should be used sparingly and cautiously in patients with methamphetamine-induced psychosis because of the risk of developing extrapyramidal symptoms (EPS) and because these patients are prone to develop motor complications as a result of methamphetamine abuse. Second-generation antipsychotics (e.g., *risperidone* and *olanzapine*) may be more appropriate because of the lower risks of EPS. The presence of high norepinephrine levels in some patients with recurrent methamphetamine psychosis suggests that drugs that block norepinephrine receptors (e.g., *prazosin* or *propranolol*) might be of therapeutic benefit although they have not been studied in controlled trials.

▷ *aripiprazole* (C)(G) initially 15 mg once daily; may increase to max 30 mg/day
  Pediatric: <10 years: not recommended; ≥10-17 years: initially 2 mg/day in a single dose for 2 days; then increase to 5 mg/day in a single dose for 2 days; then increase to target dose of 10 mg/day in a single dose; may increase by 5 mg/day at weekly intervals as needed to max 30 mg/day
    Abilify *Tab:* 2, 5, 10, 15, 20, 30 mg
    Abilify Discmelt *Tab:* 15 mg orally-disint (vanilla) (phenylalanine)
    Abilify Maintena *Vial:* 300, 400 mg ext-rel pwdr for IM injection after reconstitution; 300, 400 mg single-dose prefilled dual-chamber syringes w. supplies
▷ *aripiprazole lauroxil* (C) administer by IM injection in the deltoid (441 mg dose only) or gluteal (441 mg, 662 mg, 882 mg, or 1064 mg) muscle by a qualified healthcare professional; initiate at a dose of 441 mg, 662 mg, or 882 mg administered monthly, or 882 mg every 6 weeks, or 1064 mg every 2 months
  Pediatric: <18 years: not recommended; ≥18 years: same as adult
    Aristada *Prefilled syringe:* 441, 662, 882, 1064 mg single-use, ext-rel susp
    Comment: **Aristada** *(aripiprazole)* is an atypical antipsychotic available in 4 doses with 3 dosing duration options for flexible dosing. For patients naïve to *aripiprazole*, establish tolerability with oral *aripiprazole* prior to initiating treatment with **Aristada**. **Aristada** can be initiated at any of the 4 doses at the appropriate dosing duration option. In conjunction with the first injection, administer treatment with oral *aripiprazole* for 21 consecutive days for all 4 dose sizes. The most common adverse event associated with **Aristada** is akathisia. Patients are also at increased risk for developing neuroleptic malignant syndrome, tardive dyskinesia, pathological gambling or other compulsive behaviors, orthostatic hypotension, hyperglycemic, dyslipidemia, and weight gain. Hypersensitive reactions can occur and range from pruritus or urticaria to anaphylaxis. Stroke, transient ischemic attacks, and falls have been reported in elderly patients with dementia-related psychosis who were treated with *aripiprazole*. **Aristada** is not for treatment of people who have lost touch with reality (psychosis) due to confusion and memory loss (dementia). May cause extrapyramidal and/or withdrawal symptoms in neonates exposed in utero in the third trimester of pregnancy. *Aripiprazole* is present in human breast milk; however, there are insufficient data to assess the amount in human milk or the effects on the breast-fed infant. The development and health benefits of breastfeeding should be considered along with the mother's clinical need for **Aristada** and any potential adverse effects on the breastfed infant from **Aristada** or from the underlying maternal condition. For more information or to report ASEs, contact the National Pregnancy Registry for Atypical Antipsychotics at 1-866-961-2388 or visit http://womensmentalhealth.org/clinical-and-research-programs/pregnancyregistry. Limited published data on *aripiprazole* use in pregnant females are not sufficient to inform any drug-associated risks for birth defects or miscarriage.
    Aristada Initio administer a single 675 mg **Aristada Initio** injection plus a single 30 mg dose of oral *aripiprazole*; administer the IM injection into the deltoid or gluteal muscle; must be administered only by a qualified healthcare

professional; **Aristada Initio** is only to be used as a single dose and is not for repeated dosing

   Prefilled pen: 675 mg/2.4 ml ext-rel single-dose
   Comment: **Aristada Initio** (*aripiprazole lauroxil*) is a smaller particle-size version of extended-release injectable (*aripiprazole*) for adults with schizophrenia. It is the first and only long-acting atypical antipsychotic that can be initiated on day one. Combining **Aristada Initio** with a single 30 mg dose of oral *aripiprazole* provides an alternative regimen to initiate patients onto any dose of **Aristada** on day one. Previously, the initiation process for the older *aripiprazole* product was to give the first dose and to then give oral *aripiprazole* for 21 consecutive days. **Aristada Initio** releases relevant levels of *aripiprazole* within 4 days of initiation. **Aristada Initio** carries a warning that it is not approved for use by older patients with dementia-related psychosis, as this patient population is at risk for increased mortality when treated with antipsychotics. For patients naïve to *aripiprazole*, establish tolerability with oral *aripiprazole* prior to initiating treatment with **Aristada Initio**. Avoid use in known CYP2D6 poor metabolizers. Avoid use with strong CYP2D6 or CYP 3A4 inhibitors and strong CYP3A4 inducers. **Aristada Initio** is not interchangeable with **Aristada**. Most commonly observed adverse reaction (incidence ≥5%) has been akathisia. May cause extrapyramidal and/or withdrawal symptoms in neonates in females exposed during the third trimester of pregnancy. There is a pregnancy exposure registry that monitors pregnancy outcomes in women exposed to **Aristada Initio** during pregnancy. *Aripiprazole* is present in human breast milk; however, there are insufficient data to assess the amount in human milk, the effects on the breastfed infant. For more information, contact the National Pregnancy Registry for Atypical Antipsychotics at 1-866-961-2388 or visit http://womensmentalhealth.org/clinical-and-research-programs/pregnancyregistry

▷ *fluphenazine hcl* [Prolixin] (C)(G)
   Pediatric: <18 years: not studied
      Tab: 1, 2.5, 5, 10 mg; *Elixer:* 2.5 mg/5 ml; *Conc:* 5 mg/ml; *Vial:* 2.5 mg/ml
      for injection

▷ *fluphenazine decanoate* [Prolixin Decanoate] (C)(G)
   Pediatric: <18 years: not studied
      Vial: 2.5 mg/ml (5 ml)
   Comment: Previously, *fluphenazine* was marketed as **Prolixin**, but is currently only available in generic form. Optimal dose and frequency of administration of *fluphenazine* must be determined for each patient, since dosage requirements have been found to vary with clinical circumstances as well as with individual response; dosage should not exceed 100 mg; if doses > 50 mg are deemed necessary, the next dose and succeeding doses should be increased cautiously in increments of 12.5 mg. *fluphenazine decanoate injection* and *fluphenazine enanthate injection* are long-acting parenteral antipsychotic forms intended for use in the management of patients requiring prolonged parenteral neuroleptic therapy. *fluphenazine* has activity at all levels of the central nervous system (CNS) as well as on multiple organ systems. The mechanism whereby its therapeutic action is exerted is unknown. *fluphenazine* differs from other phenothiazine derivatives in several respects: it is more potent on a milligram basis, it has less potentiating effect on CNS depressants and anesthetics than do some of the phenothiazines and appears to be less sedating, and it is less likely than some of the older phenothiazines to produce hypotension (nevertheless, appropriate cautions should be observed. Neuroleptic Malignant Syndrome (NMS), a potentially fatal symptom complex, is associated with all antipsychotic drugs. Clinical manifestations of NMS are hyperpyrexia, muscle rigidity, altered mental

status and evidence of autonomic instability (irregular pulse or blood pressure, tachycardia, diaphoresis, and cardiac dysrhythmias). Anticholinergic effects may be potentiated with concomitant *atropine* and *fluphenazine.* Safety and efficacy in children have not been established. Safety during pregnancy has not been established; therefore, the possible hazards should be weighed against the potential benefits when administering this drug to pregnant patients.

▷ *haloperidol* (C)(G)
   Oral Route of Administration: Moderate Symptomology: 0.5 to 2 mg orally 2 to 3 times a day; *Severe symptomology:* 3 to 5 mg orally 2 to 3 times a day; initial doses of up to 100 mg/day have been necessary in some severely resistant cases; *Maintenance:* after achieving a satisfactory response, the dose should be adjusted as practical to achieve optimum control
   Parenteral Route of Administration: Prompt Control of Acute Agitation: 2-5 mg IM every 4-8 hours; *Maintenance:* frequency of IM administration should be determined by patient response and may be given as often as every hour; max: 20 mg/day
      Haldol *Tab:* 0.5*, 1*, 2*, 5*, 10*, 20*mg
      Haldol Lactate *Vial:* 5 mg for IM injection, single-dose

▷ *mesoridazine* (C) initially 25 mg tid; max 300 mg/day
      Serentil *Tab:* 10, 25, 50, 100 mg; *Conc:* 25 mg/ml (118 ml)

▷ *olanzapine* (C) initially 2.5-10 mg daily; increase to 10 mg/day within a few days; then by 5 mg/day at weekly intervals; max 20 mg/day
      Zyprexa *Tab:* 2.5, 5, 7.5, 10 mg
      Zyprexa Zydis *ODT:* 5, 10, 15, 20 mg (phenylalanine)

▷ *quetiapine fumarate* (C)(G)
      SeroQUEL initially 25 mg bid, titrate q 2nd or 3rd day in increments of 25-50 mg bid-tid; usual maintenance 400-600 mg/day in 2-3 divided doses
         Tab: 25, 50, 100, 200, 300, 400 mg
      SeroQUEL XR administer once daily in the PM; *Day 1:* 50 mg; *Day 2:* 100 mg; *Day 3:* 200 mg; *Day 4:* 300 mg; usual range 400-600 mg/day
         Tab: 50, 150, 200, 300, 400 mg ext-rel

▷ *risperidone* (C) 0.5 mg bid x 1 day; adjust in increments of 0.5 mg bid; usual range 0.5-5 mg/day
      Risperdal *Tab:* 1, 2, 3, 4 mg; *Oral soln:* 1 mg/ml (100 ml)
      Risperdal M-Tab *Tab:* 0.5, 1, 2 mg

▷ *thioridazine* (C)(G) 10-25 mg bid
      Mellaril *Tab:* 10, 15, 25, 50, 100, 150, 200 mg; *Oral susp:* 25 mg/5 ml, 100 mg/5 ml; *Oral conc:* 30 mg/ml, 100 mg/ml (4 oz)

⬤ MITRAL VALVE PROLAPSE (MVP)

▷ *propranolol* (C)(G)
      Inderal 10-30 mg tid-qid
         Tab: 10*, 20*, 40*, 60*, 80*mg
      Inderal LA initially 80 mg daily in a single dose; increase q 3-7 days; usual range 120-160 mg/day; max 320 mg/day in a single dose
         Cap: 60, 80, 120, 160 mg sust-rel
      InnoPran XL initially 80 mg q HS; max 120 mg/day
         Cap: 80, 120 mg ext-rel

⬤ MONONUCLEOSIS (MONO)

Opioid Analgesics *see* **Pain**
Parenteral Corticosteroids *see* Appendix M. Parenteral Corticosteroids
Oral Corticosteroids *see* Appendix L. Oral Corticosteroids

▷ **prednisone** (C) initially 40-80 mg/day, then taper off over 5-7 days
Comment: Corticosteroids are recommended in patients with significant pharyngeal edema.

MOTION SICKNESS

▷ **dimenhydrinate** (B)(OTC) 50-100 mg q 4-6 hours; start 1 hour before travel; max 400 mg/day
Pediatric: <2 years: not recommended; 2-6 years: 12.5-25 mg; max 75 mg/day; start 1 hour before travel; may repeat q 6-8 hours; 6-11 years: 25-50 mg; max 150 mg/day; start 1 hour before travel; may repeat q 6-8 hours; ≥12 years: same as adult
    Dramamine *Tab:* 50*mg; *Chew tab:* 50 mg (phenylalanine, tartrazine); *Liq:* 12.5 mg/5 ml (4 oz)

▷ **meclizine** (B)(G) 25-50 mg 1 hour before travel; may repeat q 24 hours as needed; max 50 mg/day
Pediatric: <12 years: not recommended; ≥12 years: same as adult
    Antivert *Tab:* 12.5, 25, 50*mg
    Bonine (OTC) *Cap:* 15, 25, 50 mg; *Tab:* 12.5, 25, 50 mg;
    Chew tab/Film-coat tab: 25 mg
    Dramamine II (OTC) *Tab:* 25 mg
    Zentrip *Strip:* 25 mg orally disint

▷ **prochlorperazine** (C)(G)
Pediatric: <12 years: not recommended; ≥12 years: same as adult
    Compazine 5-10 mg q 4 hours as needed
        Tab: 5 mg; *Syr:* 5 mg/5 ml (4 oz; fruit); *Rectal supp:* 2.5, 5, 25 mg
    Compazine Spansule 15 mg q AM or 10 mg q 12 hours
        Spansules: 10, 15 mg sust-rel

▷ **promethazine** (C)(G) 25 mg 30-60 minutes before travel; may repeat in 8-12 hours
Pediatric: <2 years: not recommended; ≥2 years: 12.5-25 mg 30-60 minutes before travel; may repeat in 8-12 hours
    Phenergan *Tab:* 12.5*, 25*, 50 mg; *Plain syr:* 6.25 mg/5 ml; *Fortis syr:* 25 mg/5 ml; *Rectal supp:* 12.5, 25, 50 mg
Comment: *Promethazine* is contraindicated in children with uncomplicated nausea, dehydration, Reye's syndrome, history of sleep apnea, asthma, and lower respiratory disorders in children. *Promethazine* lowers the seizure threshold in children, may cause cholestatic jaundice, anticholinergic effects, extrapyramidal effects, and potentially fatal respiratory depression.

▷ **scopolamine** (C)
Pediatric: <12 years: not recommended; ≥12 years: same as adult
    Scopace 0.4-0.8 mg 1 hour before travel; may repeat in 8 hours
        Tab: 0.4 mg
    Transderm Scop 1 patch behind ear at least 4 hours before travel; each patch is effective for 3 days
        Transdermal patch: 1.5 mg (4/carton)

MULTIPLE SCLEROSIS (MS)

NICOTINIC ACID RECEPTOR AGONIST

▷ **dimethyl fumarate** (C) initially 120 mg bid x 7 days; then maintenance 240 mg bid
Pediatric: <18 years: not recommended; ≥18 years: same as adult
    Tecfidera *Cap:* 120, 240 mg del-rel; *Starter Pack:* 14 x 120 mg, 46 x 240 mg
Comment: The mechanism by which *dimethyl fumarate* (DMF) exerts its therapeutic effect in multiple sclerosis is unknown. DMF and the metabolite,

monomethyl fumarate (MMF), have been shown to activate the nuclear factor (erythroid-derived 2)-like 2 (Nrf2) pathway in vitro and in vivo in animals and humans. The Nrf2 pathway is involved in the cellular response to oxidative stress. MMF has been identified as a nicotinic acid receptor agonist in vitro.

POTASSIUM CHANNEL BLOCKER

▷ *dalfampridine* (C)(G) 10 mg q 12 hours
   Pediatric: <18 years: not recommended; ≥18 years: same as adult
     Ampyra *Tab:* 10 mg ext-rel
   Comment: *Dalfampridine* is indicated to improve walking speed.

PURINE ANTI-METABOLITE

▷ *cladribine* swallow whole with water; do not chew; may take with or without food; separate administration from any other oral drug by at least 3 hours; swallow immediately following removal: **Mavenclad** is an uncoated oral cytotoxic tablet and, therefore, requires special handling and disposal (see comment); avoid contact with skin; wash hands thoroughly after touching; cumulative dosage of **Mavenclad** is 3.5 mg/kg divided into 2 yearly treatment courses (1.75 mg/kg per treatment course); each treatment course is divided into 2 treatment cycles; see mfr pkg insert for kilogram weight-based # of tablets per dose; administer the cycle dosage as 1 or 2 tablets once daily over 4 or 5 consecutive days; do not administer more than 2 tablets daily; if a dose is missed, do not take double or extra doses; if a dose is not taken on the scheduled day, take the missed dose on the following day and extend the number of days in that treatment cycle; if two consecutive doses are missed, extend the treatment cycle by 2 days
   First Course/First Cycle: start any time
   First Course/Second Cycle: administer 23 to 27 days after the last dose of First Course/First Cycle
   Second Course/First Cycle: administer at least 43 weeks after the last dose of First Course/Second Cycle
   Second Course/Second Cycle: administer 23 to 27 days after the last dose of Second Course/First Cycle
   Following the 2 treatment courses, do not administer additional **Mavenclad** during the next 2 years; treatment during these 2 years may further increase the risk of malignancy; safety and efficacy of re-initiating **Mavenclad** more than 2 years after completing 2 treatment courses has not been studied
  Pediatric: <18 years: safety and efficacy not studied; >18 years, <40 kg: safety and efficacy not studied; >18 years, >40 kg: same as adult
   Mavenclad *Tab:* 10 mg
Comment: **Mavenclad** *(cladribine)* is a purine anti-metabolite indicated for the treatment of highly active relapsing forms of multiple sclerosis (MS) to include relapsing-remitting disease and active secondary progressive disease, in adults. Because of its safety profile, use of **Mavenclad** is generally recommended for patients who have had an inadequate response to, or are unable to tolerate, an alternate drug indicated for the treatment of MS. **Mavenclad** is not recommended for use in patients with clinically isolated syndrome (CIS) because of its safety profile. Hands must be dry when handling the tablets and washed thoroughly afterwards. Avoid prolonged contact with skin. If a tablet is left on a surface or if a broken or fragmented tablet is released from the blister, the area must be thoroughly washed with water. Follow applicable special handling and disposal procedures. Contraindications to **Mavenclad** use: current malignancy; HIV infection, active chronic infection (e.g., hepatitis, tuberculosis), history of hypersensitivity to *cladribine*, pregnancy (embryo/fetal teratogenic), failure to use effective contraception during **Mavenclad** dosing and for 6 months after the last dose in each treatment course, breastfeeding on

a **Mavenclad** treatment day and for 10 days after the last dose. Warnings and Precautions: monitor lymphocyte counts before, during, and after treatment; screen patients for latent infections, consider delaying treatment until infection is fully controlled, and monitor for signs of developing infection; vaccinate patients antibody-negative to varicella zoster virus prior to treatment; administer anti-herpes prophylaxis in patients with lymphocyte counts less than 200 cells per microliter; measure complete blood count annually if clinically indicated after treatment; monitor for graft-versus-host-disease with blood transfusion (irradiation of cellular blood components is recommended); obtain LFTs prior to treatment and discontinue treatment if clinically significant hepatic injury is suspected. Concomitant use of immunosuppressive drugs is not recommended. Monitor patients for additive effects of hematotoxic drugs on the hematological profile. Avoid concomitant use of antiviral and antiretroviral drugs. Avoid concomitant use of BCRP or ENT/CNT inhibitors as these may alter the bioavailability of *cladribine*. The most common adverse reactions (incidence >20%) have been upper respiratory tract infection, headache, and lymphopenia.

PYRIMIDINE SYNTHESIS INHIBITOR (DMARD)

▷ *teriflunomide* (X) 7 mg or 14 mg once daily
  Pediatric: <12 years: not recommended; ≥12 years: same as adult
     Aubagio *Tab:* 7, 14 mg
  Comment: Contraindicated with severe hepatic impairment and women of childbearing potential not using reliable contraception. Co-administer *teriflunomide* with the DMARD *leflunomide* (**Arava**).

IMMUNOMODULATORS

Comment: The role of immunomodulators in the treatment of MS is to slow the progression of physical disability and to decrease frequency of clinical exacerbations.

▷ *alemtuzumab* (C) administer two treatment courses:
  First treatment course: 12 mg/day x 5 days (total 60 mg); *Second treatment course:* 12 months later, administer 12 mg/day x 3 days (total 36 mg); complete all immunizations 6 weeks prior to the first treatment; pre-medicate with 1000 mg methylprednisolone or equivalent immediately prior to the first 3 treatment days in each treatment course
  Pediatric: <18 years: not recommended; ≥18 years: same as adult
     Lemtrada *Vial:* 12 mg/1.2 ml soln for IV infusion, single-use vial
     Comment: **Lemtrada** is indicated for the treatment of patients with relapsing forms of MS. Because of its safety profile, the use of **Lemtrada** should generally be reserved for patients who have had an inadequate response to two or more drugs indicated for the treatment of MS. **Lemtrada** REMS is a restricted distribution program, which allows early detection and management of some of the serious risks associated with its use.
▷ *fingolimod* (C) 0.5 mg once daily
  Pediatric: <10 years: not recommended; ≥10 years: same as adult
     Gilenya *Cap:* 0.5 mg
  Comment: First-dose monitoring for bradycardia. In the first 2 weeks, first-dose monitoring is recommended after an interruption of 1 day or more. During weeks 3 and 4, first-dose monitoring is recommended after an interruption of more than 7 days. FDA warning: when **Gilenya** (*fingolimod*) is stopped, the MS disability can become much worse than before the medicine was started or while it was being taken. This MS worsening is rare but can result in permanent disability. Before starting treatment with **Gilenya**, patient's should be warned about the potential risk of severe increase in disability after stopping **Gilenya**.

▷ *glatiramer acetate* (B)(G)

Copaxone 20-40 mg SC once daily
Pediatric: <18 years: not recommended; ≥18 years: same as adult
    Prefilled syringe: 20, 40 mg/ml (1 ml) single-dose (mannitol 40 mg; preservative-free)

Glatopa 20 mg SC once daily or 40 mg SC 3 x/weekly at least 48 hours apart
Pediatric: <18 years: not recommended; ≥18 years: same as adult
    Prefilled syringe: 20, 40 mg/ml (1 ml) single dose (mannitol 40 mg; preservative-free)

Comment: *Glatiramer acetate* injection *(Copaxone, Glatopa)* is indicated for the treatment of patients with relapsing forms of multiple sclerosis. Mechanism(s) by which *glatiramer acetate* exerts its effects in patients with MS are not fully understood. However, *glatiramer acetate* is thought to act by modifying immune processes that are believed to be responsible for the pathogenesis of MS. The biological activity of *glatiramer acetate* is informed by its ability to block the induction of experimental autoimmune encephalomyelitis (EAE) in animal studies. Further, studies in animals and in vitro systems suggest that upon its administration, *glatiramer acetate*-specific suppressor T-cells are induced and activated in the periphery. **Glatopa** is a fully substitutable, AP-rated generic version of **Copaxone.**

▷ *interferon beta-1a* (C)
Pediatric: <18 years: not recommended; ≥18 years: same as adult

Avonex 30 mcg IM weekly; rotate sites; may titrate to reduce flu-like symptoms; may use concurrent analgesics/antipyretics on treatment days; *Titration Schedule:* 7.5 mcg week 1; 15 mcg week 2; 22.5 mcg week 3; 30 mcg week 4 and ongoing
    Vial: 30 mcg/vial pwdr for reconstitution (single-dose w. diluent, 4 vials/kit) (albumin [human], preservative-free); *Prefilled syringe:* 30 mcg single-dose (0.5 ml) (4/dose pck)

Plegridy *Recommended Therapeutic Dose:* 125 mcg SC or IM once every 14 days; dose should be titrated--*Day 1:* 63 mcg SC or IM; *Day 15:* 94 mcg SC or IM; Day 29: 125 mcg SC or IM and ongoing once every 14 days; a qualified healthcare professional should train patients in the proper technique for self-administering SC injections using the prefilled pen or syringe or SC injections using the prefilled syringe; Analgesics and/or antipyretics on treatment days may help ameliorate flu-like symptoms
    Prefilled Pen/Prefilled Syringe: 63, 94, 125 mcg/0.5 ml, single-dose w. needle for SC administration; *Prefilled syringe:* 125 mcg/0.5 ml single-dose w. needle for IM administration; *Titration Kit:* contains two titration clips--yellow clip (63 mcg/0.5 ml for dose 1) and purple clip (94 mcg/0.5 ml for dose 2)

Rebif, administer SC 3x/week (at least 48 hours apart and preferably in the late afternoon or evening); increase over 4 weeks to usual dose 22-44 mcg 3x/week; *Titration Schedule (22 mcg prescribed dose):* 4.4 mcg week 1 and 2; 11 mcg week 3 and 4; 22 mcg week 5 and ongoing; *Titration Schedule (44 mcg prescribed dose):* 8.8 mcg week 1 and 2; 22 mcg week 3 and 4; 44 mcg week 5 and ongoing
    Prefilled syringe: 22, 44 mcg/0.5 ml w. needle (12/carton) (albumin [human], preservative-free); (titration pack, 6 doses of 8.8 mcg [0.2 ml] w. needle per carton) (albumin [human], preservative-free)

Comment: Only prefilled syringes (**Rebif**) can be used to titrate to the 22 mcg prescribed dose. Prefilled syringes or autoinjectors (**Rebif Rebidose**) can be used to titrate to the 44 mcg prescribed dose.

Rebif Rebidose administer SC 3x/week (at least 48 hours apart and preferably in the late afternoon or evening) after titration to 22 mcg or 44 mcg

Titration Schedule: *see* **Rebif**.
Prefilled autoinjector: 22, 44 mcg/0.5 ml (0.5 ml, 12/carton) (titration pack, 6 doses of 8.8 mcg [0.2 ml] per carton (albumin [human], preservative-free)
Comment: Only prefilled syringes (**Rebif**) can be used to titrate to the 22 mcg prescribed dose. Prefilled syringes or autoinjectors (**Rebif Rebidose**) can be used to titrate to the 44 mcg prescribed dose.

▷ *interferon beta-1b* (C)
Pediatric: <18 years: not recommended; ≥18 years: same as adult
  Actimmune *BSA ≤0.5m²:* 1.5 mcg/kg SC in a single dose 3x weekly; *BSA ≥0.5m²:* 50 mcg/m² SC in a single dose 3x weekly *Vial:* 100 mcg/0.5 ml single-dose for SC injection
  Betaseron, Extavia 0.0625 mg (0.25 ml) SC every other day; increase over 6 weeks to 0.25 mg (1 ml) SC every other day
    Vial: 0.3 mg/vial pwdr for reconstitution (single-dose w. prefilled diluents syringes) (albumin [human], mannitol, preservative-free)

▷ *natalizumab* (C) administer 300 mg by IV infusion over 1 hour every 4 weeks; monitor during infusion and for 1 hour postinfusion
Pediatric: <18 years: not recommended; ≥18 years: same as adult
  Tysabri *Vial:* 300 mg/15 ml (15 ml)

CD20-DIRECTED CYTOLYTIC MONOCLONAL ANTIBODY

▷ *ocrelizumab* pre-medicate with corticosteroid and antihistamine, and consider antipyretic, prior to each infusion; initially administer 300 mg via IV infusion followed by another 300 mg via IV infusion 2 weeks later; then administer 600 mg every 6 months; see mfr pkg insert for infusion rates and dose modifications
Pediatric: <18 years: not recommended; ≥18 years: same as adult
  Ocrevus *Vial:* 30 mg/ml (10 ml, single-dose) for dilution (preservative-free)
  Comment: The precise mechanism of action is unknown; however, it is thought to involve binding to CD20, a cell surface antigen present on pre-B and mature B lymphocytes which results in antibody-dependent cellular cytolysis and complement-mediated lysis. **Ocrevus** is contraindicated with active HBV infection. Screen for HBV infection (HBsAg/anti-HB) prior to initiation. Concomitant live or attenuated vaccine not recommended during treatment and until B-cell repletion. Administer these at least 6 weeks prior to initiation of treatment. Additive immunosuppressive effects with other immunosupressants. Monitor for infusion reaction (pruritis, rash, urticaria, erythema, throat irritation, bronchospasm). Delay treatment with active infection. Withhold at first sign/symptom of progressive multifocal leukoencephalopathy (PMI) or HBV reactivation. Females of reproductive potential should use effective contraception during treatment and for 6 months after the last dose of **Ocrevus**. It is not known whether *ocrelizumab* is excreted in human breast milk or has any effect on the breastfed infant.

▷ *ofatumumab* initially 20 mg SC at Week 0, 1, and 2; then, 20 mg SC monthly starting at Week 4
  Pediatric: <18 years: not recommended; ≥18 years: same as adult
  Kesimpta *Prefilled Sensoready:* 20 mg/0.4 ml, single-dose; *Prefilled Syringe:* 20 mg/0.4 ml, single-dose (preservative-free)
  Comment: **Kesimpta** *(ofatumumab)* is indicated for the treatment of relapsing forms of multiple sclerosis (MS), to include clinically isolated syndrome, relapsing-remitting disease, and active secondary progressive disease, in adults. **Kesimpta** is contraindicated with active HBV infection; hepatitis B virus (HBV) and quantitative serum immunoglobulins screening required before the first dose. The most common adverse reactions (incidence >10%) are URI, headache, injection-related reactions, and local injection site reactions. Delay **Kesimpta** administration in patients with an active infection until the infection is resolved. Vaccination with live-attenuated or

live vaccines is not recommended during treatment and after discontinuation, until B-cell repletion. Management for injection-related reactions depends on the type and severity of the reaction. Monitor the level of immunoglobulins at the beginning, during, and after discontinuation of treatment until B-cell repletion. Consider discontinuing **Kesimpta** if the patient develops a serious opportunistic infection or recurrent infections if immunoglobulin levels indicate immune compromise. **Kesimpta** may cause fetal harm based on animal data. Advise females of reproductive potential of potential embryo-fetal risk and to use an effective method of contraception during treatment and for 6 months after stopping **Kesimpta**.

SPHIINGOSINE 1-PHOSPHATE RECEPTOR MODULATOR

Comment: Sphingosine 1-phosphate receptor modulators are indicated for the treatment of relapsing forms of multiple sclerosis (MS), to include clinically isolated syndrome, relapsing-remitting disease, and active secondary progressive disease, in adults. This drug class is contraindicated in patients who have experienced myocardial infarction, unstable angina, stroke, TIA, decompensated heart failure requiring hospitalization, or Class III/IV heart failure in the preceding 6 months. The presence of Mobitz type II second-degree, third-degree AV block, or sick sinus syndrome (SSS), are contraindications unless patient has a functioning pacemaker. Obtain a CBC, transaminase, and bilirubin before initiating treatment. Monitor for infection during treatment; do not initiate treatment in patients with active infection. Avoid live-attenuated vaccines during, and for up to 4 weeks after, treatment. Test patients for antibodies to varicella zoster virus (VZV) before initiating treatment. VZV vaccination of antibody-negative patients is recommended prior to commencing treatment. CYP2C9 and CYP3A4 inhibitors increase in exposure to this class; therefore, concomitant use with moderate CYP2C9 and moderate or strong CYP3A4 inhibitors is not recommended. CYP2C9 and CYP3A4 inducers decrease exposure; therefore, concomitant use with moderate CYP2C9 or strong CYP3A4 inducers is not recommended. There are no adequate data on the developmental risk associated with the use in pregnant females. However, reproductive and developmental data in animal studies have demonstrated embryo/fetal toxicity. Before initiation of treatment, females of childbearing potential should be counseled on the potential for serious risk to the fetus and the need for contraception during treatment. Because of the time it takes to eliminate the drug from the body after stopping treatment, the potential risk to the fetus may persist and females of childbearing age should also use effective contraception for 3 months after stopping. There are no data on the presence in human milk or effects on the breastfed infant.

▷ *ozanimod* initiate treatment with a 7-day titration regimen (starter pack); *Days 1-4*: 0.23 mg once daily; *Days 5-7*: 0.46 mg once daily; *Day 8 and thereafter*: 0.92 mg once daily; if a dose is missed during the first 2 weeks of treatment, re-initiate treatment using the initial titration regimen
Pediatric: safety and efficacy not established
　　Zeposia *Cap*: 0.23, 0.46, 0.92 2 mg; titration pck

▷ *siponimod* initiate treatment with a 5-day titration regimen (starter pack); *Day 1*: 0.25 mg (1 x 0.25 mg); *Day 2*: 0.25 mg (1 x 0.25 mg); *Day 3*: 0.50 mg (2 x 0.25 mg); *Day 4*: 0.75 mg (3 x 0.25 mg); *Day 5*: 1.25 mg (5 x 0.25 mg); *Day 6 and thereafter*: 2 mg ince daily; if one titration dose is missed for more than 24 hours, re-initiate using with Day 1 of the initial titration regimen; see mfr pkg insert for titration and maintenance doses for patients with CYP2C9 Genotypes *1/*3 or *2/*3
Pediatric: safety and efficacy not established
　　Mayzent *Tab*: 0.25, 2 mg film-coat; titration pck

Nrf2 PATHWAY ACTIVATOR

▷ *monomethyl fumarate Starting Dose:* 95 mg twice daily x 7 days; *Maintenance:* 190 mg (2 x 95 mg) twice daily; swallow whole and intact; do not crush, chew, or mix contents with food; take with or without food

Pediatric: not established

Bafiertam *Cap:* 95 mg del-rel

Comment: **Bafiertam** is indicated for the treatment of relapsing forms of multiple sclerosis (MS), to include clinically isolated syndrome, relapsing-remitting disease, and active secondary progressive disease, in adults. The most common adverse reactions (incidence for *dimethyl fumarate* [the prodrug of **Bafiertam**] ≥10% and ≥2% more than placebo) have been flushing, abdominal pain, diarrhea, and nausea. Co-administration of **Bafiertam** with *dimethyl fumarate* or *diroximel fumarate* is contraindicated. Blood tests are required prior to initiation of **Bafiertam**. Obtain a CBC including lymphocyte count before initiating **Bafiertam**, after 6 months, and every 6-12 months thereafter. Consider interruption of **Bafiertam** if lymphocyte counts <0.5 x 10^9/L persist for more than six months. Obtain serum aminotransferase, alkaline phosphatase, and total bilirubin levels before initiating **Bafiertam** and during treatment, as clinically indicated. Discontinue **Bafiertam** if clinically significant liver injury induced by **Bafiertam** is suspected. Discontinue and do not restart **Bafiertam** if anaphylaxis or angioedema occur. Withhold **Bafiertam** at the first sign or symptom suggestive of progressive multifocal leukoencephalopathy (PML). Consider withholding **Bafiertam** in cases of serious infection (e.g., herpes zoster and other serious opportunistic infections) until the infection has resolved. There are no adequate data on the developmental risk associated with the use of **Bafiertam** or dimethyl fumarate (the prodrug of **Bafiertam**) in pregnant females. In animals, adverse effects on offspring survival, growth, sexual maturation, and neurobehavioral function were observed when dimethyl fumarate (DMF) was administered during pregnancy and lactation at clinically relevant doses. There are no data on the presence of DMF or MMF in human milk or effects on the breastfed infant. Developmental and health benefits of breastfeeding should be considered along with the mother's clinical need for **Bafiertam** and any potential adverse effects on the breastfed infant from the drug or from the underlying maternal condition.

PSEUDOBULBAR AFFECT (PBA)

Comment: Pseudobulbar affect (PBA), emotional lability, labile affect, or emotional incontinence refers by to a neurologic disorder characterized by involuntary crying or uncontrollable episodes of crying and/or laughing, or other emotional outbursts. PBA occurs secondary to a neurologic disease or brain injury such as traumatic brain injury (TBI), stroke, Parkinson's disease, multiple sclerosis, and amyotrophic lateral sclerosis (ALS, or Lou Gehrig's disease).

▷ *dextromethorphan+quinidine* (C)(G) 1 cap once daily x 7 days; then starting on day 8, 1 cap bid

Pediatric: <12 years: not recommended; ≥12 years: same as adult

Nuedexta *Cap:* dextro 20 mg+quini 10 mg

Comment: *Dextromethorphan hydrobromide* is an uncompetitive NMDA receptor antagonist and sigma-1 agonist. *quinidine sulfate* is a CYP450 2D6 inhibitor. **Nuedexta** is contraindicated with an MAOI or within 14 days of stopping an MAOI, with prolonged QT interval, congenital long QT syndrome, history suggestive of torsades de pointes, or heart failure, complete atrioventricular (AV) block without implanted pacemaker or patients at high risk of complete AV block, and concomitant drugs that both prolong QT interval and are metabolized by CYP2D6 (e.g., *thioridazine* or *pimozide*).

Discontinue **Nuedexta** if the following occurs: hepatitis or thrombocytopenia or any other hypersensitivity reaction. Monitor ECG in patients with left ventricular hypertrophy (LVH) or left ventricular dysfunction (LVD). *desipramine* exposure increases **Nuedexta** 8-fold; reduce *desipramine* dose and adjust based on clinical response. Use of **Nuedexta** with selective serotonin reuptake inhibitors (SSRIs) or tricyclic antidepressants (TCAs) increases the risk of *serotonin syndrome*. *paroxetine* exposure increases **Nuedexta** 2-fold; therefore, reduce *paroxetine* dose and adjust based on clinical response (*digoxin* exposure may increase *digoxin* substrate plasma concentration. **Nuedexta** is not recommended in pregnancy or breastfeeding. Safety and effectiveness of **Nuedexta** in children have not been established.

ORAL FUMARATE

▷ *diroximel fumarate Starting Dose:* 231 mg twice daily x 7 days; *Maintenance Dose:* 462 mg (2 x 231 mg capsules) twice daily: swallow whole, do not crush, chew, or open capsules, and do not sprinkle contents onto food; avoid administration with a high-fat, high-calorie meal/snack; avoid co-administration with alcohol *Pediatric:* safety and efficacy not established

Vumerity *Cap:* 231 mg del-rel
Comment: **Vumerity** (*diroximel fumarate*) is a novel oral fumarate for the treatment of relapsing forms of multiple sclerosis (MS), to include clinically isolated syndrome, relapsing-remitting disease, and active secondary progressive disease, in adults. *Contraindications:* Known hypersensitivity to *diroximel fumarate, dimethyl fumarate,* or to any of the excipients of **Vumerity,** and co-administration with *dimethyl fumarate.* **Vumerity** is not recommended in patients with moderate or severe renal impairment. The most common adverse reactions have been flushing, nausea, abdominal pain, and diarrhea. Based on animal studies, Discontinue and do not restart **Vumerity** if anaphylaxis or angioedema occur. Withhold **Vumerity** at the first sign or symptom suggestive of lymphopenia or progressive multifocal leukoencephalopathy (PML). Obtain a CBC, including lymphocyte, count before initiating **Vumerity,** after 6 months, and every 6 to 12 months thereafter. Consider interruption of **Vumerity** if lymphocyte counts <0.5 × 109/L persist for more than 6 months. Obtain serum aminotransferase, alkaline phosphatase, and total bilirubin levels before initiating **Vumerity** and during treatment, as clinically indicated. Discontinue **Vumerity** if clinically significant liver injury induced by **Vumerity** is suspected. There are no adequate human data on the developmental risk associated with the use of **Vumerity** or *dimethyl fumarate* (which has the same active metabolite as **Vumerity**) in pregnancy. Animal studies have demonstrated the administration of *diroximel fumarate* during pregnancy or throughout pregnancy and lactation resulted in adverse effects on embryo/fetal and offspring development (increased incidences of skeletal abnormalities, increased mortality, decreased body weight, neurobehavioral impairment) at clinically relevant drug exposure. There are no data on the presence of *diroximel fumarate* or metabolites (MMF, HES) in human milk or effects on the breastfed infant. The developmental and health benefits of breastfeeding should be considered along with the mother's clinical need for **Vumerity** and any potential adverse effects on the breastfed infant from the drug or from the underlying maternal condition.

MUMPS (INFECTIOUS PAROTITIS, *PARAMYXOVIRUS*)

see **Childhood Immunizations**
Parenteral Corticosteroids *see* Appendix M. Parenteral Corticosteroids

Oral Corticosteroids *see* Appendix L. Oral Corticosteroids
Antipyretics *see Fever*

PROPHYLAXIS VACCINE

▷ *measles, mumps, rubella, live, attenuated, neomycin vaccine* (C)
    MMR II 25 mcg SC (preservative-free)
    Comment: Contraindications: hypersensitivity to *neomycin* or eggs, primary
    or acquired immune deficiency, immunosuppressant therapy, bone marrow or
    lymphatic malignancy, and pregnancy (within 3 months after vaccination).

 MUSCLE STRAIN

Acetaminophen for IV Infusion *see Pain*
Parenteral Corticosteroids *see* Appendix M. Parenteral Corticosteroids
Oral Corticosteroids *see* Appendix L. Oral Corticosteroids
Opioid Analgesics *see Pain*

Comment: Usual length of treatment for acute injury is approximately 5 days.

SKELETAL MUSCLE RELAXANTS

▷ *baclofen* (C)(G) 5 mg tid; titrate up by 5 mg every 3 days to 20 mg tid; max 80 mg/
    day
    Pediatric: <12 years: not recommended; ≥12 years: same as adult
        Lioresal *Tab:* 10*, 20*mg
    Comment: *Baclofen* is indicated for muscle spasm pain and chronic spasticity
    associated with multiple sclerosis and spinal cord injury or disease. Potential for
    seizures or hallucinations on abrupt withdrawal.
▷ *carisoprodol* (C)(G) 1 tab tid or qid
    Pediatric: <12 years: not recommended; ≥12 years: same as adult
        Soma *Tab:* 350 mg
▷ *chlorzoxazone* (G) 1 caplet qid; max 750 mg qid
    Pediatric: <12 years: not recommended; ≥12 years: same as adult
        Parafon Forte DSC *Cplt:* 500*mg
▷ *cyclobenzaprine* (B)(G) 10 mg tid; usual range 20-40 mg/day in divided doses;
    max 60 mg/day x 2-3 weeks or 15 mg ext-rel once daily; max 30 mg ext-rel/day x
    2-3 weeks
    Pediatric: <15 years: not recommended; ≥15 years: same as adult
        Amrix *Cap:* 15, 30 mg ext-rel
        Fexmid *Tab:* 7.5 mg
        Flexeril *Tab:* 5, 10 mg
▷ *dantrolene* (C) 25md daily x 7 days; then 25 mg tid x 7 days; then 50 mg tid x 7
    days; max 100 mg qid
    Pediatric: 0.5 mg/kg daily x 7 days; then 0.5 mg/kg tid x 7 days; then 1 mg/kg tid x
    7 days; then 2 mg/kg tid; max 100 mg qid
        Dantrium *Tab:* 25, 50, 100 mg
    Comment: *Dantrolene* is indicated for chronic spasticity associated with multiple
    sclerosis and spinal cord injury or disease.
▷ *diazepam* (C)(IV) 2-10 mg bid-qid; may increase gradually
    Pediatric: <6 months: not recommended; ≥6 months: initially 1-2.5 mg bid-qid;
    may increase gradually
        Diastat *Rectal gel delivery system:* 2.5 mg
        Diastat AcuDial *Rectal gel delivery system:* 10, 20 mg
        Valium *Tab:* 2, 5, 10 mg

Valium Intensol Oral Solution *Conc oral soln:* 5 mg/ml (30 ml w. dropper) (alcohol 19%)

Valium Oral Solution *Oral soln:* 5 mg/5 ml (500 ml) (wintergreen spice)

➤ *metaxalone* (B) 1 tab tid-qid
   Pediatric: <12 years: not recommended; ≥12 years: same as adult
      Skelaxin *Tab:* 800*mg

➤ *methocarbamol* (C)(G) initially 1.5 gm qid x 2-3 days; maintenance, 750 mg every 4 hours or 1.5 gm 3x daily; max 8 gm/day
   Pediatric: <16 years: not recommended; ≥16 years: same as adult
      Robaxin *Tab:* 500 mg
      Robaxin 750 *Tab:* 750 mg
      Robaxin Injection 10 ml IM or IV; max 30 ml/day; max 3 days; max 5 ml/ gluteal injection q 8 hours; max IV rate 3 ml/min
         Vial: 100 mg/ml (10 ml)

➤ *nabumetone* (C)
   Pediatric: <12 years: not recommended; ≥12 years: same as adult
      Relafen *Tab:* 500, 750 mg
      Relafen 500 *Tab:* 500 mg

➤ *orphenadrine citrate* (C)(G) 1 tab bid
   Pediatric: <12 years: not recommended; ≥12 years: same as adult
      Norflex *Tab:* 100 mg sust-rel

➤ *tizanidine* (C) 1-4 mg q 6-8 hours; max 36 mg/day
   Pediatric: <12 years: not recommended; ≥12 years: same as adult
      Zanaflex *Tab:* 2*, 4**mg; *Cap:* 2, 4, 6 mg

SKELETAL MUSCLE RELAXANT+NSAID COMBINATIONS

➤ *carisoprodol+aspirin* (C)(III)(G) 1-2 tabs qid
   Pediatric: <12 years: not recommended; ≥12 years: same as adult
      Soma Compound *Tab:* caris 200 mg+asp 325 mg (sulfites)

➤ *meprobamate+aspirin* (D)(IV) 1-2 tabs tid or qid
   Pediatric: <12 years: not recommended; ≥12 years: same as adult
      Equagesic *Tab:* mepro 200 mg+asp 325*mg

SKELETAL MUSCLE RELAXANT+NSAID+CAFFEINE COMBINATIONS

➤ *orphenadrine+aspirin+caffeine* (D)(G)
   Pediatric: <12 years: not recommended; ≥12 years: same as adult
      Norgesic 1-2 tabs tid-qid
         Tab: orphen 25 mg+asp 385 mg+caf 30 mg
      Norgesic Forte 1 tab tid or qid; max 4 tabs/day
         Tab: orphen 50 mg+asp 770 mg+caf 60 mg*

SKELETAL MUSCLE RELAXANT+NSAID+CODEINE COMBINATIONS

➤ *carisoprodol+aspirin+codeine* (D)(III)(G) 1-2 tabs qid prn
   Pediatric: <12 years: contraindicated; 12-<18: use extreme caution; not recommended for children and adolescents with obesity, asthma, obstructive sleep apnea, or other chronic breathing problem, or for post-tonsillectomy/ adenoidectomy pain; ≥18 years: same as adult
      Soma Compound w. Codeine
         Tab: caris 200 mg+asp 325 mg+cod 16 mg (sulfites)

TOPICAL & TRANSDERMAL ANALGESICS

➤ *capsaicin* (B)(G) apply tid-qid prn to intact skin
   Pediatric: <2 years: not recommended; ≥2 years: apply sparingly tid-qid prn
      Axsain *Crm:* 0.075% (1, 2 oz)
      Capsin *Lotn:* 0.025, 0.075% (59 ml)

> **Capzasin-HP (OTC)** *Crm*: 0.075% (1.5 oz), 0.025% (45, 90 gm); *Lotn*: 0.075% (2 oz); 0.025% (45, 90 gm)
> **Capzasin-P (OTC)** *Crm*: 0.025% (1.5 oz); *Lotn*: 0.025% (2 oz)
> **Dolorac** *Crm*: 0.025% (28 gm)
> **Double Cap (OTC)** *Crm*: 0.05% (2 oz)
> **R-Gel** *Gel*: 0.025% (15, 30 gm)
> **Zostrix (OTC)** *Crm*: 0.025% (0.7, 1.5, 3 oz)
> **Zostrix HP (OTC)** *Emol crm*: 0.075% (1, 2 oz)

▷ *capsaicin* 8% patch **(B)** apply up to 4 patches for one 60-minute application to clean dry skin; may prep area with topical anesthetic; wear non-latex gloves; patches may be cut to size/shape; treatment may be repeated every 3 months
Pediatric: <18 years: not recommended; ≥18 years: same as adult
> **Qutenza** *Patch*: 8% 1640 mcg/cm (179 mg) (1 or 2 patches w. 1-50 gm tube cleansing gel/carton)

▷ *diclofenac sodium* **(C; D ≥30 wks)** apply qid prn to intact skin
Pediatric: <12 years: not established; ≥12 years: same as adult
> **Pennsaid 1.5%** in 10 drop increments, dispense and rub into front, side, and back of knee: usually; 40 drops (40 mg) qid
> *Topical soln*: 1.5% (150 ml)
> **Pennsaid 2%** apply 2 pump actuations (40 mg) and rub into front, side, and back of knee bid
> *Topical soln*: 2% (20 mg/pump actuation, 112 gm)
> **Solaraze Gel** massage in to clean skin bid prn
> *Gel*: 3% (50 gm) (benzyl alcohol)
> **Voltaren Gel (G)(OTC)** apply qid prn to intact skin
> *Gel*: 1% (100 gm)

Comment: *Diclofenac* is contraindicated with *aspirin* allergy. As with other NSAIDs, should be avoided in late pregnancy (≥30 weeks) because it may cause premature closure of the ductus arteriosus.

▷ *doxepin* **(B)** cream apply to affected area qid at intervals of at least 3-4 hours; max 8 days
Pediatric: <12 years: not recommended; >12 years: same as adult
> **Prudoxin** *Crm*: 5% (45 gm)
> **Zonalon** *Crm*: 5% (30, 45 gm)

▷ *pimecrolimus* 1% cream **(C)(G)** <2 years: not recommended; ≥2 years: apply to affected area bid; do not apply an occlusive dressing
> **Elidel** *Crm*: 1% (30, 60, 100 gm)

Comment: *Pimecrolimus* is indicated for short-term and intermittent long-term use. Discontinue use when resolution occurs. Contraindicated if the patient is immunosuppressed. Change to the 0.1% preparation or if secondary bacterial infection is present.

▷ *trolamine salicylate* apply tid-qid
Pediatric: <2 years: not recommended; ≥2 years: same as adult
> **Mobisyl Creme** *Crm*: 10% (100 gm)

TOPICAL AND TRANSDERMAL ANESTHETICS

Comment: *Lidocaine* should not be applied to non-intact skin.

▷ *lidocaine* cream **(B)** apply to affected area bid prn
Pediatric: <12 years: not recommended; ≥12 years: same as adult
> **LidaMantle** *Crm*: 3% (1, 2 oz)
> **Lidoderm** *Crm*: 3% (85 gm)
> **ZTlido** *lidocaine* topical system 1% (30/carton)
> Comment: Compared to **Lidoderm** (*lidocaine* patch 5%), which contains 700 mg/patch, **ZTlido** only requires 35 mg per topical system to achieve the same therapeutic dose.

▷ *lidocaine* lotion (B) apply to affected area bid prn
  Pediatric: <12 years: not recommended; ≥12 years: same as adult
    LidaMantle *Lotn:* 3% (177 ml)
▷ *lidocaine* 5% patch (B)(G) apply up to 3 patches at one time for up to 12
  hours/24-hour period (12 hours on/12 hours off); patches may be cut into smaller
  sizes before removal of the release liner; do not re-use
  Pediatric: <12 years: not recommended; ≥12 years: same as adult
    Lidoderm *Patch:* 5% (10x14 cm; 30/carton)
▷ *lidocaine+dexamethasone* (B)
  Pediatric: <12 years: not recommended; ≥12 years: same as adult
    Decadron Phosphate with Xylocaine *Lotn:* dexa 4 mg+lido 10 mg per ml (5 ml)
▷ *lidocaine+hydrocortisone* (B)(G) apply to affected area bid prn
  Pediatric: <12 years: not recommended; ≥12 years: same as adult
    LidaMantle HC *Crm:* lido 3%+hydro 0.5% (1, 3 oz); *Lotn:* (177 ml)
▷ *lidocaine 2.5%+prilocaine 2.5%* apply sparingly to the burn bid-tid prn
  Pediatric: <12 years: not recommended; ≥12 years: same as adult
    Emla Cream (B) 5, 30 gm/tube

ORAL NSAIDs

For an expanded list of NSAIDs *see* Appendix J. NSAIDs online at https://connect.
springerpub.com/content/reference-book/978-0-8261-7935-7/back-matter/part02/
back-matter/bmatter10

▷ *diclofenac* (C; D ≥30 wks) take on empty stomach; 35 mg tid; *Hepatic
  Impairment:* use lowest dose
  Pediatric: <18 years: not recommended; ≥18 years: same as adult
    Zorvolex *Gelcap:* 18, 35 mg
▷ *diclofenac sodium* (C; D ≥30 wks)
  Pediatric: <18 years: not recommended; ≥18 years: same as adult
    Voltaren 50 mg bid-qid or 75 mg bid or 25 mg qid with an additional 25 mg at
    HS if necessary
      Tab: 25, 50, 75 mg ent-coat
    Voltaren XR 100 mg once daily; rarely, 100 mg bid may be used
      Tab: 100 mg ext-rel
  Comment: *Diclofenac* is contraindicated with *aspirin* allergy. As with other
  NSAIDs, should be avoided in late premature closure of the ductus arteriosus.

ORAL NSAIDs+PPI COMBINATIONS

▷ *esomeprazole+naproxen* (C)(G) 1 tab bid; use lowest effective dose for the
  shortest duration swallow whole; take at least 30 minutes before a meal
  Pediatric: <18 years: not recommended; ≥18 years: same as adult
    Vimovo *Tab:* nap 375 mg+eso 20 mg ext-rel; nap 500 mg+eso 20 mg ext-rel
    Comment: **Vimovo** is indicated to improve signs/symptoms, and risk of
    gastric ulcer in patients at risk of developing NSAID-associated gastric ulcer.

COX-2 INHIBITORS

Comment: Cox-2 inhibitors are contraindicated with history of asthma, urticaria,
and allergic-type reactions to *aspirin*, other NSAIDs, and sulfonamides, 3rd
trimester of pregnancy, and coronary artery bypass graft (CABG) surgery.

▷ *celecoxib* (C)(G) 100-400 mg daily bid; max 800 mg/day
  Pediatric: <18 years: not recommended; ≥18 years: same as adult
    Celebrex *Cap:* 50, 100, 200, 400 mg
▷ *meloxicam* (C)(G)
    Mobic <2 years, <60 kg: not recommended; ≥2, >60 kg: 0.125 mg/kg; max 7.5
    mg once daily; ≥18 years: initially 7.5 mg once daily; max 15 mg once daily;
    Hemodialysis: max 7.5 mg/day

Tab: 7.5, 15 mg; *Oral susp:* 7.5 mg/5 ml (100 ml) (raspberry)
Vivlodex <18 years: <u>not</u> established; ≥18 years: initially 5 mg qd; may increase to max 10 mg/day; *Hemodialysis:* max 5 mg/day
Cap: 5, 10 mg

▶ *meloxicam injection* administer 30 mg via IV bolus once daily; administer dose over 15 seconds; monitor analgesic response <u>and</u> administer a short-acting, non-NSAID, immediate-release analgesic if response is inadequate; patients must be well hydrated before **Anjeso** administration; use **Anjeso** for the shortest duration consistent with individual patient treatment goals
Pediatric: safety and efficacy not established
  Anjeso *Vial:* 30 mg/ml (1 ml), single dose
  Comment: **Anjeso** *(meloxicam)* is an NSAID injection indicated for use in adults for the management of moderate-to-severe pain, alone <u>or</u> in combination with non-NSAID analgesics. Because of delayed onset of analgesia, **Anjeso** as monotherapy is <u>not</u> recommended for use when rapid onset of analgesia is required. The most common adverse reactions (incidence ≥2%) in controlled clinical trials have included constipation, GGT increase, and anemia. Use of NSAIDs during the third trimester of pregnancy increases the risk of premature closure of the fetal ductus arteriosus; therefore, avoid **Anjeso** use after 30 weeks gestation. There are no human data available on whether *meloxicam* is present in human milk, <u>or</u> on the effects on breastfed infants NSAIDs are associated with reversible infertility. Consider withdrawal of **Anjeso** in women who have difficulties conceiving. **Anjeso** may also compromise fertility in males of reproductive potential; it is <u>not</u> known if this effect on male fertility is reversible.

TOPICAL & TRANSDERMAL LIDOCAINE

▶ *lidocaine* transdermal patch **(C)(G)** apply one patch to affected area for 12 hours (then off for 12 hours); remove during bathing; avoid non-intact skin
Pediatric: <12 years: not recommended; ≥12 years: same as adult
  Lidoderm *Patch:* 5% (10 cm x 14 cm; 30/carton)

 MYASTHENIA GRAVIS (MG)

COMPLEMENT INHIBITORS

▶ *eculizumab* **(C)** dilute to a final admixture concentration of 5 mg/ml using the following steps: (1) withdraw the required amount of **Soliris** from the vial into a sterile syringe; (2) transfer the dose to an infusion bag; (3) add IV fluid equal to the drug volume (0.9% NaCl <u>or</u> 0.45% NaCl <u>or</u> D5W <u>or</u> Ringer's Lactate); the final admixed **Soliris** 5 mg/ml infusion volume is: 300 mg dose (60 ml), 600 mg dose (120 ml), 900 mg dose (180 ml), 1200 mg dose (240 ml); administer 900 mg IV infusion once weekly for the first 4 weeks; then, 1200 mg IV infusion for the 5th dose 1 week after the 4th dose; then, 1200 mg IV infusion once every 2 weeks thereafter
Pediatric: <18 years: safety and effectiveness not established; ≥18 years: same as adult
  Soliris *Vial:* 300 mg (10 mg/ml, 30 ml), single-use, concentrated solution for intravenous infusion (preservative-free)
Comment: **Soliris** *(eculizumab)* is a complement inhibitor indicated for the treatment of patients with paroxysmal nocturnal hemoglobinuria (PNH) to reduce hemolysis, patients with atypical hemolytic uremic syndrome (aHUS) to inhibit complement-mediated thrombotic microangiopathy (TMA), and adult patients with generalized myasthenia gravis (gMG) who are anti-acetylcholine receptor (AchR) antibody positive. **Soliris** should be administered

for generalized MG at the above recommended dosage regimen time points or within 2 days of each time point. Supplemental dosing of **Soliris** is required in the setting of concomitant support with plasmapheresis (PI) or plasma exchange (PE) or fresh frozen plasma (FFP) infusion (see mfr pkg insert for supplemental dosing). **Soliris** is not indicated for the treatment of patients with Shiga toxin *E. coli*-related hemolytic uremic syndrome (STEC-HUS). **Soliris** is contraindicated in patients with unresolved *Neisseria meningitides* infection and patients who are not currently vaccinated against *Neisseria meningitides*, unless the risks of delaying **Soliris** treatment outweigh the risks of developing meningococcal infection. Prescribers must enroll in the **Soliris** REMS Program (1-888-SOLIRIS, 1-888-765-4747), counsel patients about the risk of meningococcal infection, provide patients with **Soliris** REMS educational materials, and ensure that patients are vaccinated with a meningococcal vaccine. There are no adequate and well-controlled human studies of **Soliris** in pregnancy or effects on the breastfed infant. Based on animal studies, **Soliris** may cause fetal harm. It is not known whether **Soliris** is excreted in human milk. IgG is excreted in human milk, so it is expected that **Soliris** will be present in human milk. However, published data suggest that antibodies in human milk do not enter the neonatal and infant circulation in substantial amounts. Caution should be exercised when **Soliris** is administered to a breastfeeding patient.

 MYELODYSPLASTIC SYNDROMES (MDS)

NUCLEOSIDE METABOLIC INHIBITOR+CYTIDINE DEAMINASE INHIBITOR

▷ *decitabine+cedazuridine* take one tablet once daily on Days 1 through 5 of each 28-day cycle; take on an empty stomach

Pediatric: not established

   Inqovi *Tab:* deci 35 mg+cedaz 100 mg film-coat

   Comment: Inqovi *(decitabine+cedazuridine)* is a nucleoside metabolic inhibitor *(decitabine)* and cytidine deaminase inhibitor *(cedazuridine)* combination indicated for the treatment of adults with intermediate and high-risk myelodysplastic syndromes (MDS), including chronic myelomonocytic leukemia (CMML). The most common adverse reactions (incidence ≥20%) have been fatigue, constipation, hemorrhage, myalgia, mucositis, arthralgia, nausea, dyspnea, diarrhea, rash, dizziness, febrile neutropenia, edema, headache, cough, decreased appetite, URI, pneumonia, and increased transaminase. The most common grade 3 or 4 laboratory abnormalities (≥50%) have been decreased leukocytes, platelet count, neutrophil count, and hemoglobin. Fatal and serious myelosuppression and infectious complications can occur. Obtain CBC counts prior to initiation of **Inqovi**, prior to each cycle, and as clinically indicated to monitor for response and toxicity (sCr ≥2 mg/dL, serum bilirubin ≥2 x ULN), AST or ALT) ≥2 x ULN, active or uncontrolled infection). Manage persistent severe neutropenia and febrile neutropenia with supportive treatment. Following resolution, delay the next cycle and resume at the same or reduced dose as indicated. See mfr pkg insert for recommended dose reductions for myelosuppression. **Inqovi** can cause fetal harm. Avoid co-administration of **Inqovi** with other drugs metabolized by cytidine deaminase. **Inqovi** can impair fertility. Advise patients of reproductive potential of potential embryo/fetal risk and to use effective contraception for 6 months (females) or 3 months (males) after the last dose. Based on animal studies of *decitabine* and *cedazuridine*, **Inqovi** may impair male fertility. Reversibility of the effect on fertility is unknown. Advise females not to breastfeed.

MYELOFIBROSIS

KINASE INHIBITORS

▷ *fedratinib* 400 mg once daily with or without food for patients with a baseline platelet count of greater than or equal to 50 x 10^9/L (2.1); reduce dose for patients taking strong CYP3A inhibitors or with severe renal impairment; avoid use in patients with severe hepatic impairment

Inrebic *Cap:* 100 mg

Comment: Inrebic *(fedratinib)* is a highly selective JAK2 inhibitor indicated for the treatment of adult patients with intermediate-2 or high-risk primary or secondary (post-polycythemia vera or post-essential thrombocythemia) myelofibrosis. Reduce Inrebic dose as recommended with concomitant use of strong CYP3A4 inhibitors. Avoid use of Inrebic when used with concomitant use of strong and moderate CYP3A4 inducers and dual CYP3A4 and CYP2C19 inhibitors. Black Box Warning (BBW): Serious and fatal encephalopathy, including Wernicke's, has occurred in patients treated with Inrebic. Wernicke's encephalopathy is a neurologic emergency; therefore, assess thiamine levels in all patients prior to starting Inrebic, periodically during treatment, and as clinically indicated. Do not start Inrebic in patients with thiamine deficiency. Replete thiamine prior to treatment initiation. If encephalopathy is suspected, immediately discontinue Inrebic and initiate parenteral thiamine. Monitor until symptoms resolve or improve and thiamine levels normalize. Warnings and precautions with use of Inbrec include anemia and thrombocytopenia (manage by dose reduction, interruption, or transfusion); gastrointestinal toxicity (manage by dose reduction or interruption if patient develops severe diarrhea, nausea, or vomiting— prophylaxis with anti-emetics and treatment with anti-diarrheal medications are recommended; hepatic toxicity (manage amylase and lipase elevation by dose reduction or interruption). There are no available data on Inrebic use in pregnant females to evaluate for a drug-associated risk of major birth defects, miscarriage or adverse maternal or fetal outcomes. However, in animal reproduction studies, oral administration of *fedratinib* during organogenesis at doses considerably lower than the recommended human daily dose of 400 mg/day resulted in adverse developmental outcomes. Consider benefits and risks of Inrebic for the mother and possible embryo/fetal risk fetus when prescribing in pregnancy. There are no data on the presence of *fedratinib* or its metabolites in human milk or effects on the breastfed infant and patients should be advised not to breastfeed during treatment with Inrebic and for at least 1 month after the last dose.

▷ *ruxolitinib Starting Dose:* based on baseline platelet count: *>200 X 10^9/L:* 20 mg twice daily; *100 X 10^9/L to 200 X 10^9/L:* 15 mg twice daily; *50 X 10^9/L to <100 X 10^9/L:* 5 mg twice daily; therapeutic dose should be individualized based on safety and efficacy; monitor CBC every 2-4 weeks until doses are stabilized, and then as clinically indicated; modify or interrupt dosing for thrombocytopenia; *Renal Impairment:* reduce starting dose or avoid use; *Hepatic Impairment:* reduce starting dose or avoid use

Pediatric: <12 years: not established; ≥12 years: same as adult

Jakafi *Tab:* 5, 10, 15, 20, 25 mg

Comment: Jakafi *(ruxolitinib)* is a kinase inhibitor indicated for treatment of adults with intermediate and high-risk myelofibrosis, including primary myelofibrosis, polycythemia vera with inadequate response to, or intolerance to, hydroxyurea, post-polycythemia vera myelofibrosis, and post-essential thrombocythemia myelofibrosis. Manage thrombocytopenia, anemia, and neutropenia with dose reduction, or treatment interruption, or transfusion.

Serious infections should be resolved before starting therapy with **Jakafi**. Assess patients for signs and symptoms of infection during **Jakafi** therapy and initiate appropriate treatment promptly. Manage symptom exacerbation following interruption or discontinuation of **Jakafi** with supportive care and then consider resuming treatment with **Jakafi**. There is risk of non-melanoma skin cancer (NMSC) with **Jakafi** use; perform periodic skin examinations. Assess lipid levels 8-12 weeks from start of **Jakafi** therapy and treat as appropriate. Avoid use of **Jakafi** with *fluconazole* doses greater than 200 mg except in patients with acute graft versus host disease (GVHD). With myelofibrosis and polycythemia vera, the most common hematologic adverse reactions (incidence >20%) have been thrombocytopenia and anemia and the most common nonhematologic adverse reactions (incidence >10%) have been bruising, dizziness, and headache. There are no studies with the use of **Jakafi** in pregnant females to inform drug-associated risks. No data are available regarding the presence of *ruxolitinib* in human milk or the effects on the breastfed infant. Patients should be advised to discontinue breastfeeding during treatment with **Jakafi** and for 2 weeks after the final dose.

⬤ NARCOLEPSY, CATAPLEXY

STIMULANTS

▷ *amphetamine sulfate* (C)(II) administer first dose on awakening, and additional doses at 4- to 6-hour intervals; usual range 5-60 mg/day
Pediatric: <6 years: not recommended; 6-12 years: 5 mg daily in the AM; may increase by 5 mg/day at weekly intervals; ≥12-18 years: initially 10 mg in the AM; may increase by 10 mg daily at weekly intervals; >18 years: same as adult
   Evekeo initially 10 mg once or twice daily at the same time(s) each day; may increase by 10 mg/day at weekly intervals; max 40 mg/day
      Tab: 5, 10 mg

▷ *armodafinil* (C)(IV)(G) *OSAHS:* 50-250 mg once daily in the AM; *SWSD:* 150 mg 1 hour before starting shift; reduce dose with severe hepatic impairment
Pediatric: <17 years: not recommended; ≥17 years: same as adult
   Nuvigil *Tab:* 50, 150, 200, 250 mg

▷ *modafinil* (C)(IV)(G) 100-200 mg q AM; max 400 mg/day
Pediatric: <17 years: not recommended; ≥17 years: same as adult
   Provigil *Tab:* 100, 200*mg
   Comment: **Provigil** also promotes wakefulness in patients with shift work sleep disorder and excessive sleepiness due to obstructive sleep apnea/hypopnea syndrome.

▷ *sodium oxybate* (B)(G)(III) initiate dosage at 4.5 gm per night orally divided into two doses; titrate to effect in increments of 1.5 gm per night at weekly intervals (0.75 gm at bedtime and 0.75 gm taken 2½ to 4 hours later)

Total Nightly Dose (gm)	4.5 gm	6 gm	7.5 gm	9 gm
Bedtime (gm)	2.25 gm	3 gm	3.75 gm	4.5 gm
2½ to 4 hours later (gm)	2.25 gm	3 gm	3.75 gm	4.5 gm

Pediatric: <7 years: not recommended; ≥7-17 years: see mfr pkg insert for weight-based (in kilograms) dosing table; ≥18 years: same as adult
   Xyrem *Oral soln:* 500 mg/ml
   Comment: **Xyrem** is used to reduce the number of cataplexy attacks (sudden and transient episode of muscle weakness coupled with full conscious awareness, typically triggered by emotions such as laughing, crying, or terror) and reduce daytime sleepiness in patients with narcolepsy. The rapid onset of sedation coupled with amnesia, particularly when combined with alcohol, has posed risks for voluntary and involuntary users (e.g., assault

victims). Contraindicated with *alcohol* and CNS depressants (may impair consciousness; may lead to respiratory depression, coma, or death), and in patients with succinic semialdehyde dehydrogenase deficiency (an inborn error of metabolism). Prepare both doses prior to bedtime and do not attempt to get out of bed after taking the first dose. Place both doses within reach at the bedside. Set the bedside clock to awaken for the second dose. Dilute each dose in 60 ml (1/4 cup, 4 tbsp) water in child resistant dosing containers. Food significantly reduces the bioavailability of *sodium oxybate*; take at least 2 hours after ingesting food. There are no adequate data on the fetal developmental risk associated with the use of *sodium oxybate* in pregnant females. GHB is excreted in human milk. There is insufficient information on risk to the breastfed infant.

Comment: Xyrem is a Schedue III controlled substance. The active ingredient of Xyrem, sodium oxybate or gamma-hydroxy-butyrate (GHB), is a Schedule I controlled substance. Xyrem is available only through a restricted distribution Xyrem REMS Program because of the risks of CNS depression and abuse and misuse, healthcare providers who prescribe Xyrem are specially certified, Xyrem is dispensed only by the central pharmacy that is specially certified, and Xyrem is dispensed and shipped only to patients who are enrolled in the Xyrem REMS Program with documentation of safe use (www.XYREMREMS. com or 1-866-XYREM88 [1-866-997-3688]).

SELECTIVE DOPAMINE AND NOREPINEPHRINE REUPTAKE INHIBITOR (DNRI)

▷ *solriamfetol* administer once daily upon awakening; avoid administration within 9 hours of planned bedtime because of the potential to interfere with sleep; *Starting Dose for Patients with Narcolepsy:* 75 mg once daily; *Starting Dose for Patients with OSA:* 37.5 mg once daily; dose may be increased at intervals of at least 3 days; max 150 mg once daily; *Moderate Renal Impairment:* starting dose 37.5 mg once daily; may increase to 75 mg once daily after at least 7 days; *Severe Renal Impairment:* Starting dose and max dose is 37.5 mg once daily; *ESRD:* not recommended.

Pediatric: safety and efficacy not established

Sunosi *Tab:* 75*, 150 mg film-coat

Comment: Sunosi *(solriamfetol)* is a dopamine and norepinephrine reuptake inhibitor (DNRI) indicated to improve wakefulness in adult patients with excessive daytime sleepiness associated with narcolepsy or obstructive sleep apnea (OSA). Sunosi is not indicated to treat the underlying airway obstruction in OSA. Ensure that the underlying airway obstruction is treated (e.g., with continuous positive airway pressure (CPAP)) for at least 1 month prior to initiating Sunosi for excessive daytime sleepiness. Modalities to treat the underlying airway obstruction should be continued during treatment with Sunosi. Sunosi is not a substitute for these modalities. Use caution when co-administering Sunosi with drugs that increase blood pressure and/or heart rate and dopaminergic drugs. Measure HR and BP prior to initiating, and periodically throughout, treatment. Control hypertension before and during therapy. Avoid use in patients with unstable cardiovascular disease, serious heart arrhythmias, or other serious heart problems. Use caution in treating patients with a history of psychosis or bipolar disorder. Consider Sunosi dose reduction or discontinuation if psychiatric symptoms develop. Sunosi is contraindicated in patients receiving treatment with a monoamine oxidase (MAO) inhibitor and within 14 days following discontinuation of an MAOI. Available data from case reports are not sufficient to determine drug-associated risks of major birth defects, miscarriage, or adverse maternal or fetal outcomes. There are no data available on the presence of *solriamfetol* or its metabolites in human milk or effects on the breastfed infant. The developmental and health benefits of breastfeeding should be considered along with the mother's clinical need for **Sunosi** and any potential adverse effects on the breastfed infant from **Sunosi** or from the underlying maternal condition. Healthcare providers are encouraged to register pregnant patients or pregnant females may enroll themselves, in the Sunosi Pregnancy Exposure Registry by calling 1-877-283-6220 or visiting www. SunosiPregnancyRegistry.com

AMPHETAMINES

▷ **dextroamphetamine sulfate** (C)(II)(G) initially start with 10 mg daily; increase by 10 mg at weekly intervals if needed; may switch to daily dose with sust-rel spansules when titrated
Pediatric: <3 years: not recommended; 3-5 years: 2.5 mg daily; may increase by 2.5 mg daily at weekly intervals if needed; 6-12 years: initially 5 mg daily-bid; may increase by 5 mg/day at weekly intervals; usual max 40 mg/day; >12 years: initially 10 mg daily; may increase by mg/day at weekly intervals; max 40 mg/day 10

Dexedrine *Tab:* 5*mg (tartrazine)
Dexedrine Spansule *Cap:* 5, 10, 15 mg sust-rel
Dextrostat *Tab:* 5, 10 mg (tartrazine)

▷ **dextroamphetamine saccharate+dextroamphetamine sulfate+amphetamine aspartate+amphetamine sulfate** (C)(II)(G)

Adderall initially 10 mg daily; may increase weekly by 10 mg/day; usual max 60 mg/day in 2-3 divided doses; first dose on awakening and then q 4-6 hours prn
Pediatric: <6 years: not indicated; 6-12 years: initially 5 mg daily; may increase weekly by 5 mg/day; usual max 40 mg/day in 2-3 divided doses; >12 years: same as adult

Tab: 5**, 7.5**, 10**, 12.5**, 15**, 20**, 30**mg

Adderall XR
Pediatric: <6 years: not recommended; 6-12 years: initially 10 mg daily in the AM; may increase by 10 mg weekly; max 30 mg/day; 13-17 years: initially 10 mg daily; may increase to 20 mg/day after 1 week; max 30 mg/day;
Do not crush or chew; may sprinkle on apple sauce

Cap: 5, 10, 15, 20, 25, 30 mg ext-rel

Comment: Adderall is also indicated to improve wakefulness in patients with shift-work sleep disorder and excessive sleepiness due to obstructive sleep apnea/hypopnea syndrome.

▷ **dexmethylphenidate** (C)(II)(G) take once daily in the AM
Pediatric: <6 years: not recommended; ≥6 years: same as adult
Focalin initially 2.5 mg bid; allow at least 4 hours between doses; may increase at 1 week intervals; max 40 mg/day
Tab: 2.5, 5, 10*mg (dye-free)
Focalin XR 20-40 mg q AM; max 40 mg/day
Tab: 5, 10, 15, 20, 30, 40 mg ext-rel (dye-free)

▷ **methylphenidate (regular-acting)** (C)(II)(G)
Pediatric: <6 years: not recommended; ≥6 years: initially 5 mg bid ac (before breakfast and lunch); may gradually increase by 5-10 mg at weekly intervals as needed; max 60 mg/day
Methylin, Methylin Chewable, Methylin Oral Solution usual dose 20-30 mg/day in 2-3 divided doses 30-45 minutes before a meal; may increase to 60 mg/day
Ritalin 10-60 mg/day in 2-3 divided doses 30-45 minutes ac; max 60 mg/day
Tab: 5, 10*, 20*mg

▷ **methylphenidate (long-acting)** (C)(II)
Adhansia XR recommended starting is 25 mg once daily in the morning; may be increased in increments of 10-15 mg at intervals of at least 5 days; dosage ≥85 mg daily (in adults) and ≥70 mg daily (children) are associated with disproportionate increases in the incidence of certain adverse reactions;

administer with or without food; may be swallowed whole or opened and the capsule contents sprinkled onto a tablespoon of applesauce or yogurt; do not crush or chew capsule contents

Cap: 25, 35, 45, 55, 70, 85 mg ext-rel

Concerta initially 18 mg q AM; may increase in 18 mg increments as needed; max 54 mg/day; do not crush or chew

Tab: 18, 27, 36, 54 mg sust-rel

Metadate CD (G) 1 cap daily in the AM; may sprinkle on food; do not crush or chew

Pediatric: <6 years: not recommended; ≥6 years: initially 20 mg daily; may gradually increase by 20 mg/day at weekly intervals as needed; max 60 mg/day

Cap: 10, 20, 30, 40, 50, 60 mg immed- and ext-rel beads

Metadate ER 1 tab daily in the AM; do not crush or chew

Pediatric: <6 years: not recommended; ≥6 years: use in place of regular-acting *methylphenidate* when the 8-hour dose of **Metadate-ER** corresponds to the titrated 8-hour dose of regular-acting *methylphenidate*

Tab: 10, 20 mg ext-rel (dye-free)

Ritalin LA 1 cap daily in the AM

Pediatric: <6 years: not recommended; ≥6 years: use in place of regular-acting *methylphenidate* when the 8-hour dose of **Ritalin LA** corresponds to the titrated 8-hour dose of regular-acting *methylphenidate*; max 60 mg/day

Cap: 10, 20, 30, 40 mg ext-rel (immed- and ext-rel beads)

Ritalin SR 1 cap daily in the AM

Pediatric: <6 years: not recommended; ≥6 years: use in place of regular-acting *methylphenidate* when the 8-hour dose of **Ritalin SR** corresponds to the titrated 8-hour dose of regular-acting *methylphenidate*; max 60 mg/day

Tab: 20 mg sust-rel (dye-free)

▷ *methylphenidate (transdermal patch)* (C)(II)(G) 1 patch daily in the AM
Pediatric: <6 years: not recommended; ≥6 years: initially 10 mg patch daily in the AM; may increase by 5-10 mg/week; max 60 mg/day

Transdermal patch: 10, 15, 20, 30 mg

▷ *pemoline* (B)(IV) 18.75-112.5 mg/day; usually start with 37.5 mg in AM; increase weekly by 18.75 mg/day if needed; max 112.5 gm/day
Pediatric: <6 years: not recommended; ≥6 years: same as adult

Cylert *Tab:* 18.75*, 37.5*, 75*mg

Cylert Chewable *Chew tab:* 37.5*mg

Comment: Monitor baseline serum ALT and repeat every 2 weeks thereafter.

HISTAMINE-3 (H3) RECEPTOR ANTAGONIST/INVERSE AGONIST

▷ *pitolisant* administer once daily in the morning upon wakening; recommended range is 17.8 mg to 35.6 mg once daily; titrate dose as follows:

Week 1: initially 8.9 mg once daily

Week 2: increase to 17.8 mg once daily

Week 3: may increase to max 35.6 mg once daily

Moderate Hepatic Impairment: initially 8.9 mg once daily; titrate to max 17.8 mg once daily after 14 days

Severe Hepatic Impairment: contraindicated

Moderate/Severe Renal Impairment: initially 8.9 mg once daily; titrate to max 17.8 mg once daily after 7 days

ESRD: not recommended

Poor Metabolizers of CYP2D6: max 17.8 mg once daily

Strong CYP2D6 Inhibitors: max 17.8 mg once daily

Strong CYP3A4 Inducers: decrease exposure to **Wakix**; consider dose adjustment

Sensitive CYP3A4 Substrates (including hormonal contraceptives): **Wakix** may reduce effectiveness of sensitive CYP3A4 substrates; recommend using an alternative non-hormonal contraceptive method during treatment with **Wakix** and for at least 21 days after discontinuation of treatment

Wakix *Tab:* 4.45, 17.8 mg

Comment: **Wakix** (*pitolisant*) is a first-in-class drug, a histamine-3 (H$_3$) receptor antagonist/inverse agonist, for the treatment of excessive daytime sleepiness (EDS) in adult patients with narcolepsy. The most common adverse reactions (incidence ≥5%) have been insomnia, nausea, and anxiety. Avoid use of **Wakix** with drugs that also increase the QT interval and in patients with risk factors for prolonged QT interval and monitor patients with hepatic or renal impairment for increased QTc. There is a pregnancy exposure registry that monitors pregnancy outcomes in women who are exposed to **Wakix** during pregnancy. Patients should be encouraged to enroll in the **Wakix** pregnancy registry if they become pregnant. To enroll or obtain information from the registry, patients can call 1-800-833-7460. There are no data on the presence of *pitolisant* in human milk or effects on the breastfed infant; however, *pitolisant* is present in the milk of lactating rats. The developmental and health benefits of breastfeeding should be considered along with the mother's clinical need for treatment with **Wakix**.

CNS DEPRESSANT

▷ *calcium, magnesium, potassium, and sodium oxybates oral solution (CIII)* prepare 2 doses prior to bedtime; dilute each dose with approximately ¼ cup of water in pharmacy-provided containers; take the first nightly dose at least 2 hours after eating; take each dose while in bed and lie down after dosing; see mfr pkg insert for adult dosing

Pediatric: <7 years: not established; ≥7 years: recommended starting dose, titration regimen, and maximum total nightly dose is based on body weight (see mfr pkg insert for dosing by weight table)

Xywav *Oral soln:* 0.5 gm/ml total salts (equivalent to 0.413 gm/ml of oxybate)

Comment: **Xywav** is a CNS depressant indicated for the treatment of cataplexy or excessive daytime sleepiness (EDS) in patients ≥7 years-of-age with narcolepsy. The most common adverse reactions in adults (incidence ≥5%) have been headache, nausea, dizziness, decreased appetite, parasomnia, diarrhea, hyperhidrosis, anxiety, and vomiting. In a pediatric study with sodium oxybate, (same active moiety as **Xywav**), the most common adverse reactions (incidence ≥5%) were enuresis, nausea, headache, vomiting, weight decreased, decreased appetite, and dizziness. **Xywav** is contraindicated in combination with sedative hypnotics or alcohol or when the patient has succinic semialdehyde dehydrogenase deficiency. When used with concomitant *divalproex sodium*, an initial reduction in **Xywav** dose of at least 20% is recommended. If transitioning from **Xyrem** to **Xywav**, initiate **Xywav** at the same dose and regimen as **Xyrem** (gram for gram) and titrate as needed based on efficacy and tolerability. If the patient has hepatic impairment, the recommended starting dosage of **Xywav** is one-half of the original dosage per night administered orally, divided into two doses. Use caution when considering the concurrent use of **Xywav** with other CNS depressants and caution patients against hazardous activity requiring complete mental alertness or motor coordination within the first 6 hours of dosing or after first initiating treatment until certain that **Xywav** does not affect them adversely. Monitor patients for emergent or increased depression and suicidality. Monitor for impaired motor/cognitive function. Evaluate episodes of sleepwalking (Parasomnia). Based on animal data, **Xywav** may cause embryo/fetal harm. Advise females of reproductive potential of the potential embryo/fetal risk and to use an effective method of contraception during treatment. GHB is excreted in human milk after oral administration of *sodium oxybate*.

There is insufficient information on risk to a breastfed infant. Developmental and health benefits of breastfeeding should be considered along with the mother's clinical need for **Xywav**, and any potential adverse effects on the breastfed infant from **Xywav**, or from the underlying maternal condition.

NAUSEA/VOMITING: CHEMOTHERAPY-INDUCED (CINV)

SUBSTANCE P/NEUROKININ-1 (NK-1) RECEPTOR ANTAGONIST AND SEROTONIN-3 (5-HT3) RECEPTOR ANTAGONIST COMBINATION

▷ *fosnetupitant* and *palonosetron*

Akynzeo capsule: one cap administered approximately 1 hour prior to the start of chemotherapy, with or without food

Akynzeo for injection: one vial reconstituted in 50 ml of D5W or 0.9% NS administered as 30-minute IV infusion starting approximately 30 minutes prior to the start of chemotherapy.

Pediatric: <18 years: not established; ≥18 years: same as adult

Akynzeo *Cap:* 300 mg netu+palo 0.5 mg

Akynzeo for injection *Vial:* fosnetu 235 mg+palo 0.25 mg, single-dose, pwdr for reconstitution and IV infusion

Comment: **Akynzeo for Injection** is indicated in combination with *dexamethasone* for the prevention of acute and delayed nausea and vomiting associated with initial and repeat courses of highly emetogenic cancer chemotherapy. **Akynzeo for injection** has not been studied for the prevention of nausea and vomiting associated with *anthracycline* plus *cyclophosphamide* chemotherapy. **Akynzeo** capsules are indicated in combination with *dexamethasone* for prevention of acute and delayed nausea and vomiting associated with initial and repeat courses of cancer chemotherapy, including, but not limited to, highly emetogenic chemotherapy. Avoid in patients with severe hepatic impairment and patients with severe renal disease and end stage renal disease (ESRD). May cause fetal harm.

NAUSEA/VOMITING: POST-ANESTHESIA

Rx ANTIEMETICS

▷ *amisulpride* Prevention of PONV (either alone or in combination with another antiemetic): 5 mg as a single IV dose infused over 1-2 minutes at the time of induction of anesthesia; *Treatment of PONV:* 10 mg as a single IV dose infused over 1-2 minutes in the event of nausea and/or vomiting after a surgical procedure; dilution is not required prior to administration

Pediatric: safety and efficacy not established

Barhemsys *Vial:* 5 mg/2 ml (2 ml), single-dose

Comment: **Barhemsys** *(amisulpride)* is a dopamine-2 (D2) antagonist for the management of post-operative nausea/vomiting (PONV). The most common adverse reactions (incidence ≥2%) have been: *Prevention of PONV:* increased blood prolactin concentrations, chills, hypokalemia, procedural hypotension, and abdominal distension; *Treatment of PONV:* infusion site pain. QT prolongation occurs in a dose- and concentration-dependent manner. Avoid use in patients with congenital long QT syndrome and in patients taking *droperidol.* ECG monitoring is recommended in patients with preexisting arrhythmias/cardiac conduction disorders, electrolyte abnormalities (e.g., hypokalemia or hypomagnesemia), congestive heart failure, and in patients taking other medicinal products (e.g., *ondansetron*) or with other medical conditions known to prolong the QT interval. There are no reports of adverse effects on the breastfed infant. A lactating woman may pump and discard breast milk for 48 hours after **Barhemsys** administration to reduce infant exposure.

▷ *ondansetron* (C)(G) 8 mg q 8 hours x 2 doses; then 8 mg q 12 hours
  Pediatric: <4 years: not recommended; 4-11 years: 4 mg q 4 hours x 3 doses; then
  4 mg q 8 hours
    Zofran *Tab:* 4, 8, 24 mg
    Zofran ODT *ODT:* 4, 8 mg (strawberry) (phenylalanine)
    Zofran Oral Solution *Oral soln:* 4 mg/5 ml (50 ml) (strawberry)
      (phenyl-alanine); *Parenteral form:* see mfr pkg insert
    Zofran Injection *Vial:* 2 mg/ml (2 ml single-dose); 2 mg/ml (20 ml multi-
      dose); 32 mg/50 ml (50 ml multi-dose); *Prefilled syringe:* 4 mg/2 ml, single-
      use (24/carton)
    Zuplenz Oral Soluble Film: 4, 8 mg oral-dis (10/carton) (peppermint)
  Comment: The FDA has issued a warning against *ondansetron* use in pregnancy
  ondansetron is a 5-HT3 receptor antagonist approved by the FDA for preventing
  nausea and vomiting related to cancer chemotherapy and surgery. However,
  it has been used "off label" to treat the nausea and vomiting of pregnancy. The
  FDA has cautioned against the use of *ondansetron* in pregnancy in light of
  studies of *ondansetron* in early pregnancy and associated with congenital cardiac
  malformations and oral clefts (i.e., cleft lip and cleft palate). Further, there are
  potential maternal risks in pregnancy with electrolyte imbalance caused by
  severe nausea and vomiting (as with hyperemesis gravidarum). These risks
  include *serotonin syndrome* (a triad of cognitive and behavioral changes including
  confusion, agitation, autonomic instability, and neuromuscular changes).
  Therefore, *ondansetron* should not be taken during pregnancy.
▷ *palonosetron* (B)(G) administer 0.25 mg IV over 30 seconds; max 1 dose/week
  Pediatric: <1 month: not recommended; 1 month to 17 years: 20 mcg/kg; max 1.5
  mg/single dose; infuse over 15 minutes beginning 30 minutes
    Aloxi *Vial (single-use):* 0.075 mg/1.5 ml; 0.25 mg/5 ml (mannitol)
▷ *promethazine* (C)(G) 25 mg PO or rectally q 4-6 hours prn
  Pediatric: <2 years: not recommended; ≥2 years: 0.5 mg/lb or 6.25-25 mg q 4-6
  hours prn
    Phenergan *Tab:* 12.5*, 25*, 50 mg; *Plain syr:* 6.25 mg/5 ml; *Fortis syr:* 25 mg/5
      ml; *Rectal supp:* 12.5, 25, 50 mg
  Comment: *Promethazine* is contraindicated in children with uncomplicated nausea,
  dehydration, Reye's syndrome, history of sleep apnea, asthma, and lower respiratory
  disorders in children. *Promethazine* lowers the seizure threshold in children, may
  cause cholestatic jaundice, anticholinergic effects, extrapyramidal effects, and
  potentially fatal respiratory depression.

NERVE AGENT POISONING

▷ *atropine sulfate* (G) 2 mg IM
  Pediatric: <15 lb: not recommended; ≥15-40 lb: 0.5 mg IM; ≥40-90 lb: 1 mg IM;
  >90 lb: same as adult
    AtroPen *Pen (single-use):* 0.5, 1, 2 mg (0.5 ml)

NEUROGENIC DETRUSER OVERACTIVITY (NDO)

Comment: *Solifenesin* is a muscarinic receptor antagonist. **VESIcare** *(solifenacin)*
and **VESIcare LS** *(solifenacin succinate)* are FDA-approved to be taken in
combination with **Myrbetriq** *(mirabegron)* for the treatment of overactive bladder
(OAB) with symptoms of frequency, urgency, and urge urinary incontinence.

▷ *solifenacin* initially 25 mg once daily; max 50 mg once daily; severe renal
  impairment, 25 mg once daily
    VESIcare *Tab:* 5, 10 mg 5-10 mg once daily

▷ **solifenacin succinate** see weight-based chart for once daily dosing; follow with a liquid drink (e.g., water or milk); initiate at recommended starting dose; titrate to the lowest effective dose; do not exceed max recommended dose
Pediatric: <2 years: not established; ≥2 years: see mfr pkg insert for weight-based once daily dosing; follow with a liquid drink (e.g., water or milk); initiate at recommended starting dose; titrate to the lowest effective dose; do not exceed max recommended dose

    VESIcare LS *Oral susp:* 5 mg/5 ml (1 mg/ml, 150 ml) (orange)
    Comment: Do not exceed the recommended starting dose of **VESIcare LS** in patients with severe renal impairment (CrCl <30 mL/min), moderate hepatic impairment (Child-Pugh B) or concomitant use of strong CYP3A4 inhibitors. **VESIcare LS** is contraindicated in patients with severe hepatic impairment (ChildPugh C), gastric retention, and uncontrolled narrow-angle glaucoma. The most common adverse reactions (incidence > 2%) have been constipation, dry mouth, and UTI. Somnolence has been reported. **VESIcare LS** is not recommended for use in patients at high risk of QT prolongation, including patients with a known history of QT prolongation and patients taking medications known to prolong the QT interval. The most common adverse reactions (incidence >2%) have been constipation, dry mouth, and UTI.

NEUROFIBROMATOSIS TYPE 1

MITOGEN-ACTIVATED PROTEIN KINASE 1 AND 2 (MEK1/2) INHIBITOR

▷ **selumetinib** 25 mg/m² twice daily; do not consume food 2 hours before each dose or 1 hour after each dose; *Moderate Hepatic Impairment (Child-Pugh Class B):* 20 mg/m² twice daily; *Severe Hepatic Impairment (Child-Pugh Class C):* not established
Pediatric: <2 years: not established; ≥2 years: same as adult

    Koselugo *Cap:* 10, 25 mg
    Comment: **Koselugo** *(selumetinib)* is an kinase inhibitor (inhibitor of mitogen-activated protein kinase 1 and 2 [MEK1/2]) indicated for the treatment of pediatric patients 2 years-of-age and older with neurofibromatosis type 1 (NF1) who have symptomatic, inoperable plexiform neurofibromas (PN). Withhold, reduce dose, or permanently discontinue **Koselugo** based on severity of any adverse reaction. Assess ejection fraction prior to initiating treatment, every 3 months during the first year, then every 6 months thereafter and as clinically indicated. Conduct ophthalmic assessments prior to initiating **Koselugo**, at regular intervals during treatment and for new or worsening visual changes. Permanently discontinue **Koselugo** for retinal vein occlusion (RVO). Withhold **Koselugo** for retinal pigment epithelial detachment (RPED), monitor with optical coherence tomography assessments until resolution, and resume at reduced dose. Advise patients to start an anti-diarrheal agent immediately after the first episode of loose stool and to increase fluid intake. Monitor for severe skin rashes. Increased Creatinine Phosphokinase (CPK) and rhabdomyolysis can occur. Obtain serum CPK prior to initiating **Koselugo**, periodically during treatment, and as clinically indicated. If increased CPK occurs, evaluate for rhabdomyolysis or other causes. **Koselugo** capsules contain vitamin E and daily intake of vitamin E that exceeds the recommended or safe limits may increase the risk of bleeding. An increased risk of bleeding may occur in patients co-administered vitamin K antagonists or anti-platelet agents. Avoid co-administration of strong or moderate CYP3A4 inhibitors or *fluconazole* with **Koselugo**. If co-administration with strong or moderate CYP3A4 inhibitors or *fluconazole* cannot be avoided, reduce the dose of **Koselugo**. Avoid concomitant use of strong and moderate CYP3A4 inducers. The most common adverse

reactions (incidence ≥40%) are vomiting, rash (all), abdominal pain, diarrhea, nausea, dry skin, fatigue, musculoskeletal pain, pyrexia, acneiform rash, stomatitis, headache, paronychia, and pruritus. Based on findings from animal studies and its mechanism of action **Koselugo** can cause fetal harm when administered to a pregnant woman. There are <u>no</u> available data on the use of **Koselugo** in pregnant females to evaluate drug-associated risk. There are <u>no</u> data on the presence of *selumetinib* <u>or</u> its active metabolite in human milk <u>or</u> effects on the breastfed infant. Due to potential for adverse reactions, advise women <u>not</u> to breastfeed during treatment with **Koselugo** and for 1 week after the last dose. To report suspected adverse reactions, contact AstraZeneca at 1-800-236-9933 <u>or</u> FDA at 1-800-FDA-1088 <u>or</u> visit www.fda.gov/medwatch.

NEUROMYELITIS OPTICA SPECTRUM DISORDER (NMOSD)

COMPLEMENT INHIBITOR

▷ *eculizumab* administer 900 mg via IV infusion once weekly for the first 4 weeks; followed by a single 1200 mg dose via IV infusion 1 week later (the fifth week); then, 1200 mg via IV infusion once every 2 weeks thereafter; administer at the recommended dosage regimen time points, <u>or</u> within two days of these time points; see mfr pkg insert for dose preparation instructions
Pediatric: safety and efficacy not established

    Soliris *Vial:* 10 mg/ml (30 ml) single-dose (preservative-free) solution for dilution and IV infusion

    Comment: **Soliris** *(eculizumab)* is indicated for the treatment of neuromyelitis optica spectrum disorder (NMOSD) in adult patients who are anti-aquaporin-4 (AQP4) antibody positive. **Soliris** is available <u>only</u> through a restricted program under a Risk Evaluation and Mitigation Strategy (REMS). Under the Soliris REMS, prescribers must enroll in the program.

NEUTROPENIA: CHEMOTHERAPY-ASSOCIATED, NEUTROPENIA: FEBRILE, NEUTROPENIA: MYELOSUPPRESSION-ASSOCIATED

LEUKOCYTE GROWTH FACTOR

▷ *pegfilgrastim* <45 kg: see mfr pkg insert for weight-based dosing Table 1; ≥45 kg: *Patients with Cancer receiving Myelosuppressive Chemotherapy:* 6 mg SC once per chemotherapy cycle; do <u>not</u> administer between 14 days before and 24 hours after administration of cytotoxic chemotherapy; *Patients Acutely Exposed to Myelosuppressive Doses of Radiation.* <45 kg: see mfr pkg insert for weight-based dosing table 1; ≥45 kg: 6 mg SC x 2 doses one week apart; administer the first dose as soon as possible after suspected <u>or</u> confirmed exposure to myelosuppressive doses of radiation

    Neulasta *Prefilled syringe:* 6 mg/0.6 ml, single-dose, for manual use <u>only</u>; 6 mg/0.6 ml, single-dose, co-packaged with the on-body *Neulasta Auto-injector*

    Comment: *Pegfilgrastim* is a leukocyte growth factor, to help reduce the risk/incidence of infection, as manifested by febrile neutropenia, in patients with non-myeloid malignancies receiving myelosuppressive anti-cancer drugs and to increase survival in patients acutely exposed to myelosuppressive doses of radiation (i.e., Hematopoietic Subsyndrome of Acute Radiation Syndrome). **Neulasta** is <u>not</u> indicated for the mobilization of peripheral blood progenitor cells for hematopoietic stem cell transplantation. Warnings and precautions associated with **Neulasta** include fatal splenic rupture, acute respiratory distress syndrome (ARDS), serious allergic reaction/anaphylaxis, allergic reaction to acrylic adhesive (used to attach the autoinjector), fatal sickle cell crisis, glomerulonephritis, on-body injector failure. There are no adequate <u>or</u> well-controlled studies of **Neulasta** use in pregnancy. Based on animal data, may cause fetal harm. It is <u>not</u> known whether *pegfilgrastim* is secreted in human milk. Other recombinant G-CSF products are poorly secreted in breast milk and G-CSF is not orally absorbed by neonates. Caution should be exercised when administered to a nursing female.

▶ *pegfilgrastim-bmez* <45 kg: see mfr pkg insert for weight-based dosing table; ≥45 kg: administer 6 mg SC once per chemotherapy cycle; do not administer between 14 days before and 24 hours after administration of cytotoxic chemotherapy

    Ziextenzo *Prefilled pen:* 6 mg/0.6 ml, single-dose

    Comment: **Ziextenzo** is biosimilar to **Neulasta** *(pegfilgrastim)*.

▶ *pegfilgrastim-jmdb*

    Fulphila *Prefilled syringe:* 6 mg/0.6 ml, single-dose, for manual use only

    Comment: **Fulphila** is biosimilar to **Neulasta** *(pegfilgrastim)*.

FILGRASTIM PRODUCTS

Comment: *Filgrastim* (**Neupogen**) and *filgrastim* biosimilar products (**Nivestym, Zarxio, Granix**) are contraindicated in patients with a prior history of serious allergic reactions to human granulocyte colony-stimulating factors (e.g., *filgrastim, pegfilgrastim*). Administration to patients <18 years is not recommended. Direct administration of less than 0.3 ml is not recommended due to potential for dosing errors. Use during pregnancy only if the potential benefit justifies the potential risk to the fetus. It is not known whether *filgrastim* or biosimilar products are excreted in human milk or effects on the breastfed infant. Prior to using *filgrastim* or a *filgrastim* biosimilar product, remove the vial or prefilled syringe from the refrigerator and allow to reach room temperature for a minimum of 30 minutes and a maximum of 24 hours. Discard any vial or prefilled syringe left at room temperature for greater than 24 hours. Visually inspect for particulate matter and discoloration prior to administration (the solution is clear and colorless). Do not administer if particulates or discoloration are observed. Discard any unused portion. Do not re-enter a vial. Inject subcutaneously in the outer area of upper arms, abdomen, thighs, or upper outer areas of the buttock. Patients or caregivers may administer the SC dose after appropriate education and supervised training by a qualified healthcare provider. For IV infusion, may be diluted in D5%W USP from a concentration of 300 mcg/ml to 5 mcg/ml (do not dilute to a final concentration < 5 mcg/mL). Dilution to concentrations from 5 mcg/ml to 15 mcg/ml should be protected from adsorption to plastic materials by the addition of Albumin (Human) to a final concentration of 2 mg/ml. When diluted in D5%W USP or D5%W plus Albumin (Human), *filgrastim* and *filgrastim* biosimilar products are compatible with glass bottles, polyvinyl chloride (PVC) and polyolefin intravenous bags, and polypropylene syringes. Do not dilute with saline at any time because the product may precipitate. Warnings and precautions include splenic rupture, acute respiratory distress syndrome (ARDS), serious allergic reaction, sickle cell disorders, glomerulonephritis, alveolar hemorrhage and hemoptysis, capillary leak syndrome (CLS), thrombocytopenia, leukocytosis, and cutaneous vasculitis (see mfr pkg insert for detailed discussion of potential ASEs and complications).

▶ *filgrastim*

Patients with cancer receiving myelosuppressive chemotherapy or induction and/ or consolidation chemotherapy for AML: recommended starting dose is 5 mcg/ kg/day via SC injection, short intravenous infusion (over 15-30 minutes), or continuous intravenous infusion; see mfr pkg insert for recommended dosage adjustments and timing of administration; obtain a complete blood count (CBC) and platelet count before instituting *filgrastim* therapy and monitor twice weekly during therapy; consider dose escalation in increments of 5 mcg/ kg for each chemotherapy cycle, according to the duration and severity of the absolute neutrophil count (ANC) nadir; recommend stopping *figrastim* if the ANC increases beyond 10,000/mm^3

Patients with cancer undergoing bone marrow transplantation: 10 mcg/kg/day via IV infusion over ≤24 hour; see mfr pkg insert for recommended dosage adjustments and timing of administration based on ANC

Patients undergoing autologous peripheral blood progenitor cell collection and therapy: 10 mcg/kg/day via SC injection; administer for at least 4 days before first leukapheresis procedure and continue until last leukapheresis

Patients with severe chronic congenital neutropenia: recommended starting dose is 6 mcg/kg via SC injection twice daily

Patients with cyclic or idiopathic neutropenia: recommended starting dose is 5 mcg/kg via SC injection once daily

Patients acutely exposed to myelosuppressive doses of radiation (i.e., Hematopoietic Syndrome of Acute Radiation Syndrome [HSARS]): recommended dose is 10 mcg/kg via SC injection once daily for patients exposed to myelosuppressive doses of radiation; administer as soon as possible after suspected or confirmed exposure to radiation doses greater than 2 gray (Gy); estimate a patient's absorbed radiation dose (i.e., level of radiation exposure) based on information from public health authorities, biodosimetry if available, or clinical findings such as time to onset of vomiting or lymphocyte depletion kinetics; obtain a baseline CBC and then serial CBCs approximately every 3rd day until the ANC remains >1,000/mm³ for 3 consecutive CBCs; do not delay administration of *filgrastim* if a CBC is not readily available; continue administration until the ANC remains >1000/mm³ for 3 consecutive CBCs or exceeds 10,000/mm³ after a radiation-induced nadir

Neupogen *Vial:* 300 mcg/ml (1 ml), 480 mcg/1.6 ml (1.6 ml) single-dose (preservative-free); *Prefilled syringe:* 300 mcg/0.5 ml (0.5 ml), 480 mcg/0.8 ml (0.8 ml) single-dose (preservative-free)

▷ *filgrastim-aafi see filgastrim* (Neupogen) above for prescribing information
Nivestym *Vial:* 300 mcg/ml (1 ml), 480 mcg/1.6 ml (1.6 ml) single-dose (preservative-free); *Prefilled syringe:* 300 mcg/0.5 ml (0.5 ml), 480 mcg/0.8 ml (0.8 ml) single-dose (preservative-free)

▷ *filgrastim-cbqv* (C) *see filgastrim* (Neupogen) above for prescribing information
Udenyca *Prefilled syringe:* 6 mg/0.6 ml (0.6 ml) single-dose; the needle cap on the prefilled syringe is not made with natural rubber latex (preservative-free)

▷ *filgrastim-sndz* (C) *see filgastrim* (Neupogen) above for prescribing information
Zarxio *Vial:* 300 mcg/ml (1 ml), 480 mcg/1.6 ml (1.6 ml) single-dose (preservative-free); *Prefilled syringe:* 300 mcg/0.5 ml (0.5 ml), 480 mcg/0.8 ml (0.8 ml) single-dose (preservative-free)

▷ *tbo-filgrastim* recommended dose: 5 mcg/kg per day via SC injection; administer the first dose no earlier than 24 hours following myelosuppressive chemotherapy; do not administer within 24 hours prior to chemotherapy

Granix *Prefilled syringe:* 300 mcg/0.5 ml (0.5 ml), 480 mcg/0.8 ml (0.8 ml) single-dose (preservative-free)

Comment: Granix *(tbo-filgrastim)* is a leukocyte growth factor indicated for reduction in the duration of severe neutropenia in patients with non-myeloid malignancies receiving myelosuppressive anti-cancer drugs associated with a clinically significant incidence of febrile neutropenia. Granix should be used during pregnancy only if the potential benefit justifies the potential risk to the fetus. It is not known if *tbo-filgrastim* is excreted in human milk or effects on the breastfed infant.

● NON-24 SLEEP-WAKE DISORDER

Comment: For other drug options (stimulants, sedative hypnotics), *see* Insomnia or *see* Sleepiness: Excessive, Shift Work Sleep Disorder

MELATONIN RECEPTOR AGONIST

▷ **tasimelteon** (C) take 1 gelcap before bedtime at the same time every night; do **not** take with food

Pediatric: <12 years: not established; ≥12 years: same as adult

    Hetlioz *Gel cap:* 20 mg

OREXIN RECEPTOR ANTAGONIST

▷ **suvorexant** (C)(IV) use lowest effective dose; take 30 minutes before bedtime; do **not** take if unable to sleep for ≥7 hours; max 20 mg

Pediatric: <12 years: not recommended; ≥12 years: same as adult

    Belsomra *Tab:* 5, 10, 15, 20 mg (30/blister pck)

 OBESITY

Comment: Target BMI is 25-30 (≤27 preferred). Approximately 17% of children and adolescents in the US aged 2-19 years are obese. Almost 32% of children and adolescents are either overweight **or** obese, and the proportion of children with severe obesity continues to rise. Obesity in childhood increases the risk of having obesity as an adult and children with obesity are about 5 times more likely to have obesity as adults than children without obesity. The immediate consequences of childhood obesity include increased incidence of psychological issues, asthma, obstructive sleep apnea, orthopedic problems, high blood pressure, elevated lipid levels, and insulin resistance. The US Preventive Services Task Force (USPSTF) recommends that clinicians screen for obesity in children and adolescents 6 years and older and offer **or** refer them to comprehensive, intensive behavioral interventions (at least 26 hours of contact) to promote improvements in weight status.

STIMULANTS

▷ **amphetamine sulfate** (C)(II)

Pediatric: <12 years: not recommended; ≥12 years: same as adult

    Evekeo initially 5 mg 30-60 minutes before meals; usually up to 30 mg/day

    Tab: 5, 10 mg

LIPASE INHIBITOR

▷ **orlistat** (X)(G) 1 cap tid 1 hour before **or** during each main meal containing fat

Pediatric: <12 years: not recommended; ≥12 years: same as adult

    Alli (OTC) *Cap:* 60 mg

    Xenical *Cap:* 120 mg

Comment: For use when BMI >30 kg/m² **or** BMI >27 kg/m² in the presence of other risk factors (i.e., HTN, DM, dyslipidemia).

ANOREXIGENICS

Sympathomimetics

Comment: ASEs of sympathomimetics include hypertension, tachycardia, restlessness, insomnia, and dry mouth.

▷ **benzphetamine** (X)(III) initially 25-50 mg daily in the mid-morning **or** mid-afternoon; may increase to bid-tid as needed

Pediatric: <12 years: not recommended; ≥12 years: same as adult

    Didrex *Tab:* 50*mg

▷ **naltrexone+bupropion** (X)(G) swallow whole; avoid high-fat meals; initially 10 mg bid; evaluate weight loss after 12 weeks; discontinue if less than 5% weight loss

Pediatric: <18 years: not recommended; ≥18 years: same as adult

    Contrave *Tab:* nal 8 mg+bup 900 mg ext-rel

▷ **methamphetamine** (C)(II) 10-15 mg q AM
Pediatric: <12 years: not recommended; ≥12 years: same as adult
    Desoxyn *Tab:* 5, 10, 15 mg sust-rel

▷ **phendimetrazine** (C)(III)
Pediatric: <12 years: not recommended; ≥12 years: same as adult
    Bontril PDM 35 mg bid-tid 1 hour ac; may reduce to 17.5 mg (1/2 tab)/dose;
    max 210 mg/day in 3 divided doses
      Tab: 35*mg
    Bontril Slow-Release 105 mg in the AM 30-60 minutes before breakfast
      Cap: 105 mg slow-rel

▷ **phentermine** (X)(IV)(G)
Pediatric: <16 years: not recommended; ≥16 years: same as adult
    Adipex-P 1 cap or tab before breakfast or 1/2 tab bid ac
      Cap: 37.5 mg; *Tab:* 37.5*mg
    Fastin 1 cap before breakfast
      Cap: 30 mg
    Ionamin 1 cap before breakfast or 10-14 hours prior to HS
      Cap: 15, 30 mg
    Suprenza ODT (X)(IV) dissolve 1 tab on top of tongue once daily in the
    morning, with or without food; use lowest effective dose
      Tab: 15, 30, 37.5 mg orally-disint
Comment: Contraindicated with history of cardiovascular disease (e.g., coronary artery disease, stroke, arrhythmias, congestive heart failure, uncontrolled hypertension, during or within 14 days following the administration of an MAOI, hyperthyroidism, glaucoma, agitated states, history of drug abuse, pregnancy, and nursing).

Sympathomimetic+Antiepileptic Combination

▷ **phentermine+topiramate ext-rel** (X)(IV)(G) initially 3.75/23 daily in the AM x 14 days; then increase to 7.5/46 and evaluate weight loss on this dose after 12 weeks; if ≤3% weight loss from baseline, discontinue or increase dose to 11.25/69 x 14 days; then increase to 15/92 and evaluate weight loss on this dose after 12 weeks; if ≤5% weight loss from baseline, discontinue by taking a dose every other day for at least 1 week prior to stopping; max 7.5/46 for moderate-to-severe renal impairment or moderate hepatic impairment.
Pediatric: <16 years: not established; ≥16 years: same as adult
    Qsymia
      Cap: **Qsymia 3.75/23** phen 3.75 mg+topir 23 mg ext-rel
            Qsymia 7.5/46 phen 7.5 mg+topir 46 mg ext-rel
            Qsymia 11.25/69 phen 11.25 mg+topir 69 mg ext-rel
            Qsymia 15/92 phen 15 mg+topir 92 mg ext-rel
Comment: Side effects include hypertension, tachycardia, restlessness, insomnia, and dry mouth. Contraindicated with glaucoma, hyperthyroidism, and within 14 days of taking an MAOI. **Qsymia 3.75/23** and **Qsymia 11.25/69** are for titration purposes only.

Serotonin 2C Receptor Agonist

▷ **lorcaserin** (X)(G) 10 mg bid; discontinue if 5% weight loss is not achieved by week 12
Pediatric: <18 years: not recommended; ≥18 years: same as adult
    Belviq *Tab:* 10 mg film-coat
Comment: **Belviq** is indicated as an adjunct to a reduced-calorie diet and increased physical activity for chronic weight management in adults with an initial body mass index (BMI) of 30 kg/m² or greater (obese) or 27 kg/m² or greater (over weight) in the presence of at least one weight-related comorbid

condition (e.g., hypertension, dyslipidemia, type 2 diabetes). Serotonin 2C receptor agonists interact with serotonergic drugs (selective serotonin reuptake inhibitors (SSRIs), serotonin-norepinephrine reuptake inhibitors (SNRIs), monoamine oxidase inhibitors (MAOIs), triptans, *bupropion*, *dextromethorphan*, *St. John's wort*); therefore, use with extreme caution due to the risk of *serotonin syndrome*.

GLUCAGON-LIKE PEPTIDE-1 (GLP-1) RECEPTOR AGONIST

▶ *liraglutide* (C) administer SC in the upper arm, abdomen, or thigh once daily; escalate dose gradually over 5 weeks to 3 mg SC daily; *Week 1:* 0.6 mg SC daily; *Week 2:* 1.2 mg SC daily; *Week 3:* 1.8 mg SC daily; *Week 4:* 2.4 mg SC daily; *Week 5:* 3 mg SC daily

Pediatric: <12 years: not recommended ≥12 years, >60 kg, initial BMI ≥30 kg/m²: same as adult

> **Saxenda** Soln for SC inj: 6 mg/ml multi-dose prefilled pen (3 ml; 3, 5 pens/carton)
> Comment: **Saxenda** is indicated as an adjunct to a reduced-calorie diet and increased physical activity for chronic weight management in adults with an initial body mass index (BMI) of 30 kg/m² or greater (obese) or 27 kg/m² or greater (over weight) in the presence of at least one weight-related comorbid condition (e.g., hypertension, dyslipidemia, type 2 diabetes). Not indicated for treatment of T2DM. Do not use with **Victoza**, other GLP-1 receptor agonists, or insulin. Contraindicated with personal or family history of medullary thyroid carcinoma (MTC) and multiple endocrine neoplasia syndrome (MENS) type 2. Monitor for signs/symptoms pancreatitis. Discontinue if gastroparesis, renal, or hepatic impairment.

⦾ OBSESSIVE-COMPULSIVE DISORDER (OCD)

SELECTIVE SEROTONIN REUPTAKE INHIBITORS (SSRIs)

Comment: Co-administration of SSRIs with TCAs requires extreme caution. Concomitant use of MAOIs and SSRIs is absolutely contraindicated. Avoid other serotonergic drugs. A potentially fatal adverse event is *serotonin syndrome*, caused by serotonin excess. Milder symptoms require HCP intervention to avert severe symptoms which can be rapidly fatal without urgent/emergent medical care. Symptoms include restlessness, agitation, confusion, hallucinations, tachycardia, hypertension, dilated pupils, muscle twitching, muscle rigidity, loss of muscle coordination, diaphoresis, diarrhea, headache, shivering, piloerection, hyperpyrexia, cardiac arrhythmias, seizures, loss of consciousness, coma, and death. Abrupt withdrawal or interruption of treatment with an antidepressant medication is sometimes associated with an *Antidepressant Discontinuation Syndrome*, which may be mediated by gradually tapering the drug over a period of 2 weeks or longer, depending on the dose strength and length of treatment. Common symptoms of the *serotonin discontinuation syndrome* include flu-like symptoms (nausea, vomiting, diarrhea, headaches, sweating), sleep disturbances (insomnia, nightmares, constant sleepiness), mood disturbances (dysphoria, anxiety, agitation), cognitive disturbances (mental confusion, hyperarousal), sensory and movement disturbances (imbalance, tremors, vertigo, dizziness, and electric-shock-like sensations in the brain, often described by sufferers as "brain zaps").

▶ *fluoxetine* (C)(G)

> **Prozac** initially 20 mg daily; may increase after 1 week; doses >20 mg/day may be divided into AM and noon doses; max 80 mg/day
> *Pediatric:* <8 years: not recommended; 8-17 years: initially 10 mg/day; may increase after 2 weeks to 20 mg/day; range 20-60 mg/day; range for lower weight children 20-30 mg/day; >17: same as adult
>> *Cap:* 10, 20, 40 mg; *Tab:* 30*, 60*mg; *Oral soln:* 20 mg/5 ml (4 oz) (mint)

Prozac Weekly following daily *fluoxetine* therapy at 20 mg/day for 13 weeks, may initiate **Prozac Weekly** 7 days after the last 20 mg *fluoxetine* dose
Pediatric: <12 years: not recommended; ≥12 years: same as adult
   Cap: 90 mg ent-coat del-rel pellets

▶ *fluvoxamine* (C)(G)
   Luvox initially 50 mg q HS; adjust in 50 mg increments at 4-7 day intervals; range 100-300 mg/day; over 100 mg/day, divide into 2 doses giving the larger dose at HS
   Pediatric: <8 years: not recommended; 8-17 years: initially 25 mg q HS; a just in 25 mg increments q 4-7 days; usual range 50-200 mg/day; over 50 mg/day, divide into 2 doses giving the larger dose at HS
      Tab: 25, 50*, 100*mg
   Luvox CR initially 100 mg once daily at HS; may increase by 50 mg increments at 1 week intervals; max 300 mg/day; swallow whole; do not crush or chew
   Pediatric: <18 years: not recommended; ≥18 years: same as adult
      Cap: 100, 150 mg ext-rel

▶ *paroxetine maleate* (D)(G)
   Pediatric: <12 years: not recommended; ≥12 years: same as adult
   Paxil initially 20 mg daily in AM; may increase by 10 mg/day at weekly intervals as needed; max 60 mg/day
      Tab: 10*, 20*, 30, 40 mg
   Paxil CR initially 25 mg daily in AM; may increase by 12.5 mg at weekly intervals as needed; max 62.5 mg/day
      Tab: 12.5, 25, 37.5 mg cont-rel ent-coat
   Paxil Suspension initially 20 mg daily in AM; may increase by 10 mg/day at weekly intervals as needed; max 60 mg/day
      Oral susp: 10 mg/5 ml (250 ml) (orange)

▶ *paroxetine mesylate* (D)(G) initially 7.5 mg daily in AM; may increase by 10 mg/ day at weekly intervals as needed; max 60 mg/day
   Pediatric: <12 years: not recommended; ≥12 years: same as adult
   Brisdelle *Cap:* 7.5 mg

▶ *sertraline* (C) initially 50 mg daily; increase at 1 week intervals if needed; max 200 mg daily
   Pediatric: <6 years: not recommended; 6-12 years: initially 25 mg daily; max 200 mg/day; 13-17 years: initially 50 mg daily; max 200 mg/day; >17 years: same as adult
   Zoloft *Tab:* 15*, 50*, 100*mg; *Oral conc:* 20 mg per ml (60 ml [dilute just before administering in 4 oz water, ginger ale, lemon-lime soda, lemonade, or orange juice]) (alcohol 12%)

TRICYCLIC ANTIDEPRESSANTS (TCAs)

▶ *clomipramine* (C)(G) initially 25 mg daily in divided doses; gradually increase to 100 mg during first 2 weeks; max 250 mg/day; total maintenance dose may be given at HS
   Pediatric: <10 years: not recommended; ≥10 years: initially 25 mg daily in divided doses; gradually increase; max 3 mg/kg or 100 mg, whichever is smaller
   Anafranil *Cap:* 25, 50, 75 mg

▶ *imipramine* (C)(G)
   Tofranil initially 75 mg/day; max 200 mg/day
   Pediatric: adolescents initially 30-40 mg/day; max 100 mg/day
      Tab: 10, 25, 50 mg
   Tofranil PM initially 75 mg/day; max 200 mg/day
   Pediatric: <12 years: not recommended; ≥12 years: same as adult
      Cap: 75, 100, 125, 150 mg

ONYCHOMYCOSIS (FUNGAL NAIL)

ORAL AGENTS

▷ *griseofulvin, microsize* (C)(G) 1 gm daily for at least 4 months for fingernails and at least 6 months for toenails
  Pediatric: 5 mg/lb/day; *see* Appendix CC.25. *griseofulvin, microsize* (Grifulvin V Suspension) *for dose by weight*
    Grifulvin V *Tab:* 250, 500 mg; *Oral susp:* 125 mg/5 ml (120 ml; alcohol 0.02%)

▷ *griseofulvin, ultramicrosize* (C) 750 mg in a single or divided doses for at least 4 months for fingernails and at least 6 months for toenails
  Pediatric: <2 years: not recommended; ≥2 years: 3.3 mg/lb in a single or divided doses
    Gris-PEG *Tab:* 125, 250 mg

▷ *itraconazole* (C)(G) 200 mg daily x 12 consecutive weeks for toenails; 200 mg bid x 1 week, off 3 weeks, then 200 mg bid x 1 additional week for fingernails
  Pediatric: <12 years: not recommended; ≥12 years: same as adult
    Sporanox *Cap:* 100 mg; *Soln:* 10 mg/ml (150 ml) (cherry-caramel)
    Pulse Pack: 100 mg caps (7/pck)

▷ *terbinafine* (B)(G) 250 mg daily x 6 weeks for fingernails; 250 mg daily x 12 weeks for toenails
  Pediatric: <12 years: not recommended; ≥12 years: same as adult
    Lamisil *Tab:* 250 mg

TOPICAL AGENTS

Comment: File and trim nail while nail is free from drug. Remove unattached infected nail as frequently as monthly. For use with mild to moderate onychomycosis of the fingernails and toenails, without lunula involvement due to *Trichophyton rubrum* immunocompetent patients as part of a comprehensive treatment program. For use on nails and adjacent skin only. Apply evenly to entire onycholytic nail and surrounding 5 mm of skin daily, preferably at HS or 8 hours before washing; apply to nail bed, hyponychium, and under surface of nail plate when it is free of the nail bed; apply over previous coats, then remove with alcohol once per week; treat for up to 48 weeks.

▷ *ciclopirox* (B)
  Pediatric: <12 years: not established; ≥12 years: same as adult
    Penlac Nail Lacquer *Topical soln (lacquer):* 8% (6.6 ml w. applicator)

▷ *efinaconazole* (C)
  Pediatric: <12 years: not established; ≥12 years: same as adult
    Jublia *Topical soln:* 5% (10 ml w. brush applicator)

▷ *tavaborole* (C)(G)
  Pediatric: <12 years: not established; ≥12 years: same as adult
    Kerydin *Topical soln:* 10% (10 ml w. dropper)

 OPHTHALMIA NEONATORUM: CHLAMYDIAL

PROPHYLAXIS

▷ *erythromycin* ophthalmic ointment 0.5-1 cm ribbon into lower conjunctival sac of each eye x 1 application
    Ilotycin Ophthalmic Ointment *Ophth oint:* 5 mg/gm (1/8 oz)
  Comment: The following treatment regimens are published in the **2015 CDC Sexually Transmitted Diseases Treatment Guidelines**. Treatment regimens are presented by generic drug name first, followed by information about brands and dose forms.

RECOMMENDED TREATMENT REGIMENS

Regimen 1

▷ **erythromycin base** 50 mg/kg/day in 4 doses x 14 days

Regimen 2

▷ **erythromycin ethylsuccinate** 50 mg/kg/day in 4 doses x 14 days; *see Appendix CC.21: erythromycin ethylsuccinate* (E.E.S. Suspension, Ery-Ped Drops/Suspension) *for dose by weight*

DRUG BRANDS AND DOSE FORMS

▷ **erythromycin base** (B)(G)
   Ery-Tab *Tab:* 250, 333, 500 mg ent-coat
   PCE *Tab:* 333, 500 mg
▷ **erythromycin ethylsuccinate** (B)(G)
   EryPed *Oral susp:* 200 mg/5 ml (100, 200 ml) (fruit); 400 mg/5 ml (60, 100, 200 ml) (banana); *Oral drops:* 200, 400 mg/5 ml (50 ml) (fruit); *Chew tab:* 200 mg wafer (fruit)
   E.E.S. *Oral susp:* 200, 400 mg/5 ml (100 ml) (fruit)
   E.E.S. Granules *Oral susp:* 200 mg/5 ml (100, 200 ml) (cherry)

 OPHTHALMIA NEONATORUM: GONOCOCCAL

Comment: The following prophylaxis and treatment regimens for gonococcal conjunctivitis is published in the **2015 CDC Sexually Transmitted Diseases Treatment Guidelines.**

PROPHYLAXIS

▷ **erythromycin 0.5%** ophthalmic ointment 0.5-1 cm ribbon into lower conjunctival sac of each eye x 1 application
   Ilotycin Ophthalmic Ointment *Ophth oint:* 5 mg/gm (1/8 oz)

TREATMENT

▷ **ceftriaxone** (B)(G) 25-50 mg/kg IV or IM in a single dose, not to exceed 125 mg
   Rocephin *Vial:* 250, 500 mg; 1, 2 gm

 OPIOID DEPENDENCE, OPIOID USE DISORDER (OUD), OPIOID WITHDRAWAL SYNDROME

Comment: Safety labeling for all immediate-release (IR) opioids has been issued by the FDA. The Black Boxed Warning (BBW) includes serious risks of misuse, abuse, addiction, overdose, and death. The dosing section offers clear steps regarding administration and patient monitoring including initial dose, dose changes, and the abrupt cessation of treatment in physical dependence. Chronic maternal use of opioids during pregnancy can lead to potentially life-threatening neonatal opioid withdrawal. The American Pain Society (APS) has released new evidence-based clinical practice guidelines that include 32 recommendations related to post-op pain management in adults and children. The Transmucosal Immediate Release Fentanyl (TIRF) Risk Evaluation and Mitigation Strategy (REMS) program is an FDA-required program designed to ensure informed risk-benefit decisions before initiating treatment, and while patients are treated to ensure appropriate use of TIRF medicines. The purpose of the TIRF REMS Access program is to mitigate the risk of misuse, abuse, addiction, overdose and serious complications due to medication errors with the use of TIRF medicines. You must enroll in the TIRF REMS Access program to prescribe, dispense, or distribute TIRF medicines. To register, call the TIRF REMS Access program at 1-866-822-1483 or register online at https://www.tirfremsaccess.com/TirfUI/rems/home.action.

SELECTIVE ALPHA 2-ADRENERGIC RECEPTOR AGONIST

Comment: **Lucemyra** *(lofexidine)* is the first FDA-approved non-opioid treatment for the management of opioid withdrawal symptoms, for the mitigation of withdrawal symptoms to facilitate abrupt discontinuation of opioids in adults. While **Lucemyra** may lessen the severity of withdrawal symptoms, it may <u>not</u> completely prevent them. This oral selective alpha 2-adrenergic receptor agonist reduces the release of norepinephrine. The actions of norepinephrine in the autonomic nervous system are believed to play a role in many of the symptoms of opioid withdrawal and is <u>only</u> approved for treatment for up to 14 days.

▷ *lofexidine* (C) 0.18 mg x 3 tabs taken orally 4 x/day at 5-to 6-hour intervals; max 14 days with dosing guided by symptoms; discontinue with a gradual dose reduction over 2 to 4 days

Pediatric: <17 years: not established; ≥17 years: same as adult

Lucemyra *Tab:* 0.18 mg

Comment: **Lucemyra** is <u>not</u> a treatment for Opioid Use Disorder (OUD), per se, but can be used as part of a broader, long-term treatment plan for managing OUD. The most common side effects from treatment with **Lucemyra** include hypotension, bradycardia, somnolence, sedation, and dizziness. **Lucemyra** has also been associated with a few cases of syncope. *methadone* and **Lucymra** both prolong the QT interval. Therefore, ECG monitoring is recommended when used concomitantly. Concomitant use of oral *naltrexone* with **Lucemyra** may reduce efficacy of oral naltrexone. Concomitant use of *paroxetine* has resulted in increased plasma levels of **Lucemyra**. Monitor for symptoms of orthostasis and bradycardia with concomitant use of CYP2D6 inhibitors. The safety of **Lucymra** in pregnant females has <u>not</u> been established. There is no information regarding the presence of **Lucemyra** <u>or</u> its metabolites in human milk <u>or</u> effects on the breastfed infant.

OPIOID AGONISTS

Methadone Detoxification and Methadone Maintenance

Comment: *Methadone* is <u>not</u> indicated as an as-needed (prn) analgesic. For use in chronic moderately severe-to-severe pain management (e.g., hospice care).

▷ *methadone* (C)(II)(G) A single dose of 20 to 30 mg may be sufficient to suppress withdrawal syndrome; *Narcotic Detoxification:* 15-40 mg daily in decreasing doses <u>not</u> to exceed 21 days; *Narcotic Maintenance:* >21 days; see mfr pkg insert; clinical stability is most commonly achieved at doses between 80 to 120 mg/day; monitor patients with periodic ECGs (e.g., risk of lethal QT interval prolongation, *torsades de pointes*)

Pediatric: <12: not recommended; ≥12 years: same as adult

Dolophine *Tab:* 5, 10 mg; *Dispersible tab:* 40 mg (dissolve in 120 ml orange juice <u>or</u> other citrus drink); *Oral soln:* 5, 10 mg/ml; *Oral conc:* 10 mg/ml; *Syr:* 10 mg/30 ml; *Vial:* 10 mg/ml (200 mg/20 ml multi-dose) for injection

Comment: *Methadone* administration is allowed <u>only</u> by approved providers with strict state and federal regulations (as stipulated in 42 CFR 8.12). Black Box Warning (BBW): *Dolophine* exposes users to risks of addiction, abuse, and misuse, which can lead to overdose and death. Assess each patient's risk and monitor regularly for development of these behaviors and conditions. Serious, life-threatening, <u>or</u> fatal respiratory depression may occur. The peak respiratory depressant effect of *methadone* occurs later, and persists longer than the peak analgesic effect. Accidental ingestion, especially by children, can result in fatal overdose. QT interval prolongation and serious arrhythmia (*torsades de pointes*) have occurred during treatment with *methadone*. Closely monitor patients with risk factors for development of prolonged QT interval, a history of cardiac conduction abnormalities, and those taking medications affecting cardiac conduction. Neonatal Opioid Withdrawal Syndrome (NOWS) is an expected and treatable outcome of use of methadone use during pregnancy. NOWS may be life-threatening if not recognized and treated in the neonate. The balance between the risks of NOWS and the benefits of maternal *methadone* use should be considered and the patient advised of the risk of NOWS so that appropriate planning for management of the neonate can occur. *Methadone* has been detected in human milk. Concomitant use with CYP3A4, 2B6, 2C19, 2C9 or 2D6 inhibitors or discontinuation of concomitantly used CYP3A4 2B6, 2C19, or 2C9 inducers can result in a fatal overdose of methadone. Concomitant use of opioids with benzodiazepines or other central nervous system (CNS) depressants, including alcohol, may result in profound sedation, respiratory depression, coma, and death.

OPIOID ANTAGONIST

➢ *naltrexone* (C)
   Pediatric: <12 years: not established; ≥12 years: same as adult
      ReVia 50 mg daily
         Tab: 50 mg
      Vivitrol 380 mg IM once monthly; alternate buttocks
         Vial: 380 mg

OPIOID PARTIAL AGONIST-ANTAGONIST

Comment: **Belbuca, Butrans, Probuphine, Sublocade,** and **Subutex** maintenance are allowed only by approved providers with strict state and federal regulations. These drugs are potentiated by CYP3A4 inhibitors (e.g., azole antifungals, macrolides, HIV protease inhibitors) and antagonized by CYP3A4 inducers (monitor for opioid withdrawal). Concomitant NNRTIs (e.g., *efavirenz, nevirapine, etravirine, delavirdine*) or PIs (e.g., *atazanavir* with or without *ritonavir*): monitor. Risk of respiratory or CNS depression with concomitant opioid analgesics, general anesthetics, benzodiazepines, phenothiazines, other tranquilizers, sedative/hypnotics, alcohol, or other CNS depressants. Risk of *serotonin syndrome* with concomitant SSRIs, SNRIs, TCAs, 5-HT3 receptor antagonists, *mirtazapine, trazodone, tramadol*, MAO inhibitors.

➢ *buprenorphine* (C)(III)
      Belbuca apply buccal film to inside of cheek; do not chew or swallow; *Opioid naïve:* initially 75 mcg once daily-q 12 hours x at least 4 days; then, increase to 150 mcg q 12 hours; may increase in increments of 150 mcg q 12 hours no sooner than every 4 days; max 900 mcg q 12 hours; see mfr pkg insert for conversion from other opioids; *Severe hepatic impairment or oral mucositis:* reduce initial and titration doses by half
      Pediatric: <12 years: not established; ≥12 years: same as adult
         Buccal film: 75, 150, 300, 450, 600, 750, 900 mcg (60/pck) (peppermint)
      Butrans Transdermal System apply one patch to clean, dry, hairless, intact skin on the upper outer arm, upper chest, upper back, or side of chest every 7 days; rotate sites and do not re-use a site for at least 21 days; *Opioid naïve or oral morphine <30 mg/day or equivalent:* one 5 mcg/hour patch; *Converting from oral morphine equivalents 30-80 mg/day:* taper current opioids for up to 7 days to ≤30 mg/day oral morphine equivalents before starting; then initiate with 10 mcg/hour patch; may use a short-acting analgesic until efficacy is attained; increase dose only after exposure to previous dose x at least 72 hours; max one 20 mcg/hour patch/week; *Conversion from higher opioid doses:* not recommended
      Pediatric: <12 years: not established; ≥12 years: same as adult
         Transdermal patch: 5, 7.5, 10, 15, 20 mcg/hour (4/pck)

Probuphine initiate when stable on *buprenorphine* ≤8 mg/day; insertion site is the inner side of the upper arm; 4 implants are intended to be in place for 6 months; remove the implants by the end of the 6th month and insert four new implants on the same day in the contralateral arm; if a new implant is not inserted on the same day as removal of a previous implant, maintain the patient on the previous dose of transmucosal *buprenorphine* (i.e., the dose from which the patient was transferred to **Probuphine** treatment).

Pediatric: <16 years: not established; ≥16 years: same as adult

　Subdermal implant: 74.2 mg of *buprenorphine* (equivalent to 80 mg of *buprenorphine hydrochloride*)

Comment: Healthcare providers who prescribe, perform insertions and/or perform removals of **Probuphine** must successfully complete a live training program, and demonstrate procedural competency prior to inserting or removing the implants. Further information: visit www.ProbuphineREMS. com or call 1-844-859-6341

Subutex (G) 8 mg in a single dose on day 1; then 16 mg in a single dose on day 2; target dose is 16 mg/day in a single dose; dissolve under tongue; do not chew or swallow whole

Pediatric: <12 years: not established; ≥12 years: same as adult

　SL tab (lemon-lime) or SL film (lime): 2, 8 mg (30/pck)

Sublocade verify that patient is clinically stable on transmucosal *buprenorphine* before initiating *Sublocade*; doses must be prepared by an authorized healthcare provider and administered once monthly only by SC injection in the abdominal region; initially, 300 mg SC once monthly x the first 2 months, followed by 100 mg SC once monthly maintenance dose; increasing the maintenance dose to 300 mg once monthly may be considered for patients in which the benefits outweigh the risks

Pediatric: <12 years: not established; ≥12 years: same as adult

　Prefilled syringe: 100 mg/0.5 ml, 300 mg/1.5 ml sust-rel single-dose w. 19 gauge 5/8-inch needle

Comment: Serious harm or death could result if **Sublocade** is administered intravenously. Neonatal opioid withdrawal syndrome (NOWS) is an expected and treatable outcome of prolonged use of opioids during pregnancy. (Not recommended with moderate-to-severe hepatic impairment. Monitor liver function tests prior to and during treatment. If diagnosed with adrenal insufficiency, treat with physiologic replacement of corticosteroids, and wean patient off of the opioid. **Sublocade** is only available through the restricted SUBLOCADE REMS Program. Healthcare settings and pharmacies that order and dispense **Sublocade** must be certified in this program.

▷ *buprenorphine hcl* Initial Dose: 0.3 mg (1 ml) deep IM or slow IV (over at least 2 minutes); may repeat once (up to 0.3 mg) if required, 30-60 minutes after initial dose; usual frequency every 6 hours prn; fixed interval or "round-the-clock" dosing should not be undertaken until the appropriate inter-dose interval has been established by clinical observation

Pediatric: <2 years: not recommended; 2-12 years: 2-6 mcg/kg deep IM or slow IV every 4-6 hours or every 6-8 hours prn; >12 years: same as adult; fixed interval or "round-the-clock" dosing should not be undertaken until the appropriate inter-dose interval has been established by clinical observation

　Buprenex *Amp:* 0.3 mg/ml (1 ml) (5 ampules/carton)

OPIOID PARTIAL AGONIST-ANTAGONIST+OPIOID ANTAGONIST

Comment: **Bunabail, Cassipa, Suboxone, Sucartonone, Troxyca ER,** and **Zubsolv** maintenance may be prescribed only by Drug Addiction Treatment Act (DATA) Certified Providers with strict state and federal regulations. These drugs are potentiated by CYP3A4 inhibitors (e.g., azole antifungals, macrolides, HIV protease inhibitors) and antagonized by CYP3A4 inducers (monitor for opioid withdrawal). Concomitant NNRTIs (e.g., *efavirenz*, *nevirapine*, *etravirine*, *delavirdine*) or PIs (e.g., *atazanavir* with or without *ritonavir*): monitor. Risk of respiratory or CNS depression with concomitant opioid analgesics, general anesthetics, benzodiazepines phenothiazines, other tranquilizers, sedative/hypnotics, alcohol, or other CNS depressants. Risk of *serotonin syndrome* with concomitant SSRIs, SNRIs, TCAs, 5-HT3 receptor antagonists, *mirtazapine*, *trazodone*, *tramadol*, MAO inhibitors. *buprenorphine/naloxone* products are not recommended in patients with severe hepatic impairment and may not be appropriate for patients with moderate hepatic impairment. *buprenorphine* passes into human breast milk. Neonatal opioid withdrawal syndrome may occur in newborn infants of mothers who are receiving treatment with *buprenorphine*.

▷ *buprenorphine+naloxone* (C)(III)(G)

Bunavail administer one buccal film once daily at the same time each day; target dose is 8.4/1.4 once daily; place the side of the **Bunavail** film with the text (BN2, BN4, or BN6) against the inside of the cheek; press and hold the film in place for 5 seconds; maintenance is usually 2.1/0.3 to 12.6/2.1 once daily

Pediatric: <16 years: not recommended; ≥16 years: same as adult

   SL film:

   Bunavail 2.1/0.3 bup 2.1 mg+nal 0.3 mg (30/carton)
   Bunavail 4.2/0.7 bup 4.2 mg+nal 0.7 mg (30/carton)
   Bunavail 6.3/1 bup 6.3 mg+nal 1 mg (30/carton)

Comment: One **Bunavail** 4.2/0.7 mg buccal film provides equivalent *buprenorphine* exposure to a **Sucartonone** 8/2 mg sublingual tablet. **Cassipa** place one film under the tongue, close to the base on the left or right side, and allow to completely dissolve as a single daily dose; initiate only after induction and stabilization of the patient, and the patient has been titrated to a dose of 16 mg *buprenorphine* using another marketed product; do not cut, chew, or swallow whole

Pediatric: <12 years: not recommended; ≥12 years: adjust in 2-4 mg of *buprenorphine SL film*

   SL film: **Cassipa 16/4** bupre 16 mg+nalox 4 mg

Suboxone (G) adjust dose in increments/decrements of 2/0.5 or 4/1 once daily *buprenorphine+naloxone*, based on the patient's daily dose of *buprenorphine*, to a level that suppresses opioid withdrawal signs and symptoms;

Recommended target dosage: 16/4 as a single daily dose; *Maintenance dose:* generally in the range of 4/1 to 24/6 per day; higher once daily doses have not been demonstrated to provide any clinical advantage

Pediatric: <12 years: not established; ≥12 years: same as adult

   Suboxone

   SL tab, SL film: **Suboxone 2/0.5** bup 2 mg+nal 0.5 mg (30/bottle) (lime)
   Suboxone 4/1 bup 4 mg+nal 1 mg (30/bottle) (lime)
   Suboxone 8/2 bup 8 mg+nal 2 mg (30/bottle) (lime)
   Suboxone 12/3 bup 12 mg+nal 3 mg (30/bottle) (lime)

Sucartonone adjust in 2-4 mg of *buprenorphine*/day in a single dose; usual range is 4-24 mg/day in a single dose; target dose is 6 mg/day in a single dose; dissolve under tongue; do not chew or swallow whole

Pediatric: <16 years: not recommended; ≥16 years: same as adult

   Sucartonone

   SL film: **Sucartonone 2/0.5** bup 2 mg+nal 0.5 mg (30/pck) (lime)
   Sucartonone 4/1 bup 4 mg+nal 1 mg (30/pck) (lime)
   Sucartonone 8/2 bup 8 mg+nal 2 mg (30/pck) (lime)
   Sucartonone 12/3 bup 12 mg+nal 3 mg (30/pck) (lime)

Zubsolv initial induction with buprenorphine sublingual tabs; administer as a single dose once daily; titrate dose in increments of 1.4/0.36 or 2.9/0.72 per day; recommended target dose is 11.4/2.9 per day; usual max 17.2/4.2 per day
Pediatric: <16 years: not recommended; ≥16 years: same as adult

> **Zubsolv**
> *SL tab:* **Zubsolv 1.4/0.36** bup 1.4 mg+nal 0.36 mg
> **Zubsolv 2.9/0.72** bup 2.9 mg+nal 0.71 mg
> **Zubsolv 5.7/1.4** bup 5.7 mg+nal 1.4 mg
> **Zubsolv 8.6/2.1** bup 8.6 mg+nal 2.1 mg
> **Zubsolv 11.4/2.9** bup 11.4 mg+nal 2.9 mg

Comment: One **Subtex 5.7/1.4** SL tab is bioequivalent to one **Sucartonone 8/2** SL film.

▷ *oxycodone+naloxone* (C)(II) *Opioid-naïve and opioid non-tolerant:* initially 10/1.2 q 12 hours; *Opioid tolerant:* single doses greater than 40/4.8, or a total daily dose greater than 80/9.6 are only for use in patients for whom tolerance to an opioid of comparable potency has been established; swallow whole, or sprinkle contents on applesauce and swallow immediately without chewing
Pediatric: <18 years: not recommended; ≥18 years: same as adult

> **Troxyca ER**
> *Cap:* **Troxyca ER 10/1.2** oxy 10 mg+nalox 1.2 mg ext-rel
> **Troxyca ER 20/1.2** oxy 20 mg+nalox 2.4 mg ext-rel
> **Troxyca ER 30/1.2** oxy 30 mg+nalox 3.6 mg ext-rel
> **Troxyca ER 40/1.2** oxy 40 mg+nalox 4.8 mg ext-rel
> **Troxyca ER 60/1.2** oxy 60 mg+nalox 7.2 mg ext-rel
> **Troxyca ER 80/1.2** oxy 80 mg+nalox 9.6 mg ext-rel

Comment: Opioid tolerant patients are those taking, for 1 week or longer, at least 60 mg oral *morphine* per day, 25 mcg transdermal *fentanyl* per hour, 30 mg oral *oxycodone* per day, 8 mg oral *hydromorphone* per day, 25 mg oral *oxymorphone* per day, 60 mg oral *hydrocodone* per day, or an equianalgesic dose of another opioid.

SELECTIVE ALPHA 2-ADRENERGIC RECEPTOR AGONIST

Comment: **Lucemyra** *(lofexidine)* is the first FDA-approved non-opioid treatment for the management of opioid withdrawal symptoms, for the mitigation of withdrawal symptoms to facilitate abrupt discontinuation of opioids in adults. While **Lucemyra** may lessen the severity of withdrawal symptoms, it may not completely prevent them. This oral selective alpha 2-adrenergic receptor agonist reduces the release of norepinephrine. The actions of norepinephrine in the autonomic nervous system are believed to play a role in many of the symptoms of opioid withdrawal and is only approved for treatment for up to 14 days.

▷ *lofexidine* (C) 0.18 mg x 3 tabs taken orally 4 x/day at 5-to 6-hour intervals; max 14 days with dosing guided by symptoms; discontinue with a gradual dose reduction over 2-4 days.
Pediatric: <17 years: not recommended; ≥17 years: same as adult
Lucemyra *Tab:* 0.18 mg
Comment: **Lucemyra** is not a treatment for Opioid Use Disorder (OUD), per se, but can be used as part of a broader, long-term treatment plan for managing OUD. The most common side effects from treatment with **Lucemyra** include hypotension, bradycardia, somnolence, sedation, and dizziness. **Lucemyra** has also been associated with a few cases of syncope. *Methadone* and **Lucymra** both prolong the QT interval. Therefore, ECG monitoring is recommended when used concomitantly. Concomitant use

of oral **naltrexone** with **Lucemyra** may reduce efficacy of oral naltrexone. Concomitant use of **paroxetine** has resulted in increased plasma levels of **Lucemyra**. Monitor for symptoms of orthostasis and bradycardia with concomitant use of CYP2D6 inhibitors. The safety of **Lucymra** in pregnant females has not been established. There is no information regarding the presence of **Lucemyra** or its metabolites in human milk or effects on the breastfed infant.

OPIOID-INDUCED CONSTIPATION (OIC)

▷ *lubiprostone* (C) swallow whole; take with food and water; initially 24 mcg bid; *Moderate hepatic impairment (Child Pugh Class B):* 16 mg bid; *Severe hepatic impairment (Child Pugh Class C):* 8 mg bid

Amitiza *Cap:* 8, 24 mg

Comment: **Amitiza** increases intestinal fluid and intestinal transit time. Suspend dosing and rehydrate if severe diarrhea occurs. **Amitiza** is contraindicated with known or suspected mechanical GI obstruction. Most common adverse reactions in CIC are nausea, diarrhea, headache, abdominal pain, abdominal distension, and flatulence .

▷ *methylnaltrexone bromide* (C) one oral dose or one weight-based SC dose every other day as needed; max one dose per 24 hours; administer SC inject into the upper arm, abdomen, or thigh; rotate sites

Chronic Non-cancer Pain: 450 mg po once daily in the morning (take with water on an empty stomach at least 30 minutes before the first meal of the day) or 12 mg SC once daily in the morning; *Severe Hepatic Impairment:* <38 kg: 0.075 mg/kg; 38-<62 kg: 4 mg (0.2 ml); 62-114 kg: 6 mg (0.3 ml); >114 kg: 0.075 mg/kg

Advanced Illness, Receiving Palliative Care: <38 kg: 0.15 mg/kg; 38-<62 kg: 8 mg (0.4 ml); 62-114 kg: 12 mg (0.6 ml); >114 kg: 0.15 mg/kg; *Moderate and Severe Renal Impairment (CrCl<60 mL/min):* <38 kg: 0.075 mg/kg; 38-<62 kg: 4 mg (0.2 ml); 62-114 kg: 6 mg (0.3 ml); >114 kg: 0.075 mg/kg

Pediatric: <18 years: not established; ≥18 years: same as adult

Relistor *Tab:* 150 mg film-coat; *Vial:* 12 mg single-dose (0.6 ml, 7/carton)

Relistor Injection: *Prefilled syringe:* 8 mg (0.4 ml), 12 mg (0.6 ml) (7/carton)

Comment: **Relistor** injection is indicated for patients with advanced illness or pain caused by active cancer who require opioid dosage escalation for palliative care. Relistor is an opioid antagonist indicated for the treatment of opioid-induced constipation (OIC) in adult patients with chronic non-cancer pain, including patients with chronic pain related to prior cancer or its treatment who do not require frequent (e.g., weekly) opioid dosage escalation.

methylnaltrexone is a selective antagonist of opioid binding at the mu-opioid receptor in the gut. As a quaternary amine, the ability of **methylnaltrexone** to cross the blood-brain barrier is restricted. This allows **methylnaltrexone** to function as a peripherally-acting mu-opioid receptor antagonist in tissues such as the gastrointestinal tract, thereby decreasing the constipating effects of opioids without impacting opioid-mediated analgesic effects on the central nervous system.

The pre-filled syringe is only for patients who require a **Relistor** injection dose of 8 mg or 12 mg. Use the vial for patients who require other doses. **Relistor** is contraindicated with known or suspected GI obstruction and patients at increased risk of recurrent obstruction, due to the potential for gastrointestinal perforation. Be within close proximity to toilet facilities once **Relistor** is administered. Discontinue all maintenance laxative therapy prior to initiation. Laxative(s) can be used as needed if there is a suboptimal response after three days. Discontinue if treatment with the opioid pain medication is also discontinued. Safety and effectiveness of **Relistor** have not been established in pediatric patients. Avoid concomitant use with other opioid antagonists because of the potential for additive effects of opioid receptor antagonism and increased risk of opioid withdrawal symptoms (sweating, chills, diarrhea, abdominal pain, anxiety, and yawning). Advise females of reproductive potential, who become pregnant or are planning to become pregnant, that the use of **Relistor** during pregnancy may precipitate opioid withdrawal in a fetus due to the undeveloped blood-brain barrier. Breastfeeding is not recommended during treatment.

▷ *naldemedine* (C) <12 years: not established; ≥12 years: take 1 tab once daily; take with or without food; discontinue if opioid pain therapy discontinued
Pediatric: <12 years: not established; ≥12 years: same as adult
    Symproic *Tab:* 0.2 mg
    Comment: **Symproic** is contraindicated with known or suspected GI obstruction and patients at increased risk for recurrent obstruction. Avoid with severe hepatic impairment (Child-Pugh Class C). Not recommended in pregnancy and breastfeeding (during and 3 days after final dose). There is risk of perforation in persons with conditions associated with reduction in structural integrity the GI tract wall (e.g., peptic ulcer disease [PUD], Ogilvie's syndrome, diverticulitis disease, infiltrative GI tract malignancies, or peritoneal metastases).

▷ *naloxegol* (C) swallow whole; take on an empty stomach; initially 25 mg once daily in the AM; discontinue other laxatives; *CrCl <60 mL/min:* 12.5 mg
Pediatric: <12 years: not established; ≥12 years: same as adult
    Movantik *Tab:* 12.5, 25 mg
    Comment: **Movantik** is an opioid antagonist indicated for the treatment of opioid-induced constipation (OIC) in adult patients with chronic non-cancer pain, including patients with chronic pain related to prior cancer or treatment who do not require frequent (e.g., weekly) opioid dosage escalation. Alteration in analgesic dosing regimen prior to starting **Movantik** is not required. Patients receiving opioids for less than 4 weeks may be less responsive to **Movantik**. Take on an empty stomach at least 1 hour prior to the first meal of the day or 2 hours after the meal. For patients who are unable to swallow the **Movantik** tablet whole, the tablet can be crushed and given orally or administered via nasogastric tube. Avoid consumption of grapefruit or grapefruit juice. Discontinue if treatment with the opioid pain medication is also discontinued.

OPIOID-INDUCED NAUSEA/VOMITING (OINV)

Comment: Opioid analgesics bind to μ (mu), κ (kappa), or δ (delta) opioid receptors in the brain, spinal cord, and digestive tract. However, opioids cause adverse effects that may interfere with their therapeutic use. Opioid-induced nausea/vomiting (OINV) treatment options include serotonin receptor antagonists, dopamine receptor antagonists, and neurokinin-1 receptor antagonists.

SEROTONIN RECEPTOR ANTAGONISTS

▷ *dolasetron* (B) administer 100 mg IV over 30 seconds; max 100 mg/dose
Pediatric: <2 years: not recommended; 2-16 years: 1.8 mg/kg; >16 years: same as adult
    Anzemet *Tab:* 50, 100 mg; *Amp:* 12.5 mg/0.625 ml; *Prefilled carpuject syringe:* 12.5 mg (0.625 ml); *Vial:* 100 mg/5 ml (single-use); *Vial:* 500 mg/25 ml (multi-dose)

▷ *granisetron*
    Kytril (B) administer IV over 30 seconds, 30 min; max 1 dose/week
    Pediatric: <2 years: not recommended; ≥2 years: 10 mcg/kg
      Tab: 1 mg; *Oral soln:* 2 mg/10 ml (30 ml; orange); *Vial:* 1 mg/ml (1 ml single-dose) (preservative-free); 1 mg/ml (4 ml multi-dose) (benzyl alcohol)

Sancuso (B) apply 1 patch 24-48 hours before chemo; remove 24 hours (minimum) to 7 days (maximum) after completion of treatment
Pediatric: <12 years: not recommended; ≥12 years: same as adult
Transdermal patch: 3.1 mg/day

▷ *ondansetron* (C)(G) 8 mg q 8 hours x 2 doses; then 8 mg q 12 hours
Pediatric: <4 years: not recommended; 4-11 years: 4 mg q 4 hours x 3 doses; then 4 mg q 8 hours

Zofran *Tab:* 4, 8, 24 mg
Zofran ODT *ODT:* 4, 8 mg (strawberry) (phenylalanine)
Zofran Oral Solution *Oral soln:* 4 mg/5 ml (50 ml) (strawberry) (phenylalanine); *Parenteral form:* see mfr pkg insert
Zofran Injection *Vial:* 2 mg/ml (2 ml single-dose); 2 mg/ml (20 ml multi-dose); 32 mg/50 ml (50 ml multi-dose); *Prefilled syringe:* 4 mg/2 ml, single-use (24/carton)
Zuplenz Oral Soluble Film: 4, 8 mg oral-dis (10/carton) (peppermint)
Comment: The FDA has issued a warning against *ondansetron)* use in pregnancy *ondansetron* is a 5-HT3 receptor antagonist approved by the FDA for preventing nausea and vomiting related to cancer chemotherapy and surgery. However, it has been used "off label" to treat the nausea and vomiting of pregnancy. The FDA has cautioned against the use of *onzansetron* in pregnancy in light of studies of *ondansetron* in early pregnancy and associated with congenital cardiac malformations and oral clefts (i.e., cleft lip and cleft palate). Further, there are potential maternal risks in pregnancy with electrolyte imbalance caused by severe nausea and vomiting (as with hyperemesis gravidarum). These risks include *serotonin syndrome* (a triad of of cognitive and behavioral changes including confusion, agitation, autonomic instability, and neuromuscular changes). Therefore, *ondansetron* should not be taken during pregnancy.

▷ *palonosetron* (B)(G) administer 0.25 mg IV over 30 seconds; max 1 dose/week
Pediatric: <1 month: not recommended; 1 month to 17 years: 20 mcg/kg; max 1.5 mg/single dose; infuse over 15 minutes
Aloxi *Vial (single-use):* 0.075 mg/1.5 ml; 0.25 mg/5 ml (mannitol)

DOPAMINE RECEPTOR ANTAGONISTS

▷ *prochlorperazine* (C)(G)
Compazine 5-10 mg tid-qid prn; usual max 40 mg/day
Pediatric: <2 years or <20 lb: not recommended; 20-29 lb: 2.5 mg daily bid prn; max 7.5 mg/day; 30-39 lb: 2.5 mg bid-tid prn; max 10 mg/day; 40-85 lb: 2.5 mg tid or 5 mg bid prn; max 15 mg/day
Tab: 5, 10 mg; *Syr:* 5 mg/5 ml (4 oz) (fruit)
Compazine Suppository 25 mg rectally bid prn; usual max 50 mg/day
Pediatric: <2 years or <20 lb: not recommended; 20-29 lb: 2.5 mg daily-bid prn; max 7.5; mg/day; 30-39 lb: 2.5 mg bid-tid prn; max 10 mg/day; 40-85 lb: 2.5 mg tid or 5 mg bid prn; max 15 mg/day
Rectal supp: 2.5, 5, 25 mg
Compazine Injectable 5-10 mg tid or qid prn
Pediatric: <2 years or <20 lb: not recommended; ≥2 years or ≥20 lb: 0.06 mg/kg x 1 dose
Vial: 5 mg/ml (2, 10 ml)
Compazine Spansule 15 mg q AM prn or 10 mg q 12 hours prn usual max 40 mg/day
Pediatric: <12 years: not recommended; ≥12 years: same as adult
Spansule: 10, 15 mg sust-rel

NEUROKININ-1 RECEPTOR ANTAGONISTS

▷ *aprepitant* (B)(G) administer with 5HT-3 receptor antagonist; *Day 1:* 125 mg; *Day 2 & 3:* 80 mg in the morning

Pediatric: <6 months: years: not recommended; ≥6 months: use oral suspension (see mfr pkg insert for dose by weight

Emend *Cap:* 40, 80, 125 mg (2 x 80 mg bi-fold pck; 1 x 25 mg/2 x 80 mg tri-fold pck); *Oral susp:* 125 mg pwdr for oral suspension, single-dose pouch w. dispenser; *Vial:* 150 mg pwdr for reconstitution and IV infusion

OPIOID OVERDOSE

Comment: Patients should be transported to an emergency care facility. Seek emergency medical support (activate EMS) immediately.

Opioid Reversal Risks:

(1) *Risk of Recurrent Respiratory and CNS Depression:* Due to the duration of action of *naloxone* relative to the opioid, keep patient under continued surveillance and administer repeat doses of *naloxone* using a new administration device as necessary, while awaiting emergency medical assistance.

(2) *Risk of Limited Efficacy with Partial Agonists or Mixed Agonist/Antagonists:* Reversal of respiratory depression caused by partial agonists or mixed agonist/antagonists, such as *buprenorphine* and *pentazocine*, may be incomplete. Larger or repeat doses may be necessary.

(3) *Precipitation of Severe Opioid Withdrawal:* Use of *naloxone* in patients who are opioid-dependent may precipitate opioid withdrawal. In neonates, opioid withdrawal may be life-threatening if not recognized and properly treated. Monitor for the development of opioid withdrawal.

(4) *Risk of Cardiovascular (CV) Effects:* Abrupt postoperative reversal of opioid depression may result in adverse CV effects. These events have primarily occurred in patients who had pre-existing CV disorders or received other drugs that may have similar adverse CV effects. Monitor these patients closely in an appropriate healthcare setting after use of *naloxone* hydrochloride.

OPIOID ANTAGONISTS

▷ *nalmefene* (B) initially 0.25 mcg/kg IV, IM, or SC, then incremental doses of 0.25 mcg/kg at 2-5 minute intervals; cumulative max 1 mcg/kg; if opioid dependency suspected use 0.1 mg/70 kg initially and then proceed as usual if no response in 2 minutes

Pediatric: not recommended

Revex *Amp:* 100 mcg/ml (1 ml); 1 mg/ml (2 ml)

▷ *naloxone* (B)(G) 0.4-2 mg; repeat in 2-3 minutes if no response

Pediatric: 0.01 mg/kg initially, repeat in 2-3 minutes at 0.1 mg/kg if response inadequate

Evzio *Prefilled autoinjector:* 0.4 mg/0.4, 2 mg/0.4 ml IM/SC only

Comment: **Evzio** 2 mg/0.4 ml comes with 2 autoinjectors and one trainer. This strength is indicated for the emergency treatment of known or suspected opioid overdose manifested by CNS depression.

If the electronic voice instruction system does not operate properly, **Evzio** will still deliver the intended dose of *naloxone* when used according to the printed instructions on the flat surface of the autoinjector label. **Evzio** cannot be administered IV. Due to the short duration of action of naloxone, as compared to opioids which are longer acting, monitoring of the patient is critical as the opioid reversal effects of naloxone may wear off before the effects of the opioid.

Kloxxado administer 1 spray in one nostril; if an additional dose is needed, spray into the opposite nostril using a new **Kloxxado** nasal spray devise with each dose; if the patient does not respond or responds and then relapses into respiratory depression. Additional doses may be administered every 2 to 3 minutes until emergency medical assistance arrives

Pediatric: same as adult

Nasal spray: 8 mg/0.1 ml, single-dose (2 blisters, each containing a single dose of *naloxone* and 2 nasal spray devices and /carton)

Narcan *Vial/Amp:* 0.4 mg/ml (1 ml), 1 mg/ml (2 ml); *Prefilled syringe:* 0.4 mg/ml (1 ml), 1 mg/ml (2 ml) IV, IM, or SC (parabens-free)

Narcan Nasal Spray position supine with head tilted back; 1 spray in one nostril; if an additional dose is needed, spray into the opposite nostril

Nasal spray: 4 mg/0.1 ml, single-dose (2 blister pcks, each w a single nasal spray/carton)

 ## ORGAN TRANSPLANT REJECTION PROPHYLAXIS (OTRP)

SELECTIVE IMMUNOMODULATORY AGENTS

Comment: Selective immunosuppressive agents are drugs that suppress the immune system due to a selective point of action. They are used to reduce the risk of rejection in organ transplants, in autoimmune diseases, and can be used as cancer chemotherapy. As immunosuppressive agents lower the immunity, there is increased risk of infection.

CHIMERIC (MURINE/HUMAN) MONOCLONAL ANTIBODY

▷ *basiliximab* (B) recommended regimen is two doses of 20 mg each; the first 20-mg dose should be administered within 2 hours prior to transplantation surgery; the second dose should be administered 4 days after transplantation; the second dose should be withheld if complications such as severe hypersensitivity reactions to **Simulect** or graft loss occurs

Pediatric: <35 kg: two doses of 10 mg each; ≥35 kg: two doses of 20 mg each; the first dose should be administered within 2 hours prior to transplantation surgery; the second dose should be administered 4 days after transplantation; the second dose should be withheld if complications such as severe hypersensitivity reactions to **Simulect** or graft loss occurs

Simulect *Vial:* 10, 20 mg (6 ml) for reconstitution and IV infusion (preservative-free 10 mg vial: contains 10 mg *basiliximab*, 3.61 mg monobasic potassium phosphate, 0.50 mg disodium hydrogen phosphate (anhydrous), 0.80 mg sodium chloride, 10 mg sucrose, 40 mg mannitol, 20 mg glycine, to be reconstituted in 2.5 ml of sterile water for injection, USP 20 mg *vial; contains* 20 mg *basiliximab*, 7.21 mg monobasic potassium phosphate, 0.99 mg disodium hydrogen phosphate (anhydrous), 1.61 mg sodium chloride, 20 mg sucrose, 80 mg mannitol and 40 mg glycine, to be reconstituted in 5 ml of sterile water for injection

INOSINE MONOPHOSPHATE DEHYDROGENASE (IMPDH) INHIBITOR)

▷ *mycophenolate mofetil (MMF)* (D) <3 years: not recommended: 3 months-18 years: recommended dose of **CellCept** oral suspension is 600 mg/m2 administered bid (up to total max 2 gm daily); patients with BSA 1.25 m2 to 1.5 m2 may be dosed with **CellCept** capsules at 750 mg bid (total 1.5 gm daily); patients with BSA >1.5 m2 may be dosed with **CellCept** capsules or tablets at 1 gm bid (total 2 gm daily); >18 years: 1.5 gm bid orally (total 3 gm daily) or via IV infusion (infuse over no less than 2 hours; do not administer by bolus or rapid infusion)

CellCept *Cap:* 250 mg; *Cap:* 500 mg; *Oral susp:* 200 mg/ml (225 ml) after reconstitution w bottle adapter and 2 oral dispensers; *Vial:* 500 mg MMF hcl for IV infusion after reconstitution and dilution in D5W

Comment: **CellCept** (*mycophenolate mofetil, MMF*) is the 2-morpholinoethyl ester of mycophenolic acid (MPA), an inosine monophosphate dehydrogenase

(IMPDH) inhibitor. MMF has been demonstrated in experimental animal models to prolong the survival of allogeneic transplants (kidney, heart, liver, intestine, limb, small bowel, pancreatic islets, and bone marrow). MMF has demonstrated teratogenic effects in humans; however, there are no adequate and well-controlled studies in pregnancy. Females of reproductive potential must be made aware of the increased risk of first trimester pregnancy loss and congenital malformations and must be counseled regarding pregnancy prevention and planning. To prevent unplanned exposure during pregnancy, females of reproductive potential should have a serum or urine pregnancy test with a sensitivity of at least 25 mIU/ml immediately before starting **CellCept**, repeated testing 8-10 days later and during routine follow-up visits. In the event of a positive pregnancy test, females should be counseled with regard to maternal-fetal risk/benefit. Animal studies have shown mycophenolic acid to be excreted in milk. It is not known whether MMF is excreted in human milk. Because of the potential for serious adverse reactions in breastfed infants from MMF exposure, risk/benefit of breastfeeding should be discussed with the patient.

Mammalian Target of Rapamycin (mTOR) Inhibitors (mTORi)

Comment: The most frequently occurring adverse events associated with mTOR inhibitors (≥30%) include aphthous stomatitis, rash, anemia, fatigue, hyperglycemia, hypertriglyceridemia, hypercholesterolemia, decreased appetite, nausea, diarrhea, abdominal pain, headache, peripheral edema, hypertension, increased serum creatinine, fever, urinary tract infection, arthralgia, pain, thrombocytopenia, and interstitial lung disease. There are no adequate and well-controlled studies in pregnant females. Effective contraception must be initiated before mTORi therapy, continued during therapy, and for 12 weeks after therapy has been stopped. It is not known whether *serolimus*-based drugs are excreted in human milk. The pharmacokinetic and safety profiles in breastfed infants are not known; therefore, a decision should be made whether to discontinue nursing or to discontinue the drug, taking into account the importance of the drug to the mother.

▷ *everolimus* (C)(G) administer consistently with or without food at the same time as *cyclosporine* or *tacrolimus*; monitor *everolimus* concentrations: adjust just maintenance dose to achieve trough concentrations within the 3-8 ng/mL target range (using LC/MS/MS assay method); *Mild hepatic impairment:* reduce initial daily dose by one-third; *Moderate or severe hepatic impairment:* reduce initial daily dose by one-half *Kidney Transplant:* indicated for patients at low-moderate immunologic risk; use in combination with *basiliximab*, *cyclosporine* (reduced doses), and *corticosteroids;* starting dose is 0.75 mg bid; initiate as soon as possible after transplantation *Liver Transplant:* use in combination with *tacrolimus* (reduced doses) and *corticosteroids*; starting dose is 1.0 mg bid; initiate 30 days after transplantation

Pediatric: <18 years: not established/not recommended; ≥18 years: same as adult

Zortress *Tab:* 0.25, 0.5, 0.75 mg

▷ *serolimus* (C)

Generic: (for prescribing information, *see* **Rapamune**)

Tab: 1, 2 mg

Rapamune administer consistently with or without food at the same time as *cyclosporine (CsA) Low to moderate-immunologic risk: Day 1:* 6 mg as a single loading dose; *Day 2:* initiate 2 mg once daily maintenance; use initially with *cyclosporine* (CsA) and *corticosteroids*; initiate CsA withdrawal over 4-8 weeks beginning 2-4 months post-transplantation *High-immunologic risk: Day 1:* up to 15 mg as a single loading dose; *Day 2:* initiate 5 mg once daily maintenance; use with CsA for the first 12 months post-transplantation

Pediatric: <13 years: not established/not recommended; ≥13 years: same as

Tab: 0.5, 1, 2, mg; *Oral soln:* 60 mg/60 ml in amber glass bottle, one oral syringe adapter for fitting into the neck of the bottle, sufficient disposable amber oral syringes and caps for daily dosing, and a carrying case; bottles should be stored protected from light and refrigerated at 2°C to 8°C (36°F to 46°F); once the bottle is opened, the contents should be used within one month; If necessary, bottles may be stored the bottles at room temperatures up to 25°C (77°F) for a short period of time (not more than 15 days)

CALCINEURIN-INHIBITOR IMMUNOSUPPRESSANTS

Comment: *Tacrolimus* products are available in immediate-release (capsule, granules, parenteral form for IV administration) and extended-release tablet form, The forms are not interchangeable. Consider dose reduction or discontinuation in the event of myocardial hypertrophy and discontinue in the event of pure red cell aplasia. Avoid live vaccines during treatment with *tacrolimus*. Monitor for new onset diabetes after transplant. Monitor for acute and/or chronic nephrotoxicity and consider dosage reduction with concomitant nephrotoxic drugs and/or neurotoxic drugs. The most common adverse reactions (incidence 10-15%) have included diarrhea, constipation, anemia, UTI, hypertension, tremor, peripheral edema, hyperkalemia, diabetes mellitus, and headache. Monitor for hypertension, hyperkalemia, other abnormal electrolytes, and QT prolongation. Data from postmarketing surveillance and the TPRI suggest that infants exposed to *tacrolimus* *in utero* are at risk for prematurity, birth defects/congenital anomalies, low birthweight, and fetal distress. Risk/benefit to mother and infant should be considered. Adult organ recipients and parents of pediatric organ recipients should be encouraged to enroll in The Transplant Pregnancy Registry International (TPRI) by calling 1-877-955-6877 or visiting www.transplantpregnancyregistry.org. Controlled lactation studies have not been conducted in humans; however, *tacrolimus* has been reported in human breast milk and effects on the breastfed infant are unknown. Risk/benefit of maternal health and infant health should be discussed.

▷ *tacrolimus* see mfr pkg insert for dosing table; dosing is based on: patient age (<18 years or ≥18 years), organ transplanted, whether concomitant with *azathioprine* or MMF/IL-2 receptor antagonist, dosage formulation, whole blood trough concentration range in ng/mL, and specific months in the treatment schedule; see the mfr pkg insert also for dosage adjustments for African-American patients, hepatic and patients with hepatic and/or renal impairment

Envarsus XR take once daily on an empty stomach at the same time of day, preferably in the morning

	Initial Oral Dose	Whole Blood Trough Concentration Range
De novo kidney transplantation with antibody induction	0.14 mg/kg/day	Month 1: 6-11 ng/mL >Month 1: 4-11 ng/mL
Conversion from *tacrolimus* immediate-release formulation	80% of the preconversion dose of *tacrolimus* immediate-release	Titrate to 4-11 ng/mL

Tab: 0.75, 1, 4 mg ext-rel

Comment: Envarsus XR (*tacrolimus* extended-release) is indicated to prevent organ rejection in *de novo* kidney transplant patients in combination with other immunosuppressants. Envarsus XR was initially approved for the prophylaxis of organ rejection in kidney transplant patients converted from *tacrolimus* immediate-release formulations. Envarsus XR is not interchangeable with other tacrolimus products.

Prograf *Cap:* 0.5, 1, 5 mg; *Granules:* 0.2, 1 mg unit-dose pkts for oral suspension (50 pkts/caton); *Amp:* 5 mg/ml solution for dilution and IV Infusion (1 ml, 10/box)

Comment: Prograf *(tacrolimus)* is indicated for the prophylaxis of organ rejection in patients receiving an allogenic liver, kidney, or heart transplant with other immunosuppressants. Frequent monitoring of trough concentration is recommended. Capsules and suspension should be consistently administered either with or without food. IV administration is intended for patients who are unable to swallow capsules or tablets. **Prograf** is not interchangeable with other extended-release *tacrolimus* products. Monitor for, and implement appropriate management for new onset diabetes, nephrotoxicity, neurotoxicity, hyperkalemia, hypertension, and anaphylaxis. **Prograf** is not recommended with concomitant use of *sirolimus* with liver and heart transplantation due to increased risk of adverse reactions.

OSGOOD-SCHLATTER DISEASE

Acetaminophen for IV Infusion *see Pain*
NSAIDs *see* Appendix J. NSAIDs online at https://connect.springerpub.com/content/reference-book/978-0-8261-7935-7/back-matter/part02/back-matter/bmatter10
Opioid Analgesics *see Pain*
Topical & Transdermal Analgesics *see Pain*
Parenteral Corticosteroids *see* Appendix M. Parenteral Corticosteroids
Oral Corticosteroids *see* Appendix L. Oral Corticosteroids
Topical Analgesic and Anesthetic Agents *see* Appendix I. Anesthetic Agents for Local Infiltration and Dermal/Mucosal Membrane Application online at https://connect.springerpub.com/content/reference-book/978-0-8261-7935-7/back-matter/part02/back-matter/bmatter9

OSTEOARTHRITIS, ANKYLOSING SPONDYLITIS

Acetaminophen for IV Infusion *see Pain*
NSAIDs *see* Appendix J. NSAIDs online at https://connect.springerpub.com/content/reference-book/978-0-8261-7935-7/back-matter/part02/back-matter/bmatter10
Opioid Analgesics *see Pain*
Topical & Transdermal Analgesics *see Pain*
Parenteral Corticosteroids *see* Appendix M. Parenteral Corticosteroids
Oral Corticosteroids *see* Appendix L. Oral Corticosteroids
Topical Analgesic and Anesthetic Agents *see* Appendix I. Anesthetic Agents for Local Infiltration and Dermal/Mucosal Membrane Application online at https://connect.springerpub.com/content/reference-book/978-0-8261-7935-7/back-matter/part02/back-matter/bmatter9

TOPICAL & TRANSDERMAL ANALGESICS

▷ *capsaicin* (B)(G) apply tid to qid prn to intact skin
  Pediatric: <2 years: not recommended; ≥2 years: same as adult
    Axsain *Crm:* 0.075% (1, 2 oz)
    Capsin *Lotn:* 0.025, 0.075% (59 ml)
    Capsaicin-HP (OTC) *Crm:* 0.075% (1.5 oz), 0.025% (45, 90 gm); *Lotn:* 0.075% (2 oz); 0.025% (45, 90 gm)
    Capzasin-P (OTC) *Crm:* 0.025% (1.5 oz); *Lotn:* 0.025% (2 oz)
    Dolorac *Crm:* 0.025% (28 gm)
    Double Cap (OTC) *Crm:* 0.05% (2 oz)
    R-Gel *Gel:* 0.025% (15, 30 gm)
    Zostrix (OTC) *Crm:* 0.025% (0.7, 1.5, 3 oz)
    Zostrix HP (OTC) *Emol crm:* 0.075% (1, 2 oz)

▷ *capsaicin* 8% patch **(B)** apply up to 4 patches for one 60-minute application to clean dry skin; may prep area with topical anesthetic; wear non-latex gloves; patches may be cut to size/shape; treatment may be repeated every 3 months
Pediatric: <18 years: not recommended; ≥18 years: same as adult
   Qutenza *Patch:* 8% 1640 mcg/cm (179 mg) (1 or 2 patches w. 1-50 gm tube cleansing gel/carton)

▷ *diclofenac sodium* **(C; D ≥30 wks)** apply qid prn to intact skin
Pediatric: <12 years: not established; ≥12 years: same as adult
   Pennsaid 1.5% in 10 drop increments, dispense and rub into front, side, and back of knee: usually; 40 drops (40 mg) qid
      Topical soln: 1.5% (150 ml)
   Pennsaid 2% apply 2 pump actuations (40 mg) and rub into front, side, and back of knee bid
      Topical soln: 2% (20 mg/pump actuation, 112 gm)
   Solaraze Gel massage in to clean skin bid prn
      Gel: 3% (50 gm) (benzyl alcohol)
   Voltaren Gel (G)(OTC) apply qid prn to intact skin
      Gel: 1% (100 gm)
Comment: *Diclofenac* is contraindicated with *aspirin* allergy. As with other NSAIDs, should be avoided in late pregnancy (≥30 weeks) because it may cause premature closure of the ductus arteriosus.

▷ *doxepin* **(B)** cream apply to affected area qid at intervals of at least 3-4 hours; max 8 days
Pediatric: <12 years: not recommended; >12 years: same as adult
   Prudoxin *Crm:* 5% (45 gm)
   Zonalon *Crm:* 5% (30, 45 gm)

▷ *pimecrolimus* 1% cream **(C)(G)** <2 years: not recommended; ≥2 years: apply to affected area bid; do not apply an occlusive dressing
   Elidel *Crm:* 1% (30, 60, 100 gm)
Comment: *Pimecrolimus* is indicated for short-term and intermittent long-term use. Discontinue use when resolution occurs. Contraindicated if the patient is immunosuppressed. Change to the 0.1% preparation or if secondary bacterial infection is present.

▷ *trolamine salicylate* apply tid-qid
Pediatric: <2 years: not recommended; ≥2 years: same as adult
   Mobisyl Creme *Crm:* 10% (100 gm)

ORAL SALICYLATE

▷ *indomethacin* **(C)** initially 25 mg bid to tid, increase as needed at weekly intervals by 25-50 mg/day; max 200 mg/day
Pediatric: <14 years: usually not recommended; >2 years, if risk warranted: 1-2 mg/kg/day in divided doses; max 3-4 mg/kg/day (or 150-200 mg/day, whichever is less); <14 years: ER cap not recommended
      Cap: 25, 50 mg; *Susp:* 25 mg/5 ml (pineapple-coconut, mint) (alcohol 1%);
      Supp: 50 mg; *ER Cap:* 75 mg ext-rel
Comment: *Indomethacin* is indicated only for acute painful flares. Administer with food and/or antacids. Use lowest effective dose for shortest duration.

ORAL NSAIDs

See more **Oral NSAIDs** https://connect.springerpub.com/content/reference-book/978-0-8261-7935-7/back-matter/part02/back-matter/bmatter10

▷ *diclofenac* **(C)** take on empty stomach; 35 mg tid; Hepatic impairment: use lowest dose
Pediatric: <18 years: not recommended; ≥18 years: same as adult
   Zorvolex *Gelcap:* 18, 35 mg

▷ *diclofenac sodium* (C)
  Pediatric: <18 years: not recommended; ≥18 years: same as adult
    Voltaren 50 mg bid to qid <u>or</u> 75 mg bid <u>or</u> 25 mg qid with an additional 25 mg at HS if necessary
    Tab: 25, 50, 75 mg ent-coat
    Voltaren XR 100 mg once daily; rarely, 100 mg bid may be used
    Tab: 100 mg ext-rel
  Comment: *Diclofenac* is contraindicated with *aspirin* allergy. As with other NSAIDs, should be avoided in late pregnancy (≥30 weeks) because it may cause premature closure of the ductus arteriosus.

ORAL NSAIDs+PPI

▷ *esomeprazole+naproxen* (C)(G) 1 tab bid; use lowest effective dose for the shortest duration swallow whole; take at least 30 minutes before a meal
  Pediatric: <18 years: not recommended; ≥18 years: same as adult
    Vimovo *Tab:* nap 375 mg+eso 20 mg ext-rel; nap 500 mg+eso 20 mg ext-rel
    Comment: **Vimovo** is indicated to improve signs/symptoms, and risk of gastric ulcer in patients at risk of developing NSAID-associated gastric ulcer.

COX-2 INHIBITORS

Comment: Cox-2 inhibitors are contraindicated with history of asthma, urticaria, and allergic-type reactions to *aspirin*, other NSAIDs, and sulfonamides, 3rd trimester of pregnancy, and coronary artery bypass graft (CABG) surgery.

▷ *celecoxib* (C)(G) 100-400 mg daily bid; max 800 mg/day
  Pediatric: <18 years: not recommended; ≥18 years: same as adult
    Celebrex *Cap:* 50, 100, 200, 400 mg
▷ *meloxicam* (C)(G)
    Mobic <2 years, <60 kg: not recommended; ≥2, >60 kg: 0.125 mg/kg; max 7.5 mg once daily; ≥18 years: initially 7.5 mg once daily; max 15 mg once daily; *Hemodialysis:* max 7.5 mg/day
      Tab: 7.5, 15 mg; *Oral susp:* 7.5 mg/5 ml (100 ml) (raspberry)
    Vivlodex <18 years: <u>not</u> established; ≥18 years: initially 5 mg qd; may increase to max 10 mg/day; *Hemodialysis:* max 5 mg/day
      Cap: 5, 10 mg

INTRA-ARTICULAR STEROID INJECTIONS

▷ *triamcinolone acetonide* ext-rel injectable synthetic corticosteroid indicated as an intra-articular injection for the management of osteoarthritis pain of the knee
    Zilretta *Vial:* 32 mg single-dose microsphere pwdr for injection + 5 ml diluent and vial adapter/single-use kit
    Comment: **Zilretta** is <u>not</u> intended for repeat administration. **Zilretta** is <u>not</u> interchangeable with other formulations of injectable *triamcinolone acetonide*.

INTRA-ARTICULAR SODIUM HYALURONATE INJECTIONS

Comment: *Sodium hyaluronate* intra-articular injection is indicated for the treatment of pain in osteoarthritis (OA) of the knee in patients who have failed to respond adequately to conservative non-pharmacologic therapy and simple analgesics (e.g., acetaminophen), alternative practices and procedures include nonsteroidal anti-inflammatory drugs (NSAIDs), intra-articular injection of corticosteroid, unmodified hyaluronan injections, avoidance of activities that cause joint pain, exercise, weight loss, physical therapy, and removal of excess fluid from the knee. For those patients who have failed the above treatments, surgical interventions such as arthroscopic surgery and total knee replacement surgery are also alternative treatments. Do <u>not</u> inject this product in the knees of patients with infections <u>or</u> skin diseases in the area of the injection site. Potential adverse effects occur in association with intraarticular injections: arthralgia, joint stiffness, joint effusion, joint swelling, joint warmth, injection site pain, arthritis, allergic reaction, and bleeding at the injection site. *Sodium hyaluronate* has <u>not</u> been formally assigned to a pregnancy category by the FDA. Animal studies have failed to reveal evidence of fertility impairment <u>or</u> teratogenicity. There are no controlled data in human pregnancy.

▷ *sodium hyaluronate* (B) using strict aseptic technique, administer by intra-articular injection (into the synovial space of the affected knee(s) for the prescribed number of weeks (see mfr pkg insert); after preparing the injection site and attaining local analgesia, remove joint synovial fluid <u>or</u> effusion prior to injection; do <u>not</u> inject intra-vascularly, extra-articularly, <u>or</u> in the synovial tissues <u>or</u> capsule; for at least 48 hours following an injection, avoid jogging, strenuous activity, <u>or</u> high-impact sports such as soccer <u>or</u> tennis, weight-bearing activity, <u>or</u> standing for longer than 1 hour at a time

Pediatric: <12 years: not recommended; ≥12 years: same as adult

Durolane administer a single intra-articular knee injection
Pediatric: <21 years: not recommended
   Prefilled syringe: 60 mg (20 mg/ml, 3 ml), single-use

Euflexxa administer 3-5 intra-articular knee injections 1 week apart
Pediatric: <21 years: not recommended
   Prefilled syringe: 20 mg (10 mg/ml, 2.0 ml), single-use

Gel-One administer a single intra-articular knee injection
Pediatric: <21 years: not recommended
   Prefilled syringe: 30 mg (10 mg/ml, 3 ml), single-use

GelSyn-3 administer 3-5 intra-articular injections 1 week apart
Pediatric: <21 years: not recommended
   Prefilled syringe: 16.5 mg (8.4 mg/ml, 2 ml), single-use

GenVisc 850 administer 3-5 intra-articular knee injections 1 week apart
Pediatric: <21 years: not recommended
   Prefilled syringe: 25 mg (10 mg/ml, 2.5 ml), single-use

Hyalgan administer 3 to 5 intra-articular injections 1 week apart
Pediatric: <21 years: not recommended
   Prefilled syringe: 10 mg/ml (20 mg, 2 ml), single-use

Monovisc administer a single intra-articular knee injection
Pediatric: <21 years: not recommended
   Prefilled syringe: 88 mg (22 mg/ml, 4 ml), single-use

Orthovisc administer 3 to 4 intra-articular knee injections 1 week apart
Pediatric: <21 years: not recommended
   Prefilled syringe: 30 mg (15 mg/ml, 2 ml), single-use

Spartz, Supartz FX administer 3- to 5 intra-articular knee injections one week apart
Pediatric: <21 years: not recommended
   Prefilled syringe: 25 mg (10 mg/ml, 2.5 ml), single-use

Synvisc administer 3 intra-articular knee injections 1 week apart
Pediatric: <21 years: not recommended
   Prefilled syringe: 16 mg (8 mg/ml, 2 ml), juvenile idiopathic arthritis single-use

Synvisc-One administer a single intra-articular knee injection
Pediatric: <21 years: not recommended
   Prefilled syringe: 48 mg (8 mg/ml, 6 ml), single-use

Triluron administer 3 intra-articular knee injections 1 week apart
Pediatric: <21 years: not established
   Vial: 20 mg/2 ml (2 ml); *Prefilled syringe:* 20 mg/2 ml (2 ml), single-use

TriVisc administer 3 intra-articular knee injections 1 week apart
Pediatric: <21 years: not recommended

Prefilled syringe: 30 mg (10 mg/ml, 3 ml), single-use
Visco-3 administer 3 intra-articular knee injections 1 week apart
Pediatric: <21 years: not recommended
Prefilled syringe: 25 mg (10 mg/ml, 2.5 ml), single-use

TUMOR NECROSIS FACTOR (TNF) ALPHA BLOCKERS FOR ANKYLOSING SPONDYLITIS

▷ *adalimumab* (B) 40 mg SC once every other week; may increase to once weekly; administer SC in abdomen or thigh; rotate sites
Pediatric: NA
Humira *Prefilled pen (Humira Pen):* 40 mg/0.4 ml, 40 mg/0.8 ml, 80 mg/0.8 ml, single-dose; *Prefilled glass syringe:* 10 mg/0.1 ml, 10 mg/0.2 ml, 20 mg/0.2 ml, 20 mg/0.4 ml, 40 mg/0.4 ml, 40 mg/0.8 ml, 80 mg/0.8 ml, single-dose; *Vial:* 40 mg/0.8 ml, single dose, institutional use only (preservative-free)
Comment: **Humira** may be used with *methotrexate* (MTX), DMARDs, corticosteroids, salicylates, NSAIDs, or analgesics.

▷ *adalimumab-adaz* (B) 40 mg SC every other week; some patients with RA not receiving *methotrexate* (MTX) may benefit from increasing the frequency to 40 mg SC every week
Pediatric: <18 years: not recommended; ≥18 years: same as adult
Hyrimox *Prefilled syringe:* 40 mg/0.8 ml single-dose (preservative-free)
Comment: **Hyrimox** is biosimilar to **Humira** *(adalimumab)*.

▷ *adalimumab-adbm* (B) initially 80 SC; then, 40 mg SC every other week starting one week after initial dose; inject into thigh or abdomen; rotate sites
Pediatric: <18 years: not recommended; ≥18 years: same as adult
Cyltezo *Prefilled syringe:* 40 mg/0.8 ml single-dose (preservative-free)
Comment: **Cyltezo** is biosimilar to **Humira** (*adalimumab*).

▷ *adalimumab-afzb* 40 mg SC every other week; some patients with RA not receiving *methotrexate* (MTX) may benefit from increasing the frequency to 40 mg SC every week
Abrilada *Prefilled pen:* 40 mg/0.8 ml, single-dose; *Prefilled syringe:* 40 mg/0.8 ml, 20 mg/0.4 ml, 10 mg/0.2 ml, single-dose; (for institutional use only) (preservative-free)
Comment: **Abrilada** is biosimilar to **Humira** (*adalimumab*).

▷ *adalimumab-bwwd* Initial Dose (Day 1): 160 mg SC; *Second Dose: two weeks later (Day 15):* 80 mg SC; *Two weeks later (Day 29):* begin maintenance dose of 40 mg every other week
Hadlima *Prefilled autoinjector:* 40 mg/0.8 ml, single-dose (Hadlima PushTouch); *Prefilled syringe:* 40 mg/0.8 ml, single-dose
Comment: **Hadlima** is biosimilar to **Humira** *(adalimumab)*.

▷ *etanercept* (B) inject SC into thigh, abdomen, or upper arm; rotate sites; initially 50 mg twice weekly (3-4 days apart) for 3 months; then 50 mg/week maintenance or 25 mg or 50 mg per week for 3 months; then 50 mg/week maintenance
Pediatric: <4 years: not recommended; 4-17 years: Chronic moderate-to-severe plaque psoriasis; >17 years: same as adult
Enbrel *Vial:* 25 mg pwdr for SC injection after reconstitution (4/carton w. supplies) (preservative-free, diluent contains benzyl alcohol); *Prefilled syringe:* 25, 50 mg/ml (preservative-free); *SureClick autoinjector:* 50 mg/ml (preservative-free)

▷ *etanercept-ykro* 50 mg SC once weekly
Pediatric: <4 years: not established; ≥4 years, ≥63 kg, 138 lbs: same as adult
Eticovo *Prefilled syringe:* 25 mg/0.5 ml, 50 mg/ml solution, single-dose
Comment: **Eticovo** is biosimilar to **Enbrel**. *(etanercept)*.

▷ *infliximab* must be refrigerated at 2°C to 8°C (36°F to 46°F); administer dose intravenously over a period of not less than 2 hours; do not use beyond the expiration date as this product contains no preservative; 5 mg/kg at 0, 2 and 6 weeks, then every 8 weeks.

Pediatric: <6 years: not studied; ≥6-17 years: mg/kg at 0, 2 and 6 weeks, then every 8 weeks; ≥18 years: same as adult

Remicade *Vial:* 100 mg pwdr for reconstitution to 10 ml administration volume, single-dose (presrvative-free)

Comment: **Remicade** is indicated to reduce signs and symptoms, and induce and maintain clinical remission, in adults and children ≥6 years-of-age with moderately to severely active disease who have had an inadequate response to conventional therapy <u>and</u> reduce the number of draining enterocutaneous and rectovaginal fistulas, and maintain fistula closure, in adults with fistulizing disease. Common adverse effects associated with **Remicade** included abdominal pain, headache, pharyngitis, sinusitis, and upper respiratory infections. In addition, **Remicade** might increase the risk for serious infections, including tuberculosis, bacterial sepsis, and invasive fungal infections. Available data from published literature on the use of *infliximab* products during pregnancy have <u>not</u> reported a clear association with *infliximab* products and adverse pregnancy outcomes. *Infliximab* products cross the placenta and infants exposed *in utero* should <u>not</u> be administered live vaccines for at least 6 months after birth. Otherwise, the infant may be at increased risk of infection, including disseminated infection which can become fatal. Available information is insufficient to inform the amount of *infliximab* products present in human milk <u>or</u> effects on the breastfed infant.

➤ *infliximab-abda* (B)

Renflexis *Vial:* 100 mg pwdr for reconstitution to 10 ml administration volume, single-dose

Comment: **Renflexis** is biosimilar to **Remicade**. *(infliximab).*

➤ *infliximab-dyyb* (B)

Inflectra *Vial:* 100 mg pwdr for reconstitution to 10 ml administration volume, single-dose

Comment: **Inflectra** is biosimilar to **Remicade**. *(infliximab).*

➤ *infliximab-axxq*

Avsola *Vial:* 100 mg pwdr in a 20 ml single-dose vial, for reconstitution, dilution, and IV infusion

Comment: **Avsola** is biosimilar to **Remicade** *(infliximab).*

➤ *infliximab-qbtx* (B)

Ixifi *Vial:* 100 mg pwdr for reconstitution to 10 ml administration volume, single-dose

Comment: **Ixifi** is biosimilar to **Remicade**. *(infliximab).*

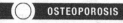 **OSTEOPOROSIS**

Comment: Indications for bone density screening include post-menopausal women <u>not</u> receiving HRT, maternal history of hip fracture, personal history of fragility fracture, presence of high serum markers of bone resorption, smoker, height >67 inches, weight <125 lb, taking a steroid, GnRH agonist, <u>or</u> antiseizure drug, immobilization, hyperthyroidism, posttransplantation, malabsorption syndrome, hyperparathyroidism, prolactinemia. The mnemonic ABONE [Age >65, Bulk (weight <140 lbs at menopause), and Never Estrogens (for more than 6 months)], represents other indications for bone density screening. Foods high in calcium include almonds, broccoli, baked beans, salmon, sardines, buttermilk, turnip greens, collard greens, spinach, pumpkin, rhubarb, and bran. Recommended Daily Calcium Intake: 1-3 years: 700 mg; 4-8 years: 1000 mg; 9-18 years: 1300 mg; 19-50 years: 1000 mg; 51-70 years (males): 1000 mg; ≥51 years (females): 1200 mg; pregnancy or nursing: 1000-1300 mg; Recommended Daily Vitamin D Intake: >1 year: 600 IU; 50+ years: 800-1000 IU. Prior to initiating, or concomitant prescribing, corticosteroids in patients at risk for, or diagnosed with, osteoporosis, referral to the following ACR guidelines is recommended: ACR Guidelines on Prevention & Treatment of Glucocorticoid-induced Osteoporosis [press release, June 7, 2017]. Atlanta, GA. American College of Rheumatology www.rheumatology.org/About-Us/Newsroom/Press-Releases/ ID/812/ACR-Releases-Guideline-on-Prevention-Treatment-of-Glucocorticoid-Induced-Osteoporosis

ESTROGEN REPLACEMENT THERAPY

Comment: Estrogen plus progesterone is indicated for post-menopausal women with an intact uterus. *Estrogen* monotherapy is indicated in women without a uterus. The following list is not inclusive; for more estrogen replacement therapies *see Menopause*.

▷ *estradiol* (X)

    Alora initially 0.05 mg/day apply patch twice weekly to lower abdomen, upper quadrant of buttocks or outer aspect of hip

      Transdermal patch: 0.025, 0.05, 0.075, 0.1 mg/day (8, 24/pck)

    Climara initially 0.025 mg/day patch once/week to trunk

      Transdermal patch: 0.025, 0.0375, 0.05, 0.075, 0.1 mg/day (4, 8, 24/pck)

    Estrace 1-2 mg daily cyclically (3 weeks on and 1 week off)

      Tab: 0.5, 1, 2*mg (tartrazine)

    Estraderm initially apply one 0.05 mg/day patch twice weekly to trunk

      Transdermal patch: 0.05, 0.1 mg/day (8, 24/pck)

    Menostar apply one patch weekly to lower abdomen, below the waist; avoid the breasts; alternate sites; *Transdermal patch:* 14 mcg/day (4/pck)

    Minivelle initially one 0.0375 mg/day patch twice weekly to trunk area; adjust after one month of therapy

      Transdermal patch: 0.025, 0.0375, 0.05, 0.075, 0.1 mg/day (8/pck)

    Vivelle initially one 0.0375 mg/day patch twice weekly to trunk area; use with an oral progestin to prevent endometrial hyperplasia

      Transdermal patch: 0.025, 0.0375, 0.05, 0.075, 0.1 mg/day (8, 48/pck)

    Vivelle-Dot initially one 0.05 mg/day patch twice weekly to lower abdomen, below the waist; use with an oral progestin to prevent endometrial hyperplasia

      Transdermal patch: 0.025, 0.0375, 0.05, 0.075, 0.1 mg/day (8, 24/pck)

▷ *estradiol+levonorgestrel* (X) apply 1 patch weekly to lower abdomen; avoid waistline; alternate sites

    Climara Pro *Transdermal patch:* estra 0.045 mg+levo 0.015 mg per day (4/pck)

▷ *estradiol+norethindrone* (X) 1 tab daily

    Activella (G) *Tab:* estra 1 mg+noreth 0.5 mg

    FemHRT 1/5 *Tab:* estra 5 mcg+noreth 1 mg

▷ *estradiol+norgestimate* (X) one x 1 mg *estradiol* tab daily x 3 days, then 1 x *estradiol* 1 mg+norgestimate 0.09 mg tab once daily x 3 days; repeat this pattern continuously

    Ortho-Prefest *Tab:* estra 1 mg+norgest 0.09 mg (30/blister pck)

▷ *estrogen, conjugated (equine)* (X)

    Premarin 1 tab daily

      Tab: 0.3, 0.45, 0.625, 0.9, 1.25, 2.5 mg

▷ *estropipate, piperazine estrone sulfate* (X)(G)

    Ogen 0.625-1.25 mg daily cyclically (3 weeks on and 1 week off)

      Tab: 0.625, 1.25, 2.5 mg

    Ortho-Est 0.75-6 mg daily cyclically (3 weeks on and 1 week off)

      Tab: 0.625, 1.25 mg

ESTROGENS, CONJUGATED+ESTROGEN AGONIST-ANTAGONIST COMBINATION

▷ *estrogen, conjugated+bazedoxifene* (X)
> **Duavee** 1 tab daily
>> *Tab:* estra, conj 0.45 mg+baze 20 mg

CALCIUM SUPPLEMENTS

Comment: Take *calcium* supplements after meals to avoid gastric upset. Dosages of calcium over 2000 mg/day have <u>not</u> been shown to have any additional benefit. *calcium* decreases *tetracycline* absorption. *calcium* absorption is decreased by corticosteroids.

▷ *calcitonin-salmon* (C)
> **Fortical** 200 IU intranasally daily; alternate nostrils each day
>> *Nasal spray:* 200 IU/actuation (30 doses, 3.7 ml)
> **Miacalcin Nasal spray** 200 IU spray in one nostril once daily; alternate nostrils each day
>> *Nasal spray:* 200 IU/actuation (30 doses, 3.7 ml)
> **Miacalcin Injection** 100 units SC <u>or</u> IM every other day
>> *Vial:* 200 units/ml (2 ml)

Comment: Supplement diet with calcium (1 gm/day) and vitamin D (400 IU/day).

▷ *calcium carbonate* (C)(OTC)(G)
> **Rolaids** chew 2 tabs bid; max 14 tabs/day
>> *Chew tab:* 550 mg
> **Rolaids Extra Strength** chew 2 tabs bid; max 8 tabs/day
>> *Chew tab:* 1000 mg
> **Tums** chew 2 tabs bid; max 16 tabs/day
>> *Chew tab:* 500 mg
> **Tums Extra Strength** chew 2 tabs bid; max 10 tabs/day
>> *Chew tab:* 750 mg
> **Tum Sultra** chew 2 tabs bid; max 8 tabs/day
>> *Chew tab:* 1000 mg
> **Os-Cal 500** (OTC) 1-2 tab bid to tid
>> *Chew tab: elemental calcium carbonate* 500 mg

▷ *calcium carbonate+vitamin D* (C)(G)
> **Os-Cal 250+D** (OTC) 1-2 tab tid
>> *Tab:* calc carb 250 mg+vit d 125 IU
> **Os-Cal 500+D** (OTC) 1-2 tab bid-tid
>> *Tab:* calc carb 500 mg+vit d 125 IU
> **Viactiv** (OTC) 1 tab tid
>> *Chew tab:* calc carb 500 mg+vit d 100 IU+vit k 40 mcg

▷ *calcium citrate* (C)(G)
> **Citracal** (OTC) 1-2 tabs bid
>> *Tab:* calc cit 200 mg

▷ *calcium citrate+vitamin D* (C)(G)
> **Citracal+D** (OTC) 1-2 cplts bid
>> *Cplt:* calc cit 315 mg+vit d 200 IU
> **Citracal 250+D** (OTC) 1-2 tabs bid
>> *Tab:* calc cit 250 mg+vit d 62.3 IU

VITAMIN D ANALOGS

Comment: Concurrent *vitamin D* supplementation is contraindicated for patients taking *calcitriol* <u>or</u> *doxercalciferol* due to the risk of *vitamin D* toxicity.

▷ *calcitriol* (C) *Predialysis:* initially 0.25 mcg daily; may increase to 0.5 mcg daily; *Dialysis:* initially 0.25 mcg daily; may increase by 0.25 mcg/day at 4-8 week intervals; usual maintenance 0.5-1 mcg/day; *Hypoparathyroidism:* initially 0.25 mcg q AM; may increase by 0.25 mcg/day at 4- to 8-week intervals; usual maintenance 0.5-2 mcg/day

Pediatric: Predialysis: <3 years: 10-15 ng/kg/day; ≥3 years: initially 0.25 mcg daily; may increase to 0.5 mcg/day; *Dialysis:* not recommended; *Hypoparathyroidism:* initially 0.25 mcg daily; may increase by 0.25 mcg/day at 2-4 week intervals; usual maintenance (1-5 years) 0.25-0.75 mcg/day, (≥6 years) 0.5-2 mcg/day

    Rocaltrol *Cap:* 0.25, 0.5 mcg

    Rocaltrol Solution *Soln:* 1 mcg/ml (15 ml, single-use dispensers)

▷ *doxercalciferol* (C) initially 0.25 mcg q AM; may increase by 0.25 mcg/day at 4-8 week intervals; usual maintenance 0.5-2 mcg/day

Pediatric: initially 0.25 mcg daily; may increase by 0.25 mcg; 0.25 mcg/day at 2-4 week intervals; usual maintenance (1-5 years) 0.25-0.75 mcg/day, (≥6 years) 0.5-2 mcg/day

    Hectorol *Cap:* 0.25, 0.5 mcg

BISPHOSPHONATES (CALCIUM MODIFIERS)

Comment: Bisphosphonates should be swallowed whole in the AM with 6-8 oz of plain water 30 minutes before first meal, beverage, or other medications of the day. Monitor serum alkaline phosphatase. Contraindications include abnormalities of the esophagus which delay esophageal emptying such as stricture or achalasia, inability to stand or sit upright for at least 30 minutes post-dose, patients at risk of aspiration, and hypocalcemia. Co-administration of bisphosphonates and *calcium*, antacids, or oral medications containing multivalent cations will interfere with absorption of the bisphosphonate. Therefore, instruct patients to wait at least half hour after taking the bisphosphonate before taking any other oral medications.

▷ *alendronate (as sodium)* (C)(G) take once weekly, in the AM, 30 minutes before the first food, beverage, or medication of the day; do not lie down (remain upright) for at least 30 minutes and after the first food of the day; *CrCl <35 mL/min:* not recommended

Pediatric: <12 years: not recommended; ≥12 years: same as adult

    Binosto dissolve the effervescent tab in 4 oz (120 ml) of plain, room temperature, water (not mineral or flavored); wait 5 minutes after the effervescence has subsided, then stir for 10 seconds, then drink

    Tab: 70 mg effervescent for buffered solution (4, 12/carton) (strawberry)

    Fosamax (G) swallow tab whole; dosing regimens are the same for men and post-menopausal women; *Prevention:* 5 mg once daily or 35 mg once weekly; *Treatment:* 10 mg once daily or 70 mg once weekly

    Tab: 5, 10, 35, 40, 70 mg

▷ *alendronate+cholecalciferol (vit d3)* (C)(G) take 1 tab once weekly, in the AM, with plain water (not mineral) 30 minutes before the first food, beverage, or medication of the day; do not lie down (remain upright) for at least 30 minutes and after the first food of the day

Pediatric: <12 years: not recommended; ≥12 years: same as adult

    Fosamax Plus D

    Tab: **Fosamax Plus D 70/2800** alen 70 mg+chole 2800 IU

    Fosamax Plus D 70/5600 alen 70 mg+chole 5600 IU

▷ *ibandronate (as monosodium monohydrate)* (C)(G)

Pediatric: <12 years: not recommended; ≥12 years: same as adult

    Boniva take 2.5 mg once daily or 150 mg once monthly on the same day; take in the AM, with plain water (not mineral) 60 minutes before the first food, beverage, or medication of the day; do not lie down (remain upright) for at least 30 minutes and after the first food of the day

    Tab: 2.5, 150 mg

    Boniva Injection administer 3 mg every 3 months by IV bolus over 15-30 seconds; if dose is missed, administer as soon as possible; then every 3 months from the date of the last dose

    Prefilled syringe: 3 mg/3 ml (5 ml)

Comment: **Boniva Injection** must be administered by a health care professional.

▷ *risedronate (as sodium)* (C)(G) take in the AM; swallow whole with a full glass of plain water (not mineral); do not lie down (remain upright) for 30 minutes afterward

Pediatric: <12 years: not recommended; ≥12 years: same as adult

Actonel take at least 30 minutes before any food or drink; *Women:* 5 mg once daily or 35 mg once weekly or 75 mg on two consecutive days monthly or 150 mg once monthly; *Men:* 35 mg once weekly

Tab: 5, 30, 35, 75, 150 mg

Atelvia 35 mg once weekly immediately after breakfast

Tab: 35 mg del-rel

▷ *risedronate+calcium* (C) 1 x 5 mg *risedronate* tab weekly plus 1 x 500 mg *calcium* tab on days 2-7 weekly

Actonel with Calcium *Tab: risedronate* 5 mg and *Tab: calcium* 500 mg (4 *risedronate* tabs + 30 *calcium* tabs/pck)

▷ *zoledronic acid* (D)(G)

Pediatric: <12 years: not recommended; ≥12 years: same as adult

Reclast administer 5 mg via IV infusion over at least 15 minutes mg once a year (for osteoporosis) or once every 2 years (for osteopenia or prophylaxis)

Bottle: 5 mg/100 ml (single-dose)

Comment: **Reclast** is indicated for the treatment of post-menopausal osteoporosis in women who are at high risk for fracture and to increase bone mass in men with primary or hypogonadal osteoporosis who are at high risk for fracture. Administered by a healthcare professional. Contraindicated in hypocalcemia.

Zometa *Bottle:* 4 mg/5 ml administer 4 mg via IV infusion over at least 15 minutes every 3-4 weeks; optimal duration of treatment not known

Vial: 4 mg/5 ml (single-dose)

Comment: **Zometa** is indicated for the treatment of hypercalcemia of malignancy. The safety and efficacy of **Zometa** in the treatment of hypercalcemia associated with hyperparathyroidism or with other nontumor-related conditions has not been established.

SELECTIVE ESTROGEN RECEPTOR MODULATOR (SERMs)

▷ *raloxifene* (X)(G) 60 mg once daily

Evista *Tab:* 60 mg

Comment: Contraindicated in women who have history of, or current, venous thrombotic event.

HUMAN PARATHYROID HORMONE RELATED PEPTIDE (PTHrP[1-34]) ANALOG

▷ *abaloparatide* 80 mcg (40 mcl) SC once daily

Tymlos *Pen:* 80 mcg/40 mcl (1.56 ml, 2000 mcg/ml) (30 doses) preassembled, single-patient use, disposable w. glass cartridge

Comment: **Tymlos** is a bone building agent for the treatment of post-menopausal women with osteoporosis at high risk for fracture. **Tymlos** is not indicated for use in females of reproductive potential. There are no human data with use in pregnant females to inform any drug associated risks and animal reproduction studies with *abaloparatide* have not been conducted. There is no information on the presence of *abaloparatide* in human milk, the effects on the breastfed infant, or the effects on milk production; however, breastfeeding is not recommended while using **Tymlos**. **Tymlos** is not recommended for use in pediatric patients with open epiphyses or hereditary disorders predisposing to osteosarcoma because of an increased baseline risk of osteosarcoma. **Tymlos** may cause hypercalciuria. It is unknown whether

Tymlos may exacerbate urolithiasis in patients with active or a history of urolithiasis. If active urolithiasis or pre-existing hypercalciuria is suspected, measurement of urinary calcium excretion should be considered. No dosage adjustment is required for patients any degree of renal impairment. Currently, there are no specific drug-drug interaction studies.

▷ *teriparatide* (C)

Forteo Multidose Pen 20 mcg SC daily in the thigh or abdomen; may treat for up to 2 years

Pediatric: <12 years: not recommended; ≥12 years: same as adult

Multi-dose pen: 250 mcg/ml (3 ml)

Comment: **Forteo** is indicated for the treatment of postmenopausal osteoporosis in women who are at high risk for fracture and to increase bone mass in men with primary or hypogonadal osteoporosis who are at high risk for fracture. **Bonsity** 20 mcg SC once daily; administer via SC injection only into the abdominal wall or thigh; initial administration under circumstances in which the patient can sit or lie down if symptoms of orthostatic hypotension occur; during the use period, time out of the refrigerator should be minimized; the dose may be delivered immediately following removal from the refrigerator

Pediatric: not recommended

Prefilled pen: 620 mcg/2.48 ml (250 mcg/ml), single-patient-use, containing 28 daily SC doses of 20 mcg

Comment: **Bonsity** *(teriparatide)* is a parathyroid hormone analog (PTH 1-34) indicated for the treatment of osteoporosis in certain patients at high risk for fracture, increase bone mass in men with primary or hypogonadal osteoporosis at high risk for fracture, and treatment of men and women with osteoporosis associated with sustained systemic glucocorticoid therapy at high risk for fracture. Use of **Bonsity** *(teriparatide)* more than 2 years during a patient's lifetime is not recommended. Patients with Paget's disease of bone, pediatric and young adult patients with open epiphyses, and patients with prior external beam or implant radiation involving the skeleton should not be treated with **Bonsity**. Use of **Bonsity** for more than 2 years during a patient's lifetime is not recommended. Patients with bone metastases, history of skeletal malignancies, metabolic bone diseases other than osteoporosis, or hypercalcemic disorders should not be treated with **Bonsity**. **Bonsity** may *increase* serum calcium, urinary calcium, and serum uric acid. Use with caution in patients with active or recent urolithiasis due to risk of exacerbation. Transient orthostatic hypotension may occur with initial doses of **Bonsity**; therefore, administer under circumstances in which the patient can sit or lie down. Use **Bonsity** with caution in patients receiving *digoxin* as transient hypercalcemia may predispose the patient to digitalis toxicity. Consider discontinuing **Bonsity** when pregnancy is recognized. Breastfeeding is not recommended during treatment with **Bonsity**. Most common adverse reactions (incidence >10%) reported have been arthralgia, pain, and nausea.

BIOENGINEERED REPLICA OF HUMAN PARATHYROID HORMONE

▷ *bioengineered replica of human parathyroid hormone* (C) initially inject mg IM into the thigh once daily; when initiating, decrease dose of active *vitamin D* by 50% if serum *calcium* is above 7.5 mg/dL; monitor serum *calcium* levels every 3-7 days after starting or adjusting dose and when adjusting either active *vitamin D* or *calcium* supplements dose

Pediatric: <18 years: not recommended; ≥18 years: same as adult

Natpara *Soln for inj:* 25, 50, 75, 100 mcg (2/pkg) multi-dose, dual-chamber glass cartridge containing a sterile powder and diluent

Comment: **Natpara** is indicated as adjunct to *calcium* and *vitamin D* in patients with parathyroidism.

OSTEOCLAST INHIBITOR (RANK LIGAND [RANKL] INHIBITOR)

▷ *denosumab* (X)

Pediatric: <18 years: not established; treatment with **Prolia** may impair bone growth in children with open growth plates and may inhibit eruption of dentition. ≥18 years: same as adult

Prolia for SC route only; should not be administered intravenously, intramuscularly, or intradermally; 60 mcg SC once every 6 months in the upper arm, abdomen, or upper thigh

Vial/Pen: 60 mg/ml (1 ml) single-dose

Comment: **Prolia** is indicated for the treatment of post-menopausal osteoporosis in females who are at high risk for fracture defined as a history of osteoporotic fracture or multiple risk factors for fracture or patients who have failed or are intolerant to other therapy and treatment to increase bone mass in women at high risk for fracture receiving adjuvant aromatase inhibitor therapy for breast cancer.

Prolia is also indicated for treatment to increase bone mass in men at high risk for fracture receiving androgen deprivation therapy for non-metastatic prostate cancer. **Prolia** must be administered by a healthcare professional. *denosumab* contraindicated with hypocalcemia. Instruct patients to take *calcium* 1,000 mg daily and at least 400 IU *vitamin D* daily. There is no information regarding the presence of *denosumab* in human milk or effects on the breastfed invent.

Xgeva *Multiple Myeloma and Bone Metastasis from Solid Tumors: admin*ister 120 mg administer SC in the upper arm, abdomen, or upper thigh; SC every 4 weeks; *Giant Cell Tumor of Bone:* administer 120 mg SC 4 every weeks with additional 120 mg doses on Days 8 and 15 of the first month of therapy and administer calcium and vitamin D as necessary to treat or prevent hypocalcemia; *Hypercalcemia of Malignancy:* administer 120 mg every 4 weeks with additional 120 mg doses Days 8 and 15 of the first month of therapy

Pediatric: recommended only for treatment of skeletally mature adolescents with giant cell tumor of bone; treatment with **Xgeva** may impair bone growth in children with open growth plates and may inhibit eruption of dentition

Vial: 120 mg/1.7 ml (70 mg/ml) solution in a single-dose

Comment: **Xgeva** is indicated for prevention of skeletal-related events in patients with multiple myeloma and in patients with bone metastases from solid tumors, treatment of adults and skeletally mature adolescents with giant cell tumor of bone that is un-resectable or where surgical resection is likely to result in severe morbidity, and treatment of hypercalcemia of malignancy refractory to bisphosphonate therapy. CrCl < 30 mL/min or receiving dialysis are at risk for hypocalcemia. Adequately supplement with calcium and vitamin D. There is no information regarding the presence of *denosumab* in human milk or effects on the breastfed invent.

ANTI-SCLEROSTIN MONOCLONAL ANTIBODY

▷ *romosozumab-aqqg* a full dose of **Evenity** requires two single-use prefilled syringes (2 x 105 mg=210 mg) administered SC (administered one after the other) in the upper arm, abdomen, or thigh once each month for 12 full doses (12 months) along with adequately supplemented calcium and vitamin D during treatment; **Evenity** should be administered by a qualified healthcare provider; limit duration of use to 12 monthly treatments

Evenity *Prefilled syringe:* 105 mg/1.17 ml, single-use (2/carton) (no natural rubber latex)

Comment: **Evenity** *(romosozumab-aqqg)* is an anti-sclerostin monoclonal antibody for the treatment of osteoporosis in post-menopausal women at increased risk of fracture defined as a history of osteoporotic fracture or multiple risk factors for fracture or patients who have failed or are intolerant to other available osteoporosis therapy. If after the 12 monthly treatments osteoporosis therapy remains warranted, continued therapy with an anti-resorptive agent should be considered. Monitor serum calcium; patients with severe renal impairment or receiving dialysis are at greater risk of developing hypocalcemia. **Evenity** should <u>not</u> be initiated in patients who have had a myocardial infarction or stroke within the preceding year. Consider whether the benefits outweigh the risks in patients with other cardiovascular risk factors. If a patient experiences a myocardial infarction or stroke during therapy, **Evenity** should be discontinued. **Evenity** is <u>not</u> indicated for use in women of reproductive potential or pediatric patients.

 OTITIS EXTERNA

OTIC ANALGESIC

▷ *antipyrine+benzocaine+zinc acetate dihydrate* (C) fill ear canal with solution; then insert a cotton plug into meatus; may repeat every 1-2 hours prn
Pediatric: same as adult
   Otozin *Otic soln:* antipyr 5.4%+benz 1%+zinc1% per ml (10 ml w. dropper)

OTIC ANTI-INFECTIVE

▷ *chloroxylenol+pramoxine* (C) 4-5 drops tid x 5-10 days
Pediatric: <1 year: not recommended; 1-12 years: 5 drops bid x 10 days; ≥12 years: same as adult
   PramOtic *Otic drops:* chlorox+pramox (5 ml w. dropper)
▷ *finafloxacin* (C) otic 4-5 drops tid x 5-10 days
Pediatric: <1 year: not recommended; ≥1 year: same as adult
   Xtoro *Otic soln:* 0.3% (5, 8 ml)
▷ *ofloxacin* (C)(G) 10 drops bid x 10 days
Pediatric: <1 year: not recommended; 1-12 years: 5 drops bid x 10 days; ≥12 years: same as adult
   Floxin Otic *Otic soln:* 0.3% (5, 10 ml w. dropper; 0.25 ml, 5 drop singles, 20/carton)
   Comment: **Floxin Otic** is indicated for adult patients with perforated tympanic membranes and pediatric patients with PE tubes.

OTIC ANTI-INFECTIVE+CORTICOSTEROID COMBINATIONS

▷ *chloroxylenol+pramoxine+hydrocortisone* (C)(G) drops 4 drops tid-qid x 5-10 days
Pediatric: 3 drops tid-qid x 5-10 days
   Cortane B, Cortane B Aqueous *Otic soln:* chlo 1 mg+pram 10 mg+hydro 10 mg per ml (10 ml w. dropper)
   Comment: **Cortane B Aqueous** may be used to saturate a cotton wick.
▷ *ciprofloxacin+hydrocortisone* (C) susp 3 drops bid x 7 days
Pediatric: <1 year: not recommended; ≥1 year: same as adult
   Cipro HC Otic *Otic susp:* cipro 0.2%+hydro 1% (10 ml w. dropper)
▷ *ciprofloxacin+dexamethasone* (C)(G) 4 drops bid x 7 days
Pediatric: <6 months: not recommended; ≥6 months: same as adult
   Ciprodex *Otic susp:* cipro 0.3%+dexa 1% (7.5 ml)
   Comment: **Ciprodex** is indicated for the treatment of otitis media in pediatric patients with tympanostomy tubes.
▷ *colistin+neomycin+hydrocortisone+thonzonium* (C)(G) 5 drops tid <u>or</u> qid x 5-10 days
Pediatric: 4 drops tid-qid x 5-10 days
   Coly-Mycin S *Otic susp:* 5, 10 ml

> **Cortisporin-TC Otic** *Otic susp:* colis 3 mg+neo 3.3 mg+hydro 10 mg+thon 0.5 mg per ml (10 ml w. dropper) (thimerosal)

▷ *polymyxin b+neomycin+hydrocortisone* (C)(G) 4 drops tid-qid; max 10 days
Pediatric: 3 drops tid-qid; max 10 days

> **Cortisporin Otic Suspension** *Otic susp:* poly b 10,000 u+neo 3.5 mg+hydro 10 mg per 5 ml (10 ml w. dropper)

> **Cortisporin Otic Solution** *Otic soln:* poly b 10000 u+neo 3.5 mg+hydro 10 mg per 5 ml (10 ml w. dropper)

OTIC ASTRINGENTS

▷ *acetic acid 2% in aluminum sulfate* (C)(G) 4-6 drops q 2-3 hours
Pediatric: same as adult

> **Domeboro Otic** *Otic soln:* 60 ml w. dropper

▷ *acetic acid+propylene glycol+benzethonium chloride+sodium acetate* (C)(G) 3-5 drops q 4-6 hours
Pediatric: same as adult

> **VoSol** *Otic soln:* acet 2% (15, 30 ml)

▷ *acetic acid+propylene glycol+hydrocortisone+benzethonium chloride+sodium acetate* (C)(G) 3-5 drops q 4-6 hours
Pediatric: same as adult

> **VoSol HC** *Otic soln:* acet 2%+hydro 1% (10 ml)

OTIC ANESTHETIC+ANALGESIC COMBINATIONS

▷ *antipyrine+benzocaine+glycerine* (C)(G) fill ear canal and insert cotton plug; may repeat q 1-2 hours as needed
Pediatric: same as adult

> **A/B Otic** *Otic soln:* 15 ml w. dropper

▷ *benzocaine* (C)(G) 4-5 drops q 1-2 hours
Pediatric: <1 year: not recommended; ≥1 year: same as adult

> **Americaine Otic** *Otic soln:* 20% (15 ml w. dropper)

> **Benzotic** *Otic soln:* 20% (15 ml w. dropper)

SYSTEMIC ANTI-INFECTIVES

Comment: Used for severe disease *or* with culture.

▷ *amoxicillin+clavulanate* (B)(G)

> **Augmentin** 500 mg tid *or* 875 mg bid x 7-10 days
Pediatric: 40-45 mg/kg/day divided tid x 10 days *or* 90 mg/kg/day divided bid x 10 days *see* Appendix CC.4. *amoxicillin+clavulanate* (Augmentin Suspension) *for dose by weight*

> > *Tab:* 250, 500, 875 mg; *Chew tab:* 125, 250 mg (lemon-lime); 200, 400 mg (cherry-banana) (phenylalanine); *Oral susp:* 125 mg/5 ml (banana), 250 mg/5 ml (75, 100, 150 ml) (orange); 200, 400 mg/5 ml (50, 75, 100 ml) (orange) (phenylalanine)

> **Augmentin ES-600** not recommended for adults
Pediatric: <3 months: not recommended; ≥3 months, <40 kg: 90 mg/kg/day in 2 divided doses x 7-10 days; ≥40 kg: not recommended

> > *Oral susp:* 42.9 mg/5 ml (50, 75, 100, 125, 150, 200 ml) (strawberry cream) (phenylalanine)

> **Augmentin XR** 2 tabs q 12 hours x 7-10 days
Pediatric: <16 years: use other forms; ≥16 years: same as adult

> > *Tab:* 1000*mg ext-rel

▷ *cefaclor* (B)(G)

> **Ceclor** 250 mg tid *or* 375 mg bid 3-10 days
Pediatric: <1 month: not recommended; 1 month-12 years: 20-40 mg/kg divided bid or q 12 hours x 3-10 days; max 1 gm/day; see Appendix CC.8. *cefaclor* (Ceclor Suspension) for *dose by weight;* >12 years: same as adult

Tab: 500 mg; Cap: 250, 500 mg; Susp: 125 mg/5 ml (75, 150 ml)
(strawberry); 187 mg/5 ml (50, 100 ml) (strawberry); 250 mg/5 ml (75, 150 ml) (strawberry); 375 mg/5 ml (50, 100 ml) (strawberry)

Ceclor Extended Release 375-500 mg bid x 3-10 days
Pediatric: <16 years: ext-rel not recommended; ≥16 years: same as adult
Tab: 375, 500 mg ext-rel

▷ *dicloxacillin* (B) 500 mg qid x 7-10 days
Pediatric: 12.5-25 mg/kg/day in 4 divided doses x 7-10 days; see Appendix CC.18.
dicloxacillin (Dynapen Suspension) for dose by weight
Dynapen Cap: 125, 250, 500 mg; Oral susp: 62.5 mg/5 ml (80, 100, 200 ml)

▷ *trimethoprim+sulfamethoxazole (TMP-SMX)* (C)(G)
Pediatric: <2 months: not recommended; ≥2 months: 40 mg/kg/
day of *sulfamethoxazole* in 2 doses bid x 10 days; see Appendix CC.33:
trimethoprim+sulfamethoxazole (Bactrim Suspension, Septra Suspension) for dose by weight
Bactrim, Septra 2 tabs bid x 10 days
Tab: trim 80 mg+sulfa 400 mg*
Bactrim DS, Septra DS 1 tab bid x 10 days
Tab: trim 160 mg+sulfa 800 mg*
Bactrim Pediatric Suspension, Septra Pediatric Suspension
Oral susp: trim 40 mg+sulfa 200 mg per 5 ml (100 ml) (cherry) (alcohol 0.3%)

OTITIS MEDIA: ACUTE

OTIC ANALGESIC

▷ *antipyrine+benzocaine+zinc acetate dihydrate* otic (C) fill ear canal with
solution; then insert cotton plug into meatus; may repeat every 1-2 hours prn
Pediatric: same as adult
Otozin Otic soln: antipyr 5.4%+benz 1%+zinc1% per ml (10 ml w. dropper)

SYSTEMIC ANTI-INFECTIVES

▷ *amoxicillin* (B)(G) 500-875 mg bid or 250-500 mg tid x 10 days
Pediatric: <40 kg (88 lb): 20-40 mg/kg/day in 3 divided doses x 10 days or 25-45
mg/kg/day in 2 divided doses x 10 days; see Appendix CC.3. amoxicillin (Amoxil
Suspension, Trimox Suspension) for dose by weight
Amoxil Cap: 250, 500 mg; Tab: 875*mg; Chew tab: 125, 200, 250, 400 mg
(cherry-banana-peppermint) (phenylalanine); Oral susp: 125, 250 mg/5 ml
(80, 100, 150 ml) (strawberry); 200, 400 mg/5 ml (50, 75, 100 ml) (bubble
gum); Oral drops: 50 mg/ml (30 ml) (bubble gum)
Moxatag Tab: 775 mg ext-rel
Trimox Tab: 125, 250 mg; Cap: 250, 500 mg; Oral susp: 125, 250 mg/5 ml (80,
100, 150 ml) (raspberry-strawberry)
Comment: Consider 80-90 mg/kg/day in 3 divided doses for resistant for cases

▷ *amoxicillin+clavulanate* (B)(G)
Augmentin 500 mg tid or 875 mg bid x 7-10 days
Pediatric: 40-45 mg/kg/day divided tid x 10 days or 90 mg/kg/day divided bid
x 10 days see Appendix CC.4. amoxicillin+clavulanate (Augmentin Suspension) for dose by weight
Tab: 250, 500, 875 mg; Chew tab: 125, 250 mg (lemon-lime); 200, 400 mg
(cherry-banana) (phenylalanine); Oral susp: 125 mg/5 ml (banana), 250
mg/5 ml (75, 100, 150 ml) (orange); 200, 400 mg/5 ml (50, 75, 100 ml)
(orange) (phenylalanine)
Augmentin ES-600 not recommended for adults
Pediatric: <3 months: not recommended; ≥3 months, <40 kg: 90 mg/kg/day in
2 divided doses x 7-10 days; ≥40 kg: not recommended

Oral susp: 42.9 mg/5 ml (50, 75, 100, 125, 150, 200 ml) (strawberry cream) (phenylalanine)

Augmentin XR 2 tabs q 12 hours x 7-10 days
Pediatric: <16 years: use other forms; ≥16 years: same as adult
Tab: 1000*mg ext-rel

▷ *ampicillin* (B) 250-500 mg qid x 10 days
Pediatric: 50-100 mg/kg/day in 4 divided doses x 10 days; *see* Appendix CC.6.
ampicillin (Omnipen Suspension, Principen Suspension) *for dose by weight*
Omnipen, Principen *Cap:* 250, 500 mg; *Oral susp:* 125, 250 mg/5 ml (100, 150, 200 ml) (fruit)

▷ *azithromycin* (B)(G) 500 mg x 1 dose on day 1, then 250 mg daily on days 2-5 or 500 mg daily x 3 days or **Zmax** 2 gm in a single dose
Pediatric: 12 mg/kg/day x 5 days; max 500 mg/day; *see* Appendix CC.7.
azithromycin (Zithromax Suspension, Zmax Suspension) *for dose by weight*
Zithromax *Tab:* 250, 500, 600 mg; *Oral susp:* 100 mg/5 ml (15 ml); 200 mg/5 ml (15, 22.5, 30 ml) (cherry); *Pkt:* 1 gm for reconstitution (cherry-banana)
Zithromax Tri-pak *Tab:* 3 x 500 mg tabs/pck
Zithromax Z-pak *Tab:* 6 x 250 mg tabs/pck
Zmax *Oral susp:* 2 gm ext-rel for reconstitution (cherry-banana) (148 mg Na⁺)

▷ *cefaclor* (B)(G)
Ceclor 250 mg tid or 375 mg bid 3-10 days
Pediatric: <1 month: not recommended; 1 month-12 years: 20-40 mg/kg divided bid or q 12 hours x 3-10 days; max 1 gm/day; see Appendix CC.8.
cefaclor (Ceclor Suspension) for *dose by weight*; >12 years: same as adult
Tab: 500 mg; *Cap:* 250, 500 mg; *Susp:* 125 mg/5 ml (75, 150 ml) (strawberry); 187 mg/5 ml (50, 100 ml) (strawberry); 250 mg/5 ml (75, 150 ml) (strawberry); 375 mg/5 ml (50, 100 ml) (strawberry)
Ceclor Extended Release 375-500 mg bid x 3-10 days
Pediatric: <16 years: ext-rel not recommended; ≥16 years: same as adult
Tab: 375, 500 mg ext-rel

▷ *cefdinir* (B) 300 mg bid or 600 mg daily x 5-10 days
Pediatric: <6 months: not recommended; 6 months-12 years: 14 mg/kg/day in 1-2 divided doses x 10 days; >12 years: same as adult; *see* Appendix CC.10. *cefdinir* (Omnicef Suspension) *for dose by weight*
Omnicef *Cap:* 300 mg; *Oral susp:* 125 mg/5 ml (60, 100 ml) (strawberry)

▷ *cefixime* (B)(G)
Pediatric: <6 months: not recommended; 6 months-12 years, <50 kg: 8 mg/kg/day in 1-2 divided doses x 10 days; >12 years, ≥50 kg: same as adult; *see* Appendix CC.11. *cefixime* (Suprax Oral Suspension) *for dose by weight*
Suprax *Tab:* 400 mg; *Cap:* 400 mg; *Oral susp:* 100, 200, 500 mg/5 ml (50, 75, 100 ml) (strawberry)

▷ *cefpodoxime proxetil* (B) 100 mg bid x 5 days
Pediatric: <2 months: not recommended; 2 months-12 years: 10 mg/kg/day (max 400 mg/dose) or 5 mg/kg/day bid (max 200 mg/dose) x 5 days; >12 years: same as adult; *see* Appendix CC.12. *cefpodoxime proxetil* (Vantin Suspension) *for dose by weight*
Vantin *Tab:* 100, 200 mg; *Oral susp:* 50, 100 mg/5 ml (50, 75, 100 ml) (lemon creme)

▷ *cefprozil* (B) 250-500 mg bid or 500 mg daily x 10 days
Pediatric: <2 years: same as adult; 2-12 years: 7.5 mg/kg bid x 10 days; *see* Appendix CC.13. *cefprozil* (Cefzil Suspension) *for dose by weight;* >12 years: same as adult
Cefzil *Tab:* 250, 500 mg; *Oral susp:* 125, 250 mg/5 ml (50, 75, 100 ml) (bubble gum) (phenylalanine)

▷ *ceftibuten* (B) 400 mg daily x 10 days
  Pediatric: 9 mg/kg daily x 10 days; max 400 mg/day; *see* Appendix CC.14.
  ceftibuten (Cedax Suspension) *for dose by weight*
    Cedax *Cap:* 400 mg; *Oral susp:* 90 mg/5 ml (30, 60, 90, 120 ml); 180 mg/5 ml
    (30, 60, 120 ml) (cherry)
▷ *ceftriaxone* (B)(G) 1-2 gm IM x 1 dose; max 4 gm
  Pediatric: 50 mg/kg IM x 1 dose
    Rocephin *Vial:* 250, 500 mg; 1, 2 gm
▷ *cephalexin* (B)(G) 250 mg qid x 10 days
  Pediatric: 25-50 mg/kg/day in 4 doses x 10 days; *see* Appendix CC.15. *cephalexin*
  (Keflex Suspension) *for dose by weight*
    Keflex *Cap:* 250, 333, 500, 750 mg; *Oral susp:* 125, 250 mg/5 ml (100, 200 ml)
    (strawberry)
▷ *clarithromycin* (C)(G) 500 mg bid or 500 mg ext-rel once daily x 10 days
  Pediatric: <6 months: not recommended; ≥6 months: 7.5 mg/kg divided bid x 7
  days; *see* Appendix CC.16. *clarithromycin* (Biaxin Suspension) *for dose by weight*
    Biaxin *Tab:* 250, 500 mg
    Biaxin Oral Suspension *Oral susp:* 125, 250 mg/5 ml (50, 100 ml) (fruit-punch)
    Biaxin XL *Tab:* 500 mg ext-rel
▷ *erythromycin+sulfisoxazole* (C)(G)
  Pediatric: <2 months: not recommended; ≥2 months: 50 mg/kg/day in 3 divided
  doses x 10 days; *see* Appendix CC.22. *erythromycin+sulfamethoxazole* (Eryzole,
  Pediazole) *for dose by weight*
    Eryzole *Oral susp:* eryth 200 mg+sulfa 600 mg per 5 ml (100, 150, 200, 250 ml)
    Pediazole *Oral susp:* eryth 200 mg+sulfa 600 mg per 5 ml (100, 150, 200 ml)
    (strawberry-banana)
▷ *loracarbef* (B) 400 mg bid x 10 days
  Pediatric: 30 mg/kg/day in divided bid x 7 days; *see* Appendix CC.27. *loracarbef*
  (Lorabid Suspension) *for dose by weight*
    Lorabid *Pulvule:* 200, 400 mg; *Oral susp:* 100 mg/5 ml (50, 100 ml); 200 mg/5
    ml (50, 75, 100 ml) (strawberry bubble gum)
▷ *trimethoprim+sulfamethoxazole (TMP-SMX])* (C)(G)
  Pediatric: <2 months: not recommended; >2 months: 40 mg/kg/day of
  sulfamethoxazole in divided doses bid x 10 days; *see Appendix CC.33: trimethoprim+*
  sulfamethoxazole (Bactrim Suspension, Septra Suspension) *for dose by weight*
    Bactrim, Septra 2 tabs bid x 10 days
      Tab: trim 80 mg+sulfa 400 mg*
    Bactrim DS, Septra DS 1 tab bid x 10 days
      Tab: trim 160 mg+sulfa 800 mg*
    Bactrim Pediatric Suspension, Septra Pediatric Suspension
      Oral susp: trim 40 mg+sulfa 200 mg per 5 ml (100 ml) (cherry) (alcohol
      0.3%)

OTIC ANTI-INFECTIVE

▷ *ofloxacin* (C)(G) 10 drops bid x 14 days
  Pediatric: <6 months: not recommended; 6 months-12 years: 5 drops bid x 14
  days; >12 years: same as adult
    Floxin Otic *Otic soln:* 0.3% (5, 10 ml w. dropper)

OTIC ANTI-INFECTIVE+CORTICOSTEROID COMBINATIONS

Comment: *Neomycin* may cause ototoxicity. Do not use with known or suspected
tympanic membrane rupture.
▷ *chloroxylenol+pramoxine+hydrocortisone* (C) 4 drops tid-qid x 5-10 days
  Pediatric: 3 drops tid-qid x 5-10 days
    Cortane Ear Drops, *Otic drops:* 10 ml

▷ *ciprofloxacin+hydrocortisone* (C) otic susp 3 drops bid x 7 days
  Pediatric: <1 year: not recommended; ≥1 year: same as adult
    Cipro HC *Otic susp:* cipro 0.3%+dexa 0.1% (10 ml)
▷ *ciprofloxacin+dexamethasone* (C)(G) otic susp 4 drops bid x 7 days
  Pediatric: <6 months: not recommended; ≥6 months: same as adult
    Ciprodex *Otic susp:* cipro 0.3%+dexa 1% (7.5 ml)
    Comment: **Ciprodex** is indicated for the treatment of otitis media in pediatric patients with tympanostomy tubes (PE tubes).
▷ *colistin+neomycin+hydrocortisone+thonzonium* (C) 5 drops tid-qid x 5-10 days
  Pediatric: 4 drops tid-qid x 5-10 days
    Coly-Mycin S *Otic susp:* 5, 10 ml
▷ *polymyxin b+neomycin+hydrocortisone* (C)(G) 4 drops tid-qid; max 10 days
  Pediatric: 3 drops tid-qid; max 10 days
    Cortisporin *Otic susp:* 10 ml w. dropper; *Otic soln:* 10 ml w. dropper
    PediOtic *Otic susp:* 7.5 ml w. dropper
▷ *polymyxin b+neomycin+hydrocortisone+surfactant* (C) 4 drops tid-qid
  Pediatric: 3 drops tid-qid; max 10 days
    Cortisporin-TC *Otic susp:* 10 ml w. dropper

OTIC ANESTHETIC+ANALGESIC COMBINATIONS

▷ *antipyrine+benzocaine+glycerine* (C) fill ear canal and insert cotton plug; may repeat q 1-2 hours as needed
  Pediatric: same as adult
    A/B Otic *Otic soln:* antipy 5.4%+benzo 1.4% 15 ml w. dropper
▷ *benzocaine* (C)(OTC) 4-5 drops q 1-2 hours
  Pediatric: <1 year: not recommended; ≥1 year: same as adult
  benzocaine Otic drops: 20% (15 ml dropper-top bottle)
    Americaine Otic *Otic soln:* 15 ml w. dropper
    Benzotic *Otic soln:* 20% (15 ml w. dropper)

⬤ OTITIS MEDIA: SEROUS (SOM), OTITIS MEDIA WITH EFFUSION

Anti-infectives *see* **Otitis Media: Acute**
Antihistamines & Decongestants *see* Appendix AA. Drugs for the Management of Allergy, Cough, and Cold Symptoms online at https://connect.springerpub.com/content/reference-book/978-0-8261-7935-7/back-matter/part02/back-matter/bmatter27
Oral Corticosteroids *see* Appendix L. Oral Corticosteroids

INTRA-TYMPANIC AGENT

▷ *ciprofloxacin otic suspension* <6 months: not recommended; ≥6 months: instill 0.1 ml in each ear, via intra-tympanic administration <u>only</u> by a qualified healthcare professional, following suctioning of the middle ear effusion
    Otiprio *Vial:* 6% otic suspension (6 mg/ml, 1 ml) single-patient use with two 0.1 ml doses in each vial (preservative-free)
    Comment: **Otiprio** is *ciprofloxacin,* a synthetic fluoroquinolone antibacterial, indicated for the treatment of acute otitis media (AOM) due to *Pseudomonas aeruginosa* and *Staphylococcus aureus* and for intra-tympanic administration in pediatric patients ≥6 months-of-age with bilateral AOM with effusion undergoing tympanostomy tube placement. The bactericidal action of *ciprofloxacin* results from interference with the enzyme DNA gyrase, which is needed for the synthesis of bacterial DNA. *ciprofloxacin* has been shown to be active against most isolates of the following bacteria: Gram-positive Bacteria (i.e., *Staphylococcus aureus, Streptococcus pneumoniae*) and Gram-negative Bacteria (*Haemophilus influenza, Moraxella catarrhalis, Pseudomonas aeruginosa*). **Otiprio** is for intra-tympanic administration <u>only</u>.

The most frequently occurring adverse reactions (incidence > 3 %) were nasopharyngitis and irritability. Because of the negligible systemic exposure associated with clinical administration of **Otiprio**, this product is expected to be of minimal risk for maternal and fetal toxicity during pregnancy and nursing infants of mothers receiving **Otiprio** should not be affected.

OVARIAN CANCER

POLY ADP-RIBOSE POLYMERASE (PARP) INHIBITORS

▷ *niraparib tosolate* 300 mg (3 x 100 mg) once daily, with or without food
  Pediatric: safety and efficacy not established
  Zejula *Cap:* 100 mg
  Comment: **Zejula** *(niraparib)* is indicated for the maintenance treatment of adult patients with recurrent epithelial ovarian, fallopian tube, or primary peritoneal cancer who are in a complete or partial response to platinum-based chemotherapy, and for late-line treatment recurrent ovarian cancer. Continue treatment until disease progression or unacceptable adverse reaction; for adverse reactions, consider interruption of treatment, dose reduction, or dose discontinuation. The most common adverse reactions (incidence ≥10%) have been anemia, thrombocytopenia, neutropenia, leukopenia, hypertension, palpitations, nausea, vomiting, abdominal pain/distention, diarrhea, constipation, mucositis/stomatitis, dry mouth, fatigue/asthenia, dyspepsia, decreased appetite, urinary tract infection, AST/ALT elevation, back pain, myalgia, arthralgia, headache, dizziness, dysgeusia, insomnia, anxiety, nasopharyngitis, dyspnea, cough, and rash. Monitor CBC weekly for the first month, monitor CBC monthly for the next 11 months, and then periodically thereafter. Monitor BP and HR monthly for the first year and periodically thereafter. Manage BP and HR with appropriate medication as indicated and adjust the **Zejula** dose if necessary. Because myelodysplastic syndrome (MDS) and acute myeloid leukemia (AML) have occurred in patients exposed to **Zejula,** with some cases being fatal, monitor patients for hematological toxicity and discontinue **Zejula** if MDS/AML is confirmed. **Zejula** can cause embryo/fetal toxicity; therefore, advise females of reproductive potential of the potential risk and to use effective contraception. Advise women not to breastfeed during treatment with **Zejula** and for 1 month after receiving the final dose.

▷ *rucaparib* 600 mg twice daily with or without food
  Pediatric: safety and efficacy not established
  Rubraca *Tab:* 200, 250, 300 mg
  Comment: **Rubraca** *(rucaparib)* is indicated for the treatment of adult patients with a deleterious BRCA mutation (germline and/or somatic)-associated metastatic castration-resistant prostate cancer (mCRPC) who have been treated with androgen receptor-directed therapy and a taxane-based chemotherapy. This indication is approved under accelerated approval based on objective response rate and duration of response. Continued approval for this indication may be contingent upon verification and description of clinical benefit in confirmatory trials. Patients receiving Rubraca for mCRPC should also receive a gonadotropin-releasing hormone (GnRH) analog concurrently or should have had bilateral orchiectomy. Continue treatment until disease progression or unacceptable toxicity. For adverse reactions, consider interruption of treatment or dose reduction. The most common adverse reactions (incidence ≥20%) among patients with BRCA mutated mCRPC have been fatigue (inc asthenia), nausea, anemia, increased ALT/AST, decreased appetite, rash, constipation, thrombocytopenia, vomiting, and diarrhea. Myelodysplastic syndrome (MDS) and acute myeloid leukemia (AML) have occurred in patients exposed to **Rubraca**, and some cases have

been fatal. Monitor patients for hematological toxicity at baseline and monthly thereafter. Discontinue **Rubraca** if MDS/AML is confirmed. Adjust the dosage of CYP1A2, CYP3A, CYP2C9, and CYP2C19 substrates if clinically indicated. **Rubraca** can cause embryo/fetal harm. Advise females of reproductive potential of embryo/fetal risk and to use effective contraception. Advise females <u>not</u> to breastfeed.

PAGET'S DISEASE: BONE

Comment: Calcium decreases *tetracycline* absorption. *calcium* absorption is decreased by corticosteroids. *calcium* absorption is decreased by foods such as rhubarb, spinach, and bran.

BISPHOSPHONATES (CALCIUM MODIFIERS)

Comment: Bisphosphonates should be swallowed whole in the AM with 6-8 oz of plain water 30 minutes before first meal, beverage, <u>or</u> other medications of the day. Monitor serum alkaline phosphatase. Contraindications include abnormalities of the esophagus which delay esophageal emptying such as stricture <u>or</u> achalasia, inability to stand <u>or</u> sit upright for at least 30 minutes post-dose, patients at risk of aspiration, and hypocalcemia. Co-administration of bisphosphonates and calcium, antacids, <u>or</u> oral medications containing multivalent cations will interfere with absorption of the bisphosphonate. Therefore, instruct patients to wait at least half hour after taking the bisphosphonate before taking any other oral medications.

➤ *alendronate (as sodium)* (C)(G) take once weekly, in the AM, 30 minutes before the first food, beverage, <u>or</u> medication of the day; do <u>not</u> lie down (remain upright) for at least 30 minutes and after the first food of the day; <u>not</u> recommended with *CrCl <35 mL/min*.
Pediatric: <12 years: not recommended; ≥12 years: same as adult
  Binosto dissolve the effervescent tab in 4 oz (120 ml) of plain, room temperature, water (<u>not</u> mineral <u>or</u> flavored); wait 5 minutes after the effervescence has subsided, then stir for 10 seconds, then drink
    Tab: 70 mg effervescent for buffered solution (4, 12/carton) (strawberry)
  Fosamax (G) swallow tab whole; dosing regimens are the same for men and post-menopausal women; *Prevention:* 5 mg once daily <u>or</u> 35 mg once weekly; *Treatment:* 10 mg once daily <u>or</u> 70 mg once weekly
    Tab: 5, 10, 35, 40, 70 mg
➤ *alendronate+cholecalciferol (vit d3)* (C)(G) take 1 tab once weekly, in the AM, with plain water (<u>not</u> mineral) 30 minutes before the first food, beverage, <u>or</u> medication of the day; do <u>not</u> lie down (remain upright) for at least 30 minutes and after the first food of the day
Pediatric: <12 years: not recommended; ≥12 years: same as adult
  Fosamax Plus D
    Tab: **Fosamax Plus D 70/2800** alen 70 mg+chole 2800 IU
    Fosamax Plus D 70/5600 alen 70 mg+chole 5600 IU
➤ *ibandronate (as monosodium monohydrate)* (C)(G)
Pediatric: <12 years: not recommended; ≥12 years: same as adult
  Boniva take 2.5 mg once daily <u>or</u> 150 mg once monthly on the same day; take in the AM, with plain water (<u>not</u> mineral) 60 minutes before the first food, beverage, <u>or</u> medication of the day; do <u>not</u> lie down (remain upright) for at least 30 minutes and after the first food of the day
    Tab: 2.5, 150 mg
  Boniva Injection administer 3 mg every 3 months by IV bolus over 15-30 seconds; if dose is missed, administer as soon as possible, then every 3 months from the date of the last dose

Prefilled syringe: 3 mg/3 ml (5 ml)

Comment: Boniva Injection must be administered by a qualified healthcare professional.

▷ *risedronate (as sodium)* (C)(G) take in the AM; swallow whole with a full glass of plain water (<u>not</u> mineral) do <u>not</u> lie down (remain upright) for 30 minutes afterward

Pediatric: <12 years: not recommended; ≥12 years: same as adult

Actonel take at least 30 minutes before any food <u>or</u> drink; *Women:* 5 mg once daily <u>or</u> 35 mg once weekly <u>or</u> 75 mg on two consecutive days monthly <u>or</u> 150 mg once monthly; *Men:* 35 mg once weekly

Tab: 5, 30, 35, 75, 150 mg

Atelvia 35 mg once weekly immediately after breakfast

Tab: 35 mg del-rel

▷ *risedronate+calcium* (C) 1 x 5 mg *risedronate* tab weekly <u>and</u> 1 x 500 mg *calcium* tab on days 2-7 weekly

Actonel with Calcium *Tab: risedronate* 5 mg <u>and</u> *Tab: calcium* 500 mg (4 *risedronate* tabs + 30 *calcium* tabs/pck)

▷ *zoledronic acid* (D)(G)

Pediatric: <12 years: not recommended; ≥12 years: same as adult

Reclast administer 5 mg via IV infusion over at least 15 minutes mg once a year (for osteoporosis) <u>or</u> once every 2 years (for osteopenia <u>or</u> prophylaxis)

Bottle: 5 mg/100 ml (single-dose)

Comment: Reclast is indicated for the treatment of postmenopausal osteoporosis in women who are at high risk for fracture and to increase bone mass in men with primary <u>or</u> hypogonadal osteoporosis who are at high risk for fracture. Administered by a qualified healthcare professional. Contraindicated in hypocalcemia.

Zometa administer 4 mg via IV infusion over at least 15 minutes every 3-4 weeks; optimal duration of treatment <u>not</u> known

Bottle: 4 mg/5 ml; *Vial:* 4 mg/5 ml (single-dose)

Comment: Zometa is indicated for the treatment of hypercalcemia of malignancy. The safety and efficacy of **Zometa** in the treatment of hypercalcemia associated with hyperparathyroidism <u>or</u> with other non-tumor-related conditions has <u>not</u> been established.

 PAIN

Antidepressants *see Depression*
Skeletal Muscle Relaxants *see Muscle Strain*

ACETAMINOPHEN FOR IV INFUSION

▷ *acetaminophen* injectable (B) administer by IV infusion over 15 minutes; 1000 mg q 6 hours prn <u>or</u> 650 mg q 4 hours prn; max 4000 mg/day

Pediatric: <2 years: not recommended; 2-13 years <50 kg: 15 mg/kg q 6 hours prn <u>or</u> 2.5 mg/kg q 4 hours prn; max 750 mg/single dose; max 75 mg/kg per day; >13 years: same as adult

Ofirmev *Vial:* 10 mg/ml (100 ml) (preservative-free)

Comment: The **Ofirmev** vial is intended for single-use. If any portion is withdrawn from the vial, use within 6 hours. Discard the unused portion. For pediatric patients, withdraw the intended dose and administer via syringe pump. Do <u>not</u> admix **Ofirmev** with any other drugs.

Ofirmev is physically incompatible with *diazepam* and *chlorpromazine hydrochloride*.

IBUPROFEN FOR IV INFUSION

▷ *ibuprofen* (B) dilute dose in 0.9% NS, D5W, or Lactated Ringers (LR) solution; administer by IV infusion over at least 10 minutes; do not administer via IV bolus or IM; 400-800 mg q 6 hours prn; maximum 3,200 mg/day
Pediatric: <6 months; not recommended; 6 months-<12 years: 10 mg/kg q 4-6 hours prn; max 400 mg/dose; max 40 mg/kg or 2,400 mg/24 hours, whichever is less; 12-17 years: 400 mg q 4-6 hours prn; max 2,400 mg/24 hours
  Caldolor *Vial:* 800 mg/8 ml single-dose
  Comment: Prepare **Caldolor** solution for IV administration as follows: 100 mg dose: dilute 1 ml of **Caldolor** in at least 100 ml of diluent (IVF); 200 mg dose: dilute 2 ml of **Caldolor** in at least 100 ml of diluent; 400 mg dose: dilute 4 ml of **Caldolor** in at least 100 ml of diluent; 800 mg dose: dilute 8 ml of **Caldolor** in at least 200 ml of diluent. **Caldolor** is also indicated for management of fever. For adults with fever, 400 mg via IV infusion, followed by 400 mg q 4-6 hours or 100-200 mg q 4 hours prn.

MELOXICAM FOR IV INFUSION

▷ *meloxicam injection* administer 30 mg via IV bolus once daily; administer dose over 15 seconds; monitor analgesic response and administer a short-acting, non-NSAID, immediate-release analgesic if response is inadequate; patients must be well hydrated before **Anjeso** administration; use **Anjeso** for the shortest duration consistent with individual patient treatment goals
Pediatric: not established
  Anjeso *Vial:* 30 mg/ml (1 ml), single dose
  Comment: **Anjeso** *(meloxicam)* is an NSAID injection indicated for use in adults for the management of moderate-to-severe pain, alone or in combination with non-NSAID analgesics. Because of delayed onset of analgesia, **Anjeso** as monotherapy is not recommended for use when rapid onset of analgesia is required. The most common adverse reactions (incidence ≥ 2%) in controlled clinical trials have included constipation, GGT increase, and anemia. Use of NSAIDs during the third trimester of pregnancy increases the risk of premature closure of the fetal ductus arteriosus; therefore, avoid **Anjeso** use after 30 weeks gestation. There are no human data available on whether meloxicam is present in human milk, or on the effects on breastfed infants NSAIDs are associated with reversible infertility. Consider withdrawal of **Anjeso** in women who have difficulties conceiving. **Anjeso** may also compromise fertility in males of reproductive potential; it is not known if this effect on male fertility is reversible.

ACETAMINOPHEN+IBUPROFEN COMBINATION

▷ *ibuprofen+acetaminophen*
  Advil Dual Action with Acetaminophen (OTC) take 2 caplets every 8 hours prn pain; max 6 caplets/24 hours
Pediatric: <12 years: safety and efficacy not established; ≥12 years: 1-2 caplets every 8 hours prn pain; max 6 caplets/24 hours
  Cplt: fixed-dose combination of *ibuprofen* 125 mg (NSAID, antipyretic, analgesic) and *acetaminophen* 250 mg (antipyretic, analgesic)

OCULAR PAIN

▷ *dexamethasone ophthalmic insert* postsurgical insertion in the lower lacrimal punctum and into the canaliculus by a qualified healthcare provider; insert is resorbable (does not require removal); saline irrigation or manual expression can be performed if removal is necessary; a single insert provides sustained delivery of *dexamethasone* up to 30 days.
Pediatric: safety and efficacy not established

Dextenza 0.4 mg single dose in a foam carrier within a foil laminate pouch (preservative-free)

Comment: **Dextenza** is the first FDA-approved intra-canalicular insert delivering *dexamethasone* to treat postsurgical ocular pain for up to 30 days with a single administration.

▷ *difluprednate* (C) apply 1 drop to affected eye qid; for postop ocular pain, begin treatment 24 hours postop and continue x 2 weeks; then bid daily x 1 week; then taper

Pediatric: <12 years: not recommended; ≥12 years: same as adult

Durezol *Ophth emul:* 0.05% (5 ml)

Comment: **Durezol** is an ophthalmic steroid.

▷ *nepafenac* (C) apply 1 drop to affected eye tid; for postop ocular pain, begin treatment 24 hours before surgery and continue day of surgery and for 2 weeks post-op

Pediatric: <10 years: not recommended; ≥10 years: same as adult

Nevanac *Ophth susp:* 0.1% (3 ml) (benzalkonium chloride)

Comment: **Nevanac** is an ophthalmic NSAID.

TOPICAL & TRANSDERMAL ANALGESICS

▷ *capsaicin* (B)(G) apply tid-qid prn to intact skin

Pediatric: <2 years: not recommended; ≥2 years: apply sparingly tid-qid prn

Axsain *Crm:* 0.075% (1, 2 oz)

Capsin (OTC) *Lotn:* 0.025, 0.075% (59 ml)

Capzasin-HP (OTC) *Crm:* 0.075% (1.5 oz), 0.025% (45, 90 gm); *Lotn:* 0.075% (2 oz); 0.025% (45, 90 gm)

Capzasin-P (OTC) *Crm:* 0.025% (1.5 oz); *Lotn:* 0.025% (2 oz)

Dolorac *Crm:* 0.025% (28 gm)

Double Cap (OTC) *Crm:* 0.05% (2 oz)

R-Gel *Gel:* 0.025% (15, 30 gm)

Zostrix (OTC) *Crm:* 0.025% (0.7, 1.5, 3 oz)

Zostrix HP (OTC) *Emol crm:* 0.075% (1, 2 oz)

▷ *capsaicin* 8% patch (B) apply up to 4 patches for one 60-minute application to clean dry skin; may prep area with topical anesthetic; wear non-latex gloves; patches may be cut to size/shape; treatment may be repeated every 3 months

Pediatric: <18 years: not recommended; ≥18 years: same as adult

Qutenza *Patch:* 8% 1640 mcg/cm (179 mg) (1 or 2 patches w. 1-50 gm tube cleansing gel/carton)

▷ *diclofenac sodium* (C; D ≥30 wks) apply qid prn to intact skin

Pediatric: <12 years: not established; ≥12 years: same as adult

Pennsaid 1.5% in 10 drop increments, dispense and rub into front, side, and back of knee: usually; 40 drops (40 mg) qid

Topical soln: 1.5% (150 ml)

Pennsaid 2% apply 2 pump actuations (40 mg) and rub into front, side, and back of knee bid

Topical soln: 2% (20 mg/pump actuation, 112 gm)

Solaraze Gel massage in to clean skin bid prn

Gel: 3% (50 gm) (benzyl alcohol)

Voltaren Gel (G)(OTC) apply qid prn to intact skin

Gel: 1% (100 gm)

Comment: *Diclofenac* is contraindicated with *aspirin* allergy. As with other NSAIDs, should be avoided in late pregnancy (≥30 weeks) because it may cause premature closure of the ductus arteriosus.

▷ *doxepin* (B) cream apply to affected area qid at intervals of at least 3-4 hours; max 8 days

Pediatric: <12 years: not recommended; >12 years: same as adult

Prudoxin *Crm:* 5% (45 gm)
Zonalon *Crm:* 5% (30, 45 gm)

▷ *pimecrolimus* 1% cream (C)(G) <2 years: not recommended; ≥2 years: apply to affected area bid; do not apply an occlusive dressing
Elidel *Crm:* 1% (30, 60, 100 gm)
Comment: *Pimecrolimus* is indicated for short-term and intermittent long-term use. Discontinue use when resolution occurs. Contraindicated if the patient is immunosuppressed. Change to the 0.1% preparation or if secondary bacterial infection is present.

▷ *trolamine salicylate* apply tid-qid
Pediatric: <2 years: not recommended; ≥2 years: same as adult
Mobisyl Creme *Crm:* 10% (100 gm)

TOPICAL AND TRANSDERMAL ANESTHETICS

Comment: *Lidocaine* should not be applied to non-intact skin.

▷ *lidocaine* cream (B) apply to affected area bid prn
Pediatric: <12 years: not recommended; ≥12 years: same as adult
LidaMantle *Crm:* 3% (1, 2 oz)
Lidoderm *Crm:* 3% (85 gm)
ZTlido *lidocaine* topical system 1% (30/carton)
Comment: Compared to **Lidoderm** (*lidocaine* patch 5%) which contains 700 mg/patch, **ZTlido** only requires 35 mg per topical system to achieve the same therapeutic dose.

▷ *lidocaine* lotion (B) apply to affected area bid prn
Pediatric: <12 years: not recommended; ≥12 years: same as adult
LidaMantle *Lotn:* 3% (177 ml)

▷ *lidocaine* 5% patch (B)(G) apply up to 3 patches at one time for up to 12 hours/24-hour period (12 hours on/12 hours off); patches may be cut into smaller sizes before removal of the release liner; do not re-use
Pediatric: <12 years: not recommended; ≥12 years: same as adult
Lidoderm *Patch:* 5% (10x14 cm; 30/carton)

▷ *lidocaine+dexamethasone* (B)
Pediatric: <12 years: not recommended; ≥12 years: same as adult
Decadron Phosphate with Xylocaine *Lotn:* dexa 4 mg+lido 10 mg per ml (5 ml)

▷ *lidocaine+hydrocortisone* (B)(G) apply to affected area bid prn
Pediatric: <12 years: not recommended; ≥12 years: same as adult
LidaMantle HC *Crm:* lido 3%+hydro 0.5% (1, 3 oz); *Lotn:* (177 ml)

▷ *lidocaine 2.5%+prilocaine 2.5%* apply sparingly to the burn bid-tid prn
Pediatric: <12 years: not recommended; ≥12 years: same as adult
Emla Cream (B) 5, 30 gm/tube

OPIOID ANALGESICS

Comment: According to the American Society of Interventional Pain Physicians (ASIPP), presumptive urine drug testing (UDT) should be performed when opioid therapy for chronic pain is initiated, along with subsequent use as adherence monitoring, using in-office point of service testing, to identify patients who are non-compliant or abusing prescription drugs or illicit drugs.

Opiate agonists may produce significant central nervous system and respiratory depression of varying duration, particularly when given in high dosages and/or by rapid intravenous administration. Apnea may result from decreased respiratory drive as well as increased airway resistance, and rigidity of respiratory muscles may occur during rapid IV administration or when these agents are used in the induction of anesthesia. At therapeutic analgesic dosages, the respiratory effects are usually not clinically important except in patients with pre-existing pulmonary impairment. Therapy with opiate agonists should be avoided or administered with extreme caution and initiated at reduced dosages in patients with severe CNS depression (e.g., sleep apnea, hypoxia, anoxia, or hypercapnia, upper airway obstruction, chronic pulmonary insufficiency, limited ventilatory reserve, and other respiratory disorders). In the presence of excessive respiratory secretions, the use of opiate agonists may also be problematic because they decrease ciliary activity and reduce the cough reflex. Caution is also advised in patients who may be at increased risk for respiratory depression, such as comatose patients or those with head injury, intracranial lesions, or intracranial hypertension. Clinical monitoring of pulmonary function is recommended, and equipment for resuscitation should be immediately available if parenteral or neuraxial routes are used. *naloxone* may be administered to reverse clinically significant respiratory depression, which may be prolonged depending on the opioid agent, cumulative dose, and route of administration.

▷ *benzhydrocodone+acetaminophen* (II) <18 years: not recommended; ≥18 years: initiate treatment with at 1-2 tabs every 4-6 hours prn; max 12 tabs/24 hours; max 14 days

    Apadaz *Tab:* benz 6.12 mg+acet 325 mg

    Comment: *Benzhydrocodone* 6.12 mg is equivalent to 4.54 mg *hydrocodone* or 7.5 mg *hydrocodone bitartrate*. If switching from immediate-release *hydrocodone bitartrate+acetaminophen*, substitute **Apadaz** 6.12 mg/325 mg for 7.5 mg/325 mg *hydrocodone bitartrate+acetaminophen*. Dosage of **Apadaz** should be adjusted according to the severity of the pain and the response of the patient. Do not stop **Apadaz** abruptly in the physically-dependent patient.

▷ *butalbital+acetaminophen* (C)(G) 1 tab q 4 hours prn; max 6 tabs/day
  Pediatric: <12 years: not recommended; ≥12 years: same as adult
    Phrenilin 1-2 tabs q 4 hours prn; max 6 tabs/day
      Tab: but 50 mg+acet 325 mg
    Phrenilin Forte 1 tab or cap q 4 hours prn; max 6 caps/day
      Cap: but 50 mg+acet 325 mg; *Tab:* but 50 mg+acet 325 mg

▷ *butalbital+acetaminophen+caffeine* (C)(G)
  Pediatric: <12: not recommended; ≥12 years: same as adult
    Fioricet 1-2 tabs q 4 hours prn; max 6/day
      Tab: but 50 mg+acet 325 mg+caf 40 mg
    Zebutal 1 cap q 4 hours prn; max 5/day
      Cap: but 50 mg+acet 325 mg+caf 40 mg

▷ *butalbital+aspirin+caffeine* (C)(III)(G)
  Pediatric: <12 years: not recommended; ≥12 years: same as adult
    Fiorinal 1-2 tabs or caps q 4 hours prn; max 6 caps/day
      Tab/Cap: but 50 mg+asp 325 mg+caf 40 mg

▷ *butalbital+aspirin+codeine+caffeine* (C)(III)(G)
  Pediatric: <18 years: not recommended; ≥18 year: same as adult
    Fiorinal with Codeine 1-2 caps q 4 hours prn; max 6 caps/day
      Cap: but 50 mg+asp 325 mg+cod 30 mg+caf 40 mg

▷ *codeine sulfate* (C)(III)(G) 15-60 q 4-6 hours prn; max 60 mg/day
  Pediatric: <18 years: not recommended; ≥18 year: same as adult
    Tab: 15, 30, 60 mg

▷ *codeine+acetaminophen* (C)(III)(G) 15-60 mg of *codeine* q 4 hours prn; max 360 mg of *codeine*/day
  Pediatric: <18 years: not recommended; ≥18 year: same as adult
    Tab: **Tylenol #1** cod 7.5 mg+acet 300 mg (sulfites)
         Tylenol #2 cod 15 mg+acet 300 mg (sulfites)
         Tylenol #3 cod 30 mg+acet 300 mg (sulfites)
         Tylenol #4 cod 60 mg+acet 300 mg (sulfites)
         Tylenol with Codeine Elixir (C)(III)
    Elix: cod 12 mg+acet 120 mg per 5 ml (cherry) (alcohol)

▷ *dihydrocodeine+acetaminophen+caffeine* (C)(III)(G)
   Pediatric: <18 years: not recommended; ≥18 years: same as adult
     Panlor DC 1-2 caps q 4-6 hours prn; max 10 caps/day
       Cap: dihydro 16 mg+acet 325 mg+caf 30 mg
     Panlor SS 1 tab q 4 hours prn; max 5 tabs/day
       Tab: dihydro 32 mg+acet 325 mg+caf 60*mg
▷ *dihydrocodeine+aspirin+caffeine* (D)(III)(G) 1-2 caps q 4 hours prn
   Pediatric: <18 years: not recommended; ≥18 years: same as adult
     Synalgos-DC
       Cap: dihydro 16 mg+asp 356.4 mg+caf 30 mg
▷ *hydrocodone bitartrate* (C)(II)
   Pediatric: <18 years: not recommended; ≥18 years: same as adult
     Hysingla ER swallow whole; 1 tab once daily at the same time each day
       Tab: 20, 30, 40, 60, 80, 100, 120 mg ext-rel
     Vantrela ER swallow whole; 1 tab once daily at the same time each day
       Tab: 15, 30, 45, 60, 90 mg ext-rel
     Zohydro ER swallow whole; *Opioid naïve:* 10 mg q 12 hours; may increase by 10 mg
     q 12 hours every 3-7 days; when discontinuing, titrate downward every 2-4 days
       Cap: 10, 15, 20, 30, 40, 50 mg ext-rel
▷ *hydrocodone bitartrate+acetaminophen* (C)(II)(G)
   Pediatric: <18: not recommended; ≥18 years: same as adult
     Hycet 5/325 1-2 tabs q 4-6 hours prn; max 8 tabs/day
       Tab: hydro 5 mg+acet 325 mg*
     Hycet 7.5/325 1 tab q 4-6 hours prn; max 6 tabs/day
       Tab: hydro 7.5 mg+acet 325 mg*
     Hycet 10/325 1 tab q 4-6 hours prn; max 6 tab/day
       Tab: hydro 10 mg+acet 325 mg*
     Hycet Oral Solution 2.5/325 3 tsp (15 ml) q 4-6 hours prn; max 24 tsp (90
     ml)/day (alcohol 7%)
       Liq: hydro 2.5 mg+acet 108 mg per 15 ml (alcohol 7%)
     Hycet Oral Solution 7.5/325 1 tsp (5 ml) q 4-6 hours prn; max 8 tsp (90 ml)/
     day (alcohol 7%)
       Liq: hydro 7.5 mg+acet 325 mg per 15 ml (alcohol 7%)
     Lorcet 1-2 tabs q 4-6 hours prn; max 8 caps/day*
       Tab: hydro 5 mg+acet 325 mg
     Lorcet Plus 1 tab q 4-6 hours prn; max 6 tabs/day*
       Tab: hydro 7.5 mg+acet 325 mg
     Lorcet-HD 1 cap q 4-6 hours prn; max 6 tabs/day*
       Tab: hydro 10 mg+acet 325 mg
     Lortab 5/325 1-2 tabs q 4-6 hours prn; max 8 tabs/day
       Tab: hydro 5 mg+acet 325 mg*
     Lortab 7.5/325 1 tab q 4-6 hours prn; max 6 tabs/day
       Tab: hydro 7.5 mg+acet 325 mg*
     Lortab 10/500 1 tab q 4-6 hours prn; max 6 tabs/day
       Tab: hydro 10 mg+acet 500 mg*
     Maxidone 1 tab q 4-6 hours prn; max 5 tabs/day
       Tab: hydro 10 mg+acet 750 mg*
     Norco 5/325 1-2 tab2 q 4-6 hours prn; max 8 tabs/day
       Tab: hydro 5 mg+acet 325 mg*
     Norco 7.5/325 1 tab q 4-6 hours prn; max 6 tabs/day
       Tab: hydro 7.5 mg+acet 325 mg*
     Norco 10/325 1 tab q 4-6 hours prn; max 6 tabs/day
       Tab: hydro 10 mg+acet 325 mg*
     Vicodin 1-2 tabs q 4-6 hours prn; max 8 tabs/day

Tab: hydro 5 mg+acet 300 mg*

Vicodin ES 1 tab q 4-6 hours prn; max 6 tabs/day
Tab: hydro 7.5 mg+acet 300 mg*

Vicodin HP 1 tab q 4-6 hours prn; max 6 tabs/day
Tab: hydro 10 mg+acet 300 mg*

Xodol 5/300 1-2 tabs q 4-6 hours prn; max 8 tabs/day
Tab: hydro 5 mg+acet 300 mg*

Xodol 7.5/300 1 tab q 4-6 hours prn; max 6 tabs/day
Tab: hydro 7.5 mg+acet 300 mg*

Xodol 10/300 1 tab q 4-6 hours prn; max 6 tabs/day
Tab: hydro 10 mg+acet 300 mg*

Zamicet Oral Solution 5/163 3 tsp (15 ml) q 4-6 hours prn; max 24 tsp (90 ml)/day (alcohol 7.7%)
Liq: hydro 5 mg+acet 325 mg per 163 ml (alcohol 7%)

Zamicet Oral Solution 10/325 3 tsp (15 ml) q 4-6 hours prn; max 24 tsp (90 ml)/day (alcohol 7.7%)
Liq: hydro 10 mg+acet 325 mg per 15 ml (alcohol 7%)

Zydone 5/400 1-2 tabs q 4-6 hours prn; max 8 tabs/day
Tab: hydro 5 mg+acet 400 mg

Zydone 7.5/400 1 tab q 4-6 hours prn; max 6 tabs/day
Tab: hydro 7.5 mg+acet 400 mg

Zydone 10/400 1 tab q 4-6 hours prn; max 6 tabs/day
Tab: hydro 10 mg+acet 400 mg

▶ *hydrocodone+ibuprofen* (C; <u>not</u> for use in 3rd)(II)(G)
Pediatric: <18: not recommended; ≥18 years: same as adult

Ibudone 5/200 1 tab q 4-6 hours prn; max 5 tabs/day
Tab: hydro 5 mg+ibup 200 mg

Ibudone 10/200 1 tab q 4-6 hours prn; max 5 tabs/day
Tab: hydro 10 mg+ibup 200 mg

Reprexain 1 tab q 4-6 hours prn; max 5 tabs/day
Tab: hydro 5 mg+ibup 200 mg

Vicoprofen 1 tab q 4-6 hours prn; max 5 tabs/day
Tab: hydro 7.5 mg+ibup 200 mg

▶ *hydromorphone* (C)(II)(G)
Pediatric: <18: not recommended; ≥18 years: same as adult

Dilaudid initially 2-4 mg q 4-6 hours prn
Tab: 2, 4, 8 mg (sulfites)

Dilaudid Oral Liquid 2.5-10 mg q 3-6 hours prn
Liq: 5 mg/5 ml (sulfites)

Dilaudid Rectal Suppository 2.5-10 mg q 6-8 hours prn
Rectal supp: 3 mg

Dilaudid Injection initially 1-2 mg SC <u>or</u> IM q 4-6 hours prn
Amp: 1, 2, 4 mg/ml (1 ml)

Dilaudid-HP Injection initially 1-2 mg SC <u>or</u> IM q 4-6 hours prn
Amp: 10 mg/ml (1 ml)

Exalgo initially 8-64 mg once daily
Tab: 8, 12, 16, 32 mg ext-rel (sulfites)

▶ *meperidine* (C; D in 2nd, 3rd)(II)(G) 50-150 mg q 3-4 hours prn
Pediatric: 0.5-0.8 mg/lb q 3-4 hours prn; max adult dose

Demerol *Tab:* 50, 100 mg; *Syr:* 50 mg/5 ml (banana) (alcohol-free)

▶ *meperidine+promethazine* (C; D in 2nd, 3rd)(II)(G)
Pediatric: <18: not recommended; ≥18 years: same as adult

Mepergan 1-2 tsp q 3-4 hours prn
Syr: mep 25 mg+prom 25 mg per ml

Mepergan Fortis 1-2 tsp q 4-6 hours prn
Tab: mep 50 mg+prom 25 mg

▷ *methadone* (C)(II)(G) 2.5-10 mg PO, SC, or IM q 3-4 hours; for use only in chronic moderately severe-to-severe pain management (e.g., hospice care). For opioid naïve patients, initiate **Dolophine** tablets with 2.5 mg every 8-12 hours; unlike other opioid analgesics, *methadone* is not indicated as an as-needed (prn) analgesic, per se; titrate slowly with dose increases no more frequent than every 3 to 5 days; to convert to **Dolophine** tablets from another opioid, use available conversion factors to obtain estimated dose (see mfr pkg insert); do not abruptly discontinue **Dolophine** in a physically dependent patient
Pediatric: <18: not recommended; ≥18 years: same as adult

Dolophine *Tab:* 5, 10 mg; *Dispersible tab:* 40 mg (dissolve in 120 ml orange juice or other citrus drink); *Oral soln:* 5, 10 mg/ml; *Oral conc:* 10 mg/ml; *Syr:* 10 mg/30 ml; *Vial:* 10 mg/ml (200 mg/20 ml multi-dose) for injection

Comment: *Methadone* administration is allowed only by approved providers with strict state and federal regulations (as stipulated in 42 CFR 8.12). Black Box Warning (BBW): *Dolophine* exposes users to risks of addiction, abuse, and misuse, which can lead to overdose and death. Assess each patient's risk and monitor regularly for development of these behaviors and conditions. Serious, life-threatening, or fatal respiratory depression may occur. The peak respiratory depressant effect of *methadone* occurs later, and persists longer than the peak analgesic effect. Accidental ingestion, especially by children, can result in fatal overdose. QT interval prolongation and serious arrhythmias (*torsades de pointes*) have occurred during treatment with *methadone*. Closely monitor patients with risk factors for development of prolonged QT interval, a history of cardiac conduction abnormalities, and those taking medications affecting cardiac conduction. Neonatal Opioid Withdrawal Syndrome (NOWS) is an expected and treatable outcome of use of methadone use during pregnancy. NOWS may be life-threatening if not recognized and treated in the neonate. The balance between the risks of NOWS and the benefits of maternal *methadone* use should be considered and the patient advised of the risk of NOWS so that appropriate planning for management of the neonate can occur. *methadone* has been detected in human milk. Concomitant use with CYP3A4, 2B6, 2C19, 2C9 or 2D6 inhibitors or discontinuation of concomitantly used CYP3A4 2B6, 2C19, or 2C9 inducers can result in a fatal overdose of *methadone*. Concomitant use of opioids with benzodiazepines or other central nervous system (CNS) depressants, including alcohol, may result in profound sedation, respiratory depression, coma, and death.

▷ *morphine sulfate (immed-release)* (C)(II)(G) usually 15-30 mg q 4 hours prn; solution, usually 10-20 mg q 4 hours prn
Pediatric: <18: not recommended; ≥18 years: same as adult

Tab: 15*, 30*mg; *Oral soln:* 10 mg/5 ml, 20 mg/5 ml (100, 500 ml), 100 mg/5 ml (30, 120 ml)

▷ *morphine sulfate (immed- and sust-rel)* (C)(II)
Comment: Dosage dependent upon previous opioid dosage; see mfr pkg insert for conversion guidelines; not for prn use; swallow whole or sprinkle contents of caps on applesauce (do crush, chew, or dissolve). Generic *morphine sulfate* is available in the following forms: *Tab:* 15*, 30*mg; *Oral soln:* 10, 20 mg/5 ml (100 ml); 100 mg/5 ml (30, 120 ml w. oral syringe)
Pediatric: <18 years: not recommended; ≥18 years: same as adult

Arymo ER swallow whole; 1 tab once daily at the same time each day
Tab: 15, 30, 60 mg ext-rel
Duramorph administer per anesthesia
IV/Intrathecal/Epidural: 0.5, 1 mg/ml

Infumorph administer per anesthesia
Intrathecal/Epidural: 10, 20 mg/ml
Kadian (G) 1 cap every 12-24 hours
Cap: 10, 20, 30, 50, 60, 80, 100, 200 mg sust-rel
MS Contin (G) 1 tab every 24 hours
Tab: 15, 30, 60, 100, 200 mg sust-rel
MSIR 5-30 mg q 4 hours prn
Tab: 15*, 30*mg; *Cap:* 15, 30 mg
MSIR Oral Solution 5-30 mg q 4 hours prn
Oral soln: 10, 20 mg/5 ml (120 ml)
MSIR Oral Solution Concentrate 5-30 mg q 4 hours prn
Oral conc: 20 mg/ml (30, 120 ml w. dropper)
Oramorph SR 1 cap every 12-24 hours
Tab: 15, 30, 60, 100 mg sust-rel
Roxanol Oral Solution 10-30 mg q 4 hours prn
Oral soln: 20 mg/ml (1, 4, 8 oz)
Roxanol Rescudose
Oral soln: 10 mg/2.5 ml (25 single-dose)

▷ *morphine sulfate (ext-rel)* (C)(II)
Pediatric: <18 years: not recommended; ≥18 years: same as adult
MorphaBond ER *Tab:* 15, 30, 60, 100 mg ext-rel
Comment: **MorphaBond** may be prescribed only by a qualified healthcare providers knowledgeable in use of potent opioids for management of chronic pain. Do not abruptly discontinue in a physically dependent patient. Instruct patients to swallow **MorphaBond ER** tablets intact and not to cut, break, crush, chew, or dissolve **MorphaBond ER** to avoid the risk of release and absorption of potentially fatal dose of morphine. **MorphaBond ER** 100 mg tablets, a single dose greater than 60 mg, or a total daily dose >120 mg, are only for use in patients in whom tolerance to an opioid of comparable potency has been established. Patients considered opioid-tolerant are those taking, for one week or longer, at least 60 mg oral *morphine* per day, 25 mcg transdermal *fentanyl* per hour, 30 mg oral *oxycodone* per day, 8 mg oral *hydromorphone* per day, 25 mg oral *oxymorphone* per day, 60 mg oral *hydrocodone* per day, or an equianalgesic dose of another opioid. Use the lowest effective dosage for the shortest duration consistent with individual patient treatment goals. Individualize dosing based on the severity of pain, patient response, prior analgesic experience, and risk factors for addiction, abuse, and misuse.

▷ *morphine sulfate+naltrexone* (C)(II)
Pediatric: <18 years: not recommended; ≥18 years: same as adult
Embeda 1 cap q 12-24 hours
Cap: **Embeda 20/0.8** morph 20 mg+nal 0.8 mg ext-rel
Embeda 30/1.2 morph 30 mg+nal 1.2 mg ext-rel
Embeda 50/2 morph 50 mg+nal 2 mg ext-rel
Embeda 60/2.4 morph 60 mg+nal 2.4 mg ext-rel
Embeda 80/3.2 morph 80 mg+nal 3.2 mg ext-rel
Embeda 100/4 morph 100 mg+nal 4 mg ext-rel
Comment: **Embeda** is not for prn use; for use in opioid-tolerant patients only; swallow whole or sprinkle contents of caps on applesauce (do not crush, chew, or dissolve); do not administer via NG or gastric tube (PEG tube).

▷ *oxycodone* (B)(II) 5-15 mg q 4-6 hours prn
Comment: Concomitant use of CYP3A4 inhibitors may increase opioid effects and CYP3A4 inducers may decrease effects or possibly cause development of an abstinence syndrome (withdrawal symptoms) in patients who are physically *oxycodone* dependent/addicted.
Pediatric: <18 years: not recommended; ≥18 years: same as adult

Oxaydo *Tab:* 5, 7.5 mg

Comment: **Oxaydo** is the first and <u>only</u> immediate-release oral *oxycodone* that discourages intranasal abuse. **Oxaydo** is formulated with sodium lauryl sulfate, an inactive ingredient that may cause nasal burning and throat irritation when snorted and, thus potentially reducing abuse liability. There is no generic equivalent.

Oxecta *Tab:* 5, 7.5 mg

Oxycodone Oral Solution (G) *Oral soln:* 5 mg/5 ml (15, 30 ml)

OxyIR (G) *Cap:* 5 mg

RoxyBond *Tab:* 5, 15, 30 mg

Comment: The FDA recently approved **RoxyBond** immediate-release tablets for the management of severe pain that does <u>not</u> respond to alternative treatment and requires an opioid analgesic. **RoxyBond** is the first immediate-release opioid analgesic to received FDA approval with a label describing its abuse-deterrent properties under the FDA 2015 Guidance for Industry: Abuse-Deterrent Opioids Evaluation and Labeling. The drug is formulated with inactive ingredients making it more difficult to misuse and abuse. When compared with another approved immediate-release tablet, **RoxyBond** was shown to be more resistant to cutting, crushing, grinding, <u>or</u> breaking, and more resistant to extraction. Adverse events associated with **RoxyBond** include nausea, constipation, vomiting, headache, pruritus, insomnia, dizziness, asthenia, somnolence, and addiction.

Roxycodone *Tab:* 5, 15*, 30*mg; *Oral soln:* 5 mg/ml

Roxycodone Intensol *Oral soln:* 20 mg/ml

▶ *oxycodone cont-rel* **(B)(II)(G)** dosage dependent upon previous opioid dosages; see mfr pkg insert: <11 years: not recommended; 11-16 years: the child's pain must be severe enough to require around-the-clock, long-term treatment <u>not</u> managed well by other treatments; must already be taking and tolerating minimum opium dose equal to *oxycodone* 20 mg/day x 5 consecutive days; >16 year: same as adult; no previous treatment with *oxycodone* required

    OxyContin dose q 12 hours

      Tab: 10, 15, 20, 30, 40, 60, 80 mg cont-rel

    OxyFast dose q 6 hours

      Oral conc: 20 mg/ml (30 ml w. dropper)

    Xtampza ER dose q 12 hours

      Cap: 10, 15, 20, 30, 40 mg ext-rel

    Comment: May open the **Xtampza ER** capsule and sprinkle in water <u>or</u> on soft food.

▶ *oxycodone+acetaminophen* **(C)(II)(G)**

Comment: Maximum 4 gm acetaminophen per day.

Pediatric: not recommended

    Magnacet 2.5/400 1 tab q 6 hours prn; max 10 tabs/day

      Tab: oxy 2.5 mg+acet 325 mg

    Magnacet 5/400 1 tab q 6 hours prn; max 10 tabs/day

      Tab: oxy 5 mg+acet 325 mg

    Magnacet 7.5/400 1 tab q 6 hours prn; max 8 tabs/day

      Tab: oxy 7.5 mg+acet 325 mg

    Magnacet 10/400 1 tab q 6 hours prn; max 6 tabs/day

      Tab: oxy 10 mg+acet 325 mg

    Percocet 2.5/325 1 tab q 6 hours prn; max 4 gm acet/day

      Tab: oxy 2.5 mg+acet 325 mg

    Percocet 5/325 1 tab q 6 hours prn; max 4 gm acet/day

      Tab: oxy 5 mg+acet 325*mg

    Percocet 7.5/325 1 tab q 6 hours prn; max 4 gm acet/day

      Tab: oxy 7.5 mg+acet 325 mg

Percocet 7.5/500 1 tabs q 6 hours prn; max 4 gm acet/day
    Tab: oxy 7.5 mg+acet 325 mg
Percocet 10/325 1 tabs q 6 hours prn; max 4 gm acet/day
    Tab: oxy 10 mg+acet 325 mg
Percocet 10/650 1 tab q 6 hours prn; max 4 gm acet/day
    Tab: oxy 10 mg+acet 325 mg
Roxicet 5/325 1 tab/tsp q 6 hours prn
    Tab: oxy 5 mg+acet 325 mg; *Oral soln:* oxy 5 mg+acet 325 mg per 5 ml
Roxicet 5/500 1 caplet q 6 hours prn
    Cplt: oxy 5 mg+acet 325 mg
Roxicet Oral Solution 1 tsp q 6 hours prn
    Oral soln: oxy 5 mg+acet 325 mg per 5 ml (alcohol 0.4%)
Tylox 1 cap q 6 hours prn
    Cap: oxy 5 mg+acet 325 mg
Xartemis XR 2 tabs q 12 hours prn
    Tab: oxy 7.5 mg+acet 325 mg

▷ *oxycodone+aspirin* (D)(II)(G)
    Percodan 1 tab q 6 hours prn
      Pediatric: not recommended
      Tab: oxy 4.8355 mg+asp 325*mg
    Percodan-Demi 1-2 tabs q 6 hours prn
      Pediatric: 6-12 years: 1/4 tab q 6 hours prn; >12-18 years: 1/2 tab q 6 hours prn
      Tab: oxy 2.25 mg+asp 325 mg

▷ *oxycodone+ibuprofen* (C)(II)(G)
    Pediatric: <14 years: not recommended; ≥14 years: same as adult
    Combunox 1 tab q 6 hours prn
      Tab: oxy 5 mg+ibu 400*mg

▷ *oxycodone+naloxone* (C)(II) 1 tab q 3-4 hours prn
    Pediatric: <12 years: not recommended; ≥12 years: same as adult
    Targiniq
      Tab: **Targiniq 10/5** oxy 10 mg+nal 5 mg
          Targiniq 20/10 oxy 20 mg+nal 10 mg
          Targiniq 40/20 oxy 40 mg+nal 20 mg

▷ *oxymorphone* (C)(II)(G)
    Pediatric: <18 years: not recommended; ≥18 years: same as adult
    Numorphan 1 supp q 4-6 hours prn
      Rectal supp: 5 mg; *Vial:* 1 mg/ml (1 ml), *Amp:* 1.5 mg/ml (10 ml);
      Comment: Store in refrigerator in original package. 1 mg of **Numorphan** is approximately equivalent in analgesic activity to 10 mg of *morphine sulfate.*
    Opana 1-1 tab q 4-6 hours prn
      Tab: 5, 10 mg
    Opana ER 1 tab q 12 hours prn
      Tab: 5, 7.5, 10, 15, 20, 30, 40 mg ext-rel crush-resist
    Opana Injection initially 0.5 mg IV or IM; 1 x 1 mg IM or IV q 4-6 hours prn
      Amp: 1 mg/ml (1 ml) (paraben/sodium dithionite-free)

▷ *pentazocine+aspirin* (D)(IV) 2 cplts tid or qid prn
    Pediatric: <12 years: not recommended; ≥12 years: same as adult
    Talwin Compound *Cplt:* pent 12.5 mg+asp 325 mg

▷ *pentazocine+naloxone* (C)(IV) 1 tab q 3-4 hours prn
    Pediatric: <12 years: not recommended; ≥12 years: same as adult
    Talwin NX *Tab:* pent 50 mg+nal 0.5*mg

▷ *pentazocine lactate* (C)(IV) 30 mg IM, SC, or IV q 3-4 hours; max 360 mg/day
    Pediatric: <1 year: not recommended; ≥1 year: 0.5 mg/kg IM
    Talwin Injectable *Amp:* pent 30 mg/ml (1, 1.5, 2 ml)

▷ *propoxyphene napsylate+acetaminophen* (C)(IV)(G)
  Comment: Maximum 4 gm acetaminophen per day.
  Pediatric: <12 years: not recommended; ≥12 years: same as adult
    Balacet 325 1 tab q 4 hours prn; max 6 tabs/day
      Tab: prop 100 mg+acet 325 mg
▷ *tramadol* (C)(IV)(G)
    Conzip initially 100 mg once daily; may titrate up by 100 mg increments every 5 days according to need and tolerance; max 300 mg once daily
      Cap: 100, 150, 200, 300 mg ext-rel
    Comment: **Conzip** is an opioid agonist indicated for the management of pain severe enough to require daily, around-the-clock, long-term opioid treatment and for which alternative treatment options are inadequate. **Conzip** is not indicated as an as-needed (prn) analgesic. **Conzip** is contraindicated in children <12 years-of-age, post-operative pain management of patients <18 years-of-age following tonsillectomy and/or adenoidectomy, acute or severe bronchial asthma in an unmonitored setting or in absence of resuscitative equipment, known or suspected GI obstruction, including paralytic ileus, and concurrent use of monoamine oxidase inhibitors (MAOIs) or use within the previous 14 days. Potentially life-threatening *serotonin syndrome* can result from concomitant serotonergic drug administration. Risk of seizure is present within the recommended dose range; risk is increased with higher than recommended doses and concomitant use of SSRIs, SNRIs, anorectics, TCAs and other tricyclic compounds, other opioids, MAOIs, neuroleptics, other drugs that reduce seizure threshold, and patients with epilepsy or at risk for seizures. Do not use **Conzip** in suicidal or addiction-prone patients. If adrenal insufficiency is diagnosed, treat with physiologic replacement of corticosteroids, and wean off of the opioid. Life-threatening respiratory depression can occur with COPD or patients that are elderly, cachectic, or debilitated; monitor closely, particularly during initiation and titration. Use caution in patients with increased ICP, brain tumor, head injury, or impaired consciousness. Prolonged use of opioid analgesics during pregnancy may cause neonatal opioid withdrawal syndrome. Available data within pregnant females are insufficient to inform a drug-associated risk for major birth defects and miscarriage. Based on animal data, advise pregnant females of the potential embryo/fetal *tramadol* and its metabolite, O-desmethyltramadol (M1), are present in human milk. **Conzip** is not recommended for obstetrical pre-operative medication or for post-delivery analgesia in nursing mothers because its safety in infants and newborns has not been studied.
    Rybix ODT initially 100 mg once daily; may increase by 100 mg every 5 days; max 300 mg/day; *CrCl <30 mL/min or severe hepatic impairment:* not recommended; *Cirrhosis:* max 50 mg q 12 hours
  Pediatric: <12 years: contraindicated; 12-<18: use extreme caution; not recommended for children and adolescents with obesity, asthma, obstructive sleep apnea, or other chronic breathing problem, or for post-tonsillectomy/adenoidectomy pain; ≥18 years: same as adult
      ODT: 50 mg (mint) (phenylalanine)
    Ryzolt initially 100 mg once daily; may increase by 100 mg every 5 days; max 300 mg/day; *CrCl <30 mL/min or severe hepatic impairment:* not recommended
  Pediatric: <12 years: contraindicated; 12-<18: use extreme caution; not recommended for children and adolescents with obesity, asthma, obstructive sleep apnea, or other chronic breathing problem, or for post-tonsillectomy/adenoidectomy pain; ≥18 years: same as adult
      Tab: 100, 200, 300 mg ext-rel
    Ultram 50-100 mg q 4-6 hours prn; max 400 mg/day; *CrCl <30 mL/min:* max 100 mg q 12 hours; *Cirrhosis:* max 50 mg q 12 hours

Pediatric: <12 years: contraindicated; 12-<18: use extreme caution; not recommended for children and adolescents with obesity, asthma, obstructive sleep apnea, <u>or</u> other chronic breathing problem, <u>or</u> for post-tonsillectomy/adenoidectomy pain; ≥18 years: same as adult

> *Tab:* 50*mg

Ultram ER initially 100 mg once daily; may increase by 100 mg every 5 days; max 300 mg/day; *CrCl <30 mL/min* <u>or</u> *severe hepatic impairment:* <u>not</u> recommended

Pediatric: <12 years: contraindicated; 12-<18: use extreme caution; not recommended for children and adolescents with obesity, asthma, obstructive sleep apnea, <u>or</u> other chronic breathing problem, <u>or</u> for post-tonsillectomy/adenoidectomy pain; ≥18 years: same as adult

> *Tab:* 100, 200, 300 mg ext-rel

▷ *tramadol+acetaminophen* (C)(IV)(G) 2 tabs q 4-6 hours; max 8 tabs/day; 5 days; *CrCl <30 mL/min:* max 2 tabs q 12 hours; max 4 tabs/day x 5 days

Pediatric: <12 years: contraindicated; 12-<18: use extreme caution; not recommended for children and adolescents with obesity, asthma, obstructive sleep apnea, <u>or</u> other chronic breathing problem, <u>or</u> for post-tonsillectomy/adenoidectomy pain; ≥18 years: same as adult

> **Ultracet** *Tab:* tram 37.5+acet 325 mg

▷ *buprenorphine* (C)(III) change patch every 7 days; do <u>not</u> increase the dose until previous dose has been worn for at least 72 hours; after removal, do <u>not</u> re-use the site for at least 3 weeks; do <u>not</u> expose the patch to heat

Pediatric: <16 years: not recommended; ≥16 years: same as adult

> **Butrans Transdermal System** *Transdermal patch:* 5, 10, 20 mcg/hour (4/pck)

▷ *fentanyl* transdermal system (C)(II) apply to clean, dry, non-irritated, intact, skin; hold in place for 30 seconds; start at lowest dose and titrate upward; *Opioid-naïve:* change patch every 3 days (72 hours)

Pediatric: <18 years <u>or</u> <110 lb: not recommended; ≥18 years <u>or</u> ≥110 lb: same as adult

> **Duragesic** *Transdermal patch:* 12, 25, 37.5, 50, 62.5, 75, 87.5, 100 mcg/hour (5/pck)

▷ *fentanyl iontophoretic transdermal system*

> **Ionsys** is a transdermal patient-controlled device that sticks to the arm <u>or</u> chest; it is activated when the patient pushes the button
>
> Comment: **Ionsys** is for in-hospital use <u>only</u> and should be discontinued prior to hospital discharge. It is indicated for post-op pain relief.

TRANSMUCOSAL (SUB-LINGUAL, BUCCAL) OPIOIDS

Comment: For chronic severe pain. For management of breakthrough pain in patients with cancer who are already receiving and who are tolerant to opioid therapy. Opioid-tolerant patients are those taking oral *morphine* ≥60 mg/day, transdermal *fentanyl* ≥25 mcg/hour, *oxycodone* ≥30 mg/day, oral *hydromorphone* ≥8 mg/day, <u>or</u> an equianalgesic dose of another opioid, for ≥1 week

ORAL OPIOID PARTIAL AGONIST-ANTAGONIST

▷ *buprenorphine* (C)

Pediatric: <16 years: not recommended; ≥16 year: same as adult

> **Subutex** 8 mg in a single dose on day 1; then 16 mg in a single dose on day 2; target dose is 16 mg/day in a single dose; dissolve under tongue; do <u>not</u> chew <u>or</u> swallow whole
>
> *SL tab (lemon-lime)* <u>or</u> *SL film (lime):* 2, 8 mg (30/pck)

▷ *fentanyl* buccal soluble film (C)(II) dissolve 1 film on moistened area inside cheek; initially 200 mcg; no more than 4 doses/day at least 2 hours apart; max 1200 mcg/dose; do <u>not</u> cut film

Pediatric: <18 years: not recommended; ≥18 years: same as adult

> **Onsolis** *Buccal film:* 200, 400, 600, 800, 1200 mcg (30 films/pck)

▷ *fentanyl citrate* transmucosal unit (C)(II)(G) initially one 200 mcg unit placed between cheek and lower gum; move from side to side; suck (not chew); use 6 units before titrating; titrate dose as needed; max 4 units/day
  Pediatric: <18 years: not recommended; ≥18 years: same as adult
   Actiq *Unit:* 200, 400, 600, 800, 1200, 1600 mcg (24 units/pck)
   Fentora *Unit:* 100, 200, 400, 600, 800 mcg (24 units/pck)

▷ *fentanyl* sublingual tab (C)(II) initially one 100 mcg dose; if inadequate after 30 minutes, may repeat; titrate in increments of 100 mcg; max 2 doses per episode, up to 4 episodes per day; wait at least 2 hours before treating another episode; *Maintenance:* use only one tablet of appropriate strength; do not chew, suck, or swallow tablets; do not convert from other *fentanyl* products on a mcg-per-mcg basis or interchange with other *fentanyl* products
  Pediatric: <18 years: not recommended; ≥18 years: same as adult
   Abstral *SL tab:* 100, 200, 300, 400, 600, 800 mcg (32 tabs/pck)

▷ *fentanyl sublingual spray* (C)(II)
  Pediatric: <18 years: not recommended; ≥18 years: same as adult
   Subsys 100, 200, 400, 600, 800 mcg/S L spray
   Comment: **Subsys** is not bioequivalent with other *fentanyl* products. Do not convert patients from other *fentanyl* products to **Subsys** on a mcg-per-mcg basis. There are no conversion directions available for patients on any other *fentanyl* products other than **Actiq**. (Note: This includes oral, transdermal, or parenteral formulations of *fentanyl*.)

▷ *sufentanil* 30 mcg sublingually prn; minimum 1 hour between doses; max 12 tablets/24 hours; max 72 hours
  Pediatric: <18 years: not established; ≥18 years: same as adult
   Dsuvia *SL tab:* 30 mcg in a single use applicator (SDA)
   Comment: **Dsuvia** *(sufentanil)* is a synthetic opioid analgesic formulation for the management of acute severe pain that is severe enough to require an opioid analgesic, and for which alternative treatments are inadequate. **Dsuvia** is indicated for use only in adults in a certified medically supervised healthcare settings, such as hospitals, surgical centers, and emergency departments. **Dsuvia** is only available through the **Dsuvia** REMS Program; **Dsuvia** is not for home use or for use in children; discontinue treatment with **Dsuvia** before patients leave the certified medically supervised healthcare setting; Do not discontinue **Dsuvia** abruptly in the physically-dependent patient. Concomitant use with CYP3A4 inhibitors (or discontinuation of CYP3A4 inducers) can result in a fatal overdose of *sufentanil*. The most commonly reported adverse reactions (incidence ≥ 2%) have been nausea, headache, vomiting, dizziness, and hypotension.

PARENTERAL OPIOID AGONIST-ANTAGONISTS

▷ *buprenorphine hcl Initial Dose:* 0.3 mg (1 ml) deep IM or slow IV (over at least 2 minutes); may repeat once (up to 0.3 mg) if required, 30-60 minutes after initial dose; usual frequency every 6 hours prn; fixed interval or "round-the-clock" dosing should not be undertaken until the appropriate inter-dose interval has been established by clinical observation
  Pediatric: <2 years: not recommended; 2-12 years: 2-6 mcg/kg deep IM or slow IV every 4-6 hours or every 6-8 hours prn; >12 years: same as adult; fixed interval or "round-the-clock" dosing should not be undertaken until the appropriate inter-dose interval has been established by clinical observation
   Buprenex *Amp:* 0.3 mg/ml (1 ml) (5 ampules/carton)

▷ *nalbuphine* (B)(G) 10 mg/70 kg IM, SC, or IV q 3-6 hours prn
  Pediatric: <18 years: not recommended; ≥18 years: same as adult
   Nubain *Amp:* 10, 20 mg/ml (1 ml) (sulfite-free, parabens-free)

▷ *pentazocine+naloxone* (C)(IV) 1-2 tabs q 3-4 hours prn; max 12 tabs/day
  Pediatric: <12 years: not recommended; ≥12 year: same as adult
    Talwin-NX *Tab:* pent 50 mg+nal 0.5*mg

TRANSMUCOSAL (INTRA-NASAL) OPIOIDS

▷ *butorphanol tartrate* nasal spray (C)(IV) initially 1 spray (1 mg) in one nostril
  and may repeat after 60-90 minutes (*Elderly* 90-120 minutes) in opposite nostril if
  needed or 1 spray in each nostril and may repeat q 3-4 hours prn
  Pediatric: <18 years: not recommended; ≥18 years: same as adult
    Butorphanol Nasal Spray *Nasal spray:* 1 mg/actuation (10 mg/ml, 2.5 ml)
    Stadol Nasal Spray *Nasal spray:* 1 mg/actuation (10 mg/ml, 2.5 ml)
▷ *fentanyl* nasal spray (C)(II) initially 1 spray (100 mcg) in one nostril and may
  repeat after 2 hours; when adequate analgesia is achieved, use that dose for
  subsequent breakthrough episodes
  Titration steps: 100 mcg using 1 x 100 mcg spray; 200 mcg using 2 x 100 mcg
  spray (1 in each nostril); 400 mcg using 1 x 400 mcg spray; 800 mcg using 2 x 400
  mcg (1 in each nostril); max 800 mcg; limit to ≤4 doses per day
  Pediatric: <18 years: not recommended; ≥18 years: same as adult
    Lazanda Nasal Spray *Nasal spray:* 100, 400 mcg/100 mcl (8 sprays/bottle)
    Comment: **Lazanda Nasal Spray** is available by restricted distribution program.
    To enroll, call 855-841-4234 or visit https://www.fda.gov/downloads/drugs/
    drugsafety/postmarketdrugsafetyinformationforpatientsandproviders/
    ucm261983.pdf. **Lazanda Nasal Spray** is indicated for the management of
    breakthrough pain in cancer patients who are already receiving and who are
    tolerant to opioid therapy for their underlying persistent cancer pain. Patients
    considered opioid tolerant are those who are taking at least 60 mg of oral
    morphine/day, 25 mcg of transdermal *fentanyl*/hour, 30 mg oral *oxycodone*/
    day, 8 mg oral *hydromorphone*/day, 25 mg oral *oxymorphone*/day, or an
    equianalgesic dose of another opioid for a week or longer. Patients must remain
    on around-the-clock opioids when using **Lazanda Nasal Spray**. As such, it
    is contraindicated in the management of acute or post-op pain, including
    headache/migraine, or dental pain.

INTRATHECAL OPIOID

▷ *ziconotide* intrathecal (IT) infusion (C) initially no more than 2.4 mcg/day (0.1
  mcg/hour) and titrate to upward by up to 2.4 mcg/day (0.1 mcg/day at intervals of
  no more than 2-3 times per week, up to a recommended maximum of 19.2 mcg/
  day (0.8 mcg/hour) by Day 21; dose increases in increments of less than 2.4 mcg/
  day (0.1 mcg/hour) and increases in dose less frequently than 2-3 times per week
  may be used.
  Pediatric: <12 years: not recommended; ≥12 years: same as adult
    Prialt *Vial:* 25 mcg/ml (20 ml), 100 mcg/ml (1, 2, 5 ml)
    Comment: Patients with a pre-existing history of psychosis should not be treated
    with *ziconotide*. Contraindications to the use of IT analgesia include conditions
    such as the presence of infection at the microinfusion injection site, uncontrolled
    bleeding diathesis, and spinal canal obstruction that impairs circulation of CSF.

◯ PANCREATIC ENZYME INSUFFICIENCY

Comment: Seen in chronic pancreatitis, post-pancreatectomy, cystic fibrosis,
steatorrhea, post-GI tract bypass surgery, and ductal obstruction from neoplasia.
May sprinkle cap; however, do not crush or chew cap or tab. May mix with
applesauce or other acidic food; follow with water or juice. Do not let any drug
remain in mouth. Take dose just prior to each meal or snack. Base dose on lipase

units; adjust per diet and clinical response (i.e., steatorrhea). Pancrelipase products are interchangeable. Contraindicated with pork protein hypersensitivity.

PANCRELIPASE PRODUCTS

▷ *pancreatic enzymes* (C)

Creon 500 units/kg per meal; max 2500 units/kg per meal or <10,000 units/kg per day or <4,000 units/gm fat ingested per day
Pediatric: <12 months: 2000-4000 units per 120 ml formula or per breastfeeding (do not mix directly into formula or breast milk; 12 months to 4 years: 1000 units/kg per meal; max 2500 units/kg per meal <10,000 units/kg per day; >4 years: same as adult

   Cap: **Creon 3000** lip 3000 units+pro 9,500 units+amyl 15,000 units del-rel
      Creon 6000 lip 6000 units+pro 19,000 units+amyl 30,000 units del-rel
      Creon 12000 lip 12,000 units+pro 38,000 units+amyl 60,000 units del-rel
      Creon 24000 lip 24,000 units+pro 76,000 units+amyl 120,000 units del-rel
      Creon 36000 lip 36,000 units+pro 114,000 units+amyl 180,000 units del-rel

Cotazym 1-3 tabs just prior to each meal or snack
Pediatric: <12 years: not recommended; ≥12 years: same as adult

   Tab: **Cotazym** lip 1000 units+pro 12,500 units+amyl 12,500 units del-rel
      Cotazym-S lip 5000 units+pro 20,000 units+amyl 20,000 units del-rel

Donnazyme 1-3 caps just prior to each meal or snack
Pediatric: <12 years: not recommended; ≥12 years: same as adult

   Cap: **Donnazyme** lip 5000 units+pro 20,000 units+amyl 20,000 units del-rel

Ku-Zyme 1-2 caps just prior to each meal or snack
Pediatric: <12 years: not recommended; ≥12 years: same as adult

   Cap: **Ku-Zyme:** lip 12,000 units+pro 15,000 units+amyl 15,000 units del-rel

Kutrase 1-2 caps just prior to each meal or snack
Pediatric: <12 years: not recommended; ≥12 years: same as adult

   Cap: **Kutrase:** lip 12,000 units+pro 30,000 units+amyl 30,000 units del-rel

Pancreaze 2500 lipase units/kg per meal or <10,000 lipase units/kg per day or <4,000 lipase units/gm fat ingested per day
Pediatric: <12 months: 2000-4000 lipase units per 120 ml formula or per breastfeeding; >12 months to <4 years 1000 lipase units/kg per meal; >4 years: 500 lipase units/kg per meal; max: adult dose

   Cap: **Pancreaze 4200** lip 4200 units+pro 10,000 units+amyl 17,500 units ec-microtabs
      Pancreaze 10500 lip 10,500 units+pro 25,000 units+amyl 43,750 units ec-microtabs
      Pancreaze 16800 lip 16,800 units+pro 40,000 units+amyl 70,000 units ec-microtabs
      Pancreaze 21000 lip 21,000 units+pro 37,000 units+amyl 61,000 units ec-microtabs

Pertyze *12 months to 4 years and ≥8 kg:* initially 1,000 lipase units/kg per meal; *≥4 years and ≥16 kg:* initially 500 lipase units/kg per meal; *Both:* 2,500 lipase units/kg per meal or <10,000 units/kg per day or <4000 units/gm fat ingested per day

   Cap: **Pertyze 8000** lip 8000 units+pro 28,750 units+amyl 30,250 units del-rel

Pertyze 16000 lip 16,000 units+pro 57,500 units+amyl 65,000 units del-rel

Ultrase 1-3 tabs just prior to each meal or snack
Pediatric: same as adult

   Cap: **Ultrase** lip 4500 units+pro 20,000 units+amyl 25,000 units del-rel

Ultrase MT lip 12,000 units+pro 39,000 units+amyl 39,000 units del-rel

Ultrase MT 18 lip 18,000 units+pro 58,500 units+amyl 58,500 units del-rel

Ultrase MT 20 lip 20,000 units+pro 65,000 units+amyl 65,000 units del-rel

Viokace initially 500 lip units/kg per meal; max 2500 lipase units/kg per meal, or <10,000 lipase units/kg per meal, or <4,000 units/gm fat ingested per day

Pediatric: same as adult

Tab: **Viokace 8** lip 8000 units+pro 30,000 units+amyl 30,000 units

Viokace 16 lip 16,000 units+pro 60,000 units amyl 60,000 units

Viokace 0440 lip 10,440 units+pro 39,150 units amyl 39,150 units

Viokace 20880 lip 20,880 units+pro 78,300 units amyl 78,300 units

Comment: Viokace 10440 and **Viokase 20880** should be taken with a daily proton pump inhibitor (PPI).

Viokace Powder 1/4 tsp (0.7 gm) with meals

Viokace Powder lip 16,800 units+pro 70,000 units+amyl 70,000 units per 1/4 tsp (8 oz)

Zenpep initially 500 lipase units/kg per meal; max 2500 lipase units/kg per meal or <10,000 units/kg per day or <4000 units/gm fat ingested per day

Pediatric: Infant-12 months: infants may be given 3000 lipase units (one capsule) per 120 ml of formula or per breastfeeding; do not mix capsule contents directly into formula or breast milk prior to administration; *Children >12 months to <4 Years:* enzyme dosing should begin with 1,000 lipase units/kg of body weight per meal to a maximum of 2500 lipase units/kg of body weight per meal (or ≤10,000 lipase units/kg/day), or <4,000 lipase units/gm fat ingested per day; *Children ≥4 Years:* same as adult

Cap: **Zenpep 3000** lip 3000 units+pro 10,000 units+amyl 14,000 units del-rel

Zenpep 5000 lip 5000 units+pro 17,000 units+amyl 24,000 units

Zenpep 10000 lip 10,000 units+pro 32,000 units+amyl 42,000 units del-rel

Zenpep 15000 lip 15,000 units+pro 47,000 units+amyl 63,000 units del-rel

Zenpep 20000 lip 20,000 units+pro 63,000 units+amyl 84,000 units del-rel

Zenpep 25000 lip 25,000 units+pro 79,000 units+amyl 105,000 units del-rel

Zenpep 40000 lip 40,000 units+pro 126,000 units+amyl 168,000 units del-rel

Comment: Zenpep is not interchangeable with any other pancrelipase product. Dosing should not exceed the recommended maximum dosage set forth by the Cystic Fibrosis Foundation Consensus Conferences Guidelines. **Zenpep** should be swallowed whole. For infants or patients unable to swallow intact capsules, the contents may be sprinkled on soft acidic food, e.g., applesauce.

Zymase 1-3 caps just prior to each meal or snack

Pediatric: <12 years: not recommended; ≥12 years: same as adult

Cap: **Zymase** lip 12,000 units+prot 24,000 units+amyl 24,000 units del-rel

◯ PANIC DISORDER

Comment: If possible when considering a benzodiazepine to treat anxiety, a short-acting benzodiazepines should be used only prn to avert intense anxiety and panic for the least time necessary while a different non-addictive anti-anxiety regimen (e.g., SSRI, SNRI, TCA, *buspirone*, beta-blocker) is established and effective treatment goals achieved. Co-administration of SSRIs with TCAs requires extreme caution. Concomitant use of MAOIs and SSRIs is absolutely contraindicated. Avoid other serotonergic drugs. A potentially fatal adverse event is *serotonin syndrome*, caused by serotonin excess. Milder symptoms require HCP intervention to avert severe symptoms which can be rapidly fatal without urgent/emergent medical care. Symptoms include restlessness, agitation, confusion, hallucinations, tachycardia, hypertension, dilated pupils, muscle twitching, muscle rigidity, loss of muscle coordination, diaphoresis, diarrhea, headache, shivering, piloerection, hyperpyrexia, cardiac arrhythmias, seizures, loss of consciousness, coma, and death. Abrupt withdrawal or interruption of treatment with an antidepressant medication is sometimes associated with an *antidepressant discontinuation syndrome,* which may be mediated by gradually tapering the drug over a period of 2 weeks or longer, depending on the dose strength and length of treatment. Common symptoms of the *serotonin discontinuation syndrome* include flu-like symptoms (nausea, vomiting, diarrhea, headaches, sweating), sleep disturbances (insomnia, nightmares, constant sleepiness), mood disturbances (dysphoria, anxiety, agitation), cognitive disturbances (mental confusion, hyperarousal), sensory and movement disturbances (imbalance, tremors, vertigo, dizziness, electric-shock-like sensations in the brain, often described by sufferers as "brain zaps").

SELECTIVE SEROTONIN REUPTAKE INHIBITORS (SSRIs)

▷ *escitalopram* (C)(G) initially 10 mg daily; may increase to 20 mg daily after 1 week; *Elderly or hepatic impairment*: 10 mg once daily
  Pediatric: <12 years: <12 years: not recommended; ≥12 years: same as adult; 12-17 years: initially 10 mg once daily; may increase to 20 mg once daily after 3 weeks
    Lexapro *Tab:* 5, 10*, 20*mg
    Lexapro Oral Solution *Oral soln:* 1 mg/ml (240 ml) (peppermint) (parabens)
▷ *fluoxetine* (C)(G)
    Prozac initially 20 mg daily; may increase after 1 week; doses >20 mg/day should be divided into AM and noon doses; max 80 mg/day
    Pediatric: <8 years: not recommended; 8-17 years: initially 10 mg/day; may increase after 2 weeks to 20 mg/day; range 20-60 mg/day; range for lower weight children 20-30 mg/day; >17 years: same as adult
      Cap: 10, 20, 40 mg; *Tab:* 30*, 60*mg; *Oral soln:* 20 mg/5 ml (4 oz) (mint)
    Prozac Weekly following daily *fluoxetine* therapy at 20 mg/day for 13 weeks, may initiate **Prozac Weekly** 7 days after the last 20 mg *fluoxetine* dose
    Pediatric: <12 years: not recommended; ≥12 years: same as adult
      Cap: 90 mg ent-coat del-rel pellets
▷ *paroxetine maleate* (D)(G)
    Pediatric: <12 years: not recommended; ≥12 years: same as adult
    Paxil initially 20 mg daily in AM; may increase by 10 mg/day at weekly intervals as needed; max 60 mg/day
      Tab: 10*, 20*, 30, 40 mg
    Paxil CR initially 25 mg daily in AM; may increase by 12.5 mg at weekly intervals as needed; max 62.5 mg/day
      Tab: 12.5, 25, 37.5 mg cont-rel ent-coat
    Paxil Suspension initially 20 mg daily in AM; may increase by 10 mg/day at weekly intervals as needed; max 60 mg/day
      Oral susp: 10 mg/5 ml (250 ml) (orange)
▷ *paroxetine mesylate* (D)(G) initially 7.5 mg daily in AM; may increase by 10 mg/day at weekly intervals as needed; max 60 mg/day
    Pediatric: <12 years: not recommended; ≥12 years: same as adult
      Brisdelle *Cap:* 7.5 mg
▷ *sertraline* (C) initially 50 mg daily; increase at 1 week intervals if needed; max 200 mg daily
    Pediatric: <6 years: not recommended; 6-12 years: initially 25 mg daily; max 200 mg/day; 13-17 years: initially 50 mg daily; max 200 mg/day; ≥17 years: same as adult

Zoloft *Tab*: 15*, 50*, 100*mg; *Oral conc*: 20 mg per ml (60 ml, dilute just before administering in 4 oz water, ginger ale, lemon-lime soda, lemonade, or orange juice) (alcohol 12%)

SEROTONIN-NOREPINEPHRINE REUPTAKE INHIBITORS (SNRIs)

▷ *desvenlafaxine* (C)(G) swallow whole; initially 50 mg once daily; max 120 mg/day
 Pediatric: <12 years: not recommended; ≥12 years: same as adult
  Pristiq *Tab*: 50, 100 mg ext-rel

▷ *venlafaxine* (C)(G)
  Effexor initially 75 mg/day in 2-3 doses; may increase at 4 day intervals in 75 mg increments to 150 mg/day; max 375 mg/day
  Pediatric: <18 years: not recommended; ≥18 years: same as adult
   Tab: 25, 37.5, 50, 75, 100 mg
  Effexor XR initially 75 mg q AM; may start at 37.5 mg daily x 4-7 days, then increase by increments of up to 75 mg/day at intervals of at least 4 days; usual max 375 mg/day
  Pediatric: <18 years: not recommended; ≥18 years: same as adult
   Cap: 37.5, 75, 150 mg ext-rel

TRICYCLIC ANTIDEPRESSANTS (TCAs)

▷ *doxepin* (C)(G)
 Pediatric: <12 years: not recommended; ≥12 years: same as adult
  Cap: 10, 25, 50, 75, 100, 150 mg; *Oral conc*: 10 mg/ml (4 oz w. dropper)

▷ *imipramine* (C)(G)
 Pediatric: <12 years: not recommended; ≥12 years: same as adult
  Tofranil initially 75 mg daily (max 200 mg); *Adolescents*: initially 30-40 mg daily (max 100 mg/day); if maintenance dose exceeds 75 mg daily, may switch to **Tofranil PM** for divided or bedtime dose
   Tab: 10, 25, 50
  Tofranil PM initially 75 mg daily 1 hour before HS; max 200 mg
   Cap: 75, 100, 125, 150
  Tofranil Injection 50 mg IM; lower dose for adolescents; switch to oral form as soon as possible
   Amp: 25 mg/2 ml (2 ml)

FIRST GENERATION ANTIHISTAMINE

▷ *hydroxyzine* (C)(G) 50-100 mg qid; max 600 mg/day
 Pediatric: <6 years: 50 mg/day divided qid; ≥6 years: 50-100 mg/day divided qid
  Atarax *Tab*: 10, 25, 50, 100 mg; *Syr*: 10 mg/5 ml (alcohol 0.5%)
  Vistaril *Cap*: 25, 50, 100 mg; *Oral susp*: 25 mg/5 ml (4 oz) (lemon)
 Comment: *Hydroxyzine* is contraindicated in early pregnancy and in patients with a prolonged QT interval. It is not known whether this drug is excreted in human milk; therefore, *hydroxyzine* should not be given to nursing mothers.

AZAPIRONES

▷ *buspirone* (B) initially 7.5 mg bid; may increase by 5 mg/day q 2-3 days; max 60 mg/day
 Pediatric: <6 years: not recommended; 6-17 years: same as adult
  BuSpar *Tab*: 5, 10, 15*, 30*mg

BENZODIAZEPINES
Short Acting

▷ *alprazolam* (D)(IV)(G)
 Pediatric: <18 years: not recommended; ≥18 years: same as adult
  Niravam initially 0.25-0.5 mg tid; may titrate every 3-4 days; max 4 mg/day
   Tab: 0.25*, 0.5*, 1*, 2*mg orally-disint

Xanax initially 0.25-0.5 mg tid; may titrate every 3-4 days; max 4 mg/day
Tab: 0.25*, 0.5*, 1*, 2*mg

Xanax XR initially 0.5-1 mg once daily, preferably in the AM; increase at intervals of at least 3-4 days by up to 1 mg/day. Taper no faster than 0.5 mg every 3 days; max 10 mg/day. When switching from immediate-release **alprazolam**, give total daily dose of immediate-release once daily.
Tab: 0.5, 1, 2, 3 mg ext-rel

▷ *oxazepam* (C)(IV)(G) 10-15 mg tid-qid for moderate symptoms; 15-30 mg tid-qid for severe symptoms
Pediatric: <12 years: not recommended; ≥12 years: same as adult
oxazepam Tab: 15 mg; *Cap:* 10, 15, 30 mg

Intermediate-Acting

▷ *lorazepam* (D)(IV)(G) 1-10 mg/day in 2-3 divided doses
Pediatric: <12 years: not recommended; ≥12 years: same as adult
Ativan *Tab:* 0.5, 1*, 2*mg
Lorazepam Intensol *Oral conc:* 2 mg/ml (30 ml w. graduated dropper)

Long-Acting

▷ *chlordiazepoxide* (D)(IV)(G)
Pediatric: <6 years: not recommended; ≥6 years: 5 mg bid-qid; increase to 10 mg bid-tid
Librium 5-10 mg tid-qid for moderate symptoms; 20-25 mg tid-qid for severe symptoms
Cap: 5, 10, 25 mg
Librium Injectable 50-100 mg IM or IV; then 25-50 mg IM tid-qid prn; max 300 mg/day
Inj: 100 mg

▷ *chlordiazepoxide+clidinium* (D)(IV) 1-2 caps tid-qid; max 8 caps/day
Pediatric: <12 years: not recommended; ≥12 years: same as adult
Librax *Cap:* chlor 5 mg+clid 2.5 mg

▷ *clonazepam* (D)(IV)(G) initially 0.25 mg bid; increase to 1 mg/day after 3 days
Pediatric: <18 years: not recommended; ≥18 years: same as adult
Klonopin *Tab:* 0.5*, 1, 2 mg
Klonopin Wafers dissolve in mouth with or without water
Wafer: 0.125, 0.25, 0.5, 1, 2 mg orally-disint

▷ *clorazepate* (D)(IV)(G) 30 mg/day in divided doses; max 60 mg/day
Pediatric: <9 years: not recommended; ≥9 years: same as adult
Tranxene *Tab:* 3.75, 7.5, 15 mg
Tranxene SD do not use for initial therapy
Tab: 22.5 mg ext-rel
Tranxene SD Half Strength do not use for initial therapy
Tab: 11.25 mg ext-rel
Tranxene T-Tab *Tab:* 3.75*, 7.5*, 15*mg

▷ *diazepam* (D)(IV)(G) 2-10 mg bid to qid
Pediatric: <12 years: not recommended; ≥12 years: same as adult
Diastat *Rectal gel delivery system:* 2.5 mg
Diastat AcuDial *Rectal gel delivery system:* 10, 20 mg
Valium *Tab:* 2*, 5*, 10*mg
Valium Injectable *Vial:* 5 mg/ml (10 ml); *Amp:* 5 mg/ml (2 ml); *Prefilled syringe:* 5 mg/ml (5 ml)
Valium Intensol Oral Solution *Conc oral soln:* 5 mg/ml (30 ml w. dropper) (alcohol 19%)
Valium Oral Solution *Oral soln:* 5 mg/5 ml (500 ml) (wintergreen spice)

PHENOTHIAZINES

▷ *prochlorperazine* (C)(G)
Pediatric: <12 years: not recommended; ≥12 years: same as adult
 Compazine 5 mg tid-qid
  Tab: 5 mg; *Syr:* 5 mg/5 ml (4 oz) (fruit); *Rectal supp:* 2.5, 5, 25 mg
 Compazine Spansule 15 mg q AM <u>or</u> 10 mg q 12 hours
  Spansule: 10, 15 mg sust-rel

▷ *trifluoperazine* (C)(G) 1-2 mg bid; max 6 mg/day; max 12 weeks
Pediatric: <12 years: not recommended; ≥12 years: same as adult
 Stelazine *Tab:* 1, 2, 5, 10 mg

 PARKINSON'S DISEASE (PD)

Parkinson's Disease-Associated Dementia, *see* **Dementia**
Comment: When administering *carbidopa* and *levodopa* separately, administer each at the same time. Titrate daily dose ratio of 1:10 *carbidopa* to *levodopa*. Max daily *carbidopa* 200 mg. Most patients will require *levodopa* 400-1600 mg/day in divided doses every 4-8 hours. After titrating both drugs to the desired effects without intolerable side effects, switch to a *carbidopa+levodopa* combination form.

DOPAMINE PRECURSOR (LEVODOPA)

▷ *levodopa* (C)(G)
 Tab: 125, 150, 200 mg

DECARBOXYLASE INHIBITOR (CARBIDOPA)

▷ *carbidopa* (C)(G)
 Lodosyn *Tab:* 25 mg

TREATMENT OF DOPAMINE OFF EPISODES

▷ *levodopa inhalation powder* for oral inhalation <u>only</u>; do <u>not</u> swallow capsules; administer capsules <u>only</u> with the **Inhibra** inhaler; max 1 dose (2 capsules) for any OFF period; max 5 doses (10 capsules , 420 mg)/day
 Inbrija *Inhal cap:* 42 mg inhal pwdr (60 caps; 4 caps/foil blister card, 15 cards/carton) w. **Inbrija** inhaler
 Comment: **Inbrija** is an aromatic amino acid oral inhalation powder for the intermittent (on-demand) treatment of OFF episodes in people with Parkinson's disease treated with *carbidopa/levodopa*. OFF episodes, also known as OFF periods, are defined as the return of Parkinson's symptoms that result from low levels of dopamine between doses of oral carbidopa/levodopa, the standard oral baseline Parkinson's treatment. **Inbrija** is <u>not</u> recommended for patients with asthma, COPD, <u>or</u> other chronic underlying lung disease. **Inbrija** is contraindicated within 14 days before <u>and</u> 7 days after taking a non-selective monoamine oxidase inhibitor (MOAI). Monitor patients on MAO-B inhibitors for orthostatic hypotension. Concomitant dopamine D2 antagonists, respiratory tract infection, and discolored sputum.

NON-ERGOLINE DOPAMINE AGONIST

▷ *apomorphine sublingual film* 10-30 mg SL as a single dose prn; do <u>not</u> cut,chew, <u>or</u> swallow; separate doses by at least 2 hours; max single dose 30 mg; max 5 doses per day; initiation and titration should be supervised by an appropriate healthcare provider; a concomitant anti-emetic (e.g. *trimethobenzamide*) is recommended beginning 3 days prior to initial dose
 Kynmobi *SL film:* 10, 15, 20, 25, 30 mg, single-dose in an individual foil pouch
 Comment: **Kynmobi** *(apomorphine sublingual film)* is a novel formulation of the approved dopamine agonist *apomorphine* for the on-demand

management of OFF episodes associated with Parkinson's disease (PD). Contraindictions include concomitant use with 5HT3 antagonists and hypersensitivity to *apomorphine* or any of its ingredients (including sodium metabisulfite). The most common adverse reactions (incidence ≥10%) have been nausea, oral/pharyngeal soft tissue swelling, oral/pharyngeal soft tissue pain and paraesthesia, dizziness, and somnolence. Discontinue if falling asleep during activities of daily living and daytime somnolence occurs at lowest dose. Syncope and hypotension/orthostatic hypotension may occur; monitor blood pressure. Oral mucosal irritation may require pausing or discontinuation. Falls may occur or increase. If hallucinations and psychotic-like behavior, loss of impulse control, or impulsive behaviors occur; consider dose reduction or discontinuation. Withdrawal-emergent hyperpyrexia and confusion may occur with rapid dose reduction or withdrawal. May prolong QTc and cause torsades de pointes or sudden death; consider risk factors prior to initiation. Concomitant use of antihypertensive medications and vasodilators may increase risk for hypotension, myocardial infarction, falls, and injuries. Avoid use of **Kynmobi** in patients with severe hepatic impairment (Child-Pugh Class C). No dosage adjustment is required for patients with mild or moderate hepatic impairment (Child-Pugh Class A or B). Avoid use of **Kynmobi** in patients with severe and end-stage renal disease (ESRD, CrCl <30 ml/min). No dosage adjustment is required for patients with mild or moderate renal impairment. Concomitant dopamine antagonists may diminish effectiveness of **Kynmobi**. *apomorphine* is not a controlled substance. In premarketing clinical experience, **Kynmobi** did not reveal any tendency for a withdrawal syndrome or any drug-seeking behavior. However, there are rare postmarketing reports of abuse of medications containing *apomorphine*. Advise patients that **Kynmobi** may cause prolonged painful erections (priapism) and if this occurs to seek immediate medical attention. Based on animal data, **Kynmobi** may cause fetal harm. There are no data on the presence of *apomorphine* in human milk or effects on the breastfed infant.

DOPAMINE RECEPTOR AGONISTS

▷ *amantadine* (C)

Gocovri take once daily at bedtime; initially 137 mg; after 1 week, increase to the recommended daily dosage of 274 mg; swallow whole; may sprinkle contents on soft food; take with or without food; avoid use with alcohol; a lower dosage is recommended for patients with moderate or severe renal impairment; Contraindicated in patients with end-stage renal disease

    Cap: 68.5, 137 mg ext-rel

Comment: **Gocovri** is a chrono-synchronous *amantadine* therapy indicated for the treatment of dyskinesia in patients with Parkinson's disease receiving *levodopa*-based therapy, with or without concomitant dopaminergic medications, as adjunctive treatment to *levodopa/carbidopa* in patients with Parkinson's disease experiencing "off" episodes. The most commonly observed adverse reactions (incidence ≥10%) have been hallucination, dizziness, dry mouth, peripheral edema, constipation, fall, and orthostatic hypotension. Advise patients prior to treatment about the potential to fall asleep during activities of daily living; discontinue if this occurs. Monitor patients for depressed mood, depression, or suicidal ideation or behavior. Patients with major psychotic disorder should ordinarily not be treated with **Gocovri**; observe patients for the occurrence of hallucinations throughout treatment, especially at initiation and after dose increases. Monitor patients for dizziness and orthostatic hypotension, especially after starting **Gocovri** and after dose increases. Avoid sudden discontinuation, which can result in withdrawal-emergent hyperpyrexia and confusion. Impulse control and compulsive behaviors may occur, such as gambling urges, sexual urges, uncontrolled spending; consider dose reduction or discontinuation if any occur. Increased risk of anticholinergic effects may require reduction of **Gocovri** or dose of the anticholinergic drug(s). Excretion of *amantadine* increases with acidic urine resulting in possible accumulation with urine change towards alkaline. Live attenuated vaccines (LAVs) are not recommended during treatment with **Gocovri**. Concomitant use of alcohol is not recommended due to increased potential for CNS effects. There are no adequate data on embryo/fetal risk associated with use of *amantadine* in pregnant females. Animal studies suggest a potential risk for fetal harm with *amantadine*. *Amantadine* is excreted in human milk, but amounts have not been quantified. There is no information on the risk to the breastfed infant.

Osmolex ER initial dose 129 mg orally once daily in the morning; may be increase dose in weekly intervals; max daily dose 322 mg in the morning; dose frequency reduction and monitoring required for renal impairment; swallow whole; do not chew, crush, or divide

    Tab: 129, 193, 258 mg ext-rel

Comment: **Osmolex ER** is not interchangeable with other *amantadine* immediate- or extended-release products. Most common adverse reactions (incidence ≥5%) are nausea, dizziness/ lightheadedness, and insomnia. **Osmolex ER** is contraindicated in patients with end-stage renal disease (ESRD). Advise patients prior to treatment about potential for falling asleep during activities of daily living (ADLs) and somnolence and discontinue **Osmolex ER** if occurs. Monitor patients for depressed mood, depression, and suicidal ideation or behavior. Patients with major psychotic disorder should ordinarily not be treated with **Osmolex ER**; observe patients throughout treatment for the occurrence of hallucinations, especially at initiation and after dose increases. Monitor patients for dizziness and orthostatic hypotension, especially after starting **Osmolex ER** or increasing the dose. Avoid sudden withdrawal/discontinuation due to risk of withdrawal-emergent hyperpyrexia and confusion. Monitor patient for development of impulse control/compulsive behaviors. Ask patients about increased gambling urges, sexual urges, uncontrolled spending or other urges and consider dose reduction or discontinuation if any occur. Increased risk of anticholinergic effects may require reduction of **Osmolex ER** or dose of the anticholinergic drug(s). Excretion of *amantadine* increases with acidic urine resulting in possible accumulation with urine change towards alkaline. Live attenuated vaccines (LAVs) are not recommended during treatment with **Osmolex ER**. Concomitant use of alcohol is not recommended due to increased potential for CNS effects. There are no adequate data on the developmental risk associated with use of *amantadine* in pregnant females. Animal studies suggest a potential risk for fetal harm with *amantadine*. *Amantadine* is excreted in human milk, but amounts have not been quantified. There is no information on the risk to the breastfed infant.

Symadine (G) initially 100 mg bid; may increase after 1-2 weeks by 100 mg/day; max 400 mg/day in divided doses; for extrapyramidal effects, 100 mg bid; max 300 mg/day in divided doses

    Cap: 100 mg

Symmetrel (G) initially 100 mg bid; may increase after 1-2 weeks by 100 mg/day; max 400 mg/day in divided doses; for extrapyramidal effects, 100 mg bid; max 300 mg/day in divided doses

    Cap: 100 mg; *Syr:* 50 mg/5 ml (16 oz) (raspberry)

▷ **bromocriptine (B)(G)** initially 1.25 mg bid to 2.5 mg tid with meals; increase as needed every 2-4 weeks by 2.5 mg/day; max 100 mg/day

Parlodel *Tab:* 2.5*mg; *Cap:* 5 mg

▷ **pramipexole (C)(G)** initially 0.125 mg tid; increase at intervals q 5-7 days; max 1.5 mg tid

Mirapex *Tab:* 0.125, 0.25*, 0.5*, 1*, 1.5*mg

▷ **ropinirole (C)** initially 0.25 mg tid for first week; then 0.5 mg tid for second week; then 0.75 mg tid for third week; then 1 mg tid for fourth week; may increase by 1.5 mg/day at 1 week intervals to 9 mg/day; then increase up to 3 mg/day at 1 week intervals; max 24 mg/day

Requip *Tab:* 0.25, 0.5, 1, 2, 4, 5 mg

▷ **rotigotine** transdermal patch **(C)** apply to clean, dry, intact skin on abdomen, thigh, hip, flank, shoulder, or upper arm; rotate sites and allow 14 days before reusing site; if hairy, shave site at least 3 days before application to site; avoid abrupt cessation; taper by 2 mg/24 hr every other day; *Early stage:* initially 2 mg/24 hr patch once daily; may increase weekly by 2 mg/24 hr if needed; max 6 mg/24 hr once daily; *Advanced stage:* initially 4 mg/24 hr patch once daily; may increase weekly by 2 mg/24 hr if needed; max 8 mg/24 hr once daily

Neupro *Trans patch:* 1 mg/24 hr, 2 mg/24 hr, 3 mg/24 hr, 4 mg/24 hr, 6 mg/24 hr, 8 mg/24 hr (30/carton) (sulfites)

DOPA-DECARBOXYLASE INHIBITORS

Comment: Contraindicated in narrow-angle glaucoma. Use with caution with sympathomimetics and antihypertensive agents.

▷ **carbidopa+levodopa (C)(G)** usually 400-1600 mg *levodopa*/day

Duopa *Ent susp:* carb 4.63 mg+levo 20 mg single-use cassettes for use w. CADD Legacy 1400 Pump

Sinemet 10/100 initially 1 tab tid-qid; increase if needed daily or every other day up to qid

Tab: carb 10 mg+levo 100 mg*

Sinemet 25/100 initially 1 tab bid-tid; increase if needed daily or every other day up to qid

Tab: carb 25 mg+levo 100 mg*

Sinemet 25/250 1 tab tid-qid

Tab: carb 25 mg+levo 250 mg*

Sinemet CR 25/100 initially one 25/100 tab bid; allow 3 days between dosage adjustments

Tab: carb 25 mg+levo 100 mg cont-rel

Sinemet CR 50/200 initially one 50/200 tab bid; allow 3 days between dosage adjustments

Tab: carb 50 mg+levo 200 mg cont-rel*

DOPA-DECARBOXYLASE INHIBITOR+DOPAMINE PRECURSOR+COMT INHIBITOR COMBINATION

▷ **carbidopa+levodopa+entacapone (C)** titrate individually with separate components; then switch to corresponding strength *levodopa* and *carbidopa*; max 8 tabs/day

Tab: **Stalevo 50** carb 12.5 mg+levo 50 mg+enta 200 mg

Stalevo 75 carb 12.5 mg+levo 75 mg+enta 200 mg

Stalevo 100 carb 12.5 mg+levo 100 mg+enta 200 mg

Stalevo 125 carb 12.5 mg+levo 125 mg+enta 200 mg

Stalevo 150 carb 12.5 mg+levo 150 mg+enta 200 mg

Stalevo 200 carb 12.5 mg+levo 200 mg+enta 200 mg

MONOAMINE OXIDASE INHIBITORS (MAOIs)

▷ **rasagiline (C)(G)** usual maintenance: 0.5-1 mg/day; max: 1 mg/day; initial dose for patients on concomitant *levodopa*: 0.5 mg daily; initial dose for patients not on concomitant *levodopa*: 1 mg daily

Azelect *Tab*: 0.5, 1 mg

Comment: **Azelect** is indicated as monotherapy or as adjunct to *levodopa*. With mild hepatic dysfunction (Child-Pugh 5-6), limit **Azelect** dose to 0.5 mg daily. With moderate-to-severe hepatic dysfunction (Child-Pugh 7-15), **Azelect** is not recommended. Contraindications include co-administration with *meperidine, methadone, mirtazapine, propoxyphene, tramadol, dextromethorphan, St. John's wort, cyclobenzaprine, methylphenidate, dexmethylphenidate,* or other MAOIs.

▷ *selegiline* (C)(G) 5 mg at breakfast and at lunch; max 10 mg/day
    Tab/Cap: 5 mg
▷ *selegiline* (C)(G) 1.25 mg daily; max 2.5 mg/day
    Zelapar *ODT*: 1.25 mg orally-disint (phenylalanine)

MONOAMINE OXIDASE TYPE B (MOA-B) INHIBITOR

▷ *safinamide* (C) initially 50 mg once daily at the same time each day; after 2 weeks, dose may be increased to 100 mg once daily based on individual need and tolerability; *Moderate Hepatic Impairment:* do not exceed 50 mg once daily; *Severe Hepatic Impairment:* contraindicated

Xadago *Tab*: 50, 100 mg

Comment: **Xadago** *(safinamide)* has not been shown to be effective as monotherapy; it is adjunctive treatment to *levodopa/carbodopa* in patients experiencing OFF episodes. **Xadago** drug interactions: SSRIs (monitor for *serotonin syndrome*); sympathomimetics (monitor for hypertension); tyramine: (monitor for severe hypertension); substrates of breast cancer resistance protein [BCRP]); potential for increase plasma concentration of BRCP substrate. **Xadago** is contraindicated with concomitant use of other MAOIs or other drugs that are potent inhibitors of monoamine oxidase (e.g., *linezolid; isoniazid* has some monoamine oxidase inhibiting activity), opioids and their derivatives, SNRIs, tri- or tetra-cyclic or triazolopyridine antidepressants, *cyclobenzaprine, methylphenidate,* and *amphetamine* and their derivatives, *dextromethorphan,* St. John's Wort, and severe hepatic impairment (Child-Pugh Class C). The most common adverse effects (incidence ≥2%) are dyskinesia, fall, nausea, and insomnia. Other adverse side effects include falling asleep during activities of daily living (ADLs), hallucinations, psychotic behavior, compulsive and impulsive behaviors, and withdrawal-emergent hyperpyrexia and confusion. Dopaminergic antagonists (e.g., antipsychotics, *metoclopramide*) may decrease the effectiveness of **Xadago** and exacerbate symptoms of Parkinson's disease. Dopaminergic antagonists (e.g., antipsychotics, *metoclopramide*) may decrease the effectiveness of **Xadago** and exacerbate symptoms of Parkinson's disease. There are no adequate and well-controlled human studies of **Xadago** use in pregnancy. Based on animal studies, **Xadago** may cause fetal harm. It is not known whether **Xadago** is present in human milk or effects on the breastfed infant. Mothers should be advised regarding the risk/benefit to mother and infant, and decide whether or not to discontinue the **Xadago** or breastfeeding.

ADENOSINE A₂ₐ RECEPTOR ANTAGONIST

▷ *istradefylline* 20 mg once daily; may increase to max 40 mg once daily; may take with or without food; *Moderate Hepatic Impairment:* max 20 mg once daily; *Severe Hepatic Impairment:* avoid; *Smokers (≥20 cigarettes/day or the equivalent of another tobacco product):* recommend 40 mg once daily

Nourianz *Tab*: 20, 40 mg

Comment: **Nourianz** *(istradefylline)* is an adenosine A₂ₐ receptor antagonist intended for use as adjunctive treatment to *levodopa/carbidopa* in adult patients with Parkinson's disease (PD) experiencing "OFF" episodes. Recommended maximum dosage with concomitant use of strong CYP

3A4 inhibitors is 20 mg once daily. Avoid use of **Nourianz** with strong CYP 3A4 inducers. Monitor patients for dyskinesia or exacerbation of existing dyskinesia. Consider dosage reduction or stopping **Nourianz** if hallucinations or other signs/symptions of psychosis occur, loss of impulse control, or compulsive behaviors occur. The most common adverse reactions (incidence ≥5% have been dyskinesia, dizziness, constipation, nausea, hallucination, and insomnia. Based on data from animal studies, **Nourianz** may cause embryo/fetal harm in pregnancy. There are no data on the presence of *istradefylline* in human milk or effects on the breastfed infant.

CATECHOL-O-METHYLTRANSFERASE (COMT) INHIBITORS

▷ *entacapone* (C) 1 tab with each dose of *levodopa* or *carbidopa*; max 8 tabs/day
Comtan *Tab*: 200 mg
Comment: **Comtan** is an adjunct to *levodopa+carbidopa* in patients with end-of-dose wearing off.

▷ *opicapone* 50 mg once daily at bedtime; *Moderate Hepatic Impairment*: 25 mg once daily at bedtime; *Severe Hepatic Impairment*: avoid use; do not eat food for 1 hour before and for at least 1 hour after taking dose
Ongentys *Cap*: 25, 50mg
Comment: **Ongentys** *(opicapone)* is an adjunctive treatment to levodopa/carbidopa in patients experiencing "off" episodes.

▷ *tolcapone* (C)(G) 100-200 mg tid; max 600 mg/day
Tasmar *Tab*: 100, 200 mg
Comment: Monitor LFTs every 2 weeks. Withdraw **Tasmar** if no substantial improvement in the first 3 weeks of treatment.

CENTRALLY-ACTING ANTICHOLINERGICS

▷ *benztropine mesylate* (C) initially 0.5-1 mg q HS, increase if needed; for extrapyramidal disorders 1-4 mg once daily-bid; max 6 mg/day
Cogentin *Tab*: 0.5*, 1*, 2*mg

▷ *biperiden hydrochloride* (C) initially 1 tab tid or qid, then increase as needed; max 8 tabs/day
Akineton *Tab*: 2 mg

▷ *procyclidine* (C) initially 2.5 mg tid; may increase as needed to 5 mg tid-qid every 3-5 days; max 15 mg/day
Kemadrin *Tab*: 5 mg

▷ *trihexyphenidyl* (C)(G) initially 1 mg; increase as needed by 2 mg every 3-5 days; max 15 mg/day
Artane *Tab*: 2*, 5*mg

PSEUDOBULBAR AFFECT (PBA)

Comment: Pseudobulbar affect (PBA), emotional lability, labile affect, or emotional incontinence refers by to a neurologic disorder characterized by involuntary crying or uncontrollable episodes of crying and/or laughing, or other emotional outbursts. PBA occurs secondary to a neurologic disease or brain injury such as traumatic brain injury (TBI), stroke, Parkinson's disease, multiple sclerosis, and amyotrophic lateral sclerosis (ALS, or Lou Gehrig's disease).

▷ *dextromethorphan+quinidine* (C)(G) 1 cap once daily x 7 days; then starting on day 8, 1 cap bid
Pediatric: <12 years: not recommended; ≥12 years: same as adult
Nuedexta *Cap*: dextro 20 mg+quini 10 mg
Comment: *Dextromethorphan hydrobromide* is an uncompetitive NMDA receptor antagonist and sigma-1 agonist. *quinidine sulfate* is a CYP450 2D6 inhibitor. **Nuedexta** is contraindicated with an MAOI or within 14 days of stopping an MAOI, with prolonged QT interval, congenital long QT

syndrome, history suggestive of torsades de pointes, or heart failure, complete atrioventricular (AV) block without implanted pacemaker or patients at high risk of complete AV block, and concomitant drugs that both prolong QT interval and are metabolized by CYP2D6 (e.g., *thioridazine* or *pimozide*). Discontinue **Nuedexta** if the following occurs: hepatitis or thrombocytopenia or any other hypersensitivity reaction. Monitor ECG in patients with left ventricular hypertrophy (LVH) or left ventricular dysfunction (LVD). *desipramine* exposure increases **Nuedexta** 8-fold; reduce *desipramine* dose and adjust based on clinical response. Use of **Nuedexta** with selective serotonin reuptake inhibitors (SSRIs) or tricyclic antidepressants (TCAs) increases the risk of *serotonin syndrome*. *paroxetine* exposure increases **Nuedexta** 2-fold; therefore, reduce **paroxetine** dose and adjust based on clinical response (*digoxin* exposure may increase *digoxin* substrate plasma concentration. **Nuedexta** is not recommended in pregnancy or breastfeeding. Safety and effectiveness of **Nuedexta** in children have not been established.

PARKINSON'S PSYCHOSIS
Atypical Anti-Psychotic

▷ *pimavanserin* take 34 mg once daily with or without food; no titration is needed
  Nuplazid *Tab:* 10 (2 x 17 mg tabs); *Cap:* 34 mg
  Comment: **Nuplazid** (*pimavanserin*) is an atypical antipsychotic indicated for the treatment of hallucinations and delusions associated with Parkinson's disease psychosis. **Nuplazid** is not indicated for dementia-related psychosis unrelated to Parkinson's disease as elderly patients with dementia-related psychosis treated with antipsychotic drugs are at increased risk of death. There is risk of QT interval prolongation with **Nuplazid**; therefore, avoid use in patients with risk factors for prolonged QT interval and concomitant use of other drugs that also increase the QT interval. **Nuplazid** does not affect motor function. Reduce **Nuplazid** dose by one-half with strong CYP3A4 inhibitors (e.g., *ketoconazole*). Strong CYP3A4 inducers may reduce efficacy of **Nuplazid**; increase in **Nuplazid** dosage may be needed. No **Nuplazid** dose adjustment is needed in patients with mild-to-moderate renal impairment. **Nuplazid** is not recommended for use in patients with severe renal impairment or hepatic impairment. There are no data on **Nuplazid** use in pregnancy that would allow assessment of the drug-associated risk of major congenital malformations or miscarriage, presence of *pimavanserin* in human milk, or effects on the breastfed infant. The most common adverse reactions (incidence ≥5%) are peripheral edema and confusional state.

PARONYCHIA (PERIUNGUAL ABSCESS)

▷ *cephalexin* (B)(G) 500 mg bid x 10 days
  Pediatric: 25-50 mg/day in 2 divided doses x 10 days
    Keflex *Cap:* 250, 333, 500, 750 mg; *Oral susp:* 125, 250 mg/5 ml (100, 200 ml) (strawberry)
▷ *clindamycin* (B)(G) 150-300 mg q 6 hours x 10 days
  Pediatric: 8-16 mg/kg/day in 3-4 divided doses x 10 days
    Cleocin *Cap:* 75 (tartrazine), 150 (tartrazine), 300 mg
    Cleocin Pediatric Granules *Oral susp:* 75 mg/5 ml (100 ml) (cherry)
▷ *dicloxacillin* (B)(G) 500 mg q 6 hours x 10 days
  Pediatric: 12.5-25 mg/kg/day in 4 divided doses x 10 days; *see* Appendix CC.18.
  dicloxacillin (Dynapen Suspension) *for dose by weight*
    Dynapen *Cap:* 125, 250, 500 mg; *Oral susp:* 62.5 mg/5 ml (80, 100, 200 ml)

➤ *erythromycin base* (B)(G) 500 mg q 6 hours x 10 days
  Pediatric: <45 kg: 30-50 mg in 2-4 doses x 10 days; ≥45 kg: same as adult
    Ery-Tab *Tab:* 250, 333, 500 mg ent-coat
    PCE *Tab:* 333, 500 mg
➤ *erythromycin ethylsuccinate* (B)(G) 400 mg q 6 hours x 10 days
  Pediatric: 30-50 mg/kg/day in 4 divided doses q 6 hours x 10 days; may double
  dose with severe infection; max 100 mg/kg/day; *see Appendix CC.21: erythromycin
  ethylsuccinate* (E.E.S. Suspension, Ery-Ped Drops/Suspension) *for dose by weight*
    EryPed *Oral susp:* 200 mg/5 ml (100, 200 ml) (fruit); 400 mg/5 ml (60, 100,
    200 ml) (banana); *Oral drops:* 200, 400 mg/5 ml (50 ml) (fruit); *Chew tab:*
    200 mg wafer (fruit)
    E.E.S. *Oral susp:* 200, 400 mg/5 ml (100 ml) (fruit)
    E.E.S. Granules *Oral susp:* 200 mg/5 ml (100, 200 ml) (cherry)
    E.E.S. 400 Tablets *Tab:* 400 mg

◯ PAROXYSMAL NOCTURNAL HEMOGLOBINURIA (PNH)

COMPLEMENT INHIBITOR

➤ *eculizumab* (C) dilute to a final admixture concentration of 5 mg/ml using the
  following steps: (1) withdraw the required amount of **Soliris** from the vial into
  a sterile syringe; (2) transfer the dose to an infusion bag; (3) add IV fluid equal
  to the drug volume (0.9% NaCl or 0.45% NaCl or D5W or Ringer's Lactate); the
  final admixed **Soliris** 5 mg/ml infusion volume is: 300 mg dose (60 ml), 600 mg
  dose (120 ml), 900 mg dose (180 ml), 1200 mg dose (240 ml)
  Pediatric: <18 years: safety and effectiveness not established
    Soliris *Vial:* 300 mg (10 mg/ml, 30 ml), single-use, concentrated solution for
    intravenous infusion (preservative-free)
    Comment: **Soliris** *(eculizumab)* is a complement inhibitor indicated for the
    treatment of patients with paroxysmal nocturnal hemoglobinuria (PNH) to
    reduce hemolysis, patients with atypical hemolytic uremia syndrome (aHUS)
    to inhibit complement-mediated thrombotic microangiopathy (TMA), and
    adult patients with generalized myasthenia gravis (gMG) who are anti-
    acetylcholine receptor (AchR) antibody positive. **Soliris** *(eculizumab)* should
    be administered at the above recommended dosage regimen time points or
    within 2 days of each time point. Supplemental dosing of **Soliris** is required
    in the setting of concomitant support with plasmapheresis (PI) or plasma
    exchange (PE) or fresh frozen plasma (FFP) infusion. See mfr pkg insert for
    supplemental dosing. **Soliris** is not indicated for the treatment of patients
    with Shiga toxin *E. coli*-related hemolytic uremic syndrome (STEC-HUS).
    Soliris is contraindicated in patients with unresolved *Neisseria meningitides*
    infection and patients who are not currently vaccinated against *Neisseria
    meningitides*, unless the risks of delaying **Soliris** treatment outweigh the
    risks of developing meningococcal infection. Prescribers must enroll in the
    Soliris REMS Program (1-888-SOLIRIS, 1-888-765-4747), counsel patients
    about the risk of meningococcal infection, provide patients with **Soliris**
    REMS educational materials, and ensure that patients are vaccinated with a
    meningococcal vaccine. The most frequently reported adverse reactions in
    the PNH randomized trial (incidence ≥10%) are headache, nasopharyngitis,
    back pain, and nausea. The most frequently reported adverse reactions in
    aHUS single-arm prospective trials (incidence ≥15%) are hypertension, URI,
    diarrhea, headache, anemia, vomiting, nausea, UTI, and leukopenia. There
    are no adequate and well-controlled human studies of **Soliris** in pregnancy
    or effects on the breastfed infant. Based on animal studies, **Soliris** may cause
    fetal harm. It is not known whether Soliris is excreted in human milk. IgG is
    excreted in human milk, so it is expected that **Soliris** will be present in human

milk. However, published data suggest that antibodies in human milk do not enter the neonatal and infant circulation in substantial amounts. Caution should be exercised when **Soliris** is administered to the breastfeeding patient.

▷ *ravulizumab-cwvz* withdraw the calculated volume of **Ultomiris** from the appropriate number of vials (according to the weight-based reference table) and dilute in an infusion bag using 0.9%NS to a final concentration of 5 mg/ml; administer all doses via IV infusion only; starting 2 weeks after administration of the loading dose, begin maintenance doses at once every 8-week intervals; the dosing schedule is allowed to occasionally vary within 7 days of the scheduled infusion day (except for the first maintenance dose of **Ultomiris**) but the subsequent dose should be administered according to the original schedule; for patients switching from *eculizumab* (**Soliris**) to **Ultomiris**, administer the loading dose of **Ultomiris** 2 weeks after the last *eculizumab* (**Soliris**) infusion, and then administer maintenance doses once every 8 weeks, starting 2 weeks after loading dose administration; dilute the appropriate number of vials to a final concentration of 5 mg/ml prior to administration

Weight-Based Dosing Regimen		
	Loading	Maintenance
≥40-<60 mg/kg:	2,400 mg	3,000 mg
≥60-<100 mg/kg:	2,700 mg	3,300 mg
≥100 mg/kg:	3,000 mg	3,600 mg

Pediatric: <18 years: not recommended; ≥18 years: same as adult

Ultomiris *Vial:* 300 mg/30 ml (10 mg/ml) in a single-dose

Comment: **Ultomiris** *(ravulizumab-cwvz)* is a long-acting C5 complement inhibitor for the treatment of paroxysmal nocturnal hemoglobinuria (PNH). Vaccinate patients for meningococcal disease according to current ACIP guidelines to reduce the risk of serious infection. Provide 2 weeks of antibacterial drug prophylaxis to patients if **Ultomoris** must be initiated immediately and vaccines are administered less than 2 weeks before starting **Ultomiris** therapy. There are no available data on **Ultomiris** use in pregnant females to inform a drug-associated risk of major birth defects, miscarriage, or adverse maternal or fetal outcomes (PNH in pregnancy is associated with adverse maternal outcomes, including worsening cytopenias, thrombotic events, infections, bleeding, miscarriages, and increased maternal mortality, and adverse fetal outcomes, including fetal death and premature delivery). There are no data on the presence of *ravulizumab-cwvz* in human milk or effect on the breastfed infant. However, breastfeeding should be discontinued during treatment and for 8 months after the final dose. Healthcare professionals who prescribe **Ultomiris** must enroll in the **Ultomiris** REMS program by telephone at 1-888-765-4747 or by visiting www.ultomirisrems.com.

⊙ PEANUT (ARACHIS HYPOGAEA) ALLERGY

ORAL IMMUNOTHERAPY

▷ *arachis hypogaea allergen powder-dnfp* open capsule(s) or sachet and empty the entire dose onto refrigerated or room temperature semi-solid food; mix well; consume the entire volume do not swallow capsule(s); do not inhale powder

Initial Dose Escalation (Day 1): the first 5 doses, and all new dose escalations, must be administered by a qualified health care provider, on a single day, under continuous observation by qualified health care staff, in an appropriate health care setting with epinephrine and other emergency support readily available to treat anaphylaxis

Up-Dosing Phase: begins Day 2; 11 up-dosing levels starting with Level 1 (3 mg) and finishing with Level 11 (300 mg); see mfr pkg insert for level dosing regimen); remain at each dose level for a period of at least 2 weeks; a dose level cannot be skipped

Maintenance Therapy: 300 mg/day; all doses must be taken daily, at the same time each day, to maintain treatment effect; patients must be co-prescribed injectable epinephrine for home use, provided with instruction and training on appropriate use, and instruction to seek immediate medical care upon its use

Pediatric: <4 years: not established; ≥4 years: same as adult

Palforzia *Cap:* 0.5 ,1, 10, 20, 100 mg; *Sachet:* 300 mg

Comment: **Palforzia** is an oral immunotherapy indicated to help reduce the severity of allergic reactions, including anaphylaxis, that may occur with accidental exposure to peanut. **Palforzia** does not treat allergic reactions and should not be taken during an allergic reaction. Patients must maintain a strict peanut-free diet while taking **Palforzia.** The first dose, and all dose increases, must be administered in a healthcare setting under the observation of trained healthcare staff for at least one hour. The most common adverse reactions reported in subjects treated with Palforzia (incidence ≥5%) have been abdominal pain, vomiting, nausea, oral pruritus, oral paresthesia, throat irritation, cough, rhinorrhea, sneezing, throat tightness, wheezing, dyspnea, pruritus, urticaria, anaphylactic reaction, and ear pruritus. Patients should be advised to stop taking **Palforzia** and seek emergency medical treatment right away if they have any of the following symptoms after taking **Palforzia**: trouble breathing or wheezing, chest discomfort or tightness, throat tightness, difficulty swallowing or speaking, swelling of the face, lips, eyes, or tongue, dizziness or fainting, severe stomach cramps or pain, vomiting, or diarrhea, hives, severe flushing of the skin. Contraindications to **Palforzia** are uncontrolled asthma, history of eosinophilic esophagitis (EoE) or other eosinophilic gastrointestinal disease. No human or animal data are available to establish the presence or absence of the risks due to **Palforzia** in pregnancy. Anaphylaxis can cause a dangerous decrease in blood pressure, which could result in compromised placental perfusion and significant risk to a fetus. There is a pregnancy exposure registry that monitors pregnancy outcomes in women exposed to **Palforzia** during pregnancy. Women exposed to **Palforzia** during pregnancy or their healthcare professionals are encouraged to contact Aimmune by calling 1-833-246-2566. There are no data available on the presence of **Palforzia** in human milk or effects on the breastfed infant. The developmental and health benefits of breastfeeding should be considered, along with the mother's clinical need for **Palforzia** and any other potential adverse effects on the breastfed infant from **Palforzia** or from the underlying maternal condition. **Palforzia** is available only through a restricted program under a Risk Evaluation and Mitigation Strategy (REMS) called the Palforzia REMS. **Palforzia** is only dispensed and distributed to certified healthcare settings and only administered to patients in certified healthcare settings.

PEDICULOSIS HUMANUS CAPITIS (HEAD LICE), PEDICULOSIS PHTHIRUS (PUBIC LICE)

► *abametapir* shake well before use; apply to dry hair in an amount sufficient (up to the full content of one bottle) to thoroughly coat the hair and scalp; avoid contact with eyes; massage into scalp and throughout the hair; leave on the hair and scalp for 10 minutes, and then rinse off with warm water

Pediatric: <6 months: not established; ≥6 months: same as adult

Xeglyze Lotion *Lotn:* 0.74% (approx 7 oz or 210 ml), single-use, amber glass bottle

Comment: **Xeglyze** is a pediculicide indicated for the topical treatment of head lice infestation. Systemic exposure to benzyl alcohol has been associated with serious adverse reactions and death in neonates and low birth-weight infants. **Xeglyze** use is not recommended in pediatric patients under <6 months-of-age because of the potential for increased systemic absorption. Direct supervision of children by an adult is required due to the risk of accidental ingestiion. Treatment involves a single application. Discard any unused product. Do not flush contents down sink or toilet. The most common adverse reactions (incidence of ≥1%) have been erythema, rash, skin burning sensation, contact dermatitis, vomiting, eye irritation, pruritus, and hair color changes. Other than age, there are no contraindications to **Xeglyze** use. For 2 weeks after a **Xeglyze** application, avoid taking drugs that are substrates of CYP3A4, CYP2B6 or CYP1A2. There are no available data on **Xeglyze** use in pregnancy to evaluate for a drug associated risk of major birth defects, miscarriage, or adverse maternal or fetal outcomes. In animal embryo/fetal development studies conducted with oral administration of *abametapir* during organogenesis there was no evidence of fetal harm or malformations. No data are available regarding the presence of *abametapir* in human milk or effects on the breastfed infant.

▷ *ivermectin* (C)(G) thoroughly wet hair; leave on for 10 minutes; then rinse off with water; do not re-treat
Pediatric: <6 months, <33 lbs: not recommended; ≥6 months, ≥33 lbs: same as adult
   Sklice *Lotn:* 0.5% (4 oz, 117 gm, laminate tube)

▷ *lindane* (C)(G) apply, leave on for 4 minutes, then thoroughly wash off
Pediatric: <2 years: not recommended; ≥2 years: same as adult
   Kwell Shampoo *Shampoo:* 1% (60 ml)

▷ *malathion* (B)(G) thoroughly wet hair; allow to dry naturally; shampoo and rinse after 8-12 hours; use a fine tooth comb to remove lice and nits; if lice persist after 7-9 days, may repeat treatment
Pediatric: same as adult
   Ovide (OTC) *Lotn:* 59% (2 oz)

▷ *permethrin* (B)(G) apply to washed and towel-dried hair; allow to remain on for 10 minutes, then rinse off; repeat after 7 days if needed
Pediatric: <2 months: not recommended; ≥2 months: same as adult
   Nix (OTC) *Crm rinse:* 1% (2 oz w. comb)

▷ *pyrethrins with piperonyl butoxide* (C)(G) apply and leave on for 10 minutes, then wash off
   A-200 *Shampoo:* pyr 0.33%+pip but 3%
   Rid Mousse *Shampoo:* pyr 0.33%+pip but 4%
   Rid Shampoo *Shampoo:* pyr 0.33%+pip but 3%
Comment: To remove nits, soak hair in equal parts white vinegar and water for 15-20 minutes.

▷ *spinosad* shake bottle well; apply a sufficient amount to cover dry scalp, then apply to dry hair; rinse off with warm water after 10 minutes; repeat treatment only if live lice are seen 7 days after the first treatment
Pediatric: <6 months years: safety and efficacy not established >6 months: same as adult
   Natroba *Topical susp:* 0.9% (9 mg/gm; 120ml)
Comment: **Natroba** is a pediculicide/scabicide, indicated for the topical treatment of head lice infestation in patients ≥6 months and (2) scabies infestation in patients ≥4 years. The most common adverse reactions (incidence (>1%) have been application site erythema and ocular erythema. *Spinosad*, the active ingredient in **Natroba**, is not absorbed systemically following topical application, and maternal use is not expected to result in

embryo/fetal exposure to the drug. **Natroba** contains benzyl alcohol. Topical benzyl alcohol is unlikely to be absorbed through the skin in clinically relevant amounts; therefore, maternal use is not expected to result in embryo/fetal exposure to the drug. Breastfeeding is <u>not</u> expected to result in the exposure of the infant to *spinosad*.

 PELVIC INFLAMMATORY DISEASE (PID)

Comment: The following treatment regimens are published in the **2015 CDC Sexually Transmitted Diseases Treatment Guidelines.** Treatment regimens are presented by generic drug name first, followed by information about brands and dose forms. Treat all sexual partners. Because of the high risk for maternal morbidity and preterm delivery, pregnant females who have suspected PID should be hospitalized and treated with parenteral antibiotics. HIV-infected women with PID respond equally well to standard parenteral and antibiotic regimens as HIV-negative women.

OUTPATIENT REGIMENS
Regimen 1
▷ *ceftriaxone* 250 mg IM in a single dose <u>plus</u> *doxycycline*
▷ *doxycycline* 100 mg bid x 14 days with <u>or</u> without *metronidazole*
▷ *metronidazole* 500 mg PO bid x 14 days

Regimen 2
▷ *cefoxitin* 2 gm IM in a single dose <u>plus</u> *probebecid*
▷ *probenecid* 1 gm PO in a single dose administered concurrently <u>plus</u> *doxycycline* 100 mg bid x 14 days with <u>or</u> without *metronidazole*
▷ *metronidazole* 500 mg PO bid x 14 days

Regimen 3
▷ Other parenteral third-generation cephalosporin (e.g., *ceftizoxime* <u>or</u> *cefotaxime*) in a single dose) <u>plus</u> *doxycycline*
▷ *doxycycline* 100 mg bid x 14 days with <u>or</u> without *metronidazole*
▷ *metronidazole* 500 mg PO bid x 14 days

DRUG BRANDS AND DOSE FORMS
▷ *cefoxitin* (B)(G)
    Mefoxin *Vial*: 1, 2 g
▷ *ceftriaxone* (B)(G)
    Rocephin *Vials* 250, 500 mg; 1, 2 gm
▷ *doxycycline* (D)(G)
    Acticlate *Tab*: 75, 150**mg
    Adoxa *Tab*: 50, 75, 100, 150 mg ent-coat
    Doryx *Tab*: 50, 75, 100, 150, 200 mg del-rel
    Doxteric *Tab*: 50 mg del-rel
    Monodox *Cap*: 50, 75, 100 mg
    Oracea *Cap*: 40 mg del-rel
    Vibramycin *Tab*: 100 mg; *Cap*: 50, 100 mg; *Syr*: 50 mg/5 ml (raspberry-apple) (sulfites); *Oral susp*: 25 mg/5 ml (raspberry)
    Vibra-Tab *Tab*: 100 mg film-coat
▷ *metronidazole* (<u>not</u> for use in 1st; B in 2nd, 3rd)
    Flagyl *Tab*: 250*, 500*mg
    Flagyl 375 *Cap*: 375 mg
    Flagyl ER *Tab*: 750 mg ext-rel
▷ *probenecid* (B)(G)
    Benemid *Tab*: 500*mg; *Cap*: 500 mg

PEMPHIGUS VULGARIS (PV), PEMPHIGUS FOLIACEUS (PF)

Comment: Pemphigus is a rare bullous autoimmune disorder that has no cure and is fatal if left untreated. It is characterized by auto-antibody-mediated blistering of the skin (primarily affecting the chest and back; usually sparing the palms and soles of the feet) and oral mucosa. There are two histologic subtypes. Pemphigus vulgaris (PV), accounting for 70% of pemphigus cases, affects the mid-to-deep layers of the epidermis. The hallmark of PV is involvement of the oral mucosa. Pemphigus foliaceus (PF) affects the superficial skin layers and does not affect the oral mucosa. Systemic administration of corticosteroids is the standard first-line treatment to suppress the immune response. Adjuvant nonsteroidal immunosuppressants may be used (e.g., *azathioprine, cyclophosphamide, mycophenolate mofetil* [MMF], *dapsone*).

GLUCOCORTICOSTEROID

▷ *prednisone* 1.0-1.5 mg/kg (oral or parenteral) daily with slow tapering and discontinuation after lesions have resolved

MYCOPHENOLIC ACID

▷ *azathioprine* (D) 1 mg/kg/day in a single or divided doses; may increase by 0.5 mg/kg/day q 4 weeks; max 2.5 mg/kg/day; minimum trial to ascertain effectiveness is 12 weeks; administer IV doses over no less than 2 hours
  Pediatric: <12 years: not recommended; >12 years: same as adult
    Azasan *Tab* 75*, 100*mg
    Imuran *Tab* 50*mg
▷ *cyclophosphamide* (D)(G) *Oral:* Usually 1 mg per kg per day to 5 mg per kg per day for both initial and maintenance dosing; *Intravenous:* initial course for patients with no hematologic deficiency: 40 mg/kg to 50 mg/kg in divided doses over 2 to 5 days; *Other regimens include:* 10 mg/kg to 15 mg/kg every 7-10 days or 3 mg/kg to 5 mg/kg twice weekly
    Tab: 25, 50 mg; *Vial:* 500 mg; 1, 2 gm pwdr for reconstitution and IV infusion

SULFONE

▷ *dapsone* topical (C)(G) apply to affected area bid
  Pediatric: <12 years: not recommended; ≥12 years: same as adult
    Aczone *Gel:* 5, 7.5% (30, 60, 90 gm pump)

CD20-DIRECTED CYTOLYTIC MONOCLONAL ANTIBODY

▷ *rituximab* initially (Month 0) 1000 mg x 2 IV infusions separated by 2 weeks in combination with a tapering course of glucocorticoids; then a 500 mg IV infusion at Month 12 and every 6 months thereafter or based on clinical evaluation; *Relapse:* 1000 mg IV infusion with considerations to resume or increase the glucocorticoid dose based on clinical evaluation; subsequent infusions may be no sooner than 16 weeks after the previous infusion; methylprednisolone 100 mg IV or equivalent glucocorticoid recommended 30 minutes prior to each infusion
  Pediatric: <6 years: not recommended; ≥6 years: same as adult
    Rituxan *Vial:* 100 mg/10 ml (10 mg/ml), 500 mg/50 ml (10 mg/ml), single-use, (preservative-free)
    Comment: Rituxan *(rituximab)* is a CD20-targeting cytolytic monoclonal antibody that received FDA Breakthrough Therapy Designation for treatment of PV in 2017. Safety and efficacy in recalcitrant PV has been demonstrated in approximately 500 patients across several small trials and case studies, with clinical remission occurring within six weeks in up to 95% of cases. In a recent

phase 2 trial comparing *rituximab* plus *prednisone* with *prednisone* alone in patients with newly diagnosed PV, a 55% increase in 2-year remission rate (89% vs 34%) was observed in those receiving *rituximab* plus *prednisone*. Consider intravenous immunoglobulin (e.g., IVIG).

INTERLEUKIN-6 (IL-6) RECEPTOR ANTAGONIST

▷ *tocilizumab* (B) *<100 kg:* 162 mg SC every other week on the same day followed by an increase according to clinical response; *≥100 kg:* 162 mg SC once weekly on the same day; SC injections may be self-administered after being trained and supervised by a qualified healthcare provider

Actemra *Vial:* 80 mg/4 ml, 200 mg/10 ml, 400 mg/20 ml, single-use, for IV infusion after dilution; *Prefilled syringe:* 162 mg (0.9 ml, single-dose)

Comment: Actemra *(tocilizumab)* has received FDA Orphan Drug Designation in PV and is currently being investigated in a phase 2 trial. It is indicated for active recalcitrant pemphigus vulgaris has that has failed 2 lines of prior treatment comprising *prednisone, mycophenolate mofetil MMF)*, and IV immunoglobulin.

B-LYMPHOCYTE STIMULATOR (BLyS)-SPECIFIC INHIBITOR

▷ *belimumab SC administration:* 200 mg SC once weekly; may be self-administered by the patient in the home setting; *IV infusion:* 10 mg/kg at 2-week intervals by a qualified healthcare provider
Pediatric: <5 years: not established; ≥5 years: same as adult

Benlysta *Prefilled syringe:* 200 mg/ml (1 ml) single-dose (4/carton); *Auto injector:* 200 mg (1 ml) single-dose (4/carton); *Vial:* 120 mg/5 ml, 400 mg/20 ml, single-dose, pwdr for reconstitution and IV infusion (4/carton)

Comment: Benlysta *(belimumab)* is an IgG1-lambda monoclonal antibody that prevents the survival of B lymphocytes by blocking the binding of soluble human B lymphocyte stimulator protein (BLyS) to receptors on B lymphocytes. This reduces the activity of B-cell mediated immunity and the autoimmune response. Benlysta was initially approved as an intravenous formulation administered in a hospital or clinic setting as a weight-dosed IV infusion every four weeks. Patients can now self-administer Benlysta as a once weekly SC injection after being trained and supervised by a qualified healthcare provider.

⬭ PEPTIC ULCER DISEASE (PUD)

Helicobacter pylori Eradication Regimens *see Helicobacter Pylori (H. Pylori)* Infection
Antacids *see* GERD

H2 ANTAGONISTS

▷ *cimetidine* (B)(G)
Pediatric: <16 years: not recommended; ≥16 years: same as adult
Tagamet 800 mg bid or 400 mg qid; max 2.4 gm/day
Tab: 300, 400*, 800*mg
Tagamet HB (OTC) *Prophylaxis:* 1 tab ac; *Treatment:* 1 tab bid
Tab: 200 mg
Tagamet HB Oral Suspension (OTC) *Prophylaxis:* 1 tsp ac; *Treatment:* 1 tsp bid
Oral susp: 200 mg/20 ml (12 oz)
Tagamet Liquid *Liq:* 300 mg/5 ml (mint-peach) (alcohol 2.8%)
▷ *famotidine* (B)(G) 20 mg bid or 40 mg q HS; *max* 6 weeks
Pediatric: 0.5 mg/kg/day q HS or in 2 divided doses; max 40 mg/day

Pepcid *Tab:* 20, 40 mg; *Oral susp:* 40 mg/5 ml (50 ml)
Pepcid AC (OTC) 1 tab ac; max 2 doses/day
Tab/Rapid dissolv tab: 10 mg
Pepcid Complete (OTC) 1 tab ac; max 2 doses/day
Tab: fam 10 mg+CaCO2 800 mg+mag hydrox 165 mg
Pepcid RPD
Tab: 20, 40 mg rapid-dissolv

▷ *nizatidine* (B)(G) 150 mg bid; max 12 weeks
Pediatric: <12 years: not recommended; ≥12 years: same as adult
Axid *Cap:* 150, 300 mg
Axid AR (OTC) 1 tab ac; max 150 mg/day
Tab: 75 mg

▷ *ranitidine* (B)(G)
Pediatric: <1 month: not recommended; 1 month-16 years: 2-4 mg/kg/day in 2 divided doses; max 300 mg/day; *Duodenal/Gastric Ulcer:* 2-4 mg/kg/day divided bid; max 300 mg/day; *Erosive Esophagitis:* 5-10 mg/kg/day divided bid; max 300 mg/day; >16 years: same as adult
Zantac 150 mg bid or 300 mg q HS
Tab: 150, 300 mg
Zantac 75 (OTC) 1 tab ac
Tab: 75 mg
Zantac EFFERdose dissolve 25 mg tab in 5 ml water; dissolve 150 mg tab in 6-8 oz water
Efferdose: 25, 150 mg effervescent (phenylalanine)
Zantac Syrup *Syr:* 15 mg/ml (peppermint) (alcohol 7.5%)

▷ *ranitidine bismuth citrate* (C) 400 mg bid
Pediatric: <12 years: not recommended; ≥12 years: same as adult
Tritec *Tab:* 400 mg

PROTON PUMP INHIBITORS (PPIs)

Comment: If hepatic impairment, or if patient is Asian, consider reducing the PPI dosage. Research has demonstrated associations between PPI use and fractures of the hip, wrist, and spine, hypomagnesemia, kidney injuries and chronic kidney disease, possible cardiovascular drug interactions, and infections (e.g., *Clostridioides difficile* and pneumonia). Reducing the acidity of the stomach allows bacteria to thrive and spread to other organs like the lungs and intestines. This risk is increased with high dose and chronic use and greatest in the elderly. The most recent class-wide FDA warning cites reports of cutaneous and systemic lupus erythematosis (CLS/SLE) associates with PPIs in patients with both new onset and exacerbation of existing autoimmune disease. PPI treatment should be discontinued and the patient should be referred to a specialist (http://www.fda.gov/Drugs/DrugSafety/InformationbyDrugClass/ucm213259.htm).

▷ *dexlansoprazole* (B)(G) 30-60 mg daily for up to 4 weeks
Pediatric: <18 years: not recommended; ≥18 years: same as adult
Dexilant *Cap:* 30, 60 mg ent-coat del-rel granules; may open and sprinkle on applesauce; do not crush or chew granules
Dexilant SoluTab *Tab:* 30 mg del-rel orally-disint

▷ *esomeprazole* (B)(OTC)(G) 20-40 mg daily; max 8 weeks; take 1 hour before food; swallow whole or mix granules with food or juice and take immediately; do not crush or chew granules
Pediatric: <1 year: not recommended; 1-11 years: <20 kg: 10 mg; ≥20 kg: 10-20 mg once daily; 12-17 years: 20-40 mg once daily; max 8 weeks; >17 years: same as adult
Nexium *Cap:* 20, 40 mg ent-coat del-rel pellets

Nexium for Oral Suspension *Oral susp:* 10, 20, 40 mg ent-coat del-rel granules/pkt (30 pkt/carton); mix in 2 tbsp water and drink immediately

▷ *lansoprazole* **(B)(OTC)(G)** 15-30 mg daily for up to 8 weeks; may repeat course; take before eating
Pediatric: <1 year: not recommended; 1-11, <30 kg: 15 mg once daily; ≥12 years: same as adult

Prevacid *Cap:* 15, 30 mg ent-coat del-rel granules; swallow whole or mix granules with food or juice and take immediately; do not crush or chew granules; follow with water
Prevacid for Oral Suspension *Oral susp:* 15, 30 mg ent-coat del-rel granules/pkt (30 pkt/carton); mix in 2 tbsp water and drink immediately; (strawberry)
Prevacid SoluTab *ODT:* 15, 30 mg (strawberry) (phenylalanine)
Prevacid 24HR 15 mg ent-coat del-rel granules; swallow whole or mix granules with food or juice and take immediately; do not crush or chew granules; follow with water

▷ *omeprazole* **(C)(OTC)(G)** 20-40 mg daily; take before eating; swallow whole or mix granules with applesauce and take immediately; do not crush or chew; follow with water
Pediatric: <1 year: not recommended; 5-<10 kg: 5 mg daily; 10-<20 kg: 10 mg daily; ≥20 kg: same as adult

Prilosec *Cap:* 10, 20, 40 mg ent-coat del-rel granules
Prilosec OTC *Tab:* 20 mg del-rel (regular, wild berry)

▷ *pantoprazole* **(B)(G)** initially 40 mg bid
Pediatric: <12 years: not recommended; ≥12 years: same as adult

Protonix *Tab:* 40 mg ent-coat del-rel
Protonix for Oral Suspension *Oral susp:* 40 mg ent-coat del-rel granules/pkt; mix in 1 tsp apple juice for 5 seconds or sprinkle on 1 tsp apple sauce, and swallow immediately; do not mix in water or any other liquid or food; take approximately 30 minutes prior to a meal; 30 pkt/carton

▷ *rabeprazole* **(B)(OTC)(G)** initially 20 mg daily; then titrate; may take 100 mg daily in divided doses or 60 mg bid
Pediatric: <12 years: not recommended; ≥12 years: 20 mg once daily; max 8 weeks

AcipHex *Tab:* 20 mg ent-coat del-rel
AcipHex Sprinkle *Cap:* 5, 10 mg del-rel

OTHER AGENTS

▷ *glycopyrrolate* **(B)(G)** initially 1-2 mg bid-tid; *Maintenance:* 1 mg bid; max 8 mg/day
Pediatric: <12 years: not recommended; ≥12 years: same as adult

Robinul *Tab:* 1 mg (dye-free)
Robinul Forte *Tab:* 2 mg (dye-free)
Comment: *Glycopyrrolate* is an anticholinergic adjunct to PUD treatment.

▷ *mepenzolate* **(B)(G)** 25-50 mg divided qid, with meals and at HS
Cantil *Tab:* 25 mg

▷ *sucralfate* **(B)(G)** **Active ulcer:** 1 gm qid; *Maintenance:* 1 gm bid
Carafate *Tab:* 1*g; *Oral susp:* 1 gm/10 ml (14 oz)

PROPHYLAXIS

▷ *misoprostol* **(X)** 200 mg qid with food for prevention of NSAID-induced gastric ulcers
Cytotec *Tab:* 100, 200 mg
Comment: *Misoprostol* is a prostaglandin E1 analog indicated for the prevention of NSAID-induced gastric ulcers. Females of childbearing potential should have a negative serum pregnancy test within 2 weeks before starting and first dose on the 2nd or 3rd day of next the menstrual period. A contraceptive method should be maintained during therapy. Risks to pregnant females include: spontaneous abortion, premature birth, fetal anomalies, and uterine rupture.

PERIPHERAL NEURITIS, DIABETIC NEUROPATHIC PAIN, PERIPHERAL NEUROPATHIC PAIN

▷ **Acetaminophen for IV Infusion** *see Pain*
▷ **Ibuprophen for IV Infusion** *see Pain*

▷ *acetaminophen* (B)(G) *see Fever*

▷ *aspirin* (D)(G) *see Fever*

ALPHA-2 DELTA LIGAND

▷ *pregabalin (GABA analog)* (C)(G)(V) initially 150 mg daily divided bid-tid; may titrate within 1 week; max 600 mg divided bid-tid; discontinue over 1 week
Pediatric: <18 years: not recommended; ≥18 years: same as adult
 Lyrica *Cap:* 25, 50, 75, 100, 150, 200, 225, 300 mg; *Oral soln:* 20 mg/ml

SEROTONIN-NOREPINEPHRINE REUPTAKE INHIBITOR (SNRI)

▷ *duloxetine* (C) swallow whole; 30-60 mg once daily; may increase by 30 mg at 1 week intervals; usual target 60 mg daily; max 120 mg/day
Pediatric: <12 years: not recommended; ≥12 years: same as adult
 Cymbalta *Cap:* 20, 30, 60 mg ent-coat pellets
 Comment: **Cymbalta** is indicated for chronic pain syndromes (e.g., arthritis, fibromyalgia, lowback pain).

TOPICAL & TRANSDERMAL ANALGESICS

▷ *capsaicin* (B)(G) apply tid-qid prn to intact skin
Pediatric: <2 years: not recommended; ≥2 years: apply sparingly tid-qid prn
 Axsain *Crm:* 0.075% (1, 2 oz)
 Capsin *Lotn:* 0.025, 0.075% (59 ml)
 Capzasin-HP (OTC) *Crm:* 0.075% (1.5 oz), 0.025% (45, 90 gm); *Lotn:* 0.075% (2 oz); 0.025% (45, 90 gm)
 Capzasin-P (OTC) *Crm:* 0.025% (1.5 oz); *Lotn:* 0.025% (2 oz)
 Dolorac *Crm:* 0.025% (28 gm)
 Double Cap (OTC) *Crm:* 0.05% (2 oz)
 R-Gel *Gel:* 0.025% (15, 30 gm)
 Zostrix (OTC) *Crm:* 0.025% (0.7, 1.5, 3 oz)
 Zostrix HP (OTC) *Emol crm:* 0.075% (1, 2 oz)
▷ *capsaicin* 8% patch (B) apply up to 4 patches for one 60-minute application to clean dry skin; may prep area with topical anesthetic; wear non-latex gloves; patches may be cut to size/shape; treatment may be repeated every 3 months
Pediatric: <18 years: not recommended; ≥18 years: same as adult
 Qutenza *Patch:* 8% 1640 mcg/cm (179 mg) (1 or 2 patches w. 1-50 gm tube cleansing gel/carton)
▷ *diclofenac sodium* (C; D ≥30 wks) apply qid prn to intact skin
Pediatric: <12 years: not established; ≥12 years: same as adult
 Pennsaid 1.5% in 10 drop increments, dispense and rub into front, side, and back of knee: usually; 40 drops (40 mg) qid
  Topical soln: 1.5% (150 ml)
 Pennsaid 2% apply 2 pump actuations (40 mg) and rub into front, side, and back of knee bid
  Topical soln: 2% (20 mg/pump actuation, 112 gm)
 Solaraze Gel massage in to clean skin bid prn
  Gel: 3% (50 gm) (benzyl alcohol)
 Voltaren Gel (G)(OTC) apply qid prn to intact skin
  Gel: 1% (100 gm)

Comment: *Diclofenac* is contraindicated with *aspirin* allergy. As with other NSAIDs, should be avoided in late pregnancy (≥30 weeks) because it may cause premature closure of the ductus arteriosus.

▷ *doxepin* (B) cream apply to affected area qid at intervals of at least 3-4 hours; max 8 days

Pediatric: <12 years: not recommended; >12 years: same as adult

    Prudoxin *Crm:* 5% (45 gm)

    Zonalon *Crm:* 5% (30, 45 gm)

▷ *pimecrolimus* 1% cream (C)(G) <2 years: not recommended; ≥2 years: apply to affected area bid; do not apply an occlusive dressing

    Elidel *Crm:* 1% (30, 60, 100 gm)

Comment: *Pimecrolimus* is indicated for short-term and intermittent long-term use. Discontinue use when resolution occurs. Contraindicated if the patient is immunosuppressed. Change to the 0.1% preparation or if secondary bacterial infection is present.

▷ *trolamine salicylate* apply tid-qid

Pediatric: <2 years: not recommended; ≥2 years: same as adult

    Mobisyl Creme *Crm:* 10% (100 gm)

TOPICAL AND TRANSDERMAL ANESTHETICS

Comment: *Lidocaines* should not be applied to non-intact skin.

▷ *lidocaine* cream (B) apply to affected area bid prn

Pediatric: <12 years: not recommended; ≥12 years: same as adult

    LidaMantle *Crm:* 3% (1, 2 oz)

    Lidoderm *Crm:* 3% (85 gm)

    ZTlido *lidocaine* topical system 1% (30/carton)

    Comment: Compared to **Lidoderm** (*lidocaine* patch 5%), which contains 700 mg/patch, **ZTlido** requires 35 mg per topical system to achieve the same therapeutic dose.

▷ *lidocaine* lotion (B) apply to affected area bid prn

Pediatric: <12 years: not recommended; ≥12 years: same as adult

    LidaMantle *Lotn:* 3% (177 ml)

▷ *lidocaine* 5% patch (B)(G) apply up to 3 patches at one time for up to 12 hours/24-hour period (12 hours on/12 hours off); patches may be cut into smaller sizes before removal of the release liner; do not re-use

Pediatric: <12 years: not recommended; ≥12 years: same as adult

    Lidoderm *Patch:* 5% (10x14 cm; 30/carton)

▷ *lidocaine+dexamethasone* (B)

Pediatric: <12 years: not recommended; ≥12 years: same as adult

    Decadron Phosphate with Xylocaine *Lotn:* dexa 4 mg+lido 10 mg per ml (5 ml)

▷ *lidocaine+hydrocortisone* (B)(G) apply to affected area bid prn

Pediatric: <12 years: not recommended; ≥12 years: same as adult

    LidaMantle HC *Crm:* lido 3%+hydro 0.5% (1, 3 oz); *Lotn:* (177 ml)

▷ *lidocaine* 2.5%+*prilocaine* 2.5% apply sparingly to the burn bid-tid prn

Pediatric: <12 years: not recommended; ≥12 years: same as adult

    Emla Cream (B) 5, 30 gm/tube

ORAL ANALGESICS

▷ *tramadol* (C)(IV)(G)

    Rybix ODT initially 100 mg once daily; may increase by 100 mg every 5 days; max 300 mg/day; *CrCl <30 mL/min or severe hepatic impairment:* not recommended; *Cirrhosis:* max 50 mg q 12 hours

    Pediatric: <12 years: contraindicated; 12-<18: use extreme caution; not recommended for children and adolescents with obesity, asthma, obstructive sleep apnea, or other chronic breathing problem, or for post-tonsillectomy/adenoidectomy pain; ≥18 years: same as adult

   ODT: 50 mg (mint) (phenylalanine)

Ryzolt initially 100 mg once daily; may increase by 100 mg every; 5 days; max 300 mg/day; *CrCl <30 mL/min or severe hepatic impairment:* not recommended

Pediatric: <18 years: not recommended; ≥18 years: same as adult

   Tab: 100, 200, 300 mg ext-rel

Ultram 50-100 mg q 4-6 hours prn; max 400 mg/day; *CrCl <30 mL/min:* max 100 mg q 12 hours; *Cirrhosis:* max 50 mg q 12 hours

Pediatric: <18 years: not recommended; ≥18 years: same as adult

   Tab: 50 mg

Ultram ER initially 100 mg once daily; may increase by 100 mg every 5 days; max 300 mg/day; *CrCl <30 mL/min or severe hepatic impairment:* not recommended

Pediatric: <18 years: not recommended; ≥18 years: same as adult

   Tab: 100, 200, 300 mg ext-rel

▷ *tramadol+acetaminophen* (C)(IV)(G) 2 tabs q 4-6 hours; max 8 tabs/day; 5 days; *CrCl <30 mL/min:* max 2 tabs q 12 hours; max 4 tabs/day x 5 days

Pediatric: <18 years: not recommended; ≥18 years: same as adult

   Ultracet *Tab:* tram 37.5+acet 325 mg

OPIOID AGONIST

▷ *tapentadol* (C)(II)

Pediatric: <18 years: not recommended; ≥18 years: same as adult

   Nucynta 50-100 mg q 4-6 hours prn; max 700 mg/day on the first day; 600 mg/day on subsequent days

     Tab: 50, 75, 100 mg

   Nucynta ER *Opioid-naïve:* initially 50 mg q 12 hours, then titrate to optimal dose within therapeutic range; usual therapeutic range 100-250 mg q 12 hours; doses >500 mg not recommended; *Converting from Nucynta:* divide total **Nucynta** daily dose into 2 **Nucynta ER** doses and administer q 12 hours; converting from *oxycodone CR* and other opioids, see mfr recommendations

     Tab: 50, 100, 150, 200, 250 mg ext-rel

PERIPHERAL VASCULAR DISEASE (PVD, ARTERIAL INSUFFICIENCY, INTERMITTENT CLAUDICATION)

ANTIPLATELET THERAPY

▷ *aspirin* (D)(OTC) usually 81 mg once daily; range 75-325 mg once daily

   Ecotrin *Tab/Cap:* 81, 325, 500 mg ent-coat

▷ *cilostazol* (C) 100 mg bid 1/2 hour before or 2 hours after breakfast or dinner; may reduce to 50 mg bid if used with CYP 3A4 (e.g., azole antifungals, macrolides, *diltiazem, fluvoxamine, fluoxetine, nefazodone, sertraline*) or CYP 2C19 (e.g., *omeprazole*) inhibitors

   Tab: 50, 100 mg

Comment: *Cilostazol* may be used with *aspirin.* Cautious use with other antiplatelet agents and anticoagulants.

clopidogrel (B) 75 mg daily

   Plavix *Tab:* 75 mg

▷ *dipyridamole* (B)(G) 25-100 mg tid-qid

   Persantine *Tab:* 25, 50, 75 mg

Comment: *Dipyridamole* does not potentiate *warfarin* and may be taken concomitantly. Do not administer *dipyridamole* concomitantly with *aspirin.*

▷ *pentoxifylline* (C) 400 mg tid with food
    PentoPak *Tab:* 400 mg ext-rel
    Trental *Tab:* 400 mg sust-rel
▷ *ticlopidine* (B) 250 mg bid with food
    Ticlid *Tab:* 250 mg
    Comment: Monitor for neutropenia; resolves after discontinuation.
▷ *warfarin* (X) adjust dose to maintain INR in recommended range; *see*
    Anticoagulation Therapy see Appendix T. Anticoagulants
    Coumadin *Tab:* 1*, 2*, 2.5*, 5*, 7.5*, 10*mg
    Coumadin for Injection *Vial:* 2 mg/ml (5 mg) pwdr for reconstitution
    Comment: Treatment for over-anticoagulation with *warfarin* is *vitamin K*.

PERLECHE (ANGULAR STOMATITIS)

Comment: Perleche is a form of intertrigo. This localized tissue inflammation and maceration is characterized by constant exposure to saliva, which normally contains bacteria, yeast, and other organisms, in the natural anatomical furrow at the corners of the mouth. Perleche is often misdiagnosed as yeast infection, but almost never responds to anti-yeast agents. Patients with severe vitamin deficiencies (e.g., chronic alcoholism, malnutrition) are often at increased risk. Sensitivities or allergies to toothpaste may be contributing irritants.

Treatment: apply a small amount of a combination of 2.5% *hydrocortisone* cream and *miconazole* cream (which kills yeast, fungi, and many bacteria) to the affected area twice a day. Once the area is clear, recurrence can be prevented with local application of petroleum jelly.

PERTUSSIS (WHOOPING COUGH)

Prophylaxis *see Childhood Immunizations*

POST-EXPOSURE PROPHYLAXIS & TREATMENT

Comment: Antibiotics do <u>not</u> alter the course of illness, but they do prevent transmission. Infected persons should be isolated until after the fifth day of antibiotic treatment.
▷ *azithromycin* (B)(G) 500 mg x 1 dose on day 1, then 250 mg daily on days 2-5 <u>or</u>
    500 mg daily x 3 days
    Pediatric: 12 mg/kg/day x 5 days; max 500 mg/day; *see* Appendix CC.7.
    azithromycin (Zithromax Suspension, Zmax Suspension) *for dose by weight*
    Zithromax *Tab:* 250, 500, 600 mg; *Oral susp:* 100 mg/5 ml (15 ml); 200 mg/5
    ml (15, 22.5, 30 ml) (cherry); *Pkt:* 1 gm for reconstitution (cherry-banana)
    Zithromax Tri-pak *Tab:* 3 x 500 mg tabs/pck
    Zithromax Z-pak *Tab:* 6 x 250 mg tabs/pck
    Zmax *Oral susp:* 2 gm ext-rel for reconstitution (cherry-banana) (148 mg Na+)
    Comment: *Azithromycin* is the drug of choice for infants <1 month-of-age.
▷ *clarithromycin* (C)(G) 250 mg bid <u>or</u> 500 mg ext-rel once daily x 10 days
    Pediatric: <6 months: not recommended; ≥6 months: 7.5 mg/kg divided bid x 10
    days; *see* Appendix CC.16. *clarithromycin* (Biaxin Suspension) *for dose by weight*
    Biaxin *Tab:* 250, 500 mg
    Biaxin Oral Suspension *Oral susp:* 125, 250 mg/5 ml (50, 100 ml)
    (fruit-punch)
    Biaxin XL *Tab:* 500 mg ext-rel
▷ *erythromycin base* (B)(G) 1 gm/day divided qid x 14 days
    Pediatric: 40 mg/kg/day in divided doses x 14 days
    Ery-Tab *Tab:* 250, 333, 500 mg ent-coat
    PCE *Tab:* 333, 500 mg

▷ *erythromycin ethylsuccinate* (B)(G) 1 gm/day in 4 divided doses x 14 days
Pediatric: 40-50 mg/kg/day in 4 divided doses x 7 days; may double dose
with severe infection; max 100 mg/kg/day; *see Appendix CC.21: erythromycin
ethylsuccinate (E.E.S. Suspension, Ery-Ped Drops/Suspension) for dose by weight*

    EryPed *Oral susp:* 200 mg/5 ml (100, 200 ml) (fruit); 400 mg/5 ml (60, 100,
200 ml) (banana); *Oral drops:* 200, 400 mg/5 ml (50 ml) (fruit); *Chew tab:* 200
mg wafer (fruit)

    E.E.S. *Oral susp:* 200, 400 mg/5 ml (100 ml) (fruit)

    E.E.S. Granules *Oral susp:* 200 mg/5 ml (100, 200 ml) (cherry)

    E.E.S. 400 Tablets *Tab:* 400 mg

▷ *trimethoprim+sulfamethoxazole (TMP-SMX)* (C)(G)
Pediatric: <2 months: not recommended; ≥2 months: 40 mg/kg/day of
sulfamethoxazole in 2 doses bid x 10 days; *see Appendix CC.33. trimethoprim+
sulfamethoxazole (Bactrim Suspension, Septra Suspension) for dose by weight*

    Bactrim, Septra 2 tabs bid x 10 days

        Tab: trim 80 mg+sulfa 400 mg*

    Bactrim DS, Septra DS 1 tab bid x 10 days

        Tab: trim 160 mg+sulfa 800 mg

    Bactrim Pediatric Suspension, Septra Pediatric Suspension

        Oral susp: trim 40 mg+sulfa 200 mg per 5 ml (100 ml) (cherry) (alcohol
0.3%)

PHARYNGITIS: GONOCOCCAL

Comment: Treat all sexual contacts. Empiric therapy requires concomitant
treatment for *Chlamydia.* Posttreatment culture recommended with PMHx history
rheumatic fever.

PRIMARY THERAPY

▷ *azithromycin* (B)(G) 1 gm x 1 dose
Pediatric: 12 mg/kg/day x 5 days; max 500 mg/day; *see Appendix CC.7.*
azithromycin (Zithromax Suspension, Zmax Suspension) for dose by weight

    Zithromax *Tab:* 250, 500, 600 mg; *Oral susp:* 100 mg/5 ml (15 ml); 200 mg/5
ml (15, 22.5, 30 ml) (cherry); *Pkt:* 1 gm for reconstitution (cherry-banana)

    Zithromax Tri-pak *Tab:* 3 x 500 mg tabs/pck

    Zithromax Z-pak *Tab:* 6 x 250 mg tabs/pck

    Zmax *Oral susp:* 2 gm ext-rel for reconstitution (cherry-banana) (148 mg Na⁺)

    Comment: Per the CDC 2015 STD Treatment Guidelines, *azithromycin* should be
used <u>with</u> *ceftriaxone* 250 mg.

▷ *ceftriaxone* (B)(G) 250 mg IM x 1 dose
Pediatric: <45 kg: 125 mg IM x 1 dose; ≥45 kg: same as adult

    Rocephin *Vial:* 250, 500 mg; 1, 2 gm

PHARYNGITIS: STREPTOCOCCAL (STREP THROAT)

Comment: Acute rheumatic fever is a rare but serious autoimmune disease that may
occur following a group A *streptococcal* throat infection. It causes inflammatory
lesions in connective tissue, especially that of the heart, kidneys, joints, blood
vessels, and subcutaneous tissue. Prior to the broad availability of penicillin,
rheumatic fever was a leading cause of death in children and one of the leading
causes of acquired heart disease in adults. Strep throat is highly responsive to the
penicillins and cephalosporins.

▷ *amoxicillin* (B)(G) 500-875 mg bid <u>or</u> 250-500 mg tid x 10 days
Pediatric: <40 kg (88 lb): 20-40 mg/kg/day in 3 divided doses x 10 days <u>or</u> 25-45
mg/kg/day in 2 divided doses x 10 days; ≥40 kg: same as adult; *see Appendix CC.3.*
amoxicillin (Amoxil Suspension, Trimox Suspension) for dose by weight

Amoxil *Cap:* 250, 500 mg; *Tab:* 875*mg; *Chew tab:* 125, 200, 250, 400 mg (cherry-banana-peppermint) (phenylalanine); *Oral susp:* 125, 250 mg/5 ml (80, 100, 150 ml) (strawberry); 200, 400 mg/5 ml (50, 75, 100 ml) (bubble gum); *Oral drops:* 50 mg/ml (30 ml) (bubble gum)

Moxatag *Tab:* 775 mg ext-rel

Trimox *Tab:* 125, 250 mg; *Cap:* 250, 500 mg; *Oral susp:* 125, 250 mg/5 ml (80, 100, 150 ml) (raspberry-strawberry)

▷ *amoxicillin+clavulanate* (B)(G)

Augmentin 500 mg tid or 875 mg bid x 7-10 days

Pediatric: 40-45 mg/kg/day divided tid x 10 days or 90 mg/kg/day divided bid x 10 days *see* Appendix CC.4. *amoxicillin+clavulanate* (Augmentin Suspension) *for dose by weight*

Tab: 250, 500, 875 mg; *Chew tab:* 125, 250 mg (lemon-lime); 200, 400 mg (cherry-banana) (phenylalanine); *Oral susp:* 125 mg/5 ml (banana), 250 mg/5 ml (75, 100, 150 ml) (orange); 200, 400 mg/5 ml (50, 75, 100 ml) (orange) (phenylalanine)

Augmentin ES-600 not recommended for adults

Pediatric: <3 months: not recommended; ≥3 months, <40 kg: 90 mg/kg/day in 2 divided doses x 7-10 days; ≥40 kg: not recommended

Oral susp: 42.9 mg/5 ml (50, 75, 100, 125, 150, 200 ml) (strawberry cream) (phenylalanine)

Augmentin XR 2 tabs q 12 hours x 7-10 days

Pediatric: <16 years: use other forms; ≥16 years: same as adult

Tab: 1000*mg ext-rel

▷ *azithromycin* (B)(G) 500 mg x 1 dose on day 1, then 250 mg daily on days 2-5 or 500 mg daily x 3 days

Pediatric: 12 mg/kg/day x 5 days; max 500 mg/day; *see* Appendix CC.7. *azithromycin* (Zithromax Suspension, Zmax Suspension) *for dose by weight*

Zithromax *Tab:* 250, 500, 600 mg; *Oral susp:* 100 mg/5 ml (15 ml); 200 mg/5 ml (15, 22.5, 30 ml) (cherry); *Pkt:* 1 gm for reconstitution (cherry-banana)

Zithromax Tri-pak *Tab:* 3 x 500 mg tabs/pck

Zithromax Z-pak *Tab:* 6 x 250 mg tabs/pck

Zmax *Oral susp:* 2 gm ext-rel for reconstitution (cherry-banana) (148 mg Na⁺)

▷ *cefaclor* (B)(G)

Ceclor 250 mg tid or 375 mg bid 3-10 days

Pediatric: <1 month: not recommended; 1 month-12 years: 20-40 mg/kg divided bid or q 12 hours x 3-10 days; max 1 gm/day; *see* Appendix CC.8. *cefaclor* (Ceclor Suspension) *for dose by weight*; >12 years: same as adult

Tab: 500 mg; *Cap:* 250, 500 mg; *Susp:* 125 mg/5 ml (75, 150 ml) (strawberry); 187 mg/5 ml (50, 100 ml) (strawberry); 250 mg/5 ml (75, 150 ml) (strawberry); 375 mg/5 ml (50, 100 ml) (strawberry)

Cefaclor Extended Release 375-500 mg bid x 3-10 days

Pediatric: <16 years: ext-rel not recommended; ≥16 years: same as adult

Tab: 375, 500 mg ext-rel

▷ *cefadroxil* (B) 1 gm in 1-2 doses x 10 days

Pediatric: 30 mg/kg/day in 2 divided doses x 10 days; *see* Appendix CC.9. *cefadroxil* (Duricef Suspension) *for dose by weight*

Duricef *Cap:* 500 mg; *Tab:* 1 gm; *Oral susp:* 250 mg/5 ml (100 ml); 500 mg/5 ml (75, 100 ml) (orange-pineapple)

▷ *cefdinir* (B) 300 mg bid x 10 days

Pediatric: <6 months: not recommended; 6 months-12 years: 14 mg/kg/day in 1-2 doses x 10 days; *see* Appendix CC.10. *cefdinir* (Omnicef Suspension) for dose by weight; >12 years: same as adult

Omnicef *Cap:* 300 mg; *Oral susp:* 125 mg/5 ml (60, 100 ml) (strawberry)

▷ *cefditoren pivoxil* (**B**) 200 mg bid x 10 days
Pediatric: <12 years: not recommended; ≥12 years: same as adult
Spectracef *Tab*: 200 mg
Comment: **Spectracef** is contraindicated with milk protein allergy or carnitine deficiency.

▷ *cefixime* (**B**)(**G**) 400 mg daily x 5 days
Pediatric: <6 months: not recommended; 6 months-12 years, <50 kg: 8 mg/kg/day in 1-2 divided doses x 10 days; *see* Appendix CC.11. *cefixime* (Suprax Oral Suspension) *for dose by weight*; >12 years, ≥50 kg: same as adult
Suprax *Tab*: 400 mg; *Cap*: 400 mg; *Oral susp*: 100, 200, 500 mg/5 ml (50, 75, 100 ml) (strawberry)

▷ *cefpodoxime proxetil* (**B**) 100 mg bid x 5-7 days
Pediatric: <2 months: not recommended; 2 months-12 years: 10 mg/kg/day in 2 divided doses x 5-7 days; *see* Appendix CC.12. *cefpodoxime proxetil* (Vantin Suspension) *for dose by weight*; >12 years: same as adult
Vantin *Tab*: 100, 200 mg; *Oral susp*: 50, 100 mg/5 ml (50, 75, 100 ml) (lemon creme)

▷ *cefprozil* (**B**) 500 mg daily x 10 days
Pediatric: <2 years: not recommended; 2-12 years: 7.5 mg/kg divided bid x 10 days; *see* Appendix CC.13. *cefprozil* (Cefzil Suspension) *for dose by weight*; >12 years: same as adult
Cefzil *Tab*: 250, 500 mg; *Oral susp*: 125, 250 mg/5 ml (50, 75, 100 ml) (bubble gum) (phenylalanine)

▷ *ceftibuten* (**B**) 400 mg daily x 5 days
Pediatric: 9 mg/kg daily x 5 days; *see* Appendix CC.14. *ceftibuten* (Cedax Suspension) *for dose by weight*
Cedax *Cap*: 400 mg; *Oral susp*: 90 mg/5 ml (30, 60, 90, 120 ml); 180 mg/5 ml (30, 60, 120 ml) (cherry)

▷ *cephalexin* (**B**)(**G**) 500 mg bid x 10 days
Pediatric: 25-50 mg/kg/day in 2 divided doses x 10 days; *see* Appendix CC.15. *cephalexin* (Keflex Suspension) *for dose by weight*
Keflex *Cap*: 250, 333, 500, 750 mg; *Oral susp*: 125, 250 mg/5 ml (100, 200 ml) (strawberry)

▷ *clarithromycin* (**C**)(**G**) 250 mg bid or 500 mg ext-rel once daily x 10 days
Pediatric: <6 months: not recommended; ≥6 months: 7.5 mg/kg divided bid x 10 days; *see* Appendix CC.16. *clarithromycin* (Biaxin Suspension) *for dose by weight*
Biaxin *Tab*: 250, 500 mg
Biaxin Oral Suspension *Oral susp*: 125, 250 mg/5 ml (50, 100 ml) (fruit punch)
Biaxin XL *Tab*: 500 mg ext-rel

▷ *dirithromycin* (**C**)(**G**) 500 mg daily x 10 days
Pediatric: <12 years: not recommended; ≥12 years: same as adult
Dynabac *Tab*: 250 mg

▷ *erythromycin base* (**B**)(**G**) 500 mg qid x 10 days
Pediatric: <45 kg: 30-50 mg divided bid-qid x 10 days; ≥45 kg: same as adult
Ery-Tab *Tab*: 250, 333, 500 mg ent-coat
PCE *Tab*: 333, 500 mg

▷ *erythromycin estolate* (**B**)(**G**) 250-500 mg qid x 10 days
Pediatric: 20-50 mg/kg divided q 6 hours x 10 days; *see* Appendix CC.20. *erythromycin* estolate (Ilosone Suspension) *for dose by weight*
Ilosone *Pulvule*: 250 mg; *Tab*: 500 mg; *Liq*: 125, 250 mg/5 ml (100 ml)

▷ *erythromycin ethylsuccinate* (**B**)(**G**) 400 mg qid or 800 mg bid x 10 days
Pediatric: 30-50 mg/kg/day in 4 divided doses x 7 days; may double dose with severe infection; max 100 mg/kg/day; *see Appendix CC.21: erythromycin ethylsuccinate* (E.E.S. Suspension, Ery-Ped Drops/Suspension) *for dose by weight*

EryPed *Oral susp:* 200 mg/5 ml (100, 200 ml) (fruit); 400 mg/5 ml (60, 100, 200 ml) (banana); *Oral drops:* 200, 400 mg/5 ml (50 ml) (fruit); *Chew tab:* 200 mg wafer (fruit)

E.E.S. *Oral susp:* 200, 400 mg/5 ml (100 ml) (fruit)

E.E.S. Granules *Oral susp:* 200 mg/5 ml (100, 200 ml) (cherry)

E.E.S. 400 Tablets *Tab:* 400 mg

▷ *loracarbef* (B) 200 mg bid x 5 days
Pediatric: 15 mg/kg/day in 2 divided doses x 5 days; *see* Appendix CC.27.
loracarbef (Lorabid Suspension) *for dose by weight*

Lorabid *Pulvule:* 200, 400 mg; *Oral susp:* 100 mg/5 ml (50, 100 ml); 200 mg/5 ml (50, 75, 100 ml) (strawberry bubble gum)

▷ *penicillin g (benzathine)* (B)(G) 1.2 million units IM x 1 dose
Pediatric: <60 lb: 300,000-600,000 units IM x 1 dose; ≥60 lb: 900,000 units x 1 dose

Bicillin L-A *Cartridge-needle unit:* 600,000 units (1 ml); 1.2 million units (2 ml)

▷ *penicillin g (benzathine and procaine)* (B)(G) 2.4 million units IM x 1 dose
Pediatric: <30 lb: 600,000 units IM x 1 dose; 30-60 lb: 900,000-1.2 million units IM x 1 dose; >60 lb: same as adult

Bicillin C-R *Cartridge-needle unit:* 600,000 units (1 ml); 1.2 million units; (2 ml); 2.4 million units (4 ml)

▷ *penicillin v potassium* (B)(G) 500 mg bid or 250 mg qid x 10 days
Pediatric: <12 years: 25-50 mg/kg day in 4 divided doses x 10 days; *see* Appendix CC.29. *penicillin v potassium* (Pen-Vee K Solution, Veetids Solution) *for dose by weight;* >12 years: same as adult

Pen-Vee K *Tab:* 250, 500 mg; *Oral soln:* 125 mg/5 ml (100, 200 ml); 250 mg/5 ml (100, 150, 200 ml)

Veetids *Tab:* 250, 500 mg; *Oral soln:* 125, 250 mg/5 ml (100, 200 ml)

◯ PHENYLKETONURIA (PKU)

PHENYLALANINE-METABOLIZING ENZYME

Comment: **Palynziq** (*pegvaliase epbx*) is a phenylalanine-metabolizing enzyme indicated to reduce blood phenylalanine (PHa) concentrations in adult patients with phenylketonuria who have uncontrolled blood phenylalanine concentrations >600 micromol/L on existing management. **Palynziq** is to be used in conjunction with a Pha-restricted diet.

▷ *pegvaliase epbx* recommended initial dosage is 2.5 mg SC once weekly x 4 weeks; titrate dosage in a step-wise manner over at least 5 weeks based on tolerability to achieve a dosage of 20 mg SC once daily; see mfr pkg insert for titration regimen; consider increasing the dosage to max 40 mg SC once daily in patients who have been on 20 mg once daily continuously for at least 24 weeks and who have not achieved either a 20% reduction in blood phenylalanine concentration from pre-treatment baseline or a blood phenylalanine concentration ≤600 micromol/L; discontinue **Palynziq** in patients who have not achieved at least a 20% reduction in blood phenylalanine concentration from pre-treatment baseline or a blood phenylalanine concentration ≤ 600 micromol/L after 16 weeks of continuous treatment with the maximum dosage of 40 mg once daily; reduce the dosage and/or modify dietary protein and phenylalanine intake, as needed, to maintain blood phenylalanine concentrations within a clinically acceptable range and >30 micromol/L *ALWAYS co-prescribe auto-injectable epinephrine.*
Pediatric: <18 years: not recommended; ≥18 years: same as adult

Palynziq *Prefilled syringe:* 2.5, 10 mg/0.5 ml; 20 mg/ml, single-dose (preservative-free)

Comment: Obtain blood phenylalanine concentrations every 4 weeks until a maintenance dosage is established. After a maintenance dosage is established, periodically monitor blood phenylalanine concentrations. Counsel patients to monitor dietary protein and phenylalanine intake, and adjust as directed by their healthcare provider. Anaphylaxis has been reported after administration of **Palynziq** and may occur at any time during treatment. Administer the initial dose under the supervision of a healthcare provider equipped to manage anaphylaxis, and closely observe patients for at least 60 min following injection. Prior to self-injection, confirm patient competency with self-administration, and the patient's and observer's (if applicable) ability to recognize signs and symptoms of anaphylaxis and to administer auto-injectable epinephrine, if needed. *Prescribe auto-injectable epinephrine.* Prior to first dose, instruct the patient and observer (if applicable) on its appropriate use. Instruct the patient to seek immediate medical care upon its use. Instruct patients to carry auto-injectable epinephrine with them at all times during **Palynziq** treatment. **Palynziq** is available only through the restricted Palynziq REMS program. **Palynziq** may cause fetal harm when administered to a pregnant woman. Limited available data with *pegvaliase-pqpz* use in pregnant females are insufficient to inform a drug-associated risk of adverse developmental outcomes. There are risks to the fetus associated with poorly controlled phenylalanine concentrations in women with PKU during pregnancy including increased risk for miscarriage, major birth defects (including microcephaly, major cardiac malformations), intrauterine fetal growth retardation, and future intellectual disability with low IQ; therefore, phenylalanine concentrations should be closely monitored in women with PKU during pregnancy. There are no data on the presence of *pegvaliase-pqpz* in human milk or the effects on the breastfed infant.

PENYLALANINE HYDROXYLASE ACTIVATOR (PHA)

Comment: **Kuvan** *(sapropterin)* is a phenylalanine hydroxylase activator (PHA) indicated to reduce blood phenylalanine (Phe) levels in patients with hyperphenylalaninemia (HPA) due to tetrahydrobiopterin- (BH4-) responsive Phenylketonuria (PKU). **Kuvan** is to be used in conjunction with a Phe-restricted diet.

▷ *sapropterin* (G) recommended starting dose is 10 mg/kg/day taken once daily; doses may be adjusted in the range of 5 to 20 mg/kg taken once daily. Blood Phe must be monitored regularly; take with food to increase absorption; tabs may be swallowed whole or dissolved in 4 to 8 oz (120-240 ml) of water or apple juice; once dissolved, dose should be taken within 15 minutes; pwdr for oral soln should be dissolved in 4 to 8 oz (120-240 m) of water or apple juice and consumed within 30 minutes of preparation
Pediatric: <18 years: not recommended; ≥18 years: same as adult
   Kuvan *Tab:* 100 mg; *Pwdr for Oral Soln:* 100 mg/unit dose pkt

◯ PHEOCHROMOCYTOMA (ADRENAL GLAND TUMOR)

▷ *metyrosine* (C)(G) initially, 250 mg 4 x/day; may increase by 250 mg to 500 mg every day; max 4 g/day in divided doses; *Preoperative Preparation:* the optimally effective dose should be administered for at least 5-7 days prior to surgery.
Pediatric: <12 years: not established; ≥12 years: same as adult
   Demser Capsules *Cap:* 250 mg
   Comment: **Demser** is indicated in the treatment of patients with pheochromocytoma for: pre-operative preparation of patients for surgery; management of patients when surgery is contraindicated; chronic treatment of patients with malignant pheochromocytoma. **Demser** is not recommended for the control of essential hypertension. When **Demser** is used pre-operatively,

alone or especially in combination with alpha-adrenergic blocking drugs, adequate intravascular volume must be maintained intraoperatively (especially after tumor removal) and postoperatively to avoid hypotension and decreased perfusion of vital organs resulting from vasodilatation and expanded volume capacity. Following tumor removal, large volumes of plasma may be needed to maintain blood pressure and central venous pressure within the normal range. In addition, life-threatening arrhythmias may occur during anesthesia and surgery, and may require treatment with a beta-blocker or lidocaine. During surgery, patients should have continuous BP and ECG monitoring. While the pre-operative use of **Demser** in patients with pheochromocytoma is thought to decrease intraoperative problems with blood pressure control, **Demser** does not eliminate the danger of hypertensive crises or arrhythmias during manipulation of the tumor, and the alpha-adrenergic blocking drug, *phentolamine*, may be needed. **Demser** may add to the sedative effects of alcohol and other CNS depressants, e.g., hypnotics, sedatives, and tranquilizers. *metyrosine* crystalluria and urolithiasis have been found in animal studies with **Demser** at doses similar to those used in humans, and crystalluria has also been observed in a few patients. To minimize the risk of crystalluria, patients should be urged to maintain water intake sufficient to achieve a daily urine volume of 2000 ml or more, particularly with doses greater than 2 gm per day. Routinely monitor urine clarity. *Metyrosine* will crystallize as needles or rods, causing the urine will appear cloudy. If *metyrosine* crystalluria occurs, fluid intake should be increased further. If crystalluria persists, the dose regimen should be reduced or the drug discontinued. Caution should be observed when administering **Demser** to patients receiving phenothiazines or *haloperidol* because the extrapyramidal effects of these drugs can be expected to be potentiated by inhibition of catecholamine synthesis. Common side effects of **Demser** may include drowsiness or involuntary muscle movement. Adverse side effects requiring urgent/emergent medical intervention include drooling, trouble speaking, confusion, hallucinations; tremors, muscle spasms, painful or difficult urination, cloudy urine, severe, or ongoing diarrhea. If patients are not adequately controlled by the use of **Demser**, an alpha-adrenergic blocking agent *(phenoxybenzamine)* should be added. It is not known whether **Demser** can cause embryo/fetal harm when administered in pregnancy or can affect reproduction capacity. **Demser** should be used in pregnancy only if clearly needed after a risk/benefit assessment. It is not known whether **Demser** is excreted in human milk or if it may have effect on the breastfeed infant.

ALPHA-BLOCKER

▷ *phenoxybenzamine* (C) initially 10 mg bid; increase every other day as needed; usually 20-40 mg bid-tid

Pediatric: <18 years: not established; ≥18 years: same as adult

Dibenzyline *Cap:* 10 mg

Comment: Dibenzyline *(phenoxybenzamine hydrochloride)* is a long-acting, adrenergic, alpha-receptor blocking agent, which can produce and maintain "chemical sympathectomy" by oral administration. It increases blood flow to the skin, mucosa and abdominal viscera, and lowers both supine and erect blood pressures. It has no effect on the parasympathetic system. Dibenzyline is indicated in the treatment of pheochromocytoma, to control episodes of hypertension and sweating. If tachycardia is excessive, it may be necessary to use a *beta*-blocking agent concomitantly. Dibenzyline-induced *alpha*-adrenergic blockade leaves *beta*-adrenergic receptors unopposed. Compounds that stimulate both types of receptors may, therefore, produce an exaggerated hypotensive response and tachycardia.

PHEOCHROMOCYTOMA: UNRESECTABLE, LOCALLY ADVANCED, OR METASTATIC

ALPHA-BLOCKER

▷ *phenoxybenzamine* (C) initially 10 mg bid; increase every other day as needed; usually 20-40 mg bid-tid
Pediatric: <18 years: not established; ≥18 years: same as adult
   Dibenzyline *Cap:* 10 mg
(see **Pheochromocytoma** for comment)

ANTINEOPLASIA AGENT

▷ *iobenguane I 131* to be administered only by a qualified healthcare professional; verify pregnancy status in females of reproductive potential prior to administration; initiate thyroid-blocking medication prior to **Azedra** administration and continue after each dose. do not administer if platelet count <80,000/mcL or absolute neutrophil count <1,200/mcL; administer intravenously as a dosimetric dose followed by two therapeutic doses administered 90 days apart
   Recommended **Dosimetric** *Dose:*
      >*50 kg:* 185 to 222 MBq (5 to 6 mCi)
      ≤*50 kg:* 3.7 MBq/kg (0.1 mCi/kg)
   Recommended Therapeutic Dose for each of the 2 doses:
      > *62.5 kg:* 18,500 MBq (500 mCi)
      ≤*62.5 kg:* 296 MBq/kg (8 mCi/kg)
   Adjust therapeutic doses based on radiation dose estimates results from dosimetry, if needed
   Pediatric: <12 years: not established; ≥12 years: same as adult
      Azedra *Vial:* 555 MBq/ml (15 mCi/ml) single-dose for IV infusion
   Comment: Azedra *(iobenguane I 131)* is a radioactive therapeutic agent indicated for the treatment of patients with iobenguane scan-positive, unresectable, locally advanced, or metastatic pheochromocytoma or paraganglioma who require systemic anti-cancer therapy. Monitor for hypothyroidism and thyroid-stimulating hormone (TSH) before starting **Azedra** and annually thereafter. Monitor blood pressure frequently during the first 24 hours after each dose. **Azendra** can cause fetal harm; advise females and males of reproductive potential of the potential risk to a fetus and to use effective contraception. **Azendra** may cause infertility. Advise women not to breastfeed.

 PINWORM (*ENTEROBIUS VERMICULARIS*)

Comment: Treatment of all family members is recommended.

ANTHELMINTICS

Comment: Oral bioavailability of anthelmintics is enhanced when administered with a fatty meal (estimated fat content 40 gm). Treatment of all family members is recommended. Some clinicians recommend all household contacts of infected patients receive treatment, especially when multiple or repeated symptomatic infections occur, since such contacts commonly also are infected; retreatment after 14-21 days may be needed.

▷ *albendazole* (C) 400 mg x 1 dose; may repeat in 2-3 weeks if needed; take with a meal
Pediatric: <20 kg: 200 mg as a single dose; ≥20 kg: same as adult
   Albenza *Tab:* 200 mg

▷ *mebendazole* (C) chew, swallow, or mix with food; 100 mg x 1 dose; may repeat in 3 weeks if needed; take with a meal

Pediatric: <2 years: not recommended; ≥2 years: same as adult
> **Emverm** *Chew tab*: 100 mg
> **Vermox (G)** *Chew tab*: 100 mg

▷ *pyrantel pamoate* (C) 11 mg/kg x 1 dose; max 1 gm/dose; may repeat in 2-3 weeks if needed; take with a meal

Pediatric: 25-37 lb: 1/2 tsp x 1 dose; 38-62 lb: 1 tsp x 1 dose; 63-87 lb: 1 tsp x 1 dose; 88-112 lb: 2 tsp x 1 dose; 113-137 lb: 2 tsp x 1 dose; 138-162 lb: 3 tsp x 1 dose; 163-187 lb: 3 tsp x 1 dose; >187 lb: 4 tsp x 1 dose
> **Pin-X (OTC)**; *Cap:* 180 mg; *Liq:* 50 mg/ml (30 ml); 144 mg/ml (30 ml); *Oral susp:* 50 mg/ml (30 ml)

▷ *thiabendazole* (C) 50 mg/kg x 1 dose after a meal; max 3 gm; may repeat in 2-3 weeks if needed; take with a meal

Pediatric: same as adult
> **Mintezol** *Chew tab*: 500*mg (orange); *Oral susp:* 500 mg/5 ml (120 ml) (orange)

Comment: *Thiabendazole* is <u>not</u> for prophylaxis and should <u>not</u> be used as first-line therapy for pinworms. May impair mental alertness. May <u>not</u> be available in the US.

◑ PITYRIASIS ALBA

Topical Corticosteroids *see* Appendix K. Topical Corticosteroids by Potency

Comment: Pityriasis alba is a chronic skin disorder seen in children with a genetic predisposition to atopic disease. Treatment is directed toward controlling roughness and pruritus. There is no known treatment for the associated skin pigment changes. Pityriasis alba resolves spontaneously and permanently in the 2nd <u>or</u> 3rd decade of life.

COAL TAR PREPARATIONS

▷ *coal tar* (C)
Pediatric: same as adult
> **Scytera (OTC)** apply qd-qid; use lowest effective dose
> *Foam:* 2%
> **T/Gel Shampoo Extra Strength (OTC)** use every other day; max 4 x/week; massage into affected area for 5 minutes; rinse; repeat
> *Shampoo:* 1%
> **T/Gel Shampoo Original Formula (OTC)** use every other day; max 7 x/week; massage into affected area for 5 minutes; rinse; repeat
> *Shampoo:* 0.5%
> **T/Gel Shampoo Stubborn Itch Control (OTC)** use every other day; max 7 x/week; massage into affected area for 5 minutes; rinse; repeat
> *Shampoo:* 0.5%

EMOLLIENTS AND OTHER MOISTURIZING AGENTS
see **Dermatitis: Atopic**

◑ PITYRIASIS ROSEA

Topical Corticosteroids *see* Appendix K. Topical Corticosteroids by Potency
Antihistamines *see* Appendix AA. Drugs for the Management of Allergy, Cough, and Cold Symptoms online at https://connect.springerpub.com/content/reference-book/978-0-8261-7935-7/back-matter/part02/back-matter/bmatter27

PLAGUE (*YERSINIA PESTIS*)

Comment: *Yersinia pestis* is transmitted via the bite of a flea from an infected rodent or the bite, lick, or scratch of an infected cat. Untreated bubonic plague may progress to secondary pneumonic plague, which may be transmitted via contaminated respiratory droplet spread.

▶ *streptomycin* (C)(G) 15 mg/kg IM bid x 10 days
   Pediatric: same as adult
   Amp: 1 gm/2.5 ml or 400 mg/ml (2.5 ml)
   Comment: For patients with renal impairment, reduce dose of *streptomycin* to 20 mg/kg/day if mild and 8 mg/kg/day q 3 days if advanced). For patients who are pregnant or who have hearing impairment, shorten the course of treatment to 3 days after fever has resolved.

▶ *moxifloxacin* (C)(G) 400 mg daily x 10 days
   Pediatric: <18 years: not recommended; ≥18 years: same as adult
   Avelox *Tab:* 400 mg; IV soln: 400 mg/250 mg (latex-free, preservative-free)

▶ *tetracycline* (D)(G) 500 mg qid or 25-50 mg/kg/day divided q 6 hours x 10 days
   Pediatric: <8 years: not recommended; ≥8 years: same as adult

PNEUMONIA: BACTERIAL, HOSPITAL-ACQUIRED (HABP)

PARENTERAL CEPHALOSPORIN ANTIBACTERIAL+BETA-LACTIMASE INHIBITOR

▶ *ceftazidime+avibactam* (B) infuse dose over 2 hours; recommended duration of treatment: 5 to 4 days; *CrCl 31-50 mL/min:* 1.25 gm every 8 hours; *CrCl 16-30 mL/min:* 0.94 gm every 12 hours; *CrCl 6-15 mL/min:* 0.94 gm every 24 hours; *CrCl ≤5 mL/min:* 0.94 gm every 48 hours; both *ceftazidime* and *avibactam* are hemodialyzable; thus, administer **Avycaz** after hemodialysis on hemodialysis days
   Pediatric: <18 years: not recommended; ≥18 years: same as adult
   Avycaz *Vial:* 2.5 gm, single-dose, pwdr for reconstitution and IV infusion
   Comment: **Avycaz** 2.5 gm contains *ceftazidime* (a cephalosporin) 2 grams (equivalent to 2.635 grams of *ceftazidime pentahydrate/sodium carbonate powder*) and *avibactam* (a beta lactam inhibitor) 0.5 grams (equivalent to 0.551 grams of *avibactam sodium*). As only limited clinical safety and efficacy data for **Avycaz** are currently available, reserve **Avycaz** for use in patients who have limited or no alternative treatment options. To reduce the development of drug-resistant bacteria and maintain the effectiveness of **Avycaz** and other antibacterial drugs, **Avycaz** should be used only to treat infections that are proven or strongly suspected to be caused by susceptible bacteria. Seizures and other neurologic events may occur, especially in patients with renal impairment. Adjust dose in patients with renal impairment. Decreased efficacy in patients with baseline CrCl 30--≤50 mL/min. Monitor CrCl at least daily in patients with changing renal function and adjust the dose of **Avycaz** accordingly. Monitor for hypersensitivity reactions, including anaphylaxis and serious skin reactions. Cross-hypersensitivity may occur in patients with a history of penicillin allergy. If an allergic reaction occurs, discontinue **Avycaz**. *Clostridioides difficile*-associated diarrhea (CDAD) has been reported with nearly all systemic antibacterial agents, including **Avycaz**. There are no adequate and well-controlled studies of **Avycaz**, *ceftazidime*, or *avibactam* in pregnant females. *ceftazidime* is excreted in human milk in low concentrations. It is not known whether *avibactam* is excreted into human milk. There are no studies to inform effects on the breastfed infant.

▶ *ceftolozane+tazobactam* administer 3 gm every 8 hours via IV infusion over 1 hour x 8-14 days; *CrCl 30-50 ml/min:* 1.5 gm via IV infusion every 8 hours; *CrCl 15-29 ml/min:* 750 mg via IV infusion every 8 hours; *ESRD:* a single loading dose of 2.25 gm via IV infusion, followed by 450 mg via IV infusion every 8 hours for the remainder of the treatment period (on hemodialysis days, administer the dose at the earliest possible time following completion of dialysis)

Pediatric: <18: not established; ≥18 years: same as adult

Zerbaxa *Vial:* 1.5 gm (*ceftolozane* 1 gm+*tazobactam* 0.5 gm), single-dose, pwdr for reconstitution and IV infusion

Comment: For doses >1.5 gm, reconstitute a second vial in the same manner as the first one, withdraw an appropriate volume (see Table 3 in the mfr pkg insert) and add to the same infusion bag. The most common adverse reactions in patients with HABP (incidence ≥5%) have been increase in hepatic transaminases, renal impairment/renal failure, and diarrhea.

PARENTERAL PENEM ANTIBACTERIAL + RENAL DEHYDROPEPTIDASE INHIBITOR + BETA-LACTAMASE INHIBITOR

▷ *imipenem+cilastatin+relebactam)* administer dose via IV infusion over 30 minutes every 6 hours; *CrCL* ≥90 *mL/min:* 1.25 gm/dose (*imipenem* 500 mg, *cilastatin* 500 mg, *relebactam* 250 mg); *CrCL* 60-89 *mL/min:* 1 gm/dose (*imipenem* 400 mg, *cilastatin* 400 mg, *relebactam* 200 mg); *CrCL* 30-59 *mL/min:* 0.75 gm/dose (*imipenem* 300 mg, *cilastatin* 300 mg, *relebactam* 150 mg); *CrCL* 15-29 *mL/min:* 0.5 gm/dose (*imipenem* 200 mg, *cilastatin* 200 mg, *relebactam* 100 mg); *ESRD/Dialysis:* 0.5 gm/dose (*imipenem* 200 mg, *cilastatin* 200 mg, *relebactam* 100 mg)

Pediatric: <18 years: not established; ≥18 years: same as adult

Recarbrio *Vial:* imipen 500 mg+cilast 500 mg+relebac 250 mg, single-dose, pwdr for reconstitution, dilution, and IV infusion

Comment: **Recarbrio** *(imipenem+cilastatin+relebactam)* is a fixed-dose triple combination of *imipenem* (a penem antibacterial), *cilastatin* (a renal dehydropeptidase inhibitor), and *relebactam* (a beta-lactamase inhibitor) indicated for the treatment of complicated urinary tract infection (cUTI), including pyelonephritis, complicated intra-abdominal infection (cIAI) caused by susceptible gram-negative bacteria in patients who have limited or no alternative treatment options, hospital-acquired bacterial pneumonia (HABP), and ventilator-associated bacterial pneumonia (VABP) in adults. Avoid concomitant use of **Recarbrio** with *ganciclovir, valproic acid, or divalproex sodium.* Based on clinical reports on patients treated with imipenem/cilastatin plus relebactam 250 mg, the most frequent adverse reactions (incidence ≥2%) have been diarrhea, nausea, headache, vomiting, alanine aminotransferase increased, aspartate aminotransferase increased, phlebitis/infusion site reactions, pyrexia, and hypertension. There are insufficient human data to establish whether there is a drug-associated risk for major birth defects, miscarriage, or adverse maternal or fetal outcomes with *imipenem, cilastatin,* or *relebactam* in pregnancy. However, embryonic loss has been observed in monkeys treated with *imipenem/cilastatin,* and fetal abnormalities have been observed in *relebactam*-treated mice; therefore, advise pregnant females of the potential risks to pregnancy and the fetus. There are insufficient data on the presence of *imipenem/cilastatin* and *relebactam* in human milk, and no data on the effects on the breastfed infant; However, *relebactam* is present in the milk of lactating rats and, therefore, developmental and health benefits of breastfeeding should be considered along with the mother's clinical need for **Recarbrio** and any potential adverse effects on the breastfed infant from **Recarbrio** or from the underlying maternal condition.

SIDEROPHORE CEPHALOSPORIN

▷ *cefiderocol* administer 2 gm via IV infusion every 8 hours; infuse dose over 3 hours in patients with CrCl 60-119 mL/min; see mfr pkg insert for dose adjustments required in patients with CrCl <60 mL/min and ≥CrCl 120 mL/min; see mfr pkg insert for dose preparation

Fetroja *Vial:* 1 gm pwdr for reconstitution and IV infusion, single-dose
Comment: Fetroja *(cefi derocol)* is a siderophore cephalosporin for the treatment of complicated urinary tract infection (cUTI), including pyelonephritis, caused by susceptible Gram-negative microorganisms, in patients ≥18 years-of-age with limited or no alternative treatment options. Approval of this indication is based on limited clinical safety and efficacy data. An increase in all-cause mortality was observed in Fetroja-treated patients compared to those treated with best available therapy (BAT). Closely monitor the clinical response to therapy in patients with cUTI. Serious and occasionally fatal hypersensitivity (anaphylactic) reactions have been reported in patients receiving betalactam antibacterial drugs. Hypersensitivity was observed with Fetroja. Cross-hypersensitivity may occur in patients with a history of penicillin allergy. If an allergic reaction occurs, discontinue Fetroja. *Clostridioides Difficile*-Associated Diarrhea (CDAD) has been reported with nearly all systemic antibacterial agents, including Fetroja. Seizures and other CNS adverse reactions have been reported with Fetroja. If focal tremors, myoclonus, or seizures occur, evaluate patients to determine whether Fetroja should be discontinued. The most frequently occurring adverse reactions (incidence ≥2% of patients treated with Fetroja have been diarrhea, infusion site reactions, constipation, rash, candidiasis, cough, elevations in liver tests, headache, hypokalemia, nausea, and vomiting. There are no available data on Fetroja use in pregnant females to evaluate for a drug-associated risk of major birth defects, miscarriage, or adverse maternal or fetal outcomes. Available data from published prospective cohort studies, case series, and case reports over several decades with cephalosporin use in pregnant women have not established drug-associated risks of major birth defects, miscarriage, or adverse maternal or fetal outcomes. Developmental toxicity studies with *cefiderocol* administered during organogenesis in animal studies showed no evidence of embryo/fetal toxicity, including drug-induced fetal malformations. It is not known whether *cefiderocol* is excreted into human milk. No information is available on the effects of Fetroja on the breastfed infant. Developmental and health benefits of breastfeeding should be considered along with the mother's clinical need for Fetroja and any potential adverse effects on the breastfed infant or from the underlying maternal condition.

PNEUMONIA: BACTERIAL, VENTILATOR-ASSOCIATED (VABP)

PARENTERAL CEPHALOSPORIN ANTIBACTERIAL+BETA-LACTIMASE INHIBITOR

▷ *ceftazidime+avibactam* (B) infuse dose over 2 hours; recommended duration of treatment: 5 to 4 days; *CrCl 31-50 mL/min:* 1.25 gm every 8 hours; *CrCl 16-30 mL/min:* 0.94 gm every 12 hours; *CrCl 6-15 mL/min:* 0.94 gm every 24 hours; *CrCl ≤5 mL/min:* 0.94 gm every 48 hours; both *ceftazidime* and *avibactam* are hemodialyzable; thus, administer Avycaz after hemodialysis on hemodialysis days *Pediatric:* <18 years: not recommended; ≥18 years: same as adult

Avycaz *Vial:* 2.5 gm, single-dose, pwdr for reconstitution and IV infusion
Comment: Avycaz 2.5 gm contains *ceftazidime* (a cephalosporin) 2 gm (equivalent to 2.635 gm of *ceftazidime pentahydrate/sodium carbonate powder*) and *avibactam* (a beta lactam inhibitor) 0.5 gm (equivalent to 0.551 gm of *avibactam sodium*). As only limited clinical safety and efficacy data for Avycaz are currently available, reserve Avycaz for use in patients who have limited or no alternative treatment options. To reduce the development of drug-resistant bacteria and maintain the effectiveness of Avycaz and other

antibacterial drugs, **Avycaz** should be used only to treat infections that are proven or strongly suspected to be caused by susceptible bacteria. Seizures and other neurologic events may occur, especially in patients with renal impairment. Adjust dose in patients with renal impairment. Decreased efficacy in patients with baseline CrCL 30--≤50 mL/min. Monitor CrCl at least daily in patients with changing renal function and adjust the dose of **Avycaz** accordingly. Monitor for hypersensitivity reactions, including anaphylaxis and serious skin reactions. Cross-hypersensitivity may occur in patients with a history of penicillin allergy. If an allergic reaction occurs, discontinue **Avycaz**. *Clostridioides difficile*-associated diarrhea CDAD) has been reported with nearly all systemic antibacterial agents, including **Avycaz**. There are no adequate and well-controlled studies of **Avycaz**, *ceftazidime*, or *avibactam* in pregnant females. *ceftazidime* is excreted in human milk in low concentrations. It is not known whether *avibactam* is excreted into human milk. There are no studies to inform effects on the breastfed infant.

▷ *ceftolozane+tazobactam* administer 3 gm every 8 hours via IV infusion over 1 hour x 8-14 days; *CrCl 30-50 ml/min:* 1.5 gm via IV infusion every 8 hours; *CrCl 15-29 ml/min:* 750 mg via IV infusion every 8 hours; *ESRD:* a single loading dose of 2.25 gm via IV infusion, followed by 450 mg via IV infusion every 8 hours for the remainder of the treatment period (on hemodialysis days, administer the dose at the earliest possible time following completion of dialysis)
Pediatric: <18: not established; ≥18 years: same as adult

> **Zerbaxa** *Vial:* 1.5 gm (*ceftolozane* 1 gm+*tazobactam* 0.5 gm), single-dose, pwdr for reconstitution and IV infusion
> Comment: For doses >1.5 gm, reconstitute a second vial in the same manner as the first one, withdraw an appropriate volume (see Table 3 in the mfr pkg insert) and add to the same infusion bag. The most common adverse reactions in patients with VABP (incidence ≥5%) have been increase in hepatic transaminases, renal impairment/renal failure, and diarrhea.

PARENTERAL PENEM ANTIBACTERIAL + RENAL DEHYDROPEPTIDASE INHIBITOR + BETA-LACTAMASE INHIBITOR

▷ *imipenem+cilastatin+relebactam)* administer dose via IV infusion over 30 minutes every 6 hours; *CrCL ≥90 mL/min:* 1.25 gm/dose (*imipenem* 500 mg, *cilastatin* 500 mg, *relebactam* 250 mg); *CrCL 60-89 mL/min:* 1 gm/dose (*imipenem* 400 mg, *cilastatin* 400 mg, *relebactam* 200 mg); *CrCL 30-59 mL/min:* 0.75 gm/dose (*imipenem* 300 mg, *cilastatin* 300 mg, *relebactam* 150 mg); *CrCL 15-29 mL/min:* 0.5 gm/dose (*imipenem* 200 mg, *cilastatin* 200 mg, *relebactam* 100 mg); *ESRD/Dialysis:* 0.5 gm/dose (*imipenem* 200 mg, *cilastatin* 200 mg, *relebactam* 100 mg)
Pediatric: <18 years: not established; ≥18 years: same as adult

> **Recarbrio** *Vial:* imipen 500 mg+cilast 500 mg+relebac 250 mg, single-dose, pwdr for reconstitution, dilution, and IV infusion
> Comment: **Recarbrio** (*imipenem+cilastatin+relebactam*) is a fixed-dose triple combination of *imipenem* (a penem antibacterial), *cilastatin* (a renal dehydropeptidase inhibitor), and *relebactam* (a beta-lactamase inhibitor) indicated for the treatment of complicated urinary tract infection (cUTI), including pyelonephritis, complicated intra-abdominal infection (cIAI) caused by susceptible gram-negative bacteria in patients who have limited or no alternative treatment options, hospital-acquired bacterial pneumonia (HABP), and ventilator-associated bacterial pneumonia (VABP) in adults. Avoid concomitant use of **Recarbrio** with *ganciclovir*, *valproic acid*, or *divalproex sodium*. Based on clinical reports on patients treated with imipenem/cilastatin plus relebactam 250 mg, the most frequent adverse reactions (incidence ≥2%) have been diarrhea, nausea, headache, vomiting, alanine aminotransferase

increased, aspartate aminotransferase increased, phlebitis/infusion site reactions, pyrexia, and hypertension. There are insufficient human data to establish whether there is a drug-associated risk for major birth defects, miscarriage, or adverse maternal or fetal outcomes with *imipenem, cilastatin*, or *relebactam* in pregnancy. However, embryonic loss has been observed in monkeys treated with *imipenem/cilastatin*, and fetal abnormalities have been observed in *relebactam*-treated mice; therefore, advise pregnant females of the potential risks to pregnancy and the fetus. There are insufficient data on the presence of *imipenem/cilastatin* and *relebactam* in human milk, and no data on the effects on the breastfed infant; However, *relebactam* is present in the milk of lactating rats and, therefore, developmental and health benefits of breastfeeding should be considered along with the mother's clinical need for **Recarbrio** and any potential adverse effects on the breastfed infant from **Recarbrio** or from the underlying maternal condition.

SIDEROPHORE CEPHALOSPORIN

▷ *cefiderocol* administer 2 gm via IV infusion every 8 hours; infuse dose over 3 hours in patients with CrCl 60-119 mL/min; see mfr pkg insert for dose adjustments required in patients with CrCl <60 mL/min and ≥CrCl 120 mL/min; see mfr pkg insert for dose preparation

Fetroja *Vial:* 1 gram pwdr for reconstitution and IV infusion, single-dose

Comment: Fetroja *(cefiderocol)* is a siderophore cephalosporin for the treatment of complicated urinary tract infection (cUTI), including pyelonephritis, caused by susceptible Gram-negative microorganisms, in patients ≥18 years-of-age with limited or no alternative treatment options. Approval of this indication is based on limited clinical safety and efficacy data. An increase in all-cause mortality was observed in **Fetroja**-treated patients compared to those treated with best available therapy (BAT). Closely monitor the clinical response to therapy in patients with cUTI. Serious and occasionally fatal hypersensitivity (anaphylactic) reactions have been reported in patients receiving betalactam antibacterial drugs. Hypersensitivity was observed with **Fetroja**. Cross-hypersensitivity may occur in patients with a history of penicillin allergy. If an allergic reaction occurs, discontinue **Fetroja**. *Clostridioides Difficile*-Associated Diarrhea (CDAD) has been reported with nearly all systemic antibacterial agents, including **Fetroja**. Seizures and other CNS adverse reactions have been reported with **Fetroja**. If focal tremors, myoclonus, or seizures occur, evaluate patients to determine whether **Fetroja** should be discontinued. The most frequently occurring adverse reactions (incidence ≥2% of patients treated with **Fetroja** have been diarrhea, infusion site reactions, constipation, rash, candidiasis, cough, elevations in liver tests, headache, hypokalemia, nausea, and vomiting. There are no available data on **Fetroja** use in pregnant females to evaluate for a drug-associated risk of major birth defects, miscarriage, or adverse maternal or fetal outcomes. Available data from published prospective cohort studies, case series, and case reports over several decades with cephalosporin use in pregnant women have not established drug-associated risks of major birth defects, miscarriage, or adverse maternal or fetal outcomes. Developmental toxicity studies with *cefiderocol* administered during organogenesis in animal studies showed no evidence of embryo/fetal toxicity, including drug-induced fetal malformations. It is not known whether *cefiderocol* is excreted into human milk. No information is available on the effects of **Fetroja** on the breastfed infant. Developmental and health benefits of breastfeeding should be considered along with the mother's clinical need for **Fetroja** and any potential adverse effects on the breastfed infant or from the underlying maternal condition.

PNEUMONIA: CHLAMYDIAL

RECOMMENDED REGIMEN

▷ *erythromycin base* (B)(G) 500 mg qid hours x 10-14 days
  Pediatric: <45 kg: 50 mg in 4 divided doses x 10-14 days; ≥45 kg: same as adult
      Ery-Tab *Tab:* 250, 333, 500 mg ent-coat
      PCE *Tab:* 333, 500 mg

▷ *erythromycin ethylsuccinate* (B)(G) 400 mg qid x 10-14 days
  Pediatric: <45 kg: 50 mg/kg/day in 4 divided doses x 10-14 days; ≥45 kg: same
  as adult; *see Appendix CC.21. erythromycin ethylsuccinate* (E.E.S. Suspension, Ery-
  Ped Drops/Suspension) *for dose by weight*
      EryPed *Oral susp:* 200 mg/5 ml (100, 200 ml) (fruit); 400 mg/5 ml (60, 100,
      200 ml) (banana); *Oral drops:* 200, 400 mg/5 ml (50 ml) (fruit); *Chew tab:*
      200 mg wafer (fruit)
      E.E.S. *Oral susp:* 200, 400 mg/5 ml (100 ml) (fruit)
      E.E.S. Granules *Oral susp:* 200 mg/5 ml (100, 200 ml) (cherry)
      E.E.S. 400 Tablets *Tab:* 400 mg

ALTERNATE REGIMENS

▷ *azithromycin* (B)(G) 500 mg once daily x 10 days
  Pediatric: 20 mg/kg per dose once daily x 3 days; max 500 mg/day; *see* Appendix
  CC.7. *azithromycin* (Zithromax Suspension, Zmax Suspension) *for dose by weight*
      Zithromax *Tab:* 250, 500, 600 mg; *Oral susp:* 100 mg/5 ml (15 ml); 200 mg/5 ml
      (15, 22.5, 30 ml) (cherry); Pkt: 1 gm for reconstitution (cherry-banana)
      Zithromax Tri-pak *Tab:* 3 x 500 mg tabs/pck
      Zithromax Z-pak *Tab:* 6 x 250 mg tabs/pck
      Zmax *Oral susp:* 2 gm ext-rel for reconstitution (cherry-banana) (148 mg Na⁺)

▷ *levofloxacin* (C) *Uncomplicated:* 500 mg daily x 7 days; *Complicated:* 750 mg
  daily x 7 days
  Pediatric: <18 years: not recommended; ≥18 years: same as adult
      Levaquin *Tab:* 250, 500, 750 mg; *Oral soln:* 25 mg/ml (480 ml) (benzyl
      alcohol); *Inj conc:* 25 mg/ml for IV infusion after dilution (20, 30 ml single-use
      vial) (preservative-free); *Premix soln:* 5 mg/ml for IV infusion (50, 100, 150
      ml) (preservative-free)

PNEUMONIA: COMMUNITY ACQUIRED (CAP) AND
COMMUNITY ACQUIRED BACTERIAL PNEUMONIA (CABP)

Comment: Over 70% of patients with uncomplicated community-acquired
pneumonia (CAP) received prescriptions for antibiotics that exceeded
national duration recommendations, according to a retrospective study that
included 22,128 patients from 18 to 64 years-of-age with private insurance and
130,746 patients aged >65 years with Medicare, who were hospitalized with
uncomplicated CAP. Length of antibiotic therapy (LOT) during hospital stay was
estimated using the MarketScan Hospital Drug Database and outpatient LOT
was determined using prescriptions filled at discharge. The researchers defined
excessive duration as a LOT of more than 3 days.

ANTI-INFFECTIVES

▷ *amoxicillin* (B)(G) 500-875 mg bid or 250-500 mg tid x 3-10 days
  Pediatric: <40 kg (88 lb): 20-40 mg/kg/day in 3 divided doses x 3-10 days or 25-45
  mg/kg/day in 2 divided doses x 3-10 days; ≥40 kg: same as adult
      Amoxil *Cap:* 250, 500 mg; *Tab:* 875 mg; *Chew tab:* 125, 200, 250, 400 mg
      (cherry-banana-peppermint) (phenylalanine); *Oral susp:* 125, 250 mg/5 ml
      (80, 100, 150 ml) (strawberry); 200, 400 mg/5 ml (50, 75, 100 ml) (bubble
      gum); *Oral drops:* 50 mg/ml (30 ml) (bubble gum)

    Moxatag *Tab:* 775 mg ext-rel

    Trimox *Tab:* 125, 250 mg; *Cap:* 250, 500 mg; *Oral susp:* 125, 250 mg/5 ml (80, 100, 150 ml) (raspberry-strawberry)

▶ *amoxicillin+clavulanate* (B)(G) 500 mg tid or 875 mg bid x 3-10 days

    Augmentin 500 mg tid or 875 mg bid x 3-10 days

    Pediatric: 40-45 mg/kg/day divided tid x 10 days or 90 mg/kg/day divided bid x 10 days *see* Appendix CC.4. *amoxicillin+clavulanate* (Augmentin Suspension) *for dose by weight*

        Tab: 250, 500, 875 mg; *Chew tab:* 125, 250 mg (lemon-lime); 200, 400 mg (cherry-banana) (phenylalanine); *Oral susp:* 125 mg/5 ml (banana), 250 mg/5 ml (75, 100, 150 ml) (orange); 200, 400 mg/5 ml (50, 75, 100 ml) (orange) (phenylalanine)

    Augmentin ES-600 not recommended for adults

    Pediatric: <3 months: not recommended; ≥3 months, <40 kg: 90 mg/kg/day in 2 divided doses x 3-10 days; ≥40 kg: not recommended

    Oral susp: 42.9 mg/5 ml (50, 75, 100, 125, 150, 200 ml) (strawberry cream) (phenylalanine)

    Augmentin XR 2 tabs q 12 hours x 3-10 days

    Pediatric: <16 years: use other forms; ≥16 years: same as adult

        Tab: 1000*mg ext-rel

▶ *azithromycin* (B)(G) *Day 1,* 500 mg as a single dose and *Days 2-5,* 250 mg once daily or 500 mg once daily x 3 days

    Pediatric: <6 months: not recommended; ≥6 months: 10 mg/kg x 1 dose on day 1; then 5 mg/kg/day on days 2-5; max 500 mg/day; *see* Appendix CC.7. *azithromycin* (Zithromax Suspension, Zmax Suspension) *for dose by weight*

    Zithromax *Tab:* 250, 500, 600 mg; *Oral susp:* 100 mg/5 ml (15 ml); 200 mg/5 ml (15, 22.5, 30 ml) (cherry); *Pkt:* 1 gm for reconstitution (cherry-banana)

    Zithromax Tri-pak *Tab:* 3 x 500 mg tabs/pck

    Zithromax Z-pak *Tab:* 6 x 250 mg tabs/pck

    Zmax *Oral susp:* 2 gm ext-rel for reconstitution (cherry-banana) (148 mg Na$^+$)

▶ *cefaclor* (B)(G)

    Ceclor 250 mg tid or 375 mg bid 3-10 days

    Pediatric: <1 month: not recommended; 1 month-12 years: 20-40 mg/kg divided bid or q 12 hours x 3-10 days; max 1 gm/day; *see* Appendix CC.8. *cefaclor* (Ceclor Suspension) *for dose by weight;* >12 years: same as adult

        Tab: 500 mg; *Cap:* 250, 500 mg; *Susp:* 125 mg/5 ml (75, 150 ml) (strawberry); 187 mg/5 ml (50, 100 ml) (strawberry); 250 mg/5 ml (75, 150 ml) (strawberry); 375 mg/5 ml (50, 100 ml) (strawberry)

    Cefaclor Extended Release 375-500 mg bid x 3-10 days

    Pediatric: <16 years: ext-rel not recommended; ≥16 years: same as adult

        Tab: 375, 500 mg ext-rel

▶ *cefdinir* (B) 300 mg bid or 600 mg daily x 3-10 days

    Pediatric: <6 months: not recommended; 6 months-12 years: 14 mg/kg/day in a single or 2 divided doses x 3-10 days; *see* Appendix CC.10. *cefdinir* (Omnicef Suspension) *for dose by weight;* >12 years: same as adult

    Omnicef *Cap:* 300 mg; *Oral susp:* 125 mg/5 ml (60, 100 ml) (strawberry)

▶ *cefpodoxime proxetil* (B) 200 mg bid x 3-10 days

    Pediatric: 2 months-12 years: 10 mg/kg/day in 2 divided doses x 3-5 days; *see* Appendix CC.12. *cefpodoxime proxetil* (Vantin Suspension) *for dose by weight;* >12 years: same as adult

    Vantin *Tab:* 100, 200 mg; *Oral susp:* 50, 100 mg/5 ml (50, 75, 100 ml) (lemon creme)

▶ *ceftaroline fosamil* (B) administer by IV infusion after reconstitution every 12 hours x 3-10 days; *CrCl ≥50 mL/min:* 600 mg; *CrCl >30-<50 mL/min:* 400 mg; *CrCl: >15-<30 mL/min:* 300 mg; ES RD: 200 mg

Pediatric: <18 years: not recommended; ≥18 years: same as adult

    Teflaro *Vial:* 400, 600 mg

▷ **ceftriaxone** (B)(G) 1-2 gm IM daily; x 1-3 days

Pediatric: 50-75 mg/kg IM in 2 divided doses; max 2 gm/day x 1-3 days

    Rocephin *Vial:* 250, 500 mg; 1, 2 gm

▷ **clarithromycin** (C)(G) 500 mg bid <u>or</u> 500 mg ext-rel once daily x 3-10 days

Pediatric: <6 months: not recommended; ≥6 months: 7.5 mg/kg bid x 3-10 days

    Biaxin *Tab:* 250, 500 mg

    Biaxin Oral Suspension *Oral susp:* 125, 250 mg/5 ml (50, 100 ml) (fruit punch)

    Biaxin XL *Tab:* 500 mg ext-rel

▷ **dirithromycin** (C)(G) 500 mg daily x 3-10 days

Pediatric: <12 years: not recommended; ≥12 years: same as adult

    Dynabac *Tab:* 250 mg

▷ **doxycycline** (D)(G) 100 mg bid x 3-10 days

Pediatric: <8 years: not recommended; ≥8 years, ≤100 lb: 2 mg/lb on first day in 2 divided doses, followed by 1 mg/lb/day in 1-2 divided doses; ≥8 years, >100 lb: same as adult; *see Appendix CC.19. doxycycline* (Vibramycin Syrup/Suspension) *for dose by weight*

    Acticlate *Tab:* 75, 150**mg

    Adoxa *Tab:* 50, 75, 100, 150 mg ent-coat

    Doryx *Tab:* 50, 75, 100, 150, 200 mg del-rel

    Doxteric *Tab:* 50 mg del-rel

    Monodox *Cap:* 50, 75, 100 mg

    Oracea *Cap:* 40 mg del-rel

    Vibramycin Tab: 100 mg; *Cap:* 50, 100 mg; *Syr:* 50 mg/5 ml (raspberry-apple) (sulfites); *Oral susp:* 25 mg/5 ml (raspberry)

    Vibra-Tab *Tab:* 100 mg film-coat

▷ **ertapenem** (B)(G) 1 gm daily; *CrCl <30 mL/min:* 500 mg daily x 3-10 days; may switch to an oral antibiotic after 3 days if warranted; *IV infusion:* administer over 30 minutes; *IM injection:* reconstitute with **lidocaine** <u>only</u>

    Invanz *Vial:* 1 gm pwdr for reconstitution

▷ **erythromycin base** (B)(G) 500 mg q 6 hours x 14-21 days; <45 kg: 30-50 mg in 2-4 doses x 3-10 days; ≥45 kg: same as adult

    Ery-Tab *Tab:* 250, 333, 500 mg ent-coat

    PCE *Tab:* 333, 500 mg

▷ **erythromycin estolate** (B) 500 mg q 6 hours x 3-10 days

    Ilosone *Pulvule:* 250 mg; *Tab:* 500 mg; *Liq:* 125, 250 mg/5 ml (100 ml)

▷ **gemifloxacin** (C)(G) 320 mg daily x 3-10 days

Pediatric: <18 years: not recommended; ≥18 years: same as adult

    Factive *Tab:* 320*mg

▷ **levofloxacin** (C) 250 mg once daily x 3-10 days

Pediatric: <18 years: not recommended; ≥18 years: same as adult

    Levaquin *Tab:* 250, 500, 750 mg; *Oral soln:* 25 mg/ml (480 ml) (benzyl alcohol); *Inj conc:* 25 mg/ml for IV infusion after dilution (20, 30 ml single-use vial) (preservative-free); *Premix soln:* 5 mg/ml for IV infusion (50, 100, 150 ml) (preservative-free)

▷ **linezolid** (C)(G) 400-600 mg q 12 hours x 10-14 days

Pediatric: <5 years: 10 mg/kg q 8 hours x 10-14 days; 5-11 years: 10 mg/kg q 12 hours x 10-14 days; >11 years: same as adult

    Zyvox *Tab:* 400, 600 mg; *Oral susp:* 100 mg/5 ml (150 ml) (orange) (phenylalanine)

Comment: *Linezolid* is indicated to treat susceptible vancomycin-resistant *E. faecium* infections.

▷ *loracarbef* (B) 400 mg bid x 3-10 days
  Pediatric: <12 years: 15 mg/kg/day in 2 divided doses x 7 days; *see* Appendix
  CC.27. loracarbef (Lorabid Suspension) *for dose by weight table;* ≥12 years: 200
  mg bid x 7 days
    Lorabid *Pulvule:* 200, 400 mg; *Oral susp:* 100 mg/5 ml (50, 100 ml); 200 mg/5
    ml (50, 75, 100 ml) (strawberry bubble gum)
▷ *moxifloxacin* (C)(G) 400 mg daily x 3-10 days
  Pediatric: <18 years: not recommended; ≥18 years: same as adult
    Avelox *Tab:* 400 mg; *IV soln:* 400 mg/250 mg (latex-free, preservative-free)
▷ *ofloxacin* (C)(G) 400 mg bid x 3-10 days
  Pediatric: <18 years: not recommended; ≥18 years: same as adult
    Floxin *Tab:* 200, 300, 400 mg
▷ *penicillin v potassium* (B) 250-500 mg q 6 hours x 3-10 days
  Pediatric: <12 years: 25-75 mg/kg day divided q 6-8 hours x 5-7 days; *see*
  Appendix CC.29. *penicillin v potassium* (Pen-Vee K Solution, Veetids Solution)
  for dose by weight table; ≥12 years: same as adult
    Pen-VK *Tab:* 250, 500 mg; *Oral soln:* 125 mg/5 ml (100, 200 ml); 250 mg/5 ml
    (100, 150, 200 ml)
▷ *tedizolid phosphate* (B) administer 200 mg once daily x 6 days, via PO or IV
  infusion over 1 hour
    Sivextro *Tab:* 200 mg (6/blister pck)
    Comment: **Sivextro** is indicated for the treatment of community-acquired
    bacterial pneumonia (CABP).
▷ *telithromycin* (C) 2 x 400 mg tabs in a single dose once daily x 3-5 days
  Pediatric: <8 years: not recommended; ≥8 years: same as adult
    Ketek *Tab:* 300, 400 mg
  Comment: *Telithromycin* is contraindicated with PMHx hepatitis or jaundice
  associated with macrolide use.
▷ *tigecycline* (D)(G) 100 mg once; then 50 mg q 12 hours x 3-5 days; *Severe hepatic
  impairment (Child-Pugh Class C):* 100 mg once; then 25 mg q 12 hours x 3-5
  days
  Pediatric: <18 years: not recommended; ≥18 years: same as adult
    Tygacil *Vial:* 50 mg pwdr for reconstitution and IV infusion (preservative-
      free)
    Comment: **Tygacil** is indicated only for the treatment of adults (≥18 years-
    of-age) with community-acquired bacterial pneumonia (CABP). *tigecycline*
    is contraindicated in pregnancy, and lactation (discolors developing tooth
    enamel). A side effect may be photo-sensitivity (photophobia). Do not give
    with antacids, calcium supplements, milk or other dairy, or within 2 hours of
    taking another drug.
▷ *trimethoprim+sulfamethoxazole (TMP-SMX)* (C)(G)
  Pediatric: <2 months: not recommended; ≥2 months: 40 mg/kg/day of
  sulfamethoxazole in 2 doses bid x 3-10 days; *see Appendix CC.33: trimethoprim+
  sulfamethoxazole* (Bactrim Suspension, Septra Suspension) *for dose by weight*
    Bactrim, Septra 2 tabs bid x 3-10 days
      Tab: trim 80 mg+sulfa 400 mg*
    Bactrim DS, Septra DS 1 tab bid x 3-10 days
      Tab: trim 160 mg+sulfa 800 mg*
    Bactrim Pediatric Suspension, Septra Pediatric Suspension 160/800 bid x 3-10
    days
      Oral susp: trim 40 mg+sulfa 200 mg per 5 ml (100 ml) (cherry) (alcohol
      0.3%)

AMINOMETHYLCYCLINE TETRACYCLINE

▷ *omadacycline Loading Dose, Day 1:* 200 mg via IV infusion over 60 minutes or 100 mg via IV infusion over 30 minutes twice; *Maintenance:* 100 mg via IV infusion over 30 minutes once daily or 300 mg orally once daily; total treatment duration 7-14 days; before oral dosing, fast x at least 4 hours and then take tablets with water; after oral dosing, no food or drink (except water) x 2 hours and no dairy products, antacids, or multivitamins x 4 hours
Pediatric: <18 years: not recommended; ≥18 years: same as adult

Nuzyra *Tab:* 150 mg; *Vial:* 100 mg single dose for reconstitution, dilution, and IV infusion

Comment: **Nuzyra** *(omadacycline)* is an aminomethylcycline tetracycline antibiotic for the treatment of community-acquired bacterial pneumonia (CABP) and acute bacterial skin and skin structure infection (ABSSSI). The most common adverse reactions (incidence ≥2%) are nausea, vomiting, infusion site reactions, alanine aminotransferase (ALT) increased, aspartate aminotransferase (AST) increased, gamma-glutamyl transferase (GGT) increased, hypertension, headache, diarrhea, insomnia, and constipation. Like other tetracycline-class antibacterial drugs, **Nuzyra** may cause discoloration of deciduous teeth and reversible inhibition of bone growth when administered during the second and third trimester of pregnancy. The limited available data of **Nuzyra** use in pregnancy is insufficient to inform drug-associated risk of major birth defects and miscarriages. There is no information on the presence of *omadacycline* in human milk or effects on the breastfed infant.

SEMI-SYNTHETIC PLEUROMUTILIN ANTIBIOTIC

▷ *lefamulin Tab:* 600 mg every 12 hours x 5 days; take at least 1 hour before or 2 hours after a meal; swallow whole with 6-8 ounces of water; *Moderate-to-Severe Hepatic Impairment (Child-Pugh Class B/C):* tablets have not been studied in, and are not recommended; *IV Infusion:* 150 mg every 12 hours x 5-7 days; infuse over 60 minutes; *Severe Hepatic Impairment (Child-Pugh Class C):* reduce the IV infusion dose to 150 mg every 24 hours
Pediatric: <18 years: not established; ≥18 years: same as adult

Xenleta *Tab:* 600 mg; Vial: 150 mg/15 ml 0.9%NS, single dose, for dilution and IV infusion

Comment: **Xenleta** *(lefamulin)* is a first-in-class, semi-synthetic pleuromutilin antibiotic for the treatment of community-acquired bacterial pneumonia (CABP). To reduce the development of drug resistant bacteria and maintain effectiveness of **Xenleta** and other antibacterial drugs, **Xenleta** should be used only to treat or prevent infections that are proven or strongly suspected to be caused by bacteria. *IV Infusion:* avoid use of **Xenleta** via IV infusion with concomitant strong or moderate CYP3A inducers or P-gp inducers, unless benefit outweighs risk, and monitor for reduced **Xenleta** efficacy. *Tablet:* concomitant use of **Xenleta** tablets with CYP3A substrates that prolong the QT interval is contraindicated. Avoid use of **Xenleta** tablet in patients with known QT prolongation, ventricular arrhythmias including torsades de pointes, and patients receiving drugs that prolong the QT interval such as antiarrhythmic agents. Avoid **Xenleta** tablet with strong CYP3A inhibitors or P-gp inhibitors; monitor for adverse reactions with concomitant CYP3A inhibitors or P-gp inhibitors, *midazolam* (**Versed**), and other sensitive CYP3A substrates. The most common adverse reactions (incidence ≥2%) have been *(tab)* diarrhea, nausea, vomiting, hepatic enzyme elevation, and *(IV infusion)* administration site reactions, hepatic enzyme elevation, nausea, hypokalemia, insomnia, and headache. Evaluate patients who develop diarrhea for *Clostridium difficile* (CDAD). **Xenleta** may cause embryo/fetal toxicity. Verify pregnancy status prior to initiation of treatment and advise females of reproductive potential of the potential risk and to use effective contraception for the duration of treatment and for 2 days after the final dose. There is a pregnancy pharmacovigilance program. If **Xenleta** is inadvertently administered during pregnancy or if a patient becomes pregnant while receiving **Xenleta**, healthcare providers should report **Xenleta** exposure by calling 1-855-5NABRIVA to enroll. Lactating females should pump and discard breast milk for the duration of treatment with **Xenleta** and for 2 days after the final dose.

PNEUMONIA: LEGIONELLA

ANTI-INFECTIVES

▷ *ciprofloxacin* (C) 500 mg bid x 14-21 days
Pediatric: <18 years: not recommended; ≥18 years: same as adult
    Cipro (G) *Tab:* 250, 500, 750 mg; *Oral susp:* 250, 500 mg/5 ml (100 ml) (strawberry)
    Cipro XR *Tab:* 500, 1000 mg ext-rel
    ProQuin XR *Tab:* 500 mg ext-rel

▷ *clarithromycin* (C)(G) 500 mg bid or 500 mg ext-rel once daily x 14-21 days
    Biaxin *Tab:* 250, 500 mg
    Biaxin Oral Suspension *Oral susp:* 125, 250 mg/5 ml (50, 100 ml) (fruit punch)
    Biaxin XL *Tab:* 500 mg ext-rel

▷ *dirithromycin* (C)(G) 500 mg once daily x 14-21 days
    Dynabac *Tab:* 250 mg

▷ *erythromycin base* (B)(G) 500 mg qid x 14-21 days
Pediatric: <45 kg: 30-50 mg in 2-4 divided doses x 14-21 days; ≥45 kg: same as adult
    Ery-Tab *Tab:* 250, 333, 500 mg ent-coat
    PCE *Tab:* 333, 500 mg

▷ *erythromycin estolate* (B)(G) 1-2 gm daily in divided doses x 14-21 days
Pediatric: 30-50 mg/kg/day in divided doses x 14-21 days; *see Appendix CC.20:* erythromycin estolate (Ilosone Suspension) *for dose by weight*
    Ilosone *Pulvule:* 250 mg; *Tab:* 500 mg; *Liq:* 125, 250 mg/5 ml (100 ml)

▷ *trimethoprim+sulfamethoxazole (TMP-SMX)* (C)(G)
Pediatric: <2 months: not recommended; ≥2 months: 40 mg/kg/day of *sulfamethoxazole* in 2 doses bid x 10 days
    Bactrim, Septra 2 tabs bid x 10 days
      Tab: trim 80 mg+sulfa 400 mg*
    Bactrim DS, Septra DS 1 tab bid x 10 days
      Tab: trim 160 mg+sulfa 800 mg*
    Bactrim Pediatric Suspension, Septra Pediatric Suspension
      Oral susp: trim 40 mg+sulfa 200 mg per 5 ml (100 ml) (cherry) (alcohol 0.3%)

PNEUMONIA: MYCOPLASMA

ANTI-INFECTIVES

▷ *azithromycin* (B)(G) 500 mg x 1 dose on day 1, then 250 mg daily on days 2-5 or 500 mg daily x 3 days or **Zmax** 2 gm in a single dose
Pediatric: 12 mg/kg/day x 5 days; max 500 mg/day; *see* Appendix CC.7. *azithromycin* (Zithromax Suspension, Zmax Suspension) *for dose by weight*
    Zithromax *Tab:* 250, 500, 600 mg; *Oral susp:* 100 mg/5 ml (15 ml); 200 mg/5 ml (15, 22.5, 30 ml) (cherry); *Pkt:* 1 gm for reconstitution (cherry-banana)
    Zithromax Tri-pak *Tab:* 3 x 500 mg tabs/pck
    Zithromax Z-pak *Tab:* 6 x 250 mg tabs/pck
    Zmax *Oral susp:* 2 gm ext-rel for reconstitution (cherry-banana) (148 mg Na⁺)

▷ *clarithromycin* (C)(G) 500 mg bid or 500 mg ext-rel once daily x 14-21 days
   Pediatric: <6 months: not recommended; ≥6 months: 7.5 mg/kg bid x 7 days; *see*
   Appendix CC.16. *clarithromycin* (Biaxin Suspension) *for dose by weight*
      Biaxin *Tab:* 250, 500 mg
      Biaxin Oral Suspension *Oral susp:* 125, 250 mg/5 ml (50, 100 ml) (fruit-punch)
      Biaxin XL *Tab:* 500 mg ext-rel
▷ *erythromycin base* (B)(G) 500 mg q 6 hours x 14-21 days
   Pediatric: <45 kg: 30-50 mg in 2-4 doses x 14-21 days; ≥45 kg: same as adult
      Ery-Tab *Tab:* 250, 333, 500 mg ent-coat
      PCE *Tab:* 333, 500 mg
▷ *erythromycin ethylsuccinate* (B)(G) 400 mg qid x 14-21 days
   Pediatric: 30-50 mg/kg/day in 4 divided doses x 14-21 days; may double dose
   with severe infection; max 100 mg/kg/day; *see Appendix CC.21. erythromycin*
   ethylsuccinate (E.E.S. Suspension, Ery-Ped Drops/Suspension) *for dose by weight*
      EryPed *Oral susp:* 200 mg/5 ml (100, 200 ml) (fruit); 400 mg/5 ml (60, 100,
      200 ml) (banana); *Oral drops:* 200, 400 mg/5 ml (50 ml) (fruit); *Chew tab:*
      200 mg wafer (fruit)
      E.E.S. *Oral susp:* 200, 400 mg/5 ml (100 ml) (fruit)
      E.E.S. Granules *Oral susp:* 200 mg/5 ml (100, 200 ml) (cherry)
      E.E.S. 400 Tablets *Tab:* 400 mg
▷ *tetracycline* (D)(G) 500 mg qid
   Pediatric: <8 years: not recommended; ≥8 years, <100 lb: 25-50 mg/kg/day in 2-4
   divided doses; ≥8 years, ≥100 lb: same as adult; *see Appendix CC.31. tetracycline*
   (Sumycin Suspension) *for dose by weight*
      Achromycin V *Cap:* 250, 500 mg
      Sumycin *Tab:* 250, 500 mg; *Cap:* 250, 500 mg; *Oral susp:* 125 mg/5 ml (100,
      200 ml) (fruit) (sulfites)

◯ PNEUMONIA: PNEUMOCOCCAL

PNEUMOCOCCAL VACCINATION

ACIP recommends a routine single dose of **PPSV23** (pneumococcal 23-valent
polysaccharide vaccine) in adults age ≥65 years. If not previously administered
PCV13, PCV13 is recommended by shared clinical decision-making in persons age
≥65 years. who do not have an immunocompromising condition, cerebrospinal fluid
leak, or cochlear implant. If **PCV13** is to be administered, it should be administered
first, followed by **PPSV23** at least 1 year later.

TREATMENT
see CAP/CABP

PROPHYLAXIS
▷ *pneumococcal* vaccine (C) 0.5 ml IM or SC in deltoid x 1 dose
      Pneumovax
      Pediatric: <2 years: not recommended; ≥2 years: same as adult
         Vial: 25 mcg/0.5 ml (single-dose, 10/pck; multi-dose, 2.5 ml, 10/pck)
      Pnu-Imune 23
      Pediatric: <2 years: not recommended; ≥2 years: same as adult
         Vial: 25 mcg/0.5 ml (0.5 ml single-dose, 5/pck; 2.5 ml)
      Prevnar 13 for adults ≥50 years of age
      Pediatric: total 4 doses: 2, 4, 6, and 12-15 months-of-age; may start at 6 weeks
      of age; administer first 3 doses 4-8 weeks apart and the 4th dose at least 2
      months after the 3rd dose
         Vial: 25 mcg/0.5 ml (single-dose, 10/pck); *Prefilled syringe:* (single-dose,
         10/pck; 2.5 ml, multi-dose)

Comment: Pneumococcal vaccine contains 23 polysaccharide isolates representing approximately 85-90% of common U.S. isolates. Administer the pneumococcal vaccine in the anterolateral aspect of the thigh for infants and the deltoid for toddlers, children, and adults.

PNEUMONIA (*PNEUMOCYSTIS JIROVECI*)

QUINONE ANTIMICROBIAL

▷ *atovaquone* (C)(G) take as a single dose with food or a milky drink at the same time each day; repeat dose if vomited within 1 hour; *Prophylaxis:* 1500 mg once daily; *Treatment:* 750 mg bid x 21 days

Pediatric: <12 years: not recommended; ≥12 years: same as adult

Mepron *Susp:* 750 mg/5 ml (210 ml; 5 ml pouches) (citrus)

Comment: **Mepron** *(atovaquone)* suspension is a quinone antimicrobial drug indicated for the prevention of *Pneumocystis jiroveci* pneumonia (PCP), and treatment of mild-to-moderate PCP, in adults and adolescents ≥13 years-of-age who cannot tolerate *trimethoprim+sulfamethoxazole* (TMP-SMX). Treatment of severe PCP (alveolar arterial oxygen diffusion gradient [(A-a) DO2] >45 mm Hg) with **Mepron**, and the efficacy of **Mepron** in subjects who are failing therapy with TMPSMX, have not been studied. Elevated liver chemistry tests and cases of hepatitis and fatal liver failure have been reported. Failure to administer **Mepron** suspension with food may result in lower plasma *atovaquone* concentrations and may limit response to therapy. Patients with gastrointestinal disorders may have limited absorption resulting in suboptimal *atovaquone* concentrations. Concomitant administration of the following drugs reduce *atovaquone* concentrations: *rifampin* and *rifabutin*, *tetracyclines*, *metoclopramide*. Concomitant administration of *indinavir* reduces *indinavir* trough concentrations. The most frequent adverse reactions (≥25% that required discontinuation) attributed to **Mepron** taken for prophyllaxis have been diarrhea, rash, headache, nausea, and fever. The most frequent adverse reactions (≥14% that required discontinuation) attributed to **Mepron** taken for prophylaxis have been rash (including maculopapular), nausea, diarrhea, headache, vomiting, and fever. There are no adequate and well-controlled studies of **Mepron** use in pregnancy. *atovaquone* was not teratogenic and did not cause reproductive toxicity in animal studies at plasma concentrations up to 2-3 times the estimated human exposure (dose of 1000 mg/kg/day). However, **Mepron** should be used during pregnancy only if the potential benefit justifies the potential risk to the fetus. It is not known whether *atovaquone* is excreted into human milk or effects on the breastfed infant. In an animal study (with doses of 10 and 250 mg/kg), *atovaquone* concentrations in milk were 30% of the concurrent *atovaquone* concentrations in maternal plasma at both doses; therefore, caution should be exercised when **Mepron** is administered to patients who are breastfeeding.

▷ *trimethoprim+sulfamethoxazole (TMP-SMX)* (C)(G) Prophylaxis: 1 tab 3 x/week; *Treatment:* 1 tab daily x 3 weeks; *Septra* can be given if intolerable to *Bactrim*

Pediatric: <2 months: not recommended; ≥2 months: 40 mg/kg/day of *sulfamethoxazole* in 2 doses bid x 10 days

Bactrim, Septra 2 tabs bid x 10 days

Tab: trim 80 mg+sulfa 400 mg*

Bactrim DS, Septra DS 1 tab bid x 10 days

Tab: trim 160 mg+sulfa 800 mg*

Bactrim Pediatric Suspension, Septra Pediatric Suspension

Oral susp: trim 40 mg+sulfa 200 mg per 5 ml (100 ml) (cherry) (alcohol 0.3%)

POLIOMYELITIS

PROPHYLAXIS

▷ **trivalent poliovirus vaccine, inactivated (type 1, 2, and 3)** (C)
  Pediatric: <6 weeks: not recommended; ≥6 weeks: one dose at 2, 4, 6-18 months
  and 4-6 years of age
  Ipol 0.5 ml SC or IM in deltoid area

POLYANGIITIS

CD20-DIRECTED CYTOLYTIC ANTIBODY

▷ **rituximab** *Induction:* 375 mg/m^2 via IV infusion once weekly x 4 weeks, in
  combination with glucocorticoids; *Follow up, patients who have achieved disease
  control with induction treatment, in combination with glucocorticoids:* two 500
  mg IV infusions separated by two weeks, followed by one 500 mg IV infusion
  every 6 months thereafter, based on clinical evaluation; **Rituxan** should only be
  administered by a qualified healthcare professional with appropriate medical
  support to manage severe infusion-related reactions that can be fatal if they occur
  Pediatric: <2 years: safety and efficacy not established; ≥2 years: *Induction:*
  375 mg/m^2 via IV infusion once weekly x 4 weeks, in combination with
  glucocorticoids; *Follow up, patients who have achieved disease control with
  induction treatment, in combination with glucocorticoids:* two 250 mg/m^2 via IV
  infusions separated by two weeks, followed by one 250 mg/m^2 via IV infusion
  every 6 months thereafter, based on clinical evaluation; **Rituxan** should only be
  administered by a qualified healthcare professional with appropriate medical
  support to manage severe infusion-related reactions that can be fatal if they occur
    Rituxan *Vial:* 100 mg/10 ml (10 mg/ml), 500 mg/50 ml (10 mg/ml), single-
    dose, soln for dilution and IV infusion (preservative-free)
    Comment: **Rituxan** is indicated for the treatment of Wegener's
    Granulomatosis, in combination with glucocorticoids, for adults and pediatric
    patients ≥2 years-of-age. The most adverse common reactions (incidence
    ≥15%) in clinical trials have been infections, nausea, diarrhea, headache,
    muscle spasms, anemia, peripheral edema, infusion-related reactions.
    For tumor lysis syndrome, administer aggressive IV hydration, anti-
    hyperuricemic agents, and monitor renal function. Monitor for infections;
    withhold **Rituxan** and institute appropriate anti-infective therapy. For cardiac
    adverse reactions, discontinue infusions in case of serious or life-threatening
    events. Discontinue **Rituxan** in patients with rising serum creatinine or
    oliguria. Bowel obstruction and perforation can occur; consider and evaluate
    for abdominal pain, vomiting, or related symptoms. Live virus vaccinations
    prior to or during **Rituxan** treatment is not recommended. **Rituxan** is
    embryo/fetal toxic. Advise males and females of reproductive potential of
    the potential risk and to use effective contraception. Advise women not to
    breastfeed during treatment and for at least 6 months after the last dose.
▷ **rituximab-arrx** *Induction:* 375 mg/m^2 once weekly x 4 weeks; *then, If Disease
  Control Achieved:* 500 mg via IV infusion x 2 doses separated by two weeks;
  then, 500 mg via IV infusion once every 6 months based on clinical evaluation;
  administer all doses of **Riabni** in combination with glucocorticoids; **Riabni**
  should only be administered by a qualified healthcare professional with
  appropriate medical support to manage severe infusion-related reactions that can
  be fatal
  Pediatric: safety and efficacy not established
    Riabni *Vial:* 100 mg/10 ml (10 mg/ml), 500 mg/50 ml (10 mg/ml) soln, single-
    dose

Comment: **Riabni** *(rituximab-arrx)* is a biosimilar to **Rituxan** indicated for the treatment of adult patients with microscopic polyangiitis (MPA) in combination with glucocorticoids. The most common adverse reactions in MPA clinical trials with MPA (incidence ≥15%) have been infections, nausea, diarrhea, headache, muscle spasms, anemia, peripheral edema, and infusion-related reactions. Monitor renal function. Discontinue **Riabni** in patients with rising serum creatinine or oliguria. If tumor lysis syndrome (TLS) is suspected, administer aggressive IV hydration and anti-hyperuricemic agents. If infection occurs, withhold **Riabni** and institute appropriate anti-infective therapy. Bowel obstruction and perforation can occur; evaluate for abdominal pain, vomiting, and related symptoms. Live virus vaccine administration prior to or during treatment with **Riabni** is not recommended. **Riabni** is embryo/fetal toxic. Advise females of reproductive potential of embryo/fetal risk and to use effective contraception. Advise not to breastfeed.

POLYCYSTIC KIDNEY DISEASE, AUTOSOMAL DOMINANT (ADPKD)

SELECTIVE VASOPRESSIN V2 RECEPTOR ANTAGONIST

▶ *tolvaptan* usual starting dose is 15 mg once daily with or without food; may titrate the dose once daily after at least 24 hours to 30 mg; then may titrate once daily dose to 60 mg as needed to achieve the desired level of serum sodium; do not administer for more than 30 days to minimize the risk of liver injury; initiation and re-initiation of therapy too should occur in a hospital environment to evaluate the therapeutic response and because too rapid correction of hyponatremia can cause osmotic demyelination resulting in dysarthria, mutism, dysphagia, lethargy, affective changes, spastic quadriparesis, seizures, coma and death; avoid fluid restriction during the first 24 hours of therapy. Patients receiving *tolvaptan* should be advised that they can continue ingestion of fluid in response to thirst; following discontinuation from *tolvaptan*, patients should be advised to resume fluid restriction and should be monitored for changes in serum sodium and volume status
Pediatric: <18 years: not established; ≥18 years: same as adult

Jynarque *Tab:* 15, 30, 45, 60, 90 mg (7, 28/pck)

Samsca *Tab:* 15, 30 mg

Comment: *Tolvaptan* is indicated to slow kidney function decline patients at risk of rapidly progressing autosomal dominant polycystic kidney disease (ADPKD). Further, *tolvaptan* is indicated for the treatment of clinically significant hypervolemic and euvolemic hyponatremia (serum sodium <125 mEq/L or less marked hyponatremia that is symptomatic and has resisted correction with fluid restriction), including patients with heart failure and Syndrome of Inappropriate Antidiuretic Hormone (SIAD). Contraindications to *tolvaptan* include use in in patients with autosomal dominant polycystic kidney disease (ADPKD) outside of FDA-approved REMS, patients requiring intervention to raise serum sodium urgently to prevent or to treat serious neurological symptoms, patients unable to respond appropriately to thirst, hypovolemic hyponatremia, concomitant use of strong CYP 3A inhibitors, anuria, and hypersensitivity to the drug. Avoid use in patients with underlying liver disease; if hepatic injury is suspected, discontinue. Avoid use with CYP 3A inducers and moderate CYP 3A inhibitors. Dehydration and hypovolemia may require intervention. Avoid use with hypertonic saline. Consider dose reduction if co-administered with P-gp inhibitors. Monitor serum K^+ in patients with potassium >5 mEq/L or on drugs known to increase potassium. Based on animal data, *tolvaptan* may cause fetal harm. Discontinue *tolvaptan* or breastfeeding taking into consideration importance of the drug to mother.

POLYCYSTIC OVARIAN SYNDROME (PCOS, STEIN-LEVENTHAL DISEASE)

See **Contraceptives**
See **Type 2 Diabetes Mellitus**

POLYCYTHEMIA VERA

▷ *ruxolitinib* initially 10 mg twice daily; therapeutic dose should be individualized based on safety and efficacy; *Renal Impairment:* reduce starting dose or avoid use; *Hepatic Impairment:* reduce starting dose or avoid use
Pediatric: safety and efficacy not established

Jakafi *Tab:* 5, 10, 15, 20, 25 mg

Comment: Jakafi *(ruxolitinib)* is a kinase inhibitor indicated for treatment of adults with intermediate and high-risk myelofibrosis, including primary myelofibrosis, polycythemia vera with inadequate response to, or intolerance to, hydroxyurea, post-polycythemia vera myelofibrosis, and post-essential thrombocythemia myelofibrosis. Manage thrombocytopenia, anemia, and neutropenia with dose reduction, or treatment interruption, or transfusion. Serious infections should be resolved before starting therapy with **Jakafi**. Assess patients for signs and symptoms of infection during **Jakafi** therapy and initiate appropriate treatment promptly. Manage symptom exacerbation following interruption or discontinuation of **Jakafi** with supportive care and then consider resuming treatment with **Jakafi**. There is risk of non-melanoma skin cancer (NMSC) with **Jakafi** use; perform periodic skin examinations. Assess lipid levels 8-12 weeks from start of **Jakafi** therapy and treat as appropriate. Avoid use of **Jakafi** with *fluconazole* doses greater than 200 mg except in patients with acute graft versus host disease (GVHD). With myelofibrosis and polycythemia vera, the most common hematologic adverse reactions (incidence >20%) have been thrombocytopenia and anemia and the most common nonhematologic adverse reactions (incidence >10%) have been bruising, dizziness, and headache. There are no studies with the use of **Jakafi** in pregnant females to inform drug-associated risks. No data are available regarding the presence of *ruxolitinib* in human milk or the effects on the breastfed infant. Patients should be advised to discontinue breastfeeding during treatment with **Jakafi** and for 2 weeks after the final dose.

POLYMYALGIA RHEUMATICA

Oral Corticosteroids *see* Appendix L. Oral Corticosteroids
Calcium and Vitamin D Supplementation *see* **Hypocalcemia**

Comment: Initial treatment is low-dose prednisone at 12-25 mg/day. May attempt a very slow tapering regimen after 2-4 weeks. If relapse occurs, increase the daily dose of corticosteroid to the previous effective dose. Most people with polymyalgia rheumatica need to continue corticosteroid treatment for at least a year. Approximately 30%-60% of people will have at least one relapse during corticosteroid tapering. Joint guidelines from the American Academy of Rheumatology (AAR) and the European League Against Rheumatism (ELAR) suggest using concomitant *methotrexate* (MTX) along with corticosteroids in some patients. It may be useful early in the course of treatment or later, if the patient relapses or does not respond to corticosteroids. The American Academy of Rheumatology (AAR) recommends the following daily doses for anyone on a chronic oral corticosteroid regimen: Calcium 1200-1500 mg/day and vitamin D 800-1000 IU/day.

METHOTREXATE

▷ *methotrexate* (MTX)(X) 7.5 mg x 1 dose per week <u>or</u> 2.5 mg x 3 at 12 hour intervals once a week; max 20 mg/week; therapeutic response begins in 3-6 weeks; administer *methotrexate* (MTX) injection SC <u>only</u> into the abdomen <u>or</u> thigh

Pediatric: <2 years: not recommended; ≥2 years: 10 mg/m² once weekly; max 20 mg/m²

    Rasuvo *Autoinjector:* 7.5 mg/0.15 ml, 10 mg/0.20 ml, 12.5 mg/0.25 ml, 15 mg/0.30 ml, 17.5 mg/0.35 ml, 20 mg/0.40 ml, 22.5 mg/0.45 ml, 25 mg/0.50 ml, 27.5 mg/0.55 ml, 30 mg/0.60 ml (solution concentration for SC injection is 50 mg/ml)

    Rheumatrex *Tab:* 2.5*mg (5, 7.5, 10, 12.5, 15 mg/week, 4/card unit dose pack)

    TrexallR *Tab:* 5*, 7.5*, 10*, 15*mg (5, 7.5, 10, 12.5, 15 mg/week, 4/card unit dose pack)

Comment: *Methotrexate* (MTX) is contraindicated with immunodeficiency, blood dyscrasias, alcoholism, and chronic liver disease.

◯ POLYNEUROPATHY, CHRONIC INFLAMMATORY DEMYELINATING (CIDP)

IMMUNE GLOBULIN, HUMAN

▷ *immune globulin subcutaneous [human] 20% liquid* <18 years: not recommended; ≥18 years: administer once weekly via SC infusion <u>only</u>; *Infusion sites:* abdomen, thigh, upper arm, <u>and/or</u> lateral hip; may use up to 8 injection sites simultaneously, with at least 2 inches between sites; *Infusion volume:* for the first infusion, up to 15 ml per injection site; may increase to 20 ml per site after the fourth infusion; max 25 ml per site as tolerated; *Infusion rate:* first infusion, up to 15 ml/hr per site; may increase, to max 25 ml/hr per site as tolerated; however, maximum flow rate is <u>not</u> to exceed a total of 50 ml/hr for all sites combined; before switching to **Hizentra**, obtain the patient's serum IgG trough level to guide subsequent dose adjustments; adjust the dose: based on clinical response and serum IgG trough levels; initiate therapy 1 week after the last IGIV infusion; recommended subcutaneous dose is 0.2 g/kg (1 ml/kg) per week; in the clinical study after transitioning from IGIV to **Hizentra**, a dose of 0.4 g/kg (2 ml/kg) per week was also safe and effective to prevent CIDP relapse; If CIDP symptoms worsen, consider re-initiating treatment with an IGIV approved for the treatment of CIDP, while discontinuing **Hizentra**; if improvement and stabilization are observed during IGIV treatment, consider re-initiating **Hizentra** at 0.4 gm/kg per week, while discontinuing IGIV; if CIDP symptoms worsen on 0.4 gm/kg per week, consider reinitiating **Hizentra** therapy with IGIV, while discontinuing **Hizentra**; monitor patient's clinical response and adjust duration of therapy based on patient need

    Hizentra *Vial:* 0.2 mg/ml (20%; 5, 10, 20, 50 ml)

    Comment: IgA-deficient patients with anti-IgA antibodies are at greater risk of severe hypersensitivity and anaphylactic reactions. Thrombosis may occur following treatment with immune globulin products, including **Hizentra**. Aseptic meningitis syndrome has been reported with IGIV and IGSC, including **Hizentra**. Monitor renal function in patients at risk of acute renal failure (ARF). Monitor for clinical signs and symptoms of hemolysis. Monitor for pulmonary adverse reactions (transfusion-related acute lung injury [TRALI]). **Hizentra** is made from human blood and may contain infectious agents (e.g., viruses, the variant Creutzfeldt-Jakob disease (vCJD) agent and, theoretically, the Creutzfeldt-Jakob disease (CJD) agent). Monitor for clinical signs and symptoms of hemolysis. The most common adverse reactions observed in ≥5% of study subjects were local infusion site reactions, headache, diarrhea, fatigue, back pain, nausea, pain in extremity, cough, upper respiratory tract infection, rash, pruritus, vomiting, abdominal pain (upper), migraine, arthralgia, pain, fall, and nasopharyngitis. No human or animal reproduction studies have not been conducted with **Hizentra**. It is not known whether **Hizentra** can cause fetal harm when administered during pregnancy. No human data are available to inform maternal use of **Hizentra** on the breastfed infant. Safety and effectiveness of weekly **Hizentra** administration have not been established in children <2 years of age.

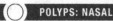
POLYPS: NASAL

LONG-ACTING CORTICOSTEROID SINUS IMPLANT
▷ *mometasone furoate* the **Sinuva Sinus Implant** must be inserted by a physician trained in otolaryngology; the implant is loaded into a sterile delivery system supplied with the implant and placed in the ethmoid sinus under endoscopic visualization; the implant is left in the sinus to gradually release the corticosteroid over 90 days; the implant is removed at Day 90 or earlier at the physician's discretion using standard surgical instruments; repeat administration has not been studied.
Pediatric: <18 years: not established: ≥18 years: same as adult
   Sinuva Sinus Implant *Sinus implant:* 1350 mcg w. sterile delivery system
   Comment: **Sinuva** is a corticosteroid-eluting sinus implant indicated for the treatment of recurrent nasal polyp disease in patients who have ethmoid sinus surgery. Monitor nasal mucosa adjacent to the **Sinuva Sinus Implant** for any signs of bleeding (epistaxis), irritation, infection, or perforation. Avoid use in patients with nasal ulcers or trauma. Monitor patients with a change in vision or with a history of increased intraocular pressure, glaucoma, and/or cataracts closely. Potential worsening of existing tuberculosis; fungal, bacterial, viral, parasitic infection, or ocular herpes simplex. More serious or even fatal course of chickenpox or measles in susceptible patients. If corticosteroid effects such as hypercorticism and adrenal suppression appear in patients, consider sinus implant removal.

NASAL SPRAY CORTICOSTEROIDS
▷ *beclomethasone dipropionate* (C)
   Beconase 1 spray in each nostril bid-qid
   Pediatric: <6 years: not recommended; 6-12 years: 1 spray in each nostril tid; >12 years: same as adult
      Nasal spray: 42 mcg/actuation (6.7 gm, 80 sprays; 16.8 gm, 200 sprays)
   Beconase AQ 1-2 sprays in each nostril bid
   Pediatric: <6: not recommended; ≥6 years: same as adult
      Nasal spray: 42 mcg/actuation (25 gm, 180 sprays)
   Beconase Inhalation Aerosol 1-2 sprays in each nostril bid to qid
   Pediatric: <6: not recommended; 6-12 years: 1 spray in each nostril tid; >12 years: same as adult
      Nasal spray: 42 mcg/actuation (6.7 gm, 80 sprays; 16.8 gm, 200 sprays)
   Vancenase AQ 1-2 sprays in each nostril bid
   Pediatric: <6 years: not recommended; ≥6 years: same as adult
      Nasal spray: 84 mcg/actuation (25 gm, 200 sprays)
   Vancenase AQ DS 1-2 sprays in each nostril once daily
   Pediatric: <6 years: not recommended; ≥6 years: same as adult
      Nasal spray: 84, 168 mcg/actuation (19 gm, 120 sprays)
   Vancenase Pockethaler 1 spray in each nostril bid or qid
   Pediatric: <6: not recommended; ≥6 years: 1 spray in each nostril tid
      Pockethaler: 42 mcg/actuation (7 gm, 200 sprays)

QNASL Nasal Aerosol 2 sprays, 80 mcg/spray, in each nostril once daily
Pediatric: <12 years: 2 sprays, 40 mcg/spray, in each nostril once daily; ≥12 years: same as adult

> *Nasal spray:* 40 mcg/actuation (4.9 gm, 60 sprays); 80 mcg/actuation (8.7 gm, 120 sprays)

▷ *budesonide* (C)

Rhinocort initially 2 sprays in each nostril bid in the AM and PM, or 4 sprays in each nostril in the AM; max 4 sprays each nostril/day; use lowest effective dose
Pediatric: <6 years: not recommended; ≥6 years: same as adult

> *Nasal spray:* 32 mcg/actuation (7 gm, 200 sprays)

Rhinocort Aqua Nasal Spray initially 1 spray in each nostril once daily; max 4 sprays in each nostril once daily
Pediatric: <6 years: not recommended; ≥6-12 years: initially 1 spray in each nostril once daily; max 2 sprays in each nostril once daily

> *Nasal spray:* 32 mcg/actuation (10 ml, 60 sprays)

▷ *ciclesonide* (C)

Pediatric: <6 years: not recommended; ≥6 years: same as adult

Omnaris 2 sprays in each nostril once daily

> *Nasal spray:* 50 mcg/actuation (12.5 gm, 120 sprays)

Zetonna 1-2 sprays in each nostril once daily

> *Nasal spray:* 37 mcg/actuation (6.1 gm, 60 sprays) (HFA)

▷ *dexamethasone* (C) 2 sprays in each nostril bid-tid; max 12 sprays/day; maintain at lowest effective dose
Pediatric: <6 years: not recommended; ≥6-12 years: 1-2 sprays in each nostril bid; max 8 sprays/day; maintain at lowest effective dose; >12 years: same as adult

Dexacort Turbinaire *Nasal spray:* 84 mcg/actuation (12.6 gm, 170 sprays)

▷ *flunisolide* (C) 2 sprays in each nostril bid; may increase to 2 sprays in each nostril tid; max 8 sprays/nostril/day
Pediatric: <6 years: not recommended; 6-14 years: initially 1 spray in each nostril tid or 2 sprays in each nostril bid; max 4 sprays/nostril/day; >14 years: same as adult

Nasalide *Nasal spray:* 25 mcg/actuation (25 ml, 200 sprays)
Nasarel *Nasal spray:* 25 mcg/actuation (25 ml, 200 sprays)

▷ *fluticasone furoate* (C) 2 sprays in each nostril once daily; may reduce to 1 spray each nostril once daily
Pediatric: <2 years: not recommended; ≥2-11 years: 1 spray in each nostril once daily; ≥12 years: same as adult

Veramyst *Nasal spray:* 27.5 mcg/actuation (10 gm, 120 sprays) (alcohol-free)

▷ *fluticasone propionate* (C)

Flonase (OTC)(G) initially 2 sprays in each nostril once daily or 1 spray bid; maintenance 1 spray once daily
Pediatric: <4 years: not recommended; ≥4 years: initially 1 spray in each nostril once daily; may increase to 2 sprays in each nostril once daily; maintenance 1 spray in each nostril once daily; max 2 sprays in each nostril/day

> *Nasal spray:* 50 mcg/actuation (16 gm, 120 sprays)

Xhance 1 spray per nostril bid (total daily dose 372 mcg); 2 sprays per nostril bid may also be effective in some patients (total daily dose 744 mcg)
Pediatric: <12 years: not established; ≥12 years: same as adult

> *Nasal spray:* 93 mcg/actuation (16 ml, 120 metered sprays)

Comment: Available data from published literature on the use of inhaled or intranasal *fluticasone propionate* in pregnant females have not reported a clear association with adverse developmental outcomes. There are no available data on the presence of *fluticasone propionate* in human milk or effects on the breastfed infant. The safety and efficacy of **Xhance** in pediatric patients have not been established.

▷ *mometasone furoate* (C)(G) 2 sprays in each nostril once daily
Pediatric: <2 years: not recommended; 2-11 years: 1 spray in each nostril once daily; max 2 sprays in each nostril once daily; >11 years: same as adult
    Nasonex *Nasal spray:* 50 mcg/actuation (17 gm, 120 sprays)

▷ *olopatadine* (C) 2 sprays in each nostril bid
Pediatric: <6 years: not recommended; 6-11 years: 1 spray in each nostril bid; >11 years: same as adult
    Patanase *Nasal spray:* 0.6%; 665 mcg/actuation (30.5 gm, 240 sprays) (benzalkonium chloride)

▷ *triamcinolone acetonide* (C)(G) initially 2 sprays in each nostril once daily; max 4 sprays in each nostril once daily or 2 sprays in each nostril bid or 1 spray in each nostril qid; maintain at lowest effective dose
Pediatric: <6 years: not recommended; ≥6 years: 1 spray in each nostril once daily; max 2 sprays in each nostril once daily
    Nasacort Allergy 24HR (OTC) *Nasal spray:* 55 mcg/actuation (10 gm, 120 sprays)
    Tri-Nasal *Nasal spray:* 50 mcg/actuation (15 ml, 120 sprays)

POLYURIA: NOCTURNAL

VASOPRESSIN ANALOG

▷ **desmopressin acetate** administer a single sublingual dose 1 hour prior to bedtime
Females: 27.7 mcg; *Males:* 55.3 mcg
    Nocdurna *SL tab:* 27.7, 55.3 mcg
    Comment: Nocdurna (*desmopressin acetate*) a vasopressin analog and the first sublingual tab indicated for the treatment of nocturia due to nocturnal polyuria in adults. **Nocdurna** is indicated for patients ≥18 years-of-age with nocturnal polyuria who awaken at least 2 x/night to void. **Nocdurna** is available in two strengths: 27.7 mcg of *desmopressin acetate* (equivalent to 25 mcg of *desmopressin*) and 55.3 mcg of *desmopressin acetate* and dose is gender-based. **Nocdurna** is contraindicated with the following conditions: hyponatremia or a history of hyponatremia, polydipsia, concomitant use with loop diuretics or systemic or inhaled glucocorticoids, eGFR <50 mL/min/1.73 m², syndrome of inappropriate antidiuretic hormone secretion (SIADH), during illnesses that can cause fluid or electrolyte imbalance, heart failure (HF), uncontrolled hypertension. **Nocdurna** can cause hyponatremia, which may be life-threatening if severe. Ensure serum sodium concentration is normal before starting or resuming **Nocdurna**. Measure serum sodium within one week and approximately 1 month after initiating therapy and periodically during treatment. Monitor serum sodium more frequently in patients ≥65 years-of-age and in patients at increased risk of hyponatremia. Monitor serum sodium more frequently when **Nocdurna** is concomitantly used with drugs that may increase the risk of hyponatremia (e.g., tricyclic antidepressants (TCAs), selective serotonin re-uptake inhibitors (SSRIs), *chlorpromazine*, opiate analgesics, thiazide diuretics, NSAIDs, *lamotrigine*, *chlorpropamide* and, *carbamazepine*). **Nocdurna** is not recommended in patients at risk of increased intracranial pressure or history of urinary retention. Limit fluid intake to a minimum from 1 hour before until 8 hours after administration; treatment without concomitant reduction of fluid intake may lead to fluid retention and hyponatremia. If hyponatremia occurs, **Nocdurna** may need to be temporarily or permanently discontinued. Use of **Nocdurna** is not recommended and **Nocdurna** is not recommended for the treatment of nocturia in pregnancy (nocturia is usually related to normal, physiologic

changes during pregnancy that do <u>not</u> require treatment). There are no data with **Nocdurna** use in pregnancy to inform any drug-associated risks. ***desmopressin*** is present in small amounts in human milk; however, there is no information on the effects of desmopressin on the breastfed infant.

 POST-HERPETIC NEURALGIA (PHN)

Acetaminophen for IV Infusion *see Pain*
Oral Analgesics *see Pain*

GAMMA AMINOBUTYRIC ACID ANALOGS

Comment: The gabapentinoids (*gabapentin* [**Gralise, Neurontin, Horizant**] and *pregabalin* [**Lyrica**]) have respiratory depression risk potential. Therefore, when co-prescribed with other CNS depressant agents, initiate the gabapentinoid at the lowest possible dose and monitor the patient for respiratory depression (especially elders and patients with compromised pulmonary function). Side effects include fatigue, somnolence/sedation, dizziness, vertigo, feeling drunk, headache, nausea, and dry mouth. To discontinue a gabapentinoid, withdraw gradually over 1 week <u>or</u> longer.

▷ *gabapentin (C) CrCl 30-60 mL/min:* 600-1800 mg; *CrCl <30 mL/min or on hemodialysis:* <u>not</u> recommended
 Gralise initially 300 mg on Day 1; then 600 mg on Day 2; then 900 mg on Days 3-6; then 1200 mg on Days 7-10; then 1500 mg on Days 11-14; titrate up to 1800 mg on Day 15; take entire dose once daily with the evening meal; do <u>not</u> crush, split, <u>or</u> chew
 Pediatric: <18 years: not recommended; ≥18 years: same as adult
  Tab: 300, 600 mg
 Neurontin (G) 300 mg daily x 1 day, then 300 mg bid x 1 day, then 300 mg tid continuously; max 1800 mg/day in 3 divided doses; taper over 7 days
 Pediatric: <3 years: not recommended; 3-12 years: initially 10-15 mg/kg/day in 3 divided doses; max 12 hours between doses; titrate over 3 days; 3-4 years: titrate to 40 mg/kg/day; 5-12 years: titrate to 25-35 mg/kg/day; max 50 mg/kg/day
  Tab: 600*, 800*mg; *Cap:* 100, 300, 400 mg; **Neurontin Oral Solution (G)** *Oral soln:* 250 mg/5 ml (480 ml) (strawberry-anise)
▷ *gabapentin enacarbil (C)* 600 mg once daily at about 5:00 PM; if dose <u>not</u> taken at recommended time, next dose should be taken the following day; swallow whole; take with food; *CrCl 30-59 mL/min:* 600 mg on Day 1, Day 3, and every day thereafter; *CrCl <30 mL/min:* <u>or</u> on hemodialysis: <u>not</u> recommended
 Pediatric: <18 years: not recommended; ≥18 years: same as adult
  Horizant *Tab:* 300, 600 mg ext-rel
▷ *pregabalin (GABA analog) (C)(V)*
 Pediatric: <12 years: not recommended; ≥12 years: same as adult
  Lyrica initially 50 mg tid; may titrate to 100 mg tid within 1 week; max 600 mg divided tid; discontinue over 1 week
   Cap: 25, 50, 75, 100, 150, 200, 225, 300 mg; *Oral soln:* 20 mg/ml
  Lyrica CR *Tab:* usual dose: 165 mg once daily; may increase to 330 mg/day within 1 week; max 660 mg/day
   Tab: 82.5, 165, 330 mg ext-rel

Tricyclic Antidepressants (TCAs)

Comment: Co-administration of SSRIs and TCAs requires extreme caution.

▷ *amitriptyline (C)(G)* initially 75 mg/day in divided doses of 50-100 mg/day q HS; max 300 mg/day
 Pediatric: <12 years: not recommended; ≥12 years: same as adult
  Tab: 10, 25, 50, 75, 100, 150 mg

▷ *amoxapine* (C) initially 50 mg bid-tid; after 1 week may increase to 100 mg bid-tid; usual effective dose 200-300 mg/day; if total dose exceeds 300 mg/day, give in divided doses (max 400 mg/day); may give as a single bedtime dose (max 300 mg q HS)
  Pediatric: <12 years: not recommended; ≥12 years: same as adult
    Tab: 25, 50, 100, 150 mg
▷ *desipramine* (C)(G) 100-200 mg/day in single or divided doses; max 300 mg/day
  Pediatric: <12 years: not recommended; ≥12 years: same as adult
    Norpramin *Tab:* 10, 25, 50, 75, 100, 150 mg
▷ *doxepin* (C)(G) 75 mg/day; max 150 mg/day
  Pediatric: <12 years: not recommended; ≥12 years: same as adult
    Cap: 10, 25, 50, 75, 100, 150 mg; Oral conc: 10 mg/ml (4 oz w. dropper)
▷ *imipramine* (C)(G)
  Pediatric: <12 years: not recommended; ≥12 years: same as adult
    Tofranil initially 75 mg daily (max 200 mg); adolescents initially 30-40 mg daily (max 100 mg/day); if maintenance dose exceeds 75 mg daily, may switch to **Tofranil PM** for divided or bedtime dose
      Tab: 10, 25, 50 mg
    Tofranil PM initially 75 mg daily 1 hour before HS; max 200 mg
      Cap: 75, 100, 125, 150 mg
    Tofranil Injection 50 mg IM; lower dose for adolescents; switch to oral form as soon as possible
      Amp: 25 mg/2 ml (2 ml)
▷ *nortriptyline* (D)(G) initially 25 mg tid-qid; max 150 mg/day
  Pediatric: <12 years: not recommended; ≥12 years: same as adult
    Pamelor *Cap:* 10, 25, 50, 75 mg; *Oral soln:* 10 mg/5 ml (16 oz)
▷ *protriptyline* (C) initially 5 mg tid; usual dose 15-40 mg/day in 3-4 divided doses; max 60 mg/day
  Pediatric: <12 years: not recommended; ≥12 years: same as adult
    Vivactil *Tab:* 5, 10 mg
▷ *trimipramine* (C) initially 75 mg/day in divided doses; max 200 mg/day
  Pediatric: <12 years: not recommended; ≥12 years: same as adult
    Surmontil *Cap:* 25, 50, 100 mg

ALPHA-2 DELTA LIGAND

▷*pregabalin (GABA analog)* (C)(G)(V) initially 150 mg daily divided bid-tid and may titrate within one week; max 600 mg divided bid-tid; discontinue over one week
  Pediatric: <18 years: not recommended; ≥18 years: same as adult
    Lyrica *Cap:* 25, 50, 75, 100, 150, 200, 225, 300 mg; *Oral soln:* 20 mg/ml

TOPICAL AND TRANSDERMAL ANALGESICS

▷ *capsaicin* 8% patch (B) apply up to 4 patches for one 60-minute application to clean dry skin; may prep area with topical anesthetic; wear non-latex gloves; patches may be cut to size/shape; treatment may be repeated every 3 months
  Pediatric: <18 years: not recommended; ≥18 years: same as adult
    Qutenza *Patch:* 8% 1640 mcg/cm (179 mg) (1 or 2 patches w. 1-50 gm tube cleansing gel/carton)
▷ *diclofenac sodium* (C; D ≥30 wks) apply qid prn to intact skin
  Pediatric: <12 years: not established; ≥12 years: same as adult
    Pennsaid 1.5% in 10 drop increments, dispense and rub into front, side, and back of knee: usually; 40 drops (40 mg) qid
      Topical soln: 1.5% (150 ml)
    Pennsaid 2% apply 2 pump actuations (40 mg) and rub into front, side, and back of knee bid

> *Topical soln:* 2% (20 mg/pump actuation, 112 gm)
> **Solaraze Gel** massage in to clean skin bid prn
> *Gel:* 3% (50 gm) (benzyl alcohol)
> **Voltaren Gel (G)(OTC)** apply qid prn to intact skin
> *Gel:* 1% (100 gm)

Comment: *Diclofenac* is contraindicated with *aspirin* allergy. As with other NSAIDs, should be avoided in late pregnancy (≥30 weeks) because it may cause premature closure of the ductus arteriosus.

> *doxepin* (B) cream apply to affected area qid at intervals of at least 3-4 hours; max 8 days
> *Pediatric:* <12 years: not recommended; >12 years: same as adult
> **Prudoxin** *Crm:* 5% (45 gm)
> **Zonalon** *Crm:* 5% (30, 45 gm)

> *pimecrolimus* 1% cream (C)(G) <2 years: not recommended; ≥2 years: apply to affected area bid; do not apply an occlusive dressing
> **Elidel** *Crm:* 1% (30, 60, 100 gm)

Comment: *Pimecrolimus* is indicated for short-term and intermittent long-term use. Discontinue use when resolution occurs. Contraindicated if the patient is immunosuppressed. Change to the 0.1% preparation or if secondary bacterial infection is present.

> *trolamine salicylate* apply tid-qid
> *Pediatric:* <2 years: not recommended; ≥2 years: same as adult
> **Mobisyl Creme** *Crm:* 10% (100 gm)

TOPICAL & TRANSDERMAL ANESTHETICS

Comment: *Lidocaine* should not be applied to non-intact skin.

> *lidocaine* cream (B) apply to affected area bid prn
> *Pediatric:* <12 years: not recommended; ≥12 years: same as adult
> **LidaMantle** *Crm:* 3% (1, 2 oz)
> **Lidoderm** *Crm:* 3% (85 gm)
> **ZTlido** *lidocaine* topical system 1% (30/carton)
> Comment: Compared to **Lidoderm** (*lidocaine* patch 5%), which contains 700 mg/patch, **ZTlido** requires 35 mg per topical system to achieve the same therapeutic dose.

> *lidocaine* lotion (B) apply to affected area bid prn
> *Pediatric:* <12 years: not recommended; ≥12 years: same as adult
> **LidaMantle** *Lotn:* 3% (177 ml)

> *lidocaine* 5% patch (B)(G) apply up to 3 patches at one time for up to 12 hours/24-hour period (12 hours on/12 hours off); patches may be cut into smaller sizes before removal of the release liner; do not re-use
> *Pediatric:* <12 years: not recommended; ≥12 years: same as adult
> **Lidoderm** *Patch:* 5% (10x14 cm; 30/carton)
> *lidocaine+dexamethasone* (B)
> *Pediatric:* <12 years: not recommended; ≥12 years: same as adult
> **Decadron Phosphate with Xylocaine** *Lotn:* dexa 4 mg+lido 10 mg per ml (5 ml)

> *lidocaine+hydrocortisone* (B)(G) apply to affected area bid prn
> *Pediatric:* <12 years: not recommended; ≥12 years: same as adult
> **LidaMantle HC** *Crm:* lido 3%+hydro 0.5% (1, 3 oz); *Lotn:* (177 ml)

> *lidocaine* 2.5%+*prilocaine* 2.5% apply sparingly to the burn bid-tid prn
> *Pediatric:* <12 years: not recommended; ≥12 years: same as adult
> **Emla Cream** (B) 5, 30 gm/tube

ORAL ANALGESICS

> *acetaminophen* (B)(G) *see Fever*

▷ *aspirin* (D)(G) *see Fever*
▷ *tramadol* (C)(IV)(G)

    Rybix ODT initially 100 mg once daily; may increase by 100 mg every 5 days; max 300 mg/day; *CrCl <30 mL/min* or *severe hepatic impairment:* not recommended; *Cirrhosis:* max 50 mg q 12 hours
    Pediatric: <18 years: not recommended; ≥18 years: same as adult
      ODT: 50 mg (mint) (phenylalanine)
    Ryzolt initially 100 mg once daily; may increase by 100 mg every 5 days; max 300 mg/day; *CrCl <30 mL/min* or *severe hepatic impairment:* not recommended
    Pediatric: <18 years: not recommended; ≥18 years: same as adult
      Tab: 100, 200, 300 mg ext-rel
    Ultram 50-100 mg q 4-6 hours prn; max 400 mg/day; *CrCl <30 mL/min:* max 100 mg q 12 hours; *Cirrhosis:* max 50 mg q 12 hours
    Pediatric: <18 years: not recommended; ≥18 years: same as adult
      Tab: 50*mg
    Ultram ER initially 100 mg once daily; may increase by 100 mg every 5 days; max 300 mg/day; *CrCl <30 mL/min:* or *severe hepatic impairment:* not recommended
    Pediatric: <18 years: not recommended; ≥18 years: same as adult
      Tab: 100, 200, 300 mg ext-rel

▷ *tramadol+acetaminophen* (C)(IV)(G) 2 tabs q 4-6 hours; max 8 tabs/day; 5 days; *CrCl <30 mL/min:* max 2 tabs q 12 hours; max 4 tabs/day x 5 days
    Pediatric: <18 years: not recommended; ≥18 years: same as adult
    Ultracet *Tab:* tram 37.5+acet 325 mg

TRICYCLIC ANTIDEPRESSANTS (TCAs)

Comment: Co-administration of TCAs with SSRIs requires extreme caution.

▷ *amitriptyline* (C)(G) titrate to achieve pain relief; max 300 mg/day
    Pediatric: <12 years: not recommended; ≥12 years: same as adult
    Tab: 10, 25, 50, 75, 100, 150 mg
▷ *amoxapine* (C) titrate to achieve pain relief; if total dose exceeds 300 mg/day, give in divided doses; max 400 mg/day
    Pediatric: <12 years: not recommended; ≥12 years: same as adult
    Tab: 25, 50, 100, 150 mg
▷ *desipramine* (C)(G) titrate to achieve pain relief; max 300 mg/day
    Pediatric: <12 years: not recommended; ≥12 years: same as adult
    Norpramin *Tab:* 10, 25, 50, 75, 100, 150 mg
▷ *doxepin* (C)(G) titrate to achieve pain relief; max 150 mg/day
    Pediatric: <12 years: not recommended; ≥12 years: same as adult
    Cap: 10, 25, 50, 75, 100, 150 mg; *Oral conc:* 10 mg/ml (4 oz w. dropper)
▷ *imipramine* (C)(G)
    Pediatric: <12 years: not recommended; ≥12 years: same as adult
    Tofranil titrate to achieve pain relief; max 200 mg/day; adolescents max 100 mg/day; if maintenance dose exceeds 75 mg/day, may switch to **Tofranil PM** at bedtime
      Tab: 10, 25, 50 mg
    Tofranil PM titrate to achieve pain relief; initially 75 mg at HS; max 200 mg at HS
      Cap: 75, 100, 125, 150 mg
    Tofranil Injection 50 mg IM; lower dose for adolescents; switch to oral form as soon as possible
      Amp: 25 mg/2 ml (2 ml)
▷ *nortriptyline* (D)(G) titrate to achieve pain relief; initially 10-25 mg tid-qid; max 150 mg/day; lower doses for elderly and adolescents
    Pediatric: <12 years: not recommended; ≥12 years: same as adult
    Pamelor titrate to achieve pain relief; max 150 mg/day
      Cap: 10, 25, 50, 75 mg; *Oral soln:* 10 mg/5 ml (16 oz)

▷ *protriptyline* (C) titrate to achieve pain relief; initially 5 mg tid; max 60 mg/day
   Pediatric: <12 years: not recommended; ≥12 years: same as adult
      Vivactil *Tab:* 5, 10 mg
▷ *trimipramine* (C) titrate to achieve pain relief; max 200 mg/day
   Pediatric: <12 years: not recommended; ≥12 years: same as adult
      Surmontil *Cap:* 25, 50, 100 mg

POST-TRAUMATIC STRESS DISORDER (PTSD)

Comment: No one pharmacological agent has emerged as the best treatment for PTSD. A combination of pharmacological agents (e.g., antidepressants, non-adrenergic agents, antipsychosis drugs) may comprise an individualized treatment plan to successfully manage core symptoms of PTSD, as well as associated anxiety, depression, sleep disturbances, and co-occurring psychiatric disorders.

SELECTIVE SEROTONIN REUPTAKE INHIBITORS (SSRIs)

Comment: The FDA has approved two SSRIs for the treatment of PTSD: *paroxetine* and *sertraline*. However, the safety and efficacy of other SSRIs (*fluoxetine, citalopram, escitalopram, fluvoxamine*) have been tested in clinical practice. Co-administration of SSRIs with TCAs requires extreme caution. Concomitant use of MAOIs and SSRIs is absolutely contraindicated. Avoid St. John's wort and other serotonergic agents. A potentially fatal adverse event is *serotonin syndrome*, caused by serotonin excess. Milder symptoms require HCP intervention to avert severe symptoms which can be rapidly fatal without urgent/emergent medical care. Symptoms include restlessness, agitation, confusion, hallucinations, tachycardia, hypertension, dilated pupils, muscle twitching, muscle rigidity, loss of muscle coordination, diaphoresis, diarrhea, headache, shivering, piloerection, hyperpyrexia, cardiac arrhythmias, seizures, loss of consciousness, coma, death. Abrupt withdrawal or interruption of treatment with an antidepressant medication is sometimes associated with an *Antidepressant Discontinuation Syndrome* which may be mediated by gradually tapering the drug over a period of two weeks or longer, depending on the dose strength and length of treatment. Common symptoms of the *serotonin discontinuation syndrome* include flu-like symptoms (nausea, vomiting, diarrhea, headaches, sweating), sleep disturbances (insomnia, nightmares, constant sleepiness), mood disturbances (dysphoria, anxiety, agitation), cognitive disturbances (mental confusion, hyperarousal) sensory and movement disturbances (imbalance, tremors, vertigo, dizziness, electric-shock-like sensations in the brain, often described by sufferers as "brain zaps").

▷ *paroxetine maleate* (D)(G)
   Pediatric: <12 years: not recommended; ≥12 years: same as adult
      Paxil initially 20 mg daily in AM; may increase by 10 mg/day at weekly intervals as needed; max 60 mg/day
         Tab: 10*, 20*, 30, 40 mg
      Paxil CR initially 25 mg daily in AM; may increase by 12.5 mg at weekly intervals as needed; max 62.5 mg/day
         Tab: 12.5, 25, 37.5 mg cont-rel ent-coat
      Paxil Suspension initially 20 mg daily in AM; may increase by 10 mg/day at weekly intervals as needed; max 60 mg/day
         Oral susp: 10 mg/5 ml (250 ml; orange)
▷ *paroxetine mesylate* (D)(G) initially 7.5 mg daily in AM; may increase by 10 mg/day at weekly intervals as needed; max 60 mg/day
   Pediatric: <12 years: not recommended; ≥12 years: same as adult
      Brisdelle *Cap:* 7.5 mg

▶ *sertraline* (C) initially 50 mg daily; increase at 1 week intervals if needed; max 200 mg daily
Pediatric: <6 years: not recommended; 6-12 years: initially 25 mg daily; max 200 mg/day; 13-17 years: initially 50 mg daily; max 200 mg/day; ≥17 years: same as adult
   Zoloft *Tab:* 15*, 50*, 100*mg; *Oral conc:* 20 mg per ml (60 ml [dilute just before administering in 4 oz water, ginger ale, lemon-lime soda, lemonade, or orange juice]) (alcohol 12%)

ATYPICAL ANTIPSYCHOSIS DRUGS

▶ *olanzapine* (C)(G) initially 2.5-5 mg once daily at HS; increase by 5 mg every week to 20 mg at HS; usual maintenance 10-20 mg/day
   Zyprexa *Tab:* 2.5, 5, 7.5, 10, 15, 20 mg
   Zyprexa Zydis *ODT:* 5, 10, 15, 20 mg (phenylalanine)
▶ *quetiapine* (C)(G) initially 25 mg bid; increase total daily dose by 50 mg, as needed and tolerated, to max 300-600 mg/day
   Seroquel *Tab:* 25, 100, 200, 300 mg
   Seroquel XR *Tab:* 50, 150, 200, 300, 400 mg ext-rel
▶ *risperidone* (C)(G) initially 0.5-1 mg bid; titrate to 3 mg bid by the end of the first week; usual maintenance 4-6 mg/day
   Risperdal *Tab:* 0.25, 0.5, 1, 2, 3, 4 mg; *Soln:* 1 mg/ml (30 ml w. pipette); *Consta* (*Inj*): 25, 37.5, 50 mg
   Risperdal M-Tabs *M-tab:* 0.5, 1, 2, 3, 4 mg orally-disint (phenylalanine)

NON-ADRENERGIC AGENTS
ALPHA-1 ANTAGONISTS

Comment: *Prazosin* is useful in reducing combat-trauma nightmares, normalizing dreams for combat veterans, and mediating other sleep disturbances.
▶ *prazosin* (C)(G) first dose at HS, 1 mg bid-tid; increase dose slowly; usual range 6-15 mg/day in divided doses; max 20-40 mg/day
Pediatric: <12 years: not recommended; ≥12 years: same as adult
   Minipress *Cap:* 1, 2, 5 mg

CENTRAL ALPHA-2 AGONISTS

Comment: *Clonidine* is useful to reduce nightmares, hypervigilance, startle reactions, and outbursts of rage.
▶ *clonidine* (C)
Pediatric: <12 years: not recommended; ≥12 years: same as adult
   Catapres initially 0.1 mg bid; usual range 0.2-0.6 mg/day in divided doses; max 2.4 mg/day *Tab:* 0.1*, 0.2*, 0.3*mg
   Catapres-TTS initially 0.1 mg patch weekly; increase after 1-2 weeks if needed; max 0.6 mg/day
      Patch: 0.1, 0.2 mg/day (12/carton); 0.3 mg/day (4/carton)
   Kapvay (G) initially 0.1 mg bid; usual range 0.2-0.6 mg/day in divided doses; max 2.4 mg/day *Tab:* 0.1, 0.2 mg
   Nexiclon XR initially 0.18 mg (2 ml) suspension or 0.17 mg tab once daily; usual max 0.52 mg (6 ml suspension) once daily
      Tab: 0.17, 0.26 mg ext-rel; *Oral susp:* 0.09 mg/ml ext-rel (4 oz)

BETA-ADRENERGIC BLOCKER (NON-CARDIOSELECTIVE)

Comment: *Propranolol* is useful to mediate hyperarousal. For other non-cardioselective beta-adrenergic blockers, *see* **Hypertension**
▶ *propranolol* (C)(G) 40-240 mg daily
Pediatric: <12 years: not recommended; ≥12 years: same as adult

Inderal *Tab:* 10*, 20*, 40*, 60*, 80*mg
Inderal LA initially 80 mg daily in a single dose; increase q 3-7 days; usual range 120-160 mg/day; max 320 mg/day in a single dose

SEROTONIN-NOREPINEPHRINE REUPTAKE INHIBITORS (SNRIs)

▷ *desvenlafaxine* (C)(G) swallow whole; initially 50 mg once daily; max 120 mg/day
  Pediatric: <12 years: not recommended; ≥12 years: same as adult
  Pristiq *Tab:* 50, 100 mg ext-rel
▷ *duloxetine* (C)(G) swallow whole; initially 30 mg once daily x 1 week; then increase to 60 mg once daily; max 120 mg/day
  Pediatric: <12 years: not recommended; ≥12 years: same as adult
  Cymbalta *Cap:* 20, 30, 40, 60 mg del-rel
▷ *venlafaxine* (C)(G)
  Effexor initially 75 mg/day in 2-3 divided doses; may increase at 4-day intervals in 75 mg increments to 150 mg/day; max 225 mg/day
  Pediatric: <18 years: not recommended; ≥18 years: same as adult
  Tab: 37.5, 75, 150, 225 mg
  Effexor XR initially 75 mg q AM; may start at 37.5 mg daily x 4-7 days, then increase by increments of up to 75 mg/day at intervals of at least 4 days; usual max 375 mg/day
  Pediatric: <18 years: not recommended; ≥18 years: same as adult
  Tab/Cap: 37.5, 75, 150 mg ext-rel

5HT2/3 RECEPTOR BLOCKERS

▷ *mirtazapine* (C) initially 15 mg q HS; increase at intervals of 1-2 weeks; 1-2 weeks; usual range 15-60 mg/day; max 60 mg/day
  Pediatric: <12 years: not recommended; ≥12 years: same as adult
  Remeron *Tab:* 15*, 30*, 45*mg
  Remeron SolTab *ODT:* 15, 30, 45 mg (orange) (phenylalanine)

SERTONIN+ACETYLCHOLINE+NOREPINEPHRINE+DOPAMINE BLOCKER

▷ *trazodone* (C)(G) initially 150 mg/day in divided doses with food; increase by 50 mg/day q 3-4 days; max 400 mg/day in divided doses or 50-400 mg at HS
  Pediatric: <18 years: not recommended; ≥18 years: same as adult
  Oleptro *Tab:* 50, 100*, 150*, 200, 250, 300 mg

TRICYCLIC ANTIDEPRESSANTS (TCAs)

▷ *amitriptyline* (C)(G) 10-20 mg at HS
  Pediatric: <12 years: not recommended; ≥12 years: same as adult
  Tab: 10, 25, 50, 75, 100, 150 mg
▷ *doxepin* (C)(G) 10-200 mg at HS
  Pediatric: <12 years: not recommended; ≥12 years: same as adult
  Cap: 10, 25, 50, 75, 100, 150 mg; *Oral conc:* 10 mg/ml (4 oz w. dropper)
▷ *imipramine* (C)(G) 10-200 mg q HS
  Tofranil 100-300 mg at HS or divided bid or tid
  Pediatric: <6 years: not recommended; 6-12 years: initially 25 mg; >12 years: 50 mg max 2.5 mg/kg/day
  Tab: 10, 25, 50 mg
  Tofranil PM initially 75 mg daily 1 hour before HS; max 200 mg
  Pediatric: <12 years: not recommended; ≥12 years: same as adult
  Cap: 75, 100, 125, 150 mg
  Tofranil Injection 50 mg IM; lower dose for adolescents; switch to oral form as soon as possible
  Amp: 25 mg/2 ml (2 ml)

▷ *nortriptyline* (D)(G) 10-150 mg q HS
  Pediatric: <12 years: not recommended; ≥12 years: same as adult
    Pamelor *Cap:* 10, 25, 50, 75 mg; *Oral soln:* 10 mg/5 ml

MONOAMINE OXIDASE INHIBITORS (MAOIs)

Comment: Many drug and food interactions with this class of drugs, use cautiously. MAOIs should be reserved for refractory depression that has not responded to other classes of antidepressants. Concomitant use of MAOIs and SSRIs is contraindicated. See mfr pkg insert for drug and food interactions. MAOIs have been used to reduce recurrent recollections of the trauma, nightmares, flashbacks, numbing, sleep disturbances, and social withdrawal in PTSD.

▷ *phenelzine* (C)(G) initially 15 mg tid; max 90 mg/day
  Pediatric: <16 years: not recommended; ≥16 years: same as adult
    Nardil *Tab:* 15 mg

▷ *selegiline* (C) initially 10 mg tid; max 60 mg/day
  Pediatric: <12 years: not recommended; ≥12 years: same as adult
    Emsam *Transdermal patch:* 6 mg/24 hrs, 9 mg/24 hrs, 12 mg/24 hrs
    Comment: At the **Emsam** transdermal patch 6 mg/24 hrs dose, the dietary restrictions commonly required when using nonselective MAOIs are not necessary.

PRECOCIOUS PUBERTY, CENTRAL (CPP)

Comment: GnRH-dependent CPP is defined by pubertal development occurring before the age of 8 years in girls and 9 years in boys. It is characterized by early pubertal changes such as breast development and start of menses in girls and increased testicular and penile growth in boys, appearance of pubic hair, as well as acceleration of growth velocity and bone maturation and tall stature during childhood, which often results in reduced adult height due to premature fusion of the growth plates.

GONADOTROPIN RELEASING HORMONE (GnRH) AGONIST

▷ *leuprolide acetate*
  Pediatric: <2 years: safety and efficacy not established; ≥2 years: 45 mg SC once every 6 months in the abdomen, upper buttocks, or another location with adequate amounts of subcutaneous tissue that does not have excessive pigment, nodules, lesions, or hair; avoid areas with brawny or fibrous subcutaneous tissue or locations that could be rubbed or compressed (e.g., by a belt or clothing waistband); rotate sites; refrigerate the kit; if the kit remains sealed, may remain at room temperature for up to 8 weeks; allow to reach room temperature before reconstitution; administer within 30 minutes of reconstitution or discard; must be administered by a qualified healthcare professional
    Fensolvi *Administration kit:* 45 mg/pwdr (prefilled syringe) for reconstitution w. diluent (prefilled syringe), single-dose
    Comment: **Fensolvi** *(leuprolide acetate)* is a gonadotropin releasing hormone (GnRH) agonist indicated for the treatment of pediatric patients 2 years of age and older with central precocious puberty. Monitor response to **Fensolvi** with a GnRH agonist stimulation test, basal serum luteinizing hormone (LH) levels or serum concentration of sex steroid levels at 1 to 2 months following initiation of therapy and as needed to confirm adequate suppression of pituitary gonadotropins, sex steroids, and progression of secondary sexual characteristics. Measure height every 3-6 months and monitor bone age periodically. The most common adverse reactions (incidence ≥5%) have been injection site pain, nasopharyngitis, pyrexia, headache, cough,

abdominal pain, injection site erythema, nausea, constipation, vomiting, upper respiratory tract infection, bronchospasm, productive cough, and hot flush. Initial rise of gonadotropins and sex steroid levels are expected during the early phase of therapy because of the initial stimulatory effect of the drug. Therefore, an increase in clinical signs and symptoms of puberty, including vaginal bleeding, may be observed during the first weeks of therapy or after subsequent doses. Instruct patients and caregivers to notify the healthcare provider if these symptoms continue beyond the second month after **Fensolvi** administration. Psychiatric events have been reported in patients taking GnRH agonists including emotional lability, such as crying, irritability, impatience, anger, and aggression. Monitor for development or worsening of psychiatric symptoms. Convulsions have been observed in patients with or without a history of seizures, epilepsy, cerebrovascular disorder, central nervous system anomalies or tumors, and in patients on concomitant medications that have been associated with convulsions. Non-compliance with drug regimen or inadequate dosing may lead to gonadotropins and/or sex steroids increasing above prepubertal levels resulting in inadequate control of the pubertal process. If the dose of **Fensolvi** is not adequate, switching to an alternative GnRH agonist for the treatment of CPP with the ability for dose adjustment may be necessary. Discontinue **Fensolvi** treatment at the appropriate age of onset of puberty. Anaphylactic reactions to synthetic GnRH or GnRH agonists have been reported. **Fensolvi** is contraindicated in pregnancy; may cause embryo/fetal harm. Exclude pregnancy in females of reproductive potential prior to initiating **Fensolvi** if clinically indicated. Fensolvi is not a contraceptive. If contraception is indicated, advise females of reproductive potential to use a non-hormonal method of contraception during treatment. Based on its pharmacodynamic effects of decreasing secretion of gonadal steroids, fertility is expected to be decreased while on treatment with **Fensolvi**. Clinical and pharmacologic studies in adults (>18 years) with *leuprolide acetate* and similar analogs have shown reversibility of fertility suppression when the drug is discontinued after continuous administration for periods of up to 24 weeks. There are no data on the presence of *leuprolide acetate* in either animal or human milk or effects on the breastfed infant. Developmental and health benefits of breastfeeding should be considered along with the mother's clinical need for **Fensolvi** and any potential adverse effects on the breastfed infant from **Fensolvi** or from the underlying maternal condition.

▷ *triptorelin* (X)
Pediatric: <2 years: not recommended; ≥2 years: administer as a single 22.5 mg IM injection once every 24 weeks; must be administered under the supervision of a physician; monitor response with LH levels after a GnRH or GnRH agonist stimulation test, basal LH, or serum concentration of sex steroid levels beginning 1-2 months following initiation of therapy, during therapy as necessary to confirm maintenance of efficacy, and with each subsequent dose; measure height every 3-6 months and monitor bone age periodically; see mfr pkg insert for reconstitution and administration instructions

Triptodur Single-use kit: 1 single-dose vial of **triptorelin** 22.5 mg w. Flip-Off seal containing sterile lyophilized white to slightly yellow powder cake, 1 sterile, glass syringe prefilled with 2 ml of sterile water for injection, 2 sterile 21 gauge, 1½" needles (thin-wall) with safety cover

Comment: Triptodur is contraindicated in females who are pregnant since expected hormonal changes that occur with *triptorelin* treatment increase the risk for pregnancy loss. Available data with *triptorelin* use in pregnant females are insufficient to determine a drug-associated risk of adverse developmental outcomes. Based on mechanism of action in humans and findings of increased pregnancy loss in animal studies, *triptorelin* may cause fetal harm when administered to pregnant females. Advise pregnant females of the potential risk to a fetus. The estimated background risk of major birth defects and miscarriage is unknown. There are no data on the presence of *triptorelin* in human milk or the effects of the drug on the breastfed infant. The developmental and health benefits of breastfeeding should be considered along with the mother's clinical need for *triptorelin* and any potential adverse effects on the breastfed infant from *triptorelin* or from the underlying maternal condition. During the early phase of therapy, gonadotropins and sex steroids rise above baseline because of the initial stimulatory effect of the drug. Therefore, a transient increase in clinical signs and symptoms of puberty, including vaginal bleeding, may be observed during the first weeks of therapy. Post-marketing reports with this class of drugs include symptoms of emotional lability, such as crying, irritability, impatience, anger, and aggression. Monitor for development or worsening of psychiatric symptoms during treatment with **Triptodur**. Postmarketing reports of convulsions have been observed in patients receiving GnRH agonists, including *triptorelin.* These included patients with a history of seizures, epilepsy, cerebrovascular disorders, central nervous system anomalies or tumors, and patients on concomitant medications that have been associated with convulsions such as bupropion and SSRIs. Convulsions have also been reported in patients in the absence of any of the conditions mentioned above.

 PREGNANCY

See **Prescription Prenatal Vitamins**
Comment: Prenatal vitamins should have at least 400 mcg of folic acid content. Take one dose once daily. It is recommended that prenatal vitamins be started at least 3 months prior to conception to improve preconception nutritional status, and continued throughout pregnancy and the postnatal period, in lactating and nonlactating women, and throughout the childbearing years.

NAUSEA/VOMITING

▷ *doxyalamine succinate+pyridoxine* (A)(G) do not crush or chew; take on an empty stomach with water; initially 2 tabs at HS on day 1; may increase to 1 tab AM and 2 tabs at HS day 2; may increase to 1 tab AM, 1 tab mid-afternoon, 2 tabs at HS; max 4 tabs/day
  Diclegis *Tab:* doxyl 10 mg+pyri 10 mg del-rel
  Comment: **Diclegis** is the only FDA-approved drug for the treatment of morning sickness. It has not been studied in women with hyperemesis gravidarum.
▷ *promethazine* (C)(G) 12.5-50 mg PO/IM/rectally q 4-6 hours prn
  Phenergan *Tab:* 12.5*, 25*, 50 mg; *Plain syr:* 6.25 mg/5 ml; *Fortis syr:* 25 mg/5 ml; *Rectal supp:* 12.5, 25, 50 mg; *Amp:* 25, 50 mg/ml (1 ml)
  Comment: *Promethazine* is contraindicated in children with uncomplicated nausea, dehydration, Reye's syndrome, history of sleep apnea, asthma, and lower respiratory disorders in children. *promethazine* lowers the seizure threshold in children, may cause cholestatic jaundice, anticholinergic effects, extrapyramidal effects, and potentially fatal respiratory depression.

 PREMENSTRUAL DYSPHORIC DISORDER (PMDD)

NSAIDs *see* Appendix J. NSAIDs online at https://connect.springerpub.com/content/reference-book/978-0-8261-7935-7/back-matter/part02/back-matter/bmatter10
Opioid Analgesics *see* **Pain**
Oral Contraceptives *see* Appendix H. Contraceptives

ORAL ESTROGEN+PROGESTERONE COMBINATIONS

Comment: Rajani (a generic form of **Beyaz**) and **Yaz**; also available in generic Forms (**Gianvi, Ocella, Syeda, Vestura, Yasmin, Zarah**) have an FDA indication for treatment of PMDD in females who choose to use an OCP. Contraindicated with renal and adrenal insufficiency. Monitor K⁺ level during the first cycle if the patient is at risk for hyperkalemia for any reason. If the patient is taking a drug that increase serum potassium (e.g., ACEIs, ARBS, NSAIDs, K⁺ sparing diuretics), the patient is at risk for hyperkalemia.

➤ *ethinyl estradiol+drospirenone* (X)(G) Pre-menarchal: not indicated; Post-menarchal: 1 tab once daily x 28 days; repeat cycle; start on first Sunday after menses begins or on first day of next menses

    Yaz *Tab:* ethin estra 20 mcg+drospir 3 mg

➤ *ethinyl+estradiol+drospirenone+levomefolate calcium* (X)(G) Pre-menarchal: not indicated; Post-menarchal: 1 tab once daily x 28 days; repeat cycle; start on first Sunday after menses begins or on first day of next menses preceded by a negative pregnancy test

    Beyaz *Tab:* ethin estra 20 mcg+drospir 3 mg+levo 0.451 mg

    Rajani *Tab:* ethin estra 20 mcg+drospir 3 mg+levo 0.451 mg

DIURETICS

➤ *spironolactone* (D)(G) initially 50-100 mg once daily or in divided doses; titrate at 2-week intervals

Pediatric: <12 years: not recommended; ≥12 years: same as adult

    Aldactone *Tab:* 25, 50*, 100*mg

ANTIDEPRESSANTS

➤ *fluoxetine* (C)(G)

    Prozac initially 20 mg daily; may increase after 1 week; doses >20 mg/day should be divided into AM and noon doses; max 80 mg/day

    Pediatric: <8 years: not recommended; 8-17 years: initially 10 or 20 mg/ day; start lower weight children at 10 mg/day; if starting at 10 mg/day, may increase after 1 week to 20 mg/day; ≥17 years: same as adult

      Tab: 10*mg; *Cap:* 10, 20, 40 mg; *Oral soln:* 20 mg/5 ml (4 oz) (mint)

    Prozac Weekly following daily *fluoxetine* therapy at 20 mg/day for 13 weeks, may initiate **Prozac Weekly** 7 days after the last 20 mg *fluoxetine* dose

    Pediatric: <12 years: not recommended; ≥12 years: same as adult

      Cap: 90 mg ent-coat del-rel pellets

    Sarafem administer daily or 14 days before expected menses and through first full day of menses; initially 20 mg/day; max 80 mg/day

    Pediatric: <8 years: not recommended; 8-17 years: initially 10 or 20 mg/ day; start lower weight children at 10 mg/day; if starting at 10 mg/day, may increase after 1 week to 20 mg/day

      Tab: 10, 15, 20 mg; *Cap:* 20 mg

➤ *paroxetine maleate* (D)(G)

    Pediatric: <12 years: not recommended; ≥12 years: same as adult

    Paxil initially 20 mg daily in AM; may increase by 10 mg/day at weekly intervals as needed; max 60 mg/day

      Tab: 10*, 20*, 30, 40 mg

    Paxil CR initially 25 mg daily in AM; may increase by 12.5 mg at weekly intervals as needed; max 62.5 mg/day; may start 14 days before and continue through day one of menses

      Tab: 12.5, 25, 37.5 mg cont-rel ent-coat

Paxil Suspension initially 20 mg daily in AM; may increase by 10 mg/day at weekly intervals as needed; max 60 mg/day
  Oral susp: 10 mg/5 ml (250 ml) (orange)
▷ *paroxetine mesylate* (D)(G) initially 7.5 mg daily in AM; may increase by 10 mg/day at weekly intervals as needed; max 60 mg/day
  Pediatric: <12 years: not recommended; ≥12 years: same as adult
    Brisdelle *Cap:* 7.5 mg
▷ *sertraline* (C)
    For 2 weeks prior to onset of menses: initially 50 mg daily x 3; then increase to 100 mg daily for remainder of the cycle; *For full cycle:* initially 50 mg daily; then may increase by 50 mg/day each cycle to max 150 mg/day
    Pediatric: <12 years: not recommended; ≥12 years: same as adult
    Zoloft *Tab:* 25*, 50*, 100*mg; *Oral conc:* 20 mg per ml (60 ml) (alcohol 12%); dilute just before administering in 4 oz water, ginger ale, lemon-lime soda, lemonade, or orange juice
▷ *nortriptyline* (D)(G) initially 25 mg tid-qid; max 150 mg/day
    Pediatric: <12 years: not recommended; ≥12 years: same as adult
    Pamelor *Cap:* 10, 25, 50, 75 mg; *Oral soln:* 10 mg/5 ml

CALCIUM SUPPLEMENTS

▷ *calcium* (C) 1200 mg/day
see Osteoporosis

 PROCTITIS: ACUTE (PROCTOCOLITIS, ENTERITIS)

Comment: The following regimen for the treatment of proctitis, proctocolitis, and enteritis is published in the **2015 CDC Sexually Transmitted Diseases Treatment Guidelines.**

RECOMMENDED REGIMEN

▷ *ceftriaxone* (B)(G) 250 mg IM in a single dose
    Rocephin *Vial:* 250, 500 mg; 1, 2 gm
      plus
▷ *doxycycline* 100 mg bid x 7 days
    Acticlate *Tab:* 75, 150**mg
    Adoxa *Tab:* 50, 75, 100, 150 mg ent-coat
    Doryx *Tab:* 50, 75, 100, 150, 200 mg del-rel
    Doxteric *Tab:* 50 mg del-rel
    Monodox *Cap:* 50, 75, 100 mg
    Oracea *Cap:* 40 mg del-rel
    Vibramycin *Tab:* 100 mg; *Cap:* 50, 100 mg; *Syr:* 50 mg/5 ml (raspberry-apple) (sulfites); *Oral susp:* 25 mg/5 ml (raspberry)
    Vibra-Tab *Tab:* 100 mg film-coat

 PROSTATITIS: ACUTE

ANTI-INFECTIVES

▷ *ciprofloxacin* (C) 500 mg bid x 4-6 weeks
    Pediatric: <18 years: not recommended; ≥18 years: same as adult
    Cipro (G) *Tab:* 250, 500, 750 mg; *Oral susp:* 250, 500 mg/5 ml (100 ml) (strawberry)
    Cipro XR *Tab:* 500, 1000 mg ext-rel
    ProQuin XR *Tab:* 500 mg ext-rel
▷ *norfloxacin* (C) 400 mg bid x 28 days
    Pediatric: <18 years: not recommended; ≥18 years: same as adult
    Noroxin *Tab:* 400 mg

▷ *ofloxacin* (C)(G) 300 mg x bid x 6 weeks
   Pediatric: <18 years: not recommended; ≥18 years: same as adult
     Floxin *Tab:* 200, 300, 400 mg
▷ *trimethoprim+sulfamethoxazole (TMP-SMX)* (C)(G)
   Pediatric: <12 years: not recommended; ≥12 years: same as adult
     Bactrim, Septra 2 tabs bid x 10 days
      Tab: trim 80 mg+sulfa 400 mg*
     Bactrim DS, Septra DS 1 tab bid x 10 days
      Tab: trim 160 mg+sulfa 800 mg*
     Bactrim Pediatric Suspension, Septra Pediatric Suspension
      Oral susp: trim 40 mg+sulfa 200 mg per 5 ml (100 ml) (cherry) (alcohol 0.3%)

PROSTATITIS: CHRONIC

ANTI-INFECTIVES

▷ *carbenicillin* (B) 2 tabs qid x 4-12 weeks
     Geocillin *Tab:* 382 mg
▷ *ciprofloxacin* (C) 500 mg bid x 3 or more months
   Pediatric: <18 years: not recommended; ≥18 years: same as adult
     Cipro (G) *Tab:* 250, 500, 750 mg; *Oral susp:* 250, 500 mg/5 ml (100 ml) (strawberry)
     Cipro XR *Tab:* 500, 1000 mg ext-rel
     ProQuin XR *Tab:* 500 mg ext-rel
▷ *norfloxacin* (C) 400 mg bid x 4-12 weeks
   Pediatric: <18 years: not recommended; ≥18 years: same as adult
     Noroxin *Tab:* 400 mg
▷ *ofloxacin* (C)(G) 300 mg bid x 4-12 weeks
   Pediatric: <18 years: not recommended; ≥18 years: same as adult
     Floxin *Tab:* 200, 300, 400 mg
▷ *trimethoprim+sulfamethoxazole* (C)(G)
   Pediatric: <18 years: See *Appendix O.33: trimethoprim+sulfamethoxazole* (Bactrim Suspension, Septra Suspension) for dose by weight; ≥18 years: same as adult
     Bactrim, Septra 2 tabs bid x 10 days
      Tab: trim 80 mg+sulfa 400 mg*
     Bactrim DS, Septra DS 1 tab bid x 10 days
      Tab: trim 160 mg+sulfa 800 mg
     Bactrim Pediatric Suspension, Septra Pediatric Suspension 20 ml bid x 10 days
      Oral susp: trim 40 mg+sulfa 200 mg per 5 ml (100 ml) (cherry) (alcohol 0.3%)

SUPPRESSION THERAPY

▷ *trimethoprim+sulfamethoxazole (TMP-SMX)* (C)(G)
   Pediatric: <18 years: not recommended; ≥18 years: same as adult
     Bactrim, Septra 2 tabs bid x 10 days
      Tab: trim 80 mg+sulfa 400 mg*
     Bactrim DS, Septra DS 1 tab bid x 10 days
      Tab: trim 160 mg+sulfa 800 mg*
     Bactrim Pediatric Suspension, Septra Pediatric Suspension 20 ml bid x 10 days
      Oral susp: trim 40 mg+sulfa 200 mg per 5 ml (100 ml) (cherry) (alcohol 0.3%)

PRURITUS

Antihistamines *See* Drugs for the Management of Allergy, Cough, and Cold Symptoms online at https://connect.springerpub.com/content/reference-book/978-0-8261-7935-7/back-matter/part02/back-matter/bmatter27

Topical Corticosteroids *see* Appendix K. Topical Corticosteroids by Potency
Parenteral Corticosteroids *see* Appendix M. Parenteral Corticosteroids
Oral Corticosteroids *see* Appendix L. Oral Corticosteroids
OTC Antihistamines
OTC Eucerin Products
OTC Lac-Hydrin Products
OTC Lubriderm Products
OTC Aveeno Products

TOPICAL OIL

▷ *fluocinolone acetonide* 0.01% topical oil (C)
  Pediatric: <6 years: not recommended; ≥6 years: apply sparingly bid for up to
  4 weeks
  Derma-Smoothe/FS Topical Oil apply sparingly tid
    Topical oil: 0.01% (4 oz) (peanut oil)

TOPICAL AND TRANSDERMAL ANALGESICS

▷ *capsaicin* (B)(G) apply tid-qid prn to intact skin
  Pediatric: <2 years: not recommended; ≥2 years: same as adult
  Axsain *Crm:* 0.075% (1, 2 oz)
  Capsin (OTC) *Lotn:* 0.025, 0, 075% (59 ml)
  Capzasin-HP (OTC) *Crm:* 0.075% (1.5 oz); Lotn: 0.075% (2 oz) 0.025% (45,
  90 gm)
  Capzasin-P (OTC) *Crm:* 0.025% (1.5 oz); Lotn: 0.025% (2 oz)
  Dolorac *Crm:* 0.025% (28 gm)
  Double Cap (OTC) *Crm:* 0.05% (2 oz)
  R-Gel *Gel:* 0.025% (15, 30 gm)
  Zostrix (OTC) *Crm:* 0.025% (0.7, 1.5, 3 oz) **Zostrix HP (OTC)** *Emol crm:*
  0.075% (1, 2 oz)
▷ *capsaicin* 8% patch (B) apply up to 4 patches for one 60-minute application to
  clean dry skin; may prep area with topical anesthetic; wear non-latex gloves;
  patches may be cut to size/shape; treatment may be repeated every 3 months
  Pediatric: <18 years: not recommended; ≥18 years: same as adult
  Qutenza *Patch:* 8% 1640 mcg/cm (179 mg) (1 or 2 patches w. 1-50 gm tube
  cleansing gel/carton)
▷ *diclofenac sodium* (C; D ≥30 wks) apply qid prn to intact skin
  Pediatric: <12 years: not established; ≥12 years: same as adult
  Pennsaid 1.5% in 10 drop increments, dispense and rub into front, side, and
  back of knee: usually; 40 drops (40 mg) qid
    Topical soln: 1.5% (150 ml)
  Pennsaid 2% apply 2 pump actuations (40 mg) and rub into front, side, and
  back of knee bid
    Topical soln: 2% (20 mg/pump actuation, 112 gm)
  Solaraze Gel massage in to clean skin bid prn
    Gel: 3% (50 gm) (benzyl alcohol)
  Voltaren Gel (G)(OTC) apply qid prn to intact skin
    Gel: 1% (100 gm)
  Comment: *Diclofenac* is contraindicated with *aspirin* allergy. As with other
  NSAIDs, should be avoided in late pregnancy (≥30 weeks) because it may cause
  premature closure of the ductus arteriosus.
▷ *doxepin* (B) cream apply to affected area qid at intervals of at least 3-4 hours; max
  8 days
  Pediatric: <12 years: not recommended; >12 years: same as adult
  Prudoxin *Crm:* 5% (45 gm)
  Zonalon *Crm:* 5% (30, 45 gm)

▷ *pimecrolimus* 1% cream (C)(G) <2 years: not recommended; ≥2 years: apply to affected area bid; do not apply an occlusive dressing

    Elidel *Crm:* 1% (30, 60, 100 gm)

Comment: *Pimecrolimus* is indicated for short-term and intermittent long-term use. Discontinue use when resolution occurs. Contraindicated if the patient is immunosuppressed. Change to the 0.1% preparation or if secondary bacterial infection is present.

▷ *trolamine salicylate* apply tid-qid

    Pediatric: <2 years: not recommended; ≥2 years: same as adult

    Mobisyl Creme *Crm:* 10% (100 gm)

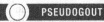 **PSEUDOBULBAR AFFECT (PBA) DISORDER**

Comment: Pseudobulbar affect (PBA), emotional lability, labile affect, or emotional incontinence refers by to a neurologic disorder characterized by involuntary crying or uncontrollable episodes of crying and/or laughing, or other emotional outbursts. PBA occurs secondary to a neurologic disease or brain injury such as traumatic brain injury (TBI), stroke, Parkinson's disease, multiple sclerosis, amyotrophic lateral sclerosis (ALS, Lou Gehrig's disease).

▷ *dextromethorphan+quinidine* (C)(G) 1 cap once daily x 7 days; then starting on day 8, 1 cap bid

    Pediatric: <12 years: not recommended; ≥12 years: same as adult

    Nuedexta *Cap:* dextro 20 mg+quini 10 mg

Comment: *dextromethorphan hydrobromide* is an uncompetitive NMDA receptor antagonist and sigma-1 agonist. *quinidine sulfate* is a CYP450 2D6 inhibitor. **Nuedexta** is contraindicated with an MAOI or within 14 days of stopping an MAOI, with prolonged QT interval, congenital long QT syndrome, history suggestive of torsades de pointes, or heart failure, complete atrioventricular (AV) block without implanted pacemaker or patients at high risk of complete AV block, and concomitant drugs that both prolong QT interval and are metabolized by CYP2D6 (e.g., *thioridazine* or *pimozide*). Discontinue **Nuedexta** if the following occurs: hepatitis or thrombocytopenia or any other hypersensitivity reaction. Monitor ECG in patients with left ventricular hypertrophy (LVH) or left ventricular dysfunction (LVD). *desipramine* exposure increases **Nuedexta** 8-fold; reduce *desipramine* dose and adjust based on clinical response. Use of **Nuedexta** with selective serotonin reuptake inhibitors (SSRIs) or tricyclic antidepressants (TCAs) increases the risk of *serotonin syndrome. paroxetine* exposure increases **Nuedexta** 2-fold; therefore, reduce **paroxetine** dose and adjust based on clinical response (*digoxin* exposure may increase *digoxin* substrate plasma concentration. **Nuedexta** is not recommended in pregnancy or breastfeeding. Safety and effectiveness of **Nuedexta** in children have not been established.

PSEUDOGOUT

Injectable Acetaminophen *see Pain*

NSAIDs *see* Appendix J. NSAIDs online at https://connect.springerpub.com/content/reference-book/978-0-8261-7935-7/back-matter/part02/back-matter/bmatter10

Opioid Analgesics *see Pain*

Topical and Transdermal Analgesics *see Pain*

Parenteral Corticosteroids *see* Appendix M. Parenteral Corticosteroids

Oral Corticosteroids *see* Appendix L. Oral Corticosteroids

Topical Analgesic and Anesthetic Agents *see* Appendix I. Anesthetic Agents for Local Infiltration and Dermal/Mucosal Membrane Application online at https://connect.springerpub.com/content/reference-book/978-0-8261-7935-7/back-matter/part02/back-matter/bmatter9

PSEUDOMEMBRANOUS COLITIS

Comment: Staphylococcal enterocolitis and antibiotic-associated pseudomembranous colitis caused by *C. difficile*.

ANTI-INFECTIVES

▷ *metronidazole* (not for use in 1st; B in 2nd, 3rd)(G) 500 mg tid x 14 days
    Flagyl *Tab:* 250*, 500*mg
    Flagyl 375 *Cap:* 375 mg
    Flagyl ER *Tab:* 750 mg ext-rel
▷ *vancomycin hcl capsule* (B)(G) 500 mg to 2 gm in 3-4 doses x 7-10 days; max 2 gm/day
    Pediatric: 40 mg/kg/day in 3-4 doses x 7-10 days; max 2 gm/day; use caps or oral solution as appropriate
    Vancocin *Cap:* 125, 250 mg

GLYCOPEPTIDE ANTIBACTERIAL AGENT

Comment: Firvanq *(vancomycin hcl oral solution)* is a glycopeptide antibacterial agent FDA approved to treat *C. difficile*-associated diarrhea (CDAD) and entercolitis caused by *Staphylococcus aureus*, including methicillin-resistant strains (MRSA). Firvanq should be used only to treat or prevent infections that are proven or strongly suspected to be caused by susceptible bacteria. Orally administered *vancomycin hcl* is not effective for treatment of other types of infections. Prescribing Firvanq in the absence of a proven or strongly suspected bacterial infection is unlikely to provide benefit to the patient and increases the risk of the development of drug-resistant bacteria.

▷ *vancomycin hcl oral solution* see mfr pkg insert for preparation and important
    administration information; *CDAD* 125 mg orally 4 x/day x 10 days;
    Staphylococcal enterocolitis: 500 mg to 2 gm orally in 3 or 4 divided doses x
    7-10 days
    Pediatric: <18 years: *CDAD and Staphylococcal enterocolitis:* 40 mg/kg orally in 3
    or 4 divided doses x 7-10 days; total daily dosage max 2 gm; ≥18 years: same as
    adult
        Firvanq *Kit w. pwdr for oral soln:* 25, 50 mg/ml (150, 300 ml) equivalent to
        3.75, 7.5, 10.5, or 15 gm *vancomycin hcl*, and grape-flavored diluent
    Comment: Nephrotoxicity has occurred following oral *vancomycin hcl* therapy and can occur either during or after completion of therapy. The risk is increased in geriatric patients. Monitor renal function. Ototoxicity has occurred in patients receiving *vancomycin hcl*. Assessment of auditory function may be appropriate in some instances. The most common adverse reactions (≥10%) have been nausea (17%), abdominal pain (15%), and hypokalemia (13%). There are no available data on Firvanq use in pregnant females to inform a drug-associated risk of major birth defects or miscarriage. Available published data on *vancomycin hcl* use in pregnancy during the second and third trimesters have not shown an association with adverse pregnancy related outcomes. There are insufficient data to inform the levels of *vancomycin hcl* in human milk. However, systemic absorption of *vancomycin hcl* following oral administration is expected to be minimal. There are no data on the effects of Firvanq on the breastfed infant.

 PSITTACOSIS

ANTI-INFECTIVES

▷ *tetracycline* (D)(G) 250 mg qid or 500 mg tid x 7-14 days
    Pediatric: <8 years: not recommended; ≥8 years, <100 lb: 25-50 mg/kg/day in 4
    doses x 7-14 days; ≥8 years, ≥100 lb: same as adult

Achromycin V *Cap:* 250, 500 mg
Sumycin *Tab:* 250, 500 mg; *Cap:* 250, 500 mg; *Oral susp:* 125 mg/5 ml (100, 200 ml) (fruit) (sulfites)

PSORIASIS, PLAQUE PSORIASIS

Emollients *see* **Dermatitis: Atopic**
Topical Corticosteroids *see* Appendix K. Topical Corticosteroids by Potency

VITAMIN D-3 DERIVATIVES

▷ *calcipotriene* (C)
  Pediatric: <12 years: not recommended; ≥12 years: same as adult
    Dovonex apply bid to lesions and gently rub in completely
      Crm: 0.005% (30, 120 gm)
    Sorilux Foam *Foam:* 0.005% (60, 120 gm)

VITAMIN D-3 DERIVATIVE+CORTICOSTEROID COMBINATIONS

▷ *calcipotriene+betamethasone dipropionate* (C)(G)
  Pediatric: <18 years: not recommended; ≥18 years: same as adult
    Enstilar apply to affected area and gently rub in once daily x up to 4 weeks; limit treatment area to 30% of body surface area; do not cover with occlusive dressing; do not use on face, axillae, groin, or atrophic skin; max 100 gm/week
      Foam: calci 0.005%+beta 0.064% (60 gm spray can)
    Taclonex apply to affected area and gently rub in once daily as needed, up to 4 weeks
    Taclonex Ointment apply bid to lesions and gently rub in completely; limit treatment area to 30% of body surface area; do not cover with occlusive dressing; do not use on face, axillae, groin, or atrophic skin; max 100 gm/week
      Oint: calci 0.005%+beta 0.064% (60, 100 gm)
    Taclonex Scalp Topical Suspension apply to affected area and gently rub in once daily x 2 weeks or until cleared; max 8 weeks; limit treatment area to 30% of body surface area; do not cover with occlusive dressing; do not use on face, axillae, groin, or atrophic skin; max 100 gm/week
      Bottle: (30, 60 gm; 120 gm [2 x 60 gm])
    Wynzora Cream apply to affected areas once daily for up to 8 weeks; discontinue when control is achieved; max 100 gm/week; do not cover with occlusive dressing; do not use on face, axillae, groin, or atrophic skin; max 100 gm/week
      Cream: calci 0.005%+beta 0.064% (60 gm)
▷ *calcitriol* (C) apply bid to lesions and gently rub in completely; do not cover with occlusive dressing; do not use on face, axillae, groin, or atrophic skin; max weekly dose should not exceed 200 gm
  Pediatric: <18 years: not recommended; ≥18 years: same as adult
    Vectical *Oint:* 3 mcg/gm (100 gm)

HIGH-POTENCY TOPICAL STEROID

For other high-potency Topical Corticosteroids *see* Appendix K. Topical Corticosteroids by Potency

▷ *clobetasol propionate* apply a thin layer to the affected skin areas bid; rub in gently and completely; wash hands after each application; discontinue when control is achieved; max 50 gm/week; max 2 consecutive weeks per treatment course; do not use if atrophy is present at the treatment site; do not bandage, cover, or wrap the treated skin area; avoid use on the face, scalp, axilla, groin, or other intertriginous areas; topical use only; not for oral, ophthalmic, or intravaginal use

Pediatric: <18 years: not recommended; ≥18 years: same as adult
Impoyz *Crm:* 0.025% (60, 112 gm)
Comment: **Impoyz** *(clobetasol propionate 0.025%)* cream is a high potency corticosteroid specifically indicated for the treatment of moderate-to-severe plaque psoriasis.

▷ *halobetasol propionate*
Pediatric: <18 years: not recommended; ≥18 years: same as adult
Bryhali apply a thin layer to the affected skin areas bid; rub in gently and completely; wash hands after each application; discontinue when control is achieved; max 50 gm/week; max 2 consecutive weeks per treatment course; do <u>not</u> use if atrophy is present at the treatment site; do <u>not</u> bandage, cover, <u>or</u> wrap the treated skin area; avoid use on the face, scalp, axilla, groin, <u>or</u> other intertriginous areas; topical use <u>only</u>; <u>not</u> for oral, ophthalmic, <u>or</u> intravaginal use
Lotn: 0.01% (60, 112 gm)
Comment: **Bryhali** *(halobetasol propionate 0.01%)* cream is a high potency corticosteroid specifically indicated for the treatment of moderate-to-severe plaque psoriasis.
Lexette Foam apply a thin layer of foam to affected areas once daily
Can: 0.05% (50 gm)
Comment: **Lexette Foam** *(halobetasol propionate)* is a potent corticosteroid specifically indicated for the topical treatment of plaque psoriasis in adult patients.

HIGH-POTENCY TOPICAL STEROID+RETINOID PRODRUG

▷ *halobetasol propionate+tazarotene*
Pediatric: safety and efficacy not established
Duobrii *Lotn:* halo prop 0.01%+tara 0.045% per gm (100 gm tube)

IMMUNOSUPPRESSANTS

▷ *alefacept* (B) 7.5 mg IV bolus <u>or</u> 15 mg IM once weekly x 12 weeks; may re-treat x 12 weeks
Pediatric: <12 years: not recommended; ≥12 years: same as adult
Amevive *IV dose pack:* 7.5 mg single-use (w. 10 ml sterile water diluents [use 0.6 ml]; 1, 4/pck); *IM dose pack:* 15 mg single-use (w. 10 ml sterile water diluent [use 0.6 ml]; 1, 4/pck
Comment: CD4+ and T-lymphocyte count should be checked prior to initiating treatment with *alefacept* and then monitored. Treatment should be withheld if CD4+ T-lymphocyte counts are below 250 cells/mcl.
▷ *cyclosporine* (C) 1.25 mg/kg bid; may increase after 4 weeks by 0.5 mg/kg/day; then adjust at 2-week intervals; max 4 mg/kg/day; administer with meals
Pediatric: <18 years: not recommended; ≥18 years: same as adult
Neoral *Cap:* 25, 100 mg (alcohol)
Neoral Oral Solution *Oral soln:* 100 mg/ml (50 ml) may dilute in room temperature apple juice <u>or</u> orange juice (alcohol)

ANTIMITOTICS

▷ *anthralin* (C) apply once daily
Pediatric: <12 years: not recommended; ≥12 years: same as adult
Zithranol-RR *Crm:* 1.2% (15, 45 gm)

RETINOIDS

▷ *acitretin* (X)(G) 25-50 mg once daily with main meal
Pediatric: <12 years: not recommended; ≥12 years: same as adult
Soriatane *Cap:* 10, 25 mg

▷ *tazarotene* (X)(G) apply once daily at HS
  Pediatric: <12 years: not recommended; ≥12 years: same as adult
    Avage Cream *Crm:* 0.1% (30 gm)
    Tazorac Cream *Crm:* 0.05, 0.1% (15, 30, 60 gm)
    Tazorac Gel *Gel:* 0.05, 0.1% (30, 100 gm)

COAL TAR PREPARATIONS

▷ *coal tar* (C)(G)
  Pediatric: same as adult
    Scytera (OTC) apply qd-qid; use lowest effective dose
      Foam: 2%
    T/Gel Shampoo Extra Strength (OTC) use every other day; max 4 x/week; massage into affected areas for 5 minutes; rinse; repeat *Shampoo:* 1%
    T/Gel Shampoo Original Formula (OTC) use every other day; max 7 x/week; massage into affected areas for 5 minutes; rinse; repeat *Shampoo:* 0.5%
    T/Gel Shampoo Stubborn Itch Control (OTC) use every other day; max 7 x/week; massage into affected areas for 5 minutes; rinse; repeat *Shampoo:* 0.5%

HUMANIZED INTERLEUKIN-17A ANTAGONIST

▷ *brodalumab* (B) inject SC into the upper arm, abdomen, or thigh; rotate sites; administer 210 mg SC (as two separate 150 mg SC injections) at weeks 0, 1, and 2; then 210 mg every 2 weeks
  Pediatric: <18 years: not recommended; ≥18 years: same as adult
    Siliq *Prefilled pen:* 210 mg/1.5 ml solution, single-use (2/carton) (preservative-free)
    Comment: **Siliq** is currently indicated for plaque psoriasis only. **Siliq** is contraindicated with Crohn's disease. *Black Box Warning (BBW):* Suicidal ideation and behavior, including completed suicides, have occurred in patients treated with **Siliq**. Prior to prescribing, weigh potential risks and benefits in patients with a history of depression and/or suicidal ideation or behavior. Patients with new or worsening suicidal thoughts and behavior should be referred to a mental health professional, as appropriate. Advise patients and caregivers to seek medical attention for manifestations of suicidal ideation or behavior, new onset or worsening depression, anxiety, or other mood changes. Avoid using live vaccines concurrently with **Siliq** therapy. There are no human data on **Siliq** use in pregnant females to inform a drug associated risk. Human IgG antibodies are known to cross the placental barrier; therefore, **Siliq** may be transmitted from the mother to the developing fetus. There are no data on the presence of *brodalumab* in human milk or effects on the breastfed infant. **Siliq** is available only through the restricted **Siliq** REMS Program.

▷ *ixekizumab* <18 years: not recommended; ≥18 years: recommended dose is 160 mg (2 x 80 mg injections) SC at Week 0, followed by 80 mg at weeks 2, 4, 6, 8, 10, and 12, then 80 mg SC every 4 weeks
  Pediatric: <18 years: not recommended; ≥18 years: same as adult
    Taltz *Prefilled pen/Prefilled autoinjector:* 80 mg/ml (1 ml) single-dose
    Comment: **Taltz** injection the first and only treatment approved by the FDA for moderate-to-severe plaque psoriasis involving the genital area. This indication is based upon positive results from a randomized, double-blind, placebo-controlled study in moderate-to-severe psoriasis involving the genital area which involved 149 patients with plaque psoriasis who were candidates for phototherapy or systemic therapy but failed to respond to or were intolerant to at least 1 topical therapy. There are no available data on **Taltz** use in pregnancy to inform any drug associated risks. Human IgG is

known to cross the placental barrier; therefore, **Taltz** may be transmitted from the mother to the developing fetus. There are no data on the presence of *ixekizumab* in human milk or effects on the breastfed infant.

▷ *secukinumab* (**B**) inject SC into the upper arm, abdomen, or thigh; rotate sites; administer 300 mg SC (as two separate 150 mg SC injections) at weeks 0, 1, 2, 3, and 4; then 300 mg every 4 weeks; for some patients, 150 mg/dose may be sufficient

Pediatric: <18 years: not recommended; ≥18 years: same as adult

Cosentyx *Vial:* 150 mg/ml pwdr for SC inj after reconstitution single-use (preservative-free)

Comment: **Cosentyx** may be used as monotherapy or in combination with *methotrexate* (MTX). Avoid using live vaccines concurrently with **Siliq** therapy. For professional preparation and administration only.

INTERLEUKIN-23 ANTAGONIST

▷ *guselkumab* **injection** administer 100 mg SC at Week 0, Week 4 and every 8 weeks thereafter

Tremfya *Prefilled syringe:* 100 mg/ml (1 ml) single-dose; *OnePress:* 100 mg/ml (1 ml), single-use, patient-controlled injector

Comment: **Tremfya** is indicated for the treatment of patients >18 years-of-age with moderate-to-severe plaque psoriasis who are candidates for systemic therapy or phototherapy. Evaluate for TB prior to initiating treatment with **Tremfya**. **Tremfya** may increase the risk of infection. Instruct patients to seek medical advice if signs or symptoms of clinically important chronic or acute infection occur. If a serious infection develops, discontinue **Tremfya** until the infection resolves. Avoid use of live vaccines in patients treated with **Tremfya**. The most common (≥1%) adverse reactions associated with **Tremfya** include upper respiratory infections, headache, injection site reactions, arthralgia, diarrhea, gastroenteritis, tinea infections, and herpes simplex infections. The safety and efficacy of **Tremfya** in pediatric patients (<18 years-of-age) have not been established. There are no available data on **Tremfya** use in pregnancy to inform a drug-associated risk of adverse developmental outcomes, presence of *guselkumab* in human milk, or effects on the breastfed infant.

▷ *risankizumab-rzaa* administer 150 mg (2 x 75 mg injections) via SC injection at Week 0, Week 4 and every 12 weeks thereafter

Pediatric: <18 years: not established: ≥18 years: same as adult

Skyrizi *Prefilled syringe:* 75 mg/0.83 ml (1 ml) single-use (2 glass syringes/kit with fixed 29 g 1/2 inch needle and needle guard) (preservative-free)

Comment: **Skyrizi** (*risankizumab-rzaa*) is an interleukin-23 antagonist indicated for the treatment of moderate-to-severe plaque psoriasis in adults who are candidates for systemic therapy or phototherapy. Evaluate the patient for TB prior to initiating treatment. Treatment with **Skyrizi** may increase the risk of infection. Instruct patients to seek medical advice if signs or symptoms of clinically important infection occur. If such an infection develops, do not administer **Skyrizi** until the infection resolves. Avoid use of live vaccines in patients treated with **Skyrizi**. Limited available data with **Skyrizi** use in pregnant females are insufficient to evaluate a drug-associated risk of major birth defects, miscarriage, or adverse maternal or fetal outcomes. However, human IgG is known to cross the placental barrier and, therefore, **Skyrizi** may be transmitted from the mother to the developing fetus. There are no data on the presence of *risankizumab-rzaa* in human milk or effects on the breastfed infant. Maternal IgG is known to be present in human milk. The developmental and health benefits of breastfeeding should be considered along with the mother's clinical need for **Skyrizi** and any potential adverse effects on the breastfed infant from **Skyrizi** or from the underlying maternal condition. The safety and efficacy of **Skyrizi** in patients <18 years- of-age have not yet been established. The most common adverse reactions (incidence ≥ 1%) have been upper respiratory infections, headache, fatigue, injection site reactions, and tinea infections.

▷ *tildrakizumab-asmn* inject SC; rotate sites; recommended dose is 100 mg at Weeks 0, 4, and every 12 weeks thereafter.

Pediatric: <18 years: not recommended; ≥18 years: same as adult

Ilumya *Prefilled syringe:* 100 mg/ml (1 ml) single-use (preservative-free)

Comment: **Ilumya** is an interleukin-23 (IL-23) antagonist indicated for the treatment of adults with moderate-to-severe plaque psoriasis who are candidates for systemic therapy or phototherapy. **Ilumya** acts by selectively binding to the p19 subunit of IL-23 and inhibiting its interaction with the Il-23 receptor, blocking the release of pro-inflammatory cytokines and chemokines. Most common adverse reactions associated with **Ilumya** treatment are upper respiratory infections, injection site reactions, and diarrhea. Avoid use of live vaccines in patients treated with **Ilumya**. If a serious allergic reaction occurs, discontinue **Ilumya** immediately and initiate appropriate therapy. **Ilumya** may increase the risk of infection. Evaluate for TB prior to initiating treatment. Instruct patients to seek medical advice if signs or symptoms of clinically important chronic or acute infection occur. If a serious infection develops, consider discontinuing females until the infection resolves. Limited available data with **Ilumya** use in pregnant women are insufficient to inform a drug associated risk of adverse developmental outcomes. Human IgG is known to cross the placental barrier; therefore, **Ilumya** may be transferred from the mother to the fetus. There are no data on the presence of *tildrakizumab- asmn* in human milk or effects on the breastfed infant.

INTERLEUKIN-23 ANTAGONIST

▷ *guselkumab* 100 mg SC at Week 0, Week 4 and every 8 weeks thereafter; can be used alone or in combination with a conventional DMARD (e.g. *methotrexate* [MTX])

Pediatric: <18 years: not established; ≥18 years: same as adult

Tremfya *Prefilled syringe:* 100 mg/ml (1 ml), single-dose; *OnePress:* 100 mg/ml (1 ml), single-use, patient-controlled injector

Comment: **Tremfya** is an interleukin-23 blocker indicated for active plaque psoriasis. Evaluate for TB prior to initiating treatment. **Tremfya** may increase the risk of infection. Instruct patients to seek medical advice if signs or symptoms of clinically important chronic or acute infection occur. If a serious infection develops, discontinue **Tremfya** until the infection resolves. Avoid use of live vaccines in patients treated with **Tremfya**. The most common (incidence ≥1%) adverse reactions have been URI, headache, injection site reaction, arthralgia, diarrhea, gastroenteritis, tinea infection, and herpes simplex infection. There are no available data on **Tremfya** use in pregnancy to inform a drug-associated risk of adverse developmental outcomes, presence of *guselkumab* in human milk, or effects on the breastfed infant.

INTERLEUKIN-12+INTERLEUKIN-23 ANTAGONIST

▷ *ustekinumab* (B) rotate sites; ≤100 kg: 45 mg SC once; then 45 mg SC once 4 weeks later; then 45 mg SC once every 12 weeks thereafter; >100 kg: 90 mg SC once; then 90 mg SC once 4 weeks later; then 90 mg SC once every 12 weeks thereafter

Pediatric: <12 years: not recommended; ≥12 years: same as adult

Stelara *Prefilled syringe:* 45 mg/0.5 ml, single dose; *Vial:* 45 mg/0.5 ml, 90 mg/ml, single-dose, 130 mg/26 ml, single-dose (preservative-free)

Comment: **Stelara** is indicated for patients with moderate-to-severe psoriatic arthritis and may be used as monotherapy <u>or</u> with *methotrexate* (MTX).

TUMOR NECROSIS FACTOR (TNF) BLOCKERS

▷ *adalimumab* (B) initially 80 mg SC once followed by 40 mg once every other week starting one week after initial dose; inject into thigh <u>or</u> abdomen; rotate sites
Pediatric: <18 years: not recommended; ≥18 years: same as adult
Humira *Prefilled syringe:* 20 mg/0.4 ml; 40 mg/0.8 ml single-dose (2/pck; 2, 6/ starter pck) (preservative-free)

▷ *adalimumab-adaz* (B) initially 80 SC; then, 40 mg SC every other week starting one week after initial dose; inject into thigh <u>or</u> abdomen; rotate sites
Pediatric: <18 years: not recommended; ≥18 years: same as adult
Hyrimoz *Prefilled syringe/Prefilled pen:* 40 mg/0.8 ml, single-dose (preservative-free)
Comment: **Hymirox** is biosimilar to **Humira** *(adalimumab)*.

▷ *adalimumab-adbm* (B) initially 80 SC; then, 40 mg SC every other week starting one week after initial dose; inject into thigh <u>or</u> abdomen; rotate sites
Pediatric: <18 years: not recommended; ≥18 years: same as adult
Cyltezo *Prefilled syringe:* 40 mg/0.8 ml single-dose (preservative-free)
Comment: **Cyltezo** is biosimilar to **Humira** *(adalimumab)*.

▷ *adalimumab-afzb* 40 mg SC every other week; some patients with RA <u>not</u> receiving *methotrexate* (MTX) may benefit from increasing the frequency to 40 mg SC every week
Abrilada *Prefilled pen:* 40 mg/0.8 ml, single-dose; *Prefilled syringe:* 40 mg/0.8 ml, 20 mg/0.4 ml, 10 mg/0.2 ml, single-dose; (for institutional use only) (preservative-free)
Comment: **Abrilada** is biosimilar to **Humira** *(adalimumab)*.

▷ *adalimumab-bwwd* *Initial Dose (Day 1):* 160 mg SC; *Second Dose: two weeks later (Day 15):* 80 mg SC; *Two weeks later (Day 29):* begin maintenance dose of 40 mg every other week
Hadlima *Prefilled autoinjector:* 40 mg/0.8 ml, single-dose (Hadlima PushTouch); *Prefilled syringe:* 40 mg/0.8 ml, single-dose
Comment: **Hadlima** is biosimilar to **Humira** *(adalimumab)*.

▷ *etanercept* (B) inject SC into thigh, abdomen, <u>or</u> upper arm; rotate sites; initially 50 mg twice weekly (3-4 days apart) for 3 months; then 50 mg/week maintenance <u>or</u> 25 mg <u>or</u> 50 mg per week for 3 months; then 50 mg/week maintenance
Pediatric: <4 years: not recommended; 4-17 years: Chronic moderate-to-severe plaque psoriasis; >17 years: same as adult
Enbrel *Vial:* 25 mg pwdr for SC injection after reconstitution (4/carton w. supplies) (preservative-free, diluent contains benzyl alcohol); *Prefilled syringe:* 25, 50 mg/ml (preservative-free); *SureClick autoinjector:* 50 mg/ml (preservative-free)

▷ *etanercept-ykro* 50 mg SC once weekly
Pediatric: <4 years: not established; ≥4 years, ≥63 kg, 138 lbs: same as adult
Eticovo *Prefilled syringe:* 25 mg/0.5 ml, 50 mg/ml solution, single-dose
Comment: **Eticovo** is biosimilar to **Enbrel** *(etanercept)*.

▷ *golimumab* (B) administer SC <u>or</u> IV infusion
Pediatric: <18 years: not recommended; ≥18 years: same as adult
Simponi 50 mg SC once monthly; rotate sites
Prefilled syringe, SmartJect autoinjector: 50 mg/0.5 ml, single-use (preservative-free)
Simponi Aria 2 mg/kg IV infusion week 0 and week 4; then every 8 weeks thereafter
Vial: 50 mg/4 ml, single-use, soln for IV infusion after dilution (latex-free, preservative-free)

▷ *infliximab* (B) must be refrigerated at 2°C to 8°C (36°F to 46°F); administer dose intravenously over a period of not less than 2 hours; do not use beyond the expiration date as this product contains no preservative; administer in conjunction with *methotrexate* (MTX), infuse 3 mg/kg at 0, 2, and 6 weeks; then every 8 weeks; some patients may benefit from increasing the dose up to 10 mg/kg or treatment as often as every 4 weeks

Pediatric: <6 years: not studied; ≥6-17 years: 3 mg/kg at 0, 2 and 6 weeks, then every 8 weeks; ≥18 years: same as adult

Remicade *Vial:* 100 mg for reconstitution to 10 ml administration volume, single-dose pwdr (presrvative-free)

Comment: **Remicade** is indicated to reduce signs and symptoms, and induce and maintain clinical remission, in adults and children ≥6 years-of-age with moderately to severely active disease who have had an inadequate response to conventional therapy and reduce the number of draining enterocutaneous and rectovaginal fistulas, and maintain fistula closure, in adults with fistulizing disease. Common adverse effects associated with **Remicade** included abdominal pain, headache, pharyngitis, sinusitis, and upper respiratory infections. In addition, **Remicade** might increase the risk for serious infections, including tuberculosis, bacterial sepsis, and invasive fungal infections. Available data from published literature on the use of *infliximab* products during pregnancy have not reported a clear association with *infliximab* products and adverse pregnancy outcomes. *Infliximab* products cross the placenta and infants exposed *in utero* should not be administered live vaccines for at least 6 months after birth. Otherwise, the infant may be at increased risk of infection, including disseminated infection which can become fatal. Available information is insufficient to inform the amount of *infliximab* products present in human milk or effects on the breastfed infant.

▷ *infliximab-abda* (B)
Renflexis *Vial:* 100 mg pwdr for reconstitution to 10 ml administration volume, single-dose
Comment: **Renflexis** is biosimilar to **Remicade** (*infliximab*).

▷ *infliximab-dyyb* (B)
Inflectra *Vial:* 100 mg pwdr for reconstitution to 10 ml administration volume, single-dose
Comment: **Inflectra** is biosimilar to **Remicade** (*infliximab*).

▷ *infliximab-axxq*
Avsola *Vial:* 100 mg pwdr in a 20 ml single-dose vial; for reconstitution, dilution, and IV infusion
Comment: **Avsola** is biosimilar to **Remicade** *(infliximab)*.

▷ *infliximab-qbtx* (B)
Ixifi *Vial:* 100 mg pwdr for reconstitution to 10 ml administration volume, single-dose
Comment: **Ixifi** is biosimilar to **Remicade** (*infliximab*).

MOISTURIZING AGENTS

Aquaphor Healing Ointment (OTC) *Oint:* (1.75, 3.5, 14 oz) (alcohol)
Eucerin Daily Sun Defense (OTC) *Lotn:* 6 oz (fragrance-free)
Comment: **Eucerin Daily Sun Defense** is a moisturizer with SPF 15.
Eucerin Facial Lotion (OTC) *Lotn:* 4 oz
Eucerin Light Lotion (OTC) *Lotn:* 8 oz
Eucerin Lotion (OTC) *Lotn:* 8, 16 oz
Eucerin Original Creme (OTC) *Crm:* 2, 4, 16 oz (alcohol)
Eucerin Plus Creme *Crm:* 4 oz
Eucerin Plus Lotion (OTC) *Lotn:* 6, 12 oz
Eucerin Protective Lotion (OTC) *Lotn:* 4 oz (alcohol)

Comment: Eucerin Protective Lotion is a moisturizer with SPF 25.
Lac-Hydrin Cream (OTC) *Crm:* 280, 385 gm
Lac-Hydrin Lotion (OTC) *Lotn:* 225, 400 gm
Lubriderm Dry Skin Scented (OTC) *Lotn:* 6, 10, 16, 32 oz
Lubriderm Dry Skin Unscented (OTC) *Lotn:* 3.3, 6, 10, 16 oz (fragrance-free)
Lubriderm Sensitive Skin Lotion (OTC) *Lotn:* 3.3, 6, 10, 16 oz (lanolin-free)
Lubriderm Dry Skin (OTC) *Lotn (scented):* 2.5, 6, 10, 16 oz;
Lotn (fragrance-free): 1, 2.5, 6, 10, 16 oz
Lubriderm Bath 1-2 capfuls in bath or rub onto wet skin as needed; then rinse
(8 oz)

PSORIATIC ARTHRITIS

Injectable Acetaminophen *see Pain*
NSAIDs *see* Appendix J. NSAIDs online at https://connect.springerpub.com/content/
reference-book/978-0-8261-7935-7/back-matter/part02/back-matter/bmatter10
Opioid Analgesics *see Pain*
Topical & Transdermal Analgesics *see Pain*
Parenteral Corticosteroids *see* Appendix M. Parenteral Corticosteroids
Oral Corticosteroids *see* Appendix L. Oral Corticosteroids
Topical Analgesic and Anesthetic Agents *see* Appendix I. Anesthetic Agents for
Local Infiltration and Dermal/Mucosal Membrane Application online at https://
connect.springerpub.com/content/reference-book/978-0-8261-7935-7/back-matter/
part02/back-matter/bmatter9

TOPICAL AND TRANSDERMAL ANALGESICS

▷ *capsaicin* (B)(G) apply tid-qid prn to intact skin
  Pediatric: <2 years: not recommended; ≥2 years: same as adult
    Axsain *Crm:* 0.075% (1, 2 oz)
    Capsin *Lotn:* 0.025, 0.075% (59 ml)
    Capzasin-HP (OTC) *Crm:* 0.075% (1.5 oz), 0.025% (45, 90 gm); *Lotn:* 0.075%
    (2 oz); 0.025% (45, 90 gm)
    Capzasin-P (OTC) *Crm:* 0.025% (1.5 oz); *Lotn:* 0.025% (2 oz)
    Dolorac *Crm:* 0.025% (28 gm)
    Double Cap (OTC) *Crm:* 0.05% (2 oz)
    R-Gel *Gel:* 0.025% (15, 30 gm)
    Zostrix (OTC) *Crm:* 0.025% (0.7, 1.5, 3 oz)
    Zostrix HP (OTC) *Emol crm:* 0.075% (1, 2 oz)
▷ *capsaicin* 8% patch (B) apply up to 4 patches for one 60-minute application
  to clean dry skin; may prep area with topical anesthetic; wear non-latex
  gloves; patches may be cut to size/shape; treatment may be repeated every 3
  months
  Pediatric: <18 years: not recommended; ≥18 years: same as adult
    Qutenza *Patch:* 8% 1640 mcg/cm (179 mg) (1 or 2 patches w. 1-50 gm tube
    cleansing gel/carton)
▷ *diclofenac sodium* (C; D ≥30 wks) apply qid prn to intact skin
  Pediatric: <12 years: not established; ≥12 years: same as adult
    Pennsaid 1.5% in 10 drop increments, dispense and rub into front, side, and
    back of knee: usually; 40 drops (40 mg) qid
      Topical soln: 1.5% (150 ml)
    Pennsaid 2% apply 2 pump actuations (40 mg) and rub into front, side, and
    back of knee bid
      Topical soln: 2% (20 mg/pump actuation, 112 gm)
    Solaraze Gel massage in to clean skin bid prn
      Gel: 3% (50 gm) (benzyl alcohol)

Voltaren Gel (G)(OTC) apply qid prn to intact skin
   Gel: 1% (100 gm)
Comment: *Diclofenac* is contraindicated with *aspirin* allergy. As with other NSAIDs, should be avoided in late pregnancy (≥30 weeks) because it may cause premature closure of the ductus arteriosus.

▷ *doxepin* (B) cream apply to affected area qid at intervals of at least 3-4 hours; max 8 days
   Pediatric: <12 years: not recommended; >12 years: same as adult
     Prudoxin *Crm:* 5% (45 gm)
     Zonalon *Crm:* 5% (30, 45 gm)

▷ *pimecrolimus* 1% cream (C)(G) <2 years: not recommended; ≥2 years: apply to affected area bid; do not apply an occlusive dressing
     Elidel *Crm:* 1% (30, 60, 100 gm)
Comment: *Pimecrolimus* is indicated for short-term and intermittent long-term use. Discontinue use when resolution occurs. Contraindicated if the patient is immunosuppressed. Change to the 0.1% preparation or if secondary bacterial infection is present.

▷ *trolamine salicylate* apply tid-qid
   Pediatric: <2 years: not recommended; ≥2 years: same as adult
     Mobisyl Creme *Crm:* 10% (100 gm)

ORAL SALICYLATE

▷ *indomethacin* (C) initially 25 mg bid-tid, increase as needed at weekly intervals by 25-50 mg/day; max 200 mg/day
   Pediatric: <14 years: usually not recommended; >2 years, if risk warranted: 1-2 mg/kg/day in divided doses; max 3-4 mg/kg/day or 150-200 mg/day, whichever is less; <14 years: ER cap not recommended
     Cap: 25, 50 mg; *Susp:* 25 mg/5 ml (pineapple-coconut, mint) (alcohol 1%); *Supp:* 50 mg; *ER Cap:* 75 mg ext-rel
Comment: *Indomethacin* is indicated only for acute painful flares. Administer with food and/or antacids. Use lowest effective dose for shortest duration.

ORAL NSAIDs

See more **Oral NSAIDs** NSAIDs online at https://connect.springerpub.com/content/reference-book/978-0-8261-7935-7/back-matter/part02/back-matter/bmatter10

▷ *diclofenac* (C) take on empty stomach; 35 mg tid; Hepatic impairment: use lowest dose
   Pediatric: <18 years: not recommended; ≥18 years: same as adult
     Zorvolex *Gelcap:* 18, 35 mg

▷ *diclofenac sodium* (C)
   Pediatric: <18 years: not recommended; ≥18 years: same as adult
     Voltaren 50 mg bid to qid or 75 mg bid or 25 mg qid with an additional 25 mg at HS if necessary
       Tab: 25, 50, 75 mg ent-coat
     Voltaren XR 100 mg once daily; rarely, 100 mg bid may be used
       Tab: 100 mg ext-rel
Comment: *Diclofenac* is contraindicated with *aspirin* allergy. As with other NSAIDs, should be avoided in late pregnancy (≥30 weeks) because it may cause premature closure of the ductus arteriosus.

NSAID+PPI

▷ *esomeprazole+naproxen* (C)(G) 1 tab bid; use lowest effective dose for the shortest duration swallow whole; take at least 30 minutes before a meal
   Pediatric: <18 years: not recommended; ≥18 years: same as adult
     Vimovo *Tab:* nap 375 mg+eso 20 mg ext-rel; nap 500 mg+eso 20 mg ext-rel

Comment: **Vimovo** is indicated to improve signs/symptoms, and risk of gastric ulcer in patients at risk of developing NSAID-associated gastric ulcer.

COX-2 INHIBITORS

Comment: Cox-2 inhibitors are contraindicated with history of asthma, urticaria, and allergic-type reactions to *aspirin*, other NSAIDs, and sulfonamides, 3rd trimester of pregnancy, and coronary artery bypass graft (CABG) surgery.

▷ *celecoxib* (C)(G) 50-400 mg once daily-bid; max 800 mg/day
   Pediatric: <18 years: not recommended; ≥18 years: same as adult
      Celebrex *Cap:* 50, 100, 200, 400 mg
▷ *meloxicam* (C)(G)
   Pediatric: <18 years: not recommended; ≥18 years: same as adult
      Mobic <2 years, <60 kg: not recommended; ≥2, ≥60 kg: 0.125 mg/kg; max 7.5 mg once daily; ≥18 years: initially 7.5 mg once daily; max 15 mg once daily; *Hemodialysis:* max 7.5 mg/day
      Tab: 7.5, 15 mg; *Oral susp:* 7.5 mg/5 ml (100 ml) (raspberry)
      Vivlodex <18 years: <u>not</u> established; ≥18 years: initially 5 mg qd; may increase to max 10 mg/day; *Hemodialysis:* max 5 mg/day
      Cap: 5, 10 mg

PHOSPHODIESTERASE 4 (PDE4) INHIBITOR

▷ *apremilast* (C)(G) swallow whole; initial titration over 5 days; maintenance 30 mg bid; *Day 1:* 10 mg in AM; *Day 2:* 10 mg AM and 10 mg PM; *Day 3:* 10 mg AM and 20 mg PM; *Day 4:* 20 mg AM and 20 mg PM; *Day 5:* 20 mg AM and 30 mg PM; *Day 6 and ongoing:* 30 mg AM and 30 mg PM
   Pediatric: <12 years: not recommended; ≥12 years: same as adult
      Otezla *Tab:* 10, 20, 30 mg; *2-Week Starter Pack*
   Comment: Register pregnant patients exposed to **Otezla** by calling 877-311-8972.

INTERLEUKIN-23 ANTAGONIST

▷ *guselkumab* 100 mg SC at Week 0, Week 4, and every 8 weeks thereafter; can be used alone <u>or</u> in combination with a conventional DMARD (e.g. *methotrexate* [MTX])
   Pediatric: <18 years: not established; ≥18 years: same as adult
      Tremfya *Prefilled syringe:* 100 mg/ml (1 ml), single-dose; *OnePress:* 100 mg/ml (1 ml), single-use, patient-controlled injector
   Comment: **Tremfya** is an interleukin-23 blocker indicated for active psoriatic arthritis. Evaluate for TB prior to initiating treatment. **Tremfya** may increase the risk of infection. Instruct patients to seek medical advice if signs <u>or</u> symptoms of clinically important chronic <u>or</u> acute infection occur. If a serious infection develops, discontinue **Tremfya** until the infection resolves. Avoid use of live vaccines in patients treated with **Tremfya**. The most common (incidence ≥1%) adverse reactions have been URI, headache, injection site reaction, arthralgia, diarrhea, gastroenteritis, tinea infection, and herpes simplex infection. There are <u>no</u> available data on **Tremfya** use in pregnancy to inform a drug-associated risk of adverse developmental outcomes, presence of *guselkumab* in human milk, <u>or</u> effects on the breastfed infant.

INTERLEUKIN-12 & INTERLEUKIN-23 ANTAGONIST

▷ *ustekinumab* (B) inject SC; rotate sites; <100 kg: 45 mg once; then 4 weeks later; then every 12 weeks; ≥100 kg: 90 mg once; then 4 weeks later; then every 12 weeks
   Pediatric: <18 years: not recommended; ≥18 years: same as adult
      Stelara *Prefilled syringe:* 45 mg/0.5 ml, single dose; *Vial:* 45 mg/0.5 ml, 90 mg/ml, single-dose, 130 mg/26 ml, single-dose (preservative-free)
   Comment: **Stelara** may be used as monotherapy <u>or</u> in combination with *methotrexate* (MTX).

TUMOR NECROSIS FACTOR (TNF) BLOCKERS

▷ *adalimumab* (B) 40 mg SC once every other week; may increase to once weekly without *methotrexate* (MTX); administer in abdomen or thigh; rotate sites; 2-17 years, supervise first dose

Pediatric: <5 years, <20 kg: not recommended; 5-18 years, living with moderate-to-severe UC, weight-based: 20 kg (44 lb) to <40 kg (<88 lb): *Day 1:* 80 mg; Day 8: 40 mg; *Day 15:* 20 mg; Starting on *Day 29:* 20 mg every week or 40 mg every other week; >40 kg (>88 lb): *Day 1:* 160 mg (as a single dose or split over two consecutive days); *Day 8:* 80 mg; Day 15: 80 mg; *Starting on Day 29:* 40 mg every week or 80 mg every other week; It is recommended to continue the recommended pediatric dosage in patients who turn 18 years-of-age and who are well-controlled on their **Humira** regimen.

   Humira *Prefilled syringe:* 20 mg/0.4 ml; 40 mg/0.8 ml single-dose (2/pck; 2, 6/ starter pck) (preservative-free)

   Comment: **Humira** may use with *methotrexate* (MTX), DMARDS, corticoids, salicylates, NSAIDs, or analgesics.

▷ *adalimumab-adaz* (B) 40 mg SC every other week; some patients with RA not receiving *methotrexate* (MTX) may benefit from increasing the frequency to 40 mg SC every week

Pediatric: <18 years: not recommended; ≥18 years: same as adult

   Hyrimox *Prefilled syringe/Prefilled pen:* 40 mg/0.8 ml single-dose (preservative-free)

Comment: **Hyrimox** is biosimilar to **Humira** *(adalimumab)*.

▷ *adalimumab-adbm* (B) initially 80 SC; then, 40 mg SC every other week starting one week after initial dose; inject into thigh or abdomen; rotate sites

Pediatric: <18 years: not recommended; ≥18 years: same as adult

   Cyltezo *Prefilled syringe:* 40 mg/0.8 ml single-dose (preservative-free)

   Comment: **Cyltezo** is biosimilar to **Humira** *(adalimumab)*.

▷ *adalimumab-afzb* 40 mg SC every other week; some patients with RA not receiving *methotrexate* (MTX) may benefit from increasing the frequency to 40 mg SC every week

   Abrilada *Prefilled pen:* 40 mg/0.8 ml, single-dose; *Prefilled syringe:* 40 mg/0.8 ml, 20 mg/0.4 ml, 10 mg/0.2 ml, single-dose; (for institutional use only) (preservative-free)

   Comment: **Abrilada** is biosimilar to **Humira** *(adalimumab)*.

▷ *adalimumab-bwwd* Initial Dose (Day 1): 160 mg SC; *Second Dose: two weeks later (Day 15):* 80 mg SC; *Two weeks later (Day 29):* begin maintenance dose of 40 mg every other week

   Hadlima *Prefilled autoinjector:* 40 mg/0.8 ml, single-dose (Hadlima PushTouch); *Prefilled syringe:* 40 mg/0.8 ml, single-dose

   Comment: **Hadlima** is biosimilar to **Humira** *(adalimumab)*.

▷ *etanercept* (B) 25 mg SC twice weekly (72-96 hours apart) or 50 mg SC weekly; rotate sites

Pediatric: <4 years: not recommended; 4-17 years: 0.4 mg/kg SC twice weekly, 72-96 hours apart (max 25 mg/dose) or 0.8 mg/kg SC weekly (max 50 mg/dose); >17 years: same as adult

   Enbrel *Vial:* 25 mg pwdr for SC injection after reconstitution (4/carton w. supplies) (preservative-free; diluent contains benzyl alcohol); *Prefilled syringe:* 25, 50 mg/ml (preservative-free); *SureClick Autoinjector:* 50 mg/ml (preservative-free)

Comment: *Etanercept* reduces pain, morning stiffness, and swelling. May be administered in combination with *methotrexate* (MTX). Live vaccines should not be administered concurrently. Do not administer with active infection.

▷ *etanercept-ykro* 50 mg SC once weekly

Pediatric: <4 years: not established; ≥4 years, ≥63 kg, 138 lbs: same as adult

Eticovo *Prefilled syringe:* 25 mg/0.5 ml, 50 mg/ml solution, single-dose
Comment: Eticovo *(etanercept-ykro)* is biosimilar to Enbrel.

▷ *golimumab* (B) administer SC or IV infusion
Simponi 50 mg SC once monthly; rotate sites
Pediatric: <18 years: not recommended; ≥18 years: same as adult
Prefilled syringe, SmartJect autoinjector: 50 mg/0.5 ml, single-use
(preservative-free)
Simponi Aria 2 mg/kg IV infusion week 0 and week 4; then every 8 weeks
thereafter
Pediatric: <2 years: not recommended; ≥2 years, with active (PsA): 80 mg/m²
via IV infusion over 30 minutes at weeks 0 and 4, and every 8 weeks thereafter
Vial: 50 mg/4 ml, single-use, soln for IV infusion after dilution (latex-free,
preservative-free)
Comment: Corticosteroids, non-biologic DMARDs, and/or NSAIDs may be
continued during treatment with *golimumab.*

▷ *infliximab* must be refrigerated at 2ºC to 8ºC (36ºF to 46ºF); administer dose
intravenously over a period of not less than 2 hours; do not use beyond the
expiration date as this product contains no preservative; 5 mg/kg at 0, 2, and
6 weeks, then every 8 weeks; some adult patients who initially respond to
treatment may benefit from increasing the dose to 10 mg/kg if response is lost
later
Pediatric: <6 years: not studied; ≥6-17 years: mg/kg at 0, 2, and 6 weeks, then
every 8 weeks; ≥18 years: same as adult
Remicade *Vial:* 100 mg pwdr for reconstitution to 10 ml administration
volume, single-dose (presrvative-free)
Comment: Remicade is indicated to reduce signs and symptoms, and induce
and maintain clinical remission, in adults and children ≥6 years-of-age
with moderately to severely active disease who have had an inadequate
response to conventional therapy and reduce the number of draining
enterocutaneous and rectovaginal fistulas, and maintain fistula closure, in
adults with fistulizing disease. Common adverse effects associated with
Remicade included abdominal pain, headache, pharyngitis, sinusitis, and
upper respiratory infections. In addition, Remicade might increase the risk
for serious infections, including tuberculosis, bacterial sepsis, and invasive
fungal infections. Available data from published literature on the use of
infliximab products during pregnancy have not reported a clear association
with *infliximab* products and adverse pregnancy outcomes. *Infliximab*
products cross the placenta and infants exposed *in utero* should not be
administered live vaccines for at least 6 months after birth. Otherwise, the
infant may be at increased risk of infection, including disseminated infection
which can become fatal. Available information is insufficient to inform the
amount of *infliximab* products present in human milk or effects on the
breastfed infant.

▷ *infliximab-abda* (B)
Renflexis *Vial:* 100 mg pwdr for reconstitution to 10 ml administration
volume, single-dose
Comment: Renflexis is biosimilar to Remicade. (*infliximab*).

▷ *infliximab-dyyb* (B)
Inflectra *Vial:* 100 mg pwdr for reconstitution to 10 ml administration
volume, single-dose
Comment: Inflectra is biosimilar to Remicade. (*infliximab*).

▷ *infliximab-axxq*
Avsola *Vial:* 100 mg pwdr in a 20 ml single-dose vial, for reconstitution, dilution,
and IV infusion
Comment: Avsola is biosimilar to Remicade. (*infliximab*).

▷ *infliximab-qbtx* (B)

    Ixifi *Vial:* 100 mg pwdr for reconstitution to 10 ml administration volume, single-dose

    Comment: **Ixifi** is biosimilar to **Remicade**. (*infliximab*).

Selective Costimulation Modulator

▷ *abatacept* (C) administer as an IV infusion over 30 minutes at weeks 0, 2, and 4; then every 4 weeks thereafter; <60 kg, administer 500 mg/dose; 60-100 kg, administer 750 mg/dose; >100 kg, administer 1 gm/dose

    Pediatric: <6 years: not recommended; 6-17 years: administer as an IV infusion over 30 minutes at weeks 0, 2, and 4; then every 4 weeks thereafter; <75 kg, administer 10 mg/kg; same as adult (max 1 gm); >17 years: same as adult

    Orencia *Vial:* 250 mg pwdr for IV infusion after reconstitution (silicone-free) (preservative-free); *Prefilled syringe:* 125 mg/ml soln for SC injection (preservative-free); *ClickJect Autoinjector:* 125 mg/ml soln for SC injection

CD20-DIRECTED CYTOLYTIC MONOCLONAL ANTIBODY

▷ *rituximab* (C) administer corticosteroid 30 minutes prior to each infusion; concomitant *methotrexate* (MTX) therapy, administer a 1000 mg IV infusion at 0 and 2 weeks; then every 24 weeks <u>or</u> based on response, but <u>not</u> sooner than every 16 weeks.

    Pediatric: <6 years: not recommended; ≥6 years: same as adult

    Rituxan *Vial:* 100 mg/10 ml (10 mg/ml), 500 mg/50 ml (10 mg/ml), single-use (preservative-free)

    Comment: *Rituximab* is a B-cell targeting chimeric monoclonal antibody that acts against CD20 and reduces antibody titers. B-cell depletion by *rituximab* may also set the stage for production of interleukin 10–secreting B cells that do <u>not</u> interact with T cells, which further reduces production of antidesmoglein antibodies. *Rituximab* carries a black box warning regarding fatal infusion reactions, severe mucocutaneous reactions, hepatitis B virus reactivation, and progressive multifocal leukoencephalopathy. However, serious adverse events are rare. There was no evidence of increased mortality with longer exposure to **rituximab** <u>or</u> to multiple courses of therapy.

◯ PULMONARY ARTERIAL HYPERTENSION (PAH) (WHO GROUP I)

ENDOTHELIAL RECEPTOR ANTAGONIST (ERA)

▷ *bosentan* (G) initiate at 62.5 mg orally twice daily; for patients weighing greater than 40 kg, increase to 125 mg orally twice daily after 4 weeks

    Pediatric: <3 years: not established; 3-12: initiate at 62.5 mg orally twice daily; for patients weighing > 40 kg, increase to 125 mg orally twice daily after 4 weeks; >12 years: same as adult

    Tracleer *Tab:* 62.5, 125 mg film-coat; *Tab for oral suspension:* 32 mg

    Comment: *Bosentan* is an endothelin receptor antagonist (ERA) indicated for the treatment of pulmonary arterial hypertension (PAH) (WHO Group 1). **Tracleer** is the first ERA indicated for the treatment of PAH in patients aged 3 years and older with idiopathic <u>or</u> congenital PAH to improve pulmonary vascular resistance (PVR), which is expected to result in an improvement in exercise ability. The most common adverse events associated with **Tracleer** in clinical trials include respiratory tract infections, headache, edema, chest pain, syncope, flushing, hypotension, sinusitis, arthralgia, abnormal serum aminotransferases, palpitations, and anemia. Monitor hemoglobin levels after 1 and 3 months of treatment, then every 3 months thereafter. If signs of pulmonary edema occur, consider the diagnosis of associated pulmonary veno-occlusive disease (PVOD) and consider discontinuing **Tracleer**. Measure liver aminotransferases prior to initiation of treatment and then monthly. Reduce the dose and closely monitor patients developing aminotransferase elevations >3 x ULN. Co-administration of **Tracleer** with drugs metabolized by CYP2C9 and CYP3A can increase exposure to **Tracleer** and/or the co-administered drug. **Tracleer** use decreases contraceptive exposure and reduces effectiveness. There are no data on the presence of *bosentan* in human milk or the effects on the breastfed infant. However, because of the potential for serious adverse reactions, such as fluid retention and hepatotoxicity in breastfed infants, advise women not to breastfeed during treatment with **Tracleer** and pregnancy is contraindicated while taking **Tracleer**. To prevent pregnancy, females of reproductive potential must use two reliable forms of contraception during treatment and for one month after stopping **Tracleer** Due to the risks of hepatotoxicity and birth defects, **Tracleer** includes a boxed warning and is only available through the restricted **Tracleer** Risk Evaluation and Mitigation Strategy REMS Program, a restricted distribution program. Patients, prescribers, and pharmacies must enroll in the program to receive and administer **Tracleer**: www.tracleerrems.com/prescribers.aspx.

PROSTACYCLIN RECEPTOR AGONIST

▶ *macitentan* (G) 10 mg once daily; doses higher than 10 mg once daily have not been studied in patients with PAH and are not recommended
Pediatric: safety and efficacy not established
    Opsumit *Tab:* 10 mg film-coat
    Comment: **Opsumit** is an endothelin receptor antagonist (ERA) indicated for the treatment of (PAH, WHO Group I) to reduce the risks of disease progression and hospitalization. The most common adverse reactions (more frequent than placebo by ≥3%) have been anemia, nasopharyngitis/pharyngitis, bronchitis, headache, influenza, and UTI. ERAs cause hepatotoxicity and liver failure. Obtain baseline liver enzymes and monitor as clinically indicated. Fluid retention may require intervention. Pulmonary edema in patients with pulmonary veno-occlusive disease; if confirmed, discontinue treatment. Decreases in sperm count have been observed in patients taking ERAs. Monitor for decreases in hemoglobin. Strong CYP3A4 inducers (e.g., *rifampin*) reduce exposure to *macitentan*; avoid co-administration with **Opsumit**. Strong CYP3A4 inhibitors (e.g., *ketoconazole, ritonavir*) increase exposure to *macitentan*; avoid co-administration with **Opsumit**. BBW: embryo/fetal toxicity; therefore, do not administer **Opsumit** to a pregnant female. For females of reproductive potential, exclude pregnancy before start of treatment, monthly during treatment, and 1 month after stopping treatment. Advise males and females of reproductive potential regarding contraception. Advise not to breastfeed. For all female patients, **Opsumit** is available only through the **Opsumit** Risk Evaluation and Mitigation Strategy (REMS) program. Further information is available at www.OPSUMITREMS.com or 1-866-228-3546. Information on **Opsumit**-certified pharmacies or wholesale distributors is available through Actelion Pathways at 1-866-228-3546.

▶ *selexipag* (X) initially 200 mcg bid; increase by 200 mcg bid to highest tolerated dose up to 1600 mcg bid; *Moderate hepatic impairment (Child-Pugh Class B):* initially 200 mcg once daily; increase by 200 mcg once daily at weekly intervals as tolerated; swallow whole; may take with food to improve tolerability
Pediatric: <12 years: not recommended; ≥12 years: same as adult
    Uptravi
        Tab: 200, 400, 600, 800, 1000, 1200, 1400, 1600 mcg; *Titration pck:* 140 x 200 mcg + 60 x 800 mcg)
    Comment: Discontinue **Uptravi** if pulmonary veno-occlusive disease is confirmed or severe hepatic impairment (Child-Pugh Class C). May be

potentiated by concomitant strong CYP2C8 inhibitors (e.g., *gemfibrozil*); *Nursing mothers:* not recommended. Discontinue breastfeeding or discontinue the drug.

ENDOTHELIN RECEPTOR ANTAGONIST, SELECTIVE FOR THE ENDOTHELIN TYPE-A (ETA) RECEPTOR

▷ *ambrisentan* (X)(G) initiate treatment at 5 mg once daily, with or without *tadalafil* 20 mg once daily; at 4-week intervals, either the dose of **Letairis** or *tadalafil* can be increased, as needed and tolerated, to **Letairis** 10 mg or *tadalafil* 40 mg; do not split, crush, or chew

Pediatric: <12 years: not recommended; ≥12 years: same as adult

Letairis *Tab:* 5, 10 mg film-coat

Comment: In patients with PAH, plasma ET-1 concentrations are increased as much as 10-fold and correlate with increased mean right atrial pressure and disease severity. ET-1 and ET-1 mRNA concentrations are increased as much as 9-fold in the lung tissue of patients with PAH, primarily in the endothelium of pulmonary arteries. These findings suggest that ET-1 may play a critical role in the pathogenesis and progression of PAH. When taken with *tadalafil*, **Letairis** is indicated to reduce the risk of disease progression and hospitalization, to reduce the risk of hospitalization due to worsening PAH, and to improve exercise tolerance. **Letairis** is contraindicated in idiopathic pulmonary fibrosis (IPF). Exclude pregnancy before the initiation of treatment with **Letairis.** Females of reproductive potential must use acceptable methods of contraception during treatment with **Letairis** and for one month after treatment. Obtain monthly pregnancy tests during treatment and 1 month after discontinuation of treatment. Females can only receive **Letairis** through the **Letairis** Risk Evaluation and Mitigation Strategy (REMS) Program, a restricted distribution program, because of the risk of embryo/fetal toxicity: www.Letairisrems.com or 1-866-664-5327.

Guanylate Cyclase Stimulator

▷ *riociguat* (X) initially 0.5-1 mg tid; titrate every 2 weeks as tolerated (SBP ≥95 and absence of hypotensive symptoms) to highest tolerated dose; max 2.5 mg tid

Pediatric: <12 years: not recommended; ≥12 years: same as adult

Adempas *Tab:* 0.5, 1, 1.5, 2, 2.5 mg

Comment: If **Adempas** is interrupted for ≥3 days, re-titrate. Consider titrating to dosage higher than 2.5 mg tid, if tolerated, in patients who smoke. Consider a starting dose of 0.5 mg tid when initiating **Adempas** in patients receiving strong cytochrome P450 (CYP) and P-glycoprotein/breast cancer resistance protein (P-gp/BCRP) inhibitors such as azole antimycotics (e.g., *ketoconazole, itraconazole*) or HIV protease inhibitors (e.g., *ritonavir*). Monitor for signs and symptoms of hypotension with strong CYP and P-gp/BCRP inhibitors. Obtain pregnancy tests prior to initiation and monthly during treatment. **Adempas** has consistently shown to have teratogenic effects when administered to animals. Females can only receive **Adempas** through the Adempas Risk Evaluation and Mitigation Strategy (REMS) Program, a restricted distribution program: www.AdempasREMS.com or 855-4 ADEMPAS. It is not known if **Adempas** is present in human milk; however, *riociguat* or its metabolites were present in the milk of rats. Because of the potential for serious adverse reactions in nursing infants from *riociguat*, discontinue nursing or **Adempas**. In placebo-controlled clinical trials, serious bleeding has occurred (including hemoptysis, hematemesis, vaginal hemorrhage, catheter site hemorrhage, subdural hematoma, and intra-abdominal hemorrhage. Safety and efficacy have not been demonstrated in patients with creatinine clearance <15 mL/min or on dialysis or severe hepatic impairment (Child-Pugh Class C).

PHOSPHODIESTERASE TYPE 5 (PDE5) INHIBITORS, CGMP-SPECIFIC DRUGS

▷ *sildenafil citrate* (B)(G) *Orally:* initially 5 or 20 mg tid, 4-6 hours apart; max 20 mg tid; *IV bolus:* 2.5 mg or 10 mg bolus injection tid, 4-6 hours apart; max 10 mg tid; the dose does not need to be adjusted for body weight

Pediatric: <12 years: not recommended; ≥12 years: same as adult

Revatio *Tab:* 20 mg film-coat; *Oral susp:* 10 mg/ml pwdr for reconstitution (1.12 gm, 112 ml) (grape) (sorbitol); *Vial:* 10 mg/12.5 ml (0.8 mg/ml)

Comment: A 10 mg IV dose is predicted to provide pharmacological effect equivalent to the 20 mg oral dose. **Revatio** is contraindicated with concomitant nitrate drugs including *nitroglycerin*, *isosorbide dinitrate*, isosorbide mononitrate, and some recreational drugs such as "poppers." Taking **Revatio** with a nitrate can cause a sudden and serious decrease in blood pressure. **Revatio** is contraindicated with concomitant guanylate cyclase stimulator drugs such as *riociguat* (**Adempas**). Avoid the use of grapefruit products while taking **Revatio**. Stop **Revatio** and get emergency medical help if sudden vision loss. **Revatio** is contraindicated with other phosphodiesterase type 5 (PDE5) Inhibitors, cGMP-specific drugs such as *avanafil* (**Stendra**), *tadalafil* (**Cialis**) or *vardenafil* (**Levitra**). Caution with history of recent MI, stroke, life-threatening arrhythmia, hypotension, hypertension, cardiac failure, unstable angina, retinitis pigmentosa, CYP3A4 inhibitors (e.g., *cimetidine*, the azoles, *erythromycin*, protease inhibitors (e.g., *ritonavir*), CYP3A4 inducers (e.g., *rifampin*, *carbamazepine*, *phenytoin*, *phenobarbital*), alcohol, antihypertensive agents. Side effects include headache, flushing, nasal congestion, rhinitis, dyspepsia, and diarrhea. Use **Revatio** with caution in patients with anatomical deformation of the penis (e.g., angulation, cavernosal fibrosis, or Peyronie's disease) or in patients who have conditions, which may predispose them to priapism (e.g., sickle cell anemia, multiple myeloma, or leukemia). In the event of an erection that persists longer than 4 hours, the patient should seek immediate medical assistance. If priapism (painful erection greater than 6 hours in duration) is not treated immediately, penile tissue damage, and permanent loss of potency could result.

▷ *tadalafil* (B)(G) 40 mg once daily; *CrCl 31-80 mL/min:* initially 20 mg once daily; increase to 40 mg once daily if tolerated; *CrCl <30 mL/min:* not recommended; *Mild or moderate hepatic cirrhosis (Child-Pugh Class A or B):* initially 20 mg once daily. *Severe hepatic cirrhosis (Child-Pugh Class C):* not recommended; *use with ritonavir; Receiving ritonavir for at least 1 week:* initiate *tadalafil* at 20 mg once daily; may increase to 40 mg once daily if tolerated; *Already on tadalafil:* stop *tadalafil* at least 24 hours prior to initiating *ritonavir;* resume *tadalafil* at 20 mg once daily after at least 1 week; may increase to 40 mg once daily if tolerated

Pediatric: <12 years: not recommended; ≥12 years: same as adult

Adcirca *Tab:* 20 mg

Comment: Contraindicated with concomitant organic nitrates and guanylate cyclase stimulators (e.g., *riociguat*).

▷ *treprostinil* (B) swallow whole; take with food

Orenitram *Tab:* 0.125, 0.25, 1, 2.5 mg ext-rel

Comment: **Orenitram** is indicated to improve exercise capacity. It is contraindicated with severe hepatic impairment (Child-Pugh Class C). **Orenitram** inhibits platelet aggregation and increases the risk of bleeding. Concomitant administration of **Orenitram** with diuretics, antihypertensive agents, or other vasodilators increases the risk of symptomatic hypotension.

 PULMONARY FIBROSIS, IDIOPATHIC (IPF)

Parenteral Corticosteroids *see* Appendix M. Parenteral Corticosteroids
Oral Corticosteroids *see* Appendix L. Oral Corticosteroids

Comment: Idiopathic pulmonary fibrosis (IPF) is a chronic, progressive, interstitial lung disease of unknown etiology. There are few effective therapies and the mortality rate is high. New treatments for IPF are urgently needed. Antiinflammatory therapy with corticosteroids or immunosuppressants fails to significantly improve the survival time of patients with IPF. Other pharmacological interventions, which *nintedanib* (Ofev), *etanercept* (Enbrel), *warfarin, imatinib mesylate* (Gleevec), and *bosentan* (Tracleer) remain controversial. *pirfenidone* was approved by the European Medicines Agency in 2011. In a 2016 study, *N-Acetylcysteine* was found to have a significant effect only on decreases in percentage of predicted vital capacity and 6 minutes walking test distance. *N*-acetylcysteine showed no beneficial effect on changes in forced vital capacity, changes in predicted carbon monoxide diffusing capacity, rates of adverse events, or death rates.

▶ *azathioprine* (D) 1 mg/kg/day in a single or divided doses; may increase by 0.5 mg/kg/day q 4 weeks; max 2.5 mg/kg/day; minimum trial to ascertain effectiveness is 12 weeks
Pediatric: <12 years: not recommended; ≥12 years: same as adult
  Azasan *Tab* 75*, 100*mg
  Imuran *Tab* 50*mg

▶ *nintedanib* (D) recommended dose is 150 mg bid, approximately 12 hours apart, with food; *Mild Hepatic Impairment (Child-Pugh Class A):* 100 mg bid, approximately 12 hours apart, with food; *Moderate or Severe Hepatic Impairment (Child-Pugh Class B or C):* not recommended; consider temporary dose reduction to 100 mg, treatment interruption, or discontinuation for management of adverse reactions; prior to initiation of treatment, perform a pregnancy test; monitor LFTs and bilirubin before and during treatment
Pediatric: <12 years: not established; ≥12 years: same as adult
  Ofev *Cap* 100, 150 mg
  Comment: Monitor liver enzymes. If elevated LFTs (3 <AST/ALT< 5 XULN) without severe liver damage, interrupt therapy or reduce dose to 100 mg bid. When liver enzymes return to baseline, restart at 100 mg bid and titrate up. Diarrhea, nausea, and vomiting have occurred with **Ofev**. Treat patients at first signs with adequate hydration and antidiarrheal medicine (e.g., *loperamide*) or anti-emetics. Discontinue **Ofev** if severe diarrhea, nausea, or vomiting persists despite symptomatic treatment. Gastrointestinal perforation has been reported. Use **Ofev** with caution when treating patients with recent abdominal surgery. Discontinue **Ofev** in patients who develop gastrointestinal perforation. Only use **Ofev** in patients with known risk of gastrointestinal perforation if the anticipated benefit outweighs the potential risk. Arterial thromboembolic events have been reported. Use caution when treating patients at higher cardiovascular risk including known coronary artery disease (CAD). Bleeding events have been reported. Use **Ofev** in patients with known bleeding risk only if anticipated benefit outweighs the potential risk. There are no human data to inform safety on the use of **Ofev** in pregnancy; however, based on animal studies and the mechanism of action, the use of **Ofev** in pregnancy can cause fetal harm (structural damage during organogenesis and embryo/fetal death). Advise patients of the potential risks to the developing fetus vs patient need/benefit and advise females of reproductive potential to use effective contraception. There is no information on the presence of *nintedanib* in human milk or effects on the breastfed infant; breastfeeding is not recommended. Safety and efficacy of **Ofev** have not been studied in patients with severe renal impairment and end-stage renal disease (ESRD). Decreased exposure has been noted in smokers which may alter the efficacy profile of **Ofev**. The most common adverse reactions (≥5%) are: diarrhea, nausea, abdominal pain, vomiting, liver enzyme elevation, decreased appetite, headache, weight decreased, and hypertension.

▷ **pirfenidone** (C) take with food at the same time each day; *Days 1-7:* 267 mg
3 x/day (801 mg/day); *Days 8-14:* 534 mg 3 x/day (1602 mg/day); *Days 15 and
ongoing:* 801 mg 3 x/day (2403 mg/day)
  Pediatric: <12 years: not established; ≥12 years: same as adult
    Esbriet *Gelcap:* 267, 801 mg
    Comment: Esberet (*pirfenidone*) is a pyridone. In the post-marketing setting,
    non-serious and serious cases of drug-induced liver injury, including severe
    liver injury with fatal outcomes, have been reported. Monitor ALT, AST,
    and bilirubin before and during treatment. Photosensitivity and rash have
    been noted with **Esbriet**. Avoid exposure to sunlight and sunlamps. **Esbriet**
    is not recommended for use in patients with severe hepatic impairment
    or patients with ESRD on dialysis. Advise patients to wear sunscreen and
    protective clothing. Nausea, vomiting, diarrhea, dyspepsia, gastroesophageal
    reflux disease, and abdominal pain have occurred with **Esbriet**. Temporary
    dosage reductions or discontinuations may be required for any of these
    ASEs. The most common adverse reactions (incidence ≥10%) have been,
    anorexia, gastro-esophageal reflux disease, abdominal pain, dyspepsia, nausea,
    vomiting, diarrhea, weight loss, URI, sinusitis, fatigue, headache, dizziness,
    insomnia, rash and arthralgia. Moderate (e.g., *ciprofloxacin*) and strong (e.g.,
    fluvoxamine) inhibitors of CYP1A2 increase systemic exposure of **Esbriet** and
    may alter the adverse reaction profile of **Esbriet**. Discontinue *fluvoxamine*
    prior to administration of **Esbriet** or reduce **Esbriet** dose to 267 mg 3 x/day
    (801 mg/day). Consider dosage reduction with use of *ciprofloxacin*. Decreased
    exposure has been noted in smokers which may alter the efficacy profile of
    Esbriet.

PYELONEPHRITIS: ACUTE

URINARY TRACT ANALGESIA

▷ **phenazopyridine** (B)(G) 95-200 mg q 6 hours prn; max 2 days
  Pediatric: <12 years: not recommended; ≥12 years: same as adult
    AZO Standard, Prodium, Uristat (OTC) *Tab:* 95 mg
    AZO Standard Maximum Strength (OTC) *Tab:* 97.5 mg
    Pyridium, Urogesic *Tab:* 100, 200 mg
    Urogesic *Tab:* 100, 200 mg

OUTPATIENT ANTI-INFECTIVE TREATMENT

Comment: Acute pyelonephritis can be treated with a single IM antibiotic
administration followed by a PO antibiotic regimen and close follow up. Example:
Rocephin 1 gm IM followed by **Bactrim DS,** *cephalexin, ciprofloxacin, levofloxacin,* or
loracarbef.

▷ **cephalexin** (B)(G) 1-4 gm/day in 4 divided doses x 10-14 days
  Pediatric: 25-50 mg/kg/day in 4 divided doses x 10-14 days; *see* Appendix CC.15.
  cephalexin (Keflex Suspension) *for dose by weight*
    Keflex *Cap:* 250, 333, 500, 750 mg; *Oral susp:* 125, 250 mg/5 ml (100, 200 ml)
    (strawberry)
▷ **ciprofloxacin** (C) 500 mg bid or 1000 mg XR once daily x 3-14 days
  Pediatric: <18 years: not recommended; ≥18 years: same as adult
    Cipro (G) *Tab:* 250, 500, 750 mg; *Oral susp:* 250, 500 mg/5 ml (100 ml)
    (strawberry)
    Cipro XR *Tab:* 500, 1000 mg ext-rel
    ProQuin XR *Tab:* 500 mg ext-rel

▷ *levofloxacin* (C) *Uncomplicated:* 500 mg once daily x 10 days; *Complicated:* 750 mg once daily x 10 days
Pediatric: <18 years: not recommended; ≥18 years: same as adult
    Levaquin *Tab:* 250, 500, 750 mg; *Oral soln:* 25 mg/ml (480 ml) (benzyl alcohol); *Inj conc:* 25 mg/ml for IV infusion after dilution for IV infusion (50, 100, 150 ml) (preservative-free)

▷ *loracarbef* (B) 400 mg bid x 14 days
Pediatric: 15 mg/kg/day in 2 divided doses x 14 days; *see* Appendix CC.27. *loracarbef* (Lorabid Suspension) *for dose by weight*
    Lorabid *Pulvule:* 200, 400 mg; *Oral susp:* 100 mg/5 ml (50, 100 ml); 200 mg/5 ml (50, 75, 100 ml) (strawberry bubble gum)

▷ *trimethoprim+sulfamethoxazole (TMP-SMX)* (D)(G) bid x 10 days
Pediatric: <2 months: not recommended; ≥2 months: 40 mg/kg/day of *sulfamethoxazole* in 2 divided doses x 10 days; *see Appendix CC.33. trimethoprim+ sulfamethoxazole* (Bactrim Suspension, Septra Suspension) *for dose by weight*
    Bactrim, Septra 2 tabs bid x 10 days
        Tab: trim 80 mg+sulfa 400 mg*
    Bactrim DS, Septra DS 1 tab bid x 10 days
        Tab: trim 160 mg+sulfa 800 mg*
    Bactrim Pediatric Suspension, Septra Pediatric Suspension
        Oral susp: trim 40 mg+sulfa 200 mg per 5 ml (100 ml) (cherry) (alcohol 0.3%)

PYELONEPHRITIS: ACUTE, COMPLICATED (ACP)

PARENTERAL CEPHALOSPORIN ANTIBACTERIAL+BETA-LACTIMASE INHIBITOR

▷ *ceftazidime+avibactam* (B) infuse dose over 2 hours; recommended duration of treatment: 5 to 4 days; *CrCl 31-50 mL/min:* 1.25 gm every 8 hours; *CrCl 16-30 mL/min:* 0.94 gm every 12 hours; *CrCl 6-15 mL/min:* 0.94 gm every 24 hours; *CrCl ≤5 mL/min:* 0.94 gm every 48 hours; both *ceftazidime* and *avibactam* are hemodializable; thus, administer **Avycaz** after hemodialysis on hemodialysis days
Pediatric: <18 years: not recommended; ≥18 years: same as adult
    Avycaz *Vial:* 2.5 gm, single-dose, pwdr for reconstitution, dilution, and IV infusion
    Comment: Avycaz 2.5 gm contains *ceftazidime* (a cephalosporin) 2 gm (equivalent to 2.635 gm of *ceftazidime pentahydrate/sodium carbonate powder*) and *avibactam* (a beta lactam inhibitor) 0.5 grams (equivalent to 0.551 grams of *avibactam sodium*). As only limited clinical safety and efficacy data for **Avycaz** are currently available, reserve **Avycaz** for use in patients who have limited or no alternative treatment options. To reduce the development of drug-resistant bacteria and maintain the effectiveness of **Avycaz** and other antibacterial drugs, **Avycaz** should be used only to treat infections that are proven or strongly suspected to be caused by susceptible bacteria. Seizures and other neurologic events may occur, especially in patients with renal impairment. Adjust dose in patients with renal impairment. Decreased efficacy in patients with baseline CrCl 30-≤50 mL/min. Monitor CrCl at least daily in patients with changing renal function and adjust the dose of **Avycaz** accordingly. Monitor for hypersensitivity reactions, including anaphylaxis and serious skin reactions. Cross-hypersensitivity may occur in patients with a history of penicillin allergy. If an allergic reaction occurs, discontinue **Avycaz**. Clostridioides difficile-associated diarrhea CDAD) has been reported with nearly all systemic antibacterial agents, including **Avycaz**. There are no adequate and well-controlled studies of **Avycaz**, *ceftazidime*, or

avibactam in pregnant females. *ceftazidime* is excreted in human milk in low concentrations. It is not known whether *avibactam* is excreted into human milk. There are no studies to inform effects on the breastfed infant.

PARENTERAL PENEM ANTIBACTERIAL+RENAL DEHYDROPEPTIDASE INHIBITOR+ BETA-LACTAMASE INHIBITOR

▷ *imipenem+cilastatin+relebactam* administer dose via IV infusion over 30 minutes every 6 hours; *CrCl ≥90 mL/min*: 1.25 gm/dose (*imipenem* 500 mg, *cilastatin* 500 mg, *relebactam* 250 mg); *CrCl 60-89 mL/min*: 1 gm/dose (*imipenem* 400 mg, *cilastatin* 400 mg, *relebactam* 200 mg); *CrCl 30-59 mL/min*: 0.75 gm/dose (*imipenem* 300 mg, *cilastatin* 300 mg, *relebactam* 150 mg); *CrCl 15-29 mL/min*: 0.5 gm/dose (*imipenem* 200 mg, *cilastatin* 200 mg, *relebactam* 100 mg); *ESRD/Dialysis*: 0.5 gm/dose (*imipenem* 200 mg, *cilastatin* 200 mg, *relebactam* 100 mg)

Pediatric: <18 years: not established; ≥18 years: same as adult

Recarbrio *Vial:* imipen 500 mg+cilast 500 mg+relebac 250 mg, single-dose, pwdr for reconstitution, dilution, and IV infusion

Comment: Recarbrio *(imipenem+cilastatin+relebactam)* is a fixed-dose triple combination of *imipenem* (a penem antibacterial), *cilastatin* (a renal dehydropeptidase inhibitor), and *relebactam* (a beta-lactamase inhibitor) indicated for the treatment of complicated urinary tract infection (cUTI), including pyelonephritis, and complicated intra-abdominal infection (cIAI) caused by susceptible gram-negative bacteria in patients who have limited or no alternative treatment options, hospital-acquired bacterial pneumonia (HABP), and ventilator-associated bacterial pneumonia (VABP) in adults. Avoid concomitant use of **Recarbrio** with *ganciclovir, valproic acid,* or *divalproex sodium*. Based on clinical reports on patients treated with imipenem/cilastatin plus relebactam 250 mg, the most frequent adverse reactions (incidence ≥2 %) have been diarrhea, nausea, headache, vomiting, alanine aminotransferase increased, aspartate aminotransferase increased, phlebitis/infusion site reactions, pyrexia, and hypertension. There are insufficient human data to establish whether there is a drug-associated risk for major birth defects, miscarriage, or adverse maternal or fetal outcomes with *imipenem, cilastatin,* or *relebactam* in pregnancy. However, embryonic loss has been observed in monkeys treated with *imipenem/cilastatin,* and fetal abnormalities have been observed in *relebactam*-treated mice; therefore, advise pregnant females of the potential risks to pregnancy and the fetus. There are insufficient data on the presence of *imipenem/cilastatin* and *relebactam* in human milk, and no data on the effects on the breastfed infant; However, *relebactam* is present in the milk of lactating rats and, therefore, developmental and health benefits of breastfeeding should be considered along with the mother's clinical need for **Recarbrio** and any potential adverse effects on the breastfed infant from **Recarbrio** or from the underlying maternal condition.

PARENTERAL AMINOGLYCOSIDE ANTIBACTERIAL

▷ *plazomicin* recommended dose is 15 mg/kg once every 24 hours by IV infusion over 30 minutes x 4-7 days in patients with CrCl ≥90 mL/min; *CrCl ≥60 to <90 mL/min*: 15 mg/kg once every 24 hours; *CrCl ≥30 to <60 mL/min*: 10 mg/kg every 24 hours; CrCl ≥15 to <30 mL/min: 10 mg/kg every 48 hours

Pediatric: <18 years: not recommended; ≥18 years: same as adult

Zemdri Injection *Vial:* 500 mg/10 ml (50 mg/ml) single-dose

Comment: Zemdri *(plazomicin)* is an aminoglycoside antibacterial for the treatment of complicated urinary tract infection (cUTI) including pyelonephritis. As <u>only</u> limited clinical safety and efficacy data are available, reserve **Zemdri** for use in patients who have limited <u>or</u> no alternative treatment options. Assess creatinine clearance in all patients prior to initiating therapy and daily during therapy. Adjustment of initial dose and therapeutic drug monitoring (TDM) is recommended in patients with renal impairment. There is insufficient information to recommend a dosing regimen in patients with CrCl <15 mL/min <u>or</u> on hemodialysis <u>or</u> continuous renal replacement therapy. For patients with CrCl ≥15 mL/min and <90 mL/min, TDM is recommended in order to avoid *plazomicin*-induced nephrotoxicity. Monitor *plazomicin* trough concentrations and adjust **Zemdri** as described in the mfr pkg insert. BBW: Aminoglycosides are associated with nephrotoxicity, ototoxicity, and neuromuscular blockade; therefore, administer **Zamdri** no faster than 30 minutes, monitor for adverse reactions, and stop the infusion if any of these adverse events occur. Aminoglycosides can cause fetal harm in pregnancy. There are <u>no</u> available data on the use of **Zamdri** in pregnancy to inform a drug-related risk of adverse developmental outcomes. *streptomycin*, an aminoglycoside, can cause total and irreversible in children whose mothers received *streptomycin* in pregnancy. There are <u>no</u> data on the presence of **Zemdri** in human milk <u>or</u> effects on the breastfed infant; therefore, potential risk/benefit should be discussed with the mother. The most common adverse reactions (incidence ≥1%) are decreased renal function, diarrhea, hypertension, headache, nausea, vomiting, and hypotension.

RABIES (LYSSAVIRUS)

PRE-EXPOSURE PROPHYLAXIS (PrEP) AND POST-EXPOSURE PROPHYLAXIS (PEP)

Comment: Have *epinephrine* 1:1000 readily available. Every exposure to possible rabies infection must be individually evaluated. Rabies vaccine and **Rabies Immune Globulin (Human) (HRIG)** should be given to all persons suspected of exposure to rabies with one exception: persons who have been previously immunized with rabies vaccine and have a confirmed adequate rabies antibody titer should receive <u>only</u> vaccine. Recommendations for use of passive and active immunization after exposure to an animal suspected of having rabies have been detailed by the Health Canada National Advisory Committee on Immunization19 and the U.S. Public Health Service Immunization Practices Advisory Committee (ACIP). HRIG should be used in conjunction with rabies vaccine and can be administered through the seventh day after the first dose of vaccine is administered. Beyond the seventh day, HRIG is <u>not</u> indicated since an antibody response to cell culture vaccine is presumed to have occurred. If the patient has previously received HRIG, and has a confirmed adequate rabies antibody titer, administer <u>only</u> the vaccine. HRIG should be administered as promptly as possible after exposure, but can be administered up to the eighth day after the first dose of vaccine is administered. Repeated doses of rabies immune globulin should <u>not</u> be administered once vaccine treatment has been initiated as this could prevent the full expression of active immunity expected from the rabies vaccine. Administer HRIG via IM injection <u>only</u>. Do <u>not</u> give intravenously. The recommended HRIG dose 20 IU/kg (0.133 ml/kg) of body weight administered at the time of the first vaccine dose. It may also be given through the seventh day after the first dose of vaccine is given. If anatomically feasible, up to one-half the HRIG dose should be thoroughly infiltrated in the area around the wound and the rest should be administered intramuscularly in the gluteal area <u>or</u> lateral thigh muscle using a separate syringe and needle. Because of risk of injury to the sciatic nerve, <u>only</u> the upper, outer quadrant should be used. **HRIG** should never be administered in the same syringe <u>or</u> needle <u>or</u> in the same anatomical site as vaccine. Because of interference with active antibody production, the recommended dose should not be exceeded. It is not known whether rabies immune globulin can cause fetal harm when administered to a pregnant female or can affect reproduction capacity. It should be administered in pregnancy only if clearly needed. Safety and effectiveness in the pediatric population have not been established.

PRE-EXPOSURE PROPHYLAXIS (PrEP)

Comment: Postpone pre-exposure prophylaxis during acute febrile illness or infection. Have *epinephrine* 1:1000 readily available.

▷ *rabies vaccine, human diploid cell [HDVC]* (C) *Infants and Young Children:* administer IM in the vastus lateralis; *All others:* administer IM in the deltoid; do not inject the vaccine into the gluteal area as administration in this area may result in lower neutralizing antibody titers; *Not previously immunized: Day 0,* administer 1 ml IM as soon as possible after exposure; then repeat on days 7, and 21 or 28; administer 1st dose with rabies immune globulin, human (HRIG); *Previously immunized:* only 2 doses are administered; Day 0, Administer 1 ml IM immediately after exposure and again 3 days later; no HRIG is needed

Imovax, RabAvert *Vial:* 2.5 IU/ml (1 ml) (2.5 IU of freeze-dried vaccine w. diluent) for IM injection after reconstitution (preservative-free)

Comment: Administer vaccine immediately after reconstitution. If not used, discard. It is also not known whether rabies vaccine can cause fetal harm when administered to a pregnant female or can affect reproductive capacity. Rabies vaccine 10 should be given to a pregnant woman only if potential benefits outweigh potential risks. All serious systemic neuroparalytic or anaphylactic reactions to a rabies vaccine should be immediately reported to VAERS at 1-800-822-7967 (http://vaers.hhs.gov) or Sanofi Pasteur at 1-800-VACCINE (1-800-822-2463).

POST-EXPOSURE PROPHYLAXIS (PEP)
Rabies Immune Globulin, Human (HRIG)

▷ *rabies immune globulin, human (HRIG)* (C) administer 20 IU/kg infiltrated into wound area as much as feasible, then remaining dose administered IM at site remote from vaccine administration

BayRab, KamRAB, Imogam Rabies HT *Vial:* 150 IU/ml (2, 10 ml)

Comment: Administer *rabies immune globulin, human (HRIG)* concurrently with a full course of rabies vaccine if the patient have not previously received the rabies vaccine and has confirmed adequate antibodies, administer only the vaccine.

HyperRAB S/D *Vial:* 300 IU/2 ml (2 ml); 1500 IU/10 ml (10 ml), single-dose

Comment: HyperRAB S/D is a high-potency rabies immunoglobulin.

Comment: If the patient has previously received rabies vaccine, and has a confirmed adequate rabies antibody titer, administer only the vaccine. Repeated dosing of *immune globulin, human (HRIG)* after administration of rabies vaccine may suppress the immune response to the vaccine. If the patient has not previously received rabies vaccine, administer **HRIG** concurrently with a full course of rabies vaccine. Defer live vaccine (measles, mumps, rubella) administration for 4 months. There are no data with **HRIG** use in pregnant females to inform a drug-associated risk. There is no information regarding the presence of HRIG in human milk or effect on the breastfed infant.

TETANUS PROPHYLAXIS VACCINE

See *Tetanus* for patients not vaccinated within the past 5 years.

RESPIRATORY SYNCYTIAL VIRUS (RSV)

PROPHYLAXIS

▷ *palivizumab* 15 mg/kg IM administered monthly throughout the RSV season
   Synagis *Vial:* 100 mg/ml

TREATMENT

See Bronchiolitis

 RESTLESS LEGS SYNDROME (RLS)

GAMMA AMINOBUTYRIC ACID ANALOGS

Comment: The gabapentinoids (*gabapentin* [**Gralise, Neurontin, Horizant**] and *pregabalin* [**Lyrica**]) have respiratory depression risk potential. Therefore, when co-prescribed with other CNS depressant agents, initiate the gabapentinoid at the lowest possible dose and monitor the patient for respiratory depression (especially elders and patients with compromised pulmonary function). Side effects include fatigue, somnolence/sedation, dizziness, vertigo, feeling drunk, headache, nausea, and dry mouth. To discontinue a gabapentinoid, withdraw gradually over 1 week or longer.

▷ *gabapentin* (C) 100 mg once daily x 1 day; then 100 mg bid x 1 day; then 100 mg tid thereafter; max 900 mg tid
   Gralise (C) initially 300 mg on Day 1; then 600 mg on Day 2; then 900 mg on Days 3-6; then 1200 mg on Days 7-10; then 1500 mg on Days 11-14; titrate up to 1800 mg on Day 15; take entire dose once daily with the evening meal; do not crush, split, or chew
   Pediatric: <12 years: not recommended; ≥12 years: same as adult
      Tab: 300, 600 mg
   Neurontin (G)(OTC) 100 mg daily x 1 day, then 100 mg bid x 1 day, then 100 mg tid continuously; max 900 mg tid
   Pediatric: <3 years: not recommended; 3-12 years: initially 10-15 mg/kg/day in 3 divided doses; max 12 hours between doses; titrate over 3 days; 3-4 years: titrate to 40 mg/kg/day; 5-12 years: titrate to 25-35 mg/kg/day; max 50 mg/kg/day

▷ *gabapentin enacarbil* (C) 600 mg once daily at about 5:00 PM; if dose not taken at recommended time, next dose should be taken the following day; swallow whole; take with food; *CrCl 30-59 mL/min:* 600 mg on Day 1, Day 3, and every day thereafter; *CrCl <30 mL/min* or on hemodialysis: not recommended
   Pediatric: <12 years: not recommended; ≥12 years: same as adult
   Horizant *Tab:* 300, 600 mg ext-rel

▷ *pregabalin* (*GABA analog*) (C)(V)
   Pediatric: <12 years: not recommended; ≥12 years: same as adult
   Lyrica initially 50 mg tid; may titrate to 100 mg tid within one week; max 600 mg divided tid; discontinue over 1 week
      Cap: 25, 50, 75, 100, 150, 200, 225, 300 mg; *Oral soln:* 20 mg/ml
   Lyrica CR *Tab:* usual dose: 165 mg once daily; may increase to 330 mg/day within 1 week; max 660 mg/day
      Tab: 82.5, 165, 330 mg ext-rel

DOPAMINE RECEPTOR AGONISTS

▷ *pramipexole dihydrochloride* (C)(G) initially 0.125 mg once daily 2-3 hours before bedtime; may double dose every 4-7 days; max 0.75 mg/day
   Pediatric: <12 years: not recommended; ≥12 years: same as adult
   Mirapex *Tab:* 0.125, 0.25*, 0.5*, 0.75*, 1*, 1.5*mg

▷ **ropinirole** (C) take once daily 1-3 hours prior to bedtime; initially 0.25 mg on days 1 and 2; then 0.5 mg on days 3-7; increase by 0.5 mg/day at 1 week intervals to 3 mg; max 4 mg/day
Pediatric: <12 years: not recommended; ≥12 years: same as adult
 Requip *Tab:* 0.25, 0.5, 1, 2, 3, 4, 5 mg

▷ **rotigotine** transdermal patch (C) apply to clean, dry, intact skin on abdomen, thigh, hip, flank, shoulder, or upper arm; initially 1 mg/24 Hrs patch once daily; may increase weekly by 1 mg/24 Hrs if needed; max 3 mg/24 Hrs once daily; rotate sites and allow 14 days before reusing site; if hairy, shave site at least 3 days before application to site; avoid abrupt cessation; reduce by 1 mg/24 Hrs every other day
Pediatric: <12 years: not recommended; ≥12 years: same as adult
 Neupro *Trans patch:* 1 mg/24 Hrs, 2 mg/24 Hrs, 3 mg/24 Hrs, 4 mg/24 Hrs, 6 mg/24 Hrs, 8 mg/24 Hrs (30/carton) (sulfites)

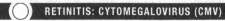

RETINITIS: CYTOMEGALOVIRUS (CMV)

Comment: *cidofovir* and *valganciclovir* are nucleoside analogs and prodrugs of *ganciclovir* indicated for the treatment of AIDS-related *cytomegalovirus* (CMV) retinitis and prevention of CMV disease in adult kidney, heart, and kidney-pancreas transplant patients at high risk, and for prevention of CMV disease in pediatric kidney and heart transplant patients at high risk. *Letermovir* is a CMV DNA terminase complex inhibitor indicated for prophylaxis of CMV infection and disease in adult CMV-seropositive recipients [R+] of an allogeneic hemato-poietic stem cell transplant (HSCT).

▷ **cidofovir** (C) administer via IV infusion over 1 hour; pre-treat with oral **probenecid** (2 gm, 3 hours prior to starting the *cidofovir* infusion and 1 gm, 2 and 8 hours after the infusion is ended) and 1 liter of IV NaCl should be infused immediately before each dose of *cidofovir* (a 2nd liter of NaCl should also be infused either during or after each dose of *cidofovir* if a fluid load is tolerable); *Induction:* 5 mg/kg once weekly for 2 consecutive weeks; *Maintenance:* 5 mg/kg once every 2 weeks; reduce to 3 mg/kg if serum creatinine (sCr) increases 0.3-0.4 mg/dL above baseline; discontinue if sCr increases to >0.5 mg/dL above baseline or if >3+ proteinuria develops
Pediatric: <12 years: not recommended; ≥12 years: same as adult
 Vistide *Vial:* 75 mg/ml (5 ml) (preservative-free)
Comment: *Cidofovir* is a nucleoside analog indicated for treatment of AIDS-related *cytomegalovirus* (CMV) retinitis.

▷ **valganciclovir** (C)(G) take with food; *Induction:* 900 mg bid x 21 days; *Maintenance:* 900 mg daily; *CrCl <60 mL/min:* reduce dose (see mfr pkg insert; hemodialysis or *CrCl <10 mL/min* not recommended (use **ganciclovir**)
Pediatric: <4 months: not recommended; 4 months-16 years: see mfr pkg insert for dosing calculation equation
 Valcyte *Tab:* 450 mg (preservative-free); *Oral pwdr for reconstitution:* 50 mg/ml (tutti-frutti)

CMV DNA TERMINASE VOMPLRX INHIBITOR

Comment: *Letermovir* is a CMV DNA terminase complex inhibitor indicated for prophylaxis of CMV infection and disease in adult CMV-seropositive recipients [R+] of an allogeneic hemato-poietic stem cell transplant (HSCT).

▷ **cidofovir** (C) administer via IV infusion over 1 hour; pre-treat with oral **probenecid** (2 gm, 3 hours prior to starting the *cidofovir* infusion and 1 gm, 2 and 8 hours after the infusion is ended) and 1 liter of IV NaCl should be infused immediately before each dose of cidofovir (a 2nd liter of NaCl should also be infused either during or after each dose of *cidofovir* if a fluid load is tolerable); Induction: 5 mg/kg once weekly for 2 consecutive weeks; Maintenance: 5 mg/kg once every 2 weeks; reduce to 3 mg/kg if serum creatinine (sCr) increases 0.3-0.4 mg/dL above baseline; discontinue if sCr increases to >0.5 mg/dL above baseline or if >3+ proteinuria develops

Pediatric: <12 years: not recommended; >12 years: same as adult

> **Vistide** *Vial:* 75 mg/ml (5 ml) (preservative-free)

Comment: *Cidofovir* is a nucleoside analog indicated for treatment of AIDS-related cytomegalovirus (CMV) retinitis.

▷ *letermovir* administer dose orally or as an IV infusion over 1 hour; dose is 480 mg once daily through 100 days post-transplant; if co-administered with *cyclosporine*, decrease the *letermovir* dose to 240 mg once daily

Pediatric: <18 years: not recommended; ≥18 years: same as adult

> **Prevymis** *Tab:* 240, 450 mg; *Vial:* 240 mg/12 ml (20 mg/ml), 480 mg/24 ml (20 mg/ml), single-dose

Comment: Closely monitor serum creatinine levels in patients with CrCL <50 mL/min using **Prevymis** injection for IV infusion. **Prevymis** is not recommended for patients with severe (Child-Pugh Class C) hepatic impairment. **Prevymis** is contraindicated with *pimozide*, ergot alkaloids, and *pitavastatin* and *simvastatin* when co-administered with *cyclosporine*. Most common adverse events (10%) have been nausea, diarrhea, vomiting, peripheral edema, cough, head ache, fatigue, and abdominal pain. No adequate human data are available to inform whether **Prevymis** poses a risk to pregnancy outcomes. It is not known whether *letermovir* is present in human breast milk or effects the breastfed infant.

▷ *valganciclovir* (C)(G) take with food; Induction: 900 mg bid x 21 days; Maintenance: 900 mg daily; CrCl <60 mL/min: reduce dose (see mfr pkg insert; hemodialysis or CrCl <10 mL/min not recommended (use ganciclovir)

Pediatric: <4 months: not recommended; 4 months-16 years: see mfr pkg insert for dosing calculation equation

> **Valcyte** *Tab:* 450 mg (preservative-free); Oral pwdr for reconstitution: 50 mg/ml (tutti-frutti)

RHEUMATOID ARTHRITIS (RA)

Injectable Acetaminophen *see Pain*
NSAIDs *see* Appendix J. NSAIDs online at https://connect.springerpub.com/content/reference-book/978-0-8261-7935-7/back-matter/part02/back-matter/bmatter10
Opioid Analgesics *see Pain*
Topical & Transdermal Analgesics *see Pain*
Parenteral Corticosteroids *see* Appendix M. Parenteral Corticosteroids
Oral Corticosteroids *see* Appendix L. Oral Corticosteroids
Topical Analgesic and Anesthetic Agents *see* Appendix I. Anesthetic Agents for Local Infiltration and Dermal/Mucosal Membrane Application online at https://connect.springerpub.com/content/reference-book/978-0-8261-7935-7/back-matter/part02/back-matter/bmatter9

TOPICAL AND TRANSDERMAL ANALGESICS

▷ *capsaicin* cream (B)(G) apply tid-qid prn to intact skin

Pediatric: <2 years: not recommended; ≥2 years: same as adult

> **Axsain** *Crm:* 0.075% (1, 2 oz)
> **Capsin** *Lotn:* 0.025, 0.075% (59 ml)
> **Capzasin-HP** (OTC) *Crm:* 0.075% (1.5 oz), 0.025% (45, 90 gm); *Lotn:* 0.075% (2 oz); 0.025% (45, 90 gm)
> **Capzasin-P** (OTC) *Crm:* 0.025% (1.5 oz); *Lotn:* 0.025% (2 oz)

Dolorac *Crm:* 0.025% (28 gm)
Double Cap (OTC) *Crm:* 0.05% (2 oz)
R-Gel *Gel:* 0.025% (15, 30 gm)
Zostrix (OTC) *Crm:* 0.025% (0.7, 1.5, 3 oz)
Zostrix HP (OTC) *Emol crm:* 0.075% (1, 2 oz)

▷ *capsaicin* 8% patch (B) apply up to 4 patches for one 60-minute application to clean dry skin; may prep area with topical anesthetic; wear non-latex gloves; patches may be cut to size/shape; treatment may be repeated every 3 months
Pediatric: <18 years: not recommended; ≥18 years: same as adult
Qutenza *Patch:* 8% 1640 mcg/cm (179 mg) (1 or 2 patches w. 1-50 gm tube cleansing gel/carton)

▷ *diclofenac sodium* (C; D ≥30 wks) apply qid prn to intact skin
Pediatric: <12 years: not established; ≥12 years: same as adult
Pennsaid 1.5% in 10 drop increments, dispense and rub into front, side, and back of knee: usually; 40 drops (40 mg) qid
Topical soln: 1.5% (150 ml)
Pennsaid 2% apply 2 pump actuations (40 mg) and rub into front, side, and back of knee bid
Topical soln: 2% (20 mg/pump actuation, 112 gm)
Solaraze Gel massage in to clean skin bid prn
Gel: 3% (50 gm) (benzyl alcohol)
Voltaren Gel (G)(OTC) apply qid prn to intact skin
Gel: 1% (100 gm)
Comment: *Diclofenac* is contraindicated with *aspirin* allergy. As with other NSAIDs, should be avoided in late pregnancy (≥30 weeks) because it may cause premature closure of the ductus arteriosus.

▷ *doxepin* (B) cream apply to affected area qid at intervals of at least 3-4 hours; max 8 days
Pediatric: <12 years: not recommended; >12 years: same as adult
Prudoxin *Crm:* 5% (45 gm)
Zonalon *Crm:* 5% (30, 45 gm)

▷ *pimecrolimus* 1% cream (C)(G) <2 years: not recommended; ≥2 years: apply to affected area bid; do not apply an occlusive dressing
Elidel *Crm:* 1% (30, 60, 100 gm)
Comment: *Pimecrolimus* is indicated for short-term and intermittent long-term use. Discontinue use when resolution occurs. Contraindicated if the patient is immunosuppressed. Change to the 0.1% preparation or if secondary bacterial infection is present.

▷ *trolamine salicylate* apply tid-qid
Pediatric: <2 years: not recommended; ≥2 years: same as adult
Mobisyl Creme *Crm:* 10% (100 gm)

ORAL SALICYLATE

▷ *indomethacin* (C) initially 25 mg bid-tid, increase as needed at weekly intervals by 25-50 mg/day; max 200 mg/day
Pediatric: <14 years: usually not recommended; >2 years, if risk warranted: 1-2 mg/kg/day in divided doses; max 3-4 mg/kg/day (or 150-200 mg/day, whichever is less; <14 years: ER cap not recommended
Cap: 25, 50 mg; *Susp;* 25 mg/5 ml (pineapple-coconut, mint) (alcohol 1%); *Supp:* 50 mg; *ER Cap:* 75 mg ext-rel
Comment: *Indomethacin* is indicated only for acute painful flares. Administer with food and/or antacids. Use lowest effective dose for shortest duration.

ORAL NSAID

See more **Oral NSAIDs** NSAIDs online at https://connect.springerpub.com/content/reference-book/978-0-8261-7935-7/back-matter/part02/back-matter/bmatter10

▷ *diclofenac* (C) take on empty stomach; 35 mg tid; Hepatic impairment: use lowest dose

Pediatric: <18 years: not recommended; ≥18 years: same as adult

Zorvolex *Gelcap:* 18, 35 mg

▷ *diclofenac sodium* (C)(G)

Pediatric: <18 years: not recommended; ≥18 years: same as adult

Voltaren 50 mg bid to qid or 75 mg bid or 25 mg qid with an additional 25 mg at HS if necessary

Tab: 25, 50, 75 mg ent-coat

Voltaren XR 100 mg once daily; rarely, 100 mg bid may be used

Tab: 100 mg ext-rel

Comment: *Diclofenac* is contraindicated with *aspirin* allergy. As with other NSAIDs, should be avoided in late pregnancy (≥30 weeks) because it may cause premature closure of the ductus arteriosus.

ORAL NSAID+PPI

▷ *esomeprazole+naproxen* (C)(G) 1 tab bid; use lowest effective dose for the shortest duration swallow whole; take at least 30 minutes before a meal

Pediatric: <18 not recommended; ≥18 years: same as adult

Vimovo *Tab:* nap 375 mg+eso 20 mg ext-rel; nap 500 mg+eso 20 mg ext-rel

Comment: Vimovo is indicated to improve signs/symptoms, and risk of gastric ulcer in patients at risk of developing NSAID-associated gastric ulcer.

COX-2 INHIBITORS

Comment: Cox-2 inhibitors are contraindicated with history of asthma, urticaria, and allergic-type reactions to *aspirin*, other NSAIDs, and sulfonamides, 3rd trimester of pregnancy, and coronary artery bypass graft (CABG) surgery.

▷ *celecoxib* (C)(G) 50-400 mg once daily-bid; max 800 mg/day

Pediatric: <18 years: not recommended; ≥18 years: same as adult

Celebrex *Cap:* 50, 100, 200, 400 mg

▷ *meloxicam* (C)(G)

Mobic <2 years, <60 kg: not recommended; ≥2, ≥60 kg: 0.125 mg/kg; max 7.5 mg once daily; ≥18 years: initially 7.5 mg once daily; max 15 mg once daily;

Hemodialysis: max 7.5 mg/day

Tab: 7.5, 15 mg; *Oral susp:* 7.5 mg/5 ml (100 ml) (raspberry)

Vivlodex <18 years: not established; ≥18 years: initially 5 mg qd; may increase to max 10 mg/day; Hemodialysis: max 5 mg/day

Cap: 5, 10 mg

JANUS KINASE (JAK) INHIBITOR (JAKI)

▷ *baricitinib* recommended dose is 2 mg once daily; avoid initiation or interrupt Olumiant in patients with Hgb <8 gm/dL and/or absolute lymphocyte count (ALC) <500 cells/mm³, and/or absolute neutropenia count (ANC)

Olumiant *Tab:* 2 mg <1000 cells/mm³.

Comment: Olumiant *(baricitinib)* is indicated for the treatment pf patients ≥18 years-of-age with moderate-to-severe active RA who have had an inadequate response to one or more TNF antagonist therapies. Olumiant may be used as monotherapy or in combination with *methotrexate* (MTX) or other DMARDs; Olumiant is not recommended in combination with other JAK inhibitors, biologic DMARDs, potent immunosuppressants (e.g., *azathioprine*, *cyclosporine*), or strong organic anion transporter 3 (OAT3) inhibitors (e.g., probenecid). Olumiant is not recommended with moderate-to-severe renal impairment or severe hepatic impairment. Adverse reactions (incidence ≥1%) include nausea, upper respiratory infections (URIs), herpes simplex, and herpes zoster. Laboratory assessments are recommended due to potential for changes in lymphocytes, neutrophils, hemoglobin, liver enzymes, and lipids. Avoid use of **Olumiant** with active serious infection including localized infection or tuberculosis (TB). If infection occurs, halt the **Olumiant** until the infection is controlled or resolved. Avoid use of **Olumiant** with live vaccines. Use caution in patients who might be at risk for thrombosis or gastrointestinal perforation. Limited human data on use of **Olumiant** in pregnancy are not sufficient to inform drug-associated risk for major birth defects or miscarriage. No information is available on the presence of **Olumiant** in human milk or effects on the breastfed infant.

▷ *tofacitinib* (C) 5 mg twice daily or 11 mg once daily; discontinue after 16 weeks if adequate therapeutic benefit is not achieved; use the lowest effective dose to maintain response; see mfr pkg insert for dosage adjustments for patients receiving CYP2C19 and/or CYP3A4 inhibitors; in patients with moderate or severe renal impairment or moderate hepatic impairment, and patients with lymphopenia, neutropenia, or anemia; use of **Xeljanz/Xeljanz XR** in patients with severe hepatic impairment is not recommended in any patient population
Comment: FDA has issued a MedWatch Alert to the public that a recent safety clinical trial found an increased risk of blood clots in the lungs and death when a 10 mg twice daily dose of *tofacitinib* (**Xeljanz, Xeljanz XR**) was administered to patients with rheumatoid arthritis (RA). FDA has not approved the 10 mg twice daily dosing regimen for RA; this dosing regimen is only approved for patients with ulcerative colitis (UC).
Pediatric: safety and efficacy not established
    Xeljanz *Tab:* 5 mg film-coat
    Xeljanz Oral Solution *Oral soln:* 1 mg/ml (240 ml) with press-in bottle adapter and oral dosing syringe (no latex)
    Xeljanz XR *Tab:* 11 mg film-coat
Comment: **Xeljanz** is indicated for moderate-to-severe RA as monotherapy in patients who have inadequate response or intolerance to *methotrexate* (MTX) and/or in combination with other non-biologic DMARDs.
Use **Xeljanz** with caution in patients that may be at increased risk for gastrointestinal perforation. The most common adverse events associated with **Xeljanz** treatment are diarrhea, elevated cholesterol level, headache, herpes zoster (shingles), increased blood creatine phosphokinase, nasopharyngitis, rash, and upper respiratory tract infection (URI). Avoid use of **Xeljanz/Xeljanz XR** during an active serious infection, including localized infection. Patients treated with **Xeljanz** are at increased risk for developing serious infections that may lead to hospitalization or death. **Xeljanz** has a BBW for serious infections (e.g., opportunistic infections) and malignancy (e.g., lymphoma). Use of **Xeljanz** in combination with biological therapies or with potent immunosuppressants, such as *azathioprine* and *cyclosporine*, is not recommended. Avoid live vaccine administration during treatment with **Xeljanz**. Prior to starting **Xeljanz**, perform a test for latent tuberculosis; if it is positive, start treatment for tuberculosis latent tuberculosis test is negative. Recommend lab monitoring due to potential for changes in lymphocytes, neutrophils, hemoglobin, liver enzymes, and lipids. Do not initiate **Xeljanz** if absolute lymphocyte count <500 cells/mm³, an absolute neutrophil count (ANC) <1000 cells/mm3 or Hgb <9 gm/dL. The safety and effectiveness of **Xeljanz/Xeljanz XR** in pediatric patients have not been established. Available data with **Xeljanz** use in pregnancy are insufficient to establish a drug associated risk of major birth defects, miscarriage, or adverse maternal or fetal outcomes. In animal reproduction studies, fetocidal, and teratogenic effects were noted. There is a pregnancy exposure registry that monitors pregnancy outcomes in females exposed

to **Xeljanz/Xeljanz XR** during pregnancy. Consider pregnancy planning and prevention for females of reproductive potential. Patients should be encouraged to enroll in the **Xeljanz/Xeljanz XR** pregnancy registry if they become pregnant. To enroll or obtain information from the registry, patients can call the toll free number 1-877-311-8972. There are no data on the presence of *tofacitinib* in human milk or the effects on a breastfed infant; however, patients should be advised not to breastfeed.

▷ *upadacitinib* 15 mg once daily; may be used as monotherapy or in combination with *methotrexate* (MTX) or other nonbiologic DMARDs; avoid initiation or interrupt **Rinvoq** if absolute lymphocyte count is <500 cells/mm^3, absolute neutrophil count <1000 cells/mm^3, or Hgb <8 gm/dL.

Pediatric: <18 years: not established; ≥18 years: same as adult

Rinvoq Extended-Release Tablets *Tab:* 15 mg ext-rel

Comment: **Rinvoq** *(upadacitinib)* is a Janus kinase (JAK) inhibitor for the treatment of adult patients with moderate-to-severe active RA who have had an inadequate response or intolerance to *methotrexate* (MTX). Use of **Rinvoq** in combination with other JAK inhibitors, biologic DMARDs, or with potent immunosuppressants such as *azathioprine* and *cyclosporine* is not recommended. Use of **Rinvoq** in patients with severe hepatic impairment (Child-Pugh Class C) is not recommended. Co-administration of **Rinvoq** with strong CYP3A4 inducers (e.g., *rifampin*) is not recommended. Use with caution in patients receiving chronic treatment with strong CYP3A4 inhibitors (e.g., *ketoconazole*). Avoid use of **Rinvoq** with live vaccines. Serious infections leading to hospitalization or death, including tuberculosis and bacterial, invasive fungal, viral, and other opportunistic infections, have occurred in patients receiving **Rinvoq**. Avoid use of **Rinvoq** in patients with active, serious infection, including localized infection. If a serious infection develops, interrupt **Rinvoq** until the infection is controlled. Prior to starting **Rinvoq**, test for latent tuberculosis; if the test is positive, start treatment for tuberculosis. Monitor all patients for active tuberculosis during treatment, even if the initial latent tuberculosis testis negative. Lymphoma and other malignancies have been observed in patients treated with **Rinvoq**. Thrombosis, including deep vein thrombosis, pulmonary embolism, and arterial thrombosis, have occurred in patients treated with Janus kinase inhibitors (JAKIs) used to treat inflammatory conditions. Consider risk/benefit prior to initiating **Rinvoq** in patients with a known malignancy, patients who may be at increased risk of thrombosis or gastrointestinal perforation. Monitor for potential changes in lymphocytes, neutrophils, Hgb, liver enzymes, and lipids. **Rinvoq** may cause embryo/fetal toxicity; therefore, advise females of reproductive potential to use effective contraception during treatment and for 4 weeks following the final dose. Advise lactating women that breastfeeding is not recommended during treatment with *upadacitinib*, and for 6 days (approximately 10 half-lives) after the last dose.

DISEASE MODIFYING ANTI-RHEUMATIC DRUGS (DMARDs)

Comment: DMARDs are first-line treatment options for RA. DMARDs include penicillamine, gold salts (*auranofin, aurothio-glucose*), immunosuppressants, and *hydroxychloroquine*. The DMARDs reduce ESR, reduce RF, and favorably affect the outcome of RA. Immunosuppressants may require 6 weeks to affect benefits and 6 months for full improvement.

▷ *auranofin (gold salt)* (C) 3 mg bid or 6 mg once daily; if inadequate response after 6 months, increase to 3 mg tid

Pediatric: <12 years: not recommended; ≥12 years: same as adult

Ridaura *Vial:* 100 mg/20 ml

▷ *azathioprine* (D) 1 mg/kg/day in a single or divided doses; may increase by 0.5 mg/kg/day q 4 weeks; max 2.5 mg/kg/day; minimum trial to ascertain effectiveness is 12 weeks
Pediatric: <12 years: not recommended; ≥12 years: same as adult
  Azasan *Tab* 75*, 100*mg
  Imuran *Tab* 50*mg

▷ *cyclosporine (immunosuppressant)* (C) 1.25 mg/kg bid; may increase after 4 weeks by 0.5 mg/kg/day; then adjust at 2 week intervals; max 4 mg/kg/day; administer with meals
Pediatric: <12 years: not recommended; ≥12 years: same as adult
  Neoral *Cap:* 25, 100 mg (alcohol)
  Neoral Oral Solution *Oral soln:* 100 mg/ml (50 ml) may dilute in room temperature apple juice or orange juice (alcohol)
  Comment: **Neoral** is indicated for RA unresponsive to *methotrexate* (MTX).

▷ *hydroxychloroquine* (C) 400-600 mg/day
Pediatric: <12 years: not recommended; ≥12 years: same as adult
  Plaquenil *Tab:* 200 mg
  Comment: May require several weeks to achieve beneficial effects. If no improvement in 6 months, discontinue.

▷ *leflunomide* (X)(G) initially 100 mg once daily x 3 days; maintenance dose 20 mg once daily; max 20 mg daily
Pediatric: <18 years: not recommended; ≥18 years: same as adult
  Arava *Tab:* 10, 20, 100 mg
  Comment: **Arava** is contraindicated with breastfeeding.

▷ *methotrexate* (MTX) (X) 7.5 mg x 1 dose per week or 2.5 mg x 3 at 12 hour intervals once a week; max 20 mg/week; therapeutic response begins in 3-6 weeks; administer *methotrexate* (MTX) injection SC only into the abdomen or thigh
Pediatric: <2 years: not recommended; ≥2 years: 10 mg/m² once weekly; max 20 mg/m²
  Rasuvo *Autoinjector:* 7.5 mg/0.15 ml, 10 mg/0.20 ml, 12.5 mg/0.25 ml, 15 mg/0.30 ml, 17.5 mg/0.35 ml, 20 mg/0.40 ml, 22.5 mg/0.45 ml, 25 mg/0.50 ml, 27.5 mg/0.55 ml, 30 mg/0.60 ml (solution concentration for SC injection is 50 mg/ml)
  Rheumatrex *Tab:* 2.5*mg (5, 7.5, 10, 12.5, 15 mg/week, 4/card unit-of-use dose pack)
  Trexall *Tab:* 5*, 7.5*, 10*, 15*mg (5, 7.5, 10, 12.5, 15 mg/week, 4/card unit-of-use dose pack)
  Comment: *methotrexate* (MTX) is contraindicated with immunodeficiency, blood dyscrasias, alcoholism, and chronic liver disease.

▷ *penicillamine* administer on an empty stomach, at least 1 hour before meals or 2 hours after meals, and at least 1 hour apart from any other drug, food, milk, antacid, zinc or iron-containing preparation; maintenance dosage must be individualized, and may require adjustment during the course of treatment. *initially,* a single daily dose of 125-250 mg; then, increase at 1-3 month intervals by 125-250 mg/day, as patient response and tolerance indicate; if a satisfactory remission of symptoms is achieved, the dose associated with the remission should be continued as the patient's maintenance therapy; if there is no improvement, and there are no signs of potentially serious toxicity after 2-3 months of treatment with doses of 500-750 mg/day, increase by 250 mg/day at 2-3 month intervals until a satisfactory remission occurs or signs of toxicity develop; if there is no discernible improvement after 3-4 months of treatment with 1000-1500 mg/day, discontinue **Cuprimine**. Changes in maintenance dosage levels may not be reflected clinically or in the erythrocyte sedimentation rate (ESR) for 2-3 months after each dosage adjustment.

Cuprimine *Cap:* 125, 250 mg
Depen: 250 mg
Comment: The use of *penicillamine* has been associated with fatalities due to certain diseases such as aplastic anemia, agranulocytosis, thrombocytopenia, Goodpasture's syndrome, and myasthenia gravis. Because of the potential for serious hematological and renal adverse reactions to occur at any time, routine urinalysis, white and differential blood cell count, hemoglobin, and direct platelet count must be checked twice weekly, together with monitoring of the patient's skin, lymph nodes and body temperature, during the first month of therapy, every 2 weeks for the next 5 months, and monthly thereafter. Patients should be instructed to report promptly the development of signs and symptoms of granulocytopenia and/or thrombocytopenia, such as fever, sore throat, chills, bruising or bleeding; the above laboratory studies should then be promptly repeated.

▷ *sulfasalazine* (C; D in 2nd, 3rd)(G) initially 0.5 gm once daily bid; gradually increase every 4 days; usual maintenance 2-3 gm/day in equally divided doses at regular intervals; max 4 gm/day
Pediatric: <6 years: not recommended; 6-16 years: initially 1/4 to 1/3 of maintenance dose; increase weekly; maintenance 30-50 mg/kg/day in 2 divided doses at regular intervals; max 2 gm/day; >16 years: same as adult
Azulfidine *Tab:* 500 mg
Azulfidine EN *Tab:* 500 mg ent-coat

TUMOR NECROSIS FACTOR (TNF) BLOCKERS

▷ *adalimumab* (B) 40 mg SC once every other week; may increase to once weekly without *methotrexate* (MTX); administer in abdomen or thigh; rotate sites; 2-17 years, supervise first dose
Pediatric: <2 years, <10 kg: not recommended; 10-<15 kg: 10 mg every other week; 15-<30 kg: 20 mg every other week; ≥30 kg: 40 mg every other week
Humira *Prefilled pen (Humira Pen):* 40 mg/0.4 ml, 40 mg/0.8 ml, 80 mg/0.8 ml, single-dose; *Prefilled glass syringe:* 10 mg/0.1 ml, 10 mg/0.2 ml, 20 mg/0.2 ml, 20 mg/0.4 ml, 40 mg/0.4 ml. 40 mg/0.8 ml, 80 mg/0.8 ml, single-dose; *Vial:* 40 mg/0.8 ml, single dose, institutional use only (preservative-free)
Comment: **Humira** may be used with *methotrexate* (MTX), DMARDs, corticosteroids, salicylates, NSAIDs, or analgesics.

▷ *adalimumab-adbm* (B) initially 80 SC; then, 40 mg SC every other week starting one week after initial dose; inject into thigh or abdomen; rotate sites
Pediatric: <18 years: not recommended; ≥18 years: same as adult
Cyltezo *Prefilled syringe:* 40 mg/0.8 ml single-dose (preservative-free)
Comment: **Cyltezo** is biosimilar to **Humira** (*adalimumab*).

▷ *adalimumab-afzb* 40 mg SC every other week; some patients with RA not receiving *methotrexate* (MTX) may benefit from increasing the frequency to 40 mg SC every week
Abrilada *Prefilled pen:* 40 mg/0.8 ml, single-dose; *Prefilled syringe:* 40 mg/0.8 ml, 20 mg/0.4 ml, 10 mg/0.2 ml, single-dose; (for institutional use only) (preservative-free)
Comment: **Abrilada** is biosimilar to **Humira** (*adalimumab*).

▷ *adalimumab-bwwd Initial Dose (Day 1):* 160 mg SC; *Second Dose: two weeks later (Day 15):* 80 mg SC; *Two weeks later (Day 29):* begin maintenance dose of 40 mg every other week
Hadlima *Prefilled autoinjector:* 40 mg/0.8 ml, single-dose (Hadlima PushTouch); *Prefilled syringe:* 40 mg/0.8 ml, single-dose
Comment: **Hadlima** is biosimilar to **Humira** (*adalimumab*).

▷ *certolizumab pegol* (B) 400 mg SC on day 1, at week 2, and at week 4; then 200 mg every other week; rotate sites

Pediatric: <12 years: not recommended; ≥12 years: same as adult

Cimzia *Vial:* 200 mg single-dose w. supplies (2/pck, 2, 6/starter pck); *Prefilled syringe:* 200 mg single-dose w. supplies (2/pck, 2, 6/starter pck) (preservative-free)

▶ *etanercept* (B) 25 mg SC twice weekly, 72-96 hours apart <u>or</u> 50 mg SC weekly; rotate sites

Pediatric: <4 years: not recommended; 4-17 years: 0.4 mg/kg SC twice weekly, 72-96 hours apart (max 25 mg/dose) <u>or</u> 0.8 mg/kg SC weekly (max 50 mg/dose)

Enbrel *Vial:* 25 mg pwdr for SC injection after reconstitution (4/carton w. supplies) (preservative-free; diluent contains benzyl alcohol); *Prefilled syringe:* 50 mg/ml (preservative-free); *SureClick autoinjector:* 50 mg/ml (preservative-free)

Comment: *Etanercept* reduces pain, morning stiffness, and swelling. May be administered in combination with *methotrexate* (MTX). Live vaccines should <u>not</u> be administered concurrently. Do <u>not</u> administer with active infection.

▶ *etanercept-ykro* 50 mg SC once weekly

Pediatric: <4 years: not established; ≥4 years, ≥63 kg, 138 lbs: same as adult

Eticovo *Prefilled syringe:* 25 mg/0.5 ml, 50 mg/ml solution, single-dose

Comment: **Eticovo** is biosimilar to **Enbrel** (*etanercept*).

▶ *golimumab* (B) administer SC <u>or</u> IV infusion (in combination with *methotrexate* [MTX])

Pediatric: <18 years: not recommended; ≥18 years: same as adult

Simponi 50 mg SC once monthly; rotate sites

Prefilled syringe, SmartJect autoinjector: 50 mg/0.5 ml, single-use (preservative-free)

Simponi Aria 2 mg/kg IV infusion week 0 and week 4; then every 8 weeks thereafter

Vial: 50 mg/4 ml, single-use, soln for IV infusion after dilution (latex-free, preservative-free)

Comment: Corticosteroids, non-biologic DMARDs, and/or NSAIDs may be continued during treatment with *golimumab*.

▶ *infliximab* must be refrigerated at 2°C to 8°C (36°F to 46°F); administer dose intravenously over a period of <u>not</u> less than 2 hours; do <u>not</u> use beyond the expiration date as this product contains no preservative; 5 mg/kg at 0, 2, and 6 weeks, then every 8 weeks.

Pediatric: <6 years: not studied; ≥6-17 years: mg/kg at 0, 2 and 6 weeks, then every 8 weeks; ≥18 years: same as adult

Remicade *Vial:* 100 mg pwdr for reconstitution to 10 ml administration volume, single-dose (presrvative-free)

Comment: Use *infliximab* concomitantly with *methotrexate* (MTX) when there has been insufficient response to *methotrexate* (MTX) alone. **Remicade** is indicated to reduce signs and symptoms, and induce and maintain clinical remission, in adults and children ≥6 years-of-age with moderately to severely active disease who have had an inadequate response to conventional therapy <u>and</u> reduce the number of draining enterocutaneous and rectovaginal fistulas, and maintain fistula closure, in adults with fistulizing disease. Common adverse effects associated with **Remicade** included abdominal pain, headache, pharyngitis, sinusitis, and upper respiratory infections. In addition, **Remicade** might increase the risk for serious infections, including tuberculosis, bacterial sepsis, and invasive fungal infections. Available data from published literature on the use of *infliximab* products during pregnancy have <u>not</u> reported a clear association with *infliximab* products and adverse pregnancy outcomes. *Infliximab* products cross the placenta and infants exposed *in utero* should <u>not</u> be administered live vaccines for at least 6 months after birth. Otherwise, the infant may be at increased risk of infection, including disseminated infection which can become fatal. Available information is insufficient to inform the amount of *infliximab* products present in human milk <u>or</u> effects on the breastfed infant.

▷ *infliximab-abda* (B)
Renflexis *Vial:* 100 mg pwdr for reconstitution to 10 ml administration volume, single-dose
Comment: **Renflexis** is biosimilar to **Remicade**. (*infliximab*).

▷ *infliximab-dyyb* (B)
Inflectra *Vial:* 100 mg pwdr for reconstitution to 10 ml administration volume, single-dose
Comment: **Inflectra** is biosimilar to **Remicade**. (*infliximab*).

▷ *infliximab-axxq* (B)
Avsola *Vial:* 100 mg pwdr in a 20 ml single-dose vial, for reconstitution, dilution, and IV infusion
Comment: **Avsola** is biosimilar to **Remicade** (*infliximab*). **Avsola** is indicated for the treatment of RA, in combination with *methotrexate*, for reducing signs and symptoms, inhibiting the progression of structural damage, and improving physical function in patients with moderate-to-severe active disease. See *infliximab* (**Remicade**) above for prescribing information.

▷ *infliximab-qbtx* (B)
Ixifi *Vial:* 100 mg pwdr for reconstitution to 10 ml administration volume, single-dose
Comment: **Ixifi** is biosimilar to **Remicade**. (*infliximab*).

Interleukin-1 Receptor Antagonist

▷ *anakinra (interleukin-1 receptor antagonist)* (B) 100 mg SC once daily; discard any unused portion
Pediatric: <12 years: not recommended; ≥12 years: same as adult
Kineret *Prefilled syringe:* 100 mg/single-dose syringe (7, 28/pck) (preservative-free)

Interleukin-6 Receptor Antagonists

▷ *sarilumab* 200 mg SC every 2 weeks on the same day; if necessary, the dosage can be reduced 150 mg every 2 weeks to manage potential laboratory abnormalities, such as neutropenia, thrombocytopenia, and liver enzyme elevations; SC injections may be self-administered
Pediatric: <18 years: not recommended; ≥18 years: same as adult
Kevzara *Prefilled syringe:* 150, 200 mg (1.4 ml, single-use)
Comment: *Sarilumab* is a human monoclonal antibody that binds to the interleukin-6 receptor (IL-6R), and has been shown to inhibit IL-6R-mediated signaling. IL-6 is a cytokine in the body that, in excess and over time, can contribute to the inflammation associated with RA. **Kevzara** received FDA approval in May, 2017 for use in patients with active moderate-to-severe rheumatoid arthritis (RA) in adults who have had an inadequate response or intolerance to one or more disease modifying antirheumatic drugs (DMARDs). **Kevzara** may be used as monotherapy or in combination with *methotrexate* (MTX) or other conventional DMARDs. Monitor patient for dose related laboratory changes including elevated LFTs, neutropenia, and thrombocytopenia. **Kevzara** should not be initiated in patients with an absolute neutrophil count (ANC) <2000/mm³, platelet count <150,000/mm³, or liver transaminases above 1.5 times the upper limit of normal (ULN). Registration in the Pregnancy Exposure Registry (1-877-311-8972) is encouraged for monitoring pregnancy outcomes in women exposed to **Kevzara** during pregnancy. Negative side effects of **Kevzara** should be reported to the FDA at www.fda.gov/medwatch or call 1-800-FDA-1088 or call Sanofi-Aventis at 1-800-633-1610. The limited available data with **Kevzara** in pregnant females are not sufficient to determine whether there is a drug-associated risk for major birth defects and miscarriage. Monoclonal antibodies, such as *sarilumab*, are actively transported across the placenta during the third trimester of pregnancy and may

affect immune response in the infant exposed *in utero*. It is not known whether *sarilumab* passes into breast milk; therefore, breastfeeding is not recommended while using **Kevzara**.

▷ *tocilizumab* (**B**) *IV Infusion:* administer over 1 hour; do not administer as bolus or IV push; *Adults, PJIA, and SJIA, ≥30 kg:* dilute to 100 mL in 0.9% or 0.45% NaCl. *PJIA and SJIA, <30 kg:* dilute to 50 mL in 0.9% or 0.45% NaCl.

    Adults: IV Infusion: Whether used in combination with DMARDs or as monotherapy, the recommended IV infusion starting dose is 4 mg/kg IV every 4 weeks followed by an increase to 8 mg/kg IV every 4 weeks based on clinical response; Max 800 mg per infusion in RA patients; *SC Administration:* ≥100 kg: 162 mg SC once weekly on the same day; <100 kg: 162 mg SC every other week on the same day followed by an increase according to clinical response; SC injections may be self-administered

    Pediatric: <2 years: not recommended; ≥2 years: weight-based dosing according to diagnosis: *PJIA:* ≥30 kg: 8 mg/kg SC every 4 weeks; <30 kg: 10 mg/kg SC every 4 weeks; *SJIA:* ≥30 kg: 8 mg/kg SC every 2 weeks; <30 kg: 12 mg/kg SC every 2 weeks

    Actemra *Vial:* 80 mg/4 ml, 200 mg/10 ml, 400 mg/20 ml, single-use, for IV infusion after dilution; *Prefilled syringe:* 162 mg (0.9 ml, single-dose)

Comment: *Tocilizumab* is an interleukin-6 receptor-α inhibitor indicated for use in moderate-to-severe rheumatoid arthritis (RA) that has not responded to conventional therapy, and also for some subtypes of juvenile idiopathic arthritis (JIA). **Actemra** may be used alone or in combination with *methotrexate* (MTX) and in RA, other DMARDs may be used. Monitor patient for dose related laboratory changes including elevated LFTs, neutropenia, and thrombocytopenia. **Actemra** should not be initiated in patients with an absolute neutrophil count (ANC) below 2000 per mm³, platelet count below 100,000 per mm³, or who have ALT or AST above 1.5 times the upper limit of normal (ULN). Registration in the Pregnancy Exposure Registry (1-877-311-8972) is encouraged for monitoring pregnancy outcomes in women exposed to **Actemra** during pregnancy. The limited available data with **Actemra** in pregnant females are not sufficient to determine whether there is a drug-associated risk for major birth defects and miscarriage. Monoclonal antibodies, such as *tocilizumab*, are actively transported across the placenta during the third trimester of pregnancy and may affect immune response in the infant exposed *in utero*. It is not known whether *tocilizumab* passes into breast milk; therefore, breastfeeding is not recommended while using **Actemra**.

Selective Co-stimulation Modulator

▷ *abatacept* (**C**) administer as an IV infusion over 30 minutes at weeks 0, 2, and 4; then every 4 weeks thereafter; <60 kg, administer 500 mg/dose; 60-100 kg, administer 750 mg/dose; >100 kg, administer 1 gm/dose

Pediatric: <6 years: not recommended; 6-17 years: administer as an IV infusion over 30 minutes at weeks 0, 2, and 4; then every 4 weeks thereafter; <75 kg, administer 10 mg/kg; same as adult (max 1 gm)

    Orencia *Vial:* 250 mg pwdr for IV infusion after reconstitution (silicone-free) (preservative-free); *Prefilled syringe:* 125 mg/ml soln for SC injection (preservative-free); *ClickJect Autoinjector:* 125 mg/ml soln for SC injection

CD20 ANTIBODY

▷ *rituximab* (**C**) administer corticosteroid 30 minutes prior to each infusion; concomitant *methotrexate* (MTX) therapy, administer a 1000 mg IV infusion at 0 and 2 weeks; then every 24 weeks or based on response, but not sooner than every 16 weeks.

Pediatric: <6 years: not recommended; ≥6 years: same as adult

Rituxan *Vial:* 100 mg/10 ml (10 mg/ml), 50 mg/50 ml (10 mg/ml). single-use (preservative-free)

INTRA-ARTICULAR INJECTION

▷ **sodium hyaluronate** 20 mg as intra-articular injection weekly x 5 weeks
  Pediatric: <12 years: not recommended; ≥12 years: same as adult
    Hyalgan *Prefilled syringe:* 20 mg/2 ml
  Comment: Remove joint effusion and inject with **lidocaine** if possible before injecting **Hyalgan**.

 RHINITIS/SINUSITIS: ALLERGIC

see Appendix AA. Drugs for the Management of Allergy, Cough, and Cold Symptoms online at https://connect.springerpub.com/content/reference-book/978-0-8261-7935-7/back-matter/part02/back-matter/bmatter27
Parenteral Corticosteroids *see* Appendix M. Parenteral Corticosteroids
Oral Corticosteroids *see* Appendix L. Oral Corticosteroids

Comment: The Joint Task Force on Practice Parameters, which comprises representatives of the American Academy of Allergy, Asthma and Immunology (AAAAI) and the American College of Allergy, Asthma and Immunology (ACAAI), has provided guidance to healthcare providers on the initial pharmacologic treatment of seasonal allergic rhinitis in patients aged ≥12 years. For initial treatment of seasonal allergic rhinitis in persons aged ≥12 years: routinely prescribe monotherapy with an intranasal corticosteroid rather than an intranasal corticosteroid in combination with an oral antihistamine. For initial treatment of seasonal allergic rhinitis in persons aged ≥15 years: recommend an intranasal corticosteroid over a leukotriene. For initial treatment of seasonal allergic rhinitis in persons aged ≥15 years: recommend an intranasal corticosteroid over a leukotriene receptor antagonist. For initial treatment of moderate-to-severe seasonal allergic rhinitis in persons aged ≥12 years: recommend a combination of an intranasal corticosteroid and an intranasal antihistamine.

SECOND-GENERATION ANTIHISTAMINES

Comment: The following drugs are second-generation antihistamines. As such they minimally sedating, much less so than the first generation antihistamines. All antihistamines are excreted into breast milk.

▷ **cetirizine** (C)(OTC)(G) initially 5-10 mg once daily; 5 mg once daily; ≥65 years: use with caution
  Pediatric: <6 years: not recommended; ≥6 years: same as adult
    cetirizine *Cap:* 10 mg
    Children's Zyrtec Chewable *Chew tab:* 5, 10 mg (grape)
    Children's Zyrtec Allergy Syrup *Syr:* 1 mg/ml (4 oz) (grape, bubble gum) (sugar-free, dye-free)
    Zyrtec *Tab:* 10 mg
    Zyrtec Hives Relief *Tab:* 10 mg
    Zyrtec Liquid Gels *Liq gel:* 10 mg
▷ **desloratadine** (C)
    Clarinex 1/2-1 tab once daily
  Pediatric: <6 years: not recommended; ≥6 years: same as adult
    Tab: 5 mg
    Clarinex RediTabs 5 mg once daily
  Pediatric: <6 years: not recommended; 6-12 years: 2.5 mg once daily; ≥12 years: same as adult
    ODT: 2.5, 5 mg (tutti-frutti) (phenylalanine)
    Clarinex Syrup 5 mg (10 ml) once daily

Pediatric: <6 months: not recommended; 6-11 months: 1 mg (2 ml) once daily; 1-5 years: 1.25 mg (2.5 ml) once daily; 6-11 years: 2.5 mg (5 ml) once daily; ≥12 years: same as adult

  Syr: 0.5 mg per ml (4 oz) (tutti-frutti) (phenylalanine)

Desloratadine ODT 1 tab once daily

Pediatric: <6 years: not recommended; 6-11 years: 1/2 tab once daily; ≥12 years: same as adult

  ODT: 5 mg

▷ *fexofenadine* **(C)(OTC)(G)** 60 mg once daily-bid or 180 mg once daily; *CrCl <90 mL/min:* 60 mg once daily

Pediatric: <6 months: not recommended; 6 months-2 years: 15 mg bid; *CrCl ≤90 mL/min:* 15 mg once daily; 2-11 years: 30 mg bid; *CrCl ≤90 mL/min:* 30 mg once daily; ≥12 years: same as adult

  Allegra *Tab:* 30, 60, 180 mg film-coat

  Allegra Allergy *Tab:* 60, 180 mg film-coat

  Allegra ODT *ODT:* 30 mg (phenylalanine)

  Allegra Oral Suspension *Oral susp:* 30 mg/5 ml (6 mg/ml) (4 oz)

▷ *levocetirizine* **(B)(OTC)(G)** administer dose in the PM; *Seasonal Allergic Rhinitis:* <2 years: not recommended; may start at ≥2 years; *Chronic Idiopathic Urticaria (CIU), Perennial Allergic Rhinitis:* <6 months: not recommended; may start at ≥ 6 months; *Dosing by Age:* 6 months-5 years: max 1.25 mg once daily; 6-11 years: max 2.5 mg once daily; ≥12 years: 2.5-5 mg once daily; *Renal Dysfunction <12 years:* contraindicated; *Renal Dysfunction ≥12 years:* CrCl 50-80 ml/min: 2.5 mg once daily; CrCl 30-50 mL/min: 2.5 mg every other day; CrCl: 10-30 mL/min: 2.5 mg twice weekly (every 3-4 days); CrCl <10 mL/min, ESRD or hemodialysis: contraindicated

  Children's Xyzal Allergy 24HR *Oral Soln:* 0.5 mg/ml (150 ml)

  Xyzal Allergy 24HR *Tab:* 5*mg

▷ *loratadine* **(C)(OTC)(G)** 5 mg bid or 10 mg once daily; *Hepatic or Renal Insufficiency:* see mfr pkg insert

Pediatric: <2 years: not recommended; 2-5 years: 5 mg once daily; ≥6 years: same as adult

  Children's Claritin Chewables *Chew tab:* 5 mg (grape) (phenylalanine)

  Children's Claritin Syrup 1 mg/ml (4 oz) (fruit) (sugar-free, alcohol-free, dye-free; sodium 6 mg/5 ml)

  Claritin *Tab:* 10 mg

  Claritin Hives Relief *Tab:* 10 mg

  Claritin Liqui-Gels *Lig gel:* 10 mg

  Claritin RediTabs 12 Hours *ODT:* 5 mg (mint)

  Claritin RediTabs 24 Hours *ODT:* 10 mg (mint)

FIRST GENERATION ANTIHISTAMINES

▷ *diphenhydramine* **(B)(G)** 25-50 mg q 6-8 hours; max 100 mg/day

Pediatric: <2 years: not recommended; 2-6 years: 6.25 mg q 4-6 hours; max 37.5 mg/day; >6-12 years: 12.5-25 mg q 4-6 hours; max 150 mg/day; >12 years: same as adult

  Benadryl (OTC) *Chew tab:* 12.5 mg (grape) (phenylalanine); *Liq:* 12.5 mg/5 ml (4, 8 oz); *Cap:* 25 mg; *Tab:* 25 mg; *Dye-free soft gel:* 25 mg; *Dye-free liq:* 12.5 mg/5 ml (4, 8 oz)

▷ *diphenhydramine injectable* **(B)(G)** 25-50 mg IM immediately; then q 6 hours prn

Pediatric: <12 years: *See mfr pkg insert:* 1.25 mg/kg up to 25 mg IM x 1 dose; then q 6 hours prn; ≥12 years: same as adult

  Benadryl Injectable *Vial:* 50 mg/ml (1 ml single-use); 50 mg/ml (10 ml multidose); *Amp:* 10 mg/ml (1 ml); *Prefilled syringe:* 50 mg/ml (1 ml)

▷ *hydroxyzine* (C)(G) 50-100 mg/day divided qid prn
  Pediatric: <6 years: 50 mg/day divided qid prn; ≥6 years-12 years: 50 mg/day divided qid prn; >12 years: same as adult
    Atarax *Tab:* 10, 25, 50, 100 mg; *Syr:* 10 mg/5 ml (alcohol 0.5%)
    Vistaril *Cap:* 25, 50, 100 mg; *Oral susp:* 25 mg/5 ml (4 oz) (lemon)
  Comment: *Hydroxyzine* is contraindicated in early pregnancy and in patients with a prolonged QT interval. It is not known whether this drug is excreted in human milk; therefore, *hydroxyzine* should not be given to nursing mothers.

ALLERGEN EXTRACTS

Comment: Allergen extracts (**Grastek, Oralair, Ragwitek**) are not for immediate relief of allergic symptoms. Contraindicated with severe, unstable, and uncontrolled asthma, history of eosinophilic esophagitis, and severe local or systemic reaction. First dose under supervision HCP and observe ≥30 minutes. Subsequent doses may be taken at home.

▷ *short ragweed pollen allergen extract* (C) one SL tab once daily
  Pediatric: <18 years: not established; ≥18 years: same as adult
    Ragwitek *SL tab: Ambrosia artemisiifolia 12 amb a 1-unit* (30, 90/blister pck)
    Comment: Initiate **Ragwitek** at least 12 weeks before onset of ragweed pollen season and continue throughout season.

▷ *sweet vernal, orchard, perennial rye, timothy, Kentucky blue grass mixed pollen allergen extract* (C) 300 IR once daily
  Pediatric: <10 years: not established; 10-17 years: Day 1: 100 IR; Day 2: 200 IR; Day 3 and thereafter: 300 IR once daily
    Oralair *SL tab:* 100, 300 IR (index of reactivity) (30/blister pck)
    Comment: **Oralair** is indicated for grass pollen-induced allergic rhinitis with or without conjunctivitis confirmed by positive skin test. Initiate **Oralair** at least 4 months before onset of grass pollen season and continue throughout season.

▷ *Timothy grass pollen allergen extract* (C) one SL tab once daily
  Pediatric: <5 years: not established; ≥5 years: same as adult
    Grastek *SL tab:* 2800 bioequivalent allergy units (BAUS) (30/blister pck)
    Comment: **Grastek** is indicated for grass pollen-induced allergic rhinitis with or without conjunctivitis confirmed by positive skin test. Initiate **Grastek** at least 12 weeks before onset of grass pollen season and continue throughout season.

NASAL DECONGESTANT

▷ *tetrahydrozoline* (C)
    Tyzine 2-4 drops or 3-4 sprays in each nostril q 3-8 hours prn
    Pediatric: <6 years: not recommended; ≥6 years: same as adult
      Nasal spray: 0.1% (15 ml); *Nasal drops:* 0.1% (30 ml)
    Tyzine Pediatric Nasal Drops 2-3 sprays or drops in each nostril q 3-6 hours prn
      Nasal drops: 0.05% (15 ml)

LEUKOTRIENE RECEPTOR ANTAGONISTS (LRAs)

Comment: For prophylaxis and chronic treatment only. Not for primary (rescue) treatment of acute asthma attack.

▷ *montelukast* (B)(G) 10 mg once daily in the PM; for EIB, take at least 2 hours before exercise; max 1 dose/day
  Pediatric: <12 months: not recommended; 12-23 months: one 4 mg granule pkt daily; 2-5 years: one 4 mg chew tab or granule pkt daily; 6-14 years: one 5 mg chew tab daily; ≥15 years: same as adult

Singulair *Tab:* 10 mg
Singulair Chewable *Chew tab:* 4, 5 mg (cherry, phenylalanine)
Singulair Oral Granules: 4 mg/pkt; take within 15 minutes of opening pkt; may mix with applesauce, carrots, rice, or ice cream

➢ *zafirlukast* (B)(G) 20 mg bid, 1 hour ac or 2 hours pc
Pediatric: <7 years: not recommended; 7-11 years: 10 mg bid 1 hour ac or 2 hours pc; >11 years: same as adult
Accolate *Tab:* 10, 20 mg

➢ *zileuton* (C)(G)
Pediatric: <12 years: not recommended; ≥12 years: same as adult
Zyflo 1 tab qid (total 2400 mg/day)
Tab: 600 mg
Zyflo CR 2 tab bid (total 2400 mg/day)
Tab: 600 mg ext-rel

NASAL CORTICOSTEROIDS

➢ *beclomethasone dipropionate* (C)
Beconase 1 spray in each nostril bid-qid
Pediatric: <6 years: not recommended; 6-12 years: 1 spray in each nostril tid; >12 years: same as adult
Nasal spray: 42 mcg/actuation (6.7 gm, 80 sprays; 16.8 gm, 200 sprays)
Beconase AQ 1-2 sprays in each nostril bid
Pediatric: <6: not recommended; ≥6 years: same as adult
Nasal spray: 42 mcg/actuation (25 gm, 180 sprays)
Beconase Inhalation Aerosol 1-2 sprays in each nostril bid to qid
Pediatric: <6: not recommended; 6-12 years: 1 spray in each nostril tid; >12 years: same as adult
Nasal spray: 42 mcg/actuation (6.7 gm, 80 sprays; 16.8 gm, 200 sprays)
Vancenase AQ 1-2 sprays in each nostril bid
Pediatric: <6 years: not recommended; ≥6 years: same as adult
Nasal spray: 84 mcg/actuation (25 gm, 200 sprays)
Vancenase AQ DS 1-2 sprays in each nostril once daily
Pediatric: <6 years: not recommended; ≥6 years: same as adult
Nasal spray: 84, 168 mcg/actuation (19 gm, 120 sprays)
Vancenase Pockethaler 1 spray in each nostril bid or qid
Pediatric: <6: not recommended; ≥6 years: 1 spray in each nostril tid
Pockethaler: 42 mcg/actuation (7 gm, 200 sprays)
QNASL Nasal Aerosol 2 sprays, 80 mcg/spray, in each nostril once daily
Pediatric: <12 years: 2 sprays, 40 mcg/spray, in each nostril once daily; ≥12 years: same as adult
Nasal spray: 40 mcg/actuation (4.9 gm, 60 sprays); 80 mcg/actuation (8.7 gm, 120 sprays)

➢ *budesonide* (C)
Rhinocort initially 2 sprays in each nostril bid in the AM and PM, or 4 sprays in each nostril in the AM; max 4 sprays each nostril/day; use lowest effective dose
Pediatric: <6 years: not recommended; ≥6 years: same as adult
Nasal spray: 32 mcg/actuation (7 gm, 200 sprays)
Rhinocort Aqua Nasal Spray initially 1 spray in each nostril once daily; max 4 sprays in each nostril once daily
Pediatric: <6 years: not recommended; ≥6-12 years: initially 1 spray in each nostril once daily; max 2 sprays in each nostril once daily
Nasal spray: 32 mcg/actuation (10 ml, 60 sprays)

➢ *ciclesonide* (C)
Pediatric: <6 years: not recommended; ≥6 years: same as adult

> **Omnaris** 2 sprays in each nostril once daily
> *Nasal spray:* 50 mcg/actuation (12.5 gm, 120 sprays)
> **Zetonna** 1-2 sprays in each nostril once daily
> *Nasal spray:* 37 mcg/actuation (6.1 gm, 60 sprays) (HFA)

▶ *dexamethasone* (C) 2 sprays in each nostril bid-tid; max 12 sprays/day; maintain at lowest effective dose
Pediatric: <6 years: not recommended; ≥6-12 years: 1-2 sprays in each nostril bid; max 8 sprays/day; maintain at lowest effective dose; >12 years: same as adult
> **Dexacort Turbinaire** *Nasal spray:* 84 mcg/actuation (12.6 gm, 170 sprays)

▶ *fluticasone furoate* (C) 2 sprays in each nostril once daily; may reduce to 1 spray each nostril once daily
Pediatric: <2 years: not recommended; ≥2-11 years: 1 spray in each nostril once daily; ≥12 years: same as adult
> **Veramyst** *Nasal spray:* 27.5 mcg/actuation (10 gm, 120 sprays) (alcohol-free)

▶ *fluticasone propionate* (C)(OTC)(G) initially 2 sprays in each nostril once daily or 1 spray bid; maintenance 1 spray once daily
Pediatric: <4 years: not recommended; ≥4 years: initially 1 spray in each nostril once daily; may increase to 2 sprays in each nostril once daily; maintenance 1 spray in each nostril once daily; max 2 sprays in each nostril/day
> **Flonase** *Nasal spray:* 50 mcg/actuation (16 gm, 120 sprays)

▶ *flunisolide* (C) 2 sprays in each nostril bid; may increase to 2 sprays in each nostril tid; max 8 sprays/nostril/day
Pediatric: <6 years: not recommended; 6-14 years: initially 1 spray in each nostril tid or 2 sprays in each nostril bid; max 4 sprays/nostril/day; >14 years: same as adult
> **Nasalide** *Nasal spray:* 25 mcg/actuation (25 ml, 200 sprays)
> **Nasarel** *Nasal spray:* 25 mcg/actuation (25 ml, 200 sprays)

▶ *mometasone furoate* (C)(G) 2 sprays in each nostril once daily
Pediatric: <2 years: not recommended; 2-11 years: 1 spray in each nostril once daily; max 2 sprays in each nostril once daily; >11 years: same as adult
> **Nasonex** *Nasal spray:* 50 mcg/actuation (17 gm, 120 sprays)

▶ *olopatadine* (C) 2 sprays in each nostril bid
Pediatric: <6 years: not recommended; 6-11 years: 1 spray each nostril bid; >11 years: same as adult
> **Patanase** *Nasal spray:* 0.6%; 665 mcg/actuation (30.5 gm, 240 sprays) (benzalkonium chloride)

▶ *triamcinolone acetonide* (C)(G) initially 2 sprays in each nostril once daily; max 4 sprays in each nostril once daily or 2 sprays in each nostril bid or 1 spray in each nostril qid; maintain at lowest effective dose
Pediatric: <6 years: not recommended; ≥6 years: 1 spray in each nostril once daily; max 2 sprays in each nostril once daily
> **Nasacort Allergy 24HR (OTC)** *Nasal spray:* 55 mcg/actuation (10 gm, 120 sprays)
> **Tri-Nasal** *Nasal spray:* 50 mcg/actuation (15 ml, 120 sprays)

NASAL MAST CELL STABILIZERS

▶ *cromolyn sodium* (B)(OTC) 1 spray in each nostril tid-qid; max 6 sprays in each nostril/day
Pediatric: <2 years: not recommended; ≥2 years: same as adult
> **Children's NasalCrom, NasalCrom** *Nasal spray:* 5.2 mg/spray (13 ml, 100 sprays; 26 ml, 200 sprays)
Comment: Begin 1-2 weeks before exposure to known allergen. May take 2-4 weeks to achieve maximum effect.

NASAL ANTIHISTAMINES

▷ *azelastine* (C)

Astelin Ready Spray 2 sprays in each nostril bid
Pediatric: <5 years: not recommended; ≥5-12 years: 1 spray in each nostril
once daily bid; >12 years: same as adult
  Nasal spray: 137 mcg/actuation (30 ml, 200 sprays) (benzalkonium
  chloride)
Astepro 0.15% Nasal Spray 1 or 2 sprays each nostril once daily bid
Pediatric: <12 years: not recommended; ≥12 years: same as adult
  Nasal spray: 205.5 mcg/actuation (17 ml, 106 sprays; 30 ml, 200 sprays)
  (benzalkonium chloride)

NASAL ANTIHISTAMINE+CORTICOSTEROID COMBINATION

▷ *azelastine/fluticasone* (C)(G) 1 spray in each nostril bid
Pediatric: <6 years: not recommended; ≥6 years: same as adult
  Dymista *Nasal spray:* azel 137 mcg/*flutic* 50 mcg per actuation (23 gm, 120
  sprays) (benzalkonium chloride)

NASAL ANTICHOLINERGICS

▷ *ipratropium bromide* (B)(G)

Atrovent Nasal Spray 0.03% 2 sprays in each nostril bid-tid
Pediatric: <6 years: not recommended; ≥6 years: same as adult
  Nasal spray: 21 mcg/actuation (30 ml, 345 sprays)
Atrovent Nasal Spray 0.06% 2 sprays in each nostril tid-qid; max 5-7 days
Pediatric: <5 years: not recommended; ≥5-11 years: 2 sprays in each nostril
tid; >11 years: same as adult
  Nasal spray: 42 mcg/actuation (15 ml, 165 sprays)
Comment: Avoid use with narrow-angle glaucoma, prostate hyperplasia, and
bladder neck obstruction.

CHRONIC RHINOSINUSITIS WITH NASAL POLYPS (CRSwNP)

Interleukin-4 Receptor Alpha Antagonist

▷ *dupilumab* administer SC into the upper arm, abdomen, or thigh; rotate sites; 300
mg SC once every other week; may use with or without nasal corticosteroids
Pediatric: safety and efficacy not established
  Dupixent *Prefilled syringe:* 200 mg/1.14 ml, 300 mg/2 ml, single-dose (2/pck
  without needle) (preservative-free)
Comment: *Dupilumab* is a human monoclonal IgG4 antibody that inhibits
interleukin-4 (IL-4) and interleukin-13 (IL-13) signaling by specifically binding
to the IL4Ra subunit shared by the IL-4 and IL-13 receptor complexes, thereby
inhibiting the release of pro-inflammatory cytokines, chemokines, and IgE.
dupilumab is also indicated as an add-on maintenance therapy for patients ≥12
years-of-age with moderate-to-severe asthma with an eosinophilic subtype or
with oral corticosteroid-dependent asthma, and to treat moderate-to-severe
atopic dermatitis. Avoid live vaccines.

 RHINITIS MEDICAMENTOSA

Comment: The nasal/oral regimen selected should be instituted with concurrent
weaning from the nasal decongestant.

Nasal Corticosteroids *see Rhinitis, Sinusitis: Allergic*
Oral Corticosteroids *see* Appendix L. Oral Corticosteroids
Parenteral Corticosteroids *see* Appendix M. Parenteral Corticosteroids

OTC Decongestants
OTC Antihistamine+Decongestant Combinations

NASAL ANTICHOLINERGICS

▷ *ipratropium bromide* (B)(G)
> **Atrovent Nasal Spray 0.03%** stop nasal decongestant; 2 sprays in each nostril
> bid-tid with progressive weaning as tolerated
> *Pediatric:* <6 years: not recommended; ≥6 years: same as adult
> > *Nasal spray:* 21 mcg/actuation (30 ml, 345 sprays)
> **Atrovent Nasal Spray 0.06%** stop nasal decongestant; 2 sprays in each nostril
> tid-qid with progressive weaning as tolerated
> *Pediatric:* <5 years: not recommended; ≥5-11 years: 2 sprays in each nostril
> tid; ≥11 years: same as adult
> > *Nasal spray:* 42 mcg/actuation (15 ml, 165 sprays)

Comment: Avoid use with narrow-angle glaucoma, prostate hyperplasia, and
bladder neck obstruction

NASAL ANTIHISTAMINE

▷ *azelastine* (C) 2 sprays in each nostril bid
> *Pediatric:* <5 years: not recommended; ≥5-12 years: 1 spray in each nostril bid
> **Astelin Ready Spray** *Nasal spray:* 137 mcg/actuation (30 ml, 200 sprays)

FIRST GENERATION ANTIHISTAMINES

▷ *diphenhydramine* (B)(G) 25-50 mg q 6-8 hours; max 100 mg/day
> *Pediatric:* <2 years: not recommended; 2-6 years: 6.25 mg q 4-6 hours; max 37.5
> mg/day; >6-12 years: 12.5-25 mg q 4-6 hours; max 150 mg/day; >12 years: same
> as adult
> > **Benadryl (OTC)** *Chew tab:* 12.5 mg (grape) (phenylalanine); *Liq:* 12.5 mg/5
> > ml (4, 8 oz); *Cap:* 25 mg; *Tab:* 25 mg; *Dye-free soft gel:* 25 mg; *Dye-free liq:*
> > 12.5 mg/5 ml (4, 8 oz)
▷ *diphenhydramine* injectable (B)(G) 25-50 mg IM immediately; then q 6 hours prn
> *Pediatric:* <12 years: *See mfr pkg insert:* 1.25 mg/kg up to 25 mg IM x 1 dose; then
> q 6 hours prn; ≥12 years:
> > **Benadryl Injectable** *Vial:* 50 mg/ml (1 ml single-use); 50 mg/ml (10 ml multi-
> > dose); *Amp:* 10 mg/ml (1 ml); *Prefilled syringe:* 50 mg/ml (1 ml)
▷ *hydroxyzine* (C)(G) 25 mg tid prn; max 600 mg/day
> *Pediatric:* <6 years: 50 mg/day divided qid prn; ≥6 years: 50-100 mg/day divided
> qid prn; max 600 mg/day
> > **Atarax** *Tab:* 10, 25, 50, 100 mg; *Syr:* 10 mg/5 ml (alcohol 0.5%)
> > **Vistaril** *Cap:* 25, 50, 100 mg; *Oral susp:* 25 mg/5 ml (4 oz) (lemon)

SECOND GENERATION ANTIHISTAMINES

Comment: Second generation antihistamines are sedating, but much less so than the
first generation antihistamines. All antihistamines are excreted into breast milk.
▷ *cetirizine* (C)(OTC)(G) <6 years: not recommended; ≥6-<65 years: initially 5-10
> mg once daily; ≥65 years: 5 mg once daily
> > *cetirizine Cap:* 10 mg
> > **Children's Zyrtec Chewable** *Chew tab:* 5, 10 mg (grape)
> > **Children's Zyrtec Allergy Syrup** *Syr:* 1 mg/ml (4 oz) (grape, bubble gum)
> > (sugar-free, dye-free)
> > **Zyrtec** *Tab:* 10 mg
> > **Zyrtec Hives Relief** *Tab:* 10 mg
> > **Zyrtec Liquid Gels** *Liq gel:* 10 mg

▷ *desloratadine* (C)

Clarinex <6 years: not recommended; ≥6 years: 1/2-1 tab once daily
Tab: 5 mg
Clarinex RediTabs <6 years: not recommended; 6-12 years: 2.5 mg once daily;
≥12 years: 5 mg once daily
ODT: 2.5, 5 mg (tutti-frutti) (phenylalanine)
Clarinex Syrup <6 months: not recommended; 6-11 months: 1 mg (2 ml)
once daily; 1-5 years: 1.25 mg (2.5 ml) once daily; 6-11 years: 2.5 mg (5 ml)
once daily; ≥12 years: 5 mg (10 ml) once daily
Tab: 0.5 mg per ml (4 oz) (tutti-frutti) (phenylalanine)
Desloratadine ODT

▷ *fexofenadine* (C)(OTC)(G) 6 months-2 years: 15 mg bid; *CrCl ≤90 mL/min:* 15
mg once daily; 2-11 years: 30 mg bid; *CrCl ≤90 mL/min:* 30 mg once daily ≥12
years and older: ≥12 years: 60 mg once daily-bid or 180 mg once daily; *CrCl <90
mL/min:* 60 mg once daily **Allegra** *Tab:* 30, 60, 180 mg film-coat

Allegra Allergy *Tab:* 60, 180 mg film-coat
Allegra ODT *ODT:* 30 mg (phenylalanine)
Allegra Oral Suspension *Oral susp:* 30 mg/5 ml (6 mg/ml) (4 oz)

▷ *levocetirizine* (B)(OTC)(G) administer dose in the PM; *Seasonal Allergic Rhinitis:*
<2 years: <u>not</u> recommended; may start at ≥2 years; *Chronic Idiopathic Urticaria
(CIU), Perennial Allergic Rhinitis:* <6 months: <u>not</u> recommended; may start at ≥ 6
months; *Dosing by Age:* 6 months-5 years: max 1.25 mg once daily; 6-11 years:
max 2.5 mg once daily; ≥12 years: 2.5-5 mg once daily; *Renal Dysfunction <12
years:* contraindicated; *Renal Dysfunction ≥12 years:* CrCl 50-80 ml/min: 2.5 mg
once daily; CrCl 30-50 mL/min: 2.5 mg every other day; CrCl: 10-30 mL/min:
2.5 mg twice weekly (every 3-4 days); CrCl <10 mL/min, ESRD or hemodialysis:
contraindicated

Children's Xyzal Allergy 24HR *Oral Soln:* 0.5 mg/ml (150 ml)
Xyzal Allergy 24HR *Tab:* 5*mg

▷ *loratadine* (C)(OTC)(G) 5 mg bid or 10 mg once daily; *Hepatic or Renal
Insufficiency:* see mfr pkg insert
Pediatric: <2 years: not recommended; 2-5 years: 5 mg once daily; ≥6 years:
same as adult

Children's Claritin Chewables *Chew tab:* 5 mg (grape) (phenylalanine)
Children's Claritin Syrup 1 mg/ml (4 oz) (fruit) (sugar-free, alcohol-free, dye-
free, sodium 6 mg/5 ml)
Claritin *Tab:* 10 mg
Claritin Hives Relief *Tab:* 10 mg
Claritin Liqui-Gels *Liq gel:* 10 mg
Claritin RediTabs 12 Hours *ODT:* 5 mg (mint)
Claritin RediTabs 24 Hours *ODT:* 10 mg (mint)

RHINITIS: VASOMOTOR

NASAL ANTICHOLINERGICS

Comment: Avoid use with narrow-angle glaucoma, prostate hyperplasia, and
bladder neck obstruction

▷ *ipratropium bromide* (B)(G)

Atrovent Nasal Spray 0.03% stop nasal decongestant; 2 sprays in each nostril
bid-tid with progressive weaning as tolerated
Pediatric: <6 years: not recommended; ≥6 years: same as adult
Nasal spray: 21 mcg/actuation (30 ml, 345 sprays)
Atrovent Nasal Spray 0.06% stop nasal decongestant; 2 sprays in each nostril
tid-qid with progressive weaning as tolerated

Pediatric: <5 years: not recommended; ≥5-11 years: 2 sprays in each nostril tid; >11 years: same as adult

Nasal spray: 42 mcg/actuation (15 ml, 165 sprays)

 RIVER BLINDNESS (ONCHOCERCIASIS)

ANTHELMINTIC

▷ *moxidectin* **(G)** take 8 mg (4 x 2 mg tablets) as a single dose, with *or* without food
Pediatric: <12 years: not recommended; ≥12 years: same as adult

Tab: 2 mg

Comment: *Moxidectin* is a macrocyclic lactone anthelmintic medicine indicated for the treatment of river blindness (onchocerciasis) due to *Onchocerca volvulus* in patients ≥12 years-of-age. *Moxidectin* does not kill adult *O. volvulus* parasites. Follow-up is advised. The safety and efficacy of repeat administration of *moxidectin* tablets in patients with *O. volvulus* has not been studied. Cutaneous, ophthalmological and/or systemic adverse reactions of varying severity (Mazzotti Reaction) have occurred in patients with onchocerciasis following treatment. Episodes of symptomatic orthostatic hypotension, including inability to stand without support, may occur in patients following treatment. Serious *or* even fatal encephalopathy following treatment may occur in patients co-infected with *Loa loa* (assess patients for loiasis in *Loa loa* endemic areas prior to treatment. Patients with hyper-reactive onchodermatitis (sowda) may be more likely than others to experience severe edema and aggravation of onchodermatitis. Limited available data on the use of *moxidectin* in pregnant patients are insufficient to establish whether there is a *moxidectin*-associated risk for major birth defects and miscarriage. *Moxidectin* has been detected in human milk following a single 8 mg dose. There are no data on the effects of *moxidectin* on breastfed infants. Risk/benefit of the developmental and health benefits of breastfeeding should be considered along with the mother's clinical need for *moxidectin*. The most common adverse reactions (incidence > 10%) have been eosinophilia, pruritus, musculoskeletal pain, headache, lymphopenia, tachycardia, rash, abdominal pain, hypotension, pyrexia, leukocytosis, influenza-like illness, neutropenia, cough, lymph node pain, dizziness, diarrhea, hyponatremia, and peripheral swelling.

 ROCKY MOUNTAIN SPOTTED FEVER (RMSF, *RICKETTSIA RICKETTSII*)

ANTI-INFECTIVES

▷ *doxycycline* **(D)(G)** 200 mg on first day; then 100 mg bid x 7-10 days
Pediatric: <8 years: not recommended; ≥8 years, <100 lb: 2-2.5 mg/kg q 12 hours x 7-10 days; ≥8 years, ≥100 lb: same as adult

Acticlate *Tab:* 75, 150**mg
Adoxa *Tab:* 50, 75, 100, 150 mg ent-coat
Doryx *Tab:* 50, 75, 100, 150, 200 mg del-rel
Doxteric *Tab:* 50 mg del-rel
Monodox *Cap:* 50, 75, 100 mg
Oracea *Cap:* 40 mg del-rel
Vibramycin *Tab:* 100 mg; *Cap:* 50, 100 mg; *Syr:* 50 mg/5 ml (raspberry-apple) (sulfites); *Oral susp:* 25 mg/5 ml (raspberry)
Vibra-Tab *Tab:* 100 mg film-coat

Comment: IV therapy might be indicated for more severely ill patients who require hospitalization, particularly in patients who are vomiting or obtunded. Recommended duration of therapy is at least 3 days after subsidence of fever and until evidence of clinical improvement is noted. Typically, the minimum total course of treatment is 5-7 days. Severe or complicated disease could require a longer treatment course. Diagnostic tests for rickettsial diseases, particularly for RMSF, are usually not helpful in making a timely diagnosis during the initial stages of illness and treatment decisions for rickettsial pathogens should never be delayed while awaiting laboratory confirmation. Delay in treatment can lead to severe disease and long-term sequelae or death. The American Academy of Pediatrics and CDC recommend *doxycycline* as the treatment of choice for children of all ages with suspected tick-borne rickettsial disease. Previous concerns about tooth staining in children aged <8 years stem from experience with older tetracycline-class drugs that bind more readily to calcium than newer members of the drug class, such as *doxycycline*. *Doxycycline* used at the dose and duration recommended for treatment of RMSF in children aged <8 years, even after multiple courses, did not result in tooth staining or enamel hypoplasia in a 2013 retrospective cohort study of 58 children. These results support the findings of a study published in 2007 reporting no evidence of tooth staining among 31 children with asthma exacerbation who were treated with *doxycycline*.

▷ *tetracycline* (D)(G) 500 mg q 6 hours x 7-10 days
  Pediatric: <8 years: not recommended; ≥8 years, <100 lb: 10 mg/kg/day q 6 hours x 7-10 days; ≥8 years, ≥100 lb: same as adult
    Achromycin V *Cap:* 250, 500 mg
    Sumycin *Tab:* 250, 500 mg; *Cap:* 250, 500 mg; *Oral susp:* 125 mg/5 ml (100, 200 ml) (fruit) (sulfites)

 ROSEOLA INFANTUM (EXANTHEM SUBITUM)

Antipyretics *see* **Fever**

Comment: Roseola infantum (also known as exanthem subitum, sixth disease, pseudorubella, exanthem criticum, and three-day fever) is a generally mild clinical syndrome, commonly occurring in children <3 years-of-age, characterized by sudden onset of high fever (may exceed 40°C [104°F]) that lasts 3 days and resolves abruptly, and is followed by development of a rash lasting ≤3 days. Roseola usually is caused by human herpesvirus 6 (HHV-6). Treatment is antipyretics (aspirin is contraindicated) and adequate hydration. Monitor for febrile seizures. As with the common cold, roseola spreads from person to person through contact with an infected person's respiratory secretions or saliva. The disease can occur at any time of year.

ROTAVIRUS GASTROENTERITIS

PROPHYLAXIS

Comment: RotaTeq targets the most common strains of rotavirus (G1, G2, G3, G4), which are responsible for more than 90% of rotavirus disease in the United States.

▷ *rotavirus vaccine, live* not recommended for adults
  Pediatric: <6 weeks or >32 weeks: not recommended; >6 weeks and <32 weeks: administer 1st dose at 6-12 weeks of age; administer 2nd and 3rd doses at 4-10-week intervals for a total of 3 doses; if an incomplete dose is administered, do not administer a replacement dose, but continue with the remaining doses in the recommended series
    RotaTeq *Oral susp:* 2 ml single-use tube (fetal bovine serum [trace], preservative-free, thimerosal-free)

ROUNDWORM (*ASCARIASIS*)

ANTHELMINTICS

Comment: Oral bioavailability of anthelmintics is enhanced when administered with a fatty meal (estimated fat content 40 gm).

▷ *albendazole* (C) take with a meal; swallow, chew, crush, or mix with food; 400 mg once daily x 7 days
Pediatric: <2 years: 200 mg once daily x 3 days; may repeat in 3 weeks if needed; 2-12 years: 400 mg once daily x 3 days; may repeat in 3 weeks if needed; >12 years: same as adult
  Albenza *Tab:* 200 mg

▷ *mebendazole* (C) take with a meal; swallow, chew, crush, or mix with food; 100 mg bid x 3 days; may repeat in 3 weeks if needed
Pediatric: <2 years: not recommended; ≥2 years: same as adult
  Emverm *Chew tab:* 100 mg
  Vermox (G) *Chew tab:* 100 mg

▷ *pyrantel pamoate* (C) take with a meal; may open capsule and sprinkle or mix with food; treat x 3 days; may repeat in 2-3 weeks if needed; 11 mg/kg once daily x 3 days; max 1 gm/dose
Pediatric: 25-37 lb: 1/2 tsp x 1 dose; 38-62 lb: 1 tsp x 1 dose; 63-87 lb: 1 tsp x 1 dose; 88-112 lb: 2 tsp x 1 dose; 113-137 lb: 2 tsp x 1 dose; 138-162 lb: 3 tsp x 1 dose; 163-187 lb: 3 tsp x 1 dose; >187 lb: 4 tsp x 1 dose
  Antiminth (OTC) *Cap:* 180 mg; *Liq:* 50 mg/ml (30 ml); 144 mg/ml (30 ml); *Oral susp:* 50 mg/ml (60 ml)
  Pin-X (OTC) *Cap:* 180 mg; *Liq:* 50 mg/ml (30 ml); 144 mg/ml (30 ml); *Oral susp:* 50 mg/ml (30 ml)

▷ *thiabendazole* (C) 25 mg/kg bid x 7 days; max 1.5 gm/dose; max 3000 mg/day; take with a meal
Pediatric: same as adult
  Mintezol *Chew tab:* 500*mg (orange); *Oral susp:* 500 mg/5 ml (120 ml) (orange)
  Comment: *Thiabendazole* is not for prophylaxis. May impair mental alertness. May not be available in the US.

RUBELLA (GERMAN MEASLES)

Antipyretics *see* **Fever**
See **Childhood Immunizations**

Comment: Rubella is highly contagious and highly teratogenic. Quarantine is mandatory to prevent a community outbreak. Herd immunity is the best prevention.

PROPHYLAXIS VACCINE

Comment: <12 months: not recommended; ≥12 months: 25 mcg SC; if vaccinated <12 months, re-vaccinate at 12 months; administer in the upper posterior arm.

▷ *rubella virus, live, attenuated+neomycin* vaccine (C)
Pediatric: <12 months: not recommended (if vaccinated <12 months, re-vaccinate at 12 months); ≥12 months: 25 mcg SC
  Meruvax II 25 mcg SC

▷ *measles, mumps, rubella, live, attenuated, neomycin vaccine* (C)
  MMR II 25 mcg SC (preservative-free)

Comment: Contraindications: hypersensitivity to *neomycin* or eggs, primary or acquired immune deficiency, immunosuppressant therapy, bone marrow or lymphatic malignancy, and pregnancy (within 3 months following vaccination). *see Childhood Immunizations*

PRE- AND POST-EXPOSURE PROPHYLAXIS
Immune Globulin

▷ *immune globulin (human)* administer via intramuscular injection only (never intravenously); ensure adequate hydration prior to administration

Household and Institutional Rubella Case Contacts: promptly administer 0.55 ml/kg IM as a single dose

Planned Travel to Rubella Endemic Area: administer 0.55 ml/kg as a single dose at least 6 days prior to travel

Pediatric: 0.25 ml/kg IM (0.5 mg/kg in immunocompromised children)

GamaSTAN S/D *Vial:* 2, 10 ml single-dose

Comment: **GamaSTAN S/D** is the only *gammaglobulin* product FDA-approved for measles and HAV post-exposure prophylaxis (PEP). **GamaSTAN S/D** is also FDA-approved for varicella post-exposure prophylaxis (PEP). Other **GamaSTAN S/D** indications: to prevent or modify measles in a susceptible person exposed fewer than 6 days previously; to modify varicella; to modify rubella in exposed women who will not consider a therapeutic abortion. **GamaSTAN S/D** is not indicated for routine prophylaxis or treatment of viral hepatitis B, rubella, poliomyelitis, mumps or varicella. Contraindications to **GamaSTAN S/D** include persons with cancer, chronic liver disease, and persons allergic to *gammaglobulin*, the HAV vaccine, or a component of the HAV vaccine. Dosage is higher for HAV PEP than for measles and varicella PEP based on recently observed decreasing concentrations of HAV antibodies in **GamaSTAN S/D**, attributed to the decreasing prevalence of previous HAV infection among plasma donors.

RUBEOLA (RED MEASLES)

Antipyretics *see* **Fever**
See **Childhood Immunizations**

PROPHYLAXIS VACCINE

▷ *measles, mumps, rubella, live, attenuated, neomycin vaccine* (C)
MMR II 25 mcg SC (preservative-free)
Comment: Contraindications: hypersensitivity to *neomycin* or eggs, primary or acquired immune deficiency, immunosuppressant therapy, bone marrow or lymphatic malignancy, and pregnancy (within 3 months following vaccination).

PRE- AND POST-EXPOSURE PROPHYLAXIS
Immune Globulin (Human)

▷ *immune globulin (human)* administer via intramuscular injection only (never intravenously); ensure adequate hydration prior to administration

Household and Institutional Measles Case Contacts: promptly administer 0.025 ml/kg IM as a single dose

Planned Travel to Measles Endemic Area: administer 0.025 ml/kg IM as a single dose at least 6 days prior to travel

Pediatric: 0.25 ml/kg IM (0.5 mg/kg in immunocompromised children)

GamaSTAN S/D *Vial:* 2, 10 ml single-dose

Comment: **GamaSTAN S/D** is the only *gammaglobulin* product FDA-approved for measles and HAV post-exposure prophylaxis (PEP).

GamaSTAN S/D is also FDA-approved for varicella post-exposure prophylaxis (PEP). Other **GamaSTAN S/D** indications: to prevent or modify measles in a susceptible person exposed fewer than 6 days previously; to modify varicella; to modify rubella in exposed women who will not consider a therapeutic abortion. **GamaSTAN S/D** is not indicated for routine prophylaxis or treatment of viral hepatitis B, rubella, poliomyelitis, mumps, or varicella. Contraindications to **GamaSTAN S/D** include persons with cancer, chronic liver disease, and persons allergic to *gammaglobulin*, the HAV vaccine, or a component of the HAV vaccine. Dosage is higher for HAV PEP than for measles and varicella PEP based on recently observed decreasing concentrations of HAV antibodies in **GamaSTAN S/D**, attributed to the decreasing prevalence of previous HAV infection among plasma donors.

SALMONELLOSIS

ANTI-INFECTIVES

▷ *ciprofloxacin* (C) 500 mg bid x 3-5 days
  Pediatric: <18 years: not recommended; ≥18 years: same as adult
    Cipro (G) *Tab:* 250, 500, 750 mg; *Oral susp:* 250, 500 mg/5 ml (100 ml) (strawberry)
    Cipro XR *Tab:* 500, 1000 mg ext-rel
    ProQuin XR *Tab:* 500 mg ext-rel

▷ *trimethoprim+sulfamethoxazole (TMP-SMX)* (D)(G)
  Pediatric: <2 months: not recommended; ≥2 months: 40 mg/kg/day of *sulfamethoxazole* in 2 divided doses bid x 10 days; *see Appendix CC.33: trimethoprim+ sulfamethoxazole (Bactrim Suspension, Septra Suspension) for dose by weight*
    Bactrim, Septra 2 tabs bid x 10 days
      Tab: trim 80 mg+sulfa 400 mg*
    Bactrim DS, Septra DS 1 tab bid x 10 days
      Tab: trim 160 mg+sulfa 800 mg*
    Bactrim Pediatric Suspension, Septra Pediatric Suspension
      Oral susp: trim 40 mg+sulfa 200 mg per 5 ml (100 ml) (cherry) (alcohol 0.3%)

SCABIES (*SARCOPTES SCABIEI*)

Comment: This section presents treatment regimens for scabies infestation published in the **2015 CDC Sexually Transmitted Diseases Treatment Guidelines**, as well as other available treatments.

▷ *spinosad* shake bottle well; apply product to skin by rubbing it in to completely cover the body from the neck down to the soles of the feet; patients with balding scalp should also apply product to the scalp, hairline, temples, and forehead; allow to absorb in the skin and dry for 10 minutes before getting dressed; leave on the skin for at least 6 hours before showering or bathing
  Pediatric: <4 years: safety and efficacy not established; ≥4 years: same as adult
    Natroba *Topical susp:* 0.9% (9 mg/gm; 120ml)
    Comment: **Natroba** is a pediculocide/scabicide, indicated for the topical treatment of scabies infestation in patients ≥4 years. The most common adverse reactions (incidence >1%) have been application site irritation (pain and burning) and dry skin. *Spinosad*, the active ingredient in **Natroba**, is not absorbed systemically following topical application, and maternal use is not expected to result in embryo/fetal exposure to the drug. **Natroba** contains benzyl alcohol. Topical benzyl alcohol is unlikely to be absorbed through the skin in clinically relevant amounts; therefore, maternal use is not expected to result in embryo/fetal exposure to the drug. Breastfeeding is not expected to

result in the exposure of the infant to **spinosad**. Advise breastfeeding females to remove **Natroba** from the breast with soap and water before breastfeeding to avoid direct infant exposure to **Natroba**.

RECOMMENDED REGIMEN

▷ *permethrin* (B)(G) massage into skin from head to soles of feet; leave on x 8-14 hours, then rinse off
 Pediatric: <2 months: not recommended; ≥2 months: same as adult
   Acticin, Elimite *Crm:* 5% (60 gm)

ALTERNATIVE REGIMEN

▷ *lindane* (B)(G) 1 oz of lotion or 30 gm of cream apply to all skin surfaces from neck down to the soles of the feet; leave on x 8 hours, then wash off thoroughly; may repeat if needed in 14 days
 Pediatric: <2 months: not recommended; ≥2 months: same as adult
   Kwell *Lotn:* 1% (60, 473 ml); *Crm:* 1% (60 gm); *Shampoo:* 1% (60, 473 ml)

OTHER TOPICAL TREATMENTS

▷ *crotamiton* (C) massage into skin from chin down; repeat in 24 hours
 Pediatric: <12 years: not recommended; ≥12 years: same as adult
   Eurax *Lotn:* 10% (60 gm); *Crm:* 10% (60 gm)

SCARLET FEVER (SCARLATINA)

Comment: Microorganism responsible for scarlet fever is Group A beta-hemolytic *Streptococcus* (GABHS). Strep cultures and screens will be positive.

▷ *azithromycin* (B)(G) 500 mg x 1 dose on day 1, then 250 mg once daily on days 2-5 or 500 mg once daily x 3 days
 Pediatric: 12 mg/kg/day x 5 days; max 500 mg/day; *see* Appendix CC.7.
 azithromycin (Zithromax Suspension, Zmax Suspension) *for dose by weight*
   Zithromax *Tab:* 250, 500, 600 mg; *Oral susp:* 100 mg/5 ml (15 ml); 200 mg/5 ml (15, 22.5, 30 ml) (cherry); *Pkt:* 1 gm for reconstitution (cherry-banana)
   Zithromax Tri-pak *Tab:* 3 x 500 mg tabs/pck
   Zithromax Z-pak *Tab:* 6 x 250 mg tabs/pck
   Zmax *Oral susp:* 2 gm ext-rel for reconstitution (cherry-banana) (148 mg Na⁺)

▷ *cefadroxil* (B)
 Pediatric: 15-30 mg/kg/day in 2 divided doses x 10 days; *see* Appendix CC.9.
 cefadroxil (Duricef Suspension) *for dose by weight*
   Duricef *Cap:* 500 mg; *Tab:* 1 gm; *Oral susp:* 250 mg/5 ml (100 ml); 500 mg/5 ml (75, 100 ml) (orange-pineapple)

▷ *cephalexin* (B)(G)
 Pediatric: 25-50 mg/kg/day in 2 divided doses x 10 days; *see* Appendix CC.15.
 cephalexin (Keflex Suspension) *for dose by weight*
   Keflex *Cap:* 250, 333, 500, 750 mg; *Oral susp:* 125, 250 mg/5 ml (100, 200 ml) (strawberry)

▷ *clarithromycin* (C)(G) 250 mg bid or 500 mg ext-rel once daily x 10 days
 Pediatric: <6 months: not recommended; ≥6 months: 7.5 mg/kg bid x 10 days; *see* Appendix CC.16. *clarithromycin* (Biaxin Suspension) *for dose by weight*
   Biaxin *Tab:* 250, 500 mg
   Biaxin Oral Suspension *Oral susp:* 125, 250 mg/5 ml (50, 100 ml) (fruit punch)
   Biaxin XL *Tab:* 500 mg ext-rel

▷ *clindamycin* (B)(G) 150-300 mg q 6 hours x 10 days
 Pediatric: 8-16 mg/kg/day in 3-4 divided doses x 10 days
   Cleocin *Cap:* 75 (tartrazine), 150 (tartrazine), 300 mg
   Cleocin Pediatric Granules *Oral susp:* 75 mg/5 ml (100 ml) (cherry)

▷ **erythromycin estolate (B)(G)** 250 mg q 6 hours x 10 days
Pediatric: 20-50 mg/kg q 6 hours x 10 days; *see Appendix CC.20: erythromycin* estolate (Ilosone Suspension) *for dose by weight*
   Ilosone *Pulvule:* 250 mg; *Tab:* 500 mg; *Liq:* 125, 250 mg/5 ml (100 ml)
▷ **erythromycin ethylsuccinate (B)(G)** 400 mg qid or 800 mg bid x 10 days
Pediatric: 30-50 mg/kg/day in 4 divided doses x 10 days; may double dose with severe infection; max 100 mg/kg/day; *see Appendix CC.21: erythromycin ethylsuccinate* (E.E.S. Suspension, Ery-Ped Drops/Suspension) *for dose by weight*
   EryPed *Oral susp:* 200 mg/5 ml (100, 200 ml) (fruit); 400 mg/5 ml (60, 100, 200 ml) (banana); *Oral drops:* 200, 400 mg/5 ml (50 ml) (fruit); *Chew tab:* 200 mg wafer (fruit)
   E.E.S. *Oral susp:* 200, 400 mg/5 ml (100 ml) (fruit)
   E.E.S. Granules *Oral susp:* 200 mg/5 ml (100, 200 ml) (cherry)
   E.E.S. 400 Tablets *Tab:* 400 mg
▷ **penicillin g (benzathine and procaine) (B)(G)** 2.4 million units IM x 1 dose
Pediatric: <30 lb: 600,000 units IM x 1 dose; 30-60 lb: 900,000-1.2 million units IM x 1 dose
   Bicillin C-R Cartridge-needle unit: 600,000 units (1 ml); 1.2 million units; (2 ml); 2.4 million units (4 ml)
▷ **penicillin v potassium (B)** 250 mg tid x 10 days
Pediatric: 25-50 mg/kg day in 4 divided doses x 10 days; ≥12 years: same as adult; *see* Appendix CC.29. penicillin v potassium (Pen-Vee K Solution, Veetids Solution) *for dose by weight*
   Pen-Vee K *Tab:* 250, 500 mg; *Oral soln:* 125 mg/5 ml (100, 200 ml); 250 mg/5 ml (100, 150, 200 ml)

SCHISTOSOMIASIS

TREMATODICIDE

Comment: *Praziquantel* is a trematodicide indicated for the treatment of infections due to all species of genus *Schistosoma* (e.g., *Schistosoma mekongi*, *Schistosoma japonicum*, *Schistosoma mansoni*, and *Schistosoma hematobium)* and infections due to liver flukes (i.e., *Clonorchis sinensis*, *Opisthorchis viverrini). Praziquantel* induces a rapid contraction of schistosomes by a specific effect on the permeability of the cell membrane. The drug further causes vacuolization and disintegration of the schistosome tegument.

▷ **praziquantel (B)** 20 mg/kg tid as a one-day treatment; take the 3 doses at intervals of not less than 4 hours and not more than 6 hours; swallow whole with water during meals; holding the tablets in the mouth leaves a bitter taste which can trigger gagging or vomiting.
Pediatric: <4 years: not established; ≥4 years: same as adult
   Biltricide *Tab:* 600 mg film-coat
Comment: Concomitant administration with strong Cytochrome P450 (P450) inducers, such as *rifampin*, is contraindicated since therapeutically effective blood levels of *praziquantel* may not be achieved. In patients receiving *rifampin* who need immediate treatment for schistosomiasis, alternative agents for schistosomiasis should be considered. However, if treatment with *praziquantel* is necessary, *rifampin* should be discontinued 4 weeks before administration of *praziquantel*. Treatment with *rifampin* can then be restarted one day after completion of *praziquantel* treatment.
Concomitant administration of other P450 inducers (e.g., antiepileptic drugs such as *phenytoin*, *phenobarbital*, *carbamazepine)* and *dexamethasone*, may also reduce plasma levels of *praziquantel*. Concomitant administration of P450 inhibitors (e.g., *cimetidine*, *ketoconazole*, *itraconazole*, *erythromycin)* may increase plasma levels of

praziquantel. Patients should be warned not to drive a car or operate machinery on the day of **Biltricide** treatment and the following day. There are no adequate or well-controlled studies in pregnant females. This drug should be used during pregnancy only if clearly needed. *praziquantel* appears in the milk of nursing women at a concentration of about 1/4 that of maternal serum. It is not known whether a pharmacological effect is likely to occur in children. Women should not nurse on the day of **Biltricide** treatment and during the subsequent 72 hours.

 SCHIZOPHRENIA, SCHIZOPHRENIA WITH CO-MORBID PERSONALITY DISORDER

Other Antipsychosis Drugs *see* **Antipsychosis Drugs**
see **Tardive Dyskinesia**

Comment: A team of researchers examined the effects of antipsychotics on mortality risk in schizophrenia patients. They studied data on 29,823 patients with schizophrenia in Sweden, aged 16 to 64 years and found mortality among patients with schizophrenia was 40% lower when they used antipsychotics as compared to when they did not. Long-acting injection (LAI) use was associated with an approximately 33% lower risk of death compared with the oral use of the same medication. The lowest mortality was observed with use of once-monthly *paliperidone* LAI, oral *aripiprazole*, and *risperidone* LAI.

ATYPICAL ANTIPSYCHOTICS

▷ *aripiprazole* (C)(G) initially 15 mg once daily; may increase to max 30 mg/day
Pediatric: <10 years: not recommended; ≥10-17 years: initially 2 mg/day in a single dose for 2 days; then increase to 5 mg/day in a single dose for 2 days; then increase to target dose of 10 mg/day in a single dose; may increase by 5 mg/day at weekly intervals as needed to max 30 mg/day
   Abilify *Tab:* 2, 5, 10, 15, 20, 30 mg
   Abilify Discmelt *Tab:* 15 mg orally-disint (vanilla) (phenylalanine)
   Abilify Maintena *Vial:* 300, 400 mg ext-rel pwdr for IM injection after reconstitution; 300, 400 mg single-dose prefilled dual-chamber syringes w. supplies
▷ *aripiprazole lauroxil* (C)
ALERT: aripiprazole lauroxil is available in two parenteral delivery forms, **Aristada** and **Aristada Initio,** with differing doses and frequently of administration. Therefore, **Aristada Initio** is not interchangeable with **Aristada**. **Aristada Initio** is a smaller particle-size version of extended-release injectable *aripiprazole*). It is the first and only long-acting atypical antipsychotic that can be initiated on day one. Combining **Aristada Initio** with a single 30 mg dose of oral *aripiprazole* provides an alternative regimen to initiate patients onto any dose of **Aristada** on day one. Previously, the initiation process for the older *aripiprazole* product was to give the first dose and to then give oral *aripiprazole* for 21 consecutive days. **Aristada Initio** releases relevant levels of *aripiprazole* within 4 days of initiation. **Aristada Initio** carries a warning that it is not approved for use by older patients with dementia-related psychosis, as this patient population is at risk for increased mortality when treated with antipsychotics. For patients naïve to *aripiprazole*, establish tolerability with oral *aripiprazole* prior to initiating treatment with **Aristada Initio**.
Pediatric: <18 years: not recommended; ≥18 years: same as adult
   Aristada administer by IM injection in the deltoid (441 mg dose only) or gluteal (441 mg, 662 mg, 882 mg or 1064 mg) muscle by a qualified healthcare professional; initiate at a dose of 441 mg, 662 mg or 882 mg administered monthly, or 882 mg every 6 weeks, or 1064 mg every 2 months
   Prefilled syringe: 441, 662, 882, 1064 mg single-use, ext-rel susp

Aristada Initio administer a single 675 mg **Aristada Initio** injection (plus a single 30 mg dose of oral *aripiprazole* in conjunction with the first **Aristada Initio** injection); administer the IM injection into the deltoid or gluteal muscle; must be administered only by a qualified healthcare professional; **Aristada Initio** is only to be used as a single dose and is not for repeated dosing

Prefilled pen: 675 mg/2.4 ml ext-rel single-dose

Comment: **Aristada and Aristada Initio** are atypical antipsychotics. **Aristada** is available in 4 doses with 3 dosing duration options for flexible dosing. **Aristada initio** is a single-dose *longer-acting* form of *aripiprazole lauroxil* For patients naïve to *aripiprazole*, establish tolerability with oral *aripiprazole* prior to initiating treatment with **Aristada**. **Aristada** can be initiated at any of the 4 doses at the appropriate dosing duration option. In conjunction with the first injection, administer treatment with oral *aripiprazole* for 21 consecutive days for all 4 dose sizes. The most common adverse event associated with **Aristada/Aristada Initio** is akathisia. Patients are also at increased risk for developing neuroleptic malignant syndrome, tardive dyskinesia, pathological gambling or other compulsive behaviors, orthostatic hypotension, hyperglycemic, dyslipidemia, and weight gain. Hypersensitive reactions can occur and range from pruritus or urticaria to anaphylaxis. Stroke, transient ischemic attacks, and falls have been reported in elderly patients with dementia-related psychosis who were treated with *apriprazole*. **Aristada/Aristada Initio** are not for treatment of people who have lost touch with reality (psychosis) *due to* confusion and memory loss dementia). Avoid use in known CYP2D6 poor metabolizers. Avoid use with strong CYP2D6 or CYP 3A4 inhibitors and strong CYP3A4 inducers. *aripiprazole* may cause extrapyramidal and/or withdrawal symptoms in neonates exposed in utero in the third trimester of pregnancy. *aripiprazole* is present in human breast milk; however, there are insufficient data to assess the amount in human milk or the effects on the breastfed infant. The development and health benefits of breastfeeding should be considered along with the mother's clinical need for *aripiprazole* and any potential adverse effects on the breastfed infant from **Aristada/Aristada Initio** or from the underlying maternal condition. For more information or to report suspected ASEs, contact the National Pregnancy Registry for Atypical Antipsychotics at 1-866-961-2388 or visit http://womensmentalhealth.org/clinical-and-research programs/ pregnancy registry. Limited published data on *aripiprazole* use in pregnant females are not sufficient to inform any drug-associated risks for birth defects or miscarriage.

▷ *asenapine* apply one transdermal system every 24 hours to the upper back, upper arm, abdomen, or hip; rotate sites; recommended starting dose is 3.8 mg/24 hours; may increase to 5.7 mg/24 hours or 7.6 mg/24 hours after 1 week

Pediatric: safety and efficacy not established

Secuado *Trandermal system:* 3.8 mg/24 hours, 5.7 mg/24 hours, 7.6 mg/24 hours

Comment: **Secuado** *(asenapine)* is an atypical antipsychotic indicated for the treatment schizophrenia, in a transdermal drug delivery system (TDDS) that provides sustained concentrations during wear time (24 hours). Commonly observed adverse reactions to **Secuado** (incidence ≥5%) have included extrapyramidal disorder, application site reaction, and weight gain. **Secuado** is contraindicated in patients with severe hepatic impairment (Child-Pugh C). **Secuado** is not approved for treatment of patients with dementia-related psychosis. Elderly patients with dementia-related psychosis treated with antipsychotic drugs are at an increased risk of death and increased incidence of cerebrovascular adverse reactions (e.g., stroke, TIA). Manage neuroleptic malignant syndrome (NMS) with immediate discontinuation and close monitoring. Manage tardive dyskinesia (TD) with discontinuation. Monitor for hyperglycemia/diabetes mellitus, dyslipidemia, and weight gain. Monitor for orthostatic hypotension. Monitor HR and BP and warn patients with known cardiovascular or cerebrovascular disease of risk of dehydration or syncope. Monitor for leukopenia, neutropenia, and agranulocytosis; monitor CBC in patients with pre-existing low WBC or history of leukopenia or neutropenia and consider discontinuation if a clinically significant decline in WBC occurs in the absence of other causative factors. Monitor for increases in QT interval; avoid use with drugs that also increase the QT interval and in patients with risk factors for prolonged QT interval. Use cautiously in patients with a history of seizures or with conditions that lower the seizure threshold. Use caution when operating machinery; there is potential for cognitive and motor impairment. Avoid exposing **Secuado** to external heat sources during wear because both the rate and extent of absorption are increased. During wear time or immediately after removal of **Secuado**, local skin reactions may occur; advise patient to be sure to remove the expiring transdermal patch when applying the new patch. **Secuado** may enhance the antihypertensive effects of the patient's antihertensive medications; monitor BP and adjust antihypertensive drug disage accordingly. Based on clinical response, consider **Secuado** dose reduction when co-administered with Strong CYP1A2 Inhibitors. *paroxetine* is a CYP2D6 substrate and inhibitor; therefore; reduce *paroxetine* dose by half. **Secuado** may cause extrapyramidal and/or withdrawal symptoms in neonates with third trimester exposure. In animal studies, *asenapine* increased post-implantation loss and decreased pup weight and survival at doses similar to or less than recommended clinical doses. In these studies there was no increase in the incidence of structural abnormalities caused by *asenapine*. Lactation studies have not been conducted to assess the presence of *asenapine* in human milk or effects on the breastfed infant. *asenapine* is excreted in rat milk. The development and health benefits of breastfeeding should be considered along with the mother's clinical need for **Secuado** and any potential adverse effects on the breastfed infant from **Secuado** or from the underlying maternal condition. There is a pregnancy exposure registry that monitors pregnancy outcomes in women exposed to atypical antipsychotics, including **Secuado**, during pregnancy. For more information contact the National Pregnancy Registry for Atypical Antipsychotics at 1-866-961-2388 or visit http://womensmentalhealth.org/clinical-andresearch-programs/pregnancyregistry/.

▷ *lumateperone* 42 mg once daily; no titration required; take with food
  Pediatric: safety and efficacy not established
    Caplyta *Cap:* 42 mg
    Comment: Caplyta *(lumateperone)* is first-in-class atypical antipsychotic for the treatment of schizophrenia in adults. **Caplyta** is not approved for the treatment of patients with dementia-related psychosis due to increased incidence of cerebrovascular adverse reactions (e.g., stroke, TIA) and death in these patients. Avoid **Caplyta** use with moderate-to-severe hepatic impairment. Avoid use with concomitant CYP3A4 inducers and moderate or strong CYP3A4 inhibitors. Discontinue **Caplyta** immediately, and monitor the patient closely, if signs of neuroleptic malignant syndrome (NMS) develop. Manage signs of tardive dyskinesia (TD) with discontinuation if clinically appropriate. Monitor for hyperglycemia/diabetes mellitus, dyslipidemia, and weight gain. Leukopenia, neutropenia, and agranulocytosis may develop; therefore, monitor CBC—especially in patients with preexisting low WBC or history of leukopenia or neutropenia. Consider discontinuing **Caplyta** if clinically significant decline in WBC occurs in the absence of other causative factors. Orthostatic hypotension and syncope may occur; therefore, monitor HR and BP and warn patients with known cardiovascular or cerebrovascular disease, and caution to avoid dehydration. Use caution in patients with a

history of seizure or with conditions that lower seizure threshold. There is potential for cognitive and motor impairment; therefore, advise caution when operating hazardous equipment or machinery and monitor as appropriate. The most common adverse reactions reported in clinical trials (incidence >5%) have been somnolence/sedation and dry mouth. **Caplyta** may cause extrapyramidal and/or withdrawal symptoms in neonates with third trimester exposure. Breastfeeding is *not* recommended.

▷ *lurasidone* (B)(G) initially 40 mg once daily; usual range 40 to max 160 mg/day; take with food; *CrCl <50 mL/min, moderate hepatic impairment (Child-Pugh 7-9):* max 80 mg/day; *Child-Pugh 10-15):* max 40 mg/day
Pediatric: <13 years: not established; 13-17 years: initially 40 mg once daily; may titrate up to max 80 mg/day
  Latuda *Tab:* 20, 40, 60, 80, 120 mg
  Comment: **Latuda** is contraindicated with concomitant strong CYP3A4 inhibitors (e.g., *ketoconazole, voriconazole, clarithromycin, ritonavir*) and inducers (e.g., *phenytoin, carbamazepine, rifampin, St. John's wort*); see mfr pkg insert if patient taking moderate CYP3A4 inhibitors (e.g., *diltiazem, atazanavir, erythromycin, fluconazole, verapamil*).

SEIZURE, CLUSTER

▷ *diazepam nasal spray* (IV) *Initial Dose:* 5 mg and 10 mg doses are administered as a single spray intranasally into one nostril (administration of 15 mg and 20 mg doses requires two nasal spray devices, one spray into each nostril); *Second Dose:* when required, may be administered at least 4 hours after the initial dose; if administered, use a new blister pack; *Max Dose and Treatment Frequency:* do *not* use more than 2 doses to treat a single episode; it is recommended that **Valtoco** be used to treat *no more* than one episode every 5 days and *no more* than 5 episodes per month
Pediatric: <6 years: safety and efficacy not established; ≥6 years: dosage is dependent on the patient's age and weight (see mfr pkg insert)
  Valtoco *Nasal spray:* 5, 7.5, 10 mg in 0.1 ml, single-dose
  Comment: **Valtoco** is a benzodiazepine indicated for the acute treatment of intermittent, stereotypic episodes of frequent seizure activity (i.e., seizure clusters, acute repetitive seizures) that are distinct from a patient's usual seizure pattern in patients with epilepsy 6 years-of-age and older. Benzodiazepines may cause an increased CNS-depressant effect when used with alcohol or other CNS depressants. Antiepileptic drugs increase the risk of suicidal ideation and behavior. **Valtoco** is contraindicated in patients with Acute narrow-angle glaucoma. The most common adverse reactions (incidence 4%) have been somnolence, headache, and nasal discomfort. Concomitant CYP2C19 and CYP3A4 inhibitors may increase adverse reactions to **Valtoco.** Concomitant inducers of CYP2C19 and CYP3A4 inducers may decrease *diazepam* exposure. Advise pregnant females and women of childbearing age of potentially serious embryo/fetal risk. *diazepam* is excreted in human milk. There are *no* data to assess the effects of **Valtoco** and/or its active metabolite(s) on the breastfed infant. Postmarketing experience suggests that breastfed infants of mothers taking benzodiazepines, such as **Valtoco,** may have effects of lethargy, somnolence, and poor sucking. There is a pregnancy exposure registry that monitors pregnancy outcomes in women exposed to antiepileptic drugs (AEDs), such as **Valtoco,** during pregnancy. Encourage women who are taking **Valtoco** during pregnancy to enroll in the North American Antiepileptic Drug (NAAED) Pregnancy Registry by calling 1-888-233-2334 or visiting http://www.aedpregnancyregistry.org.

SEIZURE DISORDER

Cluster Seizures *see Seizure, Clusters*
Status Epilepticus *see Status Epilepticus*
see **Anticonvulsant Drugs**

 SEXUAL ASSAULT (STD/STI/VD EXPOSURE)

Comment: The following treatment regimens for victims of sexual assault are
published in the **2015 CDC Sexually Transmitted Diseases Treatment Guidelines.**

RECOMMENDED PROPHYLAXIS REGIMEN

▷ *ceftriaxone* 250 mg IM in a single dose plus *metronidazole* 2 gm in a single dose
   plus *azithromycin* 1 gm in a single dose

ALTERNATE PROPHYLAXIS REGIMENS
Regimen 1

▷ *ceftriaxone* 250 mg IM in a single dose plus *metronidazole* 2 gm in a single dose
   plus *doxycycline* 100 mg bid x 7 days

Regimen 2

▷ *cefixime* 400 mg in a single dose plus *metronidazole* 2 gm in a single dose plus
   azithromycin 1 gm in a single dose

Regimen 3

▷ *cefixime* 400 mg in a single dose plus *metronidazole* 2 gm in a single dose plus
   doxycycline 100 mg bid x 7 days

Regimen 4

▷ *azithromycin* (B) 1 gm as a single dose plus *metronidazole* 2 gm in a single dose

DRUG BRANDS AND DOSE FORMS

▷ *azithromycin* (B)(G)
   Zithromax *Tab:* 250, 500, 600 mg; *Oral susp:* 100 mg/5 ml (15 ml); 200 mg/5 ml
   (15, 22.5, 30 ml) (cherry); *Pkt:* 1 gm for reconstitution (cherry-banana)
   Zithromax Tri-pak *Tab:* 3 x 500 mg tabs/pck
   Zithromax Z-pak *Tab:* 6 x 250 mg tabs/pck
   Zmax *Oral susp:* 2 gm ext-rel for reconstitution (cherry-banana) (148 mg Na⁺)
▷ *cefixime* (B)(G)
   Suprax *Tab:* 400 mg; *Cap:* 400 mg; *Oral susp:* 100, 200, 500 mg/5 ml (50, 75,
   100 ml) (strawberry)
▷ *ceftriaxone* (B)(G)
   Rocephin *Vial:* 250, 500 mg; 1, 2 gm
▷ *doxycycline* (D)(G)
   Acticlate *Tab:* 75, 150**mg
   Adoxa *Tab:* 50, 75, 100, 150 mg ent-coat
   Doryx *Tab:* 50, 75, 100, 150, 200 mg del-rel
   Doxteric *Tab:* 50 mg del-rel
   Monodox *Cap:* 50, 75, 100 mg
   Oracea *Cap:* 40 mg del-rel
   Vibramycin *Tab:* 100 mg; *Cap:* 50, 100 mg; *Syr:* 50 mg/5 ml (raspberry-apple)
   (sulfites); *Oral susp:* 25 mg/5 ml (raspberry)
   Vibra-Tab *Tab:* 100 mg film-coat
▷ *metronidazole* (not for use in 1st; B in 2nd, 3rd)(G)
   Flagyl *Tab:* 250*, 500*mg
   Flagyl 375 *Cap:* 375 mg
   Flagyl ER *Tab:* 750 mg ext-rel

SHIGELLOSIS (GENUS *SHIGELLA*)

ANTI-INFECTIVES

▶ *azithromycin* (B)(G) 500 mg x 1 dose on day 1, then 250 mg once daily on days 2-5 or 500 mg once daily x 3 days or **Zmax** 2 gm in a single dose
Pediatric: <6 months: not recommended; ≥6 months: 10 mg/kg x 1 dose on day 1; then 5 mg/kg/day on days 2-5; max 500 mg/day; *see* Appendix CC.7. *azithromycin* (Zithromax Suspension, Zmax Suspension) *for dose by weight*
 Zithromax *Tab:* 250, 500, 600 mg; *Oral susp:* 100 mg/5 ml (15 ml); 200 mg/5 ml (15, 22.5, 30 ml) (cherry); *Pkt:* 1 gm for reconstitution (cherry-banana)
 Zithromax Tri-pak *Tab:* 3 x 500 mg tabs/pck
 Zithromax Z-pak *Tab:* 6 x 250 mg tabs/pck
 Zmax *Oral susp:* 2 gm ext-rel for reconstitution (cherry-banana) (148 mg Na⁺)

▶ *ciprofloxacin* (C) 500 mg bid x 3 days
Pediatric: <18 years: not recommended; ≥18 years: same as adult
 Cipro (G) *Tab:* 250, 500, 750 mg; *Oral susp:* 250, 500 mg/5 ml (100 ml) (strawberry)
 Cipro XR *Tab:* 500, 1000 mg ext-rel
 ProQuin XR *Tab:* 500 mg ext-rel

▶ *ofloxacin* (C)(G) 400 mg bid x 3 days
Pediatric: <18 years: not recommended; ≥18 years: same as adult
 Floxin *Tab:* 200, 300, 400 mg

▶ *tetracycline* (D)(G) 250-500 mg qid x 5 days
Pediatric: <8 years: not recommended; ≥8 years, <100 lb: 25-50 mg/kg/day in 4 divided doses x 5 days; ≥8 years, ≥100 lb: same as adult; *see Appendix CC.31.* *tetracycline* (Sumycin Suspension) *for dose by weight*
 Achromycin V *Cap:* 250, 500 mg
 Sumycin *Tab:* 250, 500 mg; *Cap:* 250, 500 mg; *Oral susp:* 125 mg/5 ml (100, 200 ml) (fruit) (sulfites)

▶ *trimethoprim+sulfamethoxazole* (TMP-SMX) (D)(G)
 Bactrim, Septra 2 tabs bid x 10 days
  Tab: trim 80 mg+sulfa 400 mg*
 Bactrim DS, Septra DS 1 tab bid x 10 days
  Tab: trim 160 mg+sulfa 800 mg*
 Bactrim Pediatric Suspension, Septra Pediatric Suspension 20 ml bid x 10 days
  Oral susp: trim 40 mg+sulfa 200 mg per 5 ml (100 ml) (cherry) (alcohol 0.3%)

SHOCK: SEPTIC, DISTRIBUTIVE

Comment: Septic shock is the most common form of distributive shock and is characterized by considerable mortality (treated, around 30%; untreated, probably >80%). In the US, septic shock is the leading cause of non-cardiac death in intensive care units. **Giapreza (angiotensin II)** is indicated to increase blood pressure, when added to conventional interventions used to raise blood pressure, to prevent/treat dangerously low hypotension resulting from septic and other distributive shock states. There is a potential for venous and arterial thrombotic and thromboembolic events in patients who receive **Giapreza**. Therefore, use concurrent venous thromboembolism (VTE) prophylaxis.

ANGIOTENSIN II

▶ *angiotensin II* dilute in 0.9% NaCl; must be administered as an IV infusion; initial infusion rate 20 ng/kg/min; titrate as frequently as every 5 minutes by increments of up to 15 ng/kg/min as needed; during the first 3 hours, max 80 ng/kg/min; max maintenance dose 40 ng/kg/min; diluted solution may be stored at room temperature or refrigerated; discard after 24 hours.

Dilution/Concentration:

Giapreza 1 ml (2.5 mg/ml) in 500 ml 0.9%NaCl = 5,000 ng/ml

1 ml (2.5.mg/ml in 250 ml 0.9%NaCl = 10,000 ng/ml

2 ml (5 mg/ml) in 500 ml 0.9%NaCl = 10,000 ng/ml

Giapreza *Vial:* 2.5 mg in ml, 5 mg/2 ml (2.5 mg/ml)

Comment: The safety and efficacy of **Giapreza** in pediatric patients have not been established. It is not known whether **Giapreza** is present in human milk and no data are available on the effects of angiotensin II on the breastfed infant. The published data on angiotensin II use in pregnant females are not sufficient to determine a drug-associated risk of adverse developmental outcomes. However, Delaying treatment in pregnant females with hypotension associated with septic or other distributive shock is likely to increase the risk of shock-associated maternal and fetal morbidity and mortality.

SICKLE CELL DISEASE (SCD)

▷ *hydroxyurea*

Comment: *Hydroxyurea* has an FDA-approved "orphan drug" designation for the treatment of sickle cell disease SCD). It is an antimetabolite indicated to reduce the frequency of painful crises and to reduce the need for blood transfusions in patients with sickle cell anemia SCA) with recurrent moderate-to-severe painful crises. *Black Box Warning (BBW):* **hydroxyurea** may cause severe myelosuppression. Do not administer if bone marrow function is markedly depressed. Monitor blood counts at baseline and every 2 weeks throughout treatment. Blood counts within an acceptable range are defined as: *neutrophils* ≥ 2,500 cells/mm3, *platelets* ≥95,000 cells/mm3, *Hgb* ≥5.3 gm/dL, *reticulocytes* ≥95,000 cells/mm3 if the Hgb <9 gm/dL. Discontinue **hydroxyurea** until hematologic recovery if blood counts are considered toxic. Treatment may be resumed after reducing the **hydroxyurea** dose by 2.5 mg/kg/day from the dose associated with hematological toxicity. *CrCl <60 mL/min:* reduce dose by 50%. *Hydroxyurea* is carcinogenic. Advise sun protection and monitor patients for malignancies. Avoid live vaccines when using *hydroyurea*. Discontinue **hydroxyurea** if vasculitic toxicity occurs. Risks with concomitant use of antiretroviral drugs: pancreatitis, hepatotoxicity, and neuropathy. Monitor for signs and symptoms in patients with HIV infection using antiretroviral drugs. If patients with HIV infection are treated with **hydroxyurea**, and in particular, in combination with **didanosine** and/or **stavudine**, close monitoring for signs and symptoms of pancreatitis is recommended. Permanently discontinue **hydroxyurea** in patients who develop signs and symptoms of pancreatitis. *Hydroxyurea* can cause fetal harm (embryotoxic and teratogenic effects in animal studies). Advise patients regarding potential risk to a fetus and use of effective contraception during and after treatment with **hydroxyurea** for at least 6 months after therapy is ended. Advise females to immediately report pregnancy. *Hydroxyurea* may damage spermatozoa and testicular tissue, resulting in possible genetic abnormalities. Azoospermia or oligospermia, sometimes reversible, has been observed in men. Inform male patients about the possibility of sperm conservation before the initiation of *hydroxyurea* therapy. Males with female sexual partners of reproductive potential should use effective contraception during and after treatment for at least 1 year. *Hydroxyurea* is excreted in human milk. Discontinue breastfeeding during treatment.

Droxia use actual or ideal body weight (whichever is less) for dosing; initially 15 mg/kg once daily; if the blood counts are within an acceptable range, increase the dose by 5 mg/kg/day every 12 weeks to the highest dose that does not produce toxic blood counts over 24 consecutive weeks (dosage should not exceed 35 mg/kg/day)

Pediatric: <18 years: not established; ≥18 years: same as adult
   Cap: 200, 300, 400 mg
Hydrea (see **Droxia** for prescribing information)
   Tab: 500 mg
Siklos use actual or ideal body weight (whichever is less) for dosing; *initially,* 20 mg/kg once daily; may be increased by 5 mg/kg/day every 8 weeks, or sooner if a severe painful crisis occurs, until a maximum tolerated dose or 35 mg/kg/day is reached; reduce the dose of **Siklos** by 50% (10 mg) in patients with CrCl <60 mL/min or with ESRD
Pediatric: <2 years: not recommended; ≥2 years: same as adult
   Tab: 100 mg; 1,000***mg
Comment: Safety and effectiveness of **Siklos** have been established in pediatric patients aged 2-18 years with sickle cell anemia (SSA) with recurrent moderate-to-severe painful crises and is the only *hydroxyurea* approved for use in children. Use of **Siklos** in these age groups is supported by evidence from a non-interventional cohort study, the European Sickle Cell Disease prospective Cohort study, ESCORT-HU, in which 405 pediatric patients ages 2 to <18 were treated with **Siklos**: n = 274 children (2-11 years) and n = 108 adolescents 12-16 years). Pediatric patients aged 2-16 years had a higher risk of neutropenia than patients >16 years. Continuous follow-up of the growth of treated children is recommended.

AMINO ACID

▷ *L-glutamine powder* take 5-15 gm orally, twice daily, based on body weight; <30 kg, <66 lb (1 pkt bid), 30-65 kg, 66-143 lb (2 pkts bid), >65 kg, >143 lb (3 pkts bid); mix each dose in 8 oz. (240 ml) of cold or room temperature beverage or 4-6 oz of food before ingestion
Pediatric: <5 years: not established; ≥5 years: same as adult
   Endari *Oral Powder:* 5 gm/paper-foil-plastic laminate pkt (60 pkts/carton)
   Comment: **Endari** is an amino acid indicated to reduce the acute complications of sickle cell disease. Common adverse reactions include constipation, nausea, abdominal pain, headache, cough, pain in extremity, back pain, and chest pain. There are no available data on **Endari** use in pregnancy to inform a drug-associated risk of major birth defects and miscarriage. There are no data on the presence of **Endari** in human milk or effects on the breastfed infant. The developmental and health benefits from breastfeeding should be considered along with the mother's clinical need for **Endari** and any potential adverse effects on the breastfed infant from **Endari** or from the underlying maternal condition.

CHIMERIC (MURINE/HUMAN) MONOCLONAL ANTIBODY

▷ *basiliximab* (B)
Pediatric: <6 months: not recommended; 6 months-12 years: 14 mg/kg/day in a single or 2 divided doses x 10 days; 12 years: same as adult
   Simulect *Vial:* 10, 20 mg (6 ml) for reconstitution and IV infusion (preservative-free 10 mg vial: contains 10 mg *basiliximab*, 3.61 mg monobasic potassium phosphate, 0.50 mg disodium hydrogen phosphate (anhydrous), 0.80 mg sodium chloride, 10 mg sucrose, 40 mg mannitol, 20 mg glycine, to be reconstituted in 2.5 mL of Sterile Water for Injection, USP 20 mg *vial;* contains 20 mg *basiliximab*, 7.21 mg monobasic potassium phosphate, 0.99 mg disodium hydrogen phosphate (anhydrous), 1.61 mg sodium chloride, 20 mg sucrose, 80 mg mannitol and 40 mg glycine, to be reconstituted with 5 ml of Sterile Water for Injection, US
   Comment: **Simulect** is indicated for the prophylaxis of acute organ rejection in patients receiving renal transplantation when used as part of

an immunosuppressive regimen that includes *cyclosporine* (modified) and corticosteroids. The efficacy of **Simulect** for the prophylaxis of acute rejection in recipients of other solid organ allografts has not been demonstrated. No dose adjustment is necessary when Simulect is added to triple immunosuppression regimens including *cyclosporine*, corticosteroids, and either *azathioprine* or *mycophenolate mofetil*. It is not known whether **Simulect** is excreted in human milk. A decision should be made to discontinue nursing or to discontinue the drug, taking into account the importance of the drug to the mother.

P-SELECTIN INHIBITOR

▷ *crizanlizumab-tmca* administer 5 mg/kg by intravenous infusion (IVF) over a period of 30 minutes on Week 0, Week 2, and every 4 weeks thereafter; see mfr pkg insert for preparation and administration instructions
Pediatric: <16 years: not established; ≥16 years: same as adult
   Adakveo *Vial:* 100 mg/10 ml (10 mg/ml,10 ml), single-dose
   Comment: **Adakveo** (**crizanlizumab-tmca**) is a P-selectin inhibitor for the prevention of vasoocclusive crises (VOCs) in patients ≥16 years-of-age with sickle cell disease (SCD). Monitor the patient for signs and symptoms of a infusion-related reaction; discontinue **Adakveo** infusion for severe reaction and manage medically. **Adakevo** may interfere with automated platelet counts (platelet clumping); run test as soon as possible (within 4 hours of collection or use tubes containing citrate tubes (do not use tubes containing EDTA). Most common adverse reactions (incidence >10%) have been nausea, arthralgia, back pain, and pyrexia. There are insufficient human data on **Aakveo** use in pregnant females to evaluate for a drug-associated risk of major birth defects, miscarriage, or adverse maternal or fetal outcomes; however, animal studies have demonstrated potential of **Adakevo** to cause fetal harm. Advise pregnant females of the potential risk to a fetus. **Adakveo** should only be used during pregnancy if the expected benefit to the patient justifies the potential risk to the fetus. Advise women of potential embryo/risk. **Adakveo** should only be used during pregnancy if the expected benefit to the patient justifies potential embryo/fetal risk. There are no data on the presence of *crizanlizumab-tmca* in human or animal milk or effects on the breastfed infant. Maternal IgG is known to be present in human milk. The effects of local gastrointestinal exposure and limited systemic exposure in the breastfed infant to *crizanlizumab-tmca* are unknown. The developmental and health benefits of breastfeeding should be considered along with the mother's clinical need for **Adakveo** and any potential adverse effects on the breastfed infant from **Adakveo** or from the underlying maternal condition.

ORAL HEMOGLOBIN S (sHGB) POLYMERIZATION INHIBITOR

▷ *voxelotor* 1,500 mg once daily; *Severe Hepatic Impairment (Child Pugh C):* 1,000 mg once daily; take with or without food
Pediatric: <12 years: safety and efficacy not established; ≥12 years: same as adults
   Oxbryta *Tab:* 500 mg
   Comment: **Oxbryta** *(voxelotor)* is an oral hemoglobin S (sHgb) polymerization inhibitor indicated for the treatment of sickle cell disease (SSD) in patients ≥12 years-of-age. *voxelotor* interferes with the quantification of hemoglobin species laboratory test; do this test when the patient is not receiving **Oxbryta**. Observe for signs and symptoms of a hypersensitivity reaction and manage promptly. Most common adverse reactions (incidence >10%) are headache, diarrhea, abdominal pain, nausea, fatigue, rash, and pyrexia. Avoid co-administration of **Oxbryta** with sensitive CYP3A4

substrates with a narrow therapeutic index. Avoid co-administration of **Oxbryta** with strong CYP3A4 inhibitors and *fluconazole*; if unavoidable, reduce the dose of **Oxbryta**. Avoid co-administration of **Oxbryta** with strong or moderate CYP3A4 inducers; if unavoidable, increase the dose of **Oxbryta**. Consider maternal/fetal risk/benefit of **Oxbryta** use in pregnancy. Women with SSD have an increased risk of adverse pregnancy outcomes for the mother and the fetus. Pregnant females are at greater risk for vasoocclusive crises, pre-eclampsia, eclampsia, and maternal mortality. For the fetus, there is an increased risk for intrauterine growth restriction, preterm delivery, low birth weight, and perinatal mortality. In animal reproduction studies, oral administration of *voxelotor* during organogenesis resulted in no adverse developmental effects. There are no available data on **Oxbryta** use in pregnant females to evaluate for a drug-associated risk of major birth defects, miscarriage or adverse maternal or fetal outcomes. Because of the potential for serious adverse reactions in the breastfed infant, including changes in the hematopoietic system, advise patients that breastfeeding is not recommended during treatment with **Oxbryta**, and for at least 2 weeks after the last dose.

SINUSITIS, RHINOSINUSITIS: ACUTE BACTERIAL (ABRS)

ANTI-INFECTIVES

▷ *amoxicillin* (B)(G) 500-875 mg bid or 250-500 mg tid x 10 days
   Pediatric: <40 kg (88 lb): 20-40 mg/kg/day in 3 divided doses x 10 days or 25-45 mg/kg/day in 2 divided doses x 10 days; *see* Appendix CC.3. *amoxicillin* (Amoxil Suspension, Trimox Suspension) *for dose by weight*
   Amoxil *Cap:* 250, 500 mg; *Tab:* 875*mg; *Chew tab:* 125, 200, 250, 400 mg (cherry-banana-peppermint) (phenylalanine); *Oral susp:* 125, 250 mg/5 ml (80, 100, 150 ml) (strawberry); 200, 400 mg/5 ml (50, 75, 100 ml) (bubble gum); *Oral drops:* 50 mg/ml (30 ml) (bubble gum)
   Moxatag *Tab:* 775 mg ext-rel
   Trimox *Tab:* 125, 250 mg; *Cap:* 250, 500 mg; *Oral susp:* 125, 250 mg/5 ml (80, 100, 150 ml) (raspberry-strawberry)
▷ *amoxicillin+clavulanate* (B)(G)
   Augmentin 500 mg tid or 875 mg bid x 10 days
   Pediatric: 40-45 mg/kg/day divided tid x 10 days or 90 mg/kg/day divided bid x 10 days *see* Appendix CC.4. *amoxicillin+clavulanate* (Augmentin Suspension) *for dose by weight*
   Tab: 250, 500, 875 mg; *Chew tab:* 125, 250 mg (lemon-lime); 200, 400 mg (cherry-banana) (phenylalanine); *Oral susp:* 125 mg/5 ml (banana), 250 mg/5 ml (75, 100, 150 ml) (orange); 200, 400 mg/5 ml (50, 75, 100 ml) (orange) (phenylalanine)
   Augmentin ES-600 not recommended for adults
   Pediatric: <3 months: not recommended; ≥3 months, <40 kg: 90 mg/kg/day in 2 divided doses x 10 days; ≥40 kg: not recommended
   Oral susp: 42.9 mg/5 ml (50, 75, 100, 125, 150, 200 ml) (strawberry cream) (phenylalanine)
   Augmentin XR 2 tabs q 12 hours x 10 days
   Pediatric: <16 years: use other forms; ≥16 years: same as adult
   Tab: 1000*mg ext-rel
▷ *cefaclor* (B)(G)
   Ceclor 250 mg tid or 375 mg bid 3-10 days
   Pediatric: <1 month: not recommended; 1 month-12 years: 20-40 mg/kg divided bid or q 12 hours x 3-10 days; max 1 gm/day; *see* Appendix CC.8. *cefaclor* (Ceclor Suspension) *for dose by weight;* >12 years: same as adult

Tab: 500 mg; *Cap:* 250, 500 mg; *Susp:* 125 mg/5 ml (75, 150 ml) (strawberry); 187 mg/5 ml (50, 100 ml) (strawberry); 250 mg/5 ml (75, 150 ml) (strawberry); 375 mg/5 ml (50, 100 ml) (strawberry)

Cefaclor Extended Release 375-500 mg bid x 3-10 days
Pediatric: <16 years: ext-rel not recommended; ≥16 years: same as adult
Tab: 375, 500 mg ext-rel

▷ *cefdinir* (B) 300 mg bid or 600 mg once daily x 10 days
Pediatric: <6 months: not recommended; 6 months-12 years: 14 mg/kg/day in a single or 2 divided doses x 10 days; 12 years: same as adult; *see* Appendix CC.10.
cefdinir (Omnicef Suspension) *for dose by weight*
Omnicef *Cap:* 300 mg; *Oral susp:* 125 mg/5 ml (60, 100 ml) (strawberry)

▷ *cefixime* (B)(G) 400 mg once daily x 10 days
Pediatric: <6 months: not recommended; 6 months-12 years, <50 kg: 8 mg/kg/day in 1-2 divided doses x 10 days; *see* Appendix CC.11. *cefixime* (Suprax Oral Suspension) *for dose by weight;* >12 years, >50 kg: same as adult
Suprax *Tab:* 400 mg; *Cap:* 400 mg; *Oral susp:* 100, 200, 500 mg/5 ml (50, 75, 100 ml) (strawberry)

▷ *cefpodoxime proxetil* 200 mg bid x 10 days
Pediatric: <2 months: not recommended; 2 months-12 years: 10 mg/kg/day (max 400 mg/dose) or 5 mg/kg/day bid (max 200 mg/dose) x 10 days; *see* Appendix CC.12. *cefpodoxime proxetil* (Vantin Suspension) *for dose by weight*
Vantin *Tab:* 100, 200 mg; *Oral susp:* 50, 100 mg/5 ml (50, 75, 100 mg) (lemon creme)

▷ *cefprozil* (B) 250-500 mg bid x 10 days
Pediatric: <6 months: not recommended; 6 months-12 years: *Mild:* 7.5 mg/kg bid x 10 days; *Moderate/Severe:* 15 mg/kg q 12 hours x 10 days; *see* Appendix CC.13. *cefprozil* (Cefzil Suspension) *for dose by weight;* >12 years: same as adult
Cefzil *Tab:* 250, 500 mg; *Oral susp:* 125, 250 mg/5 ml (50, 75, 100 ml) (bubble gum) (phenylalanine)

▷ *ceftibuten* (B) 400 mg once daily x 10 days
Pediatric: <12 years: 9 mg/kg once daily x 10 days; max 400 mg/day; *see* Appendix CC.14. *ceftibuten* (Cedax Suspension) *for dose by weight;* ≥12 years: 400 mg once daily x 10 days
Cedax *Cap:* 400 mg; Oral susp: 90 mg/5 ml (30, 60, 90, 120 ml); 180
Cedax *Cap:* 400 mg; *Oral susp:* 90 mg/5 ml (30, 60, 90, 120 ml); 180 mg/5 ml (30, 60, 120 ml) (cherry)

▷ *ciprofloxacin* (C) 500 mg bid x 10 days
Pediatric: <18 years: not recommended; ≥18 years: same as adult
Cipro (G) *Tab:* 250, 500, 750 mg; *Oral susp:* 250, 500 mg/5 ml (100 ml) (strawberry)
Cipro XR *Tab:* 500, 1000 mg ext-rel
ProQuin XR *Tab:* 500 mg ext-rel

▷ *clarithromycin* (C)(G) 500 mg bid or 1000 mg ext-rel once daily x 10 days
Pediatric: <6 months: not recommended; ≥6 months: 7.5 mg/kg bid x 10 days; *see* Appendix CC.16. *clarithromycin* (Biaxin Suspension) *for dose by weight*
Biaxin *Tab:* 250, 500 mg
Biaxin Oral Suspension *Oral susp:* 125, 250 mg/5 ml (50, 100 ml) (fruit punch)
Biaxin XL *Tab:* 500 mg ext-rel

▷ *levofloxacin* (C) *Uncomplicated:* 500 mg once daily x 10-14 days; *Complicated:* 750 mg once daily x 10-14 days
Pediatric: <18 years: not recommended; ≥18 years: same as adult
Levaquin *Tab:* 250, 500, 750 mg; *Oral soln:* 25 mg/ml (480 ml) (benzyl alcohol); *Inj conc:* 25 mg/ml for IV infusion after dilution (20, 30 ml single-use vial) (preservative-free); *Premix soln:* 5 mg/ml for IV infusion (50, 100, 150 ml) (preservative-free)

▷ *loracarbef* (B) 400 mg bid x 10 days
  Pediatric: 15 mg/kg/day in 2 divided doses x 10 days; *see* Appendix CC.27.
  loracarbef (Lorabid Suspension) *for dose by weight*
    Lorabid *Pulvule:* 200, 400 mg; *Oral susp:* 100 mg/5 ml (50, 100 ml); 200 mg/5 ml (50, 75, 100 ml) (strawberry bubble gum)
▷ *moxifloxacin* (C)(G) 400 mg once daily x 10 days
  Pediatric: <18 years: not recommended; ≥18 years: same as adult
    Avelox *Tab:* 400 mg
▷ *trimethoprim+sulfamethoxazole (TMP-SMX)* (D)(G)
  Pediatric: <2 months: not recommended; ≥2 months: 40 mg/kg/day of
  sulfamethoxazole in 2 divided doses bid x 10 days; *see Appendix CC.33:*
  trimethoprim+sulfamethoxazole (Bactrim Suspension, Septra Suspension) *for dose by weight*
    Bactrim, Septra 2 tabs bid x 10 days
      Tab: trim 80 mg+sulfa 400 mg*
    Bactrim DS, Septra DS 1 tab bid x 10 days
      Tab: trim 160 mg+sulfa 800 mg*
    Bactrim Pediatric Suspension, Septra Pediatric Suspension
      Oral susp: trim 40 mg+sulfa 200 mg per 5 ml (100 ml) (cherry) (alcohol 0.3%)

⬤ SJÖGREN-LARSSON-SYNDROME (SLS)

Comment: Sjögren-Larsson-Syndrome is a chronic autoimmune disorder that causes the white blood cells to attack the moisture-producing glands. Sjögren's syndrome can occur in association with other autoimmune diseases, including systemic lupus erythematosus, rheumatoid arthritis, scleroderma, systemic sclerosis, cryoglobulinemia, or polyarteritis nodosa. The disease can affect the eyes, mouth, parotid gland, pancreas, gastrointestinal system, blood vessels, lungs, kidneys, skin, and nervous system. Erythrocyte sedimentation rate (ESR) is elevated in 80% of patients. Rheumatoid factor is present in 52% of primary cases and 98% of secondary-type cases. A mild normochromic normocytic anemia is present in 50% of patients, and leukopenia occurs in up to 42% of patients. Creatinine clearance is diminished in up to 50% of patients. Anti-nuclear antibody (ANA) is positive in 70% of patients. SS-A and SS-B are marker antibodies for Sjögren's syndrome; 70% of patients are positive for SS-A and 40% are positive for SS-B.

CHOLINERGIC (MUSCARINIC) AGONIST COMBINATION

▷ *cevimeline* (C)(G) 30 mg tid
    Evoxac *Cap:* 30 mg
  Comment: *Cevimeline* is contraindicated in acute iritis, narrow angle glaucoma, and uncontrolled asthma.
▷ *pilocarpine* (C)(G) 5 mg qid or 7.5 mg tid
    Salagen *Tab:* 5, 7.5 mg

ORAL ENZYME RINSE

▷ *xylitol+solazyme+selectobac* swish 5 ml for 30 seconds bid-tid
    Orazyme Dry Mouth Rinse *Oral soln:* 1.5, 16 oz

⬤ SKIN: CALLUSED

KERATOLYTICS

▷ *salicylic acid* (C)(OTC) apply lotion, cream or gel to affected area once daily-bid;
  apply patch to affected area and leave on x 48 hours with max 5 applications/14 days
  Pediatric: <12 years: not recommended; ≥12 years: same as adult

▷ *urea* (C)
Pediatric: <12 years: not recommended; ≥12 years: same as adult
Carmol 40 apply to affected area with applicator stick provided once daily-tid; smooth over until cream is absorbed; protect surrounding tissue; may cover with adhesive bandage or gauze secured with adhesive tape
Crm/Gel: 40% (30 gm)
Keratol 40 apply to affected area with applicator stick provided once daily-tid; smooth over until cream is absorbed; protect surrounding tissue; may cover with adhesive bandage or gauze secured with adhesive tape
Crm: 40% (1, 3, 7 oz); *Gel:* 40% (15 ml); *Lotn:* 40% (8 oz)
Comment: The moisturizing effect of **Carmol 40** and **Keratol 40** is enhanced by applying while the skin is still moist (after washing or bathing).

SKIN INFECTION: BACTERIAL (CARBUNCLE, FOLLICULITIS, FURUNCLE)

Comment: Abscesses usually require surgical incision and drainage.

ANTIBACTERIAL SKIN CLEANSERS

▷ *hexachlorophene* (C) dispense 5 ml into wet hand, work up into lather; then apply to area to be cleansed; rinse thoroughly
pHisoHex *Liq clnsr:* 5, 16 oz

TOPICAL ANTI-INFECTIVES

▷ *mupirocin* (B)(G) apply to lesions bid
Pediatric: same as adult
Bactroban *Oint:* 2% (22 gm); *Crm:* 2% (15, 30 gm)
Centany *Oint:* 2% (15, 30 gm)
▷ *polymyxin b+neomycin* (C) oint apply once daily-tid
Neosporin (OTC) *Oint:* 15 gm

ORAL ANTI-INFECTIVES

▷ *amoxicillin* (B)(G) 500-875 mg bid or 250-500 mg tid x 10 days
Pediatric: <40 kg (88 lb): 20-40 mg/kg/day in 3 divided doses x 10 days or 25-45 mg/kg/day in 2 divided doses x 10 days; see Appendix CC.3. *amoxicillin* (Amoxil Suspension, Trimox Suspension) *for dose by weight*
Amoxil *Cap:* 250, 500 mg; *Tab:* 875*mg; *Chew tab:* 125, 200, 250, 400 mg (cherry-banana-peppermint) (phenylalanine); *Oral susp:* 125, 250 mg/5 ml (80, 100, 150 ml) (strawberry); 200, 400 mg/5 ml (50, 75, 100 ml) (bubble gum); *Oral drops:* 50 mg/ml (30 ml) (bubble gum)
Moxatag *Tab:* 775 mg ext-rel
Trimox *Tab:* 125, 250 mg; *Cap:* 250, 500 mg; *Oral susp:* 125, 250 mg/5 ml (80, 100, 150 ml) (raspberry-strawberry)
▷ *azithromycin* (B)(G) 500 mg x 1 dose on day 1, then 250 mg once daily on days 2-5 or 500 mg once daily x 3 days or **Zmax** 2 gm in a single dose
Pediatric: 12 mg/kg/day x 5 days; max 500 mg/day; see Appendix CC.7. *azithromycin* (Zithromax Suspension, Zmax Suspension) *for dose by weight*
Zithromax *Tab:* 250, 500, 600 mg; *Oral susp:* 100 mg/5 ml (15 ml); 200 mg/5 ml (15, 22.5, 30 ml) (cherry); *Pkt:* 1 gm for reconstitution (cherry-banana)
Zithromax Tri-pak *Tab:* 3 x 500 mg tabs/pck
Zithromax Z-pak *Tab:* 6 x 250 mg tabs/pck
Zmax *Oral susp:* 2 gm ext-rel for reconstitution (cherry-banana) (148 mg Na$^+$)
▷ *cefaclor* (B)(G)
Ceclor 250 mg tid or 375 mg bid 3-10 days

Pediatric: <1 month: not recommended; 1 month-12 years: 20-40 mg/kg divided bid or q 12 hours x 3-10 days; max 1 gm/day; *see* Appendix CC.8. *cefaclor* (Ceclor Suspension) *for dose by weight;* >12 years: same as adult

 Tab: 500 mg; *Cap:* 250, 500 mg; *Susp:* 125 mg/5 ml (75, 150 ml) (strawberry); 187 mg/5 ml (50, 100 ml) (strawberry); 250 mg/5 ml (75, 150 ml) (strawberry); 375 mg/5 ml (50, 100 ml) (strawberry)

Cefaclor Extended Release 375-500 mg bid x 3-10 days

Pediatric: <16 years: ext-rel not recommended; ≥16 years: same as adult

 Tab: 375, 500 mg ext-rel

▷ *cefadroxil* (B) 1-2 gm in a single or 2 divided doses x 10 days

Pediatric: 15-30 mg/kg/day in 2 divided doses x 10 days; *see* Appendix CC.9. *cefadroxil* (Duricef Suspension) *for dose by weight*

 Duricef *Cap:* 500 mg; *Tab:* 1 gm; *Oral susp:* 250 mg/5 ml (100 ml); 500 mg/5 ml (75, 100 ml) (orange-pineapple)

▷ *cefdinir* (B) 300 mg bid x 10 days

Pediatric: <6 months: not recommended; 6 months-12 years: 14 mg/kg/day in 1-2 divided doses x 10 days; *see* Appendix CC.10. *cefdinir* (Omnicef Suspension) *for dose by weight*

 Omnicef *Cap:* 300 mg; *Oral susp:* 125 mg/5 ml (60, 100 ml) (strawberry)

▷ *cefditoren pivoxil* (B) 200 mg bid x 10 days

Pediatric: <12 years: not recommended; ≥12 years: same as adult

 Spectracef *Tab:* 200 mg

Comment: Contraindicated with milk protein allergy or carnitine deficiency.

▷ *cefpodoxime proxetil* (B) 400 mg bid x 7-14 days

Pediatric: <2 months: not recommended; 2 months-12 years: 10 mg/kg/day (max 400 mg/dose) or 5 mg/kg/day bid (max 200 mg/dose) x 7-14 days; *see* Appendix CC.12. *cefpodoxime proxetil* (Vantin Suspension) *for dose by weight*

 Vantin *Tab:* 100, 200 mg; *Oral susp:* 50, 100 mg/5 ml (50, 75, 100 mg) (lemon creme)

▷ *cefprozil* (B) 250-500 mg bid or 500 mg once daily x 10 days

Pediatric: 2-12 years: 7.5 mg/kg bid x 10 days; >12 years: same as adult; *see* Appendix CC.13. *cefprozil* (Cefzil Suspension) *for dose by weight*

 Cefzil *Tab:* 250, 500 mg; *Oral susp:* 125, 250 mg/5 ml (50, 75, 100 ml) (bubble gum) (phenylalanine)

▷ *ceftriaxone* (B)(G) 1-2 gm IM once daily; max 4 gm/day

Pediatric: 50-75 mg/kg IM in 1-2 divided doses; max 2 gm/day

 Rocephin *Vial:* 250, 500 mg; 1, 2 gm

▷ *cephalexin* (B)(G) 500 mg bid x 10 days

Pediatric: 25-50 mg/kg/day in 4 divided doses x 10 days; *see* Appendix CC.15. *cephalexin* (Keflex Suspension) *for dose by weight*

 Keflex *Cap:* 250, 333, 500, 750 mg; *Oral susp:* 125, 250 mg/5 ml (100, 200 ml) (strawberry)

▷ *clarithromycin* (C)(G) 250-500 mg bid or 500-1000 mg ext-rel once daily x 7-14 days

Pediatric: <6 months: not recommended; ≥6 months: 7.5 mg/kg bid x 7-14 days; *see* Appendix CC.16. *clarithromycin* (Biaxin Suspension) *for dose by weight*

 Biaxin *Tab:* 250, 500 mg

 Biaxin Oral Suspension *Oral susp:* 125, 250 mg/5 ml (50, 100 ml) (fruit punch)

 Biaxin XL *Tab:* 500 mg ext-rel

▷ *dicloxacillin* (B) 500 mg qid x 10 days

Pediatric: 12.5-25 mg/kg/day in 4 divided doses x 10 days; *see* Appendix CC.18. *dicloxacillin* (Dynapen Suspension) *for dose by weight*

 Dynapen *Cap:* 125, 250, 500 mg; *Oral susp:* 62.5 mg/5 ml (80, 100, 200 ml)

▷ *dirithromycin* (C)(G) 500 mg once daily x 5-7 days
　Pediatric: <12 years: not recommended; ≥12 years: same as adult
　　Dynabac *Tab:* 250 mg

▷ *doxycycline* (D)(G) 100 mg bid x 9 days
　Pediatric: <8 years: not recommended; ≥8 years, <100 lb: 1 mg/lb in a single
　dose once daily x 9 days; *see Appendix CC.19: doxycycline* (Vibramycin Syrup/
　Suspension) *for dose by weight;* >8 years, ≥100 lb: same as adult
　　Acticlate *Tab:* 75, 150**mg
　　Adoxa *Tab:* 50, 75, 100, 150 mg ent-coat
　　Doryx *Tab:* 50, 75, 100, 150, 200 mg del-rel
　　Doxteric *Tab:* 50 mg del-rel
　　Monodox *Cap:* 50, 75, 100 mg
　　Oracea *Cap:* 40 mg del-rel
　　Vibramycin *Tab:* 100 mg; *Cap:* 50, 100 mg; *Syr:* 50 mg/5 ml (raspberry-apple)
　　(sulfites); *Oral susp:* 25 mg/5 ml (raspberry)
　　Vibra-Tab *Tab:* 100 mg film-coat

▷ *erythromycin base* (B)(G) 250-500 mg tid x 10 days
　Pediatric: 30-50 mg/kg/day in 2-4 divided doses x 10 days
　　Ery-Tab *Tab:* 250, 333, 500 mg ent-coat
　　PCE *Tab:* 333, 500 mg

▷ *erythromycin estolate* (B)(G) 250-500 mg q 6 hours x 10 days
　Pediatric: 20-50 mg/kg q 6 hours x 10 days; *see Appendix CC.20: erythromycin*
　estolate (Ilosone Suspension) *for dose by weight*
　　Ilosone *Pulvule:* 250 mg; *Tab:* 500 mg; *Liq:* 125, 250 mg/5 ml (100 ml)

▷ *erythromycin ethylsuccinate* (B)(G) 400 mg qid x 10 days
　Pediatric: 30-50 mg/kg/day in 4 divided doses x 10 days; may double dose
　with severe infection; max 100 mg/kg/day; *see Appendix CC.21: erythromycin*
　ethylsuccinate (E.E.S. Suspension, Ery-Ped Drops/Suspension) *for dose by weight*
　　EryPed *Oral susp:* 200 mg/5 ml (100, 200 ml) (fruit); 400 mg/5 ml (60, 100,
　　200 ml) (banana); *Oral drops:* 200, 400 mg/5 ml (50 ml) (fruit); *Chew tab:*
　　200 mg wafer (fruit)
　　E.E.S. *Oral susp:* 200, 400 mg/5 ml (100 ml) (fruit)
　　E.E.S. Granules *Oral susp:* 200 mg/5 ml (100, 200 ml) (cherry)
　　E.E.S. 400 Tablets *Tab:* 400 mg

▷ *gemifloxacin* (C)(G) 320 mg once daily x 5-7 days
　Pediatric: <18 years: not recommended; ≥18 years: same as adult
　　Factive *Tab:* 320*mg

▷ *levofloxacin* (C) *Uncomplicated:* 500 mg once daily x 7-10 days; *Complicated:* 750
　mg once daily x 7-10 days
　Pediatric: <18 years: not recommended; ≥18 years: same as adult
　　Levaquin *Tab:* 250, 500, 750 mg; *Oral soln:* 25 mg/ml (480 ml) (benzyl
　　alcohol); *Inj conc:* 25 mg/ml for IV infusion after dilution (20, 30 ml
　　single-use vial) (preservative-free); *Premix soln:* 5 mg/ml for IV infusion
　　(50, 100, 150 ml) (preservative-free)

▷ *linezolid* (C)(G) 400-600 mg q 12 hours x 10-14 days
　Pediatric: <5 years: 10 mg/kg q 8 hours x 10-14 days; 5-11 years: 10 mg/kg q 12
　hours x 10-14 days; >11 years: same as adult
　　Zyvox *Tab:* 400, 600 mg; *Oral susp:* 100 mg/5 ml (150 ml) (orange) (phenylalanine)
　　Comment: *Linezolid* is indicated to treat susceptible *vancomycin*-resistant *E. faecium*
　　infections.

▷ *loracarbef* (B) 200 mg bid x 7 days
　Pediatric: 15 mg/kg/day in 2 divided doses x 7 days; *see* Appendix CC.27. *lora-*
　carbef (Lorabid Suspension) *for dose by weight*
　　Lorabid *Pulvule:* 200, 400 mg; *Oral susp:* 100 mg/5 ml (50, 100 ml); 200 mg/5
　　ml (50, 75, 100 ml) (strawberry bubble gum)

▷ **minocycline** (D)(G) 200 mg on first day; then 100 mg q 12 hours x 9 more days
Pediatric: <8 years: not recommended; ≥8 years, <100 lb: 2 mg/lb on first day in
2 divided doses, followed by 1 mg/lb q 12 hours x 9 more days; ≥8 years, ≥100 lb:
same as adult
    Dynacin *Cap:* 50, 100 mg
    Minocin *Cap:* 50, 75, 100 mg; *Oral susp:* 50 mg/5 ml (60 ml) (custard) (sulfites,
alcohol 5%)
▷ **moxifloxacin** (C)(G) 400 mg once daily x 10 days
Pediatric: <18 years: not recommended; ≥18 years: same as adult
    Avelox *Tab:* 400 mg
▷ **ofloxacin** (C)(G) 400 mg bid x 10 days
Pediatric: <18 years: not recommended; ≥18 years: same as adult
    Floxin *Tab:* 200, 300, 400 mg
▷ **tetracycline** (D)(G) 500 mg qid x 10 days
Pediatric: <8 years: not recommended; ≥8 years, <100 lb: 25-50 mg/kg/day in 4
divided doses x 10 days; ≥8 years, ≥100 lb: same as adult; *see Appendix CC.31:
tetracycline* (Sumycin Suspension) *for dose by weight*
    Achromycin V *Cap:* 250, 500 mg
    Sumycin *Tab:* 250, 500 mg; *Cap:* 250, 500 mg; *Oral susp:* 125 mg/5 ml (100,
200 ml) (fruit) (sulfites)

SLEEP APNEA: OBSTRUCTIVE (HYPOPNEA SYNDROME)

ANTI-NARCOLEPTIC AGENTS

▷ **armodafinil** (C)(IV)(G) *OSAHS:* 150-250 mg once daily in the AM; *SWSD:* 150 mg
1 hour before starting shift; reduce dose with severe hepatic impairment
Pediatric: <17 years: not recommended; ≥17 years: same as adult
    Nuvigil *Tab:* 50, 150, 200, 250 mg
▷ **modafinil** (C)(IV) 100-200 mg q AM; max 400 mg/day
Pediatric: <16 years: not recommended; ≥16 years: same as adult
    Provigil *Tab:* 100, 200*mg
Comment: *Modafinil* promotes wakefulness in patients with excessive sleepiness
due to obstructive sleep apnea/hypopnea syndrome.

SELECTIVE DOPAMINE AND NOREPINEPHRINE REUPTAKE INHIBITOR (DNRI)

▷ **solriamfetol** administer once daily upon awakening; avoid administration within 9
hours of planned bedtime because of the potential to interfere with sleep; *Starting
Dose for Patients with Narcolepsy:* 75 mg once daily; *Starting Dose for Patients with
OSA:* 37.5 mg once daily; dose may be increased at intervals of at least 3 days; max
150 mg once daily; *Moderate Renal Impairment:* starting dose is 37.5 mg once daily;
may increase to 75 mg once daily after at least 7 days; *Severe Renal Impairment:*
Starting dose and max dose is 37.5 mg once daily; *ESRD:* not recommended.
Pediatric: safety and efficacy not established
    Sunosi *Tab:* 75*, 150 mg film-coat
    Comment: **Sunosi** *(solriamfetol)* is a dopamine and norepinephrine reuptake
inhibitor (DNRI) indicated to improve wakefulness in adult patients with
excessive daytime sleepiness associated with narcolepsy or obstructive sleep
apnea (OSA). **Sunosi** is not indicated to treat the underlying airway obstruction
in OSA. Ensure that the underlying airway obstruction is treated (e.g., with
continuous positive airway pressure (CPAP)) for at least 1 month prior to
initiating **Sunosi** for excessive daytime sleepiness. Modalities to treat the
underlying airway obstruction should be continued during treatment with
Sunosi. **Sunosi** is not a substitute for these modalities. Use caution when co-
administering **Sunosi** with drugs that increase blood pressure and/or heart
rate and dopaminergic drugs. Measure HR and BP prior to initiating, and

periodically throughout, treatment. Control hypertension before and during therapy. Avoid use in patients with unstable cardiovascular disease, serious heart arrhythmias, or other serious heart problems. Use caution in treating patients with a history of psychosis or bipolar disorder. Consider **Sunosi** dose reduction or discontinuation if psychiatric symptoms develop. **Sunosi** is contraindicated in patients receiving treatment with a monoamine oxidase (MAO) inhibitor and within 14 days following discontinuation of an MAOI. Available data from case reports are not sufficient to determine drug-associated risks of major birth defects, miscarriage, or adverse maternal or fetal outcomes. There are no data available on the presence of *solriamfetol* or its metabolites in human milk or effects on the breastfed infant. The developmental and health benefits of breastfeeding should be considered along with the mother's clinical need for **Sunosi** and any potential adverse effects on the breastfed infant from **Sunosi** or from the underlying maternal condition. Healthcare providers are encouraged to register pregnant patients or pregnant females may enroll themselves, in the Sunosi Pregnancy Exposure Registry by calling 1-877-283-6220 or visiting www.SunosiPregnancyRegistry.com

◯ SLEEPINESS: EXCESSIVE, SHIFT WORK SLEEP DISORDER (SWSD)

ANTI-NARCOLEPTIC AGENT

➤ *armodafinil* (C)(IV)(G) *OSAHS:* 150-250 mg once daily in the AM; *SWSD:* 150 mg 1 hour before starting shift; reduce dose with severe hepatic impairment
Pediatric: <17 years: not recommended; ≥17 years: same as adult
 Nuvigil *Tab:* 50, 150, 200, 250 mg

➤ *modafinil* (C)(IV) 100-200 mg q AM; max 400 mg/day
Pediatric: <16 years: not recommended; ≥16 years: same as adult
 Provigil *Tab:* 100, 200*mg
 Comment: **Provigil** promotes wakefulness in patients with narcolepsy, shift work sleep disorder, and excessive sleepiness due to obstructive sleep apnea/hypopnea syndrome.

◯ SMALLPOX (*VARIOLA MAJOR*), MONKEYPOX

PROPHYLAXIS

➤ *smallpox and monkeypox vaccine, live, nonreplicating* administer two SC doses (0.5 ml each) 4 weeks apart
Pediatric: <18 years: not established; ≥18 years: same as above if determined to be at high risk for smallpox or monkeypox infection
 Jynneos *Vial:* 0.5 ml, single-dose
 Comment: In smallpox vaccine-naïve healthy adults, the most common (incidence >10%) solicited injection site reactions have been pain (84.9%), redness (60.8%), swelling (51.6%), induration (45.4%), and itching (43.1%). The most common solicited systemic adverse reactions have been muscle pain (42.8%), headache (34.8%), fatigue (30.4%), nausea (17.3%) and chills (10.4%). In healthy adults previously vaccinated with a smallpox vaccine, the most common (incidence >10%) solicited injection site reactions were redness (80.9%), pain (79.5%), induration (70.4%), swelling (67.2%), and itching (32.0%). The most common solicited systemic adverse reactions have been fatigue (33.5%), headache (27.6%), and muscle pain (21.5%). Frequencies of solicited local and systemic adverse reactions among adults with HIV-infection and adults with atopic dermatitis have generally been similar to those observed in healthy adults.

➤ *vaccina virus* vaccine *(dried, calf lymph type)* (C)
Pediatric: <12 months: not recommended; 12 months-18 years, non-emergency: not recommended

DRYvax

Kit: vial dried smallpox vaccine (1), 0.25 ml diluent in syringe (1), vented needle (1), 100 individually wrapped bifurcated needles (5 needles/ strip, 20 strips) (polymyxin b sulfate+dihydrostreptomycin+sulfate, chlortetracycline HCl+neomycin sulfate+glycerin+phenol)

Comment: **DRYvax** is a dried live vaccine with approximately 100 million *Infectious vaccina* viruses (pock-forming units [pfu] per ml). Contact with immunosuppressed individuals should be avoided until the scab has separated from the skin (2 to 3 weeks) and/or a protective occlusive dressing covers the inoculation site. Scarification only. Do not inject IV, IM, or SC. Revaccination is recommended every 10 years.

TREATMENT

Comment: July 11, 2018, the U.S. Food and Drug Administration approved **Tpoxx** *(tecovirimat)*, the first drug with an indication for treatment of smallpox. Though the World Health Organization declared smallpox, a contagious and sometimes fatal infectious disease, eradicated in 1980, there have been longstanding concerns that smallpox could be used as a bioweapon. To address the risk of bioterrorism, Congress has taken steps to enable the development and approval of countermeasures to thwart pathogens that could be employed as weapons. **Tpoxx** is the first product to be awarded a Material Threat Medical Countermeasure priority review voucher.

▷ *tecovirimat* 600 mg bid x 14 days; take within 30 minutes after a full meal of moderate or high fat

Pediatric: <13 kg: not recommended; 13 kg to < 25 kg: 200 mg bid x 14 days; 25 kg to < 40 kg: 400 mg bid x 14 days; ≥40 kg: 600 mg bid x 14 days

Tpoxx *Cap:* 200 mg

Comment: **Tpoxx** is an inhibitor of the orthopoxvirus VP37 envelope wrapping protein and is indicated for the treatment of human smallpox disease in adults and pediatric patients weighing ≥ 13 kg. The effectiveness of **Tpoxx** for treatment of smallpox disease has not been determined in humans because adequate and well-controlled field trials have not been feasible, and inducing smallpox disease in humans to study the drug's efficacy is not ethical. **Tpoxx** efficacy may be reduced in immunocompromised patients based on studies demonstrating reduced efficacy in immunocompromised animal models. Co-administration of **Tpoxx** with *repaglinide* may cause hypoglycemia. Monitor blood glucose and monitor for hypoglycemic symptoms during co-administration. No adequate and well-controlled studies in pregnancy have been conducted; therefore, there are no human data to establish the presence or absence of **Tpoxx** associated risk. In animal reproduction studies, no embryo fetal developmental toxicity has been observed. There are no data to assess the presence of *tecovirimat* in human milk or effects on the breastfed infant; however, *tecovirimat* has been found in animal milk. Developmental and health benefits of breastfeeding should be considered along with the mother's clinical need for **Tpoxx** and any potential adverse effects on the breastfed infant from **Tpoxx** or from the underlying maternal condition. Common adverse reactions in healthy adult subjects (incidence ≥ 2%) were headache, nausea, abdominal pain, and vomiting.

⬤ SPINAL MUSCULAR ATROPHY (SMA)

Comment: Spinal muscular atrophy (SMA) is a group of inherited disorders characterized by motor neuron loss in the spinal cord and lower brainstem, muscle weakness, and atrophy. Survival motor neuron (SMN) protein is essential for the maintenance of motor neurons. Because of a defect in, or loss of, the SMN1 gene, patients with SMA do not produce enough SMN protein. It is the most common genetic cause of death in infants, but can affect people at any age. **Spinraza** (*nusinersen*) is the first FDA-approved drug to treat SMA.

SURVIVAL MOTOR NEURON-2 (SMN2)-DIRECTED ANTISENSE OLIGONUCLEOTIDE

▷ *nusinersen* 12 mg per intrathecal administration; initially four loading doses: the first 3 loading doses administered at 14-day intervals; the 4th loading dose administered 30 days after the 3rd loading dose; the maintenance dose is administered every 4 months after the 4th loading dose; prior to administration, 5 ml cerebral spinal fluid (CSF) should be removed; the intrathecal bolus injection should be administered over 1-3 minutes using a spinal anesthetic needle.

Pediatric: same as adult

Spinraza *Vial:* 12 mg/5 ml (2.4 mg/ml) single-dose, solution for intrathecal administration (preservative-free)

Comment: At baseline and prior to each dose, obtain a platelet count and coagulation laboratory testing (there is increased risk for thrombocytopenia and coagulation abnormalities) and quantitative spot urine protein testing (to monitor for renal toxicity). Store **Spinraza** in a refrigerator between 2°C to 8°C (36°F to 46°F) in the original carton to protect from light. Do not freeze. Prior to administration, unopened vials of **Spinraza** can be removed from and returned to the refrigerator, if necessary. If removed from the original carton, the total combined time out of refrigeration should not exceed 30 hours at a temperature that does not exceed 25°C (77°F). **Spinraza** has no labeled contraindications. **Spinraza** has not been studied in pregnant or lactating females, or in patients with renal or hepatic impairment.

SURVIVAL OF MOTOR NEURON 2 (SMN2) SPLICING MODIFIER

▷ *risdiplam* administer orally once daily, after a meal, using the provided oral syringe

Pediatric: <2 months: not established; 2 months to <2 years: 0.2 mg/kg once daily; ≥2 years, <20 kg: 0.25 mg/kg once daily; ≥2 years, ≥20 kg: 5 mg once daily

Evrysdi *Oral soln:* 60 mg, pwdr for constitution to provide 0.75 mg/ml solution

Comment: **Evrysdi** *(risdiplam)* is a survival of motor neuron 2 (SMN2) splicing modifier indicated for the treatment of spinal muscular atrophy (SMA) in patients ≥2 months-of-age. **Evrysdi** must be constituted by a pharmacist prior to dispensing (see mfr pkg insert for full prescribing information for important preparation and administration instructions. The most common adverse reactions in infantile-onset SMA have been similar to those observed in later-onset SMA patients. Additionally, adverse reactions (incidence ≥10%) have been URI, pneumonia, constipation, and vomiting. The most common adverse reactions in later-onset SMA (incidence ≥10%) have been fever, diarrhea, and rash. Avoid co-administration with drugs that are substrates of multidrug and toxin extrusion (MATE) transporters. Avoid use in patients with hepatic impairment. Based on animal data, *risdiplam* may cause embryo/fetal harm. There are no data on the presence of *risdiplam* in human milk or effects on the breastfed infant. *Risdiplam* was excreted in the milk of lactating rats after orally administered *risdiplam*. Developmental and health benefits of breastfeeding should be considered along with the mother's clinical need for **Evrysdi** and any potential adverse effects on the breastfed infant from **Evrysdi** or from the underlying maternal condition.

ADENO-ASSOCIATED VIRUS VECTOR-BASED GENE THERAPY

▷ *onasemnogene abeparvovec-xioi* initially, assess baseline liver function, check PLT count and Troponin 1, and test for the presence of anti-AAV9 antibodies;

recommended dose is 1.1 × 10vector genomes (vg) per kg of body weight; administered as a one-time single IV infusion over 60 minutes via peripheral venous access, using an infusion pump primed with normal saline; dose volume of **Zolgensma** is calculated using the upper limit of the patient weight range for pediatric patients <2 years-of-age between 2.6 kg and 13.5 kg; dose volume for pediatric patients <2 years-of-age weighing ≥13.6 kg requires a combination of **Zolgensma** kits; refer to the **Zolgensma** Dosing Table (Dose Volume in ml for Weight Range in kg) in the mfr pkg insert; starting 1 day prior to the infusion, administer systemic corticosteroids equivalent to oral ***prednisolone*** at 1 mg/ kg of body weight per day and continue for a total of 30 days; then, assess liver function by clinical examination and by laboratory testing; for patients with unremarkable findings, taper the corticosteroid dose over the next 28 days; if liver function abnormalities persist, continue systemic corticosteroids (equivalent to oral ***prednisolone*** at 1 mg/kg/day) until findings become unremarkable, and then taper the corticosteroid dose over the next 28 days; consult medical expert(s) if the patient does not respond adequately to the equivalent of 1 mg/kg/day oral ***prednisolone***

> **Zolgensma** *Vial:* 5.5, 8.3 ml/vial (2-9 vials/kit); keep the kit frozen until infusion day; contents of the **Zolgensma** kit will thaw in approximately 12 hours in a refrigerator, or approximately 4 hours at room temperature; if thawed in a refrigerator, remove from refrigerator on day of dosing; do not shake
>
> Comment: **Zolgensma** *(onasemnogene abeparvovec-xioi)* is an adeno-associated virus vector-based gene therapy indicated for the treatment of pediatric patients <2 years-of-age with spinal muscular atrophy (SMA) with bi-allelic mutations in the *survival motor neuron 1* (*SMN1*) gene. **Zolgensma** is designed to address the genetic root cause of SMA Type 1. Safety and effectiveness of repeat administration of **Zolgensma** have not been evaluated. Use of **Zolgensma** in patients with advanced SMA (e.g., complete paralysis of limbs, permanent ventilator dependence) has not been evaluated.

 SPRAIN

Comment: RICE: Rest; Ice; Compression; Elevation.

Injectable Acetaminophen *see Pain*
NSAIDs *see Appendix J.* NSAIDs online at https://connect.springerpub.com/content/ reference-book/978-0-8261-7935-7/back-matter/part02/back-matter/bmatter10
Opioid Analgesics *see Pain*
Topical and Transdermal Analgesics *see Pain*
Parenteral Corticosteroids *see* Appendix M. Parenteral Corticosteroids
Oral Corticosteroids *see* Appendix L. Oral Corticosteroids
Topical Analgesic and Anesthetic Agents *see* Appendix I. Anesthetic Agents for Local Infiltration and Dermal/Mucosal Membrane Application online at https:// connect.springerpub.com/content/reference-book/978-0-8261-7935-7/back-matter/ part02/back-matter/bmatter9

 STATUS ASTHMATICUS

Inhaled Beta-2 Agonists (Bronchodilators) *see Asthma*
Oral Beta-2 Agonists (Bronchodilators) *see Asthma*
Inhaled Anticholinergics *see Asthma*
Inhaled Anticholinergic+Beta-2 Agonist Combination *see Asthma*
Methylxanthines *see Asthma*
Parenteral Corticosteroids *see* Appendix M. Parenteral Corticosteroids
Oral Corticosteroids *see* Appendix L. Oral Corticosteroids

EPINEPHRINE

▷ *epinephrine* (C)(G) 0.3-0.5 mg (0.3-0.5 ml of a 1:1000 soln) SC q 20-30 minutes as needed up to 3 doses
  Pediatric: <2 years: 0.05-0.1 ml; 2-6 years: 0.1 ml; 6-12 years: 0.2 ml; All: q 20-30 minutes as needed up to 3 doses; >12 years: same as adult

ANAPHYLAXIS EMERGENCY TREATMENT KITS

▷ *epinephrine* (C) 0.3 ml IM or SC in thigh; may repeat if needed
  Pediatric: 0.01 mg/kg SC or IM in thigh; may repeat if needed; <15 kg: not recommended; 15-30 kg: 0.15 mg; >30 kg: same as adult
    AdrenaClick *Auto-injector:* 0.15, 0.3 mg (1 mg/ml; 2/carton) (sulfites)
    Auvi-Q *Auto-injector:* 0.15, 0.3 mg (1 mg/ml; 2/carton w. 1 non active training device) (sulfites)
    EpiPen *Autoinjector* 0.3 mg (epi 1:1000, 0.3 ml (2/carton) (sulfites)
    EpiPen Jr *Autoinjector* 0.15 mg (epi 1:2000, 0.3 ml (2/carton) (sulfites)
    Twinject *Autoinjector:* 0.15, 0.3 mg (epi 1:1000, 2/carton) (sulfites)
▷ *epinephrine+chlorpheniramine* (C) epinephrine 0.3 ml SC or IM plus 4 tabs *chlorpheniramine* by mouth
  Pediatric: infants-2 years: 0.05-0.1 ml SC or IM; 2-6 years: 0.15 ml SC or IM plus 1 tab chlor; 6-12 years: 0.2 ml SC or IM plus 2 tabs chlor; >12 years: same as adult
    Ana-Kit: 0.3 ml syringes of *epi* 1:1000 (2/carton) for self-injection plus chlor 2 mg chewable tabs x 4

◯ STATUS EPILEPTICUS

Anticonvulsant Drugs *see* Appendix R. Anticonvulsant Drugs
▷ *diazepam* (D)(IV) initially 5-10 mg IV in large vein; may repeat q 10-15 minutes; max 30 mg; may repeat in 2-4 hours if needed; do not dilute; may give IM if IV not accessible
  Pediatric: 1 month-5 years: 0.2-0.5 mg IV q 2-5 minutes; max 5 mg; >5 years: 1 mg IV q 2-5 minutes; max 10 mg; may repeat in 2-4 hours if needed
    Diastat *Rectal gel delivery system:* 2.5 mg
    Diastat AcuDial *Rectal gel delivery system:* 10, 20 mg
    Valium Injectable *Vial:* 5 mg/ml (10 ml); *Amp:* 5 mg/ml (2 ml); *Prefilled syringe:* 5 mg/ml (5 ml)
    Valium Intensol Oral Solution *Conc oral soln:* 5 mg/ml (30 ml w. dropper) (alcohol 19%)
    Valium Oral Solution *Oral soln:* 5 mg/5 ml (500 ml) (wintergreen-spice)
▷ *diazepam nasal spray* (IV) *Initial Dose:* 5 mg and 10 mg doses are administered as a single spray intranasally into one nostril (administration of 15 mg and 20 mg doses requires two nasal spray devices, one spray into each nostril); *Second Dose:* when required, may be administered at least 4 hours after the initial dose; if administered, use a new blister pack; *Max Dose and Treatment Frequency:* do not use more than 2 doses to treat a single episode; it is recommended that **Valtoco** be used to treat no more than one episode every 5 days and no more than five episodes per month
  Pediatric: <6 years: not established; ≥6 years: dosage is dependent on the patient's age and weight (see mfr pkg insert)
    Valtoco *Nasal spray:* 5, 7.5, 10 mg in 0.1 ml, single-dose
    Comment: **Valtoco** is a benzodiazepine indicated for the acute treatment of intermittent, stereotypic episodes of frequent seizure activity (i.e., seizure clusters, acute repetitive seizures) that are distinct from a patient's usual seizure pattern in patients with epilepsy 6 years-of-age and older.

Benzodiazepines may cause an increased CNS-depressant effect when used with alcohol or other CNS depressants. Antiepileptic drugs increase the risk of suicidal ideation and behavior. **Valtoco** is contraindicated in patients with Acute narrow-angle glaucoma. The most common adverse reactions (incidence 4%) have been somnolence, headache, and nasal discomfort. Concomitant CYP2C19 and CYP3A4 inhibitors may increase adverse reactions to **Valtoco**. Concomitant inducers of CYP2C19 and CYP3A4 inducers may decrease *diazepam* exposure. Advise pregnant females and women of childbearing age of potentially serious embryo/fetal risk. *diazepam* is excreted in human milk. There are no data to assess the effects of **Valtoco** and/or its active metabolite(s) on the breastfed infant. Postmarketing experience suggests that breastfed infants of mothers taking benzodiazepines, such as **Valtoco**, may have effects of lethargy, somnolence, and poor sucking. There is a pregnancy exposure registry that monitors pregnancy outcomes in women exposed to antiepileptic drugs (AEDs), such as **Valtoco**, during pregnancy. Encourage women who are taking **Valtoco** during pregnancy to enroll in the North American Antiepileptic Drug (NAAED) Pregnancy Registry by calling 1-888-233-2334 or visiting http://www.aedpregnancyregistry.org.

▷ *lorazepam* injectable **(D)(IV)** 4 mg IV over 2 minutes (dilute first); may repeat in 10-15 minutes; may give IM if needed (undiluted)
 Pediatric: <18 years: not recommended; ≥18 years: same as adult
   Ativan Injectable *Vial:* 2 mg/ml (1, 10 ml); *Tubex:* 2 mg/ml (0.5 ml); *Cartridge:* 2, 4 mg/ml (1 ml)

▷ *midazolam* **(IV)** *Initial Dose:* one spray (5 mg) into one nostril; *Second Dose:* one additional spray (5 mg) into the opposite nostril may be administered after 10 minutes if the patient has not responded to the initial dose; *Maximum Dose and Treatment Frequency:* do not use more than 2 doses to treat a seizure cluster; it is recommended that Nayzilam be used to treat no more than one episode every 3 days and treat no more than five episodes per month
 Pediatric: <12 years: not established; ≥12 years: same as adult
   Nayzilam *Nasal spray:* 5 mg/0.1 ml, single dose, nasal spray unit
   Comment: **Nayzilam** *(midazolam)* is a nasally administered benzodiazepine indicated for the acute treatment of intermittent, stereotypic episodes of frequent seizure activity (i.e., seizure clusters, acute repetitive seizures) that are distinct from a patient's usual seizure pattern in patients with epilepsy 12 years-of-age and older. **Nayzilam** is contraindicated in patients with narrow-angle glaucoma. **Nayzilam** may cause an increased CNS-depressant effect when used with alcohol or other CNS depressants. Concomitant use with moderate or strong CYP3A4 inhibitors may result in prolonged sedation because of a decrease in plasma clearance of *midazolam*. Antiepileptic drugs increase the risk of suicidal ideation and behavior. *midazolam* is associated with a high incidence of partial or complete impairment of recall for the next several hours. Based on animal data, *midazolam* may cause fetal harm. *midazolam* is excreted in human milk and effects on the breastfed infant are unknown. Patients with renal impairment may have a longer elimination half-life for *midazolam* and its metabolites which may result in prolonged exposure.

▷ *phenytoin (injectable)* **(D)(G)** 10-15 mg/kg IV, not to exceed 50 mg/minute; follow with 100 mg orally or IV q 6-8 hours; do not dilute in IV fluid
 Pediatric: 15-20 mg/kg IV, not to exceed 1-2 mg/kg/minute
   Dilantin *Vial:* 50 mg/ml (2, 5 ml); *Amp:* 50 mg/ml (2 ml)
   Comment: Monitor *phenytoin* serum levels. Therapeutic serum level: 10-20 gm/ml. Side effects include gingival hyperplasia.

STYE (HORDEOLUM)

OPHTHALMIC ANTI-INFECTIVES

▷ *erythromycin* ophthalmic ointment (B) 1 cm up to 6 x/day
  Pediatric: same as adult
    Ilotycin Ophthalmic Ointment *Ophth oint:* 5 mg/gm (1/8 oz)
▷ *erythromycin* ophthalmic solution (B) initially 1-2 drops q 1-2 hours; may then
  increase dose interval
  Pediatric: same as adult
    Isopto Cetamide Ophthalmic Solution *Ophth soln:* 15% (15 ml)
▷ *gentamicin* ophthalmic ointment (C) 1 cm bid-tid
  Pediatric: same as adult
    Garamycin Ophthalmic Ointment *Ophth oint:* 3 mg/gm (3.5 gm)
    Genoptic Ophthalmic Ointment *Ophth oint:* 3 mg/gm (3.5 gm)
    Gentacidin Ophthalmic Ointment *Ophth oint:* 3 mg/gm (3.5 gm)
▷ *polymyxin b+bacitracin* ophthalmic ointment (C) apply 1/2 inch q 3-4 hours
  Pediatric: same as adult
    Polysporin *Ophth oint:* poly b 10,000 U+bac 500 units per gm (3.75 gm)
▷ *polymyxin b+bacitracin+neomycin* ophthalmic ointment (C)(G) apply 1/2 inch
  q 3-4 hours
  Pediatric: same as adult
    Neosporin Ophthalmic Ointment *Ophth oint:* poly b 10,000 U+bac 400
    U+neo 3.5 mg/gm (3.75 gm)
▷ *polymyxin b+neomycin+gramicidin* ophthalmic solution (C) 1-2 drops 2-3 times
  q 1 hour; then 1-2 drops bid-qid x 7-10 days
  Pediatric: same as adult
    Neosporin Ophthalmic Solution
      Ophth soln: poly b 10,000 U+neo 1.75 mg/gm 0.025 mg/ml (10 ml)
▷ *sodium sulfacetamide* ophthalmic solution and ointment (C)
    Bleph-10 Ophthalmic Solution 2 drops q 4 hour x 7-14 days
    Pediatric: <2 years: not recommended; ≥2 years: 1-2 drops q 2-3 hours during
    the day
      Ophth soln: 10% (2.5, 5, 15 ml; benzalkonium chloride)
    Bleph-10 Ophthalmic Ointment apply 1/2 inch qid and HS
    Pediatric: <2 years: not recommended; ≥2 years: apply 1/4-1/3 inch qid and HS
      Ophth oint: 10% (3.5 gm) (phenylmercuric acetate)

SUNBURN

▷ *prednisone* (C)(G) 10 mg qid x 4-6 days if severe and extensive
▷ *silver sulfadiazine* (C)(G) apply topically to burn once daily-bid
  Pediatric: <12 years: not recommended; ≥12 years: same as adult
    Silvadene *Crm:* 1% (20, 50, 85, 400, 1000 gm jar; 20 gm tube)
  Comment: *Silver sulfadiazine* is contradicted in sulfa allergy, late pregnancy,
  within the first 2 months after birth, premature infants.

SYPHILIS (*TREPONEMA PALLIDUM*)

Comment: The following treatment regimens for *T. pallidum* are published in the
2015 CDC Sexually Transmitted Diseases Treatment Guidelines. Treat all sexual
contacts. Consider testing for other STDs. *Penicillin g*, administered parenterally,
is the preferred drug for treating all stages of syphilis. The preparation used (i.e.,
benzathine, aqueous procaine, or aqueous crystalline), the dosage, and the length
of treatment depend on the stage and clinical manifestations of the disease.
Combinations of *benzathine penicillin*, *procaine penicillin*, and oral *penicillin*

preparations are not appropriate (e.g., **Bicillin C-R**). All women should be screened serologically for syphilis early in pregnancy. There are no proven alternatives to *penicillin* for the treatment of syphilis during pregnancy. Pregnant patients who are allergic to penicillin should be desensitized and treated with *penicillin*. Sexual transmission of *T. pallidum* is thought to occur only when mucocutaneous syphilis at any stage should be evaluated clinically and serologically and treated with a recommended regimen according to CDC guidelines.

PRIMARY, SECONDARY, AND EARLY LATENT (<1 YEAR) SYPHILIS
Regimen 1
▷ *penicillin g (benzathine)* 2.4 million units IM in a single dose

LATE LATENT, LATENT SYPHILIS OF UNKNOWN DURATION, AND TERTIARY SYPHILIS
Regimen 1
▷ *penicillin g (benzathine)* 7.2 million units total administered in 3 divided doses of 2.4 million units each IM at 1 week intervals

REGIMEN: ADULT, NEUROSYPHILIS
Regimen 1
▷ *aqueous crystalline penicillin g* 18-24 million units per day, administered as 3-4 million units IV every 4 hours or continuous IV infusion, for 10-14 days

ALTERNATIVE REGIMEN: ADULT, NEUROSYPHILIS
Regimen 1
▷ *penicillin g (procaine)* 2.4 million units IM once daily x 10-14 days plus *probenecid* 500 mg qid x 10-14 days

PRIMARY AND SECONDARY SYPHILIS IN HIV-INFECTED PERSONS
Regimen 1
▷ *penicillin g (benzathine)* 2.4 million units IM in a single dose

LATENT SYPHILIS AMONG HIV-INFECTED PERSONS
Comment: Treatment is the same as for HIV-negative persons.

CONGENITAL SYPHILIS
Regimen 1
▷ *aqueous crystalline penicillin g* 100,000-150,000 units/kg/day, administered as 50,000 units IV every 12 hours during the first 7 days of life and every 8 hours thereafter for a total of 10 days

ALTERNATE REGIMEN
Regimen 1
▷ *penicillin g (benzathine)* 50,000 units/kg IM in a single dose

Regimen 2
▷ *penicillin g (procaine)* 50,000 units/kg/dose IM, administered in a single daily dose x 10 days

OLDER INFANTS AND CHILDREN
Regimen 1
▷ *aqueous crystalline penicillin g* 200,000-300,000 units/kg/day, administered as 50,000 units IV every 12 hours during the first 7 days of life and every 4-6 hours thereafter for a total of 10 days

DRUG BRANDS AND DOSE FORMS

➤ *aqueous crystalline penicillin g* (B)(G)
➤ *penicillin g (benzathine)* (B)(G)
  Bicillin L-A *Cartridge-needle unit:* 600,000 million units (1 ml); 1.2 million units (2 ml); 2.4 million units (4 ml)
➤ *penicillin g (procaine)* (B)(G)
  Bicillin C-R Cartridge-needle unit: 600,000 units (1 ml); 1.2 million units; (2 ml); 2.4 million units (4 ml)
➤ *probenecid* (B)(G)
  Benemid *Tab:* 500*mg; *Cap:* 500 mg

SYSTEMIC LUPUS ERYTHEMATOSIS (SLE)

NSAIDs *see* Appendix J. NSAIDs online at https://connect.springerpub.com/content/reference-book/978-0-8261-7935-7/back-matter/part02/back-matter/bmatter10
Oral Corticosteroids *see* Appendix L. Oral Corticosteroids

Comment: All SLE patients should routinely be given *hydroxychloroquine* HCQ and supplemental vitamin D as low levels of vitamin D are associated with higher rates of ESRD; supplemental vitamin D reduces urine protein (the best predictor of future renal failure). Vitamin D insufficiency and deficiency are more common in patients with SLE than in the general population. Vitamin D supplementation may decrease disease activity and improve fatigue. In addition, supplementation may improve endothelial function, which may reduce cardiovascular disease. A disease-modifying anti-rheumatic drug (DMARD) should be added when a patient's prednisone dose cannot be tapered and also when hemolysis is present and hemoglobin is abnormally low in the setting of mild-to-moderate hematological involvement. Other DMARDs, such as *methotrexate* (MTX), *azathioprine*, *mycophenolate mofetil* (MMF), *cyclosporine* (CYC), and other calcineurin-inhibitors should be considered in cases of arthritis, cutaneous disease, serositis, vasculitis, or cytopaenias if HCQ is insufficient. For refractory cases, *belimumab* (Benlysta) or *rituximab* (Rituxan), may be considered. The recommended dose of *rituximab*, if required, is either 750 mg/m² (to a maximum of 1 gm per day) at day 1 and day 15, or 375 mg/m² once a week for 4 doses. In patients with SLE without major organ manifestations, glucocorticoids and antimalarial agents may be beneficial. NSAIDs may be used for short periods in patients at low risk for complications from these drugs. Consider immunosuppressive agents (e.g., *azathioprine*, MMF, MTX) in refractory cases or when steroid doses cannot be reduced to levels for long-term use.

CD20 ANTIBODY

➤ *rituximab* (C) administer corticosteroid 30 minutes prior to each infusion; concomitant *methotrexate (MTX)* therapy, administer a 1000 mg IV infusion at 0 and 2 weeks; then every 24 weeks or based on response, but not sooner than every 16 weeks.
  Pediatric: <6 years: not recommended; >6 years: same as adult
    Rituxan *Vial:* 100 mg/10 ml (10 mg/ml), 500 mg/50 ml (10 mg/ml), single-use (preservative-free)

B-LYMPHOCYTE STIMULATOR (BLyS)-SPECIFIC INHIBITOR

Comment: *Benlysta* was initially approved as an intravenous formulation administered in a hospital or clinic setting as a weight-dosed IV infusion every 4 weeks. Patients can now self-administer **Benlysta** as a once weekly SC injection after being trained by a healthcare provider.

▷ **belimumab**

SC administration: 200 mg SC once weekly. May be self-administered by the patient in the home setting.

IV infusion: 10 mg/kg at 2-week intervals for the first 3 doses and at 4-week intervals thereafter; reconstitute, dilute, and administer as an intravenous infusion over a period of 1 hour. Consider administering premedication for prophylaxis against infusion reactions and hypersensitivity reactions. Must be administered in a hospital or clinic setting by a qualified healthcare provider

Pediatric: <5 years: not established; ≥5 years: same as adult

Benlysta *Prefilled syringe:* 200 mg/ml (1 ml) single-dose (4/carton); *Autoinjector:* 200 mg (1 ml) single-dose (4/carton); *Vial:* 120 mg/5 ml, 400 mg/ 20 ml, single-dose, pwdr for reconstitution and IV infusion (4/carton)

Comment: **Benlysta** is indicated for the treatment of patients with active, autoantibody-positive, systemic lupus erythematosus who are receiving standard therapy. Common adverse reactions include nausea, diarrhea, pyrexia, nasopharyngitis, bronchitis, insomnia, pain in extremity, depression, migraine, and pharyngitis. The efficacy of **Benlysta** has <u>not</u> been evaluated in patients with severe active lupus nephritis or severe active central nervous system lupus. **Benlysta** has <u>not</u> been studied in combination with other biologics or intravenous *cyclophosphamide.* Therefore, use of Benlysta is <u>not</u> recommended in these situations. Limited data on use of **Benlysta** in pregnancy women, from observational studies, published case reports, and postmarketing surveillance, is insufficient to determine whether there is a drug-associated risk for major birth defects or miscarriage. Monoclonal antibodies, such as *belimumab,* are actively transported across the placenta during the third trimester of pregnancy and may affect immune response in the in utero-exposed infant. Monoclonal antibodies are increasingly transported across the placenta as pregnancy progresses, with the largest amount transferred during the third trimester. No information is available on the presence of *belimumab* in human milk or the effects of the drug on the breastfed infant. As there are risks to the mother and fetus associated with SLE, risks and benefits should be considered prior to administering live or live-attenuated vaccines to infants exposed to **Benlasta** in utero. Monitor the infant of a treated mother for B-cell reduction and other immune dysfunction. There is a pregnancy exposure registry that monitors pregnancy outcomes in females exposed to **Benlysta** during pregnancy. Healthcare professionals are encouraged to register patients by calling 1-877-681-6296.

DISEASE MODIFYING ANTI-RHEUMATIC DRUGS (DMARDS)

Comment: DMARDs include *penicillamine,* gold salts (*auranofin, aurothioglucose*), immunosuppressants, and *hydroxychloroquine.* The DMARDs reduce ESR, reduce RF, and favorably affect SLE symptoms. Immunosuppressants may require 6 weeks to affect benefits and 6 months for full improvement.

▷ **auranofin (gold salt)** (C) 3 mg bid or 6 mg once daily; if inadequate response after 6 months, increase to 3 mg tid

Pediatric: <12 years: not recommended; ≥12 years: same as adult

Ridaura *Vial:* 100 mg/20 ml

▷ **azathioprine** (D) 1 mg/kg/day in a single or divided doses; may increase by 0.5 mg/kg/day q 4 weeks; max 2.5 mg/kg/day; minimum trial to ascertain effectiveness is 12 weeks

Pediatric: <12 years: not recommended; ≥12 years: same as adult

Azasan *Tab* 75*, 100*mg

Imuran *Tab* 50*mg

▷ *cyclosporine (immunosuppressant)* (C) 1.25 mg/kg bid; may increase after 4 weeks by 0.5 mg/kg/day; then adjust at 2 week intervals; max 4 mg/kg/day; administer with meals
Pediatric: <12 years: not recommended; ≥12 years: same as adult
   Neoral *Cap:* 25, 100 mg (alcohol)
   Neoral Oral Solution *Oral soln:* 100 mg/ml (50 ml) may dilute in room temperature apple juice or orange juice (alcohol)
   Comment: **Neoral** is indicated for RA unresponsive to *methotrexate (MTX).*

▷ *leflunomide* (X)(G) initially 100 mg once daily x 3 days; maintenance dose 20 mg once daily; max 20 mg daily
Pediatric: <18 years: not recommended; ≥18 years: same as adult
   Arava *Tab:* 10, 20, 100 mg
   Comment: **Arava** is contraindicated with breastfeeding.

▷ *methotrexate* (MTX)(X) 7.5 mg x 1 dose per week or 2.5 mg x 3 at 12 hour intervals once a week; max 20 mg/week; therapeutic response begins in 3-6 weeks; administer *methotrexate* (MTX) injection SC only into the abdomen or thigh
Pediatric: <2 years: not recommended; ≥2 years: 10 mg/m² once weekly; max 20 mg/m²
   Rasuvo *Autoinjector:* 7.5 mg/0.15 ml, 10 mg/0.20 ml, 12.5 mg/0.25 ml, 15 mg/0.30 ml, 17.5 mg/0.35 ml, 20 mg/0.40 ml, 22.5 mg/0.45 ml, 25 mg/0.50 ml, 27.5 mg/0.55 ml, 30 mg/0.60 ml (solution concentration for SC injection is 50 mg/ml)
   Rheumatrex *Tab:* 2.5*mg (5, 7.5, 10, 12.5, 15 mg/week, 4/card unit-of-use dose pack)
   Trexall *Tab:* 5*, 7.5*, 10*, 15*mg (5, 7.5, 10, 12.5, 15 mg/week, 4/card unit-of-use dose pack)
   Comment: *Methotrexate* (MTX) is contraindicated with immunodeficiency, blood dyscrasias, alcoholism, and chronic liver disease.

▷ *penicillamine* administer on an empty stomach, at least 1 hour before meals or two hours after meals, and at least 1 hour apart from any other drug, food, milk, antacid, zinc or iron-containing preparation; maintenance dosage must be individualized, and may require adjustment during the course of treatment. *initially*, a single daily dose of 125-250 mg; then, increase at 1-3 month intervals by 125-250 mg/day, as patient response and tolerance indicate; if a satisfactory remission of symptoms is achieved, the dose associated with the remission should be continued as the patient's maintenance therapy; if there is no improvement, and there are no signs of potentially serious toxicity after 2-3 months of treatment with doses of 500-750 mg/day, increase by 250 mg/day at 2-3 month intervals until a satisfactory remission occurs or signs of toxicity develop; if there is no discernible improvement after 3-4 months of treatment with 1000-1500 mg/day, discontinue **Cuprimine**. Changes in maintenance dosage levels may not be reflected clinically or in the erythrocyte sedimentation rate (ESR) for 2-3 months after each dosage adjustment.
   Cuprimine *Cap:* 125, 250 mg
   Depen: 250 mg
Comment: The use of *penicillamine* has been associated with fatalities due to certain diseases such as aplastic anemia, agranulocytosis, thrombocytopenia, Goodpasture's syndrome, and myasthenia gravis. Because of the potential for serious hematological and renal adverse reactions to occur at any time, routine urinalysis, white and differential blood cell count, hemoglobin, and direct platelet count must be checked twice weekly, together with monitoring of the patient's skin, lymph nodes and body temperature, during the first month of therapy, every 2 weeks for the next 5 months, and monthly thereafter. Patients should be instructed to report promptly the development of signs and symptoms of

granulocytopenia <u>and/or</u> thrombocytopenia such as fever, sore throat, chills, bruising <u>or</u> bleeding; the above laboratory studies should then be promptly repeated.

▷ *sulfasalazine* (C; D in 2nd, 3rd)(G) initially 0.5 gm once daily bid; gradually increase every 4 days; usual maintenance 2-3 gm/day in equally divided doses at regular intervals; max 4 gm/day
Pediatric: <6 years: not recommended; 6-16 years: initially 1/4 to 1/3 of maintenance dose; increase weekly; maintenance 30-50 mg/kg/day in 2 divided doses at regular intervals; max 2 gm/day
  Azulfidine *Tab:* 500 mg
  Azulfidine EN *Tab:* 500 mg ent-coat

ANTIMALARIALS

▷ *atovaquone* (C)(G) take as a single dose with food <u>or</u> a milky drink at the same time each day; repeat dose if vomited within 1 hour; *Prophylaxis:* 1,500 mg once daily; *Treatment:* 750 mg bid x 21 days
Pediatric: <13 years: not established; ≥13 years: same as adult
  Mepron *Susp:* 750 mg/5 ml

▷ *atovaquone+proguanil* (C)(G) >40 kg: take as a single dose with food <u>or</u> a milky drink at the same time each day; repeat dose if vomited within 1 hour; *Prophylaxis:* 1 tab daily starting 1-2 days before entering endemic area, during stay, and for 7 days after return; *Treatment (acute, uncomplicated):* 4 tabs daily x 3 days
Pediatric: <5 kg: not recommended; 5-40 kg:
Prophylaxis: daily dose starting 1-2 days before entering endemic area, during stay, and for 7 days after return; 5-20 kg: 1 ped tab; 21-30 kg: 2 ped tabs; 31-40 kg: 3 ped tabs; ≥40 kg: same as adult; *Treatment (acute, uncomplicated):* daily dose x 3 days; 5-8 kg: 2 ped tabs; 9-10 kg: 3 ped tabs; 11-20 kg: 1 adult tab; 21-30 kg: 2 adult tabs; 31-40 kg: 3 adult tabs; >40 kg: same as adult
  Malarone *Tab:* atov 250 mg+prog 100 mg
  Malarone Pediatric *Tab:* atov 62.5 mg+prog 25 mg
Comment: *Atovaquone* is antagonized by *tetracycline* and *metoclopramide*. Concomitant *rifampin* is <u>not</u> recommended (may elevate LFTs).

▷ *chloroquine* (C)(G) *Prophylaxis:* 500 mg once weekly (on the same day of each week); start 2 weeks prior to exposure, continue while in the endemic area, and continue 4 weeks after departure; *Treatment:* initially 1 gm; then 500 mg 6 hours, 24 hours, and 48 hours after initial dose <u>or</u> initially 200-250 mg IM; may repeat in 6 hours; max 1 gm in first 24 hours; continue to 1.875 gm in 3 days
Pediatric: Suppression: 8.35 mg/kg (max 500 mg) weekly (on the same day of each week); *Treatment:* initially 16.7 mg/kg (max 1 gm); then 8.35 mg/kg (max 500 mg) 6 hours, 24 hours, and 48 hours after initial dose, <u>or</u> initially 6.25 mg/kg IM; may repeat in 6 hours; max 12.5 mg/kg/day
Pediatric:
  Aralen *Tab:* 500 mg; *Amp:* 50 mg/ml (5 ml)
Comment: There are no adequate and well-controlled studies evaluating the safety and efficacy of *chloroquine* in pregnant females. Usage of *chloroquine* during pregnancy should be avoided except in the suppression <u>or</u> treatment of malaria when the benefit outweighs the potential risk to the fetus. Because of the potential for serious adverse reactions in nursing infants from chloroquine, a decision should be made whether to discontinue nursing <u>or</u> to discontinue the drug, taking into account the potential clinical benefit of the drug to the mother. Since this drug is known to concentrate in the liver, it should be used with caution in patients with hepatic disease <u>or</u> alcoholism <u>or</u> in conjunction with known hepatotoxic drugs.

▷ *hydroxychloroquine* (C)(G) 400-600 mg/day
   Pediatric: <12 years: not recommended; ≥12 years: same as adult
      Plaquenil *Tab:* 200 mg
   Comment: May require several weeks to achieve beneficial effects. If no
   improvement in 6 months, discontinue.

▷ *mefloquine* (C) *Prophylaxis:* 250 mg once weekly (on the same day of each week);
   start 1 week prior to exposure, continue while in the endemic area, and continue
   for 4 weeks after departure; *Treatment:* 1250 mg as a single dose
   Pediatric: <6 months: not recommended; *Prophylaxis:* ≥6 months: 3-5 mg/
   kg (max 250 mg) weekly (on the same day of each week); start 1 week prior to
   exposure, continue while in the endemic area, and continue for 4 weeks after
   departure; *Treatment:* ≥6 months: 25-50 mg/kg as a single dose; max 250 mg
      Lariam *Tab:* 250*mg
   Comment: *Mefloquine* is contraindicated with active o̲r recent history of
   depression, generalized anxiety disorder, psychosis, schizophrenia o̲r any other
   psychiatric disorder o̲r history of convulsions.

▷ *quinine sulfate* (C)(G) 1 tab o̲r cap every 8 hours x 7 days
   Pediatric: <16 years: not recommended; ≥16 years: same as adult
      quinine sulfate *Tab:* 260 mg; *Cap:* 260, 300, 325 mg
      Qualaquin *Cap:* 324 mg
   Comment: *Qualaquin* is indicated in the treatment of uncomplicated
   P. falciparum malaria (including *chloroquine*-resistant strains).

TAKAYASU ARTERITIS (TA)

Comment: Takayasu Ateritis is a rare yet well-described large-vessel vasculitis
with a predilection for the aorta and its primary branches. Treatment options
focus on preventing disease progression. There is no consensus on regimen, but
high-dose pulse corticosteroid therapy is favored for induction, and long-term
therapy includes immunosuppressants and biologics such as *cyclophosphamide,
mycophenolate mofetil, methotrexate* (MTX), *infliximab,* o̲r *tocilizumab,* as well
as revascularization surgery. Disease recurrence is common, and mortality rates
can range from 16% to 40%. Therefore, prompt identification and treatment is
imperative to prevent further morbidity and mortality.

TAPEWORM (CESTODE)

ANTHELMINTICS
Comment: Oral bioavailability of anthelmintics is enhanced when administered
with a fatty meal (estimated fat content 40 gm).

▷ *albendazole* (C)(G) take with a meal; may crush and mix with food; 400 mg bid x
   7 days; may repeat in 3 weeks if needed
   Pediatric: <2 years: 200 mg once daily x 3 days; may repeat in 3 weeks; ≥2-12
   years: 400 mg once daily x 3 days; may repeat in 3 weeks; ≥12 years: same as adult
      Albenza *Tab:* 200 mg
   Comment: *Albendazole* is a broad-spectrum benzimidazole carbamate
   anthelmintic.

▷ *nitazoxanide* (B) take with a meal; may crush and mix with food; 500 mg q 12
   hours x 3 days
   Pediatric: <12 months: not recommended; ≥12 months: treat q 12 hours x 3 days;
   <11 years: [susp] 12-47 months: 5 ml; 4-11 years: 10 ml; ≥11 years: [tab/susp] 500
   mg
      Alinia *Tab:* 500 mg; *Oral susp:* 100 mg/5 ml (60 ml)

▷ *praziquantel* (B)(G) take with a meal; may crush and mix with food; 5-10 mg/kg
   as a single dose

Pediatric: <4 years: not established; ≥4 years: same as adult
  Biltricide *Tab:* 600 mg film-coat (scored for half or quarter dose)
  Comment: Therapeutically effective levels of **Biltricide** may not be achieved
  when administered concomitantly with strong P450 inducers, such as
  rifampin. Females should not breastfeed on the day of **Biltricide** treatment
  and during the subsequent 72 hours. Use caution with hepatosplenic patients
  who have moderate-to-severe liver impairment (Child-Pugh Class B and C).

TARDIVE DYSKINESIA (TD)

Comment: Tardive dyskinesia is a treatable, albeit irreversible, neurological disorder
characterized by repetitive involuntary movements, usually of the jaw, lips, and tongue,
such as grimacing, sticking out the tongue and smacking the lips. Some affected people
also experience involuntary movement of the extremities or difficulty breathing.
This condition is most often an adverse side effect associated with the older "typical"
antipsychotic drugs. Risk is decreased with the newer "atypical" antipsychotic drugs.
The first and only FDA-approved treatment for this disorder is *valbenazine* (Ingrezza),
a vesicular monoamine transporter 2 (VMAT2) inhibitor.

VESICULAR MONOAMINE TRANSPORTER 2 (VMAT2) INHIBITOR

▷ *valbenazine* initially 40 mg once daily; after 1 week, increase to the recommended
  80 mg once daily; take with or without food; recommended dose for patients
  with moderate or severe hepatic impairment is 40 mg once daily; consider
  dose reduction based on tolerability in known CYP2D6 poor metabolizers;
  concomitant use of strong CYP3A4 inducers is not recommended; avoid
  concomitant use of MAOIs
  Pediatric: <18 years: not established; ≥18 years: same as adult
  Ingrezza *Cap:* 40 mg
  Comment: Safety and effectiveness of **Ingrezza** have not been established in
  pediatric patients. No dose adjustment is required for elderly patients. The
  limited available data on **Ingrezza** use in pregnant females are insufficient
  to inform a drug-associated risk. There is no information regarding the
  presence of **Ingrezza** or its metabolites in human milk, the effects on the
  breastfed infant, or the effects on milk production. However, women are
  advised not to breastfeed during treatment and for 5 days after the final dose.

TEMPOROMANDIBULAR JOINT (TMJ) DISORDER

Injectable Acetaminophen *see Pain*
NSAIDs *see* Appendix J. NSAIDs online at https://connect.springerpub.com/content/
reference-book/978-0-8261-7935-7/back-matter/part02/back-matter/bmatter10
Opioid Analgesics *see Pain*
Topical and Transdermal Analgesics *see Pain*
Parenteral Corticosteroids *see* Appendix M. Parenteral Corticosteroids
Oral Corticosteroids *see* Appendix L. Oral Corticosteroids
Topical Analgesic and Anesthetic Agents *see* Appendix I. Anesthetic Agents for
Local Infiltration and Dermal/Mucosal Membrane Application online at https://
connect.springerpub.com/content/reference-book/978-0-8261-7935-7/back-matter/
part02/back-matter/bmatter9

SKELETAL MUSCLE RELAXANTS

▷ *baclofen* (C)(G) 5 mg tid; titrate up by 5 mg every 3 days to 20 mg tid; max 80
  mg/day
  Pediatric: <12 years: not recommended; ≥12 years: same as adult
  Lioresal *Tab:* 10*, 20*mg

Comment: *Baclofen* is indicated for muscle spasm pain and chronic spasticity associated with multiple sclerosis and spinal cord injury or disease. Potential for seizures or hallucinations on abrupt withdrawal.

▷ *carisoprodol* (C)(G) 1 tab tid or qid
 Pediatric: <12 years: not recommended; ≥12 years: same as adult
  Soma *Tab:* 350 mg

▷ *chlorzoxazone* (G) 1 caplet qid; max 750 mg qid
 Pediatric: <12 years: not recommended; ≥12 years: same as adult
  Parafon Forte DSC *Cplt:* 500*mg

▷ *cyclobenzaprine* (B)(G) 10 mg tid; usual range 20-40 mg/day in divided doses;
 max 60 mg/day x 2-3 weeks or 15 mg ext-rel once daily; max 30 mg ext-rel/day x
 2-3 weeks
 Pediatric: <15 years: not recommended; ≥15 years: same as adult
  Amrix *Cap:* 15, 30 mg ext-rel
  Fexmid *Tab:* 7.5 mg
  Flexeril *Tab:* 5, 10 mg

▷ *dantrolene* (C) 25md daily x 7 days; then 25 mg tid x 7 days; then 50 mg tid x 7
 days; max 100 mg qid
 Pediatric: 0.5 mg/kg daily x 7 days; then 0.5 mg/kg tid x 7 days; then 1 mg/kg tid x
 7 days; then 2 mg/kg tid; max 100 mg qid
  Dantrium *Tab:* 25, 50, 100 mg
 Comment: *Dantrolene* is indicated for chronic spasticity associated with multiple
 sclerosis and spinal cord injury or disease.

▷ *diazepam* (C)(IV) 2-10 mg bid-qid; may increase gradually
 Pediatric: <6 months: not recommended; ≥6 months: initially 1-2.5 mg bid-qid;
 may increase gradually
  Diastat *Rectal gel delivery system:* 2.5 mg
  Diastat AcuDial *Rectal gel delivery system:* 10, 20 mg
  Valium *Tab:* 2, 5, 10 mg
  Valium Intensol Oral Solution *Conc oral soln:* 5 mg/ml (30 ml w. dropper)
  (alcohol 19%)
  Valium Oral Solution *Oral soln:* 5 mg/5 ml (500 ml) (wintergreen spice)

▷ *metaxalone* (B) 1 tab tid-qid
 Pediatric: <12 years: not recommended; ≥12 years: same as adult
  Skelaxin *Tab:* 800*mg

▷ *methocarbamol* (C)(G) initially 1.5 gm qid x 2-3 days; maintenance, 750 mg
 every 4 hours or 1.5 gm 3 x daily; max 8 gm/day
 Pediatric: <16 years: not recommended; ≥16 years: same as adult
  Robaxin *Tab:* 500 mg
  Robaxin 750 *Tab:* 750 mg
  Robaxin Injection 10 ml IM or IV; max 30 ml/day; max 3 days; max 5 ml/
  gluteal injection q 8 hours; max IV rate 3 ml/min
   Vial: 100 mg/ml (10 ml)

▷ *nabumetone* (C)
 Pediatric: <12 years: not recommended; ≥12 years: same as adult
  Relafen *Tab:* 500, 750 mg
  Relafen 500 *Tab:* 500 mg

▷ *orphenadrine citrate* (C)(G) 1 tab bid
 Pediatric: <12 years: not recommended; ≥12 years: same as adult
  Norflex *Tab:* 100 mg sust-rel

▷ *tizanidine* (C) 1-4 mg q 6-8 hours; max 36 mg/day
 Pediatric: <12 years: not recommended; ≥12 years: same as adult
  Zanaflex *Tab:* 2*, 4**mg; *Cap:* 2, 4, 6 mg

SKELETAL MUSCLE RELAXANT+NSAID COMBINATIONS

Comment: *Aspirin*-containing medications are contraindicated with history of allergic-type reaction to *aspirin*, children and adolescents with *Varicella* or other viral illness, and 3rd trimester of pregnancy.

▷ *carisoprodol+aspirin* (C)(III)(G) 1-2 tabs qid
  Pediatric: <12 years: not recommended; ≥12 years: same as adult
    Soma Compound *Tab:* caris 200 mg+asp 325 mg (sulfites)
▷ *meprobamate+aspirin* (D)(IV) 1-2 tabs tid or qid
  Pediatric: <12 years: not recommended; ≥12 years: same as adult
    Equagesic *Tab:* mepro 200 mg+asp 325*mg

SKELETAL MUSCLE RELAXANT+NSAID+CAFFEINE COMBINATIONS

Comment: *Aspirin*-containing medications are contraindicated with history of allergic-type reaction to *aspirin*, children and adolescents with *Varicella* or other viral illness, and 3rd trimester of pregnancy.

▷ *orphenadrine+aspirin+caffeine* (D)(G)
  Pediatric: <12 years: not recommended; ≥12 years: same as adult
    Norgesic 1-2 tabs tid-qid
      Tab: orphen 25 mg+asp 385 mg+caf 30 mg
    Norgesic Forte 1 tab tid or qid; max 4 tabs/day
      Tab: orphen 50 mg+asp 770 mg+caf 60*mg

SKELETAL MUSCLE RELAXANT+NSAID+CODEINE COMBINATIONS

▷ *carisoprodol+aspirin+codeine* (D)(III)(G) 1-2 tabs qid prn
  Pediatric: <18 years: not recommended; ≥18 years: not recommended
    Soma Compound w. Codeine *Tab:* caris 200 mg+asp 325 mg+cod 16 mg (sulfites)

Comment: *Codeine* is known to be excreted in breast milk. <12 years: not recommended; 12-<18: use extreme caution; not recommended for children and adolescents with asthma or other chronic breathing problem. The FDA and the European Medicines Agency (EMA) are investigating the safety of using *codeine* containing medications to treat pain, cough, and colds in children 12-<18 years because of the potential for serious side effects, including slowed or difficult breathing. *Aspirin*-containing medications are contraindicated with history of allergic-type reaction to *aspirin*, children and adolescents with *Varicella* or other viral illness, and 3rd trimester of pregnancy.

TENOSYNOVIAL GIANT CELL TUMOR (TGCT)

KINASE INHIBITOR

▷ *pexidartinib* 400 mg (2 x 200 mg) twice daily until disease progression or unacceptable toxicity; swallow whole, do not open or chew; take on an empty stomach, at least one hour before or 2 hours after a meal/snack
  Pediatric: safety and efficacy not established
    Turalio *Cap:* 200 mg
    Comment: **Turalio** *(pexidartinib)* is a kinase inhibitor indicated for treatment of adults with symptomatic tenosynovial giant cell tumor (TGCT) associated with severe morbidity or functional limitations not amenable to improvement with surgery. *CrCl 15-89 mL/min:* 200 mg in the AM and 400 mg in the PM. **Turalio** can cause serious and potential fatal liver injury. Monitor LFTs prior to initiation and at intervals during treatment as appropriate. If hepatotoxicity develops, withhold doses, reduce doses, or permanently discontinue **Turalio**

based on severity. Reduce the dose as appropriate for patients with mild-to-severe renal impairment. Avoid coadministration of **Turalio** with other products known to cause hepatotoxicity. Reduce the dose of **Turalio** if concomitant use of strong CYP3A inhibitors cannot be avoided. Avoid concomitant use of strong CYP3A inducers. Reduce the dose of **Turalio** if concomitant use of UGT inhibitors cannot be avoided. Avoid concomitant use of PPIs; use H-2 receptor antagonists or antacids if needed. The most common adverse reactions (incidence >20%) have been increased lactate dehydrogenase, increased aspartate aminotransferase, hair color changes, fatigue, increased alanine aminotransferase, decreased neutrophils, increased cholesterol, increased alkaline phosphatase, decreased lymphocytes, eye edema, decreased hemoglobin, rash, dysgeusia, and decreased phosphate. **Turalio** may cause embryo/fetal harm; advise pregnant females of the embryo/fetal risk. Advise women not to breastfeed during treatment and for at least one week after the last dose. **Turalio** is available only through the Toralio Risk Evaluation and Mitigation Strategy (REMS) Program. Prescribers must be certified with the program by enrolling and completing training. Patients must complete and sign an enrollment for inclusion in the patient registry. Pharmacies must be certified with the program and must only dispense to patients who are authorized to receive **Turalio**. For further information, contact the Turalio REMS Program at 1-833-887-2546 or visit www.turalioREMS.com

● TESTOSTERONE DEFICIENCY, HYPOTESTOSTERONEMIA, HYPOGONADISM

Comment: *Testosterone* is contraindicated in male breast cancer and prostate cancer. *testosterone* replacement therapy is indicated in males with primary hypogonadism (congenital or acquired due to cryptorchidism, bilateral torsion, orchitis, vanishing testis syndrome, or orchidectomy), or hypogonadotropic hypogonadism (congenital or acquired), and delayed puberty not secondary to a pathological disorder (X-ray of the hand and wrist to determine bone age should be obtained every 6 months to assess the effect of treatment on the epiphyseal centers).

ORAL ANDROGENS

▷ *fluoxymesterone* (X)(III) *Hypogonadism:* <12 years: use by specialist only; Puberty: 5-20 mg once daily; *Delayed puberty:* use low dose and limit duration to 4-6 months
   Halotestin *Tab:* 2*, 5*, 10*mg (tartrazine)
▷ *methyltestosterone* (X)(III) usually 10-50 mg once daily; for delayed puberty, use low dose and limit duration to 4-6 months
   Android *Cap:* 10 mg
   Methitest *Tab:* 10*mg
   Testred *Cap:* 10 mg
▷ *testosterone* (X)(III) 30 mg q 12 hours to gum region, just above the incisor tooth on either side of the mouth; hold system in place for 30 seconds; rotate sites with each application
   Striant *Buccal tab:* 30 mg (6 blister pks; 10 buccal systems/blister pck)
   Comment: Serum total *testosterone* concentrations may be checked 4-12 weeks after initiating treatment with **Striant**. To capture the maximum serum concentration, an early morning sample (just prior to applying the AM dose) is recommended.
▷ *testosterone undecanoate* (X) *Prior to Initiating Jatenzo:* confirm the diagnosis of hypogonadism by ensuring that serum testosterone concentrations have been measured in the morning on at least two separate days and that these concentrations are below the normal range; take with food. *Starting Dose:* 237 mg orally once in the morning and once in the evening; *Dose Adjustment:* to a

minimum of 158 mg twice daily, and maximum of 396 mg twice daily, based on serum testosterone drawn 6 hours after the morning dose at least 7 days after starting treatment or following dose adjustment and periodically thereafter
Pediatric: <18 years: not established: ≥18 years: same as adult

Jatenzo *Cap:* 158, 198, 237 mg

Comment: **Jatenzo** *(testosterone undecanoate)* is an oral testosterone replacement therapy for the treatment of low testosterone in hypogonadal men. Monitor patients with benign prostatic hyperplasia (BPH) for worsening of signs and symptoms of BPH. Monitor prostate specific antigen (PSA) and lipid concentrations periodically. Edema, with or without congestive heart failure, may occur in patients with preexisting cardiac, renal, or hepatic disease. Venous thromboembolism (VTE), including deep vein thrombosis (DVT) and pulmonary embolism (PE), have been reported in patients using testosterone. Evaluate patients with signs or symptoms consistent with DVT or PE. Monitor hematocrit approximately every 3 months to detect increased RBC mass and polycythemia. Testosterone has been subject to abuse, typically at doses higher than recommended for the approved indication and in combination with other anabolic androgenic steroids. Exogenous administration of androgens may lead to azoospermia. Depression and suicidal ideation have occurred during clinical trials in patients treated with **Jatenzo**. Contraindications: men with breast cancer or known or suspected prostate cancer and women who are pregnant.

TOPICAL ANDROGENS

Comment: Wash hands after application. Allow solution to dry before it touches clothing. Do not wash site for at least 2 hours after application. Pregnant and nursing women, and children, must avoid skin contact with application sites on men. If there is contact, wash the area as soon as possible with soap and water.

▷ *testosterone* (X)(III)(G)
Pediatric: <18 years: not recommended; ≥18 years: same as adult

AndroGel 1% (G) initially apply 25 mg once daily in the AM to clean, dry, intact skin of the shoulders, upper arms, and/or abdomen; do not apply to scrotum; may increase to 75 mg/day and then to 100 mg/day if needed
Gel: 25 mg/2.5 gm pkt (30 pkts/carton); 50 mg/5 gm pkt (30 pkts/carton)

AndroGel 1.62% (G) initially apply 25 mg once daily in the AM to clean, dry, skin of the shoulders and upper arms intact skin of the upper arms; do not apply to abdomen or genitals; may adjust dose between 1 and 4 pump actuations based on the pre-dose morning serum testosterone concentration at approximately 14 and 28 days after starting treatment or adjusting dose
Gel: 20.25 mg/1.25 gm pkt; 40.5 mg/2.5 gm pkt; *20.25* mg/1.25 gm pump actuation (60 metered dose actuations)

Axiron apply to clean dry intact skin of the axillae; do not apply to the scrotum, penis, abdomen, shoulders, or upper arms; initially apply 60 mg (30 mg/axilla) once daily in the AM; adjust dose based on serum testosterone concentration 2-8 hours after applying and at least 14 days after starting therapy or following dose adjustment; may increase dose in 30 mg increments if serum testosterone <300 ng/dL up to 120 mg; reduce dose to 30 mg if levels >1050 ng/dL; discontinue if serum testosterone remains at >1050 ng/dL; to apply a 120 mg dose, apply 30 mg to each axilla and allow to dry, then repeat
Soln: 30 mg/1.5 ml pump actuation (60 metered dose actuations) (alcohol, latex-free)

Fortesta (G) initially 40 mg of testosterone (4 pump actuations) applied to the thighs once daily in the AM; may adjust between 10 mg minimum and 70 mg maximum
Gel: 10 mg/0.5 gm pump actuation (120 metered dose actuations) (ethanol)

Comment: The **Fortesta** dose should be based on the serum *testosterone* concentration 2 hours after applying **Fortesta** and at approximately 14 days and 35 days after starting treatment or following dose adjustment. Dose adjustment criteria: ≤500 ng/dL, increase daily dose by 10 mg; 500-≤1250 ng/dL, no change; 1250-≤2500 ng/dL, decrease daily dose by 10 mg; ≥2500 ng/dL, decrease daily dose by 20 mg.

Testim (G) initially apply 5 gm once daily in the AM to clean, dry, intact skin of the shoulders and/or upper arms; do not apply to the genitals or abdomen; may increase to 10 gm after 2 weeks

  Gel: 1%, clear, hydroalcoholic (5 mg/5 gm pkt, 30 pkts/carton)

Vogelxo Gel (G) 1% initially apply 5 gm once daily in the AM to clean, dry, intact skin of the shoulders, upper arms, and/or abdomen; do not apply to scrotum; may increase to 7.5 gm/day and then to 10 gm/day if needed

  Gel: 50 mg/5 gm pkt (30 pkts/carton); 50 mg/5 gm tube (30 tubes/carton);
  Pump: 12.5 mg/1.25 gm pump actuation, 60 metered dose actuations)

INTRANASAL ANDROGENS

▷ *testosterone (nasal gel)* **(X)(III)** initially one pump actuation each nostril (33 mg) 3 x/day, at least 6-8 hours apart, at the same times each day max: 6 pump actuation/day

  Pediatric: <18 years: not established; ≥18 years: same as adult

  Natesto *Gel:* 5.5 mg/0.122 gm pump actuation (60 metered dose actuations)

TRANSDERMAL ANDROGEN PATCH

▷ *testosterone* **(X)(III)**

  Androderm initially apply 4 mg nightly at approximately 10 PM to clean, dry area of the arm, back, or upper buttocks; leave on x 24 hours; may increase to 7.5 mg or decrease to 2.5 mg based on confirmed AM serum testosterone concentrations

  Pediatric: <15 years: not recommended; ≥15 years: same as adult

    Transdermal patch: 2, 4 mg/24 Hr

PARENTERAL ANDROGENS

Comment: Contraindications include males with carcinoma of the breast or known or suspected carcinoma of the prostate and women who are pregnant (exogenous testosterone may cause fetal harm). *Prior to initiation of treatment:* confirm the diagnosis of hypogonadism by ensuring that serum testosterone has been measured in the morning on at least 2 separate days and that these concentrations are below the normal range. *Starting dose:* administer 75 mg subcutaneously in the abdominal region once weekly. Avoid intramuscular and intravascular administration. *Dose Adjustment:* Based upon total testosterone trough concentrations (measured 7 days after most recent dose) obtained following 6 weeks of dosing and periodically thereafter. *testosterone enanthate* and *testosterone cypionate* are long-acting testosterone esters suspended in oil to prolong absorption. Peak levels occur about 72 hours after intramuscular injection and are followed by a slow decline during the subsequent 1-2 weeks. For complete androgen replacement, the regimen should be between 50 and 100 mg of *testosterone enanthate* administered every 7-10 days, which will achieve relatively normal levels of testosterone throughout the time interval between injections. Longer time intervals are more convenient but are associated with greater fluctuations in testosterone levels. Higher doses of testosterone produce longer-term effects but also higher peak levels and wider swings between peak and nadir circulating testosterone levels; the result is fluctuating symptoms in many patients. The use of 100-150 mg of testosterone every 2 weeks is a reasonable compromise. Use of 300 mg injections every 3 weeks is associated with wider fluctuations of testosterone levels and is generally inadequate to ensure a consistent clinical response. With use of these longer-interval regimens, many men will have pronounced symptoms during the week preceding the next injection. In such instances, a smaller dose at closer intervals should be tried. When full androgen replacement is not required, patients should receive lower doses of testosterone. One such category includes male patients with pre-pubertal onset of hypogonadism who are going through puberty for the first time during therapy and who often may require psychologic counseling, especially when a spouse is involved as well. In these patients, testosterone therapy should be initiated at 50 mg every 3-4 weeks and then gradually increased during subsequent months, as tolerated, up to full replacement within 1 year. Men with appreciable benign prostatic hypertrophy who have hypogonadism and symptoms may be given 50-100 mg of testosterone every 2 weeks as an initial regimen and maintained on this dosage with careful monitoring of urinary symptoms and prostate examinations; therapy can be withdrawn if necessary. Attaining full virilization in the patient with hypogonadism may take as long as 3-4 years. Follow-up intervals should be between 4 and 6 months to monitor progress, review compliance, and determine whether any complications or psychologic adjustment problems are present. As a guide, testosterone levels should be above the lower limit of normal, in the range of 250 to 300 ng/dl, just before the next injection. Excessive peak levels and side effects should also be monitored and used to adjust the dosing regimens. During exogenous administration of androgens, endogenous testosterone release is inhibited through feedback inhibition of pituitary luteinizing hormone (LH). At large doses of exogenous androgens, spermatogenesis may also be suppressed through feedback inhibition of pituitary follicle stimulating hormone (FSH). Androgen therapy should be used very cautiously in pediatric patients and only by specialists who are aware of the adverse effects on bone maturation. Skeletal maturation must be monitored every 6 months by an X-ray of the hand and wrist. There is a lack of substantial evidence that androgens are effective in fractures, surgery, convalescence, and functional uterine bleeding.

▷ **testosterone cypionate** (X)(III)

   Comment: *Testosterone cypionate* is the oil-soluble 17 (beta)-cyclopentyl propionate ester of the androgenic hormone testosterone. The half-life of **testosterone cypionate** when injected intramuscularly is approximately 8 days.
   Depot-Testosterone Injection (G) *Usual Starting Dose:* 75-100 mg deep IM in the gluteal muscle; *Dose/Frequency Adjustment:* dose and frequency based upon morning total testosterone trough concentrations (measured 7 days after most recent dose) periodically thereafter; *Maintenance:* usually 100-400 mg deep IM in the gluteal muscle every 4 weeks; total doses above 400 mg per month are not required because of the prolonged action of the preparation; injections more frequently than every 2 weeks are rarely indicated
   Pediatric: <12 years: not established; ≥12 years: same as adult
      Vial: 100, 200 mg/ml (5 ml) (benzyl alcohol)

▷ **testosterone enanthate** (X)(III)

   Comment: The half-life of **testosterone enanthate** when injected intramuscularly is approximately 4.5 days.
      Delatestryl (G) *Usual Starting Dose:* 75-100 mg deep IM in the gluteal muscle; *Dose/Frequency Adjustment:* dose and frequency based upon morning total testosterone trough concentrations (measured 7 days after most recent dose) periodically thereafter; *Maintenance:* usually 100-400 mg deep IM in the gluteal muscle every 4 weeks; total doses above 400 mg per month are not required because of the prolonged action of the preparation; injections more frequently than every 2 weeks are rarely indicated
      Pediatric: <12 years: not established; ≥12 years: same as adult

Vial: 100, 200 mg/ml (5 ml) (chlorobutanol [chloral derivative] as preservative)

Xyosted *Initially:* 75 mg SC in the abdominal region once weekly; *Dose Adjustment:* based upon morning total testosterone trough concentrations (measured 7 days after most recent dose) obtained following 6 weeks of dosing and periodically thereafter

Pediatric: <18 years: not established; ≥18 years: same as adult

    Autoinjector: 50, 75, 100 mg/0.5 ml single-dose (4/carton) (preservative-free)

Comment: Use **Xyosted** only for the treatment of hypogonadal conditions associated with structural or genetic etiologies. Safety and efficacy of **Xyosted** in males with "age-related hypogonadism" (also referred to as "late-onset hypogonadism") have not been established.

TETANUS (*CLOSTRIDIUM TETANI*)

Comment: For individuals who have received 3 or more doses of tetanus toxoid-containing vaccine, for clean and minor wounds, **Tdap** or **Td** should be administered if more than 10 years have passed since the last dose. For all other wounds, **Tdap** or **Td** should be administered if more than 5 years have passed since the last dose of tetanus toxoid-containing vaccine. For those who have not previously received **Tdap** or whose **Tdap** history is unknown, **Tdap** is the preferred vaccine. Additionally, **Tdap** should be used to vaccinate pregnant women if a tetanus toxoid-containing vaccine is indicated. (ACIP, 2021)s

POSTEXPOSURE PROPHYLAXIS IN PREVIOUSLY NONIMMUNIZED PERSONS

▷ *tetanus immune globulin, human* (C) 250 mg deep IM in a single dose
    Pediatric: >7 years: same as adult

    BayTET, Hyper-TET

       Vial: 250 units single-dose; *Prefilled syringe:* 250 units

▷ *tetanus toxoid* vaccine (C) 0.5 ml IM x 3 dose series

    Vial: 5 Lf units/0.5 ml (0.5, 5 ml); *Prefilled syringe:* 5 Lf units/0.5 ml (0.5 ml)

Comment: Dose of **BayTET/HyperTET** S/D is calculated as 4 units/kg. However, it may be advisable to administer the entire contents of the syringe of **BayTET/HyperTET** S/D (250 units) regardless of the child's size, since theoretically the same amount of toxin will be produced in the child's body by the infecting tetanus organism as it will in an adult's body. At the same time but in a different extremity and with a different syringe, administer Diphtheria and Tetanus Toxoids and Pertussis Vaccine Adsorbed (DTP) or Diphtheria and Tetanus Toxoids Adsorbed (For Pediatric Use) (DT), if pertussis vaccine is contraindicated, should be administered per mfr pkg insert. Tetanus immune globulin may interact with live viral vaccines such as measles, mumps, rubella, and polio. It is also unknown if **BayTET/HyperTET** can cause fetal harm when administered to a pregnant woman or can affect reproduction capacity. The single injection of tetanus toxoid only initiates the series for producing active immunity in the recipient. Impress upon the patient the need for further toxoid injections in 1 month and 1 year, otherwise the active immunization series is incomplete. If a contraindication to using tetanus toxoid-containing preparations exists for a person who has not completed a primary series of tetanus toxoid immunization, and that person has a wound that is neither clean nor minor, only passive immunization should be given using tetanus immune globulin.

THREADWORM (*STRONGYLOIDES STERCORALIS*)

ANTHELMINTICS

Comment: Oral bioavailability of anthelmintics is enhanced when administered with a fatty meal (estimated fat content 40 gm).

▷ **albendazole** (C) take with a meal; may crush and mix with food; may repeat in 3 weeks if needed; 400 mg bid x 7 days
Pediatric: <2 years: 200 mg bid x 7 days; 2-12 years: 400 mg once daily x 7 days; >12 years: same as adult
  Albenza *Tab:* 200 mg
  Comment: *Albendazole* is a broad-spectrum benzimidazole carbamate anthelmintic.

▷ **ivermectin** (C) take with water; chew or crush and mix with food; may repeat in 3 months if needed; 200 mcg/kg as a single dose
Pediatric: <15 kg: not recommended; ≥15 kg: same as adult
  Stromectol *Tab:* 3, 6*mg

▷ **mebendazole** (C)(G) take with a meal; chew or crush and mix with food; may repeat in 3 weeks if needed; 100 mg bid x 3 days
Pediatric: <2 years: not recommended; ≥2 years: same as adult
  Emverm *Chew tab:* 100 mg
  Vermox *Chew tab:* 100 mg

▷ **praziquantel** (B)(G) take with a meal; may crush and mix with food; 5-10 mg/kg as a single dose
Pediatric: <4 years: not established; ≥4 years: same as adult
  Biltricide *Tab:* 600**mg film-coat (cross-scored for half or quarter dose)
  Comment: Therapeutically effective levels of **Biltricide** may not be achieved when administered concomitantly with strong P450 inducers, such as rifampin. Females should not breastfeed on the day of **Biltricide** treatment and during the subsequent 72 hours. Use caution with hepatosplenic patients who have moderate-to-severe liver impairment (Child-Pugh Class B and C).

▷ **pyrantel pamoate** (C) take with a meal; may open capsule and sprinkle or mix with food; treat x 3 days; may repeat in 2-3 weeks if needed; treat x 3 days; 11 mg/kg/dose; max 1 gm/dose; <25 lb: not recommended; 25-37 lb: 1/2 tsp/dose; 38-62 lb: 1 tsp/dose; 63-87 lb: 1 tsp/dose; 88-112 lb: 2 tsp/dose; 113-137 lb: 2 tsp/dose; 138-162 lb: 3 tsp/dose; 163-187 lb: 3 tsp/dose; >187 lb: 4 tsp/dose
  Antiminth *Cap:* 180 mg; *Liq:* 50 mg/ml (30 ml); 144 mg/ml (30 ml); *Oral susp:* 50 mg/ml (60 ml)
  Pin-X *Cap:* 180 mg; *Liq:* 50 mg/ml (30 ml); 144 mg/ml (30 ml); *Oral susp:* 50 mg/ml (30 ml)

▷ **nitazoxanide** (B)(G) take with a meal; may crush and mix with food; <12 months: not recommended; ≥12 months: treat q 12 hours x 3 days; <11 years: [use suspension]; 1-3 years: 5 ml; 4-11 years: 10 ml; >11 years: [use tab or suspension] 500 mg
  Alinia *Tab:* 500 mg; *Oral susp:* 100 mg/5 ml (60 ml)

▷ **thiabendazole** (C) take with a meal; may crush and mix with food; treat x 7 days; <30 lb: consult mfr pkg insert; ≥30 lb: 25 mg/kg/dose bid with meals; 30-50 lb: 250 mg bid with meals; >50 lb: 10 mg/lb/dose bid with meals; max 1.5 gm/dose; max 3 gm/day
  Mintezol *Chew tab:* 500*mg (orange); *Oral susp:* 500 mg/5 ml (120 ml) (orange)
  Comment: *Thiabendazole* is not for prophylaxis. May impair mental alertness. May not be available in the US.

THROMBOCYTOPENIA PURPURA, IDIOPATHIC (IMMUNE) (ITP)

THROMBOPOIETIN (TPO) RECEPTOR AGONIST

Comment: **Doptelet** *(avatrombopage)* is the first oral thrombopoietin (TPO) receptor agonist approved by the FDA for the treatment of adults with chronic liver disease who are scheduled to undergo a procedure. **Doptelet** is a second-generation, once-daily, orally administered TPO receptor agonist that works by increasing platelet counts to the target level of greater or equal to 50,000 per microliter.

▷ *avatrombopag* <18 years: not recommended; ≥18 years: begin dosing 10-13 days prior to a scheduled procedure; the patient should undergo the procedure within 5-8 days after the last dose; take with food, as a single dose x 5 consecutive days; PLT count <40 x 10⁹/L: 60 mg (3 tabs) once daily x 5 days; PLT count 40-50 x 10⁹/L: 40 mg (2 tabs) once daily x 5 days

Doptelet *Tab:* 20 mg film-coat

Comment: TPO receptor agonists have been associated with thrombotic and thromboembolic complications in patients with chronic liver disease. Monitor platelet counts and for thromboembolic events and institute treatment promptly. Potential adverse reactions include pyrexia, abdominal pain, nausea, headache, fatigue, and peripheral edema. Based on animal studies, *avatrombopag* may cause fetal harm when administered to a pregnant female. There are no information regarding the presence of *avatrombopag* in human milk or effects on the breastfed infant. However, breastfeeding is not recommended during treatment with **Doptelet** and for at least 2 weeks after the last dose. Safety and effectiveness in patients (<18 years-of-age) have not been established.

▷ *lusutrombopag* 3 mg orally once daily with or without food x 7 days; administer first dose 8-14 days prior to the scheduled procedure; the procedure should occur 2-8 days after the last dose

Pediatric: <18 years: not established; ≥18 years: same as adult

Mulpleta *Tab:* 3 mg

Comment: **Mulpleta** *(lusutrombopag)* is a thrombopoietin (TPO) receptor agonist indicated for the treatment of thrombocytopenia in adult patients with chronic liver disease who are scheduled to undergo a procedure. TPO receptor agonists have been associated with thrombotic and thromboembolic complications in patients with chronic liver disease. Monitor platelet counts and for thromboembolic events and institute treatment promptly. The most common adverse reaction (incidence 3%) is headache. There are no available data on **Mulpleta** in pregnant females to inform drug-associated fetal risk. However, in animal reproduction studies, oral administration of *lusutrombopag* during organogenesis and the lactation period resulted in adverse developmental fetal outcomes. Advise pregnant females of the potential risk to a fetus Breastfeeding is not recommended during treatment.

SPLEEN TYROSINE KINASE (SYK) INHIBITOR

▷ *fostamatinib disodium hexahydrate* <18 years: not recommended; ≥18 years: Initially 100 mg twice daily. Increase to 150 mg twice daily if platelet count not at ≥50x10⁹/L after 4 weeks. Discontinue if insufficient increase in platelet count after 12 weeks. Dose modifications: see full labeling.

Tavalisse *Tab:* 100, 150 mg

Comment: **Tavalisse** *(fostamatinib)* is an oral spleen tyrosine kinase (SYK) inhibitor for the treatment of patients with chronic idiopathic (immune) thrombocytopenia purpura (ITP). Monitor CBCs, including platelets, monthly until stable count (≥50 x 10⁹/L) achieved, then periodically thereafter. Monitor LFTs monthly. Discontinue if AST/ALT >5XULN for ≥2 wrks or ≥3XULN and total bilirubin >2XULN. Monitor blood pressure every 2 weeks until stable dose established, then monthly thereafter. Interrupt or discontinue dose if hypertensive crisis (>180/120 mm Hg) occurs; discontinue if repeat BP >160/100 mm Hg for >4 weeks. Temporarily interrupt if severe diarrhea (Grade ≥3) occurs; resume at next lower daily dose if improved to Grade 1. Monitor ANC monthly and for infection. Temporarily interrupt if ANC <1 x 10⁹/L occurs and remains low after 72 hours until resolved; resume at next lower daily dose. Use lowest effective dose. Due to potential for embryo/fetal toxicity, use effective contraception during and for ≥1 months after last dose. Confirm negative pregnancy status prior to initiation. Breastfeeding <u>not</u> recommended (during and for ≥1 month after last dose). Concomitant strong CYP3A4 inducers: <u>not</u> recommended. Concomitant strong CYP3A4 inhibitors <u>or</u> substrates; monitor for toxicity. May potentiate concomitant BCRP (e.g., rosuvastatin) <u>or</u> P-gp (e.g., digoxin) substrates: monitor for toxicity. Adverse reactions include diarrhea, hypertension, nausea, respiratory infection, dizziness, ALT/AST increase, rash, abdominal pain, fatigue, chest pain, and neutropenia.

 THROMBOCYTOPENIA PURPURA, THROMBOTIC, ACQUIRED AUTOIMMUNE (aTTP)

VON WILLEBRAND FACTOR (vWF)-DIRECTED ANTIBODY FRAGMENT

▷ *caplacizumab-yhdp* initial administration should be upon the initiation of plasma exchange therapy, by a qualified healthcare provider
First day of treatment: 11 mg via IV bolus at least 15 minutes *prior to* plasma exchange; followed by 11 mg SC *after completion* of plasma exchange
Subsequent treatment: during daily plasma exchange: 11 mg SC once daily once daily following plasma exchange
Treatment after the plasma exchange period: 11 mg SC once daily x 30 days beyond the last plasma exchange
After initial treatment course: if signs of persistent underlying disease, such as suppressed ADAMTS13 activity levels, remain present, treatment may be extended for a maximum 28 days
Discontinue treatment with Cablivi: if the patient experiences more than 2 recurrences of aTTP
Pediatric: safety and efficacy not established
   Cablivi *Vial:* 11 mg powder, a single-dose, for reconstitution and IV <u>or</u> SC administration
   Comment: **Cablivi** (*caplacizumab-yhdp*) is indicated for the treatment of adult patients with acquired autoimmune thrombotic thrombocytopenic purpura (aTTP), in combination with plasma exchange and immunosuppressive therapy. The **ADAMTS13** gene provides instructions for making an enzyme that is involved in blood clotting. The most common adverse reactions to **Cablivi** (incidence >15%) are epistaxis, headache, and gingival bleeding. Severe bleeding can occur; risk is increased in patients with underlying coagulopathies and patients taking an anticoagulant. The most common adverse reactions (incidence >15%) are epistaxis, headache, and gingival bleeding. If clinically significant bleeding occurs, interrupt treatment. Withhold **Cablivi** for 7 days prior to elective surgery, dental procedures, <u>or</u> any other invasive intervention. Monitor pregnant patients/fetus and neonates closely for signs of bleeding. There is no information regarding the presence of *caplacizumab-yhdp* in human milk <u>or</u> effects on the breastfed infant. Developmental and health benefits of breastfeeding should be considered along with the mother's clinical need for **Cablivi,** potential adverse effects on the breastfed infant, and the underlying maternal condition.

CD20-TARGETING MONOCLONAL ANTIBODY

▷ *rituximab* initially (Month 0) 1000 mg x 2 IV infusions separated by 2 weeks in combination with a tapering course of glucocorticoids; then a 500 mg IV infusion at Month 12 and every 6 months thereafter <u>or</u> based on clinical evaluation; *Relapse:* 1000 mg IV infusion with considerations to resume <u>or</u> increase the glucocorticoid dose based on clinical evaluation; subsequent infusions may be no sooner than 16 weeks after the previous infusion; methylprednisolone 100 mg IV <u>or</u> equivalent glucocorticoid recommended 30 minutes prior to each infusion

Pediatric: <6 years: not recommended; ≥6 years: same as adult

Rituxan *Vial:* 100 mg/10 ml (10 mg/ml), 500 mg/50 ml (10 mg/ml), single-use (preservative-free)

Comment: **Rituxan** *(rituximab)* is a CD20-targeting cytolytic monoclonal antibody that received FDA Breakthrough Therapy Designation for treatment of PV in 2017. Safety and efficacy in recalcitrant PV has been demonstrated in approximately 500 patients across several small trials and case studies, with clinical remission occurring within 8 weeks in up to 95% of cases. In a recent phase 2 trial comparing *rituximab* plus *prednisone* with *prednisone* alone in patients with newly diagnosed PV, a 55% increase in 2-year remission rate (89% vs 34%) was observed in those receiving *rituximab* plus *prednisone*. Consider intravenous immunoglobulin (e.g., IVIG).

THYROID CANCER

KINASE INHIBITOR

▶ *selpercatinib* < 50 kg: 120 mg twice daily; >50 kg: 160 mg twice daily; reduce dose in patients with severe hepatic impairment

Pediatric: <12 years: not established; ≥12 years: same as adult

Retevmo *Cap:* 40, 80 mg

Comment: **Retevmo** *(selpercatinib)* is a kinase inhibitor indicated for adult patients with metastatic RET fusion-positive non-small cell lung cancer, adult and pediatric patients ≥12 years-of-age with advanced or metastatic RET-mutant medullary thyroid cancer (MTC) who require systemic therapy; adult and pediatric patients ≥12 years-of-age with advanced or metastatic RET fusion-positive thyroid cancer who require systemic therapy and who are radioactive iodine-refractory (if radioactive iodine is appropriate). The most common adverse reactions, including laboratory abnormalities, (incidence ≥25%) have been increased aspartate aminotransferase (AST), increased alanine aminotransferase (ALT), increased glucose, decreased leukocytes, decreased albumin, decreased calcium, dry mouth, diarrhea, increased creatinine, increased alkaline phosphatase, hypertension, fatigue, edema, decreased platelets, increased total cholesterol, rash, decreased sodium, and constipation. Monitor ALT and AST prior to initiating **Retevmo**, every 2 weeks during the first 3 months, then monthly thereafter and as clinically indicated. Do not initiate **Retevmo** in patients with uncontrolled hypertension; optimize BP prior to initiating **Retevmo** and monitor BP after 1 week, at least monthly thereafter and as clinically indicated. Monitor patients who are at significant risk of developing QTc prolongation. Assess QT interval, electrolytes and TSH at baseline and periodically during treatment. Monitor QT interval more frequently when **Retevmo** is concomitantly administered with strong and moderate CYP3A inhibitors or drugs known to prolong QTc interval. Permanently discontinue **Retevmo** in patients with severe or life-threatening hemorrhage. Withhold **Retevmo** and initiate corticosteroids in the occurrence of any hypersensitivity reaction and, upon resolution, resume at a reduced dose and increase dose by 1 dose level each week until reaching the dose taken prior to onset of hypersensitivity. Continue steroids until the patient reaches target dose of **Retevmo** and then taper. Withhold **Retevmo** for at least 7 days prior to elective surgery. Do not administer for at least 2 weeks following major surgery and until adequate wound healing. The safety of resumption of **Retevmo** after resolution of wound healing complications has not been established. Avoid co-administration with PPIs; if co-administration cannot be avoided, take **Retevmo** with food (with PPI) or modify its administration time (with H2 receptor antagonist or locally-acting antacid). Avoid co-administration of strong and moderate CYP3A inhibitors; if co-administration cannot be avoided, reduce the **Retevmo** dose. Avoid co-administration with strong and moderate CYP3A inducers. Avoid co-administration with CYP2C8 and CYP3A substrates; if co-administration cannot be avoided, modify the substrate dosage as recommended in its product labeling. Based on findings from animal studies, and its mechanism of action, **Retevmo** can cause fetal harm. There are no available data on **Retevmo** use in pregnant females to inform drug-associated risk. Therefore, verify pregnancy status in females of reproductive potential prior to initiating **Retevmo** and advise of the possible risk to the fetus and to use effective contraception. There are no data on the presence of *selpercatinib* or its metabolites in human milk or effects on the breastfed infant. Because of the potential for serious adverse embryo/fetal effects, advise women not to breastfeed during treatment with **Retevmo** and for 1 week after the final dose.

THYROID EYE DISEASE

▷ *teprotumumab-trbw* 10 mg/kg for the first IV infusion, followed by 20 mg/kg once every 3 weeks for 7 additional IV infusions; administer the IV infusions over 60 to 90 minutes

Tepezza *Vial:* 500 mg pwdr, single-dose, for reconstitution, dilution, and IV infusion

Comment: **Tepezza** *(teprotumumab-trbw)* is a fully human monoclonal antibody (mAb) and a targeted inhibitor of the insulin-like growth factor 1 receptor (IGF-1R) for the treatment of active thyroid eye disease (TED). The most common adverse reactions (incidence >5%) are muscle spasm, nausea, alopecia, diarrhea, fatigue, hyperglycemia, hearing impairment, dry skin, dysgeusia, and headache. If an infusion reaction occurs, interrupt or slow the rate of infusion and use appropriate medical management. Monitor patients with preexisting IBD for disease flare; discontinue **Tepezza** if IBD worsens. Monitor glucose levels in all patients; treat hyperglycemia with glycemic control medications. Appropriate forms of contraception should be implemented prior to initiation of **Tepezza**, during treatment, and for 6 months following the last dose. There is no information regarding the presence of **Tepezza** in human milk or effects on the breastfed infant.

TINEA CAPITIS

Comment: Tinea capitis must be treated with a systemic antifungal.

FOR SEVERE KERION PRURITUS

▷ *prednisone* (C) 1 mg/kg/day for 7-14 days
see Oral Corticosteroids Appendix L. Oral Corticosteroids

SYSTEMIC ANTI-FUNGALS

▷ *griseofulvin, microsize* (C)(G) 500 mg once daily x 4-6 weeks or longer; max 1 gm/day
Pediatric: <30 lb: 5 mg/lb/day; 30-50 lb: 125-250 mg/day; >50 lb: 250-500 mg/day; 5 mg/lb/day x 4-6 weeks or longer; *see* Appendix CC.25. *griseofulvin, micro-size* (Grifulvin V Suspension) *for dose by weight*
Grifulvin V *Tab:* 250, 500 mg; *Oral susp:* 125 mg/5 ml (120 ml) (alcohol 0.02%)

▷ *griseofulvin, ultramicrosize* (C)(G) 375 mg/day in a single or divided doses x 4-6 weeks or longer
Pediatric: <2 years: not recommended; ≥2 years: 3.3 mg/lb/day in a single or divided doses x 4-6 weeks or longer
Gris-PEG *Tab:* 125, 250 mg

Comment: *Griseofulvin* should be taken with fatty foods (e.g., milk, ice cream). Liver enzymes should be monitored.

➤ *ketoconazole* (C)(G) initially 200 mg once daily; max 400 mg/day x 4 weeks
Pediatric: <2 years: not recommended; ≥2 years: 3.3-6.6 mg/kg once daily x 4 weeks
　　Nizoral *Tab:* 200 mg
Comment: Caution with *ketoconazole* due to concerns about potential for hepatotoxicity.

TINEA CORPORIS

TOPICAL ANTI-FUNGALS

➤ *butenafine* (C)(G) apply bid x 1 week or once daily x 4 weeks
Pediatric: <12 years: not recommended; ≥12 years: same as adult
　　Lotrimin Ultra (OTC) *Crm:* 1% (12, 24 gm)
　　Mentax *Crm:* 1% (15, 30 gm)
Comment: *Butenafine* is a benzylamine, not an azole. Fungicidal activity continues for at least 5 weeks after last application.

➤ *ciclopirox* (B)
　　Loprox Cream apply bid; max 4 weeks
　　Pediatric: <10 years: not recommended; ≥10 years: same as adult
　　　Crm: 0.77% (15, 30, 90 gm)
　　Loprox Lotion apply bid; max 4 weeks
　　Pediatric: <10 years: not recommended; ≥10 years: same as adult
　　　Lotn: 0.77% (30, 60 ml)
　　Loprox Gel apply bid; max 4 weeks
　　Pediatric: <16 years: not recommended; ≥16 years: same as adult
　　　Gel: 0.77% (30, 45 gm)

➤ *clotrimazole* (B)(G) apply to affected area bid x 7 days
Pediatric: same as adult
　　Lotrimin *Crm:* 1% (15, 30, 45 gm)
　　Lotrimin AF (OTC) *Crm:* 1% (12 gm); *Lotn:* 1% (10 ml); *Soln:* 1% (10 ml)

➤ *econazole* (C) apply once daily x 14 days
Pediatric: same as adult
　　Spectazole *Crm:* 1% (15, 30, 85 gm)

➤ *ketoconazole* (C) apply once daily x 14 days
Pediatric: <12 years: not recommended; ≥12 years: same as adult
　　Nizoral Cream *Crm:* 2% (15, 30, 60 gm)

➤ *luliconazole* (C) apply to affected area and 1 inch into the immediate surrounding area(s) once daily
Pediatric: <18 years: not recommended; ≥18 years: same as adult
　　Luzu Cream 1% *Crm:* 1% (30, 60 gm)

➤ *miconazole 2%* (C) apply once daily-bid x 2 weeks
Pediatric: same as adult
　　Lotrimin AF Spray Liquid (OTC) *Spray liq:* 2% (113 gm) (alcohol 17%)
　　Lotrimin AF Spray Powder (OTC) *Spray pwdr:* 2% (90 gm) (alcohol 10%)
　　Monistat-Derm *Crm:* 2% (1, 3 oz); *Spray liq:* 2% (3.5 oz); *Spray pwdr:* 2% (3 oz)

➤ *naftifine* (B)(G)
Pediatric: <12 years: not recommended; ≥12 years: same as adult
　　Naftin Cream apply once daily x 14 days
　　　Crm: 1% (15, 30, 60 gm)
　　Naftin Gel apply bid x 14 days
　　　Gel: 1% (20, 40, 60 gm)

▷ *oxiconazole nitrate* (B)(G) apply once daily-bid x 2 weeks
  Pediatric: same as adult
    Oxistat *Crm:* 1% (15, 30, 60 gm); *Lotn:* 1% (30 ml)
▷ *sulconazole* (C) apply once daily-bid x 3 weeks
  Pediatric: <12 years: not recommended; ≥12 years: same as adult
    Exelderm *Crm:* 1% (15, 30, 60 gm); *Lotn:* 1% (30 mg)
▷ *terbinafine* (B)(G)
  Pediatric: <12 years: not recommended; ≥12 years: same as adult
    Lamisil Cream (OTC) apply to affected and surrounding area once daily-bid x
    1-4 weeks until significantly improved
      Crm: 1% (15, 30 gm)
    Lamisil AT Cream (OTC) apply to affected and surrounding area once
    daily-bid x 1-4 weeks until significantly improved
      Crm: 1% (15, 30 gm)
    Lamisil Solution (OTC) apply to affected and surrounding area once daily x 1
    week
      Soln: 1% (30 ml spray bottle)

TOPICAL ANTIFUNGAL+STEROID COMBINATION

▷ *clotrimazole+betamethasone* (C)(G) apply bid x 2 weeks; max 4 weeks
  Pediatric: <12 years: not recommended; ≥12 years: same as adult
    Lotrisone *Crm:* clotrim 1 mg+beta 0.5 mg (15, 45 gm); *Lotn:* clotrim 1 mg+
    beta 0.5 mg (30 ml)

SYSTEMIC ANTIFUNGALS

▷ *griseofulvin, microsize* (C)(G) 500 mg/day x 2-4 weeks; max 1 gm/day
  Pediatric: <30 lb: 5 mg/lb/day; 30-50 lb: 125-250 mg/day; >50 lb: 250-500 mg/
  day; *see* Appendix CC.25. *griseofulvin, microsize* (Grifulvin V Suspension) *for
  dose by weight*
    Grifulvin V *Tab:* 250, 500 mg; *Oral susp:* 125 mg/5 ml (120 ml) (alcohol
    0.02%)
▷ *griseofulvin, ultramicrosize* (C)(G) 375 mg/day in a single or divided doses x 2-4
  weeks
  Pediatric: <2 years: not recommended; ≥2 years: 3.3 mg/lb/day in a single or
  divided doses
    Gris-PEG *Tab:* 125, 250 mg
  Comment: *Griseofulvin* should be taken with fatty foods (e.g., milk, ice cream).
  Liver enzymes should be monitored.
▷ *ketoconazole* (C) initially 200 mg once daily; max 400 mg/day x 4 weeks
  Pediatric: <2 years: not recommended; ≥2 years: 3.3-6.6 mg/kg/day x 4 weeks
    Nizoral *Tab:* 200 mg
  Comment: Caution with *ketoconazole* due to concerns about potential for
  hepatotoxicity.

◯ TINEA CRURIS (JOCK ITCH)

TOPICAL ANTIFUNGALS

▷ *butenafine* (B)(G) apply bid x 1 week or once daily x 4 weeks
  Pediatric: <12 years: not recommended; ≥12 years: same as adult
    Lotrimin Ultra (C)(OTC) *Crm:* 1% (12, 24 gm)
    Mentax *Crm:* 1% (15, 30 gm)
  Comment: *Butenafine* is a benzylamine, not an azole. Fungicidal activity
  continues for at least 5 weeks after last application.
▷ *ciclopirox* (B)
    Loprox Cream apply bid; max 4 weeks

      Pediatric: <10 years: not recommended; ≥10 years: same as adult
      Crm: 0.77% (15, 30, 90 gm)
    Loprox Lotion apply bid; max 4 weeks
      Pediatric: <10 years: not recommended; ≥10 years: same as adult
      Lotn: 0.77% (30, 60 ml)
    Loprox Gel apply bid; max 4 weeks
      Pediatric: <16 years: not recommended; ≥16 years: same as adult
      Gel: 0.77% (30, 45 gm)

▷ ***clotrimazole*** (B)(G) apply to affected area bid x 7 days
  Pediatric: same as adult
    Lotrimin *Crm:* 1% (15, 30, 45 gm)
    Lotrimin AF (OTC) *Crm:* 1% (12 gm); *Lotn:* 1% (10 ml); *Soln:* 1% (10 ml)

▷ ***econazole*** (C) apply once daily x 2 weeks
  Pediatric: same as adult
    Spectazole *Crm:* 1% (15, 30, 85 gm)

▷ ***ketoconazole*** (C)(G) apply bid x 4 weeks
  Pediatric: <12 years: not recommended; ≥12 years: same as adult
    Nizoral Cream *Crm:* 2% (15, 30, 60 gm)

▷ ***luliconazole*** (C) apply to affected area and 1 inch into the immediate surrounding area(s) once daily
  Pediatric: <18 years: not recommended; ≥18 years: same as adult
    Luzu Cream 1% *Crm:* 1% (30, 60 gm)

▷ ***miconazole 2%*** (C)(G) apply once daily-bid x 2 weeks
  Pediatric: same as adult
    Lotrimin AF Spray Liquid (OTC) *Spray liq:* 2% (113 gm) (alcohol 17%)
    Lotrimin AF Spray Powder (OTC) *Spray pwdr:* 2% (90 gm) (alcohol 10%)
    Monistat-Derm *Crm:* 2% (1, 3 oz); *Spray liq:* 2% (3.5 oz); *Spray pwdr:* 2% (3 oz)

▷ ***naftifine*** (B)(G)
  Pediatric: <12 years: not recommended; ≥12 years: same as adult
    Naftin Cream apply once daily x 2 weeks
      Crm: 1% (15, 30, 60 gm)
    Naftin Gel apply bid x 2 weeks
      Gel: 1% (20, 40, 60 gm)

▷ ***oxiconazole nitrate*** (B)(G) apply once daily-bid x 2 weeks
  Pediatric: same as adult
    Oxistat *Crm:* 1% (15, 30, 60 gm); *Lotn:* 1% (30 ml)

▷ ***sulconazole*** (C) apply once daily-bid x 3 weeks
  Pediatric: <12 years: not recommended; ≥12 years: same as adult
    Exelderm *Crm:* 1% (15, 30, 60 gm); *Lotn:* 1% (30 mg)

▷ ***terbinafine*** (B)(G)
  Pediatric: <12 years: not recommended; ≥12 years: same as adult
    Lamisil Cream (OTC) apply bid x 1-4 weeks
      Crm: 1% (15, 30 gm)
    Lamisil AT Cream (OTC) apply to affected and surrounding area once daily-bid x 1-4 weeks until significantly improved
      Crm: 1% (15, 30 gm)
    Lamisil Solution (OTC) apply to affected and surrounding area once daily x 1 week
      Soln: 1% (30 ml spray bottle)

▷ ***tolnaftate*** (C)(OTC)(G) apply sparingly bid x 2-4 weeks
  Pediatric: <2 years: not recommended; ≥2 years: same as adult
    Tinactin *Crm:* 1% (15, 30 gm); *Pwdr:* 1% (45, 90 gm); *Soln:* 1% (10 ml);
    Aerosol liq: 1% (4 oz); *Aerosol pwdr:* 1% (3.5, 5 oz)

▷ ***undecylenic acid*** apply bid x 4 weeks
  Pediatric: same as adult
    Desenex (OTC) *Pwdr:* 25% (1.5, 3 oz); *Spray pwdr:* 25% (2.7 oz); *Oint:* 25% (0.5, 1 oz)

TOPICAL ANTIFUNGAL+ANTI-INFLAMMATORY AGENTS

▷ *clotrimazole+betamethasone* (C)(G) apply bid x 4 weeks; max 4 weeks
  Pediatric: <12 years: not recommended; ≥12 years: same as adult
  Crm: clotrim 10 mg+beta 0.5 mg (15, 45 gm); *Lotn:* clotrim 10 mg+beta 0.5 mg
  (30 ml)

SYSTEMIC ANTIFUNGALS

▷ *griseofulvin, microsize* (C)(G) 1 gm once daily x 2 weeks
  Pediatric: <30 lb: 5 mg/lb/day; 30-50 lb: 125-250 mg/day; >50 lb: 250-500 mg/
  day; 5 mg/lb/day x 4-6 weeks or longer; *see* Appendix CC.25. griseofulvin, microsize (Grifulvin V Suspension) *for dose by weight*
    Grifulvin V *Tab:* 250, 500 mg; *Oral susp:* 125 mg/5 ml (120 ml) (alcohol
    0.02%)
▷ *griseofulvin, ultramicrosize* (C) 375 mg/day in a single or divided doses x 2 weeks
  Pediatric: <2 years: not recommended; ≥2 years: 3.3 mg/lb/day in a single or divided
  doses
    Gris-PEG *Tab:* 125, 250 mg
  Comment: *Griseofulvin* should be taken with fatty foods (e.g., milk, ice cream).
  Liver enzymes should be monitored.
▷ *ketoconazole* (C) initially 200 mg once daily; max 400 mg once daily x 4 weeks
  Pediatric: <2 years: not recommended; ≥2 years: 3.3-6.6 mg/kg/day
    Nizoral *Tab:* 200 mg
  Comment: Caution with *ketoconazole* due to concerns about potential for
  hepatotoxicity.

○ TINEA PEDIS (ATHLETE'S FOOT)

TOPICAL ANTIFUNGALS

▷ *butenafine* (B)(G) apply bid x 1 week or once daily x 4 weeks
  Pediatric: <12 years: not recommended; ≥12 years: same as adult
    Lotrimin Ultra (C)(OTC) *Crm:* 1% (12, 24 gm)
    Mentax *Crm:* 1% (15, 30 gm)
  Comment: *Butenafine* is a benzylamine, not an azole. Fungicidal activity
  continues for at least 5 weeks after last application.
▷ *Burrows solution* wet dressings
▷ *ciclopirox* (B)
    Loprox Cream apply bid; max 4 weeks
      Pediatric: <10 years: not recommended; ≥10 years: same as adult
      Crm: 0.77% (15, 30, 90 gm)
    Loprox Lotion apply bid; max 4 weeks
      Pediatric: <10 years: not recommended; ≥10 years: same as adult
      Lotn: 0.77% (30, 60 ml)
    Loprox Gel apply bid; max 4 weeks
      Pediatric: <16 years: not recommended; ≥16 years: same as adult
      Gel: 0.77% (30, 45 gm)
▷ *clotrimazole* (C)(G) apply bid to affected area x 4 weeks
  Pediatric: same as adult
    Desenex *Crm:* 1% (0.5 oz)
    Lotrimin *Crm:* 1% (15, 30, 45, 90 gm); *Lotn:* 1% (30 ml); *Soln:* 1% (10, 30 ml)
    Lotrimin AF (OTC) *Crm:* 1% (15, 30, 45, 90 gm); *Lotn:* 1% (20 ml); *Soln:* 1%
    (20 ml)
▷ *econazole* (C) apply once daily x 4 weeks
  Pediatric: same as adult
    Spectazole *Crm:* 1% (15, 30, 85 gm)

▷ *ketoconazole* (C) apply once daily x 6 weeks
  Pediatric: <12 years: not recommended; ≥12 years: same as adult
    Nizoral Cream *Crm:* 2% (15, 30, 60 gm)
▷ *luliconazole* (C) apply to affected area and 1 inch into the immediate surrounding
  area(s) once daily
  Pediatric: <18 years: not recommended; ≥18 years: same as adult
    Luzu Cream 1% *Crm:* 1% (30, 60 gm)
▷ *miconazole 2%* (C)(G) apply bid x 4 weeks
  Pediatric: same as adult
    Lotrimin AF Spray Liquid (OTC) *Spray liq:* 2% (113 gm) (alcohol 17%)
    Lotrimin AF Spray Powder (OTC) *Spray pwdr:* 2% (90 gm; alcohol 10%)
    Monistat-Derm *Crm:* 2% (1, 3 oz); *Spray liq:* 2% (3.5 oz); *Spray pwdr:* 2% (3 oz)
▷ *naftifine* (B)(G)
  Pediatric: <12 years: not recommended; ≥12 years: same as adult
    Naftin Cream apply once daily x 4 weeks
      Crm: 1% (15, 30, 60 gm)
    Naftin Gel apply bid x 4 weeks
      Gel: 1% (20, 40, 60 gm)
▷ *oxiconazole nitrate* (B)(G) apply once daily-bid x 4 weeks
  Pediatric: same as adult
    Oxistat *Crm:* 1% (15, 30, 60 gm); *Lotn:* 1% (30 ml)
▷ *sertaconazole* (C) apply once daily-bid x 4 weeks
  Pediatric: <12 years: not recommended; ≥12 years: same as adult
    Ertaczo *Crm:* 2% (15, 30 gm)
▷ *sulconazole* (C) apply once daily-bid x 4 weeks
  Pediatric: <12 years: not recommended; ≥12 years: same as adult
    Exelderm *Crm:* 1% (15, 30, 60 gm); *Lotn:* 1% (30 mg)
▷ *terbinafine* (B)(G)
  Pediatric: <12 years: not recommended; ≥12 years: same as adult
    Lamisil Cream (OTC) apply bid x 1-4 weeks
      Crm: 1% (15, 30 gm)
    Lamisil AT Cream (OTC) apply to affected and surrounding area once daily-
    bid x 1-4 weeks until significantly improved
      Crm: 1% (15, 30 gm)
    Lamisil Solution (OTC) apply to affected and surrounding area bid x 1 week
      Soln: 1% (30 ml spray bottle)
▷ *tolnaftate* (C)(OTC)(G) apply sparingly bid x 2-4 weeks
  Pediatric: <2 years: not recommended; ≥2 years: same as adult
    Tinactin *Crm:* 1% (15, 30 gm); *Pwdr:* 1% (45, 90 gm); *Soln:* 1% (10 ml);
    Aerosol liq: 1% (4 oz); *Aerosol pwdr:* 1% (3.5, 5 oz)

TOPICAL ANTIFUNGAL+ANTI-INFLAMMATORY COMBINATION

▷ *clotrimazole+betamethasone* (C)(G) apply bid x 4 weeks; max 4 weeks
  Pediatric: <12 years: not recommended; ≥12 years: same as adult
    Lotrisone *Crm:* clotrim 1 mg+beta 0.5 mg (15, 45 gm); *Lotn:* clotrim 1 mg+
    beta 0.5 mg (30 ml)

SYSTEMIC ANTIFUNGALS

▷ *griseofulvin, microsize* (C)(G) 1 gm once daily x 4-8 weeks
  Pediatric: <30 lb: 5 mg/lb/day; 30-50 lb: 125-250 mg/day; >50 lb: 250-500 mg/
  day; 5 mg/lb/day x 4-6 weeks or longer; *see* Appendix CC.25. *griseofulvin, microsize* (Grifulvin V Suspension) *for dose by weight*
    Grifulvin V *Tab:* 250, 500 mg; *Oral susp:* 125 mg/5 ml (120 ml) (alcohol 0.02%)
▷ *griseofulvin, ultramicrosize* (C) 750 mg/day in a single or divided doses x 4-6
  weeks

Pediatric: <2 years: not recommended; ≥2 years: 3.3 mg/lb/day in a single or divided doses

    Gris-PEG *Tab:* 125, 250 mg

Comment: *Griseofulvin* should be taken with fatty foods (e.g., milk, ice cream). Liver enzymes should be monitored.

▷ *ketoconazole* (C) initially 200 mg once daily; max 400 mg/day x 4 weeks
Pediatric: <2 years: not recommended; ≥2 years: 3.3-6.6 mg/kg once daily x 4 weeks

    Nizoral *Tab:* 200 mg

Comment: Caution with *ketoconazole* due to concerns about potential for hepatotoxicity.

TINEA VERSICOLOR

Comment: Resolution may take 3-6 months.

TOPICAL ANTIFUNGALS

▷ *butenafine* (G) apply once daily x 2 weeks
Pediatric: <12 years: not recommended; ≥12 years: same as adult
    Lotrimin Ultra (C)(OTC) *Crm:* 1% (12, 24 gm)
    Mentax (B) *Crm:* 1% (15, 30 gm)
Comment: *Butenafine* is a benzylamine, <u>not</u> an azole. Fungicidal activity continues for at least 5 weeks after last application.

▷ *ciclopirox* (B)
    Loprox Cream apply bid; max 4 weeks
    Pediatric: <10 years: not recommended; ≥10 years: same as adult
      Crm: 0.77% (15, 30, 90 gm)
    Loprox Lotion apply bid; max 4 weeks
    Pediatric: <10 years: not recommended; ≥10 years: same as adult
      Lotn: 0.77% (30, 60 ml)
    Loprox Gel apply bid; max 4 weeks
    Pediatric: <16 years: not recommended; ≥16 years: same as adult
      Gel: 0.77% (30, 45 gm)

▷ *clotrimazole* (B)(G) apply bid x 7 days
Pediatric: same as adult
    Lotrimin *Crm:* 1% (15, 30, 45 gm)
    Lotrimin AF (OTC) *Crm:* 1% (12 gm); *Lotn:* 1% (10 ml); *Soln:* 1% (10 ml)

▷ *econazole* (C) apply once daily x 2 weeks
Pediatric: same as adult
    Spectazole *Crm:* 1% (15, 30, 85 gm)

▷ *miconazole* 2% (C)(G) apply once daily x 2 weeks
Pediatric: same as adult
    Lotrimin AF Spray Liquid (OTC) *Spray liq:* 2% (113 gm) (alcohol 17%)
    Lotrimin AF Spray Powder (OTC) *Spray pwdr:* 2% (90 gm) alcohol 10%)
    Monistat-Derm *Crm:* 2% (1, 3 oz); *Spray liq:* 2% (3.5 oz); *Spray pwdr:* 2% (3 oz)

▷ *ketoconazole* (C)(G)
Pediatric: <12 years: not recommended; ≥12 years: same as adult
    Nizoral Cream apply once daily x 2 weeks
      Crm: 2% (15, 30, 60 gm)
    Nizoral Shampoo lather into area and leave on 5 minutes x 1 application
      Shampoo: 2% (4 oz)

▷ *oxiconazole nitrate* (B)(G) apply once daily x 2 weeks
Pediatric: same as adult
    Oxistat *Crm:* 1% (15, 30, 60 gm); *Lotn:* 1% (30 ml)

▷ **selenium sulfide** shampoo **(C)(G)** apply after shower, allow to dry, leave on overnight; then scrub off vigorously in AM; repeat in 1 week and again q 3 months until resolution occurs
Pediatric: same as adult
    Selsun Blue *Shampoo:* 1% (120, 210, 240, 330 ml); 2.5% (120 ml)

▷ **sulconazole (C)** apply once daily-bid x 3 weeks
Pediatric: <12 years: not recommended; ≥12 years: same as adult
    Exelderm *Crm:* 1% (15, 30, 60 gm); *Lotn:* 1% (30 mg)

▷ **terbinafine (B)** apply bid to affected and surrounding area x 1 week
Pediatric: <12 years: not recommended; ≥12 years: same as adult
    Lamisil Solution (OTC) *Soln:* 1% (30 ml spray bottle)

ORAL ANTI-FUNGALS

▷ **ketoconazole (C)** initially 200 mg once daily; max 400 mg/day x 4 weeks
Pediatric: <2 years: not recommended; ≥2 years: 3.3-6.6 mg/kg once daily x 4 weeks
    Nizoral *Tab:* 200 mg

 TOBACCO DEPENDENCE, TOBACCO CESSATION, NICOTINE WITHDRAWAL SYNDROME

Comment: According to findings from the Population Assessment of Tobacco and Health (PATH) Study (respondents = 10, 384, mean age = 14.3), any use of e-cigarettes, hookah, non-cigarette combustible tobacco, or smokeless tobacco was independently associated with traditional cigarette smoking 1 year later and use of more than 1 of these products increases the odds of progressing to traditional cigarette use.

NON-NICOTINE PRODUCTS

Alpha4-Beta4 Nicotinic Acetylcholine Receptor Partial Agonist

▷ **varenicline (C)** set target quit date; begin therapy 1 week prior to target quit date; take after eating with a full glass of water; initially 0.5 mg once daily for 3 days; then 0.5 mg bid x 4 days; then 1 mg bid; treat x 12 weeks; may continue treatment for 12 more weeks
Pediatric: <16 years: not studied; ≥16 years: same as adult
    Chantix *Tab:* 0.5, 1 mg; *Starting Month Pak:* 0.5 mg x 11 tabs + 1 mg x 42 tabs; *Continuing Month Pak:* 1 mg x 56 tabs
    Comment: Caution with **Chantix** due to potential risk for anxiety or suicidal ideation.

AMINOKETONES

▷ **bupropion HBr (C)(G)**
Pediatric: Safety and effectiveness in the pediatric population have not been established. When considering the use of **Aplenzin** in a child or adolescent, balance the potential risks with the clinical need
    Aplenzin initially 100 mg bid for at least 3 days; may increase to 375 or 400 mg/day after several weeks; then after at least 3 more days, 450 mg in 4 divided doses; max 450 mg/day, 174 mg/single dose
    Tab: 174, 348, 522 mg

▷ **bupropion HCl (C)(G)**
Pediatric: Safety and effectiveness in the pediatric population have not been established. When considering the use of **Forfivo XL** in a child or adolescent, balance the potential risks with the clinical need
    Forfivo XL do not use for initial treatment; use immediate-release **bupropion** forms for initial titration; switch to **Forfivo XL** 450 mg once daily when total dose/day reaches 450 mg; may switch to **Forfivo XL** when total dose/day

reaches 300 mg for 2 weeks and patient needs 450 mg/day to reach therapeutic target; swallow whole, do not crush or chew

Tab: 450 mg ext-rel

Wellbutrin initially 100 mg bid for at least 3 days; may increase to 375 or 400 mg/day after several weeks; then after at least 3 more days, 450 mg in 4 divided doses; max 450 mg/day, 150 mg/single dose

Tab: 75, 100 mg

Wellbutrin SR initially 150 mg in AM for at least 3 days; may increase to 150 mg bid if well tolerated; usual dose 300 mg/day; max 400 mg/day

Tab: 100, 150 mg sust-rel

Wellbutrin XL initially 150 mg in AM for at least 3 days; increase to 150 mg bid if well tolerated; usual dose 300 mg/day; max 400 mg/day

Tab: 150, 300 mg sust-rel

Zyban 150 mg once daily x 3 days; then 150 mg bid x 7-12 weeks; max 300 mg/day

Tab: 150 mg sust-rel

Comment: Contraindications to *bupropion* include seizure disorder, eating disorder, concurrent MAOI and alcohol use. Smoking should be discontinued after the 7th day of therapy with *bupropion*. Avoid bedtime dose.

TRANSDERMAL NICOTINE SYSTEMS (D)

Habitrol (OTC) initially one 21 mg/24 hr patch/day x 4-6 weeks; then one 14 mg/24 hr patch/day x 2-4 weeks; then one 7 mg/24 hr patch/day x 2-4 weeks; then discontinue

Pediatric: <12 years: not recommended; ≥12 years: same as adult

Transdermal patch: 7, 14, 21 mg/24 hr

Nicoderm CQ (OTC) initially one 21 mg/24 hr patch/day x 6 weeks, then one 14 mg/24 hr patch/day x 2 weeks; then one 7 mg/24 hr patch/day x 2 weeks

Pediatric: <12 years: not recommended; ≥12 years: same as adult

Transdermal patch: 7, 14, 21 mg/24 hr

Comment: Nicoderm CQ is available as a clear patch.

Nicotrol Step-down Patch (OTC) 1 patch/day x 6 weeks

Pediatric: <12 years: not recommended; ≥12 years: same as adult

Transdermal patch: 5, 10, 15 mg/16 hr (7/pck)

Nicotrol Transdermal (OTC) 1 patch/day x 6 weeks

Pediatric: <12 years: not recommended; ≥12 years: same as adult

Transdermal patch: 15 mg/16 hour (7/pck)

Prostep initially one 22 mg/24 hr patch/day x 4-8 weeks; then discontinue or one 11 mg/24 hr patch/day x 2-4 additional weeks

Pediatric: <12 years: not recommended; ≥12 years: same as adult

Transdermal patch: 11, 22 mg/24 hr (7/pck)

NICOTINE GUM

▷ *nicotine polacrilex* **(D)** chew one piece of gum slowly and intermittently over 30 minutes q 1-2 hours x 6 weeks; then q 2-4 hours x 3 weeks; then q 4-8 hours x 3 weeks; max 24 pieces/day; 2 mg if smoked <25 cigarettes/day; 4 mg if smoked >24 cigarettes/day

Pediatric: <12 years: not recommended; ≥12 years: same as adult

Nicorette (OTC) *Gum squares:* 2, 4 mg (108 piece starter kit and 48 piece refill) (orange, mint, or original, sugar-free)

NICOTINE LOZENGE

▷ *nicotine polacrilex* **(X)(OTC)(G)** dissolve over 20-30 minutes; minimize swallowing; do not eat or drink for 15 min before and during use; Use 2 mg lozenge if first cigarette smoked >30 minutes after waking; Use 4 mg lozenge if first cigarette smoked within 30 min of waking; 1 lozenge q 1-2 hours (at least

9/day) x 6 weeks; then q 2-4 hours x 3 weeks; then q 4-8 hours x 3 weeks; then stop; max 5 lozenges/6 hours and 20 lozenges/day

Pediatric: <18 years: not recommended; ≥18 years: same as adult

Commit Lozenge *Loz:* 2, 4 mg (72/pck) (phenylalanine)

Nicorette Mini Lozenge (G) *Loz:* 2, 4 mg (72/pck) (mint; phenylalanine)

NICOTINE INHALATION PRODUCTS

▷ *nicotine* 0.5 mg aqueous nasal spray (D)

Pediatric: <12 years: not recommended; ≥12 years: same as adult

Nicotrol NS 1-2 doses/hour nasally; max 5 doses/hour or 40 doses/day; usual max 3 months

Nasal spray: 0.5 mg/spray; 10 mg/ml (10 ml, 200 doses)

▷ *nicotine* 10 mg inhalation system (D)

Pediatric: <12 years: not recommended; ≥12 years: same as adult

Nicotrol Inhaler individualize therapy; at least 6 cartridges/day x 3-6 weeks; max 16 cartridges/day x first 12 weeks; then reduce gradually over 12 more weeks

Inhaler: 10 mg/cartridge, 4 mg delivered (42 cartridge/pck) (menthol)

Comment: **Nicotrol Inhaler** is a smoking replacement; to be used with decreasing frequency. Smoking should be discontinued before starting therapy. Side effects include cough, nausea, mouth, or throat irritation. This system delivers nicotine, but no tars or carcinogens. Each cartridge lasts about 20 minutes with frequent continuous puffing and provides nicotine equivalent to 2 cigarettes.

⬤ TONSILLITIS: ACUTE

ANTI-INFECTIVES

▷ *amoxicillin* (B)(G) 500-875 mg bid or 250-500 mg tid x 10 days

Pediatric: <40 kg (88 lb): 20-40 mg/kg/day in 3 divided doses x 10 days or 25-45 mg/kg/day in 2 divided doses x 10 days; *see* Appendix CC.3. *amoxicillin* (Amoxil Suspension, Trimox Suspension) *for dose by weight*

Amoxil *Cap:* 250, 500 mg; *Tab:* 875*mg; *Chew tab:* 125, 200, 250, 400 mg (cherry-banana-peppermint) (phenylalanine); *Oral susp:* 125, 250 mg/5 ml (80, 100, 150 ml) (strawberry); 200, 400 mg/5 ml (50, 75, 100 ml) (bubble gum); *Oral drops:* 50 mg/ml (30 ml) (bubble gum)

Moxatag *Tab:* 775 mg ext-rel

Trimox *Tab:* 125, 250 mg; *Cap:* 250, 500 mg; *Oral susp:* 125, 250 mg/5 ml (80, 100, 150 ml) (raspberry-strawberry)

▷ *azithromycin* (B)(G) 500 mg x 1 dose on day 1, then 250 mg once daily on days 2-5 or 500 mg once daily x 3 days or **Zmax** 2 gm in a single dose

Pediatric: 12 mg/kg/day x 5 days; max 500 mg/day; *see* Appendix CC.7. *azithromycin* (Zithromax Suspension, Zmax Suspension) *for dose by weight*

Zithromax *Tab:* 250, 500, 600 mg; *Oral susp:* 100 mg/5 ml (15 ml); 200 mg/5 ml (15, 22.5, 30 ml) (cherry); *Pkt:* 1 gm for reconstitution (cherry-banana)

Zithromax Tri-pak *Tab:* 3 x 500 mg tabs/pck

Zithromax Z-pak *Tab:* 6 x 250 mg tabs/pck

Zmax *Oral susp:* 2 gm ext-rel for reconstitution (cherry-banana) (148 mg Na⁺)

▷ *cefaclor* (B)(G)

Ceclor 250 mg tid or 375 mg bid 3-10 days

Pediatric: <1 month: not recommended; 1 month-12 years: 20-40 mg/kg divided bid or q 12 hours x 3-10 days; max 1 gm/day; *see* Appendix CC.8. *cefaclor* (Ceclor Suspension) *for dose by weight;* >12 years: same as adult

Tab: 500 mg; *Cap:* 250, 500 mg; *Susp:* 125 mg/5 ml (75, 150 ml) (strawberry); 187 mg/5 ml (50, 100 ml) (strawberry); 250 mg/5 ml (75, 150 ml) (strawberry); 375 mg/5 ml (50, 100 ml) (strawberry)

Cefaclor Extended Release 375-500 mg bid x 3-10 days
Pediatric: <16 years: ext-rel not recommended; ≥16 years; same as adult
  Tab: 375, 500 mg ext-rel

▷ *cefadroxil* (B) 1 gm once daily or divided bid x 10 days
Pediatric: 30 mg/kg/day in 2 divided doses x 10 days; *see* Appendix CC.9.
cefadroxil (Duricef Suspension) *for dose by weight*
  Duricef *Cap:* 500 mg; *Tab:* 1 gm; *Oral susp:* 250 mg/5 ml (100 ml); 500 mg/5 ml (75, 100 ml) (orange-pineapple)

▷ *cefdinir* (B) 300 mg bid x 5-10 days or 600 mg once daily x 10 days
Pediatric: <6 months: not recommended; 6 months-12 years: 14 mg/kg/day in a single or 2 divided doses x 10 days; >12 years: same as adult; *see* Appendix CC.10. *cefdinir* (Omnicef Suspension) *for dose by weight*
  Omnicef *Cap:* 300 mg; *Oral susp:* 125 mg/5 ml (60, 100 ml) (strawberry)

▷ *cefditoren pivoxil* (B) 200 mg bid x 10 days
Pediatric: <12 years: not recommended; ≥12 years: same as adult
  Spectracef *Tab:* 200 mg
Comment: Contraindicated with milk protein allergy or carnitine deficiency.

▷ *ceftibuten* (B) 200 mg once daily x 10 days
Pediatric: 9 mg/kg once daily x 10 days; max 400 mg/day; *see* Appendix CC.14.
ceftibuten (Cedax Suspension) *for dose by weight*
  Cedax *Cap:* 400 mg; *Oral susp:* 90 mg/5 ml (30, 60, 90, 120 ml); 180 mg/5 ml (30, 60, 120 ml) (cherry)

▷ *cefixime* (B)(G) 400 mg once daily x 10 days
Pediatric: <6 months: not recommended; 6 months-12 years, <50 kg: 8 mg/kg/day in a single or 2 divided doses x 10 days; *see* Appendix CC.11. *cefixime* (Suprax Oral Suspension) *for dose by weight*; >12 years, >50 kg: same as adult
  Suprax *Tab:* 400 mg; *Cap:* 400 mg; *Oral susp:* 100, 200, 500 mg/5 ml (50, 75, 100 ml) (strawberry)

▷ *cefpodoxime proxetil* (B) 200 mg bid x 5-7 days
Pediatric: <2 months: not recommended; 2 months-12 years: 10 mg/kg/day (max 400 mg/dose) or 5 mg/kg/day bid (max 200 mg/dose) x 5-7 days; *see* Appendix CC.12. *cefpodoxime proxetil* (Vantin Suspension) *for dose by weight*
  Vantin *Tab:* 100, 200 mg; *Oral susp:* 50, 100 mg/5 ml (50, 75, 100 mg) (lemon creme)

▷ *cefprozil* (B) 500 mg once daily x 10 days
Pediatric: 2-12 years: 7.5 mg/kg bid x 10 days; >12 years: same as adult; *see* Appendix CC.13. *cefprozil* (Cefzil Suspension) *for dose by weight*
  Cefzil *Tab:* 250, 500 mg; *Oral susp:* 125, 250 mg/5 ml (50, 75, 100 ml) (bubble gum) (phenylalanine)

▷ *cephalexin* (B)(G) 250 mg tid x 10 days
Pediatric: 25-50 mg/kg/day in 4 divided doses x 10 days; *see* Appendix CC.15.
cephalexin (Keflex Suspension) *for dose by weight*
  Keflex *Cap:* 250, 333, 500, 750 mg; *Oral susp:* 125, 250 mg/5 ml (100, 200 ml) (strawberry)

▷ *clarithromycin* (C)(G) 250 mg bid or 500 mg ext-rel once daily x 10 days
Pediatric: <6 months: not recommended; ≥6 months: 7.5 mg/kg bid x 10 days; *see* Appendix CC.16. *clarithromycin* (Biaxin Suspension) *for dose by weight*
  Biaxin *Tab:* 250, 500 mg
  Biaxin Oral Suspension *Oral susp:* 125, 250 mg/5 ml (50, 100 ml) (fruit punch)
  Biaxin XL *Tab:* 500 mg ext-rel

▷ *dirithromycin* (C)(G) 500 mg once daily x 10 days
Pediatric: <12 years: not recommended; ≥12 years: same as adult
  Dynabac *Tab:* 250 mg

▷ *erythromycin base* (B)(G) 300-400 mg tid x 10 days
Pediatric: 30-50 mg/kg/day in 2-4 divided doses x 10 days

Ery-Tab *Tab:* 250, 333, 500 mg ent-coat
PCE *Tab:* 333, 500 mg

➤ *erythromycin ethylsuccinate* (B)(G) 400 mg qid x 7 days
Pediatric: 30-50 mg/kg/day in 4 divided doses x 7 days; may double dose with
severe infection; max 100 mg/kg/day; *see Appendix CC.21: erythromycin ethylsuccinate (E.E.S. Suspension, Ery-Ped Drops/Suspension) for dose by weight*
    EryPed *Oral susp:* 200 mg/5 ml (100, 200 ml) (fruit); 400 mg/5 ml (60, 100,
    200 ml) (banana); *Oral drops:* 200, 400 mg/5 ml (50 ml) (fruit); *Chew tab:*
    200 mg wafer (fruit)
    E.E.S. *Oral susp:* 200, 400 mg/5 ml (100 ml) (fruit)
    E.E.S. Granules *Oral susp:* 200 mg/5 ml (100, 200 ml) (cherry)
    E.E.S. 400 Tablets *Tab:* 400 mg
➤ *loracarbef* (B) 200 mg bid x 10 days
Pediatric: 15 mg/kg/day in 2 divided doses x 10 days; *see* Appendix CC.27.
loracarbef (Lorabid Suspension) *for dose by weight*
    Lorabid *Pulvule:* 200, 400 mg; *Oral susp:* 100 mg/5 ml (50, 100 ml); 200 mg/5
    ml (50, 75, 100 ml) (strawberry bubble gum)
➤ *penicillin v potassium* (B)(G) 250 mg tid x 10 days
Pediatric: 25-50 mg/kg day in 4 divided doses x 10 days; ≥12 years: same as adult;
see Appendix CC.29. *penicillin v potassium* (Pen-Vee K Solution, Veetids Solution) *for dose by weight*
    Pen-Vee K *Tab:* 250, 500 mg; *Oral soln:* 125 mg/5 ml (100, 200 ml); 250 mg/5
    ml (100, 150, 200 ml)

TOXOPLASMOSIS

➤ *pyrimethamine* 50-75 mg daily (together with 1-4 gm daily of a sulfonamide of
the sulfapyrimidine type, e.g. *sulfadoxine*) x 1 to 3 weeks, depending on patient
response and tolerance; then, reduce dose of each drug to about one-half and
continue for an additional 4-5 weeks; tolerated best with food
Pediatric: 1 mg/kg/day divided into 2 equal daily doses (together with the usual
pediatric sulfonamide dose) x 2 to 4 days; then, reduce dose of each drug to about
one-half and continue for approximately 1 month; tolerated best with food
    Daraprim *Tab:* 25*mg
    Comment: **Daraprim** *(pyrimethamine)* is indicated for the treatment of
    toxoplasmosis when used conjointly with a sulfonamide, since synergism
    exists with this combination. *pyrimethamine* is a folic acid antagonist. The
    rationale for its therapeutic action is based on the differential requirement
    between host and parasite for nucleic acid precursors involved in growth.
    This activity is highly selective against *Toxoplasma gondii.* **Daraprim** is
    contraindicated in patients with documented megaloblastic anemia due to
    folate deficiency. Doses used in toxoplasmosis may produce megaloblastic
    anemia, leukopenia, thrombocytopenia, pancytopenia, neutropenia, atrophic
    glossitis, hematuria, and disorders of cardiac rhythm. *pyrimethamine* has
    a narrow therapeutic index. If signs of folate deficiency develop reduce the
    dosage or discontinue according to the response of the patient. Folinic acid
    (leucovorin) should be administered in a dosage of 5-15 mg daily (orally,
    IV, or IM) until normal hematopoiesis is restored. A small starting dose is
    recommended for patients with a convulsive disorder to avoid potential CNS
    toxicity. **Daraprim** should be used with caution in patients with impaired
    renal or hepatic function and patients with possible folate deficiency, such
    as individuals with malabsorption syndrome, alcoholism, or pregnancy, and
    those receiving therapy, such as *phenytoin,* affecting folate levels. Patients
    should be warned that at the first appearance of a skin rash they should stop
    use of **Daraprim** and seek medical attention immediately. Patients should also

be warned that the appearance of sore throat, pallor, purpura, or glossitis may be early indications of serious disorders which require the discontinuation of **Daraprim** and immediate medical attention. *pyrimethamine* may be used with sulfonamides, quinine and other antimalarials, and with other antibiotics. However, the concomitant use of other antifolic drugs or agents associated with myelosuppression including sulfonamides or *trimethoprim-sulfamethoxazole* combinations, *proguanil*, *zidovudine*, or cytostatic agents (e.g., *methotrexate* [MTX]), while the patient is receiving *pyrimethamine*, may increase the risk of bone marrow suppression. If signs of folate deficiency develop, *pyrimethamine* should be discontinued and folinic acid *(leucovorin)* should be administered until normal hematopoiesis is restored. There are no adequate and well-controlled studies of *pyrimethamine* use in pregnant females. However, in animal studies, *pyrimethamine* has been shown to be teratogenic in oral doses 2.5 times the human dose for treatment of toxoplasmosis; a significant increase in abnormalities such as cleft palate, brachygnathia, oligodactyly, and microphthalmia have been reported. *pyrimethamine* has also been shown to produce terata such as meningocele cleft palate with oral doses 5 times the human dose for the treatment of toxoplasmosis. **Daraprim** should be used during pregnancy only if the potential benefit justifies the potential risk to the fetus. Females of childbearing potential who are taking **Daraprim** should be warned against becoming pregnant. Concurrent administration of folinic acid is strongly recommended when **Daraprim** is used during pregnancy.*pyrimethamine* is excreted in human milk. Because of the potential for serious adverse reactions in nursing infants from *pyrimethamine*, and from concurrent use of a sulfonamide with **Daraprim** for treatment of patients with toxoplasmosis, a decision should be made whether to discontinue nursing or to discontinue the drug, taking into account the importance of the drug to the mother.

TRICHINOSIS (*TRICHINELLA SPIRALIS*)

Comment: Trichinosis is caused by eating raw or undercooked pork or wild game infected with the larvae of a parasitic worm, *Trichinella spiralis*. The initial symptoms are abdominal discomfort, nausea, vomiting, diarrhea, fatigue, and fever beginning 1-2 days following ingestion. These parasites then invade other organs (e.g., muscles) causing muscle aches, itching, fever, chills, and joint pains that begins about 2-8 weeks after ingestion. The treatment is oral anthelmintics which may cause abdominal pain, diarrhea, and (rarely) hypersensitivity reactions, convulsions, neutropenia, agranulocytosis, and hepatitis.

ANTHELMINTICS

Comment: Oral bioavailability of anthelmintics is enhanced when administered with a fatty meal (estimated fat content 40 gm).

▷ *albendazole* (C) take with a meal; may crush and mix with food; may repeat in 3 weeks if needed; 400 mg as once daily x 7 days
Pediatric: <2 years: 200 mg once daily x 3 days; may repeat in 3 weeks; 2-12 years: 400 mg once daily x 3 days; may repeat in 3 weeks; >12 years: same as adult
    Albenza *Tab:* 200 mg
Comment: *Albendazole* is a broad-spectrum benzimidazole carbamate anthelmintic.

▷ *ivermectin* (C) take with water; chew or crush and mix with food; may repeat in 3 months if needed; 200 mcg/kg as a single dose
Pediatric: <15 kg: not recommended; ≥15 kg: same as adult
    Stromectol *Tab:* 3, 6*mg

▷ *mebendazole* (C)(G) take with a meal; chew or crush and mix with food; may repeat in 3 weeks if needed; <2 years: not recommended; ≥2 years: 100 mg bid x 3 days

Pediatric: <2 years: not recommended; ≥2 years: same as adult
>   **Emverm** *Chew tab:* 100 mg
>   **Vermox (G)** *Chew tab:* 100 mg

▷ *pyrantel pamoate* (C) take with a meal; may open capsule and sprinkle <u>or</u> mix with food; treat x 3 days; may repeat in 2-3 weeks if needed; treat x 3 days; 11 mg/kg/dose; max 1 gm/dose; <25 lb: not recommended; 25-37 lb: 1/2 tsp/dose; 38-62 lb: 1 tsp/dose; 63-87 lb: 1 tsp/dose; 88-112 lb: 2 tsp/dose; 113-137 lb: 2 tsp/dose; 138-162 lb: 3 tsp/dose; 163-187 lb: 3 tsp/dose; >187 lb: 4 tsp/dose
>   **Antiminth** *Cap:* 180 mg; *Liq:* 50 mg/ml (30 ml); 144 mg/ml (30 ml); *Oral susp:* 50 mg/ml (60 ml)
>   **Pin-X (OTC)** *Cap:* 180 mg; *Liq:* 50 mg/ml (30 ml); 144 mg/ml (30 ml); *Oral susp:* 50 mg/ml (30 ml)

▷ *thiabendazole* (C) take with a meal; may crush and mix with food; treat x 7 days; 25 mg/kg bid x 7 days; max 1.5 gm/dose; take with a meal
Pediatric: same as adult; <30 lb: consult mfr pkg insert; ≥30 lb: 25 mg/kg in 2 divided doses/day with meals; 30-50 lbs: 250 mg bid with meals; >50 lb: 10 mg/lb/dose bid with meals; max 3 gm/day
>   **Mintezol** *Chew tab:* 500*mg (orange); *Oral susp:* 500 mg/5 ml (120 ml) (orange)

Comment: *Thiabendazole* is <u>not</u> for prophylaxis. May impair mental alertness. May <u>not</u> be available in the US.

⊙ TRICHOMONIASIS (*TRICHOMONAS VAGINALIS*)

Comment: The following treatment regimens for *Trichomoniasis* are published in the **2015 CDC Sexually Transmitted Diseases Treatment Guidelines**. Treat all sexual contacts. A multi-dose treatment regimen should be considered in HIV-positive women.

RECOMMENDED REGIMENS (NON-PREGNANT)
Regimen 1
▷ *metronidazole* 2 gm once in a single dose

Regimen 2
▷ *tinidazole* 2 gm once in a single dose

RECOMMENDED ALTERNATE REGIMEN
Regimen 1
▷ *metronidazole* 500 mg bid x 7 days

DRUG BRANDS AND DOSE FORMS
▷ *metronidazole* (<u>not</u> for use in 1st; B in 2nd, 3rd)(G)
>   **Flagyl** *Tab:* 250*, 500*mg
>   **Flagyl 375** *Cap:* 375 mg
>   **Flagyl ER** *Tab:* 750 mg ext-rel
▷ *tinidazole* (<u>not</u> for use in 1st; B in 2nd, 3rd)
>   **Tindamax** *Tab:* 250*, 500*mg

RECOMMENDED REGIMENS: PREGNANCY/LACTATION
Comment: All pregnant females should be considered for treatment. Women can be treated with 2 gm *metronidazole* in a single dose at any stage of pregnancy. Lactating women who are administered *metronidazole* should be instructed to interrupt breastfeeding for 12-24 hours after receiving the 2 gm dose of *metronidazole*.

TRICHOTILLOMANIA

Comment: Trichotillomania is on the obsessive-compulsive spectrum within the larger DS-5 category, Anxiety Disorders, and depression is frequently a co-morbid disorder. Hence, medications used to treat OCD can be helpful in treating trichotillomania. Recommended psychotropic agents include *clomipramine* (**Anafranil**) and *fluvoxamine* (**Luvox**). Other medications that research suggests may have some benefit include the SSRIs *fluoxetine* (**Prozac**), *sertraline* (**Zoloft**), *paroxetine* (**Paxil**), the mood stabilizer *lithium carbonate* (**Lithobid, Eskalith**), the OTC supplement **N-acetylcysteine**, an amino acid that influences neurotransmitters related to mood, **olanzapine** (**Zyprexa**), an atypical anti-psychotic, and *valproate* (**Depakote**), an anticonvulsant.

TRICYCLIC ANTIDEPRESSANT (TCA) COMBINATIONS

▷ *clomipramine* (C)(G) initially 25 mg daily in divided doses; gradually increase to 100 mg during first 2 weeks; max 250 mg/day; total maintenance dose may be given at HS
Pediatric: <10 years: not recommended; ≥10 years: initially 25 mg daily in divided doses; gradually increase; max 3 mg/kg or 100 mg, whichever is smaller
　　Anafranil *Cap:* 25, 50, 75 mg

SELECTIVE SEROTONIN REUPTAKE INHIBITORS (SSRIs)

▷ *fluoxetine* (C)(G)
　　Prozac initially 20 mg daily; may increase after 1 week; doses >20 mg/day should be divided into AM and noon doses; max 80 mg/day
　　Pediatric: <8 years: not recommended; 8-17 years: initially 10 mg/day; may increase after 1 week to 20 mg/day; range 20-60 mg/day; range for lower weight children, 20-30 mg/day
　　　Cap: 10, 20, 40 mg; *Tab:* 30*, 60*mg; *Oral soln:* 20 mg/5 ml (4 oz) (mint)
　　Prozac Weekly following daily fluoxetine therapy at 20 mg/day for 13 weeks, may initiate **Prozac Weekly** 7 days after the last 20 mg fluoxetine dose
　　Pediatric: <12 years: not recommended; ≥12 years: same as adult
　　　Cap: 90 mg ent-coat del-rel pellets
▷ *fluvoxamine* (C)(G)
　　Comment: *Fluvoxamine* has a specific FDA indication for OCD.
　　Luvox initially 50 mg q HS; adjust in 50 mg increments at 4-7 day intervals; range 100-300 mg/day; over 100 mg/day, divide into 2 doses giving the larger dose at HS
　　Pediatric: <8 years: not recommended; 8-17 years: initially 25 mg q HS; adjust in 25 mg increments q 4-7 days; usual range 50-200 mg/day; over 50 mg/day, divide into 2 doses giving the larger dose at HS; >17 years: same as adult
　　　Tab: 25, 50*, 100*mg
　　Luvox CR initially 100 mg once daily at HS; may increase by 50 mg increments at 1 week intervals; max 300 mg/day; swallow whole
　　Pediatric: <18 years: not recommended; ≥18 years: same as adult
　　　Cap: 100, 150 mg ext-rel
▷ *paroxetine maleate* (D)(G)
　　Pediatric: <12 years: not recommended; ≥12 years: same as adult
　　Paxil initially 20 mg daily in AM; may increase by 10 mg/day at weekly intervals as needed; max 60 mg/day
　　　Tab: 10*, 20*, 30, 40 mg
　　Paxil CR initially 25 mg daily in AM; may increase by 12.5 mg at weekly intervals as needed; max 62.5 mg/day
　　　Tab: 12.5, 25, 37.5 mg cont-rel ent-coat

Paxil Suspension initially 20 mg daily in AM; may increase by 10 mg/day at weekly intervals as needed; max 60 mg/day
Oral susp: 10 mg/5 ml (250 ml) (orange)
➤ *paroxetine mesylate* (D)(G) <12 years: not recommended; ≥12 years: initially 7.5 mg daily in AM; may increase by 10 mg/day at weekly intervals as needed; max 60 mg/day
Brisdelle *Cap:* 7.5 mg
➤ *sertraline* (C)(G) initially 50 mg daily; increase at 1 week intervals if needed; max 200 mg daily; dilute oral concentrate immediately prior to administration in 4 oz water, ginger ale, lemon-lime soda, lemonade, or orange juice
Pediatric: <6 years: not recommended; 6-12 years: initially 25 mg daily; max 200 mg/day; 13-17 years: initially 50 mg daily; max 200 mg/day; >17 years: same as adult
Zoloft *Tab:* 25*, 50*, 100*mg; *Oral conc:* 20 mg per ml (60 ml) (alcohol 12%)

Lithium Salts Mood Stabilizer

➤ *lithium carbonate* (D)(G) swallow whole; *Usual maintenance:* 900-1200 mg/day in 2-3 divided doses
Pediatric: <12 years: not recommended; ≥12 years: same as adult
Lithobid *Tab:* 300 mg slow-rel
Comment: Signs and symptoms of *lithium* toxicity can occur below 2 mEq/L and include blurred vision, tinnitus, weakness, dizziness, nausea, abdominal pains, vomiting, diarrhea to (severe) hand tremors, ataxia, muscle twitches, nystagmus, seizures, slurred speech, decreased level of consciousness, coma, and death.

Valproate Mood Stabilizer

➤ *divalproex sodium* (D)(G) take once daily; swallow ext-rel form whole; initially 25 mg/kg/day in divided doses; max 60 mg/kg/day; *Elderly:* reduce initial dose and titrate slowly
Pediatric: <12 years: not recommended; ≥12 years: same as adult
Depakene *Cap:* 250 mg; *Syr:* 250 mg/5 ml (16 oz)
Depakote *Tab:* 125, 250 mg
Depakote ER *Tab:* 250, 500 mg ext-rel
Depakote Sprinkle *Cap:* 125 mg

ANTIPSYCHOTIC

➤ *olanzapine* (C) initially 2.5-10 mg daily; increase to 10 mg/day within a few days; then by 5 mg/day at weekly intervals; max 20 mg/day
Zyprexa *Tab:* 2.5, 5, 7.5, 10 mg
Zyprexa Zydis *ODT:* 5, 10, 15, 20 mg (phenylalanine)

TRIGEMINAL NEURALGIA (TIC DOULOUREUX)

ANTICONVULSANTS

➤ *baclofen* (C)(G) initially 5-10 mg tid with food; usual dose 10-80 mg/day
Pediatric: <12 years: not recommended; ≥12 years: same as adult
Lioresal *Tab:* 10*, 20*mg
Comment: Potential for seizures or hallucinations on abrupt withdrawal of *baclofen*.
➤ *carbamazepine* (C)
Carbatrol initially 200 mg bid; may increase weekly as needed by 200 mg/day; usual maintenance 800 mg-1.2 gm/day
Pediatric: <12 years: max <35 mg/kg/day; use ext-rel form above 400 mg/day; 12-15 years: max 1 gm/day in 2 divided doses; >15 years: usual maintenance 1.2 gm/day in 2 divided doses
Cap: 200, 300 mg ext-rel

Tegretol (G) initially 100 mg bid <u>or</u> 1/2 tsp susp qid; may increase dose by 100 mg q 12 hours <u>or</u> by 1/2 tsp susp q 6 hours; usual maintenance 400-800 mg/day; max 1200 mg/day

Pediatric: <6 years: initially 10-20 mg/kg/day in 2 divided doses; increase weekly as needed in 3-4 divided doses; max 35 mg/kg/day in 3-4 divided doses; ≥6 years: initially 100 mg bid; increase weekly as needed by 100 mg/day in 3-4 divided doses; max 1 gm/day in 3-4 divided doses

   Tab: 200*mg; *Chew tab:* 100*mg; *Oral susp:* 100 mg/5 ml (450 ml) (citrus-vanilla)

Tegretol XR (G) initially 200 mg bid; may increase weekly by 200 mg/day in 2 divided doses

Pediatric: <6 years: use other forms; ≥6 years: initially 100 mg bid; may increase weekly by 100 mg/day in 2 divided doses; max 1 gm/day

   Tab: 100, 200, 400 mg ext-rel

▷ *clonazepam* **(D)(IV)(G)** initially 0.25 mg bid; increase to 1 mg/day after 3 days

Pediatric: <10 years, <30 kg: initially 0.1-0.3 mg/kg/day; may increase up to 0.05 mg/kg/day bid-tid; usual maintenance 0.1-0.2 mg/kg/day tid

   Klonopin *Tab:* 0.5*, 1, 2 mg

   Klonopin Wafers dissolve in mouth with <u>or</u> without water

     Wafer: 0.125, 0.25, 0.5, 1, 2 mg orally-disint

▷ *divalproex sodium* **(D)** initially 250 mg bid; gradually increase to max 1000 mg/day if needed

Pediatric: <10 years: not recommended; ≥10 years: same as adult

   Depakene *Cap:* 250 mg; *Syr:* 250 mg/5 ml

   Depakote *Tab:* 125, 250 mg

   Depakote ER *Tab:* 250, 500 mg ext-rel

   Depakote Sprinkle *Cap:* 125 mg

▷ *phenytoin* **(D)** 400 mg/day in divided doses

   Dilantin *Cap:* 30, 100 mg; *Oral susp:* 125 mg/5 ml (8 oz); *Infatab:* 50 mg

Comment: Monitor *phenytoin* serum levels. Therapeutic serum level: 10-20 gm/ml. Side effects include gingival hyperplasia.

▷ *valproic acid* **(D)** initially 15 mg/kg/day; may increase weekly by 5-10 mg/kg/day; max 60 mg/kg/day <u>or</u> 250 mg/day

   Depakene *Cap:* 250 mg; *Syr:* 250 mg/5 ml

TRICYCLIC ANTIDEPRESSANTS (TCAs)

Comment: Co-administration of TCAs with SSRIs requires extreme caution.

▷ *amitriptyline* **(C)(G)** titrate to achieve pain relief; max 300 mg/day

Pediatric: <12 years: not recommended; ≥12 years: same as adult

   Tab: 10, 25, 50, 75, 100, 150 mg

▷ *amoxapine* **(C)** titrate to achieve pain relief; if total dose exceeds 300 mg/day, give in divided doses; max 400 mg/day

Pediatric: <12 years: not recommended; ≥12 years: same as adult

   Tab: 25, 50, 100, 150 mg

▷ *desipramine* **(C)(G)** titrate to achieve pain relief; max 300 mg/day

Pediatric: <12 years: not recommended; ≥12 years: same as adult

   Norpramin *Tab:* 10, 25, 50, 75, 100, 150 mg

▷ *doxepin* **(C)(G)** titrate to achieve pain relief; max 150 mg/day

Pediatric: <12 years: not recommended; ≥12 years: same as adult

   Cap: 10, 25, 50, 75, 100, 150 mg; *Oral conc:* 10 mg/ml (4 oz w. dropper)

▷ *imipramine* **(C)(G)**

Pediatric: <12 years: not recommended; ≥12 years: same as adult

   Tofranil titrate to achieve pain relief; max 200 mg/day; adolescents max 100 mg/day; if maintenance dose exceeds 75 mg/day, may switch to **Tofranil PM** at bedtime

   Tab: 10, 25, 50 mg

Tofranil PM titrate to achieve pain relief; initially 75 mg at HS; max 200 mg at HS

    Cap: 75, 100, 125, 150 mg

Tofranil Injection 50 mg IM; lower dose for adolescents; switch to oral form as soon as possible

    Amp: 25 mg/2 ml (2 ml)

▷ *nortriptyline* (D)(G) titrate to achieve pain relief; initially 10-25 mg tid-qid; max 150 mg/day; lower doses for elderly and adolescents

Pediatric: <12 years: not recommended; ≥12 years: same as adult

    Pamelor titrate to achieve pain relief; max 150 mg/day

        Cap: 10, 25, 50, 75 mg; *Oral soln:* 10 mg/5 ml (16 oz)

▷ *protriptyline* (C) titrate to achieve pain relief; initially 5 mg tid; max 60 mg/day

Pediatric: <12 years: not recommended; ≥12 years: same as adult

    Vivactil *Tab:* 5, 10 mg

▷ *trimipramine* (C) titrate to achieve pain relief; max 200 mg/day

Pediatric: <12 years: not recommended; ≥12 years: same as adult

    Surmontil *Cap:* 25, 50, 100 mg

TUBERCULOSIS (TB): PULMONARY (*MYCOBACTERIUM TUBERCULOSIS*)

SCREENING

▷ *purified protein derivative (PPD)* (C) 0.1 ml intradermally; examine inoculation site for induration at 48 to 72 hours.

Pediatric: same as adult

    Aplisol, Tubersol *Soln:* 5 US units/0.1 ml (1, 5 ml)

PROPHYLAXIS VACCINE

The <u>only</u> tuberculosis vaccine uses attenuation of the related organism *Mycobacterium bovis* by culture in bile-containing media to create the *Bacillus Calmette-Guerin* (BCG) vaccination strain. It was first used experimentally in 1921 by Albert Calmette and Camille Guerin and is currently in widespread use outside of the US. It is <u>not</u> available in the US. The BCG vaccine protects newborns against tuberculosis-related meningitis and other systemic tuberculosis infections, but it has limited protection against active pulmonary disease. Once vaccinated, the patient will be PPD positive.

Comment: Active tuberculosis in pregnancy is associated with adverse maternal and neonatal outcomes including maternal anemia, caesarean delivery, preterm birth, low birth weight, birth asphyxia, and perinatal infant death.

ANTI-TUBERCULAR AGENTS

Comment: Avoid *streptomycin* in pregnancy. *Pyridoxine* (*vitamin B6*) 25 mg once daily x 6 months should be administered concomitantly with *INH* for prevention of side effects. *Rifapentine* produces red-orange discoloration of body tissues and body fluids and may stain contact lenses.

▷ *bedaquiline* (B)(G)

    Sirturo *Tab:* 100 mg

    Comment: *Bedaquiline* is a diarylquinoline antimycobacterial ATP synthase for the treatment of pulmonary multi-drug resistant TB (MDR-TB).

▷ *ethambutol (EMB)* (B)(G)

    Myambutol *Tab:* 100, 400*mg

▷ *isoniazid (INH)* (C) *Tab:* 300*mg

▷ *pyrazinamide (PZA)* (C) *Tab:* 500*mg

▷ *rifampin (RIF)* (C)(G)

    Rifadin, Rimactane *Cap:* 150, 300 mg

▷ *rifapentine* (C)

Priftin *Tab*: 150 mg (24, 32 pck)
Comment: The 32-count packs of **Priftin** are intended for patients with active tuberculosis infection (TB). The 24-count packs are intended for patients with latent tuberculosis infection (LTBI) who are at high risk for progression to tuberculosis disease. **Priftin** for active TB is indicated for patients ≥12 years-of-age. **Priftin** for LTBI is indicated for patients ≥2 years-of-age.

▷ *rilpivirine* (C) *Tab*: 25 mg
Rifabutin *Cap*: 150 mg
▷ *streptomycin (SM)* (C)(G) *Amp*: 1 gm/2.5 ml or 400 mg/ml (2.5 ml)

COMBINATION AGENTS

▷ *rifampin+isoniazid* (C)
Rifamate *Cap*: rif 300 mg+iso 150 mg
▷ *rifampin+isoniazid+pyrazinamide* (C)
Rifater *Tab*: rif 120 mg+iso 50 mg+pyr 300 mgss

PROPHYLAXIS AFTER EXPOSURE TO TUBERCULOSIS, WITH NEGATIVE PPD

▷ *isoniazid* 300 mg once daily in a single dose x at least 6 months
Pediatric: 10-20 mg/kg/day x 9 months

PROPHYLAXIS AFTER EXPOSURE, WITH NEW PPD CONVERSION

▷ *isoniazid* 300 mg once daily in a single dose x 12 months
Pediatric: 10-20 mg/kg/day x 9 months
Tab: 100, 300*mg; *Syr*: 50 mg/5 ml; *Inj*: 100 mg/ml
▷ *rifampin* (C) 600 mg once daily + *isoniazid* 300 mg once daily x 4 months
Pediatric: *rifampin* 10-20 mg/kg + *isoniazid* 10-20 mg/kg once daily x 4 months
▷ *rifapentine* (C) 600 mg once weekly + *isoniazid* (C) 300 mg once weekly x 12 weeks
Pediatric: ≤12 years: Treat x 12 weeks; 10-14 kg: *rifapentine* 300 mg once weekly + *isoniazid* 25 mg/kg (max 900 mg) once weekly; 14.1-25 kg: *rifapentine* 450 mg once weekly + *isoniazid* 25 mg/kg (max 900 mg) once weekly; 25.1-32 kg: *rifapentine* 600 mg once weekly + *isoniazid* 25 mg/kg (max 900 mg) once weekly; 32.1-50 kg: *rifapentine* 750 mg once weekly + *isoniazid* 25 mg/kg (max 900 mg) once weekly; >50 kg: *rifapentine* 900 mg once weekly + *isoniazid* 25 mg/kg (max 900 mg) once weekly; >12 years: same as adult

TREATMENT REGIMENS (≥12 YEARS)

Regimen 1

▷ *rifampin* 600 mg + *isoniazid* 300 mg + *pyrazinamide* 2 gm + *ethambutol* (C) 15-25 mg/kg or *streptomycin* (C) 1 gm once daily x 8 weeks; then *isoniazid* (C) 300 mg + *rifampin* 600 mg once daily x 16 weeks or *isoniazid* 900 mg + *rifampin* 600 mg 2-3 x/week x 16 weeks

Regimen 2

▷ *rifampin* 600 mg + *isoniazid* 300 mg + *pyrazinamide* 2 gm + *ethambutol* 15-25 mg/kg or *streptomycin* 1 gm once daily x 2 weeks; then *rifampin* 600 mg + *isoniazid* 900 mg + *pyrazinamide* 4 gm + *ethambutol* 50 mg/kg or *streptomycin* 1.5 gm 2 x/week x 6 weeks; then *isoniazid* 300 mg + *rifampin* 600 mg once daily x 16 weeks or 2 x/week x 16 weeks *rifampin* 600 mg once daily x 16 weeks or 2 x/week x 16 weeks

Regimen 3

▷ *rifampin* 600 mg + *isoniazid* 900 mg + *pyrazinamide* 3 gm + *ethambutol* 25-30 mg/kg or *streptomycin* 1.5 gm 3 x/week x 6 months

Regimen 4 (for smear and culture negative for pulmonary TB in adult)

▷ Options 1, 2, or 3 x 8 weeks; then *isoniazid* 300 mg + *rifampin* 600 mg once daily x 16 weeks; then *rifampin* 600 mg + *isoniazid* 300 mg + *pyrazinamide* 2 gm + *ethambutol* 15-25 mg/kg or *streptomycin* 1 gm once daily x 8 weeks or 2-3 x/week x 8 weeks

Regimen 5 (for smear and culture negative for pulmonary TB in adult)

▷ *rifapentine* 600 mg twice weekly x 2 months (at least 72 hours between doses) + once daily *isoniazid* 300 mg, *ethambutol* 15-25 mg/kg + *pyrazinamide* 2 gm; then *rifapentine* 600 mg once weekly x 4 months + once daily *isoniazid* 300 mg + another appropriate anti-tuberculosis agent for susceptible organisms

Regimen 6 (when pyrazinamide is contraindicated)

▷ *rifampin* 600 mg + *isoniazid* 300 mg + *ethambutol* 15-25 mg/kg + *streptomycin* 1 gm once daily x 4-8 weeks; then *isoniazid* 300 mg + *rifampin* 600 mg once daily x 24 weeks or 2 x/week x 24 weeks

PEDIATRIC TREATMENT REGIMENS (<12 YEARS)

Regimen 1

▷ *rifampin* 10-20 mg/kg + *isoniazid* 10-20 mg/kg + *pyrazinamide* 15-20 mg/kg + *ethambutol* 15-25 mg/kg or *streptomycin* 20-40 mg/kg once daily x 8 weeks; then *isoniazid* 10-20 mg/kg + *rifampin* 10-20 mg/kg once daily x 16 weeks or *isoniazid* 20-40 mg/kg + *rifampin* 10-20 mg/kg 2-3 x/week x 16 weeks

Regimen 2

▷ *rifampin* 10-20 mg/kg + *isoniazid* 10-20 mg/kg + *pyrazinamide* 15-30 mg/kg + *ethambutol* 15-25 mg/kg or *streptomycin* 20-40 mg/kg once daily x 2 weeks; then *rifampin* 10-20 mg/kg + *isoniazid* 20-40 mg/kg + *pyrazinamide* 50-70 mg/kg + *ethambutol* 50 mg/kg or *streptomycin* 25-30 mg/kg 2 x/week x 6 weeks; then *isoniazid* 10-20 mg/kg + *rifampin* 10-20 mg/kg once daily x 16 weeks or *rifampin* 10-20 mg/kg + *isoniazid* 20-40 mg/kg 2 x/week x 16 weeks

Regimen 3

▷ *rifampin* 10-20 mg/kg + *isoniazid* 20-40 mg/kg + *pyrazinamide* 50-70 mg/kg + *ethambutol* 25-30 mg/kg or *streptomycin* 25-30 mg/kg 3 x/week x 6 months

Regimen 4 (when pyrazinamide is contraindicated)

▷ *rifampin* 10-20 mg/kg + *isoniazid* 10-20 mg/kg + *ethambutol* 15-25 mg/kg + *streptomycin* 20-40 mg/kg once daily x 4-8 weeks; then *isoniazid* 10-20 mg/kg + *rifampin* 10-20 mg/kg once daily x 24 weeks or *rifampin* 10-20 mg/kg + *isoniazid* 20-40 mg/kg 2 x/week x 24 weeks

POLYPEPTIDE ANTIBIOTIC ISOLATED FROM STREPTOMYCES CAPREOLUS

Comment: *Capreomycin sulfate* is a complex of four microbiologically active components which have been characterized in part; however, complete structural determination of all the components has not been established. **Capastat Sulfate**, which is to be used concomitantly with other appropriate anti-tuberculosis agents, is indicated in pulmonary infections caused by *capreomycin*-susceptible strains of *M. tuberculosis* when the primary agents (i.e., *isoniazid, rifampin, ethambutol, aminosalicylic acid,* and *streptomycin*) have been ineffective or cannot be used because of toxicity or the presence of resistant tubercle bacilli.

▷ *capreomycin sulfate* (C)(G) may be administered deep IM in a large muscle mass after reconstitution with 2 ml 0.9%NS or sterile water or via IV infusion over 60 minutes after reconstitution and dilution in 100 ml 0.9%NS; usual dose is 1 gm daily (not to exceed 20 mg/kg/day) via IM or IV infusion for 60 to 120 days; see mfr pkg insert for dosage table based on kg body weight and route of administration

Pediatric: <18 years: not recommended; ≥18 years: same as adult

Capastat *Vial*: 1 gm pwdr for reconstitution with 2 ml 0.9%NS or sterile water

Comment: Black Box Warning (BBW): The use of *capreomycin sulfate* in patients with renal insufficiency or preexisting auditory impairment must be undertaken with great caution, and the risk of additional cranial nerve VIII impairment or renal injury should be weighed against the benefits to be derived from therapy. Since other parenteral antituberculosis agents (e.g., *streptomycin, viomycin*) also have similar and sometimes irreversible toxic effects, particularly on cranial nerve VIII and renal function, simultaneous administration of these agents with **Capastat Sulfate** is not recommended. Use with non-antituberculosis drugs (e.g., *polymyxin A sulfate, colistin sulfate, amikacin, gentamicin, tobramycin, vancomycin, kanamycin,* and *neomycin*) having ototoxic or nephrotoxic potential should be undertaken only with great caution. Audiometric measurements and assessment of vestibular function should be performed prior to initiation of therapy with **Capastat Sulfate** and at regular intervals during treatment. Renal injury, with tubular necrosis, elevation of the blood urea nitrogen (BUN) or serum creatinine, and abnormal urinary sediment, has been noted. Slight elevation of the BUN and serum creatinine (sCr) has been observed in a significant number of patients receiving prolonged therapy. The appearance of casts, red cells, and white cells in the urine has been noted in a high percentage of these cases. The safety of the use of **Capastat Sulfate** in pregnancy has not been determined. Safety and effectiveness in pediatric patients have not been established. It is not known whether this drug is excreted in human milk.

PULMONARY MULTIDRUG-RESISTANT TUBERCULOSIS (PMRT)

▷ *bedaquiline* 400 mg (4 x 100 mg tablets or 20 x 20 mg tablets) once daily x 2 weeks; then, 200 mg (2 x 100 mg tablets or 10 x 20 mg tablets) 3 times per week (at least 48 hours between doses) x 22 weeks; administer doses via directly observed therapy (DOT); must be taken with food; if a dose is missed during the first 2 weeks of treatment, do not administer the missed dose (skip the dose and then continue the daily dosing regimen); from Week 3 onward, if a dose is missed, administer the missed dose as soon as possible, and then resume the 3 x/ week dosing regimen

Pediatric: <5 years, <15 kg: not established; ≥5 years, ≥15 kg: see mfr pkg insert for weight-based chart

Sirturo *Tab*: 20*, 100 mg

Comment: **Sirturo** *(bedaquiline)* is an oral diarylquinoline antimycobacterial drug indicated as part of combination therapy in adult and pediatric patients (≥5 years, ≥15 kg) with pulmonary multi-drug resistant tuberculosis (MDR-TB). Reserve **Sirturo** for use when an effective treatment regimen cannot otherwise be provided. This indication is approved under accelerated approval based on time to sputum culture conversion. Continued approval for this indication may be contingent upon verification and description of clinical benefit in confirmatory trials. Do not use **Sirturo** for the treatment of latent, extrapulmonary or drug-sensitive tuberculosis or for the treatment of infections caused by non-tuberculous mycobacteria. Safety and efficacy of **Sirturo** in HIV-infected patients with MDR-TB has not been established, as clinical data are limited. Emphasize need for compliance with full course of therapy. Prior to administration, obtain ECG, liver enzymes and electrolytes. Obtain susceptibility information for the background regimen against *Mycobacterium tuberculosis* isolate if possible. Only use **Sirturo** in combination with at least 3 other drugs to which the patient's MDR-TB isolate has been shown to be susceptible in vitro. If in vitro testing results are unavailable, may initiate **Sirturo** in combination with at least 4 other drugs to which patient's MDR-TB isolate is likely to be susceptible. Monitor ECGs and discontinue **Sirturo** if significant ventricular arrhythmia or QTcF interval > 500 ms develops. Monitor liver-related laboratory tests. Discontinue **Sirturo** if evidence of liver injury occurs. The most common adverse reactions reported (incidence ≥10%) of adult patients treated with **Sirturo** have been nausea, arthralgia, headache, hemoptysis and chest pain. The most common adverse reactions reported (incidence ≥10%) in patients 12 to <18 years) have been arthralgia, nausea and abdominal pain. The most common adverse reaction reported (incidence ≥10%) in patients 5 to <12 years has been elevated liver enzymes. Avoid use of strong and moderate CYP3A4 inducers with **Sirturo**. Avoid use for more than 14 consecutive days of systemic strong CYP3A4 inhibitors with **Sirturo** unless the benefit outweighs the risk. Available data from published literature of **Sirturo** use in pregnant females are insufficient to evaluate a drug-associated risk of major birth defects, miscarriage, or adverse maternal or fetal outcomes. Monitor infants exposed to *bedaquiline* through breast milk for signs of *bedaquiline*-related adverse reactions, such as hepatotoxicity.

TREATMENT-RESISTANT TUBERCULOSIS: 3-PART COMBINATION REGIMEN FOR ADULTS
Nitroimidazooxazine Antimycobacterial+Diarylquinoline Antimycobacterial+ Oxazolidinone Antibacterial

Comment: Take each drug in the 3-part regimen daily, with food, for a total of 26 weeks. Doses of the regimen missed for safety reasons can be made up at the end of treatment. Doses of *linezolid* alone missed due to *linezolid* adverse reactions should not be made up. *Pretomanid* and *bedaquiline* are indicated for use in a limited and specific population of patients with TB. *pretomanid* (a nitroimidazooxazine antimycobacterial) and *bedaquiline* (a diarylquinoline antimycobacterial ATP synthase) are indicated as part of a the 3-part combination regimen with *linezolid* (an oxazolidinone-class antibacterial), for the treatment of adults with pulmonary extensively drug resistant (XDR) and treatment-intolerant or nonresponsive multidrug-resistant (MDR) tuberculosis (TB), when an effective treatment regimen cannot otherwise be provided. Approval of this indication is based on limited clinical safety and efficacy data. *pretomanid* and *bedaquiline* are not indicated for patients with: drug-sensitive (DS) TB, latent infection due to *Mycobacterium tuberculosis* extra-pulmonary infection due to *Mycobacterium tuberculosis, and* MDR-TB that is not treatment-intolerant or nonresponsive to standard therapy. Safety and effectiveness of *pretomanid* has not been established for use in combination with any drugs other than *bedaquiline* and *linezolid* as part of the recommended dosing regimen. Administration of this medication regimen by directly observed therapy (DOT) is recommended. Emphasize the need for compliance with the full 26-day treatment regimen.

▷ *pretomanid* take 200 mg once daily; swallow whole with water; take with food; x total 26 weeks
  Pretomanid Tablet *Tab*: 200 mg
▷ *bedaquiline* take 400 mg once daily x 2 weeks; followed by 200 mg 3 x/week (separate doses by at least 48 hours), x 22 weeks; swallow whole
  Sirturo *Tab*: 100 mg
▷ *linezolid* take 1,200 mg daily, with dose adjustments for known *linezolid* toxicities, x total 26 weeks
  Zyvox *Tab*: 400, 600 mg; *Oral susp*: 100 mg/5 ml (150 ml) (orange) (phenylalanine)

◯ TYPE 1 DIABETES MELLITUS (T1DM)

Comment: Target glycosylated hemoglobin (HbA1c) is <7%. Addition of daily ACE-I and/or ARB therapy is strongly recommended for renal protection.

Insulin may be indicated in the management of Type 2 diabetes with or without concomitant oral anti-diabetic agents.

TREATMENT FOR ACUTE HYPOGLYCEMIA

▷ *glucagon (recombinant)* **(B)** administer SC, IM, or IV; if patient does not respond in 15 minutes, may administer a single dose or 2 divided doses; <20 kg: 0.5 mg or 20-30 mg/kg; ≥20 kg: 1 mg

Comment: Necrolytic Migratory Erythema (NME), a skin rash, has been reported post-marketing following continuous *glucagon* infusion and resolved with discontinuation of the *glucagon*. Should NME occur, consider whether the benefits of continuous *glucagon* infusion outweigh the risks and consider using an oral or intravenous glucose preparation instead.

Gvoke 1 mg SC; administer via SC injection only in the upper outer arm, lower abdomen, or outer thigh; call for emergency assistance immediately after administration of the dose; if there has been no response after 15 minutes, an additional weight-appropriate dose may be administered while waiting for emergency assistance; do not re-use an injection device when the patient has responded to treatment, administer oral carbohydrates
Pediatric: <2 years: not established; 2-12 years: <45 kg: 0.5 mg SC; ≥45 kg: same as adult; administer via SC injection only in the upper outer arm, lower abdomen, or outer thigh; call for emergency assistance immediately after administering the dose; if there has been no response after 15 minutes, an additional weight-appropriate dose may be administered while waiting for emergency assistance; do not re-use an injection device; when the patient has responded to treatment, administer oral carbohydrates
HypoPen auto-injector: 0.5 mg/0.1 ml, 1 mg/0.2 ml, single-use; *Pre-filled syringe:* 0.5 mg/0.1 ml, 1 mg/0.2 ml, single-use
Comment: Gvoke *(glucagon injection)* is a ready-to-use, room-temperature stable, liquid *glucagon* for the treatment of severe hypoglycemia in adult and pediatric patients ≥2 years-of-age with diabetes. Patients taking a beta-blocker may have a transient increase in pulse and blood pressure. In patients taking *indomethacin*, Gvoke may lose its ability to raise glucose or may produce hypoglycemia. Gvoke may increase the anticoagulant effect of *warfarin*. Gvoke is contraindicated in patients with pheochromocytoma because Gvoke may stimulate the release of catecholamines from the tumor. In patients with insulinoma, Gvoke administration may produce an initial increase in blood glucose; however, Gvoke may stimulate exaggerated insulin release from an insulinoma and cause hypoglycemia; if a patient develops symptoms of hypoglycemia after a dose of Gvoke, administer glucose orally or intravenously. Allergic reactions have been reported and include generalized rash, anaphylactic shock with breathing difficulties, and hypotension. Gvoke is effective in treating hypoglycemia only if sufficient hepatic glycogen is present; patients in states of starvation, with adrenal insufficiency or chronic hypoglycemia may not have adequate levels of hepatic glycogen for Gvoke to be effective (use glucose instead). *glucagon* administered to patients with glucagonoma may cause secondary hypoglycemia. Test patients suspected of having glucagonoma for blood levels of glucagon prior to treatment, and monitor blood glucose levels during treatment; if hypoglycemia develops, administer glucose orally or intravenously.

▷ *glucagon nasal powder* 3 mg administered as one actuation of the intranasal device into one nostril; administer the dose by inserting the tip into one nostril and pressing the device plunger all the way in until the green line is no longer showing; the dose does not need to be inhaled; call for emergency assistance immediately after administering the dose; when the patient responds to treatment, administer oral carbohydrates; do not attempt to re-use the device (each device contains only one dose of *glucagon*); if there has been no response after 15 minutes, administer an additional 3 mg using an unused device

Pediatric: <4 years: not approved: ≥4 years: same as adult

Basqimi *Intranasal device:* 3 mg pwdr, single-dose

Comment: **Baqsimi** is a nasally administered antihypoglycemic agent indicated for the treatment of severe hypoglycemia in diabetes patients ≥4 years-of-age. Pheochromocytoma (**Baqsimi** may stimulate the release of catecholamines from the tumor) and insulinoma (**Baqsimi** may stimulate exaggerated insulin release from an insulinoma) are contraindications to **Baqsimi** use. Patients taking a beta-blocker may experience a transient increase in HR and BP. For patients taking *indomethacin*, **Baqsimi** may lose its ability to raise glucose or may produce hypoglycemia. **Baqsimi** may increase the anticoagulant effect of *warfarin*. **Baqsimi** is effective in treating hypoglycemia only if sufficient hepatic glycogen is present. Patients in states of starvation, with adrenal insufficiency, or chronic hypoglycemia may not have adequate levels of hepatic glycogen for **Baqsimi** to be effective; therefore, patients with any of these conditions should be treated with glucose. The most common (incidence ≥10%) adverse reactions associated with **Baqsimi** are nausea, vomiting, headache, upper respiratory tract irritation (i.e., rhinorrhea, nasal discomfort, nasal congestion, cough, and epistaxis), watery eyes, redness of eyes, and itchy nose, throat; and eyes.

▷ *dasiglucagon* 0.6 mg SC into the outer upper arm, lower abdomen, thigh, or buttocks; if there has been no response after 15 minutes, an additional dose from a new device may be administered while waiting for emergency assistance; when the patient has responded to treatment, give oral carbohydrates

Pediatric: <6 years: safety and efficacy not established; ≥6 years: same as adult

Zegalogue *Prefilled syringe:* 0.6 mg/0.6 ml, single-dose; *Autoinjector:* 0.6 mg/0.6 ml, single-dose

Comment: **Zegalogue** is a glucagon analog for the treatment of severe hypoglycemia in patients with diabetes. Contraindications to **Zegaloque** include pheochromocytoma and insulinoma. In patients with pheochromocytoma, **Zegalogue** may stimulate the release of catecholamines from the tumor. In patients with insulinoma, **Zegalogue** may produce an initial increase in blood glucose, but then stimulate exaggerated insulin release from an insulinoma, causing subsequent hypoglycemia. If the patient develops symptoms of hypoglycemia after a dose of **Zegaloque**, administer glucose orally or intravenously. **Zegalogue** is effective in treating hypoglycemia only if sufficient hepatic glycogen is present. Patients in states of starvation, with adrenal insufficiency, or chronic hypoglycemia may not have adequate levels of hepatic glycogen for **Zegalogue** to be effective and patients with these conditions should be treated with glucose. Drug interactions with **Zegalogue** include beta blockers, *indomethacin*, and *warfarin*. Patients taking a beta-blocker may have a transient increase in HR and BP. With patients taking *indomethacin*, **Zegalogue** may lose its ability to raise serum glucose or may produce hypoglycemia. Co-administration of **Zegalogue** with *warfarin* may increase *warfarin's* anticoagulant effect. The most common adverse reactions (incidence ≥2%) associated with **Zegalogue** have been: *Adult:* nausea, vomiting, headache, diarrhea, and injection site pain; *Pediatric:* nausea, vomiting, headache, and injection site pain. Allergic reactions have been reported with glucagon products. These reactions may include generalized rash, and in some cases anaphylactic shock with breathing difficulties and hypotension.

NONDIURETIC BENZOTHIADIAZINE DERIVATIVE

▷ *diazoxide* (C)(G)

Proglycem *Cap:* 50 mg, Oral Suspension: 50 mg/ml (chocolate mint) (sodium benzoate) (alcohol 7.25%)

Comment: **Proglycem** is useful in the management of hypoglycemia due to hyperinsulinism associated with the following conditions: *Adults:* inoperable islet cell adenoma or carcinoma, or extrapancreatic malignancy. *Infants and Children:* Leucine sensitivity, islet cell hyperplasia, nesidioblastosis, extrapancreatic malignancy, islet cell adenoma, or adenomatosis. **Proglycem** may be used preoperatively as a temporary measure, and postoperatively, if hypoglycemia persists. Treatment with **Proglycem** should be initiated under close clinical supervision, with careful monitoring of blood glucose and clinical response until the patient's condition has stabilized. This usually requires several days. If not effective in 2-3 weeks, **Proglycem** should be discontinued. **Proglycem**-induced hyperglycemia is reversed by the administration of insulin or *tolbutamide*. The inhibition of insulin release by **Proglycem** is antagonized by alpha-adrenergic blocking agents. The antidiuretic property of *diazoxide* may lead to significant fluid retention, which in patients with compromised cardiac reserve, may precipitate CHF. The fluid retention will respond to conventional therapy with diuretics. There have been postmarketing reports of pulmonary hypertension occurring in infants and neonates treated with *diazoxide*. The cases were reversible upon discontinuation of the drug. Monitor patients, especially those with risk factors for pulmonary hypertension, for respiratory distress and discontinue *diazoxide* if pulmonary hypertension is suspected. Development of abnormal facial features in four children treated chronically (>4 years) with **Proglycem** for hypoglycemia hyperinsulinism has been reported. *diazoxide* is highly bound to serum proteins (>90%) and, therefore, may displace other substances which are also protein bound, such as bilirubin or *coumarin* and its derivatives, resulting in higher blood levels of these substances. Concomitant administration of oral *diazoxide* and *diphenylhydantoin* may result in a loss of seizure control. IV administration of **Proglycem** during labor may cause cessation of uterine contractions, and administration of oxytocic agents may be required to reinstate labor; caution is advised in administering **Proglycem** at that time. *diazoxide* crosses the placental barrier and appears in cord blood. When given to the mother prior to delivery of the infant, the drug may produce fetal or neonatal hyperbilirubinemia, thrombocytopenia, altered carbohydrate metabolism, and possibly other side effects that have occurred in adults. Alopecia and hypertrichosis lanuginosa have occurred in infants whose mothers received oral *diazoxide* during the last 19-60 days of pregnancy. Reproduction animal studies using the oral preparation have revealed increased fetal resorptions and delayed parturition, as well as fetal skeletal anomalies; evidence of skeletal and cardiac teratogenic effects have also been noted with IV administration. **Proglycem** has also been demonstrated to cross the placental barrier in animals and to cause degeneration of the fetal pancreatic beta cells. When use of **Proglycem** is considered, potential benefits to the mother must be weighed against possible harmful effects to the fetus. Information is not available concerning the passage of diazoxide in breast milk. Because many drugs are excreted in human milk and because of the potential for adverse reactions from *diazoxide* in nursing infants, a decision should be made whether to discontinue nursing or to discontinue the drug, taking into account the importance of the drug to the mother.

INHALED INSULIN

Rapid-Acting Inhalation Powder Insulin

▶ *insulin human (inhaled)* (C) one inhaler may be used for up to 15 days, then discard; dose at meal times as follows: *Insulin naïve:* initially 4 units at each meal; adjust according to blood glucose monitoring
Conversion from SC to inhaled mealtime insulin:
SC 1-4 units: inhal 4 units
SC 5-8 units: inhal 8 units
SC 9-12 units: inhal 12 units
SC 13-16 units: inhal 16 units
SC 17-20 units: inhal 20 units
SC 21-24 units: inhal 24 units
Pediatric: <18 years: not established; ≥18 years: same as adult
Afrezza Inhalation Powder administer at the beginning of the meal; *Mealtime insulin naïve:* initially 4 units at each meal; *Using SC prandial insulin:* convert dose to **Afrezza** using a conversion table (see mfr pkg insert); *Using SC pre-mixed:* divide 1/2 of total daily injected pre-mixed insulin equally among 3 meals of the day; administer 1/2 total injected pre-mixed dose as once daily injected basal insulin dose
Inhal: 4, 8, 12 unit single-inhalation color-coded cartridges (30, 60, 90/pkg w. 2 disposable inhalers)
Comment: **Afrezza** is not a substitute for long-acting insulin. **Afrezza** must be used in combination with long-acting insulin in patients with T1DM. **Afrezza** is not recommended for the treatment of diabetic ketoacidosis. **Afrezza** is contraindicated with chronic lung disease because of the risk of acute bronchospasm. The use of **Afrezza** is not recommended in patients who smoke or who have recently stopped smoking. Each card contains 5 blister strips with 3 cartridges each (total 15 cartridges). The doses are color-coded. **Afrezza** is contraindicated with chronic respiratory disease (e.g., asthma, COPD) and patients prone to episodes of hypoglycemia.

INJECTABLE INSULINS

Rapid-Acting Insulins

▶ *insulin aspart (recombinant)* (B) onset <15 minutes; peak 1-3 hours; duration 3-5 hours; administer 5-10 minutes prior to a meal; SC or infusion pump or IV infusion
Pediatric: <3 years: not recommended; ≥3 years: same as adult
Fiasp *Vial:* 1000 units/10 ml (100 units/ml, 10 ml), muli-dose; *FlexTouch pen:* 300 units/3 ml (100 units/ml, 3 ml), single-use; *PenFill:* 300 units/3 ml (100 units/ml, 3 ml), single-use
Comment: **Fiasp** is a newer formulation of **NovoLog**, in which the addition of *niacinamide* (vitamin B3) helps to increase the speed of initial insulin absorption.
NovoLog *Vial:* 100 U/ml (10 ml); *PenFill cartridge:* 100 U/ml (3 ml, 5/pck) (zinc, m-cresol)

▶ *insulin glulisine (rDNA origin)* (C) onset <15 minutes; peak 1 hour; duration 2-4 hours; administer up to 15 minutes before, or within 20 minutes after starting a meal; use with an intermediate or long-acting insulin; SC only; may administer via insulin pump; do not dilute or mix with other insulin in pump
Pediatric: <4 years: not recommended; ≥4 years: same as adult
Apidra *Vial:* 100 U/ml (10 ml); *Cartridge:* 100 U/ml (3 ml, 5/pck; m-cresol)

▶ *insulin lispro (recombinant)* (B) onset <15 minutes; peak 1 hour; duration 3.5-4.5 hours; administer up to 15 minutes before, or immediately after, a meal; SC or IV infusion pump only
Pediatric: <3 years: not recommended; ≥3 years: same as adult

Admelog *Vial:* 100 U/ml (10 ml) (zinc, m-cresol); *Prefilled disposable SoloStar pen (disposable):* 100 U/ml (3 ml) (5/carton) (zinc, m-cresol)

Humalog *Vial:* 100 U/ml (10 ml); *Prefilled disposable KwikPen:* 100 U/ml (3 ml, 5/pck) (zinc, m-cresol); *HumaPen Memoir* and *HumaPen Luxura* HD inj device for *Humulog cartridges* (100 U/ml, 3 ml 5/pck) (zinc, m-cresol)

▷ *insulin regular* (B)

Humulin R U-100 *(human, recombinant)* **(OTC)** onset 30 minutes; peak 2-4 hours; duration up to 6-8 hours; SC or IV or IM
    Vial: 100 U/ml (10 ml)

Humulin R U-500 *(human, recombinant)* onset 30 minutes; peak 1.75-4 hours; duration up to 24 hours; SC only; for in-hospital use only
    Vial: 500 U/ml (20 ml); *KwikPen:* 3 ml (2, 5/carton)

Comment: **Humulin R U-500** formulation is 5 times more concentrated than standard U-100 concentration, indicated for adults and children who require ≥200 units of insulin/day, allowing patients to inject 80% less liquid to receive the desired dose. Recommend using U-500 syringe (BD, Eli Lilly). The U-500 syringe (0.5 ml, 6 mm x 31 gauge) is marked in 5 unit increments and allows for dosing up to 250 units.

Iletin II Regular *(pork)* **(OTC)** onset 30 minutes; peak 2-4 hours; duration 6-8 hours; SC, IV or IM
    Vial: 100 U/ml (10 ml)

Novolin R *(human)* **(OTC)** onset 30 minutes; peak 2.5-5 hours; duration 8 hours; SC, IV, or IM
    Vial: 100 U/ml (10 ml); *PenFill cartridge:* 100 U/ml (1.5 ml, 5/pck); *Prefilled syringe:* 100 U/ml (1.5 ml, 5/pck)

▷ *pramlintide* *(amylin analog/amylinomimetic)* **(C)** administer immediately before major meals (≥250 kcal or ≥30 gm carbohydrates); initially 15 mcg; titrate in 15 mcg increments for 3 days if no significant nausea occurs; if nausea occurs at 45 or 60 mcg, reduce to 30 mcg; if not tolerated, consider discontinuing therapy; *Maintenance:* 60 mcg (30 mcg only if 60 mcg not tolerated)

Symlin *Vial:* 0.6 mg/ml (5 ml) (m-cresol, mannitol)

Comment: **Symlin** is indicated as adjunct to mealtime insulin with or without a sulfonylurea and/or *metformin* when blood glucose control is suboptimal despite optimal insulin therapy. Do not mix with insulin. When initiating **Symlin**, reduce preprandial short/rapid-acting insulin dose by 50% and monitor pre- and post-prandial and bedtime blood glucose. Do not use in patients with poor compliance, HgbA1c is >9%, recurrent hypoglycemia requiring assistance in the previous 6 months, or if taking a prokinetic drug. With Type 2 DM, initial therapy is 60 mcg/dose and max is 120 mcg/dose.

RAPID-ACTING+INTERMEDIATE-ACTING INSULIN
Insulin Aspart Protamine Suspension+Insulin Aspart Combinations

▷ *insulin aspart protamine suspension 70%/insulin aspart 30%* *(recombinant)* **(B)** **(G)** onset 15 min; peak 2.4 hours; duration up to 24 hours; SC only
Pediatric: not recommended

NovoLog Mix 70/30 (OTC) *Vial:* 100 U/ml (10 ml)

NovoLog Mix 70/30 FlexPen (OTC) *Prefilled disposable pen:* 100 U/ml (3 ml, 5/pck); *PenFill cartridge:* 100 U/ml (3 ml, 5/pck)

LONG-ACTING INSULINS

▷ *insulin detemir (human)* **(B)** administer SC once daily with evening meal or at HS as a basal insulin; may administer twice daily (AM/PM); administer in the deltoid, abdomen, or thigh; onset 1-2 hours; peak 6-8 hours; duration 24 hours; switching from another basal insulin, dose should be the same on a unit-to-unit basis; may need more *insulin detemir* when switching from **NPH**; *Type 1:*

starting dose 1/3 of total daily insulin requirements; rapid-acting or short-acting, pre-meal insulin should be used to satisfy the remainder of daily insulin requirements; *Type 2 (inadequately controlled on oral antidiabetic agents)*: initially 10 units or 0.1-0.2 units/kg, once daily in the evening or divided twice daily (AM/PM); do not add-mix or dilute *insulin detemir* with other insulins.

Pediatric: <2 years: not recommended; ≥2 years: same as adult

> **Levemir** *Vial:* 100 U/ml (10 ml); *FlexPen:* 100 U/ml (3 ml, 5/pck; (zinc, m-cresol)

▷ *insulin glargine (recombinant)* (C)

Basaglar administer SC once daily, at the same time each day, as a basal insulin in the deltoid, abdomen, or thigh; onset 1-1.5 hours, no pronounced peak, duration 20-24 hours; *T1DM (adults and children >6 years-of-age)*: initially 1/3 of total daily insulin dose; administer the remainder of the total dose as short- or rapid-acting pre-prandial insulin; *T2DM (adults only)*: initially 2 units/kg or up to 10 units once daily; *Switching from once daily insulin glargine 300 units/ml (i.e., Toujeo) to 100 units/ml*: initially 80% of the insulin glargine 300 units/ml; *Switching from twice daily NPH*: initially 80% of the total daily NPH dose; do not add-mix or dilute *insulin glargine* with other insulins.

Pediatric: <6 years: not established; ≥6 years: individualize and adjust as needed

> *Prefilled KwikPen (disposable),* 100 U/ml (3 ml) (5/carton) (m-cresol)

Lantus administer SC once daily at the same time each day as a basal insulin; onset 1-1.5 hours, no pronounced peak, duration 20-24 hours; initial average starting dose 10 units for insulin-naïve patients; *Switching from once daily NPH or Ultralente insulin:* initial dose of *insulin glargine* should be on a unit-for-unit basis; *Switching from twice daily NPH insulin:* start at 20% lower than the total daily *NPH* dose

Pediatric: <6 years: not recommended; ≥6 years: same as adult

> *Vial:* 100 U/ml (10 ml); *Cartridge:* 100 U/ml (3 ml, for use in the OptiPen One Insulin Delivery Device) (5/carton) (m-cresol); *SoloStar pen (disposable):* 100 U/ml (3 ml) (5/carton)

Toujeo administer SC once daily at the same time each day as a basal insulin; in the upper arm, abdomen, or thigh; onset of action 6 hours; duration 20-24 hours; *T2DM, insulin naïve:* initially 0.2 units/kg; titrate every 3-4 days; *T1DM, insulin naïve:* initially 1/3-1/2 total daily insulin dose; remainder as short-acting insulin divided between each meal; *Switch from once daily long- or intermediate-acting insulin:* on a unit-for-unit basis; *Switching from Lantus:* a higher daily dose is expected; *Switching from twice daily NPH:* reduce initial dose by 20% of total daily NPH dose

Pediatric: <18 years: not established; ≥18 years: same as adult

> *Soln for SC injection:* 450 units/1.5 ml prefilled disposable SoloStar pen (1.5 ml, 3/pck); 300 units/ml prefilled Max SoloStar pen (3 ml, 2/pck)

Comment: The **Toujeo Max SoloStar** pen contains 900 units of *insulin glargine* for administration of up to 160 units in a single injection and need for fewer prescribed pens and fewer refills.

▷ *insulin isophane suspension (NPH)* (B)

Pediatric: <18 years: not recommended; ≥18 years: same as adult

Humulin N *(human, recombinant)* (OTC) onset 1-2 hours; peak 6-12 hours; duration 18-24 hours; SC only

> *Vial:* 100 U/ml (10 ml); *Prefilled disposable pen:* 100 U/ml (3 ml, 5/pck)

Novolin N *(recombinant)* (OTC) onset 1.5 hours; peak 4-12 hours; duration 24 hours; SC only

> *Vial:* 100 U/ml (10 ml); *PenFill cartridge:* 1.5 ml (5/pck); *KwikPens:* 1.5 ml (5/pck)

Iletin II NPH *(pork)* **(OTC)** onset 1-2 hours; peak 6-12 hours; duration 18-26 hours; SC <u>only</u>
> *Vial:* 100 U/ml (10 ml)

▷ **insulin zinc suspension** *(lente)* **(B)**
Pediatric: <18 years: not recommended; ≥18 years: same as adult
Humulin L *(human)* **(OTC)** onset 1-3 hours; peak 6-12 hours; duration 18-24 hours; SC <u>only</u>
> *Vial:* 100 U/ml (10 ml)

Iletin II Lente *(pork)* **(OTC)** onset 1-3 hours; peak 6-12 hours; duration 18-26 hours; SC <u>only</u>
> *Vial:* 100 U/ml (10 ml)

Novolin L *(human)* **(OTC)** onset 2.5 hours; peak 7-15 hours; duration 22 hours; SC <u>only</u>
> *Vial:* 100 U/ml (10 ml)

Ultra Long-Acting Insulin

▷ **insulin degludec (insulin analog) (C)** administer by SC injection once daily at any time of day, with <u>or</u> without food, into the upper arm, abdomen, <u>or</u> thigh; titrate every 3-4 days; *Insulin naïve with type 1 diabetes:* initially 1/3-1/2 of total daily insulin dose, usually 0.2-0.4 units/kg; administer the remainder of the total dose as short-acting insulin divided between each daily meal; *Insulin naive with type 2 diabetes:* initially 10 units once daily; adjust dose of concomitant oral antidiabetic agent; *Already on insulin (type 1 or type 2):* initiate at same unit dose as total daily long- <u>or</u> intermediate-acting insulin unit dose
Pediatric: <1 year: not established; ≥1 year: same as adult
Tresiba FlexTouch *Pen:* 100 U/ml (3 ml, 5 pens/carton), 200 U/ml (3 ml, 3 pens/carton) (zinc, m-cresol)
Comment: Tresiba U-200 FlexTouch is the <u>only</u> long-acting insulin in a 160-unit pen allowing up to 160 units in a single injection. The U-200 dose counter always shows the desired dose (i.e., no conversion from U/100 to U-200 is required)

▷ **insulin extended zinc suspension (Ultralente) (human) (B)** onset 4-6 hours; peak 8-20 hours; duration 24-48 hours; SC <u>only</u>
Pediatric: <18 years: not recommended; ≥18 years: same as adult
Humulin U **(OTC)** *Vial:* 100 U/ml (10 ml)

Insulin Lispro Protamine+Insulin Lispro Combinations

▷ **insulin lispro protamine75%+insulin lispro 25% (B)**
Pediatric: <18 years: not recommended; ≥18 years: same as adult
Humalog Mix 75/25 *(human)* onset 15 minutes; peak 30 minutes to 1 hour; duration 24 hours; SC <u>only</u>
> *Vial:* 100 U/ml (10 ml); *Prefilled disposable KwikPen:* 100 U/ml (3 ml, 5/pck) (zinc, m-cresol); *HumaPen Memoir* and *HumaPen Luxura HD* inj device for *Humalog cartridges* (100 U/ml, 3 ml, 5/pck) (zinc, m-cresol)

▷ **insulin lispro protamine 50%+insulin lispro 50% (B)**
Pediatric: <18 years: not recommended; ≥18 years: same as adult
Humalog Mix 50/50 *(recombinant)* **(B)** onset 15 minutes; peak 2.3 hours; range 1-5 hours; SC <u>only</u>
> *Vial:* 100 U/ml (10 ml); *Prefilled disposable KwikPen:* 100 U/ml (3 ml, 5/pck) (zinc, m-cresol); *HumaPen Memoir* and *HumaPen LUXURA HD* inj device for *Humalog cartridges* (100 U/ml, 3 ml, 5/pck) (zinc, m-cresol)

Insulin Isophane Suspension (NPH)+Insulin Regular Combinations

▷ **NPH 70%+regular 30% (B)**
Pediatric: <18 years: not recommended; ≥18 years

Humulin 70/30 (*human, recombinant*) (**OTC**) onset 30 minutes; peak 2-12 hours; duration up to 24 hours; SC <u>only</u>
 Vial: 100 U/ml (10 ml)
Novolin 70/30 (*recombinant*) (**OTC**) onset 30 minutes; peak 2-12 hours; duration up to 24 hours; SC <u>only</u>
 Vial: 100 U/ml (10 ml)

▷ *NPH 50%+regular 50%* (**B**)
 Pediatric: <18 years: not recommended; ≥18 years: same as adult
 Humulin 50/50 (*human*) (**OTC**) onset 30 minutes; peak 3-5 hours; duration up to 24 hours; SC <u>only</u>
  Vial: 100 U/ml (10 ml)

Insulin Lispro Protamine+Insulin Lispro Combinations

▷ *insulin lispro protamine 75%+insulin lispro 25%* (**B**)
 Pediatric: <18 years: not recommended; ≥18 years: same as adult
 Humalog Mix 75/25 (*recombinant*) onset 15 minutes; peak 30-90 minutes; duration 24 hours; SC <u>only</u>
  Vial: 100 U/ml (10 ml); *Prefilled disposable KwikPen:* 100 U/ml (3 ml, 5/pck) (zinc, m-cresol); *HumaPen Memoir* and *HumaPen LUXURA* HD inj device for *Humalog cartridges* (100 U/ml, 3 ml 5/pck) (zinc, m-cresol)

▷ *insulin lispro protamine 50%+insulin lispro 50%* (**B**)
 Pediatric: <18 years: not recommended; ≥18 years: same as adult
 Humalog Mix 50/50 (*recombinant*) onset 15 minutes; peak 1 hour; duration up to 16 hours; SC <u>only</u>
  Vial: 100 U/ml (10 ml); *Prefilled disposable KwikPen:* 100 U/ml (3 ml, 5/pck) (zinc, m-cresol); *HumaPen Memoir* and *HumaPen LUXURA* HD inj device for *Humalog cartridges* (100 U/ml, 3 ml 5/pck) (zinc, m-cresol); U/ml (3 ml, 5/pck) (zinc, m-cresol); *HumaPen Memoir* and *HumaPen LUXURA* HD inj device for *Humalog cartridges* (100 U/ml, 3 ml 5/pck) (zinc, m-cresol); (100 U/ml, 3 ml 5/pck (zinc, m-cresol)

Basal Insulin+GLP-1 RA Combinations

▷ *insulin degludec (insulin analog)+liraglutide* (**C**) for treatment of type 2 diabetes <u>only</u> in adults inadequately controlled on <50 units of basal insulin daily <u>or</u> ≤1.8 mg of *liraglutide* daily; administer by SC injection once daily, with <u>or</u> without food, into the upper arm, abdomen, <u>or</u> thigh; titrate every 3-4 days
 Pediatric: <18 years: not recommended; ≥18 years: same as adult
 Xultophy Prefilled pen: 100/3.6 U/ml (3 ml, 5 pens/carton)

▷ *insulin glargine (insulin analog)+lixisenatide* (**C**) for treatment of type 2 diabetes <u>only</u> in adults inadequately controlled on <60 units of basal insulin daily <u>or</u> *lixisenatide*; administer by SC injection once daily, with <u>or</u> without food, into the upper arm, abdomen, <u>or</u> thigh; titrate every 3-4 days
 Pediatric: <18 years: not recommended; ≥18 years: same as adult
 Soliqua Prefilled pen: 100/33 U/ml (3 ml, 5 pens/carton) covering 15-60 mg *insulin glargine* 100 units/ml and 15-20 mcg of *lixisenatide (m-cresol)*

◯ TYPE 2 DIABETES MELLITUS (T2DM)

Comment: Normal fasting glucose is <100 mg/dL. Impaired glucose tolerance is a risk factor for type 2 diabetes and a marker for cardiovascular disease risk; it occurs early in the natural history of these two diseases. Impaired fasting glucose is >100 mg/dL and <125 mg/dL. Impaired glucose tolerance is OGTT, 2 hour post-load 75 gm glucose >140 mg/dL and <200 mg/dL. Target pre-prandial glucose is 80 mg/dL to 120 mg/dL. Target bedtime glucose is 100 mg/dL to 140 mg/dL. Target glycosylated hemoglobin (HbA1c) is <7.0%. Additional medications to be considered for initiation at onset of T2DM, particularly in the presence of hypertension, include an angiotensin-converting enzyme inhibitor (ACEI), angiotensin II receptor blocker (ARB), thiazide-like diuretic, or a calcium channel blocker (CCB). Consider diabetes screening at age 25 years for persons in high-risk groups (non-Caucasian, positive family history for DM, obesity). Hypertension and hyperlipidemia are common comorbid conditions. Macrovascular complications include cerebral vascular disease, coronary artery disease, and peripheral vascular disease. Microvascular complications include retinopathy, nephropathy, neuropathy, and cardiomyopathy. Oral hypoglycemics are contraindicated in pregnancy.

Insulins see *Type 1 Diabetes Mellitus*

TREATMENT FOR ACUTE HYPOGLYCEMIA

▷ *dasiglucagon* 0.6 mg SC into the outer upper arm, lower abdomen, thigh, or buttocks; if there has been no response after 15 minutes, an additional dose from a new device may be administered while waiting for emergency assistance; when the patient has responded to treatment, give oral carbohydrates
  Pediatric: <6 years: safety and efficacy not established; ≥6 years: same as adult
    Zegalogue *Prefilled syringe:* 0.6 mg/0.6 ml, single-dose; *Autoinjector:* 0.6 mg/0.6 ml, single-dose
  Comment: **Zegalogue** is a glucagon analog for the treatment of severe hypoglycemia in patients with diabetes.
▷ *glucagon (recombinant)* (B) administer SC, IM, or IV; if patient does not respond in 15 minutes, may administer a single or 2 divided doses
  Adults and Children: <20 kg: 0.5 mg or 20-30 mg/kg; ≥20 kg: 1 mg

SULFONYLUREAS

Comment: Sulfonylureas are secretagogues (i.e., stimulate pancreatic insulin secretion); therefore, the patient taking a sulfonylurea should be alerted to the risk for hypoglycemia. Action is dependent on functioning beta cells in the pancreatic islets.

First Generation Sulfonylureas

▷ *chlorpropamide* (C)(G) initially 250 mg/day with breakfast; max 750 mg
  Pediatric: <12 years: not recommended; ≥12 years: same as adult
    Diabinese *Tab:* 100*, 250*mg
▷ *tolazamide* (C)(G) initially 100-250 mg/day with breakfast; increase by 100-250 mg/day at weekly intervals; maintenance 100 mg 1 gm/day; max 1 gm/day
  Pediatric: <12 years: not recommended; ≥12 years: same as adult
    Tolinase *Tab:* 100, 250, 500 mg
▷ *tolbutamide* (C) initially 1-2 gm in divided doses; max 2 gm/day
  Pediatric: <12 years: not recommended; ≥12 years: same as adult
    Tab: 500 mg

Second Generation Sulfonylureas

▷ *glimepiride* (C) initially 1-2 mg once daily with breakfast; after reaching dose of 2 mg, increase by 2 mg at 1-2 week intervals as needed; usual maintenance 1-4 mg once daily; max 8 mg/day
  Pediatric: <12 years: not recommended; ≥12 years: same as adult
    Amaryl *Tab:* 1*, 2*, 4*mg
▷ *glipizide* (C)(G)
  Pediatric: <12 years: not recommended; ≥12 years: same as adult
    Glucotrol initially 5 mg before breakfast; increase by 2.5-5 mg every few days if needed; max 15 mg/day; max 40 mg/day in divided doses
      Tab: 5*, 10*mg

Glucotrol XL initially 5 mg with breakfast; usual range 5-10 mg/day; max 20 mg/day
Tab: 2.5, 5, 10 mg ext-rel

▷ *glyburide* (C)(G) initially 2.5-5 mg/day with breakfast; increase by 2.5 mg at weekly intervals; maintenance 1.25-20 mg/day in a single or 2 divided doses; max 20 mg/day
Pediatric: <12 years: not recommended; ≥12 years: same as adult
DiaBeta, Micronase *Tab:* 1.25*, 2.5*, 5*mg

▷ *glyburide, micronized* (B)
Pediatric: <12 years: not recommended; ≥12 years: same as adult
Glynase PresTab initially 1.5-3 mg/day with breakfast; increase by 1.5 mg at weekly intervals if needed; usual maintenance 0.75-12 mg/day in single or divided doses; max 12 mg/day
Tab: 1.5*, 3*, 6*mg

ALPHA-GLUCOSIDASE INHIBITORS

Comment: Alpha-glucosidase inhibitors block the enzyme that breaks down carbohydrates in the small intestine, delaying digestion and absorption of complex carbohydrates, and lowering peak post-prandial glycemic concentrations. Use as monotherapy or in combination with a sulfonylurea. Contraindicated in inflammatory bowel disease, colon ulceration, and intestinal obstruction. Side effects include flatulence, diarrhea, and abdominal pain.

▷ *acarbose* (B) initially 25 mg tid ac, increase at 4-8 week intervals; or initially 25 mg once daily, increase gradually to 25 mg tid; usual range 50-100 mg tid; max 100 mg tid
Pediatric: <12 years: not recommended; ≥12 years: same as adult
Precose *Tab:* 25, 50, 100 mg

▷ *miglitol* (B) initially 25 mg tid at the start of each main meal, titrated to 50 mg tid at the start of each main meal; max 100 mg tid
Pediatric: <12 years: not recommended; ≥12 years: same as adult
Glyset *Tab:* 25, 50, 100 mg

BIGUANIDE

Comment: The biguanides decrease gluconeogenesis by the liver in the presence of insulin. Action is dependent on the presence of circulating insulin. Lower hepatic glucose production leads to lower overnight, fasting, and pre-prandial plasma glucose levels. Common side effects include GI distress, nausea, vomiting, bloating, and flatulence which usually eventually resolve. May be used as monotherapy (in adults only) or with a sulfonylurea or insulin. The only biguanide is *metformin*.

▷ *metformin* (B)(G) take with meals
Comment: *metformin* is contraindicated with renal impairment, metabolic acidosis, ketoacidosis. *Metformin* is contraindicated in patients with decreased tissue perfusion or hemodynamic instability, alcohol abuse, advanced liver disease, acute unstable acute congestive heart failure, or any condition that may lead to lactic acidosis. Suspend *metformin*, prior to, and for 48 hours after, surgery or receiving IV iodinated contrast agents. *Metformin* is associates with weight loss. Clinicians should consider adding either a sulfonylurea, a thiazolidindione (TZD), an SGLT-2 inhibitor, or a DPP-4 inhibitor to metformin to improve glycemic control when a second oral therapy is considered.

Fortamet initially 500 mg by mouth every evening; may increase by 500 mg/day at 1 week intervals; max 2 gm/day
Pediatric: <10 years: not recommended; ≥10-16 years: use immediate release form; >16 years: same as adult
Tab: 500, 1000 mg ext-rel

Glucophage initially 500 mg bid; may increase by 500 mg/day at 1 week intervals; max 1 gm bid or 2.5 gm in 3 divided doses; or initially 850 mg once

daily in AM; may increase by 850 mg/day in divided doses at 2 week intervals; max 2000 mg/day; take with meals
Pediatric: <10 years: not recommended; ≥10-16 years: use only as monotherapy; >16 years: same as adult dose same as adult
   Tab: 500, 850, 1000*mg
Glucophage XR initially 500 mg by mouth every evening; may increase by 500 mg/day at 1 week intervals; max 2 gm/day
Pediatric: <10 years: not recommended; ≥10-16 years: use immediate release form; >16 years: same as adult
   Tab: 500, 750 mg ext-rel
Glumetza ER (G) initially 1000 mg once daily; may increase by 500 mg/day at week intervals; max 2 gm/day
Pediatric: <18 years: not recommended; ≥18 years: same as adult
   Tab: 500, 1000 mg ext-rel
Riomet XR initially 500 mg once daily; may increase by 500 mg/day at 1 week intervals; max 2 gm/day in divided doses; take with meals
Pediatric: <10 years: not recommended; ≥10 years: monotherapy only
   Oral soln: 500 mg/ml (4 oz; cherry)

MEGLITINIDES

Comment: Meglitinides are secretagogues (i.e., stimulate pancreatic insulin secretion) in response to a meal. Action is dependent on functioning beta cells in the pancreatic islets. Use as monotherapy or in combination with *metformin*.
▷ *nateglinide* (C) 60-120 mg tid ac 1-30 minutes prior to start of the meal
Pediatric: <12 years: not recommended; ≥12 years: same as adult
   Starlix *Tab:* 60, 120 mg
▷ *repaglinide* (C)(G) initially 0.5 mg with 2-4 meals/day; take 30 minutes ac; titrate by doubling dose at intervals of at least 1 week; range 0.5-4 mg with 2-4 meals/day; max 16 mg/day
Pediatric: <12 years: not recommended; ≥12 years: same as adult
   Prandin *Tab:* 0.5, 1, 2 mg

THIAZOLIDINEDIONES (TZDs)

Comment: The TZDs decrease hepatic gluconeogenesis and reduce insulin resistance (i.e., increase glucose uptake and utilization by the muscles). Liver function tests are indicated before initiating these drugs. Do not start if ALT more than 3 times greater than normal. Recheck ALT monthly for the first 6 months of therapy; then every two months for the remainder of the first year and periodically thereafter. Liver function tests should be obtained at the first symptoms suggestive of hepatic dysfunction (nausea, vomiting, fatigue, dark urine, anorexia, abdominal pain).

▷ *pioglitazone* (C)(G) initially 15-30 mg once daily; max 45 mg/day as a monotherapy; usual max 30 mg/day in combination with *metformin*, insulin, or a sulfonylurea
Pediatric: <18 years: not recommended; ≥18 years: same as adult
   Actos *Tab:* 15, 30, 45 mg
▷ *rosiglitazone* (C)(G) initially 4 mg/day in a single or 2 divided doses; may increase after 8-12 weeks; max 8 mg/day as a monotherapy or combination therapy with *metformin* or a sulfonylurea; not for use with *insulin*
Pediatric: <18 years: not recommended; ≥18 years: same as adult
   Avandia *Tab:* 2, 4, 8 mg

DIPEPTIDYL PEPTIDASE-4 (DPP-4) INHIBITOR+THIAZOLIDINEDIONE COMBINATION

Comment: The FDA has reported that *alogliptin*-containing drugs may increase the risk of heart failure, especially in patients who already have cardiovascular or renal disease. The drug **Oseni** (*alogliptin+pioglitazone*) is in this risk group.

▶ *alogliptin+pioglitazone* (C) take 1 dose once daily with first meal of the day; max: *rosiglitazone* 8 mg and max *glimepiride* per day; same precautions as *alogliptin* and *pioglitazone*
Pediatric: <18 years: not recommended; ≥18 years: same as adult
    Oseni
      Tab: **Oseni 12.5/15** alo 12.5 mg+pio 15 mg;
           Oseni 12.5/30 alo 12.5 mg+pio 30 mg
           Oseni 12.5/45 alo 12.5 mg+pio 45 mg
           Oseni 25/15 alo 25+pio 15 mg
           Oseni 25/30 alo 25+pio 30 mg
           Oseni 25/45 alo 25 mg+pio 45 mg

SECOND GENERATION SULFONYLUREA+BIGUANIDE COMBINATIONS

Comment: *Metaglip* and *Glucovance* are combination secretagogues (sulfonylureas) and insulin sensitizers (biguanides). *Sulfonylurea:* Action is dependent on functioning beta cells in the pancreatic islets; patient should be alerted to the risk for hypoglycemia. Common side effects of the biguanide include GI distress, nausea, vomiting, bloating, and flatulence which usually eventually resolve. Take with food. *metformin* is contraindicated with renal impairment, metabolic acidosis, ketoacidosis. Suspend *metformin*, prior to, and for 48 hours after, surgery or receiving IV iodinated contrast agents.

▶ *glipizide+metformin* (C) take with meals; *Primary therapy:* 2.5/250 once daily or if FBS is 280-320 mg/dL, may start at 2.5/250 bid; may increase by 1 tab/day every 2 weeks; max 10/2000 per day in 2 divided doses; *Second Line Therapy:* 2.5/500 or 5/500 bid; may increase by up to 5/500 every 2 weeks; max: 20/2000 per day; Same precautions as *glipizide* and *metformin*
Pediatric: <12 years: not recommended; ≥12 years: same as adult
    Metaglip
      Tab: **Metaglip 2.5/250** glip 2.5 mg+met 250 mg
           Metaglip 2.5/500 glip 2.5 mg+met 500 mg
           Metaglip 5/500 glip 5 mg+met 500 mg

▶ *glyburide+metformin* (B) take with meals; *Primary therapy (initial therapy if HgbA1c <9.0%):* initially 1.25/250 once daily; max *glyburide* 20 mg and *metformin* 2000 mg per day; *Primary therapy (initial therapy if HbA1c >9.0% or FBS >200):* initially 1.25/250 bid; max *glyburide* 20 mg and *metformin* 2000 mg per day; *Second line therapy (initial therapy if HbA1c >7.0%):* initially 2.5/500 or 5/500 bid; max *glyburide* 20 mg and *metformin* 2000 mg per day; *Previously treated with a sulfonylurea and metformin:* dose to approximate total daily doses of *glyburide* and *metformin* already being taken; max: *glyburide* 20 mg and *metformin* 2000 mg per day; Same precautions as *glyburide* and *metformin*
Pediatric: <12 years: not recommended; ≥12 years: same as adult
    Glucovance
      Tab: **Glucovance 1.25/250** glyb 1.25 mg+met 250 mg
           Glucovance 2.5/500 glyb 2.5 mg+met 500 mg
           Glucovance 5/500 glyb 5 mg+met 500 mg

Comment: *Metformin* is contraindicated with renal impairment, metabolic acidosis, ketoacidosis. Suspend *metformin*, prior to, and for 48 hours after, surgery or receiving IV iodinated contrast agents.

THIAZOLIDINEDIONE (TZD)+BIGUANIDE COMBINATION

▶ *pioglitazone+metformin* (C) take in divided doses with meals; *Previously on metformin alone:* initially 15 mg/500 mg or 15 mg/850 mg once or twice daily; *Previously on pioglitazone alone:* initially 15 mg/500 mg bid; *Previously on pioglitazone and metformin:* switch on a mg/mg basis; may increase after 8-12 weeks; max: *pioglitazone* 45 mg and *metformin* 2000 mg per day; Same precautions as *pioglitazone* and *metformin*

Pediatric: <12 years: not recommended; ≥12 years: same as adult
> **Actoplus Met, Actoplis Met R (G)**
>> *Tab:* **Actoplus Met 15/500** pio 15 mg+met 500 mg
>> **Actoplus Met 15/850** pio 15 mg+met 850 mg
>> **Actoplus Met XR 15/1000** pio 15 mg+met 1000 mg
>> **Actoplus Met XR 30/1000** pio 30 mg+met 1000 mg

Comment: *Metformin* is contraindicated with renal impairment, metabolic acidosis, ketoacidosis. Suspend *metformin*, prior to, and for 48 hours after, surgery or receiving IV iodinated contrast agents.

▷ *rosiglitazone+metformin* (C)(G) take in divided doses with meals; *Previously on metformin alone:* add *rosiglitazone* 4 mg/day; may increase after 8-12 weeks; *Previously on rosiglitazone alone:* add *metformin* 1000 mg/day; may increase after 1-2 weeks; *Previously on rosiglitazone and metformin:* switch on a mg/mg basis; may increase *rosiglitazone* by 4 mg and/or *metformin* by 500 mg per day; max: *rosiglitazone* 8 mg and *metformin* 2000 mg per day; Same precautions as *rosiglitazone* and *metformin*
Pediatric: <12 years: not recommended; ≥12 years: same as adult
> **Avandamet**
>> *Tab:* **Avandamet 2/500** rosi 2 mg+met 500 mg
>> **Avandamet 2/1000** rosi 2 mg+met 1000 mg
>> **Avandamet 4/500** rosi 4 mg+met 500 mg
>> **Avandamet 4/1000** rosi 4 mg+met 1000 mg

Comment: *Rosiglitazone* has been withdrawn from retail pharmacies. In order to enroll and receive *rosiglitazone*, healthcare providers and patients must enroll in the *Avandia-Rosiglitazone Medicines Access Program.* The program limits the use of *rosiglitazone* to patients already being treated successfully, and those whose blood sugar cannot be controlled with other antidiabetic medicines. *Metformin* is contraindicated with renal impairment, metabolic acidosis, ketoacidosis. Suspend *metformin*, prior to, and for 48 hours after, surgery or receiving IV iodinated contrast agents.

THIAZOLIDINEDIONE (TZD)+SULFONYLUREA COMBINATIONS

▷ *pioglitazone+glimepiride* (C)(G) take 1 dose daily with first meal of the day; *Previously on sulfonylurea alone:* initially 30 mg/2 mg; *Previously on pioglitazone and glimepiride:* switch on a mg/mg basis; max: *pioglitazone* 30 mg and *glimepiride* 4 mg per day; Same precautions as *pioglitazone* and *glimepiride*
Pediatric: <18 years: not recommended; ≥18 years: same as adult
> **Duetact**
>> *Tab:* **Duetact 30/2** pio 30 mg+glim 2 mg
>> **Duetact 304** pio 30 mg+glim 4 mg

▷ *rosiglitazone+glimepiride* (C) take 1 dose daily with first meal of the day; max: *rosiglitazone* 8 mg and *glimepiride* 4 mg per day; Same precautions as *rosiglitazone* and *glimepiride*
Pediatric: <18 years: not recommended; ≥18 years: same as adult
> **Avandaryl**
>> *Tab:* **Avandaryl 4/1** rosi 4 mg+glim 1 mg
>> **Avandaryl 4/2** rosi 4 mg+glim 2 mg
>> **Avandaryl 4/4** rosi 4 mg+glim 4 mg
>> **Avandaryl 8/2** rosi 8 mg+glim 2 mg
>> **Avandaryl 8/4** rosi 8 mg+glim 4 mg

GLUCAGON-LIKE PEPTIDE-1 (GLP-1) RECEPTOR AGONISTS

Comment: GLP-1 receptor agonists act as an agonist at the GLP-1 receptors. They have a longer half-life than the native protein allowing them to be dosed once daily. They increase intracellular cAMP resulting in *insulin* release in the presence of increased serum concentration, decrease *glucagon* secretion, and delay gastric emptying, thus, reducing fasting, pre-meal, and post-prandial glucose throughout the day. GLP-1 receptor agonists are <u>not</u> a substitute for *insulin*, <u>not</u> for treatment of DKA, and <u>not</u> for post-prandial administration.

▷ *dulaglutide* (C) administer by SC injection into the upper arm, abdomen, <u>or</u> thigh once weekly on the same day and the same time of day, with <u>or</u> without food; initially 0.75 mg SC once weekly; may increase to 1.5 mg SC once weekly
Pediatric: <18 years: not established; ≥18 years: same as adult
   Trulicity *Prefilled pen/syringe:* 0.75, 1.5, 3.0, 4.5 mg/0.5 ml single-dose disposable autoinjector (4/pck)

▷ *exenatide* (C) administer by SC injection into the upper arm, abdomen, <u>or</u> thigh once weekly
Pediatric: <12 years: not recommended; ≥12 years: same as adult
   Bydureon inject immediately after mixing; administer 2 mg SC once weekly; administer on the same day, at any time of day; with <u>or</u> without meals; if switching from **Byetta**, discontinue **Byetta** and instead administer **Bydureon** and continue the same once weekly administration schedule with **Bydureon**
      Vial: 2 mg w. 0.65 ml diluent, single-dose; *Prefilled pen:* 2 mg w. 0.65 ml diluent, single-dose
   Bydureon BCise administer 2 mg by SC injection once weekly; at any time of day; with <u>or</u> without meals; if switching from **Byetta** to **Bydureon**, discontinue **Byetta** and start **Bydureon BBCise** SC once weekly on the same day of the week
      Autoinjector: 2 mg (0.85 ml) single-dose
   Byetta inject within 60 minutes before AM and PM meals, <u>or</u> before the 2 main meals of the day, approximately ≥6 hours apart; initially 5 mcg/dose; may increase to 10 mcg/dose after one month
      Prefilled pen: 250 mcg/ml (5, 10 mcg/dose; 60 doses, needles <u>not</u> included) (m-cresol, mannitol)
   Comment: *Exenatide* is indicated as an adjunctive therapy to basal insulin among patients whose blood sugar remains uncontrolled on one <u>or</u> more antidiabetic medications, along with diet and exercise.

▷ *liraglutide* (C) administer by SC injection into the upper arm, abdomen, <u>or</u> thigh once daily; initially 0.6 mg/day for 1 week; then 1.2 mg/day; may increase to 1.8 mg/day
Pediatric: <10 years: not recommended; ≥10 years: same as adult
   Victoza *Prefilled pen:* 6 mg/ml (3 ml; needles <u>not</u> included)

▷ *lixisenatide* (C) administer SC in the upper arm, abdomen, <u>or</u> thigh once daily; initially 10 mcg SC x 14 days; maintenance: 20 mcg beginning on day 15; administer within one hour of the first meal of the day and the same meal of the day
Pediatric: <18 years: not established; ≥18 years: same as adult
   Adlyxin Soln for SC inj; *Starter Pen:* 50 mcg/ml (14 doses of 10 mcg; 3 ml); *Maintenance Pen:* 100 mcg/ml (14 doses of 20 mcg); *Starter Pack:* 1 prefilled starter pen and 1 prefilled maintenance pen; *Maintenance Pack:* 2 prefilled maintenance pens
   Comment: **Adlyxin** is indicated as an adjunct to diet and exercise for T2DM. Not indicated for treatment of T1DM. Do <u>not</u> use with **Victoza**, **Saxenda**, other GLP-1 receptor agonists, <u>or</u> insulin. Contraindicated with gastroparesis and GFR <15 mL/min. Poorly controlled diabetes in pregnancy increases the maternal risk for diabetic ketoacidosis, pre-eclampsia, spontaneous abortions, preterm delivery, stillbirth and delivery complications. Poorly controlled diabetes increases the fetal risk for major birth defects, still birth, and macrosomia related morbidity. **Adlyxin** should be used during pregnancy <u>only</u> if the potential benefit justifies the potential risk to the fetus.

Estimated background risk of major birth defects and miscarriage in clinically recognized pregnancies is 2%-4% and 15%-20%, respectively.

▷ *semaglutide*

Comment: *Semaglutide* is not recommended as first-line therapy for patients inadequately controlled on diet and exercise and is not indicated for use in patients with type 1 diabetes mellitus or treatment of diabetic ketoacidosis. *Semaglutide* is contraindicated with a personal or family history of medullary thyroid carcinoma or in patients with multiple endocrine neoplasia syndrome type 2 (MENS-2). Pancreatitis has been reported in *semaglutide* clinical trials; discontinue promptly if pancreatitis is suspected and do not restart if pancreatitis is confirmed. Diabetic retinopathy complications have been reported in a cardiovascular outcomes trial with *semaglutide* injection. Patients with a history of diabetic retinopathy should be monitored. When used with an insulin secretagogue or insulin, consider lowering the dose of the secretagogue or insulin to reduce the risk of hypoglycemia. *Semaglutide* is not recommended as first-line therapy for patients inadequately controlled on diet and exercise. There may be potential risks to the fetus from exposure to *semaglutide* during pregnancy; therefore, *semaglutide* should be used during pregnancy only if the potential benefit justifies the potential risk to the fetus. *Semaglutide* is not recommended in females or males with reproductive potential. Discontinue in women at least 2 months before a planned pregnancy due to the long washout period for *semaglutide*. There are no data on the presence of *semaglutide* in human milk or the effects on the breastfed infant.

Ozempic administer SC in the upper arm, abdomen, or thigh once weekly at any time of day, with or without meals; initially 0.25 mg once weekly; after 4 weeks, increase the dose to 0.5 mg once weekly; if after at least 4 weeks additional glycemic control is needed, increase to 1 mg once weekly (usual main-maintenance dose); if a dose is missed, administer within 5 days of the missed dose

Pediatric: <18 years: not established: ≥18 years: same as adult

Prefilled pen: 2 mg/1.5 ml (1.34 mg/ml) single-patient-use; 0.25, 0.5, 1 mg/injection

Comment: The most common adverse reactions (incidence ≥5%) have been nausea, vomiting, diarrhea, abdominal pain and constipation. Rybelsus initially 3 mg once daily x 30 days; then, increase dose to 7 mg once daily; then, dose may be increased to 14 mg once daily if additional glycemic control is needed

Pediatric: <18 years: not established: ≥18 years: same as adult

Tab: 3, 7, 14 mg

Comment: Waiting less than 30 minutes, or taking with food, beverages (other than plain water) or other oral medications will lessen the effect of Rybelsus. Waiting more than 30 minutes to eat may increase absorption. The most common adverse reactions (incidence ≥5%) have been nausea, abdominal pain, diarrhea, decreased appetite, vomiting and constipation.

BASAL INSULIN+GLP-1 RA COMBINATIONS

▷ *insulin degludec (insulin analog)+liraglutide* (C) for treatment of type 2 diabetes only when inadequately controlled on <50 units of basal *insulin* daily or ≤1.8 mg of *liraglutide* daily; administer by SC injection once daily, with or without food, into the upper arm, abdomen, or thigh; titrate every 3-4 days

Pediatric: <18 years: not recommended: ≥18 years: same as adult

Xultophy *Prefilled pen:* 100/3.6 U/ml (3 ml, 5 pens/carton)

▷ *insulin glargine (insulin analog)+lixisenatide* (C) for treatment of type 2 diabetes only when inadequately controlled on <60 units of basal *insulin* daily or *lixisenatide*; administer by SC injection once daily, with or without food, into the upper arm, abdomen, or thigh; titrate every 3-4 days

Pediatric: <18 years: not recommended: ≥18 years: same as adult

Soliqua *Prefilled pen:* 100/33 U/ml (3 ml, 5 pens/carton) covering 15-60 mg *insulin glargine* 100 units/ml and 15-20 mcg of *lixisenatide (m-cresol)*

SODIUM-GLUCOSE CO-TRANSPORTER 2 (SGLT2) INHIBITORS

Comment: SGLT2 inhibitors block the SGLT2 protein involved in 90% of glucose reabsorption in the proximal renal tubule, resulting in increased renal glucose excretion (typically >2000 mg/dL), and lower blood glucose levels (low risk of hypoglycemia), modest weight loss, and mild reduction in blood pressure (probably due to sodium loss). These agents probably also increase insulin sensitivity, decrease gluconeogenesis, and improve *insulin* release from pancreatic beta cells. SGLT2 inhibitors are contraindicated in T1DM, and are decreased or contraindicated with decreased GFR, increased SCr, renal failure, ESRD, renal dialysis, metabolic acidosis, or diabetic ketoacidosis. The most common ASEs are increased urination, UTI, and female genital mycotic infection (due to the glycosuria). These effects may be managed with adequate oral hydration and post-voiding genital hygiene. OTC **Vagisil** wet wipes are recommended to completely remove any post-voiding glucose film, and, thus, reduce potential risk of UTI and vaginal candidiasis, and reverse initial signs/symptoms of candida vaginalis. The SGLT2 inhibitors are <u>not</u> recommended in nursing women. There is potential for a hypersensitivity reaction to include angioedema and anaphylaxis. Caution with SGLT2 use due to reports of increased risk of treatment-emergent bone fractures. Serious, life-threatening cases of necrotizing fasciitis (Fournier's gangrene) have been reported in both females and males taking an SGLT2 inhibitor. Assess patients presenting with pain or tenderness, erythema, or swelling in the genital or perineal area, along with fever or malaise. If suspected, initiate prompt diagnosis and treatment.

▷ *canagliflozin* (C) take one tab before the first meal of the day; initially 100 mg; may titrate up to max 300 mg once daily; *GFR <45 mL/min:* do <u>not</u> initiate
Pediatric: <18 years: not established; ≥18 years: same as adult
   Invokana *Tab:* 100, 300 mg
   Comment: **Invokana** is contraindicated with GFR <45 mL/min; If GFR 45-≤60 mL/min, max 100 mg once daily or consider other antihyperglycemic

▷ *dapagliflozin* (C) take one tab before the first meal of the day; initially 5 mg; may increase to max 10 mg once daily
Pediatric: <18 years: not established; ≥18 years: same as adult
   Farxiga *Tab:* 5, 10 mg
   Comment: **Farxiga** is contraindicated with GFR <60 *mL/min*. **Farxiga** has an FDA-approved indication to reduce the risk of hospitalization for heart failure (HF) in adults with T2DM and established cardiovascular diaease or multiple cardiovascular risk factors.

▷ *empagliflozin* (C) take one tab before the first meal of the day; initially 10 mg; may increase to max 25 mg once daily
Pediatric: <18 years: not established; ≥18 years: same as adult
   Jardiance *Tab:* 10, 25 mg
   Comment: **Jardiance** is contraindicated with GFR <45 mL/min.

▷ *ertugliflozen* (C) take one tab before the first meal of the day; initially 5 mg; may increase to max 15 mg once daily
Pediatric: <18 years: not established; ≥18 years: same as adult
   Steglatro *Tab:* 5, 15 mg

SODIUM-GLUCOSE CO-TRANSPORTER 2 (SGLT2) INHIBITOR+BIGUANIDE COMBINATIONS

Comment: Caution with **SGLT2** use due to reports of increased risk of treatment-emergent bone fractures. *Metformin* is contraindicated with renal impairment, metabolic acidosis, ketoacidosis. Suspend *metformin*, prior to, and for 48 hours after, surgery or receiving IV iodinated contrast agents.

▷ *canagliflozin+metformin* (C) take 1 dose twice daily with meals; max daily dose 300/2000; *GFR 45–≤60 mL/min: canagliflozin* max 100 mg once daily or consider other antihyperglycemic; *GFR <45 mL/min:* do not initiate

Pediatric: <18 years: not established; ≥18 years: same as adult

Invokamet

Tab: **Invokamet 50/500** cana 50 mg+met 500 mg

Invokamet 50/1000 cana 50 mg+met 1000 mg

Invokamet 150/500 cana 150 mg+met 500 mg

Invokamet 150/1000 cana 150 mg+met 1000 mg

▷ *dapagliflozin+metformin* (C) swallow whole; do not crush or chew; take once daily first meal of the day; max daily dose 10/2000

Pediatric: <18 years: not established; ≥18 years: same as adult

Xigduo XR

Tab: **Xigduo XR 5/500** dapa 5 mg+met 500 mg ext-rel

Xigduo XR 5/1000 dapa 5 mg+met 1000 mg ext-rel

Xigduo XR 10/500 dapa 10 mg+met 500 mg ext-rel

Xigduo XR 10/1000 dapa 10 mg+met 1000 mg ext-rel

Comment: **Xigduo** is contraindicated with GFR <60 mL/min, SCr >1.5 (men) or SCr >1.4 (women)

▷ *empagliflozin+metformin* (C) take 1 dose twice daily with meals; max daily dose 25/2000

Pediatric: <18 years: not established; ≥18 years: same as adult

Synjardy

Tab: **Synjardy 5/500** empa 5 mg+met 500 mg

Synjardy 5/1000 empa 5 mg+met 1000 mg

Synjardy 12.5/500 empa 12.5 mg+met 500 mg

Synjardy 12.5/1000 empa 12.5 mg+met 1000 mg

Synjardy XR

Tab: **Synjardy XR 5/1000** empa 5 mg+met 1000 mg

Synjardy XR 12.5/1000 empa 12.5 mg+met 1000 mg

Synjardy XR 10/1000 empa 10 mg+met 1000 mg

Synjardy XR 25/1000 empa 25 mg+met 1000 mg

Comment: **Synjardy** is contraindicated with GFR <45 mL/min, SCr >1.5 (men), or SCr >1.4 (women).

▷ *ertugliflozin+metformin* (C) take 1 dose twice daily with meals; max daily dose 15/2000

Pediatric: <18 years: not established; ≥18 years: same as adult

Segluormet

Tab: **Segluormet 2.5/500** ertu 2.5 mg+met 500 mg

Segluormet 2.5/1000 ertu 2.5 mg+met 1000 mg

Segluormet 7.5/500 ertu 7.5 mg+met 500 mg

Segluormet 7.5/1000 ertu 7.5 mg+met 1000 mg

Comment: **Steglatro** is contraindicated with GFR <30 mL/min. Do not initiate or continue with eGFR <60 mL/min.

SODIUM-GLUCOSE CO-TRANSPORTER 2 (SGLT2) INHIBITOR+DIPEPTIDYL PEPTIDASE-4 (DPP-4) INHIBITOR COMBINATIONS

Comment: Caution with **SGLT2** use due to reports of increased risk of treatment-emergent bone fractures and increased risk for UTI and Candida vaginalis secondary to drug-associated glycosuria.

▷ *dapagliflozin+saxagliptin* (C) initially 5/10 once daily, at any time of day, with or without food; if a dose is missed and it is ≥12 hours until the next dose, the dose should be taken; if a dose is missed and it is <12 hours until the next dose, the missed dose should be skipped and the next dose taken at the usual time.

Pediatric: <18 years: not recommended: ≥18 years: same as adult

Qtern *Tab:* dapa 10 mg+saxa 5 mg film-coat
Comment: **Qtern** should <u>not</u> be used during pregnancy. If pregnancy is detected, treatment with **Qtern** should be discontinued. It is unknown whether **Qtern** and/or its metabolites are excreted in human milk. Do <u>not</u> use with CrCl <60 mL/min <u>or</u> eGFR <60 mL/min/1.73 m² <u>or</u> ESRD <u>or</u> severe hepatic impairment <u>or</u> history of pancreatitis.

▷ *empagliflozin+linagliptin* (C) initially 10/5 once daily with the first meal of the day; max daily dose 25/5
Pediatric: <18 years: not established; ≥18 years: same as adult
    Glyxambi
      Tab: **Glyxambi 10/5** empa 10 mg+lina 5 mg
        Glyxambi 25/5 empa 25 mg+lina 5 mgss
    Comment: **Glyxambi** is contraindicated with GFR <45 mL/min.

▷ *ertugliflozin+sitagliptin* (C) initially 5/100 once daily with the first meal of the day; max daily dose 15/100
Pediatric: <18 years: not established; ≥18 years: same as adult
    Steglujan
      Tab: **Steglujan 5/100** ertu 5 mg+sita 100 mg
        Steglujan 15/100 ertu 15 mg+sita 100 mg
    Comment: **Steglujan** is contraindicated with GFR <45 mL/min.

SODIUM-GLUCOSE CO-TRANSPORTER 2 (SGLT-2) INHIBITOR + DIPEPTIDYL PEPTIDASE-4 (DPP-4) INHIBITOR + BIGUANIDE

▷ *dapagliflozin+saxagliptin+metformin* (C) assess renal function before initiation of therapy and periodically thereafter; individualize the starting total daily dose based on the patient's current regimen, effectiveness, and tolerability; take once daily in the morning with food; for patients <u>not</u> currently taking *dapagliflozin*, the recommended starting dose is **Qternmet XR 5/5/1000** (dapa 5 mg/saxa 5 mg/met 1000 mg) once daily; max dose is **Qternmet XR 10/5/2000** (dapa 10 mg/saxa 5 mg/met 2000 mg) once daily; swallow tablet whole; do <u>not</u> crush, cut <u>or</u> chew
Pediatric: <18 years: not recommended: ≥18 years: same as adult
    Qternmet XL
      Tab: **Qternmet XL 2.5/2.5/1000** dapa 2.5 mg+saxa 2.5 mg+met 1000 mg film-coat ext-rel
        Qternmet XL 5/2.5/1000 dapa 5 mg+saxa 2.5 mg+met 1000 mg film-coat ext-rel
        Qternmet XL 5/5/1000 dapa 5 mg+saxa 5 mg+met 1000 mg film-coat ext-rel
        Qternmet XL 10/5/1000 dapa 10 mg+saxa 5 mg+met 1000 mg film-coat ext-rel
    Comment: **Qternmet XR** is <u>not</u> indicated for the treatment of T1DM <u>or</u> diabetic ketoacidosis. **Qternmet** initiation is intended only for patients currently taking *metformin*. Discontinue **Qternmet XR** at the time of <u>or</u> prior to an iodinated contrast imaging procedure. **Qternmet XR** should <u>not</u> be used during pregnancy. If pregnancy is detected, treatment with **Qternmet** should be discontinued. It is unknown whether **Qtern** and/or its metabolites are excreted in human milk. Do <u>not</u> use with CrCl <60 mL/min <u>or</u> eGFR <60 mL/min/1.73 m² <u>or</u> ESRD <u>or</u> severe hepatic impairment <u>or</u> history of pancreatitis.

▷ *empagliflozin+linagliptin+metformin* one tablet once daily with a meal; swallow whole, do <u>not</u> split, crush, dissolve, <u>or</u> chew; individualize the starting dose based on the patient's current regimen; daily max *empagliflozin* 25 mg, *linagliptin* 5 mg, *metformin* 2000 mg
    Trijardy XR
      Tab: **Trijardy XR 5/2.5/1000** empa 5 mg + lina 2.5 mg + met 1000 mg film-coat, ext-rel

Trijardy XR 10/5/1000 empa 10 mg + lina 5 mg + met 1000 mg film-coat, ext-rel

Trijardy XR 12.5/2.5/1000 empa 12.5 mg + lina 2.5 mg + met 1000 mg film-coat, ext-rel

Trijardy XR 25/5/1000 empa 25 mg, lina 5 mg, met 1000 mg

Comment **Trijardy XR** *(empagliflozin+linagliptin+metformin hydrochloride)* is a three-drug fixed-dose combination of the sodium-glucose co-transporter 2 (SGLT2) inhibitor *empagliflozin* (**Jardiance**), the dipeptidyl peptidase-4 (DPP-4) inhibitor *linagliptin* (**Tradjenta**) and the biguanide *metformin*. Assess renal function prior to initiation of **Trijardy XR** and periodically thereafter. *eGFR <45 mL/min:* do not initiate or continue. *eGFR <30 mL/min, ESRD, or dialysis:* contraindicated. **Trijardy XR** may need to be discontinued at time of, or prior to, iodinated contrast imaging procedures. Do not initiate **Trijardy XR** in patients with acute or chronic metabolic acidosis, including diabetic ketoacidosis; discontinue **Trijardy XR** immediately if risk of, or occurrence of, metabolic acidosis occurs. Hypersensitivity reactions to *empagliflozin*, *linagliptin*, *metformin* and any of the excipients in **Trijardy XR** have occurred, including anaphylaxis, angioedema, exfoliative skin conditions, urticaria, and bronchial hyperreactivity. The most common adverse reactions associated with **Trijardy XR** (incidence ≥5%) have been URI, UTI, headache, diarrhea, constipation, and gastroenteritis. *metformin* may lower serum vitamin B12 level; monitor hematologic parameters annually. Severe and disabling arthralgia has been reported in patients taking DPP-4 inhibitors; therefore consider **Trijardy XR** as a possible cause of new onset or increased severity of severe joint pain and discontinue drug if appropriate. Advise females of potential embryo/fetal risk, especially during the second and third trimesters. **Trijardy XR** is not recommended when breastfeeding.

DIPEPTIDYL PEPTIDASE-4 (DPP-4) INHIBITOR

Comment: DPP-4 is an enzyme that degrades incretin hormones glucagon-like peptide-1 (GLP-1) and glucose-dependent insulinotropic polypeptide (GIP). Thus, DPP-4 inhibitors increase the concentration of active incretin hormones, stimulating the release of *insulin* in a glucose-dependent manner and decreasing the levels of circulating *glucagon*. The FDA has reported that *saxagliptin-* and *alogliptin-*containing drugs may increase the risk of heart failure, especially in patients who already have cardiovascular or renal disease. Drugs in this risk group include **Nesina** (*alogliptin*) and **Onglyza** (*saxagliptin*)

▷ *alogliptin* (B) take twice daily with meals; max 25 mg day
    Pediatric: <18 years: not recommended; ≥18 years: same as adult
    Nesina *Tab:* 6.25, 12.5, 25 mg
▷ *linagliptin* (B) 5 mg once daily
    Pediatric: <18 years: not recommended; ≥18 years: same as adult
    Tradjenta *Tab:* 5 mg
▷ *saxagliptin* (B) 2.5-5 mg once daily
    Pediatric: <18 years: not recommended; ≥18 years: same as adult
    Onglyza *Tab:* 2.5, 5 mg
▷ *sitagliptin* (B) as monotherapy or as combination therapy with metformin or a TZD
    Pediatric: <18 years: not recommended; ≥18 years: same as adult
    Januvia 25-100 mg once daily
    Tab: 25, 50, 100 mg

DIPEPTIDYL PEPTIDASE-4 (DPP-4) INHIBITOR+BIGUANIDE COMBINATIONS

Comment: DPP-4 inhibitor+*metformin* combinations are contraindicated with renal impairment (men: SCr ≥1.5 mg/dL; women: SCr ≥1.4 mg/dL) or abnormal CrCl, metabolic acidosis, ketoacidosis, or history of angioedema. Suspend *metformin*, prior to, and for 48 hours after, surgery or receiving IV iodinated contrast agents. Avoid in the elderly, malnourished, dehydrated, or with clinical or lab evidence of hepatic disease. For other DPP-4 and/or *metformin* precautions, see mfr pkg insert. The FDA has reported that *saxagliptin*- and *alogliptin*-containing drugs may increase the risk of heart failure, especially in patients who already have cardiovascular or renal disease. These drugs include: **Onglyza** (*saxagliptin*), **Kombiglyze XR** (*saxagliptin+metformin*), **Nesina** (*alogliptin*), **Kazano** (*alogliptin+metformin*), and **Oseni** (*alogliptin+pioglitazone*).

▷ *alogliptin+metformin* (B) take twice daily with meals; max *alogliptin* 25 mg/day, max *metformin* 2000 mg/day

    Pediatric: <18 years: not recommended; ≥18 years: same as adult

    Kazano

        Tab: **Kazano 12.5/500** algo 12.5 mg+met 500 mg

            Kazano 2.5/1000 algo 12.5 mg+met 1000 mg

▷ *linagliptin+metformin* (B)

    Pediatric: <18 years: not recommended; ≥18 years: same as adult

    Jentadueto take twice daily with meals; max *linagliptin* 5 mg/day, max *metformin* 2000 mg/day

        Tab: **Jentadueto 2.5/500** lina 2.5 mg+met 500 mg film-coat

            Jentadueto 2.5/850 lina 2.5 mg+met 850 mg film-coat

            Jentadueto 2.5/1000 lina 2.5 mg+met 1000 mg film-coat

    Jentadueto XR *Currently not treated with metformin*: initiate **Jentadueto XR 5/1000** once daily; *Already treated with metformin*: initiate **Jentadueto XR** 5 mg *linagliptin* total daily dose and a similar total daily dose of *metformin* once daily; *Already treated with linagliptin and metformin or Jentadueto*: switch to **Jentadueto XR** containing 5 mg of *linagliptin* total daily dose and a similar total daily dose of *metformin* once daily; max *linagliptin* 5 mg and *metformin* 2,000 mg; take as a single dose once daily; take with food; do not crush or chew; *eGFR <30 mL/min*: contraindicated; *eGFR 30-45 mL/min*: not recommended

        Tab: **Jentadueto 2.5/1000** lina 2.5 mg+met 1,000 mg film-coat ext-rel

            Jentadueto 5/1000 lina 5 mg+met 1,000 mg film-coat ext-rel

▷ *saxagliptin+metformin* (B) take once daily with meals; max *saxagliptin* 5 mg/day, max *metformin* 2,000 mg/day; do not crush or chew

    Pediatric: <18 years: not recommended; ≥18 years: same as adult

    Kombiglyze XR

        Tab: **Kombiglyze XR 5/500** saxa 5 mg+met 500 mg

            Kombiglyze XR 2.5/1000 saxa 2.5 mg+met 1,000 mg

            Kombiglyze XR 5/1000 saxa 5 mg+met 1,000 mg

Comment: The FDA has reported that *saxagliptin*-containing drugs may increase the risk of heart failure, especially in patients who already have cardiovascular or renal disease. The drug **Kombiglyze XR** (*saxagliptin+metformin*) is in this risk group. *metformin* is contraindicated with renal impairment, metabolic acidosis, ketoacidosis. Suspend *metformin*, prior to, and for 48 hours after, surgery or receiving IV iodinated contrast agents.

▷ *sitagliptin+metformin* (B) take twice daily with meals; max *sitagliptin* 100 mg/day, max *metformin* 2000 mg/day

    Pediatric: <18 years: not recommended; ≥18 years: same as adult

    Janumet

        Tab: **Janumet 50/500** sita 50 mg+met 500 mg

            Janumet 50/1000 sita 50 mg+met 1000 mg

    Janumet XR

        Tab: **Janumet XR 50/500** sita 50 mg+met 500 mg ext-rel

            Janumet XR 50/1000 sita 50 mg+met 1000 mg ext-rel

            Janumet XR 100/1000 sita 100 mg+met 1000 mg ext-rel

Comment: *Metformin* is contraindicated with renal impairment, metabolic acidosis, ketoacidosis. Suspend *metformin*, prior to, and for 48 hours after surgery or receiving IV iodinated contrast agents.

SODIUM-GLUCOSE CO-TRANSPORTER 2 (SGLT2) INHIBITOR+DIPEPTIDYL PEPTIDASE-4 (DPP-4) INHIBITOR+BIGUANIDE COMBINATION

▷ *dapagliflozin+saxagliptin+metformin* (C) assess renal function before initiation of therapy and periodically thereafter; individualize the starting total daily dose based on the patient's current regimen, effectiveness, and tolerability; take once daily in the morning with food; for patients not currently taking dapagliflozin, the recommended starting dose is **Qternmet XR 5/5/1000** (dapa 5 mg/saxa 5 mg/met 1000 mg) once daily; max dose is **Qternmet XR 10/5/2000** (dapa 10 mg/saxa 5 mg/met 2000 mg) once daily; swallow tablet whole; do not crush, cut or chew; *Pediatric:* <18 years: not recommended: ≥18 years: same as adult

    Qternmet XL

      Tab: **Qternmet XL 2.5/2.5/1000** dapa 2.5 mg+saxa 2.5 mg+met 1000 mg film-coat ext-rel

      Qternmet XL 5/2.5/1000 dapa 5 mg+saxa 2.5 mg+met 1000 mg film-coat ext-rel

      Qternmet XL 5/5/1000 dapa 5 mg+saxa 5 mg+met 1000 mg film-coat ext-rel

      Qternmet XL 10/5/1000 dapa 10 mg+saxa 5 mg+met 1000 mg film-coat ext-rel

Comment: **Qternmet XR** is not indicated for the treatment of T1DM or diabetic ketoacidosis. **Qternmet** initiation is intended only for patients currently taking *metformin*. Discontinue **Qternmet XR** at the time of or prior to an iodinated contrast imaging procedure. **Qternmet XR** should not be used during pregnancy. If pregnancy is detected, treatment with **Qternmet** should be discontinued. It is unknown whether **Qtern** and/or its metabolites are excreted in human milk. Do not use with CrCl <60 mL/min or eGFR <60 mL/min/1.73 m² or ESRD or severe hepatic impairment or history of pancreatitis.

MEGLITINIDE+BIGUANIDE COMBINATION

▷ *repaglinide+metformin* (C)(G) take in 2-3 divided doses within 30 minutes before food; max 4/1000 per meal and 10/2000 per day
Pediatric: <18 years: not recommended; ≥18 years: same as adult

    Prandimet

      Tab: **Prandimet 1/500** repa 1 mg+met 500 mg

      Prandimet 2/500 repa 2 mg+met 500 mg

Comment: *Metformin* is contraindicated with renal impairment, metabolic acidosis, ketoacidosis. Suspend *metformin*, prior to, and for 48 hours after, surgery or receiving IV iodinated contrast agents.

SODIUM-GLUCOSE CO-TRANSPORTER 2 (SGLT2) INHIBITOR+DIPEPTIDYL PEPTIDASE-4 (DPP-4) INHIBITOR+BIGUANIDE

▷ **Qternmet EX** individualize the starting total daily dose of **Qternmet EX** based on the patient's current regimen, effectiveness, and tolerability; take once daily in the morning with food; swallow tablet whole; do not crush, cut or chew; *Patients not currently taking dapagliflozin:* recommended starting total daily dose of **Qternmet EX** is 5 mg *dapagliflozin*+5 mg *saxagliptin*+1000 mg or 2000 mg *metformin hcl* once daily; max recommended daily dose is 10 mg *dapagliflozin*, 5 mg *saxagliptin* and 2000 mg *metformin hcl*
Pediatric: <18 years: not recommended; ≥18 years: same as adult

Tab: **Qternmet EX 2.5/2.5/1000** dapa 2.5 mg+saxa 2.5 mg+met hcl 1000 mg ext-rel

Qternmet EX 5/2.5/1000 dapa 5 mg+saxa 2.5 mg+met hcl 1000 mg) ext-rel

Qternmet EX 5/5/1000 dapa 5 mg+saxa 5 mg+met hcl 1000 mg ext-rel

Qternmet EX 10/5/1000 dapa 10 mg+saxa 5 mg+met hcl 1000 mg ext-rel

Comment: **Qternmet XR** is triple fixed-dose combination indicated for adults with T2DM. Assess renal function before initiating **Qternmet EX** and periodically thereafter. Discontinue **Qternmet EX** at the time of, or prior to, an iodinated contrast imaging procedure. Contraindications to **Qternmet EX** include history of a serious hypersensitivity reaction to *dapagliflozin*, *saxagliptin*, or *metformin*, including anaphylaxis, angioedema, or exfoliative skin conditions; moderate-to-severe renal impairment (eGFR <45 mL/min/1.73 m2), end-stage renal disease (ESRD), or patient on dialysis, acute or chronic metabolic acidosis, including diabetic ketoacidosis, with or without coma. Diabetic ketoacidosis should be treated with insulin. Do not co-administer **Qternmet XR** with strong cytochrome P450 3A4/5 inhibitors. Co-administration with carbonic anhydrase inhibitors may increase the risk of lactic acidosis (consider more frequent monitoring). Drugs that reduce *metformin* clearance (such as *ranolazine*, *vandetanib*, *dolutegravir*, and *cimetidine*) may increase the accumulation of *metformin* (consider the benefits and risks of concomitant use). Alcohol can potentiate the effects of *metformin* on lactate metabolism (warn patients against excessive alcohol intake). Advise females of reproductive potential of embryo/fetal risk, especially during the second and third trimesters. **Qternmet EX** is not recommended when breastfeeding. There is a higher incidence of adverse reactions related to volume depletion and reduced renal function in the geriatric population. Avoid use of **Qternmet EX** in patients with clinical or laboratory evidence of hepatic impairment.

DIPEPTIDYL PEPTIDASE-4 (DPP-4) INHIBITOR+HMG-COA REDUCTASE INHIBITOR COMBINATION

▷ *sitagliptin+simvastatin* (B) take once daily in the PM; swallow whole; adjust dose if needed after 4 weeks; *Concomitant verapamil or diltiazem:* max 100/10 once daily; *Concomitant amiodarone, amlodipine, or ranolazine:* max 100/20 once daily; *Homogenous familial hypercholesterolemia:* max 100/40 once daily; *Chinese patients taking lipid-modifying doses (>1 gm/day niacin) of niacin-containing products:* caution with 100/40 dose; increase risk of myopathy
Pediatric: <18 years: not recommended; ≥18 years: same as adult
Juvisync
Tab: **Juvisync 100/10** sita 100 mg+simva 10 mg
Juvisync 100/20 sita 100 mg+simva 20 mg
Juvisync 100/40 sita 100 mg+simva 40 mg

DOPAMINE RECEPTOR AGONIST

▷ *bromocriptine mesylate* (B) take with food in the morning within 2 hours of waking; initially 0.8 mg once daily; may increase by 0.8 mg/week; max 4.8 mg/week; *Severe psychotic disorders:* not recommended
Pediatric: <12 years: not recommended; ≥12 years: same as adult
Cycloset *Tab:* 0.8 mg
Comment: **Cycloset** is an adjunct to diet and exercise to improve glycemic control. Contraindicated with syncopal migraines, nursing mothers, and other ergot-related drugs.

Bile Acid Sequestrant

▷ *colesevelam* (B)(G)

WelChol recommended dose is 6 tablets once daily or 3 tablets twice daily; take with a meal and liquid

Pediatric: <10 years: not recommended; ≥10 years: same as adult

Tab: 625 mg

WelChol for Oral Suspension recommended dose is one 3.75 gm packet once daily or one 1.875 gm packet twice daily; empty one packet into a glass or cup; add 1/2 to 1 cup (4-8 oz) of water, fruit juice, or diet soft drink; stir well and drink immediately; do not swallow dry form; take with meals

Pediatric: <12 years: not established; ≥12 years: same as adult

Pwdr: 3.75 gm/pkt (30 pkt/carton), 1.875 gm/pkt (60 pkt/carton) for oral suspension

Comment: **WelChol** is indicated as adjunctive therapy to improve glycemic control in adults with type 2 diabetes. It can be added to *metformin*, sulfonylureas, or insulin alone or in combination with other antidiabetic agents

TYPHOID FEVER (*SALMONELLA TYPHI*)

PRE-EXPOSURE PROPHYLAXIS

▷ *typhoid* vaccine, oral, live, attenuated strain

Vivotif Berna 1 cap every other day, 1 hour before a meal, with a lukewarm (not > body temperature) or cold drink for a total of 4 doses; do not crush or chew; complete therapy at least 1 week prior to expected exposure; re-immunization recommended every 5 years if repeated exposure

Pediatric: <6 years: not recommended; ≥6 years: same as adult

Cap: ent-coat

▷ *typhoid Vi polysaccharide* vaccine (C)

Pediatric: <2 years: not recommended; ≥2 years: same as adult

Typhim Vi 0.5 ml IM in deltoid; re-immunization recommended every 2 years if repeated exposure

Vial: 20, 50 dose; *Prefilled syringe:* 0.5 ml

Comment: Febrile illness may require delaying administration of the vaccine; have *epinephrine* 1:1000 readily available.

TREATMENT

▷ *azithromycin* (B)(G) 8-10 mg/kg/day; *Mild Illness:* treat x 7 days; *Severe Illness:* treat x 14 days

Pediatric: 8-10 mg/kg/day; max 500 mg/day; *Mild Illness:* treat x 7 days; *Severe Illness:* treat x 14 days; *see* Appendix CC.7. *azithromycin* (Zithromax Suspension, Zmax Suspension) *for dose by weight*

Zithromax *Tab:* 250, 500, 600 mg; *Oral susp:* 100 mg/5 ml (15 ml); 200 mg/5 ml (15, 22.5, 30 ml) (cherry); *Pkt:* 1 gm for reconstitution (cherry-banana)

Zithromax Tri-pak *Tab:* 3 x 500 mg tabs/pck

Zithromax Z-pak *Tab:* 6 x 250 mg tabs/pck

Zmax *Oral susp:* 2 gm ext-rel for reconstitution (cherry-banana) (148 mg Na⁺)

▷ *cefixime* (B)(G) *Mild Illness:* 15-20 mg/kg/day x 7-14 days; *Severe Illness:* 20 mg/kg/day x 10-14 days

Pediatric: <6 months: not recommended; 6 months-12 years, <50 kg: *Mild Illness:* 15-20 mg/kg/day x 7-14 days; *Severe Illness:* 20 mg/kg/day x 10-14 >50 kg: same as adult; *see* Appendix CC.11. *cefixime* (Suprax Oral Suspension) *for dose by weight*

Suprax *Tab:* 400 mg; *Cap:* 400 mg; *Oral susp:* 100, 200, 500 mg/5 ml (50, 75, 100 ml) (strawberry)

▷ *ciprofloxacin* (C) 15 mg/kg/day; *Mild Illness:* treat x 5-7 days; *Severe Illness:* treat x 10-14 days
Pediatric: <18 years: not recommended; ≥18 years: same as adult
    Cipro (G) *Tab:* 250, 500, 750 mg; *Oral susp:* 250, 500 mg/5 ml (100 ml) (strawberry)
    Cipro XR *Tab:* 500, 1000 mg ext-rel
    ProQuin XR *Tab:* 500 mg ext-rel
▷ *ofloxacin* (C) 15 mg/kg/day; *Mild Illness:* treat x 5-7 days; *Severe Illness:* treat x 10-14 days
Pediatric: <18 years: not recommended; ≥18 years: same as adult
    Floxin *Tab:* 200, 300, 400 mg
▷ *cefotaxime* 80 mg/kg/day IM/IV x 10-14 days; max 2 gm/day
Pediatrics: 80 mg/kg/day IM/IV x 10-14 days; max 2 gm/day
    Claforan *Vial:* 500 mg; 1, 2 gm
▷ *ceftriaxone* (B)(G) 75 mg/kg/day IM/IV x 10-14 days; max 2 gm/day
Pediatrics: 75 mg/kg/day IM/IV x 10-14 days; max 2 gm/day
    Rocephin *Vial:* 250, 500 mg; 1, 2 gm
▷ *trimethoprim+sulfamethoxazole (TMP-SMX)* (D)(G) 8-40 mg/kg/day x 14 days
Pediatric: <2 months: not recommended; ≥2 months: 8-40 mg/kg/day of *sulfamethoxazole* in 2 divided doses bid x 10 days; *see Appendix CC.33.*
trimethoprim+sulfamethoxazole (Bactrim Suspension, Septra Suspension) *for dose by weight*
    Bactrim, Septra 2 tabs bid x 10 days
      Tab: trim 80 mg+sulfa 400 mg*
    Bactrim DS, Septra DS 1 tab bid x 10 days
      Tab: trim 160 mg+sulfa 800 mg*
    Bactrim Pediatric Suspension, Septra Pediatric Suspension 20 ml bid x 10 days
      Oral susp: trim 40 mg+sulfa 200 mg per 5 ml (100 ml) (cherry) (alcohol 0.3%)

ULCER: DIABETIC, NEUROPATHIC (LOWER EXTREMITY); VENOUS INSUFFICIENCY (LOWER EXTREMITY)

NUTRITIONAL SUPPLEMENT

▷ *L-methylfolate calcium (as metafolin)+pyridoxyl 5-phosphate+methylcobalamin* take 1 cap daily
Pediatric: <12 years: not recommended; ≥12 years: same as adult
    Metanx *Cap:* metafo 3 mg+pyrid 35 mg+methyl 2 mg (gluten-free, yeast-free, lactose-free)
    Comment: **Metanx** is indicated as adjunct treatment of endothelial dysfunction <u>and/or</u> hyperhomocysteinemia in patients who have lower extremity ulceration.

DEBRIDING+CAPILLARY STIMULANT AGENT

▷ *trypsin+balsam peru+castor oil* apply at least twice daily; may cover with a wet bandage
    Granulex *Aerosol liq:* tryp 0.12 mg+bal peru 87 mg+cast 788 mg per 0.82 ml

GROWTH FACTOR

▷ *becaplermin* (C) apply once daily with a cotton swab <u>or</u> tongue depressor; then cover with saline moistened gauze dressing; rinse after 12 hours; then re-cover with a clean saline dressing
    Regranex *Gel:* 0.01% (2, 7.5, 15 gm) (parabens)
Comment: Store in refrigerator; do <u>not</u> freeze. <u>Not</u> for use in wounds that close by primary intention.

ULCER: PRESSURE, DECUBITUS

DEBRIDING/CAPILLARY STIMULANT AGENT

Granulex (*trypsin 0.1 mg+balsam peru 72.5 mg+castor oil 650 mg per 0.82 ml*) apply at least twice daily; may cover with a wet bandage
> *Aerosol liq:* (2, 4 oz)

GROWTH FACTOR

▷ *becaplermin* (C) apply once daily with a cotton swab or tongue depressor; then cover with saline moistened gauze dressing; rinse after 12 hours; then recover with a clean saline dressing
> **Regranex** *Gel:* 0.01% (2, 7.5, 15 gm) (parabens)

Comment: Store in refrigerator; do not freeze. Not for use in wounds that close by primary intention.

 ULCERATIVE COLITIS (UC)

Comment: Standard treatment regimen is anti-infective, anti-spasmodic, and bowel rest; progressing to clear liquids; then to high fiber.
Parenteral Corticosteroids *see* Appendix M. Parenteral Corticosteroids
Oral Corticosteroids *see* Appendix L. Oral Corticosteroids
▷ *budesonide micronized* (C)(G) 9 mg once daily in the AM for up to 8 weeks; may repeat an 8-week course; *Maintenance of remission:* 6 mg once daily for up to 3 months; taper other systemic steroids when transferring to *budesonide*
> *Pediatric:* <12 years: not recommended; ≥12 years: same as adult
> **Entocort EC** *Cap:* 3 mg ent-coat granules
> **Uceris** *Tab:* 9 mg ext-rel

RECTAL CORTICOSTEROIDS

▷ *hydrocortisone* rectal (C)
> *Pediatric:* <12 years: not recommended; ≥12 years: same as adult
> **Anusol-HC Suppositories** 1 supp rectally 3 x/day or 2 supp rectally 2 x/day for 2 weeks; max 8 weeks
>> *Rectal supp:* 25 mg (12, 24/pck)
> **Cortenema** 1 enema q HS x 21 days or until symptoms controlled
>> *Enema:* 100 mg/60 ml (1, 7/pck)
> **Cortifoam** 1 applicator full once daily-bid x 2-3 weeks and every 2nd day thereafter until symptoms are controlled
>> *Aerosol:* 80 mg/applicator (14 application/container)
> **Proctocort** 1 supp rectally in AM and PM x 2 weeks; for more severe cases, may increase to 1 supp rectally 3 times daily or 2 supp rectally twice daily; max 4-8 weeks
>> *Rectal supp:* 30 mg (12, 24/pck)

Comment: Use *hydrocortisone* foam as adjunctive therapy in the distal portion of the rectum when *hydrocortisone* enemas cannot be retained.

RECTAL CORTICOSTEROID+ANESTHETIC

Hydrocortisone+Pramoxine

Proctofoam HC apply to anal/rectal area 3-4 times daily; max 4-8 weeks
> *Rectal foam:* hydrocort 1%+pram 1% (10 gm w. applicator)

SALICYLATES

Comment: Symptoms of salicylate toxicity include hematemesis, tachypnea, hyperpnea, tinnitus, deafness, lethargy, seizures, confusion, or dyspnea. Severe intoxication may lead to electrolyte and blood pH imbalance and potentially to other organ (e.g., renal and liver) involvement. There is no specific antidote for mesalamine overdose; however, conventional therapy for salicylate toxicity may be beneficial in the event of acute overdosage. This includes prevention of further gastrointestinal tract absorption by emesis and, if necessary, by gastric lavage. Fluid and electrolyte imbalance should be corrected by the administration of appropriate intravenous therapy. Adequate renal function should be maintained.

▷ *balsalazide disodium* (B)
  Comment: *Balsalazide* 6.75 gm provides 2.4 gm of *mesalazine* to the colon.
  Colazal 3 x 750 mg caps/day (6.75 gm/day), with or without food, x 8 weeks; may require treatment for up to 12 weeks; swallow whole or may be opened and sprinkled on applesauce, then chewed or swallowed immediately
  Pediatric: <5 years: not recommended; 5-17 years: 1 x 750 mg cap 3 x/day (2.25 gm/day), with or without food for up to 8 weeks or 3 x 750 mg caps/day (6.75 gm/day), with or without food, x 8 weeks; swallow whole or may be opened and sprinkled on applesauce, then chewed or swallowed immediately
    Cap: 750 mg
  Comment: **Colazal** is a locally-acting aminosalicylate indicated for the treatment of mildly to moderately active ulcerative colitis in patients ≥5 years. Safety and effectiveness of **Colazal** >8 weeks in children (5-17 years) and >12 weeks in patients ≥18 years has not been established.
  Giazo is a locally-acting aminosalicylate indicated for the treatment of mildly to moderately active ulcerative colitis only in male patients ≥18 years; take 3 x 1.1 gm tabs bid (6.6 gm/day) for up to 8 weeks
  Pediatric: <18 years: not recommended; >18 years: same as adult
    Tab: 1.1 gm (sodium 126 mg/tab) film-coat
  Comment: Effectiveness of **Giazo** in female patients has not been demonstrated in clinical trials. Safety and effectiveness of **Giazo** > 8 weeks has not been established.

▷ *mesalamine* (B)
  Apriso *Maintenance:* of Remission 4 x 0.375 gm caps (1.5 gm/day) once daily in the morning, for maintenance of remission with or without food; do not co-administer with antacids
  Pediatric: <18 years: not recommended; ≥18 years: same as adult
    Cap: 0.375 gm ext-rel (phenylalanine 0.56 mg/cap)
  Comment: **Apriso** is a locally-acting aminosalicylate indicated for the maintenance of remission of ulcerative colitis in adults.
  Asacol HD (G) *Induction of Remission:* 2 x 800 mg tab (1600 mg) tid x 6 weeks; *Maintenance of Remission:* 1.6 gm/day in divided doses; take on an empty stomach, at least 1 hour before or 2 hours after a meal; swallow whole; do not crush, break, or chew
  Pediatric: <18 years: not recommended; ≥18 years: same as adult
    Tab: 800 mg del-rel
  Comment: **Asacol HD** is an aminosalicylate indicated for the treatment of moderately active ulcerative colitis in adults. Do not substitute one **Asacol HD 800** tablet for two **mesalamine** delayed-release 400 mg oral products
  Canasa 1 x 1000 mg suppository administered rectally once daily at bedtime for 3 to 6 weeks.
  Pediatric: <18 years: not recommended; ≥18 years: same as adult
    Rectal supp: 1 gm del-rel (30, 42/pck)
  Comment: **Canasa** is an aminosalicylate indicated in adults for the treatment of mildly to moderately active ulcerative proctitis. Safety and effectiveness of **Canasa** beyond 6 weeks have not been established.
  Delzicol *Treatment:* 2 x 400 mg caps (800 mg/day) 3 x/day x 6 weeks; *Maintenance:* 4 x 400 mg caps (1.6 gm/day) in 2-4 divided doses once daily; swallow whole; take with or without food; do not crush or chew

Pediatric: ≥5-17 years: twice daily dosing for 6 weeks; see mfr pkg insert for weight-based dosing table; ≥18 years: same as adult

    Cap: 400 mg del-rel

Comment: 2 x 400 mg **Dezlicol** caps have **not** been shown to be interchangeable or substitutable with one *mesalamine* delayed-release 80 mg tablet. Evaluate renal function prior to initiation of **Dezlicol**.

Lialda (G) *Induction of Remission:* 2-4 x 1.2 gm tabs (2.4-4.8 gm) once daily for up to 8 weeks; *Maintenance: of Remission:* 2 x 1.2 gm tabs (2.4 gm) once daily; swallow whole; do **not** crush or chew

Pediatric: <18 years: not recommended; ≥18 years: same as adult

    Tab: 1.2 gm del-rel

Comment: **Lialda** is a locally-acting 5-aminosalicylic acid (5-ASA) indicated for the induction of remission in adults with active, mild to moderate ulcerative colitis and for the maintenance of remission of ulcerative colitis. Safety and effectiveness of **Lialda** in pediatric patients have **not** been established.

Pentasa *Induction of Remission:* 1 gm qid for up to 8 weeks

Pediatric: <18 years: not recommended; ≥18 years: same as adult

    Cap: 250, 500 mg ext-rel

Comment: **Pentasa** is an aminosalicylate anti-inflammatory agent indicated for the induction of remission and for the treatment of patients with mildly to moderately active ulcerative colitis.

Rowasa Suppository 1 supp rectally bid x 3-6 weeks; retain for 1-3 hours or longer

Pediatric: <18 years: not recommended; ≥18 years: same as adult

    Rectal supp: 500 mg (12, 24/pck)

Rowasa Rectal Suspension 4 gm (60 ml) rectally by enema q HS; retain for 8 hours x 3-6 weeks (sulfite-free)

Pediatric: <18 years: not recommended; ≥18 years: same as adult

    Enema: 4 gm/60 ml (7, 14, 28/pck; kit, 7, 14, 28/pck w. wipes)

Comment: **Rowasa Rectal Suspension** enema is indicated for the treatment of active mild to moderate distal ulcerative colitis, proctosigmoiditis, and proctitis.

▷ *olsalazine* **(C) Maintenance of Remission:** 1 gm/day in 2 divided doses; take with food

Pediatric: <18 years: not recommended; ≥18 years: same as adult

    Dipentum *Cap:* 250 mg

Comment: *Osalazine* is the sodium salt of a salicylate, disodium 3,3′-azobis (6-hydroxybenzoate) a compound that is effectively bioconverted to 5-amino-salicylic acid (5-ASA), which has anti-inflammatory activity in ulcerative colitis. The conversion of *olsalazine* to *mesalamine* (5-ASA) in the colon is similar to that of *sulfasalazine*, which is converted into *sulfapyridine* and *mesalamine*. **Olsalazine** is indicated for the maintenance of remission of ulcerative colitis in patients who are intolerant of *sulfasalazine*.

▷ *sulfasalazine* **(B; D in 2nd, 3rd)(G)** *Induction of Remission:* 3-4 gm/day in evenly divided doses with dosage intervals **not** exceeding eight hours; in some cases, it is advisable to initiate therapy with a smaller dosage, e.g., 1-2 gm/day, to reduce possible gastrointestinal intolerance. If daily doses exceeding 4 gm are required to achieve desired effects, the increased risk of toxicity should be kept in mind; **Maintenance of Remission: 4 gm/day in divided doses**

Pediatric: <2 years: not recommended; 2-16 years: initially 40-60 mg/kg/day in 3 to 6 divided doses; max 30 mg/kg/day in 4 divided doses; max 2 gm/day in divided doses; >16 years: same as adult

    Azulfidine *Tab:* 500*mg

    Azulfidine EN-Tabs *Tab:* 500 mg ent-coat

TUMOR NECROSIS FACTOR (TNF) BLOCKER

▷ *adalimumab* (B) 160 mg on Day 1 (given in one day or split over two consecutive days), 80 mg on Day 15 and 40 mg every other week starting on Day 29. Discontinue in patients without evidence of clinical remission by eight weeks (Day 57) administer in abdomen or thigh; rotate sites

Pediatric: <5 years, <20 kg: not recommended; 5-18 years, living with moderate-to-severe UC, weight-based: 20 kg (44 lb) to <40 kg (<88 lb): Day 1: 80 mg; Day 8: 40 mg; Day 15: 20 mg; Starting on Day 29: 20 mg every week or 40 mg every other week: >40 kg (>88 lb): Day 1: 160 mg (as a single dose or split over two consecutive days); Day 8: 80 mg; Day 15: 80 mg; Starting on Day 29: 40 mg every week or 80 mg every other week It is recommended to continue the recommended pediatric dosage in patients who turn 18 years-of-age and who are well-controlled on their **Humira** regimen.

   Humira *Prefilled syringe:* 20 mg/0.4 ml; 40 mg/0.8 ml single-dose (2/pck; 2, 6/ starter pck) (preservative-free)

▷ *adalimumab-adbm* (B) *First dose (Day 1):* 160 mg SC (4 x 40 mg injections in one day or 2 x 40 mg injections per day for two consecutive days); *Second dose two weeks later (Day 15):* 80 mg SC; *Two weeks later (Day 29):* begin a maintenance dose of 40 mg SC every other week (only continue in patients who have shown evidence of clinical remission by eight weeks (Day 57) of therapy.

Pediatric: <18 years: not recommended; ≥18 years: same as adult

   Cyltezo *Prefilled syringe:* 40 mg/0.8 ml single-dose (preservative-free)

   Comment: **Cyltezo** is biosimilar to **Humira** (*adalimumab*).

▷ *adalimumab-afzb* 40 mg SC every other week; some patients with RA not receiving *methotrexate* (MTX) may benefit from increasing the frequency to 40 mg SC every week

   Abrilada *Prefilled pen:* 40 mg/0.8 ml, single-dose; *Prefilled syringe:* 40 mg/0.8 ml, 20 mg/0.4 ml, 10 mg/0.2 ml, single-dose; (for institutional use only) (preservative-free)

   Comment: **Abrilada** is biosimilar to **Humira** (*adalimumab*).

▷ *adalimumab-bwwd Initial Dose (Day 1):* 160 mg SC; *Second Dose: two weeks later (Day 15):* 80 mg SC; *Two weeks later (Day 29):* begin maintenance dose of 40 mg every other week

   Hadlima *Prefilled autoinjector:* 40 mg/0.8 ml, single-dose (Hadlima PushTouch); *Prefilled syringe:* 40 mg/0.8 ml, single-dose

   Comment: **Hadlima** is biosimilar to **Humira** (*adalimumab*).

▷ *infliximab* must be refrigerated at 2°C to 8°C (36°F to 46°F); administer dose via IV infusion over a period of not less than 2 hours; do not use beyond the expiration date as this product contains no preservative; 5 mg/kg at 0, 2 and 6 weeks, then every 8 weeks.

Pediatric: <6 years: not studied; ≥6-17 years: mg/kg at 0, 2 and 6 weeks, then every 8 weeks; ≥18 years: same as adult

   Remicade *Vial:* 100 mg pwdr for reconstitution to 10 ml administration volume, single-dose (presrvative-free)

   Comment: **Remicade** is indicated to reduce signs and symptoms, and induce and maintain clinical remission, in adults and children ≥6 years-of-age with moderately to severely active disease who have had an inadequate response to conventional therapy and reduce the number of draining enterocutaneous and rectovaginal fistulas, and maintain fistula closure, in adults with fistulizing disease. Common adverse effects associated with **Remicade** included abdominal pain, headache, pharyngitis, sinusitis, and upper respiratory infections. In addition, **Remicade** might increase the risk for serious infections, including tuberculosis, bacterial sepsis, and invasive fungal infections. Available data from published literature on the use of *infliximab* products during pregnancy have not reported a clear association with *infliximab* products and adverse pregnancy outcomes. *Infliximab* products cross the placenta and infants exposed *in utero* should not be administered live vaccines for at least 6 months after birth. Otherwise, the infant may be at increased risk of infection, including disseminated infection which can become fatal. Available information is insufficient to inform the amount of *infliximab* products present in human milk or effects on the breastfed infant.

▷ *infliximab-abda* (B)
Renflexis *Vial:* 100 mg for reconstitution to 10 ml administration volume, single-dose
Comment: Renflexis is biosimilar to Remicade. (*infliximab*).

▷ *infliximab-dyyb* (B)
Inflectra *Vial:* 100 mg pwdr for reconstitution to 10 ml administration volume, single-dose
Comment: Inflectra is biosimilar to Remicade. (*infliximab*).

▷ *infliximab-axxq*
Avsola *Vial:* 100 mg pwdr in a 20 ml single-dose vial, for reconstitution, dilution, and IV infusion
Comment: Avsola is biosimilar to Remicade *(infliximab)*.

▷ *infliximab-qbtx* (B)
Ixifi *Vial:* 100 mg pwdr for reconstitution to 10 ml administration volume, single-dose
Comment: Ixifi is biosimilar to Remicade. (*infliximab*).

INTERLEUKIN-12+INTERLEUKIN-23 ANTAGONIST

▷ *ustekinumab* (B) initially a single weight-based IV infusion: <*55 kg*: 260 mg (2 vials); *55-85 kg*: 390 mg (3 vials)>*85 kg*: 520 mg (4 vials); followed by 90 mg SC every a weeks thereafter
Pediatric: <18 years: not recommended; ≥18 years: same as adult
Stelara *Prefilled syringe:* 45 mg/0.5 ml, single dose; *Vial:* 45 mg/0.5 ml, 90 mg/ml, single-dose, 130 mg/26 ml, single-dose (preservative-free)

JANUS KINASE (JAK) INHIBITOR (JAKI)

▷ *tofacitinib* (C) XELJANZ *Induction:* 10 mg twice daily or XELJANZ XR 22 mg once daily for 8 weeks; transition to maintenance therapy depending on therapeutic response; if needed, continue XELJANZ 10 mg twice daily or XELJANZ XR 22 mg once daily for a maximum of 16 weeks; discontinue XELJANZ 10 mg twice daily or XELJANZ XR 22 mg once daily after 16 weeks if adequate therapeutic response is not achieved; *Maintenance:* XELJANZ 5 mg twice daily or XELJANZ XR 11 mg once daily; if loss of response during maintenance treatment, XELJANZ 10 mg twice daily or XELJANZ XR 22 mg once daily may be considered and limited to the shortest duration, with careful consideration of the benefits and risks for the individual patient; use the lowest effective dose needed to maintain response; dose adjustment is needed in patients with moderate and severe renal impairment or moderate hepatic impairment: see mfr pkg insert FDA has not approved the 10 mg twice daily dosing regimen for RA; this dosing regimen is only approved for patients with ulcerative colitis (UC).
Pediatric: safety and efficacy not established
Xeljanz *Tab:* 5 mg
Xeljanz Oral Solution *Oral soln:* 1 mg/ml (240 ml) with press-in bottle adapter and oral dosing syringe (no latex)
Xeljanz XR *Tab:* 11 mg ext-rel

Comment: **Xeljanz** is the first oral JAKI approved for chronic treatment of moderately to severely active UC. Other FDA-approved treatments for the treatment of moderately to severely active UC must be administered through an IV infusion or SC injection. Use with caution in patients that may be at increased risk for gastrointestinal perforation. The most common adverse events associated with **Xeljanz** treatment for UC are diarrhea, elevated cholesterol level, headache, herpes zoster (shingles), increased blood creatine phosphokinase, nasopharyngitis, rash, and upper respiratory tract infection (URI). Avoid use of **Xeljanz/Xeljanz XR** during an active serious infection, including localized infection. Patients treated with **Xeljanz** are at increased risk for developing serious infections that may lead to hospitalization or death. **Xeljanz** has a BBW for serious infections (e.g., opportunistic infections), and malignancy (e.g., lymphoma). Use of **Xeljanz** in combination with biological therapies for ulcerative colitis or with potent immunosuppressants, such as *azathioprine* and *cyclosporine*, is not recommended. Avoid live vaccines administration during treatment with **Xeljanz**. Prior to starting **Xeljanz**, perform a test for latent tuberculosis; if it is positive, start treatment for tuberculosis prior to starting **Xeljanz**. Monitor all patients for active tuberculosis during treatment, even if the initial latent tuberculosis test is negative. Recommend lab monitoring due to potential for changes in lymphocytes, neutrophils, hemoglobin, liver enzymes, and lipids. Do not initiate **Xeljanz** if absolute lymphocyte count <500 cells/mm^3, an absolute neutrophil count (ANC) <1000 cells/mm3 or Hgb <9 g/dL. The safety and effectiveness of **Xeljanz/Xeljanz XR** in pediatric patients have not been established. Available data with **Xeljanz** use in pregnancy are insufficient to establish a drug associated risk of major birth defects, miscarriage, or adverse maternal or fetal outcomes. In animal reproduction studies, fetocidal, and teratogenic effects were noted. There is a pregnancy exposure registry that monitors pregnancy outcomes in women exposed to **Xeljanz/Xeljanz XR** during pregnancy. Consider pregnancy planning and prevention for females of reproductive potential. Patients should be encouraged to enroll in the **Xeljanz/Xeljanz XR** pregnancy registry if they become pregnant. To enroll or obtain information from the registry, patients can call the toll free number 1-877-311-8972. There are no data on the presence of *tofacitinib* in human milk or the effects on a breastfed infant; however, patients should be advised not to breastfeed.

INTEGRIN RECEPTOR ANTAGONIST

▷ *vedolizumab* (B) administer by IV infusion over 30 minutes; 300 mg at weeks 0, 2, 6; then once every 8 weeks
   Pediatric: <12 years: not established; ≥12 years: same as adult
   Entyvio *Vial:* 300 mg (20 ml) single-dose, pwdr for IV infusion after reconstitution (preservative-free)

ANTI-DIARRHEAL AGENTS

▷ *difenoxin+atropine* (C) 2 tabs; then 1 tab after each loose stool or 1 tab q 3-4 hours; max 8 tabs/day x 2 days
   Motofen *Tab:* dif 1 mg+atro 0.025 mg
▷ *diphenoxylate+atropine* (C)(G) 2 tabs or 10 ml qid
   Lomotil *Tab:* diphen 2.5 mg+atro 0.025 mg; *Liq:* diphen 2.5 mg+atro 0.025 mg/5 ml (2 oz w. dropper)
▷ *loperamide* (B)(G)
   Imodium (OTC) 4 mg initially; then 2 mg after each loose stool; max 16 mg/day
      Cap: 2 mg

Imodium A-D (OTC) 4 mg initially; then 2 mg after each loose stool; usual max 8 mg/day x 2 days

Cplt: 2 mg; *Liq:* 1 mg/5 ml (2, 4 oz)

▷ **loperamide+simethicone (B)(G)**

Imodium Advanced (OTC) 2 tabs chewed after first loose stool; then 1 after the next loose stool; max 4 tabs/day

Chew tab: loper 2 mg+simeth 125 mg

◯ URETHRITIS: NONGONOCOCCAL (NGU)

Comment: The following treatment regimens for NGU are published in the **2015 CDC Sexually Transmitted Diseases Treatment Guidelines**. Treatment regimens are for adults only; consult a specialist for treatment of patients less than 18 years-of-age. Treatment regimens are presented by generic drug name first, followed by information about brands and dose forms. All persons who have confirmed or suspected urethritis should be tested for gonorrhea and chlamydia. Men treated for NGU should be instructed to abstain from sexual intercourse for 7 days after a single dose regimen or until completion of a 7-day regimen.

RECOMMENDED REGIMEN: UNCOMPLICATED NGU

▷ *azithromycin* 1 gm in a single dose or 100 mg orally bid x 7 days
  plus
▷ *doxycycline* 100 mg bid x 7 days

PERSISTENT-RECURRENT NGU

Men Initially Treated With Azithromycin+Doxycycline

▷ *azithromycin* 1 gm PO in a single dose

Men Who Fail a Regimen of Azithromycin

▷ *moxifloxacin* 400 mg PO once daily x 7 days

Heterosexual Men Who Live in Areas Where *T. Vaginalis* is Highly Prevalent

▷ *metronidazole* 2 gm PO in a single dose
  or
▷ *tinidazole* 2 gm PO in a single dose

ALTERNATIVE REGIMENS

▷ *erythromycin base* 500 mg PO qid x 7 days
  or
▷ *erythromycin ethylsuccinate* 800 mg PO qid x 7 days
  or
▷ *levofloxacin* 500 mg once daily x 7 days
  or
▷ *ofloxacin* 300 mg PO bid x 7 days

DRUG BRANDS AND DOSE FORMS

▷ *azithromycin* (B)(G)

Zithromax *Tab:* 250, 500, 600 mg; *Oral susp:* 100 mg/5 ml (15 ml); 200 mg/5 ml (15, 22.5, 30 ml) (cherry); *Pkt:* 1 gm for reconstitution (cherry-banana)

Zithromax Tri-pak *Tab:* 3 x 500 mg tabs/pck

Zithromax Z-pak *Tab:* 6 x 250 mg tabs/pck

Zmax *Oral susp:* 2 gm ext-rel for reconstitution (cherry-banana) (148 mg Na⁺)

▷ *doxycycline* (D)(G)
  Acticlate *Tab:* 75, 150**mg
  Adoxa *Tab:* 50, 75, 100, 150 mg ent-coat
  Doryx *Tab:* 50, 75, 100, 150, 200 mg del-rel
  Doxteric *Tab:* 50 mg del-rel
  Monodox *Cap:* 50, 75, 100 mg
  Oracea *Cap:* 40 mg del-rel
  Vibramycin *Tab:* 100 mg; *Cap:* 50, 100 mg; *Syr:* 50 mg/5 ml (raspberry-apple)
  (sulfites); *Oral susp:* 25 mg/5 ml (raspberry)
  Vibra-Tab *Tab:* 100 mg film-coat
▷ *erythromycin base* (B)
  Ery-Tab *Tab:* 250, 333, 500 mg ent-coat
  PCE *Tab:* 333, 500 mg
▷ *erythromycin ethylsuccinate* (B)(G)
  EryPed *Oral susp:* 200 mg/5 ml (100, 200 ml) (fruit); 400 mg/5 ml (60, 100,
  200 ml) (banana); *Oral drops:* 200, 400 mg/5 ml (50 ml) (fruit); *Chew tab:* 200
  mg wafer (fruit)
  E.E.S. *Oral susp:* 200, 400 mg/5 ml (100 ml) (fruit)
  E.E.S. Granules *Oral susp:* 200 mg/5 ml (100, 200 ml) (cherry)
  E.E.S. 400 Tablets *Tab:* 400 mg
▷ *levofloxacin* (C)
  Levaquin *Tab:* 250, 500, 750 mg; *Oral soln:* 25 mg/ml (480 ml) (benzyl
  alcohol); *Inj conc:* 25 mg/ml for IV infusion after dilution (20, 30 ml
  single-use vial) (preservative-free); *Premix soln:* 5 mg/ml for IV infusion (50,
  100, 150 ml) (preservative-free)
▷ *metronidazole* (**not** for use in 1st; B in 2nd, 3rd)(G)
  Flagyl *Tab:* 250*, 500*mg
  Flagyl 375 *Cap:* 375 mg
  Flagyl ER *Tab:* 750 mg ext-rel
▷ *moxifloxacin* (C)(G)
  Avelox *Tab:* 400 mg
▷ *ofloxacin* (C)(G)
  Floxin *Tab:* 200, 300, 400 mg
▷ *tinidazole* (**not** for use in 1st; B in 2nd, 3rd)
  Tindamax *Tab:* 250*, 500*mg

⬤ URINARY RETENTION: UNOBSTRUCTIVE

▷ *bethanechol* (C) 10-30 mg tid
  Urecholine *Tab:* 5, 10, 25, 50 mg
  Comment: Contraindicated in presence of urinary obstruction. *atropine* 0.4 mg
  administered SC reverses *bethanechol* toxicity.

⬤ URINARY TRACT INFECTION, COMPLICATED (cUTI)

SIDEROPHORE CEPHALOSPORIN

▷ *cefiderocol* administer 2 gm via IV infusion every 8 hours; infuse dose over
  3 hours in patients with CrCl 60-119 mL/min; see mfr pkg insert for dose
  adjustments required in patients with CrCl <60 mL/min and ≥CrCl 120 mL/min;
  see mfr pkg insert for dose preparation
  Fetroja *Vial:* 1 gram pwdr for reconstitution and IV infusion, single-dose
  Comment: **Fetroja** (*cefiderocol*) is a siderophore cephalosporin for the
  treatment of complicated urinary tract infection (cUTI), including
  pyelonephritis, caused by susceptible Gram-negative microorganisms, in

patients ≥18 years-of-age with limited or no alternative treatment options. Approval of this indication is based on limited clinical safety and efficacy data. An increase in all-cause mortality was observed in **Fetroja**-treated patients compared to those treated with best available therapy (BAT). Closely monitor the clinical response to therapy in patients with cUTI. Serious and occasionally fatal hypersensitivity (anaphylactic) reactions have been reported in patients receiving betalactam antibacterial drugs. Hypersensitivity was observed with **Fetroja**. Cross-hypersensitivity may occur in patients with a history of penicillin allergy. If an allergic reaction occurs, discontinue **Fetroja**. *Clostridioides Difficile*-Associated Diarrhea (CDAD) has been reported with nearly all systemic antibacterial agents, including **Fetroja**. Seizures and other CNS adverse reactions have been reported with **Fetroja**. If focal tremors, myoclonus, or seizures occur, evaluate patients to determine whether **Fetroja** should be discontinued. The most frequently occurring adverse reactions (incidence ≥2% of patients treated with **Fetroja** have been diarrhea, infusion site reactions, constipation, rash, candidiasis, cough, elevations in liver tests, headache, hypokalemia, nausea, and vomiting. There are no available data on **Fetroja** use in pregnant females to evaluate for a drug-associated risk of major birth defects, miscarriage or adverse maternal or fetal outcomes. Available data from published prospective cohort studies, case series, and case reports over several decades with cephalosporin use in pregnant females have not established drug-associated risks of major birth defects, miscarriage, or adverse maternal or fetal outcomes. Developmental toxicity studies with *cefiderocol* administered during organogenesis in animal studies showed no evidence of embryo/fetal toxicity, including drug-induced fetal malformations. It is not known whether *cefiderocol* is excreted into human milk. No information is available on the effects of **Fetroja** on the breastfed infant. Developmental and health benefits of breastfeeding should be considered along with the mother's clinical need for **Fetroja** and any potential adverse effects on the breastfed infant or from the underlying maternal condition.

PARENTERAL CEPHALOSPORIN ANTIBACTERIAL+BETA-LACTIMASE INHIBITOR

▷ *ceftazidime+avibactam* (B) infuse dose over 2 hours; recommended duration of treatment: 5 to 4 days; *CrCl 31-50 mL/min:* 1.25 gm every 8 hours; *CrCl 16-30 mL/min:* 0.94 gm every 12 hours; *CrCl 6-15 mL/min:* 0.94 gm every 24 hours; *CrCl ≤5 mL/min:* 0.94 gm every 48 hours; both *ceftazidime* and *avibactam* are hemodializable; thus, administer **Avycaz** after hemodialysis on hemodialysis days *Pediatric:* <18 years: not recommended; ≥18 years: same as adult

    Avycaz *Vial:* 2.5 gm, single-dose, pwdr for reconstitution and IV infusion

    Comment: **Avycaz** 2.5 gm contains *ceftazidime* (a cephalosporin) 2 gm (equivalent to 2.635 gm of *ceftazidime pentahydrate/sodium carbonate powder*) and *avibactam* (a beta lactam inhibitor) 0.5 gm (equivalent to 0.551 gm of *avibactam sodium*). As only limited clinical safety and efficacy data for **Avycaz** are currently available, reserve **Avycaz** for use in patients who have limited or no alternative treatment options. To reduce the development of drug-resistant bacteria and maintain the effectiveness of **Avycaz** and other antibacterial drugs, **Avycaz** should be used only to treat infections that are proven or strongly suspected to be caused by susceptible bacteria. Seizures and other neurologic events may occur, especially in patients with renal impairment. Adjust dose in patients with renal impairment. Decreased efficacy in patients with baseline CrCl 30--≤50 mL/min. Monitor CrCl at least daily in patients with changing renal function and adjust the dose of **Avycaz** accordingly. Monitor for hypersensitivity reactions, including anaphylaxis and serious skin reactions. Cross-hypersensitivity may occur in patients with a history of penicillin allergy. If an allergic reaction occurs, discontinue **Avycaz**. *Clostridioides difficile*-associated diarrhea CDAD) has been reported with nearly all systemic antibacterial agents, including **Avycaz**. There are no adequate and well-controlled studies of **Avycaz**, *ceftazidime*, or *avibactam* in pregnant females. *ceftazidime* is excreted in human milk in low concentrations. It is not known whether *avibactam* is excreted into human milk. There are no studies to inform effects on the breastfed infant.

➤ *ceftolozane+tazobactam* administer 1.5 gm every 8 hours via IV infusion over 1 hour x 4-14 days; *CrCl 30-50 ml/min:* 750 mg via IV infusion every 8 hours; *CrCl 15-29 ml/min:* 375 mg via IV infusion every 8 hours; *ESRD:* a single loading dose of 750 mg via IV infusion, followed by 150 mg via IV infusion every 8 hours for the remainder of the treatment period (on hemodialysis days, administer the dose at the earliest possible time following completion of dialysis)

Pediatric: <18: not established; ≥18 years: same as adult

    Zerbaxa *Vial:* 1.5 gm (*ceftolozane* 1 gm+*tazobactam* 0.5 gm), single-dose, pwdr for reconstitution and IV infusion

    Comment: For doses >1.5 gm, reconstitute a second vial in the same manner as the first one, withdraw an appropriate volume (see Table 3 in the mfr pkg insert) and add to the same infusion bag. The most common adverse reactions in patients with cIAI (incidence ≥5%) have been nausea, diarrhea, headache and pyrexia.

PARENTERAL PENEM ANTIBACTERIAL+RENAL DEHYDROPEPTIDASE INHIBITOR+ BETA-LACTAMASE INHIBITOR

➤ *imipenem+cilastatin+relebactam* administer dose via IV infusion over 30 minutes every 6 hours; *CrCL ≥90 mL/min:* 1.25 gm/dose (*imipenem* 500 mg, *cilastatin* 500 mg, *relebactam* 250 mg); *CrCL 60-89 mL/min:* 1 gm/dose (*imipenem* 400 mg, *cilastatin* 400 mg, *relebactam* 200 mg); *CrCL 30-59 mL/min:* 0.75 gm/dose (*imipenem* 300 mg, *cilastatin* 300 mg, *relebactam* 150 mg); *CrCl 15-29 mL/min:* 0.5 gm/dose (*imipenem* 200 mg, *cilastatin* 200 mg, *relebactam* 100 mg); *ESRD/Dialysis:* 0.5 gm/dose (*imipenem* 200 mg, *cilastatin* 200 mg, *relebactam* 100 mg)

Pediatric: <18 years: not established; ≥18 years: same as adult

    Recarbrio *Vial:* imipen 500 mg+cilast 500 mg+relebac 250 mg, single-dose, pwdr for reconstitution, dilution, and IV infusion

    Comment: **Recarbrio** *(imipenem+cilastatin+relebactam)* is a fixed-dose triple combination of *imipenem* (a penem antibacterial), *cilastatin* (a renal dehydropeptidase inhibitor), and *relebactam* (a beta-lactamase inhibitor) indicated for the treatment of complicated urinary tract infection (cUTI), including pyelonephritis, and complicated intra-abdominal infection (cIAI) caused by susceptible gram-negative bacteria in patients who have limited or no alternative treatment options, hospital-acquired bacterial pneumonia (HABP), and ventilator-associated bacterial pneumonia (VABP) in adults. Avoid concomitant use of **Recarbrio** with *ganciclovir*, *valproic acid*, or *divalproex sodium*. Based on clinical reports on patients treated with imipenem/cilastatin plus relebactam 250 mg, the most frequent adverse reactions (incidence ≥2 %) have been diarrhea, nausea, headache, vomiting, alanine aminotransferase increased, aspartate aminotransferase increased, phlebitis/infusion site reactions, pyrexia, and hypertension. There are insufficient human data to establish whether there is a drug-associated risk for major birth defects, miscarriage, or adverse maternal or fetal outcomes with *imipenem*, *cilastatin*, or *relebactam* in pregnancy. However, embryonic loss has been observed in monkeys treated with *imipenem/cilastatin*, and fetal abnormalities have been observed in *relebactam*-treated mice; therefore, advise pregnant females of the potential risks to pregnancy and the fetus. There are insufficient data on the presence of *imipenem/cilastatin* and *relebactam* in human milk, and no data on the effects on the breastfed infant; However, *relebactam* is present in the milk of lactating rats and, therefore, developmental and health benefits of breastfeeding should be considered along with the mother's clinical need for **Recarbrio** and any potential adverse effects on the breastfed infant from **Recarbrio** or from the underlying maternal condition.

PARENTERAL AMINOGLYCOSIDE ANTIBACTERIAL

▷ *plazomicin* recommended dose is 15 mg/kg once every 24 hours by IV infusion over 30 minutes x 4-7 days in patients with CrCl ≥90 mL/min; *CrCl ≥60 to <90 mL/min:* 15 mg/kg every 24 hours; *CrCl ≥30 to <60 mL/min:* 10 mg/kg every 24 hours; CrCl ≥15 to <30 mL/min: 10 mg/kg every 48 hours

Pediatric: <18 years: not recommended; ≥18 years: same as adult

Zemdri Injection *Vial:* 500 mg/10 ml (50 mg/ml) single-dose

Comment: **Zemdri** (*plazomicin*) is an aminoglycoside antibacterial for the treatment of complicated urinary tract infection (cUTI) including pyelonephritis. As only limited clinical safety and efficacy data are available, reserve **Zemdri** for use in patients who have limited or no alternative treatment options. Assess creatinine clearance in all patients prior to initiating therapy and daily during therapy. Adjustment of initial dose and therapeutic drug monitoring (TDM) is recommended in patients with renal impairment. There is insufficient information to recommend a dosing regimen in patients with CrCl <15 mL/min or on hemodialysis or continuous renal replacement therapy. For patients with CrCl ≥ 15 mL/min and <90 mL/min, TDM is recommended in order to avoid *plazomicin*-induced nephrotoxicity. Monitor *plazomicin* trough concentrations and adjust **Zemdri** as described in the mfr pkg insert. BBW: Aminoglycosides are associated with nephrotoxicity, ototoxicity, and neuromuscular blockade; therefore, administer **Zamdri** no faster than 30 minutes, monitor for adverse reactions, and stop the infusion if any of these adverse events occur. Aminoglycosides can cause fetal harm in pregnancy. There are no available data on the use of **Zamdri** in pregnancy to inform a drug-related risk of adverse developmental outcomes. *streptomycin*, an aminoglycoside, can cause total and irreversible in children whose mothers received *streptomycin* in pregnancy. There are no data on the presence of **Zemdri** in human milk or effects on the breastfed infant; therefore, potential risk/benefit should be discussed with the mother. The most common adverse reactions (incidence ≥1%) are decreased renal function, diarrhea, hypertension, headache, nausea, vomiting, and hypotension.

 URINARY TRACT INFECTION (UTI, CYSTITIS: ACUTE)

URINARY TRACT ANALGESIA

Comment: Except when contraindicated, *ibuprofen* or other inflammatory agent of choice is a recommended adjunct or monotherapy in the treatment of UTI dysuria, frequency, and urgency which is due to inflammation and associated smooth muscle spasms/colic.

OTC **AZO Standard**

OTC **AZO Standard Maximum Strength**

OTC **Prodium**

OTC **Uristat**

ANTISPASMODIC AGENT

➤ *flavoxate* (B)(G) 100-200 mg tid-qid
    Pediatric: <12 years: not recommended; >12 years: same as adult
      Urispas *Tab:* 100 mg
    Comment: *Flavoxate* hydrochloride tablets are indicated for symptomatic relief of dysuria, urgency, nocturia, suprapubic pain, frequency and incontinence as may occur in cystitis, prostatitis, urethritis, urethrocystitis/urethrotrigonitis. *Flavoxate* is not indicated for definitive treatment, but is compatible with drugs used for the treatment of UTI. *Flavoxate* is contraindicated in patients who have any of the following obstructive conditions: pyloric or duodenal obstruction, obstructive intestinal lesions, ileus, achalasia, GI hemorrhage, and obstructive uropathies of the lower urinary tract. Used with caution with glaucoma. It is not known whether *flavoxate* is excreted in human milk.

URINARY TRACT ANALGESIC-ANTISPASMODIC AGENTS

➤ *hyoscyamine* (C)(G)
      Anaspaz 1-2 tabs q 4 hours prn; max 12 tabs/day
        Tab: 0.125*mg
      Pediatric: <2 years: not recommended; 2-12 years: 0.0625-0.125 mg q 4 hours prn; max 0.75 mg/day; >12 years: same as adult
      Levbid 1-2 tabs q 12 hours prn; max 4 tabs/day
      Pediatric: <12 years: not recommended; ≥12 years: same as adult
        Tab: 0.375*mg ext-rel
      Levsin 1-2 tabs q 4 hours prn; max 12 tabs/day
      Pediatric: <6 years: not recommended; 6-12 years: 1 tab q 4 hours prn; ≥12 years: same as adult
        Tab: 0.125*mg
      Levsin Drops Use SL or PO forms
      Pediatric: 3.4 kg: 4 drops q 4 hours prn; max 24 drops/day; 5 kg: 5 drops q 4 hours prn; max 30 drops/day; 7 kg: 6 drops q 4 hours prn; max 36 drops/day; 10 kg: 8 drops q 4 hours prn; max 40 drops/day
        Oral drops: 0.125 mg/ml (15 ml) (orange) (alcohol 5%)
      Levsin Elixir 5 ml q 4 hours prn ←fix raised font left
      Pediatric: <10 kg: use drops; 10-19 kg: 1.25 ml q 4 hours prn; 20-39 kg: 2.5 ml q 4 hours prn; 40-49 kg: 3.75 ml q 4 hours prn; >50 kg:
        Elix: 0.125 mg/5 ml (16 oz) (orange) (alcohol 20%)
      Levsinex SL 1-2 tabs q 4 hours prn; max 12 tabs/day
      Pediatric: <2 years: not recommended; 2-12 years: 1 tab q 4 hours; max 6 tabs/day; >12 years: same as adult
        Tab: 0.125 mg sublingual
      Levsinex Timecaps 1-2 caps q 12 hours; may adjust to 1 cap q 8 hours
      Pediatric: <2 years: not recommended; 2-12 years: 1 cap q 12 hours; max 2 caps/day; >12 years: same as adult
        Cap: 0.375 mg time-rel
      NuLev dissolve 1-2 tabs on tongue, with or without water, q 4 hours prn; max 12 tabs/day
      Pediatric: <2 years: not recommended; 2-12 years: dissolve 1 tab on tongue, with or without water, q 4 hours prn; max 6 tabs/day; >12 years:
        ODT: 0.125 mg (mint) (phenylalanine)
➤ *methenamine+phenyl salicylate+methylene blue+benzoic acid+atropine sulfate+ hyoscyamine* (C)(G) 2 tabs qid prn
    Pediatric: <6 years: not recommended; ≥6 years: same as adult

Urised *Tab:* meth 40.8 mg+phenyl salic 18.1 mg+meth blue 5.4 mg+benz acid 4.5 mg+atro sulf 0.03 mg+hyoscy 0.03 mg

Comment: **Urised** imparts a blue-green color to urine which may stain fabrics.

▷ *methenamine+phenyl salicylate+methylene blue+sod phosphate monobasic+ hyoscyamine* (C) 1 cap qid prn

Pediatric: <6 years: not recommended; ≥6 years: same as adult

Uribel *Cap:* meth 118 mg+phenyl salic 36 mg+meth blue 10 mg+sod phos mono 40.8 mg+hyoscy 0.12 mg

▷ *methenamine+phenyl salicylate+methylene blue+sod biphosphate+hyoscyamine* (C) 1 tab qid prn

Pediatric: <6 years: not recommended; ≥6 years: same as adult

Urelle *Cap:* meth 81 mg+phenyl salic 32.4 mg+meth blue 10.8 mg+sod biphos 40.8 mg+hyoscy 0.12 mg

▷ *phenazopyridine* (B)(G) 100-200 mg q 6 hours prn; max 2 days

Pediatric: <12 years: not recommended; ≥12 years: same as adult

AZO Standard, Prodium, Uristat (OTC) *Tab:* 95 mg

AZO Standard Maximum Strength (OTC) *Tab:* 97.5 mg

Pyridium, Urogesic *Tab:* 100, 200 mg

Comment: *Phenazopyridine* imparts an orange-red color to urine which may stain fabrics.

ANTI-INFECTIVES

▷ *acetyl sulfisoxazole* (C)(G)

Gantrisin initially 2-4 gm in a single or divided doses; then, 4-8 gm/day in 4-6 divided doses x 3-10 days

Pediatric: <12 years: not recommended; ≥12 years: same as adult

Tab: 500 mg

Gantrisin initially 2-4 gm in a single or divided doses; then, 4-8 gm/day in 4-6 divided doses x 3-10 days

Pediatric: <2 months: not recommended; 2 months-12 years: initial dose 75 mg/kg/ day; then 150 mg/kg/day in 4-6 divided doses x 3-10 days; max 6 gm/ day; >12 years: same as adult

Oral susp: 500 mg/5 ml (4, 16 oz); *Syr:* 500 mg/5 ml (16 oz)

▷ *amoxicillin* (B)(G) 500-875 mg bid or 250-500 mg tid x 3-10 days

Pediatric: <40 kg (88 lb): 20-40 mg/kg/day in 3 divided doses x 10 days or 25-45 mg/kg/day in 2 divided doses 3-10 days; *see* Appendix CC.3. *amoxicillin* (Amoxil Suspension, Trimox Suspension) *for dose by weight table;* ≥40 kg: same as adult

Amoxil *Cap:* 250, 500 mg; *Tab:* 875*mg; *Chew tab:* 125, 200, 250, 400 mg (cherry-banana-peppermint) (phenylalanine); *Oral susp:* 125, 250 mg/5 ml (80, 100, 150 ml) (strawberry); 200, 400 mg/5 ml (50, 75, 100 ml) (bubble gum); *Oral drops:* 50 mg/ml (30 ml) (bubble gum)

Moxatag *Tab:* 775 mg ext-rel

Trimox *Tab:* 125, 250 mg; *Cap:* 250, 500 mg; *Oral susp:* 125, 250 mg/5 ml (80, 100, 150 ml) (raspberry-strawberry)

▷ *amoxicillin+clavulanate* (B)(G)

Augmentin 500 mg tid or 875 mg bid x 3-10 days

Pediatric: <40 kg: 40-45 mg/kg/day divided tid x 3-10 days or 90 mg/kg/ day divided bid x 10 days; *see* Appendix CC.4. *amoxicillin+clavulanate* (Augmentin Suspension) *for dose by weight table;* ≥40 kg: same as adult

Tab: 250, 500, 875 mg; *Chew tab:* 125, 250 mg (lemon-lime); 200, 400 mg (cherry-banana) (phenylalanine); *Oral susp:* 125 mg/5 ml (banana), 250 mg/5 ml (75, 100, 150 ml) (orange); 200, 400 mg/5 ml (50, 75, 100 ml) (orange) (phenylalanine)

Augmentin ES-600 <3 months: not recommended; ≥3 months, <40 kg: 90 mg/kg/day divided q 12 hours x 3-10 days; *see* Appendix CC.5. *amoxicillin+ clavulanate* (Augmentin ES 600 Suspension) *for dose by weight table;* ≥40 kg: not recommended

Oral susp: 600 mg/5 ml (50, 75, 100, 125, 150, 200 ml) (strawberry cream) (phenylalanine)

Augmentin XR <16 years: use other forms; ≥16 years: 2 tabs q 12 hours x 3-10 days

Tab: 1000*mg ext-rel

▷ *ampicillin* **(B)** 500 mg qid x 3-10 days
Pediatric: <12 years: 50-100 mg/kg/day in 4 divided doses x 3-10 days; *see* Appendix CC.6. *ampicillin* (Omnipen Suspension, Principen Suspension) *for dose by weight table;* ≥12 years: same as adult

Omnipen, Principen *Cap:* 250, 500 mg; *Oral susp:* 125, 250 mg/5 ml (100, 150, 200 ml) (fruit)

▷ *carbenicillin* **(B)** 1-2 tabs qid x 3-10 days
Pediatric: <12 years: not recommended; ≥12 years: same as adult

Geocillin *Tab:* 382 mg
Tab: 375, 500 mg ext-rel

▷ *cefaclor* **(B)(G)**
Ceclor 250 mg tid or 375 mg bid 3-10 days
Pediatric: <1 month: not recommended; 1 month-12 years: 20-40 mg/kg divided bid or q 12 hours x 3-10 days; max 1 gm/day; *see* Appendix CC.8. *cefaclor* (Ceclor Suspension) *for dose by weight;* >12 years: same as adult

Tab: 500 mg; *Cap:* 250, 500 mg; *Susp:* 125 mg/5 ml (75, 150 ml) (strawberry); 187 mg/5 ml (50, 100 ml) (strawberry); 250 mg/5 ml (75, 150 ml) (strawberry); 375 mg/5 ml (50, 100 ml) (strawberry)

Cefaclor Extended Release 375-500 mg bid x 3-10 days
Pediatric: <16 years: not recommended; ≥16 years: same as adult
Tab: 375, 500 mg ext-rel

▷ *cefadroxil* **(B)** 1-2 gm in a single or 2 divided doses x 3-10 days
Pediatric: <12 years: 30 mg/kg/day in 2 divided doses x 3-10 days; *see* Appendix CC.9. *cefadroxil* (Duricef Suspension) *for dose by weight table;* ≥12 years: same as adult

Duricef *Cap:* 500 mg; *Tab:* 1 gm; *Oral susp:* 250 mg/5 ml (100 ml); 500 mg/5 ml (75, 100 ml) (orange-pineapple)

▷ *cefixime* **(B)(G)** 400 mg once daily x 5 days
Pediatric: <6 months: not recommended; 6 months-12 years, <50 kg: 8 mg/kg/day in 1-2 divided doses x 5 days; *see* Appendix CC.11. *cefixime* (Suprax Oral Suspension) *for dose by weight table;* >12 years, >50 kg: same as adult

Suprax *Tab:* 400 mg; *Cap:* 400 mg; *Oral susp:* 100, 200, 500 mg/5 ml (50, 75, 100 ml) (strawberry)

▷ *cefpodoxime proxetil* **(B)** 100 mg bid x 3-10 days
Pediatric: <2 months: not recommended; 2 months-12 years: 10 mg/kg/day (max 400 mg/dose) or 5 mg/kg/day bid (max 200 mg/dose) x 3-10 days: *see* Appendix CC.12. *cefpodoxime proxetil* (Vantin Suspension) *for dose by weight table;* ≥12 years: same as adult

Vantin *Tab:* 100, 200 mg; *Oral susp:* 50, 100 mg/5 ml (50, 75, 100 mg) (lemon creme)

▷ *cephalexin* **(B)(G)** 500 mg bid x 3-10 days
Pediatric: <12 years: 25-50 mg/kg/day in 4 divided doses x 3-10 days; *see* Appendix CC.15. *cephalexin* (Keflex Suspension) *for dose by weight table;* ≥12 years:

Keflex *Cap:* 250, 333, 500, 750 mg; *Oral susp:* 125, 250 mg/5 ml (100, 200 ml) (strawberry)

▷ *ciprofloxacin* (C) 500 mg bid or 1000 mg XR once daily x 3-7 days
    Pediatric: <18 years: not recommended; ≥18 years: same as adult
        Cipro (G) *Tab:* 250, 500, 750 mg; *Oral susp:* 250, 500 mg/5 ml (100 ml)
        (strawberry)
        Cipro XR *Tab:* 500, 1000 mg ext-rel
        ProQuin XR *Tab:* 500 mg ext-rel
▷ *doxycycline* (D)(G) 100 mg bid x 3-10 days
    Pediatric: <8 years: not recommended; ≥8 years, <100 lb: 2 mg/lb on first day in 2
    divided doses, followed by 1 mg/lb/day in a single or 2 divided doses x 3-10 days;
    ≥8 years, ≥100 lb: same as adult
        Acticlate *Tab:* 75, 150**mg
        Adoxa *Tab:* 50, 75, 100, 150 mg ent-coat
        Doryx *Tab:* 50, 75, 100, 150, 200 mg del-rel
        Doxteric *Tab:* 50 mg del-rel
        Monodox *Cap:* 50, 75, 100 mg
        Oracea *Cap:* 40 mg del-rel
        Vibramycin *Tab:* 100 mg; *Cap:* 50, 100 mg; *Syr:* 50 mg/5 ml (raspberry-apple)
        (sulfites); *Oral susp:* 25 mg/5 ml (raspberry)
        Vibra-Tab *Tab:* 100 mg film-coat
▷ *enoxacin* (C) 200 mg q 12 hours x 3-10 days
    Pediatric: <18 years: not recommended; ≥18 years: same as adult
        Penetrex *Tab:* 200, 400 mg
▷ *fosfomycin* (B)(G) take as a single dose on an empty stomach; dissolve 1 sachet
    pkt in 3-4 oz cold water and drink immediately
    Pediatric: <12 years: not established; ≥12 years: same as adult
        Monurol *Single-dose sachet pkts:* 3 gm (mandarin orange) (saccharin, sucrose)
    Comment: *Fosfomycin tromethamine* is a single-dose synthetic, broad spectrum,
    bactericidal antibiotic for treatment of uncomplicated UTI. Repeat dosing does
    not improve clinical efficacy. Safety and effectiveness in children ≥12 years have
    not been established in adequate and well-controlled studies.
▷ *levofloxacin* (C) 250 mg once daily x 3-7 days
    Pediatric: <18 years: not recommended; ≥18 years: same as adult
        Levaquin *Tab:* 250, 500, 750 mg; *Oral soln:* 25 mg/ml (480 ml) (benzyl
        alcohol); *Inj conc:* 25 mg/ml for IV infusion after dilution (20, 30 ml single-use
        vial) (preservative-free); *Premix soln:* 5 mg/ml for IV infusion (50, 100, 150
        ml) (preservative-free)
▷ *lomefloxacin* (C) 400 mg once daily x 3-7 days
    Pediatric: <18 years: not recommended; ≥18 years: same as adult
        Maxaquin *Tab:* 400 mg
▷ *minocycline* (D)(G) 100 mg q 12 hours x 3-10 days
    Pediatric: <8 years: not recommended; ≥8 years, <100 lb: 1-2 mg/lb in 2 divided
    doses x 3-10 days; ≥8 years, ≥100 lb: same as adult
        Dynacin *Cap:* 50, 100 mg
        Minocin *Cap:* 50, 75, 100 mg; *Oral susp:* 50 mg/5 ml (60 ml) (custard)
        (sulfites, alcohol 5%)
▷ *nalidixic acid* (B) 1 gm qid x 3-10 days
    Pediatric: <3 months: not recommended; ≥3 months-<12 years: 25 mg/lb/day in 4
    divided doses x 3-10 days; ≥12 years: same as adult
        NegGram *Tab:* 250, 500 mg; 1 gm; *Cap:* 250, 500 mg; *Oral susp:* 250 mg/5 ml
▷ *nitrofurantoin* (B)(G)
        Furadantin 50-100 mg qid x 3-10 days
    Pediatric: <1 month: not recommended; ≥1 month-12 years: 5-7 mg/kg/ day in
    4 divided doses x 3-10 days; *see* Appendix CC.28. *nitrofurantoin* (Furadantin
    Suspension) *for dose by weight table;* >12 years: same as adult
        Oral susp: 25 mg/5 ml (60 ml)

Macrobid 100 mg q 12 hours x 3-10 days
Pediatric: <12 years: not recommended; ≥12 years: same as adult
Cap: 100 mg
Macrodantin 50-100 mg qid x 3-10 days
Pediatric: <12 years: not recommended; ≥12 years: same as adult
Cap: 25, 50, 100 mg

➤ *norfloxacin* (C) 400 mg once daily x 3-7 days
Pediatric: <18 years: not recommended; ≥18 years: same as adult
Noroxin *Tab:* 400 mg

➤ *ofloxacin* (C)(G) 200 mg q 12 hours x 3-7 days
Pediatric: <18 years: not recommended; ≥18 years: same as adult
Floxin *Tab:* 200, 300, 400 mg
Floxin UroPak *Tab:* 200 mg (6/pck)

➤ *trimethoprim* (C)(G)
Primsol 100 mg q 12 hours <u>or</u> 200 mg once daily x 10 days
Pediatric: <6 months: not recommended; ≥6 months-12 years: 10 mg/kg/ day
in 2 divided doses x 10 days; >12 years: same as adult
Oral soln: 50 mg/5 ml (bubble gum) (dye-free, alcohol-free)
Proloprim 100 mg q 12 hours <u>or</u> 200 mg once daily x 10 days
Pediatric: <12 years: not recommended; ≥12 years: same as adult
Tab: 100, 200 mg
Trimpex 100 mg q 12 hours <u>or</u> 200 mg once daily x 10 days
Pediatric: <12 years: not recommended; ≥12 years: same as adult
Tab: 100 mg

➤ *trimethoprim+sulfamethoxazole (TMP-SMX)* (D)(G)
Bactrim, Septra 2 tabs bid x 3-10 days
Pediatric: <12 years: not recommended; ≥12 years: same as adult
Tab: trim 80 mg+sulfa 400 mg*
Bactrim DS, Septra DS 1 tab bid x 3-10 days
Pediatric: <12 years: not recommended; ≥12 years: same as adult
Tab: trim 160 mg+sulfa 800 mg*
Bactrim Pediatric Suspension, Septra Pediatric Suspension use tabs
Pediatric: <2 months: not recommended; ≥2 months-12 years: 40 mg/kg/day
of *sulfamethoxazole* in 2 doses bid; >12 years: use tabs
Oral susp: trim 40 mg+sulfa 200 mg per 5 ml (100 ml) (cherry) (alcohol 0.3%)

PARENTERAL THERAPY FOR COMPLICATED cUTI

➤ *ertapenem* (B) 1 gm once daily; *CrCl <30 mL/min:* 500 mg once daily; treat x
10-14 days; may switch to an oral antibiotic after 3 days if warranted; *IV infusion:*
administer over 30 minutes; *IM injection:* reconstitute
Pediatric: <18 years: not recommended; ≥18 years same as adult
Invanz *Vial:* 1 gm pwdr for reconstitution

➤ *meropenem+vaborbactam* administer 4 gm (*meropenem* 2 gm and *vaborbactam*
2 gm) every 8 hours by IV infusion; administer over 3 hours; treat for up to 14
days; monitor urine cultures and eGFR; *eGFR 30-49 mL/min:* 2 gm (*meropenem*
1 gm and *vaborbactam* 1 gm) every 8 hours; *eGFR 15-29 mL/min:* 2 gm
(*meropenem* 1 gm and *vaborbactam* 1 gm) every 12 hours; *eGFR <15 mL/min:*
1 gm (*meropenem* 0.5 gm and *vaborbactam* 0.5 gm) every 12 hours; *ESRD:*
administer 1 gm (*meropenem* 0.5 gm and *vaborbactam* 0.5 gm) every 12 hours
after dialysis
Pediatric: <18 years: not recommended; ≥18 years same as adult
Vabomere *Vial:* mero 1 gm+vabor 1 gm pwdr for reconstitution and dilution
Comment: **Vabomere** (formerly **Carbavance**) is a carbapenem (*meropenem*)
and beta-lactamase inhibitor (*vaborbactam*) combination indicated for

the treatment of complicated urinary tract infection (cUTI) including pyelonephritis caused by *Escherichia coli*, *Klebsiella pneumoniae*, and *Enterobacter cloacae* species complex. Administer **Vabomere** with caution with history of hyper-sensitivity to penicillin, cephalosporin, other betalactams or other allergens. Discontinue immediately if allergic reaction occurs. **Vabomere** is not recommended with concomitant *valproic acid* or *divalproex sodium*. Discontinue **Vabomere** if *C. difficile*-associated diarrhea is suspected or confirmed. Monitor, and reevaluate risk/ benefit if signs of neuromotor impairment (e.g., seizures, focal tremors, myoclonus, delirium, paresthesias), renal impairment, thrombocytopenia, and/or superinfection.

LONG-TERM PROPHYLACTIC-SUPPRESSION THERAPY

▷ *methenamine hippurate* (C) 1 gm once daily
  Pediatric: <6 years: 0.25 gm/30 lb once daily; 6-12 years: 25-50 mg/kg/day once daily or 0.5-1 gm once daily; >12 years:
    Hiprex *Tab:* 1 gm; *Oral susp:* 500 mg/5 ml (480 ml)
    Urex *Tab:* 1 gm; *Oral susp:* 500 mg/5 ml (480 ml)
▷ *nitrofurantoin* (B)(G)
    Furadantin 50-100 mg as a single dose at bedtime
    Pediatric: <1 month: not recommended; ≥1 month-12 years: 1 mg/kg as a single dose at bedtime; >12 years: same as adult
      Oral susp: 25 mg/5 ml (60 ml)
    Macrobid 50-100 mg as a single dose at bedtime
    Pediatric: <12 years: not recommended; ≥12 years: same as adult
      Cap: 100 mg
    Macrodantin 50-100 mg as a single dose at bedtime
    Pediatric: <12 years: not recommended; ≥12 years: same as adult
      Cap: 25, 50, 100 mg
    Furadantin 50-100 mg as a single dose at bedtime
    Pediatric: <12 years: not recommended; ≥12 years: same as adult
      Oral susp: 25 mg/5 ml (60 ml)
    Macrobid 100 mg as a single dose at bedtime
    Pediatric: <12 years: not recommended; ≥12 years: same as adult
      Cap: 100 mg
    Macrodantin 50-100 mg as a single dose at bedtime
    Pediatric: <12 years: not recommended; ≥12 years: same as adult
      Cap: 25, 50, 100 mg

UROLITHIASIS (RENAL CALCULI, KIDNEY STONES)

Acetaminophen for IV Infusion *see Pain*
NSAIDs *see* Appendix J. NSAIDs online at https://connect.springerpub.com/content/reference-book/978-0-8261-7935-7/back-matter/part02/back-matter/bmatter10
Opioid Analgesics *see Pain*

PREVENTION OF CALCIUM STONES

▷ *chlorothiazide* (B)(G) 50 mg bid
  Pediatric: <6 months: up to 15 mg/lb/day in 2 divided doses; ≥6 months-12 years: 10 mg/lb/day in 2 divided doses; max 375 mg/day; >12 years: Same as adult
    Diuril *Tab:* 250*, 500*mg; *Oral susp:* 250 mg/5 ml (237 ml)
▷ *hydrochlorothiazide* (B)(G) 50 mg bid
  Pediatric: <12 years: not recommended; ≥12 years: same as adult
    Esidrix *Tab:* 25, 50 mg
    Microzide *Cap:* 12.5 mg

PREVENTION OF CYSTINE STONES

▷ *penicillamine* administer on an empty stomach, at least 1 hour before meals or 2 hours after meals, and at least 1 hour apart from any other drug, food, milk, antacid, zinc or iron-containing preparation; usual dose is 2000-4,000 mg/day; maintenance dosage must be individualized, and may require adjustment during the course of treatment; initially, a single daily dose of 125-250 mg; then, increase at 1-3 month intervals by 125-250 mg/day, as patient response and tolerance indicate; if a satisfactory remission of symptoms is achieved, the dose associated with the remission should be continued as the patient's maintenance therapy; if there is no improvement, and there are no signs of potentially serious toxicity after 2-3 months of treatment with doses of 500-750 mg/day, increase by 250 mg/day at 2-3 month intervals until a satisfactory remission occurs or signs of toxicity develop; if there is no discernible improvement after 3-4 months of treatment, discontinue **Cuprimine**. Changes in maintenance dosage levels may not be reflected clinically or in the erythrocyte sedimentation rate (ESR) for 2-3 months after each dosage adjustment.

    Cuprimine *Cap:* 125, 250 mg
    Depen: 250 mg

Comment: The use of *penicillamine* has been associated with fatalities due to certain diseases such as aplastic anemia, agranulocytosis, thrombocytopenia, Goodpasture's syndrome, and myasthenia gravis. Because of the potential for serious hematological and renal adverse reactions to occur at any time, routine urinalysis, white and differential blood cell count, hemoglobin, and direct platelet count must be checked twice weekly, together with monitoring of the patient's skin, lymph nodes and body temperature, during the first month of therapy, every 2 weeks for the next 5 months, and monthly thereafter. Patients should be instructed to report promptly the development of signs and symptoms of granulocytopenia and/or thrombocytopenia such as fever, sore throat, chills, bruising or bleeding; the above laboratory studies should then be promptly repeated.

▷ *potassium citrate* (C)(G) 30 mEq qid
Pediatric: <12 years: not recommended; ≥12 years: same as adult
    Urocit-K *Tab:* 5, 10, 15 mEq ext-rel

Comment: *Potassium citrate* is contraindicated in hyperkalemia. Encourage patients to limit salt intake and maintain liberal hydration (urine volume should be at least 2 liters/day). Target urine pH is 6.0-7.0 and urine citrate at least 320 mg/day and close to the normal mean of 640 mg/day. Take with food.

PREVENTION OF URIC ACID STONES

▷ *allopurinol* (C)(G) 200-300 mg in 1-3 doses; max 800 mg/day; max single dose 300 mg
Pediatric: <6 years: max 150 mg/day; 6-10 years: max 400 mg/day; max single dose 300 mg; >10 years: same as adult
    Zyloprim *Tab:* 100*, 300*mg

▷ *potassium citrate* (C)(G) 30 mEq qid
    Urocit-K *Tab:* 5, 10, 15 mEq ext-rel

Comment: *Potassium citrate* is contraindicated in hyperkalemia. Encourage patients to limit salt intake and maintain liberal hydration (urine volume should be at least 2 liters/day). Target urine pH is 6.0-7.0 and urine citrate at least 320 mg/day and close to the normal mean of 640 mg/day. Take with food.

ALPHA-1A BLOCKERS

Comment: Alpha-1A blockers facilitate stone passage.

▷ *alfuzosin* (B)(G) 10 mg once daily taken immediately after the same meal each day
    UroXatral *Tab:* 10 mg ext-rel

▷ *tamsulosin* (B)(G) initially 0.4 mg once daily; may increase to 0.8 mg once daily after 2-4 weeks if needed

Pediatric: ≤18 years: with radiopaque lower ureteral stones of 10-12 mm or smaller have received the following doses: *tamsulosin* 0.2 mg PO at bedtime (≤4 years) and 0.4 mg PO at bedtime (>4 years); administer x 28 days or until definite stone passage (i.e., evidence of stone on urine straining); >18 years:

Flomax *Cap:* 0.4 mg

Comment: *Tamsulosin* 0.4 mg may be taken with **Avodart** 0.5 mg once daily as combination therapy. *Tamsulosin* is taken with standard analgesia (e.g., ibuprofen); mild somnolence is common. If pain is controlled with oral analgesia, clear liquids are tolerated, and there is no evidence of infection, monitor closely for spontaneous passage for 3-4 weeks prior to definitive therapy, since most data demonstrate safe lower uretal stone expulsion in the first 10 days of conservative medical management.

ANTISPASMODIC AGENT

▷ *flavoxate* (B)(G) 100-200 mg tid-qid

Pediatric: <12 years: not recommended; >12 years: same as adult

Urispas *Tab:* 100 mg

Comment: *Flavoxate* hydrochloride tablets are indicated for symptomatic relief of dysuria, urgency, nocturia, suprapubic pain, frequency and incontinence as may occur in cystitis, prostatitis, urethritis, urethrocystitis/urethrotrigonitis. *Flavoxate* is not indicated for definitive treatment, but is compatible with drugs used for the treatment of UTI. flavoxate is contraindicated in patients who have any of the following obstructive conditions: pyloric or duodenal obstruction, obstructive intestinal lesions, ileus, achalasia, GI hemorrhage, and obstructive uropathies of the lower urinary tract. Used with caution with glaucoma. It is not known whether *flavoxate* is excreted in human milk.

ACETAMINOPHEN FOR IV INFUSION

▷ *acetaminophen* injectable (B) administer by IV infusion over 15 minutes; 1,000 mg q 6 hours prn or 650 mg q 4 hours prn; max 4000 mg/day

Pediatric: <2 years: not recommended; 2-13 years <50 kg: 15 mg/kg q 6 hours prn or 2.5 mg/kg q 4 hours prn; max 750 mg/single dose; max 75 mg/kg per day; >13 years: same as adult

Ofirmev *Vial:* 10 mg/ml (100 ml) (preservative-free)

Comment: The Ofirmev vial is intended for single-use. If any portion is withdrawn from the vial, use within 6 hours. Discard the unused portion. For pediatric patients, withdraw the intended dose and administer via syringe pump. Do not admix Ofirmev with any other drugs. Ofirmev is physically incompatible with *diazepam* and *chlorpromazine hydrochloride*.

IBUPROFEN FOR IV INFUSION

▷ *ibuprofen* (B) dilute dose in 0.9% NS, D5W, or Lactated Ringers (LR) solution; administer by IV infusion over at least 10 minutes; do not administer via IV bolus or IM; 400-800 mg q 6 hours prn; maximum 3,200 mg/day

Pediatric: <6 months; not recommended; 6 months-<12 years: 10 mg/kg q 4-6 hours prn; max 400 mg/dose; max 40 mg/kg or 2,400 mg/24 hours, whichever is less; 12-17 years: 400 mg q 4-6 hours prn; max 2,400 mg/24 hours

Caldolor *Vial:* 800 mg/8 ml single-dose

Comment: Prepare Caldolor solution for IV administration as follows: 100 mg dose: dilute 1 ml of Caldolor in at least 100 ml of diluent (IVF); 200 mg dose: dilute 2 ml of Caldolor in at least 100 ml of diluent; 400 mg dose: dilute 4 ml of Caldolor in at least 100 ml of diluent; 800 mg dose: dilute 8 ml of Caldolor in at least 200 ml of diluent. Caldolor is also indicated for management of fever. For adults with fever, 400 mg via IV infusion, followed by 400 mg q 4-6 hours or 100-200 mg q 4 hours prn.

MU OPIOID ANALGESICS

▷ **tramadol** (C)(IV)(G)

Rybix ODT initially 100 mg once daily; may increase by 100 mg every 5 days; max 300 mg/day; *CrCl <30 mL/min or severe hepatic impairment:* not recommended; *Cirrhosis:* max 50 mg q 12 hours

Pediatric: <12 years: contraindicated; 12-<18: use extreme caution; not recommended for children and adolescents with obesity, asthma, obstructive sleep apnea, or other chronic breathing problem, or for post-tonsillectomy/ adenoidectomy pain; ≥18 years: same as adult

  ODT: 50 mg (mint) (phenylalanine)

Ryzolt initially 100 mg once daily; may increase by 100 mg every 5 days; max 300 mg/day; *CrCl <30 mL/min or severe hepatic impairment:* not recommended

Pediatric: <12 years: contraindicated; 12-<18: use extreme caution; not recommended for children and adolescents with obesity, asthma, obstructive sleep apnea, or other chronic breathing problem, or for post-tonsillectomy/ adenoidectomy pain; ≥18 years: same as adult

  Tab: 100, 200, 300 mg ext-rel

Ultram 50-100 mg q 4-6 hours prn; max 400 mg/day; *CrCl <30 mL/min,* max 100 mg q 12 hours; cirrhosis, max 50 mg q 12 hours

Pediatric: <12 years: contraindicated; 12-<18: use extreme caution; not recommended for children and adolescents with obesity, asthma, obstructive sleep apnea, or other chronic breathing problem, or for post-tonsillectomy/ adenoidectomy pain; ≥18 years: same as adult

  Tab: 50*mg

Ultram ER initially 100 mg once daily; may increase by 100 mg every 5 days; max 300 mg/day; *CrCl <30 mL/min or severe hepatic impairment:* not recommended

Pediatric: <12 years: contraindicated; 12-<18: use extreme caution; not recommended for children and adolescents with obesity, asthma, obstructive sleep apnea, or other chronic breathing problem, or for post-tonsillectomy/ adenoidectomy pain; ≥18 years: same as adult

  Tab: 100, 200, 300 mg ext-rel

▷ **tramadol+acetaminophen** (C)(IV)(G) 2 tabs q 4-6 hours; max 8 tabs/day x 5 days; *CrCl <30 mL/min:* max 2 tabs q 12 hours; max 4 tabs/day x 5 days

Pediatric: <12 years: contraindicated; 12-<18: use extreme caution; not recommended for children and adolescents with obesity, asthma, obstructive sleep apnea, or other chronic breathing problem, or for post-tonsillectomy/ adenoidectomy pain; same as adult

  Ultracet *Tab:* tram 37.5+acet 325 mg

INTRANASAL (TRANSMUCOSAL) OPIOID ANALGESICS

▷ **butorphanol tartrate** nasal spray (C)(IV) initially 1 spray (1 mg) in one nostril and may repeat after 60-90 minutes in opposite nostril if needed or 1 spray in each nostril and may repeat q 3-4 hours prn

Pediatric: <18 years: not recommended; ≥18 years: same as adult

  Butorphanol Nasal Spray *Nasal spray:* 1 mg/actuation (10 mg/ml, 2.5 ml)
  Stadol Nasal Spray *Nasal spray:* 1 mg/actuation (10 mg/ml, 2.5 ml)

▷ **fentanyl** nasal spray (C)(II) initially 1 spray (100 mcg) in one nostril and may repeat after 2 hours; when adequate analgesia is achieved, use that dose for subsequent breakthrough episodes; *Titration steps:* 100 mcg using 1 x 100 mcg spray; 200 mcg using 2 x 100 mcg spray (1 spray in each nostril); 400 mcg using

1 x 400 mcg spray; 800 mcg using 2 x 400 mcg (1 spray in each nostril); max 800 mcg; limit to ≤4 doses per day

Pediatric: <18 years: not recommended; ≥18 years: same as adult

Lazanda Nasal Spray *Nasal spray:* 100, 400 mcg/100 mcl (8 sprays/bottle)

Comment: **Lazanda Nasal Spray** is available by restricted distribution program. Call 855-841-4234 or visit https://www.fda.gov/downloads/drugs/drugsafety/postmarketdrugsafetyinformationforpatientsandproviders/ucm261983.pdf to enroll. **Lazanda Nasal Spray** is indicated for the management of breakthrough pain in cancer patients who are already receiving and who are tolerant to opioid therapy for their underlying persistent cancer pain. Patients considered opioid tolerant are those who are taking at least 60 mg of oral morphine/day, 25 mcg of transdermal *fentanyl*/hour, 30 mg oral *oxycodone*/day, 8 mg oral *hydromorphone*/day, 25 mg oral *oxymorphone*/day, or an equianalgesic dose of another opioid for a week or longer. Patients must remain on around-the-clock opioids when using **Lazanda Nasal Spray**. As such, it is contraindicated in the management of acute or post-op pain, including headache/migraine, or dental pain.

Comment: The Transmucosal Immediate Release Fentanyl (TIRF) Risk Evaluation and Mitigation Strategy (REMS) program is an FDA-required program designed to ensure informed risk-benefit decisions before initiating treatment, and while patients are treated to ensure appropriate use of TIRF medicines. The purpose of the TIRF REMS Access program is to mitigate the risk of misuse, abuse, addiction, overdose and serious complications due to medication errors with the use of TIRF medicines. You must enroll in the TIRF REMS Access program to prescribe, dispense, or distribute TIRF medicines.

 URTICARIA: MILD-TO-ACUTE HIVES AND CHRONIC SPONTANEOUS/IDIOPATHIC URTICARIA (CSU/CIU)

Topical Corticosteroids *see* Appendix K. Topical Corticosteroids by Potency
Oral Corticosteroids *see* Appendix L. Oral Corticosteroids
Parenteral Corticosteroids *see* Appendix M. Parenteral Corticosteroids

MILD-TO-MODERATE URTICARIA (HIVES, ANGIOEDEMA)
Second Generation Oral Antihistamines

Comment: The following drugs are second-generation antihistamines. As such they minimally sedating, much less so than the first-generation antihistamines. All antihistamines are excreted into breast milk.

▷ *cetirizine* (C)(OTC)(G) initially 5-10 mg once daily; 5 mg once daily; ≥65 years: use with caution

Pediatric: <6 years: not recommended; ≥6 years: same as adult

  cetirizine Cap: 10 mg

  Children's Zyrtec Chewable *Chew tab:* 5, 10 mg (grape)

  Children's Zyrtec Allergy Syrup *Syr:* 1 mg/ml (4 oz) (grape, bubble gum) (sugar-free, dye-free)

  Zyrtec *Tab:* 10 mg

  Zyrtec Hives Relief *Tab:* 10 mg

  Zyrtec Liquid Gels *Liq gel:* 10 mg

▷ *desloratadine* (C)

  Clarinex 1/2-1 tab once daily

  Pediatric: <6 years: not recommended; ≥6 years: same as adult

    Tab: 5 mg

  Clarinex RediTabs 5 mg once daily

Pediatric: <6 years: not recommended; 6-12 years: 2.5 mg once daily; ≥12 years: same as adult

    ODT: 2.5, 5 mg (tutti-frutti) (phenylalanine)

Clarinex Syrup 5 mg (10 ml) once daily

Pediatric: <6 months: not recommended; 6-11 months: 1 mg (2 ml) once daily; 1-5 years: 1.25 mg (2.5 ml) once daily; 6-11 years: 2.5 mg (5 ml) once daily; ≥12 years: same as adult

    Syr: 0.5 mg per ml (4 oz) (tutti-frutti) (phenylalanine)

Desloratadine ODT 1 tab once daily

Pediatric: <6 years: not recommended; 6-11 years: 1/2 tab once daily; ≥12 years: same as adult

    ODT: 5 mg

▶ *fexofenadine* (C)(OTC)(G) 60 mg once daily-bid <u>or</u> 180 mg once daily; *CrCl <90 mL/min:* 60 mg once daily

Pediatric: <6 months: not recommended; 6 months-2 years: 15 mg bid; *CrCl ≤90 mL/min:* 15 mg once daily; 2-11 years: 30 mg bid; *CrCl ≤90 mL/min:* 30 mg once daily; ≥12 years: same as adult

    Allegra *Tab:* 30, 60, 180 mg film-coat

    Allegra Allergy *Tab:* 60, 180 mg film-coat

    Allegra ODT *ODT:* 30 mg (phenylalanine)

    Allegra Oral Suspension *Oral susp:* 30 mg/5 ml (6 mg/ml) (4 oz)

▶ *levocetirizine* (B)(OTC)(G) administer dose in the PM; *Seasonal Allergic Rhinitis:* <2 years: <u>not</u> recommended; may start at ≥2 years; *Chronic Idiopathic Urticaria (CIU), Perennial Allergic Rhinitis:* <6 months: <u>not</u> recommended; may start at ≥ 6 months; *Dosing by Age:* 6 months-5 years: max 1.25 mg once daily; 6-11 years: max 2.5 mg once daily; ≥12 years: 2.5-5 mg once daily; *Renal Dysfunction <12 years:* contraindicated; *Renal Dysfunction ≥12 years:* CrCl 50-80 ml/min: 2.5 mg once daily; CrCl 30-50 mL/min: 2.5 mg every other day; CrCl: 10-30 mL/min: 2.5 mg twice weekly (every 3-4 days); CrCl <10 mL/min, ESRD <u>or</u> hemodialysis: contraindicated

    Children's Xyzal Allergy 24HR *Oral Soln:* 0.5 mg/ml (150 ml)

    Xyzal Allergy 24HR *Tab:* 5*mg

▶ *loratadine* (C)(OTC)(G) 5 mg bid <u>or</u> 10 mg once daily; *Hepatic <u>or</u> Renal Insufficiency:* see mfr pkg insert

Pediatric: <2 years: not recommended; 2-5 years: 5 mg once daily; ≥6 years: same as adult

    Children's Claritin Chewables *Chew tab:* 5 mg (grape) (phenylalanine)

    Children's Claritin Syrup 1 mg/ml (4 oz) (fruit) (sugar-free, alcohol-free, dye-free; sodium 6 mg/5 ml)

    Claritin *Tab:* 10 mg

    Claritin Hives Relief *Tab:* 10 mg

    Claritin Liqui-Gels *Liq gel:* 10 mg

    Claritin RediTabs 12 Hours *ODT:* 5 mg (mint)

    Claritin RediTabs 24 Hours *ODT:* 10 mg (mint)

First Generation Oral Antihistamines

▶ *diphenhydramine* (B)(G) 25-50 mg q 6-8 hours; max 100 mg/day

Pediatric: <2 years: not recommended; 2-6 years: 6.25 mg q 4-6 hours; max 37.5 mg/day; >6-12 years: 12.5-25 mg q 4-6 hours; max 150 mg/day; >12 years: same as adult

    Benadryl (OTC) *Chew tab:* 12.5 mg (grape) (phenylalanine); *Liq:* 12.5 mg/5 ml (4, 8 oz); *Cap:* 25 mg; *Tab:* 25 mg; *Dye-free soft gel:* 25 mg; *Dye-free liq:* 12.5 mg/5 ml (4, 8 oz)

▶ *hydroxyzine* (C)(G) 50 mg/day divided qid prn; 50-100 mg/day divided qid prn

Pediatric: <6 years: 50 mg/day divided qid prn; ≥6 years: same as adult

Atarax *Tab:* 10, 25, 50, 100 mg; *Syr:* 10 mg/5 ml (alcohol 0.5%)
Vistaril *Cap:* 25, 50, 100 mg; *Oral susp:* 25 mg/5 ml (4 oz) (lemon)
Comment: *Hydroxyzine* is contraindicated in early pregnancy and in patients with a prolonged QT interval. It is not known whether this drug is excreted in human milk; therefore, *hydroxyzine* should not be given to nursing mothers.

SEVERE URTICARIA

Parenteral Antihistamine

▷ *cetirizine* **for IV injection** 10 mg IV once every 24 hours prn
Pediatric: <6 months: not established; 6 months-5 years: 2.5 mg IV; 6-11 years: 5-10 mg IV (depending on severity); ≥12 years: same as adult
Quzyttir *Vial:* 10 mg/ml (1 ml), single-use
Comment: **Quzyttir** *(cetirizine)* is a histamine-1 (H1) receptor antagonist indicated for the treatment of acute urticaria in adults and children ≥6 months-of-age. Contraindications to **Quzyttir** include known hypersensitivity to *cetirizine hcl* or any of its ingredients, *levocetirizine,* or *hydroxyzine.* Patients should be warned about potential somnolence/sedation and to exercise caution when driving a car or operating potentially dangerous machinery. The most common adverse reactions (incidence <1%) with **Quzyttir** have been dysgeusia, headache, paresthesia, presyncope, dyspepsia, feeling hot, and hyperhidrosis.

▷ *diphenhydramine* **injectable (B)(G)** 25-50 mg IM immediately; then q 6 hours prn
Pediatric: <12 years: *See mfr pkg insert:* 1.25 mg/kg up to 25 mg IM x 1 dose; then q 6 hours prn; ≥12 years: same as adult
Benadryl Injectable *Vial:* 50 mg/ml (1 ml single-use); 50 mg/ml (10 ml multi-dose);
Amp: 10 mg/ml (1 ml); *Prefilled syringe:* 50 mg/ml (1 ml)

Parenteral Epinephrine

▷ *epinephrine* **(C)** 1:1000 0.01 ml/kg SC; max 0.3 ml
Pediatric: 0.01 mg/kg SC

CHRONIC SPONTANEOUS/IDIOPATHIC URTICARIA

IgE Blocker (IgG1k Monoclonal Antibody)

Comment: **Xolair** *(omalizumab)* is a humanized monoclonal antibody that specifically binds to free immunoglobulin E in the blood and on the surface of selected B lymphocytes, but not on the surface of mast cells, antigen-presenting dendritic cells, or basophils. In the US *omalizumab* is approved for adults at 150 mg or 300 mg subcutaneously administered every 4 weeks for the treatment of CSU not responsive to high-dose antihistamines. In three published, pivotal, phase 3 randomized trials, the clinical response rate to **omalizumab** at 300 mg every 4 weeks, as defined by a weekly 7-day Urticaria Activity Score (UAS7) ≤6 at 12 weeks, was 52% in ASTERIA I, 66% in ASTERIA II, and 52% in GLACIAL. Good control of disease activity was defined as a UAS7 score of ≤6 on the 0- to 42-point UAS7, which correlates well with minimal or no patient symptoms

Comment: A multicenter open-label study of 286 patients with CSU, conducted by the Catalan and Balearic Chronic Urticaria Network (XUrCB) at 15 hospitals, found about two-thirds of patients with CSU treated with the approved dose of *omalizumab* achieved good disease control. Three-quarters of the non-responders achieved good disease control upon up-dosing to 450 or 600 mg (twice the approved dose) every 4 weeks, without increase in adverse events.

▷ *omalizumab* (B) 150-375 mg SC every 2-4 weeks based on body weight and pre-treatment serum total IgE level; max 150 mg/injection site; approved for patient self-administration after education by a qualified health care provider
Pediatric: <12 years: not recommended; ≥12 years: 30-90 kg + IgE >30-100 IU/ml 150 mg q 4 weeks; 90-150 kg + IgE >30-100 IU/ml or 30-90 kg + IgE >100-200 IU/ml or 30-60 kg + IgE >200-300 IU/ml 300 mg q 4 hours; >90-150 kg + IgE >100-200 IU/ml or >60-90 kg + IgE >200-300 IU/ml or 30-70 kg + IgE >300-400 IU/ml 225 mg q 2 weeks; >90-150 kg + IgE >200-300 IU/ml or >70-90 kg + IgE >300-400 IU/ml or 30-70 kg + IgE >400-500 IU/ml or 30-60 kg + IgE >500-600 IU/ml or 30-60 kg + IgE >600-700 IU/ml 375 mg q 2 weeks
　　Xolair *Vial:* 150 mg, single-dose, pwdr for SC injection after reconstitution; *Prefilled syringe:* 75 mg/0.5 ml, 150 mg/1 ml, single-dose (preservative-free)

UTERINE LEIOMYOMATA (FIBROIDS)

See **Progesterone-only Contraceptives**

▷ *medroxyprogesterone acetate* (X) 10 mg daily
　　Provera *Tab:* 2.5, 5, 10 mg
▷ *Oral contraceptives* (X) with 35 mcg estrogen equivalent

SELECTIVE PROGESTERONE RECEPTOR MODULATOR

▷ *ulipristal acetate (UPA)* (X)(G) 5-10 mg once daily
　　Comment: *Ulipristal acetate* is currently approved in the US as an emergency contraceptive (a single 30 mg dose), but is marketed for treating symptomatic fibroids in Canada and Europe. It is not yet available in a dose form appropriate for treatment of uterine fibroids (i.e., 5, 10 mg). The drug reduced dysfunctional uterine bleeding in about 90% of patients in the European trials. Women with uterine fibroids taking UPA experienced significant improvement of quality of life, compared with those taking placebo according to researchers' reported outcomes of VENUS II, a phase 3, prospective, randomized, double-blind, double-dummy, placebo-controlled study. Its design incorporated both parallel and crossover elements: Some patients who were on placebo crossed over to one of two doses of UPA after a washout period, and some patients on each active arm crossed over to placebo. The women (n = 432) were between 18 and 50 years and pre-menopausal. At 13 weeks, uterine bleeding was controlled in 91% of the women receiving 5 mg of *ulipristal acetate*, 92% of those receiving 10 mg of *ulipristal* acetate, and 19% of those receiving placebo (P<0.001). Of women taking 5 mg of UPA, 91% achieved control (40.5%-42% became amenorrheic); of those taking 10 mg, 92% achieved control (54.8%-57.3% became amenorrheic) (controlled in 92%). These results compared to amenorrhea rates of 0%-8% (controlled in 19%) for women on placebo (*p*< .0001 for all values).
　　Ella *Tab:* 30 mg
　　Logilia *Tab:* 30 mg

GONADOTROPIN-RELEASING HORMONE (GnRH) RECEPTOR AGONIST + ESTROGEN + PROGESTIN

▷ *elagolix* 300 mg+*estradiol* 1 mg+*norethindrone acetate* 0.5 mg plus *elagolix* 300 mg take one Morning (AM) Capsule (*elagolix* 300 mg, *estradiol* 1 mg, *norethindrone acetate* 0.5 mg) in the morning and take one Evening (PM) capsule (*elagolix* 300 mg) in the evening for up to 24 months; exclude pregnancy before starting **Oriahnn** or start **Oriahnn** within 7 days from the onset of menses take doses at approximately the same time each day; take with or without food
　　Oriahnn *Morning (AM) Cap:* (*elagolix* 300 mg+*estradiol* 1 mg+*norethindrone acetate* 0.5 mg plus *Evening (PM) Cap:* *elagolix* 300 mg (tartrazine)

Comment: **Oriahnn** gonadotropin-releasing hormone (GnRH) receptor antagonist, estrogen and progestin co-formulation indicated for the management of heavy menstrual bleeding associated with uterine leiomyomas (fibroids) in pre-menopausal women. The following are contraindications to use of **Oriahnn**: pregnancy, high risk of arterial, venous thrombotic, or thromboembolic disorder, known osteoporosis, current or history of breast cancer or other hormonally-sensitive malignancy, known liver impairment or disease, undiagnosed abnormal uterine bleeding, women over 35 years-of-age who smoke, women with uncontrolled hypertension, known hypersensitivity to ingredients of **Oriahnn**, and organic anion transporting polypeptide (OATP)1B1 inhibitors that are known or expected to significantly increase *elagolix* plasma concentrations. Use of **Oriahnn** should be limited to 24 months due to the risk of continued bone loss, which may not be reversible. The most common adverse reaction (incidence >5%) in clinical trials have been hot flushes, headache, fatigue, and metrorrhagia.Exclude pregnancy before initiating treatment with **Oriahnn** and discontinue **Oriahnn** if pregnancy occurs during treatment. There is no information on the presence of *elagolix* in human milk or effects on the breastfed infant.

UVEITIS: POSTERIOR, CHRONIC, NON-INFECTIOUS

INTRAVITREAL IMPLANT

▷ *fluocinolone acetonide* surgical intravitreal injection is administered by a qualified healthcare provider under sterile conditions in the office/clinic/hospital setting; the implant is a 36-month sustained-release system

Yutiq 0.18 mg non-bioerodible intravitreal implant, single-dose, preloaded applicator w. 25 g needle , for ophthalmic intravitreal injection

Comment: **Yutiq** is indicated for the treatment of macular edema, diabetic macular edema, and chronic non-infectious posterior uveitis. Placement of a **Yutiq** intravitreal implant is contraindicated with active infection (e.g., ocular herpes simplex, acute blepharoconjunctivitis) or glaucoma. Use of **Yutiq** may increase of risk of cataract development. Post-procedure blurring of vision which should clear within 4 weeks. Avoid driving and hazardous activity until vision returns to baseline. If both eyes require treatment, the implants should be placed on separate dates to decrease risk of infection in both eyes.

VAGINAL IRRITATION: EXTERNAL

OTC Replens Vaginal Moisturizer
OTC Vagisil Intimate Moisturizer
Comment: **Vagisil** products have no effect on condom integrity.

VARICOSE VEINS

▷ *sodium tetradecyl sulfate* (C) generally, the 1% solution will be found most useful with the 3% solution preferred for larger varicosities; volume should be kept small, using 0.5 to 2 ml per site (preferably 1 ml max); max 10 ml per treatment session

Sotradecol *Vial:* 1% (20 mg/2ml, 10 mg/ml, 2 ml); 3% (60 mg/2 ml, 30 mg/ml, 2 ml), multi-dose

Comment: **Sotradecol** *(sodium tetradecyl sulfate)* is indicated in the treatment of small uncomplicated varicose veins of the lower extremities that show simple dilation with competent valves. Benefit-to-risk ratio should be considered in selected patients who are great surgical risks. It is not known whether **Sotradecol** can cause fetal harm when administered to a pregnant female or whether **Sotradecol** is excreted in human milk.

VERTIGO

▷ *meclizine* (B)(G) 25-100 mg/day in divided doses
Pediatric: <12 years: not established; ≥12 years: same as adult
  Antivert *Tab:* 12.5, 25, 50*mg
  Bonine (OTC) *Cap:* 15, 25, 30 mg; *Tab:* 12.5, 25, 50 mg; *Chew tab/Film-coat tab:* 25 mg
  Dramamine II (OTC) *Tab:* 25*mg
  Zentrip *Strip:* 25 mg orally-disint
▷ *methscopolamine bromide* (B) 1 tab q 6 hours prn
Pediatric: <12 years: not recommended; ≥12 years: same as adult
  Pamine *Tab:* 2.5 mg
  Pamine Forte *Tab:* 5 mg
▷ *scopolamine* (C) 0.4-0.8 mg tab (may repeat in 8 hours) or 1 x 1.5 mg transdermal patch behind ear (effective x 3 days; may replace every 4th day)
Pediatric: <12 years: not recommended; ≥12 years: same as adult
  Scopace *Tab:* 0.4 mg
  Transderm Scop *Transdermal patch:* 1.5 mg (4/carton)

VITILIGO

RE-PIGMENTATION AGENTS

▷ *methoxsalen* (C) Apply to well-defined area of vitiligo; then expose area to source of UVA (ultraviolet A) or sunlight; initial exposure no more than 1/2 predicted minimal erythemal dose; repeat weekly
Pediatric: <12 years: not recommended; ≥12 years: same as adult
  Oxsoralen *Lotn:* 1% (30 ml)
Comment: *Methoxsalen* may only be applied by a healthcare provider. Do not dispense to patient.
▷ *trioxsalen* (C) 10 mg daily, taken 2-4 hours before ultraviolet light exposure; max 14 days and 28 tabs
Pediatric: <12 years: not recommended; ≥12 years: same as adult
  Trisoralen *Tab:* 5 mg

DEPIGMENTING AGENTS

▷ *hydroquinone* (C)(G) apply sparingly to affected area and rub in bid
  Lustra *Crm:* 4% (1, 2 oz) (sulfites)
  Lustra AF *Crm:* 4% (1, 2 oz) (sunscreen, sulfites)
▷ *monobenzone* (C) apply sparingly to affected area and rub in bid-tid; depigmentation occurs in 1-4 months
Pediatric: same as adult
  Benoquin *Crm:* 20% (1.25 oz)
▷ *tazarotene* (X)(G) apply daily at HS
Pediatric: <12 years: not recommended; ≥12 years: same as adult
  Avage Cream *Crm:* 0.1% (30 gm)
  Tazorac Cream *Crm:* 0.05, 0.1% (15, 30, 60 gm)
  Tazorac Gel *Gel:* 0.05, 0.1% (30, 100 gm)
▷ *tretinoin* (C) apply daily at HS
Pediatric: <12 years: not recommended; ≥12 years: same as adult
  Avita *Crm/Gel:* 0.025% (20, 45 gm)
  Renova *Crm:* 0.02% (40 gm); 0.05% (40, 60 gm)
  Retin-A Cream *Crm:* 0.025, 0.05, 0.1% (20, 45 gm)

Retin-A Gel *Gel:* 0.01, 0.025% (15, 45 gm) (alcohol 90%)
Retin-A Liquid *Liq:* 0.05% (28 ml) (alcohol 55%)
Retin-A Micro *Microspheres:* 0.04, 0.1% (20, 45 gm)

COMBINATION AGENTS

▷ *hydroquinone+fluocinolone+tretinoin* **(C)** apply sparingly to affected area and rub in daily at HS
Pediatric: <12 years: not recommended; ≥12 years: same as adult
Tri-Luma *Crm:* hydroquin 4%+fluo 0.01%+tretin 0.05% (30 gm) (parabens, sulfites)

▷ *hydroquinone+padimate o+oxybenzone+octyl methoxycinnamate* **(C)** apply sparingly to affected area and rub in bid
Pediatric: <12 years: not recommended; ≥16 years: same as adult
Glyquin *Crm:* 4% (1 oz jar)

▷ *hydroquinone+ethyl dihydroxypropyl PABA+dioxybenzone+oxybenzone* **(C)** apply sparingly to affected area and rub in bid; max 2 months
Pediatric: <12 years: not recommended; ≥12 years: same as adult
Solaquin *Crm:* hydroquin 2%+PABA 5%+dioxy 3%+oxy 2% (1 oz) (sulfites)

▷ *hydroquinone+padimate+dioxybenzone+oxybenzone* **(C)** apply sparingly to affected area and rub in bid; max 2 months
Pediatric: <12 years: not recommended; ≥12 years: same as adult
Solaquin Forte *Crm:* hydroquin 4%+pad 0.5%+dioxy 3%+oxy 2% (1oz) (sunscreen, sulfites)

▷ *hydroquinone+padimate+dioxybenzone* **(C)** apply sparingly to affected area and rub in bid; max 2 months
Pediatric: <12 years: not recommended; ≥12 years: same as adults
Solaquin Forte Gel: hydroquin 4%+pad 0.5%+dioxy 3% (1 oz) (alcohol, sulfites)

◯ WART: COMMON (*VERRUCA VULGARIS*)

▷ *salicylic acid* **(G)**
Pediatric: same as adult
Duo Film (OTC) apply daily-bid; max 12 weeks; *Liq:* 17% (1/2 oz w. applicator)
Duo Film Patch for Kids (OTC) apply 1 patch q 48 hours; max 12 weeks
Patch: 40% (18/pck)
Occlusal HP (OTC) apply daily-bid; max 12 weeks
Liq: 17% (10 ml w. applicator)
Wart-Off (OTC) apply one drop at a time to sufficiently cover wart, let dry; repeat 1-2 times daily; max 12 weeks
Liq: 17% (0.45 oz)

▷ *trichloroacetic acid* apply after wart is pared and repeat weekly

▷ Cryotherapy with liquid nitrogen or cryoprobe or cryospray; repeat applications every 1-2 weeks as needed to destroy lesion
Histofreeze (see pkg insert for application freeze time

ORAL RETINOID

▷ *acitretin* **(X)(G)** 25-50 mg once daily with main meal
Pediatric: <18 years: not recommended; ≥18 years: same as adult
Soriatane *Cap:* 10, 25 mg

◯ WART: PLANTAR (*VERRUCA PLANTARIS*)

▷ *salicylic acid* **(G)**
Duo Plant Gel (OTC) apply daily bid; max 12 weeks
Gel: 17% (1/2 oz)

Mediplast cut to size of wart and apply; remove q 1-2 days, peel keratin, and reapply; repeat as long as needed

Occlusal-HP (OTC) apply once daily-bid; max 12 weeks
Liq: 17% (10 ml w. applicator)

Wart-Off (OTC) apply one drop at a time to sufficiently cover wart, let dry; repeat 1-2 times daily; max 12 weeks
Liq: 17% (0.45 oz)

▷ *trichloroacetic acid* apply after wart is pared and repeat weekly

ORAL RETINOID

▷ *acitretin* (X)(G) 25-50 mg once daily with main meal
Pediatric: <12 years: not recommended; ≥12 years: same as adult
Soriatane *Cap:* 10, 25 mg

 WART: VENEREAL, HUMAN PAPILLOMAVIRUS (HPV), CONDYLOMA ACUMINATA

Comment: Due to the increased risk of cervical cancer with HPV, Pap smears should be done q 3 months during active disease and then q 3-6 months for the next 2 years.

PATIENT-APPLIED AGENTS
Regimen 1

▷ *imiquimod* (C)(G)
Pediatric: <12 years: not recommended; ≥12 years: same as adult
Aldara (G) rub into lesions before bedtime and remove with soap and water 6-10 hours later; treat 3 times per week; max 16 weeks
Crm: 5% (12 single-use pkts/carton)
Zyclara rub into lesions before bedtime and remove with soap and water 8 hours later; treat 3 times per week; max 1 packet per treatment; max 8 weeks
Crm: 3.75% (28 single-use pkts/carton) (parabens)

Regimen 2

▷ *podofilox 0.5% cream* (C) apply bid (q 12 hours) x 3 days; then discontinue for 4 days; may repeat if needed; max 4 treatment cycles
Condylox *Soln:* 0.5% (3.5 ml); *Gel:* 0.5% (3.5 gm)

Regimen 3

▷ *sinecatechins 15% ointment* (C) apply to each lesion tid for up to 16 weeks
Veregen *Oint:* 15% (15, 30 gm)

PROVIDER-ADMINISTERED AGENTS
Regimen 1

▷ Cryotherapy with liquid nitrogen or cryoprobe; repeat applications every 1-2 weeks as needed

Regimen 2

▷ *trichloroacetic acid (TCA) 80-90%* (C) apply to warts; repeat weekly if needed
Comment: TCA is the preferred treatment during pregnancy. Immediate application of sodium bicarbonate paste following treatment decreases pain.

Regimen 3

▷ *podofilox 0.5% cream* (C) apply bid (q 12 hours) x 3 days; then discontinue for 4 days; may repeat if needed; max 4 treatment cycles
Condylox *Soln:* 0.5% (3.5 ml); *Gel:* 0.5% (3.5 gm)

Regimen 4

▷ *interferon alfa-n3* (C) 0.05 ml injected into base of wart twice weekly for up to 8 weeks; max 0.5 ml/session (20 warts/session)

    Alferon N *Vial:* 5 million units/ml (1 ml)

Regimen 5

▷ *interferon alfa-2b* (C) 0.1 ml injected into base of wart three times weekly for up to 3 weeks; max 0.5 ml/session (5 warts/session)

    Intron A *Vial:* 1 million units/0.1 ml (0.5, 1 ml)

Regimen 6

▷ Surgical removal either by tangential scissor excision, tangential shave excision, curettage, or electrosurgery

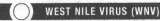

WEST NILE VIRUS (WNV)

Comment: The principal route of human infection with West Nile virus is through the bite of an infected mosquito. Additional routes of infection have become a parent during the 2002 West Nile epidemic. It is important to note that these other methods of transmission represent a very small proportion of cases. Other methods of transmission include blood transfusion, organ transplantation, mother-to-child (ingestion of breast milk and transplacental) and occupational. Symptoms of mild disease will generally last a few days. Symptoms of severe disease may last several weeks, although neurological effects may be permanent. There is no specific treatment for West Nile virus infection; treatment is symptomatic and supportive. About 8 in 10 infected with West Nile virus do not develop any symptoms. About 1 in 5 develop a fever with other symptoms such as headache, body aches, joint pains, vomiting, diarrhea, or rash. Most people with this level of disease recover completely, but fatigue and weakness can last for weeks to months. About 1 in 150 people who are infected develop a severe illness affecting the central nervous system (encephalitis meningitis). Symptoms of severe illness include high fever, headache, neck stiffness, stupor, disorientation, coma, tremors, convulsions, muscle weakness, vision loss, numbness and paralysis. About 1 in 10 who develop severe illness affecting the central nervous system die. There is currently no preventive vaccine. However, the National Institutes of Health have announced that an experimental vaccine to protect against West Nile Virus has entered human trial. The developers say because the vaccine uses inactivated virus it should be suitable for a wide range of people. The trial tested the safety of the vaccine, called **HydroVax-001**, and its ability to produce an immune response in human subjects. The randomized, placebo-controlled, double-blind clinical trial was conducted by researchers at Duke University School of Medicine, Durham, NC, and enrolled 50 healthy volunteers, men and women 18-50 years-of-age. Participants were randomly assigned to one of the three groups. One group volunteers (n = 20) received a low dose of the vaccine (1 mcg), another group (n = 20) received a higher dose (4 mcg), and a third group (n = 10) received a placebo. All participants received their doses via IM injection on day 1 and day 29 of the trial and are followed for 14 months. Results of the completed trial are pending.

WHIPWORM (TRICHURIASIS)

ANTHELMINTICS

▷ *albendazole* (C) 400 mg as a single dose; may repeat in 3 weeks; take with a meal

    Pediatric: <2 years: 200 mg daily x 3 days; may repeat in 3 weeks; 2-12 years: 400 mg daily x 3 days; may repeat in 3 weeks; >12 years: same as adult

    Albenza *Tab:* 200 mg

▷ *mebendazole* (C) chew, swallow, or mix with food; 100 mg bid x 3 days; may repeat in 3 weeks if needed; take with a meal
  Pediatric: <2 years: not recommended; ≥2 years: same as adult
    Emverm *Chew tab:* 100 mg
    Vermox (G) *Chew tab:* 100 mg
▷ *pyrantel pamoate* (C) 11 mg/kg x 1 dose; max 1 gm/dose; take with a meal
  Pediatric: 25-37 lb: 1/2 tsp x 1 dose; 38-62 lb: 1 tsp x 1 dose; 63-87 lb: 1 tsp x 1 dose; 88-112 lb: 2 tsp x 1 dose; 113-137 lb: 2 tsp x 1 dose; 138-162 lb: 3 tsp x 1 dose; 163-187 lb: 3 tsp x 1 dose; >187 lb: 4 tsp x 1 dose
    Antiminth (OTC) *Cap:* 180 mg; *Liq:* 50 mg/ml (30 ml); 144 mg/ml (30 ml); *Oral susp:* 50 mg/ml (60 ml)
    Pin-X (OTC) *Cap:* 180 mg; *Liq:* 50 mg/ml (30 ml); 144 mg/ml (30 ml); *Oral susp:* 50 mg/ml (30 ml)
▷ *thiabendazole* (C) 25 mg/kg bid x 7 days; max 1.5 gm/dose; take with a meal
  Pediatric: same as adult; <30 lb: consult mfr pkg insert; >30 lb: 2 doses/day with meals; 30-50 lb: 250 mg bid with meals; >50 lb: 10 mg/lb/dose bid with meals; max 3 gm/day
    Mintezol *Chew tab:* 500*mg (orange); *Oral susp:* 500 mg/5 ml (120 ml) (orange)
  Comment: *Thiabendazole* is not for prophylaxis. May impair mental alertness. May not be available in the US.

WILSON'S DISEASE

Comment: Wilson's disease (hepatolenticular degeneration) occurs in individuals who have inherited an autosomal recessive defect that leads to an accumulation of copper far in excess of metabolic requirements. The excess copper is deposited in several organs and tissues, and eventually produces pathological effects primarily in the liver, where damage progresses to post-necrotic cirrhosis, and in the brain, where degeneration is widespread. Copper is also deposited as characteristic, asymptomatic, golden-brown Kayser-Fleischer rings in the corneas of all patients with cerebral symptomatology. Treatment has two objectives: (1) to minimize dietary intake of copper; (2) to promote excretion and complex formation (i.e., detoxification) of excess tissue copper.

COPPER CHELATING AGENTS

▷ *penicillamine* administer on an empty stomach, at least 1 hour before meals or two hours after meals, and at least 1 hour apart from any other drug, food, milk, antacid, zinc or iron-containing preparation; dosage must be individualized, and may require adjustment during the course of treatment; initially, a single daily dose of 125-250 mg; then, increase at 1-3 month intervals by 125-250 mg/day, as patient response and tolerance indicate; if a satisfactory remission of symptoms is achieved, the dose associated with the remission should be continued as the patient's maintenance therapy; if there is no improvement, and there are no signs of potentially serious toxicity after 2-3 months of treatment with doses of 500-750 mg/day, increase by 250 mg/day at 2-3 month intervals until a satisfactory remission occurs or signs of toxicity develop; if there is no discernible improvement after 3-4 months of treatment with 1000-1500 mg/day, discontinue **Cuprimine**; changes in maintenance dosage levels may not be reflected clinically or in the erythrocyte sedimentation rate (ESR) for 2-3 months after each dosage adjustment
    Cuprimine *Cap:* 125, 250 mg
    Depen: 250 mg
  Comment: Taking *penicillamine* on an empty stomach permits maximum absorption and reduces the likelihood of inactivation by metal binding in

the GI tract. Optimal dosage can be determined by measurement of urinary copper excretion and the determination of free copper in the serum. The urine must be collected in copper-free glassware, and should be quantitatively analyzed for copper before and soon after initiation of therapy with **Cupramine**. Determination of 24-hour urinary copper excretion is of greatest value in the first week of therapy with *penicillamine*. In the absence of any drug reaction, a dose between 0.75 and 1.5 gm that results in an initial 24-hour cupriuresis of over 2 mg should be continued for about three months, by which time the most reliable method of monitoring maintenance treatment is the determination of free copper in the serum. This equals the difference between quantitatively determined total copper and ceruloplasmin-copper. Adequately treated patients will usually have less than 10 mcg free copper/dL of serum. It is seldom necessary to exceed a dosage of 2 gm/day. In patients who cannot tolerate as much as 1 g/day initially, initiating dosage with 250 mg/day, and increasing gradually to the requisite amount, gives closer control of the effects of the drug and may help to reduce the incidence of adverse reactions. If the patient is intolerant to therapy with **Cuprimine**, alternative treatment is *trientine* (**Syprine**).

The use of *penicillamine* has been associated with fatalities due to certain diseases such as aplastic anemia, agranulocytosis, thrombocytopenia, Goodpasture's syndrome, and myasthenia gravis. Because of the potential for serious hematological and renal adverse reactions to occur at any time, routine urinalysis, white and differential blood cell count, hemoglobin, and direct platelet count must be checked twice weekly, together with monitoring of the patient's skin, lymph nodes and body temperature, during the first month of therapy, every 2 weeks for the next 5 months, and monthly thereafter. Patients should be instructed to report promptly the development of signs and symptoms of granulocytopenia and/or thrombocytopenia such as fever, sore throat, chills, bruising or bleeding; the above laboratory studies should then be promptly repeated.

▷ *trientine* (C)(G) recommended initial dose is 500-750 mg/day for pediatric patients and 750-1250 mg/day for adults administered in divided doses 2, 3, or 4 x/day; may be increased to max 2000 mg/day for adults or 1500 mg/day for patients ≤12 years-of-age; the daily dose of **Syprine** should be increased only when the clinical response is not adequate or the concentration of free serum copper is persistently above 20 mcg/dL; optimal long-term maintenance dose should be determined at 6-12 month intervals; administer on an empty stomach, at least 1 hour before meals or 2 hours after meals and at least 1 hour apart from any other drug, food, or milk; swallow whole with water; do not open the cap or chew the contents

  Syprine *Cap*: 250 mg

  Comment: **Syprine** is a chelating agent indicated in the treatment of patients with Wilson's disease who are intolerant of *penicillamine*. Clinical experience with **Syprine** is limited and alternate dosing regimens have not been well-characterized; all endpoints in determining an individual patient's dose have not been well defined. **Syprine** and *penicillamine* cannot be considered interchangeable. **Syprine** should be used when continued treatment with *penicillamine* is no longer possible because of intolerable or life-endangering side effects. Unlike *penicillamine*, **Syprine** is not recommended in cystinuria or rheumatoid arthritis. The absence of a sulfhydryl moiety renders it incapable of binding cystine and, therefore, it is of no use in cystinuria. In 15 patients with rheumatoid arthritis, **Syprine** was reported not to be effective in improving any clinical or biochemical parameter after 12 weeks of treatment. The most reliable index for monitoring treatment is the determination of free copper in the serum, which equals the difference between quantitatively determined total copper and ceruloplasmin-copper. Adequately treated patients will usually have less than 10 mcg free copper/dL of serum. Therapy may be monitored with a 24-hour urinary copper analysis periodically (i.e., every 6-12 months). Urine must be collected in copper-free glassware. Since a low copper diet should keep copper absorption down to less than one milligram a day, the patient probably will be in the desired state of negative copper balance if 0.5 to 1.0 milligram of copper is present in a 24-hour collection of urine. In general, mineral supplements should not be used since they may block the absorption of **Syprine**. However, iron deficiency may develop, especially in children and menstruating or pregnant females, or as a result of the low copper diet recommended for Wilson's disease. If necessary, iron may be given in short courses, but since iron and **Syprine** each inhibit absorption of the other, two hours should elapse between administration of **Syprine** and iron. *trientine* was teratogenic in animals at doses similar to the human dose. The frequencies of both resorptions and fetal abnormalities, including hemorrhage and edema, increased while fetal copper levels decreased when *trientine* was given in the maternal diets. There are no adequate and well-controlled studies in pregnant females. **Syprine** should be used during pregnancy only if the potential benefit justifies the potential risk to the fetus. It is not known whether this drug is excreted in human milk. Caution should be exercised when **Syprine** is administered to a nursing mother. Clinical studies of **Syprine** did not include sufficient numbers of subjects ≥65 years-of-age to determine whether they respond differently from younger subjects. Other reported clinical experience is insufficient to determine differences in responses between the elderly and younger patients. In general, dose selection should be cautious, usually starting at the low end of the dosing range, reflecting the greater frequency of decreased hepatic, renal, or cardiac function, and of concomitant disease or other drug therapy. Clinical experience with **Syprine** has been limited. The following adverse reactions have been reported in a clinical study in patients with Wilson's disease who were on therapy with *trientine*: iron deficiency, systemic lupus erythematosus. In addition, the following adverse reactions have been reported in marketed use: dystonia, muscular spasm, and myasthenia gravis.

WOUND: INFECTED, NONSURGICAL, MINOR

TETANUS PROPHYLAXIS VACCINE

Previously Immunized (within previous 5 years)

▷ *tetanus toxoid* vaccine (C) 0.5 ml IM x 1 dose
Vial: 5 Lf units/0.5 ml (0.5, 5 ml); *Prefilled syringe:* 5 Lf units/0.5 ml (0.5 ml)

Not Previously Immunized

see Tetanus

TOPICAL ANTI-INFECTIVES

▷ *mupirocin* (B)(G) apply to lesions bid
Pediatric: same as adult
   Bactroban *Oint:* 2% (22 gm); *Crm:* 2% (15, 30 gm)
   Centany *Oint:* 2% (15, 30 gm)

ORAL ANTI-INFECTIVES

▷ *azithromycin* (B)(G) 500 mg x 1 dose on day 1, then 250 mg daily on days 2-5 or 500 mg daily x 3 days or Zmax 2 gm in a single dose
Pediatric: 10 mg/kg x 1 dose on day 1, then 5 mg/kg/day on days 2-5; max 500 mg/day; *see* Appendix CC.7. *azithromycin* (Zithromax Suspension, Zmax Suspension) *for dose by weight*

Zithromax *Tab:* 250, 500, 600 mg; *Oral susp:* 100 mg/5 ml (15 ml); 200 mg/5 ml (15, 22.5, 30 ml) (cherry); *Pkt:* 1 gm for reconstitution (cherry-banana)

Zithromax Tri-pak *Tab:* 3 x 500 mg tabs/pck

Zithromax Z-pak *Tab:* 6 x 250 mg tabs/pck

Zmax *Oral susp:* 2 gm ext-rel for reconstitution (cherry-banana) (148 mg Na⁺)

▷ *amoxicillin+clavulanate* (B)(G)

Augmentin 500 mg tid or 875 mg bid x 10 days

Pediatric: 40-45 mg/kg/day divided tid x 10 days or 90 mg/kg/day divided bid x 10 days *see* Appendix CC.4. *amoxicillin+clavulanate* (Augmentin Suspension) *for dose by weight*

Tab: 250, 500, 875 mg; *Chew tab:* 125, 250 mg (lemon-lime); 200, 400 mg (cherry-banana) (phenylalanine); *Oral susp:* 125 mg/5 ml (banana), 250 mg/5 ml (75, 100, 150 ml) (orange); 200, 400 mg/5 ml (50, 75, 100 ml) (orange) (phenylalanine)

Augmentin ES-600 not recommended for adults

Pediatric: <3 months: not recommended; ≥3 months, <40 kg: 90 mg/kg/day in 2 divided doses x 10 days; ≥40 kg: not recommended

Oral susp: 42.9 mg/5 ml (50, 75, 100, 125, 150, 200 ml) (strawberry cream) (phenylalanine)

Augmentin XR 2 tabs q 12 hours x 10 days

Pediatric: <16 years: use other forms; ≥16 years: same as adult

Tab: 1000*mg ext-rel

▷ *cefaclor* (B)(G)

Ceclor 250 mg tid or 375 mg bid 3-10 days

Pediatric: <1 month: not recommended; 1 month-12 years: 20-40 mg/kg divided bid or q 12 hours x 3-10 days; max 1 gm/day; *see* Appendix CC.8. *cefaclor* (Ceclor Suspension) *for dose by weight;* >12 years: same as adult

Tab: 500 mg; *Cap:* 250, 500 mg; *Susp:* 125 mg/5 ml (75, 150 ml) (strawberry); 187 mg/5 ml (50, 100 ml) (strawberry); 250 mg/5 ml (75, 150 ml) (strawberry); 375 mg/5 ml (50, 100 ml) (strawberry)

Cefaclor Extended Release 375, 500 mg bid x 3-10 days

Pediatric: <16 years: ext-rel not recommended; ≥16 years: same as adult

Tab: 375, 500 mg ext-rel

▷ *cefadroxil* 1 gm/day in 1-2 divided doses x 10 days

Pediatric: 15-30 mg/kg/day in 2 divided doses x 10 days; *see* Appendix CC.9. *cefadroxil* (Duricef Suspension) *for dose by weight*

Duricef *Cap:* 500 mg; *Tab:* 1 gm; *Oral susp:* 250 mg/5 ml (100 ml); 500 mg/5 ml (75, 100 ml) (orange-pineapple)

▷ *cefdinir* (B) 300 mg bid or 600 mg daily x 10 days

Pediatric: <6 months: not recommended; 6 months-12 years: 14 mg/kg/day in 1-2 divided doses x 10 days; *see* Appendix CC.10. *cefdinir* (Omnicef Suspension) *for dose by weight*

Omnicef *Cap:* 300 mg; *Oral susp:* 125 mg/5 ml (60, 100 ml) (strawberry)

▷ *cefpodoxime proxetil* (B) 400 mg bid x 7-14 days

Pediatric: <2 months: not recommended; 2 months-12 years: 10 mg/kg/day (max 400 mg/dose) or 5 mg/kg/day bid (max 200 mg/dose) x 7-14 days; *see* Appendix CC.12. *cefpodoxime proxetil* (Vantin Suspension) *for dose by weight*

Vantin *Tab:* 100, 200 mg; *Oral susp:* 50, 100 mg/5 ml (50, 75, 100 mg; lemon creme)

Pediatric: see Appendix CC.12. *cefpodoxime proxetil* (Vantin Suspension) *for dose by weight*

▷ *cefprozil* (B) 250-500 mg q 12 hours or 500 mg daily x 10 days

Pediatric: <2 years: not recommended; 2-12 years: 7.5 mg/kg-15 mg/kg q 12 hours x 10 days; *see* Appendix CC.13. *cefprozil* (Cefzil Suspension) *for dose by weight;* >12 years: same as adult

Cefzil *Tab*: 250, 500 mg; *Oral susp*: 125, 250 mg/5 ml (50, 75, 100 ml) (bubble gum, phenylalanine)

➤ *cephalexin* (B)(G) 2 gm 1 hour before procedure
Pediatric: 50 mg/kg/day in 4 divided doses x 10 days; *see* Appendix CC.15. *cephalexin (Keflex Suspension) for dose by weight*
Keflex *Cap*: 250, 333, 500, 750 mg; *Oral susp*: 125, 250 mg/5 ml (100, 200 ml) (strawberry)
Pediatric: see Appendix CC.15. *cephalexin (Keflex Suspension) for dose by weight*

➤ *clarithromycin* (C)(G) 500 mg bid *or* 500 mg ext-rel once daily x 7-10 days
Pediatric: see Appendix CC.16. *clarithromycin (Biaxin Suspension) for dose by weight*
Biaxin *Tab*: 250, 500 mg
Biaxin Oral Suspension *Oral susp*: 125, 250 mg/5 ml (50, 100 ml) (fruit punch)
Biaxin XL *Tab*: 500 mg ext-rel

➤ *dirithromycin* (C)(G) 500 mg daily x 7 days
Pediatric: <12 years: not recommended
Dynabac *Tab*: 250 mg

➤ *erythromycin base* (B)(G) 500 mg qid x 14 days
Pediatric: 30-50 mg/kg/day in 2-4 divided doses x 10 days
Ery-Tab *Tab*: 250, 333, 500 mg ent-coat
PCE *Tab*: 333, 500 mg

➤ *erythromycin ethylsuccinate* (B)(G) 400 mg qid x 7 days
Pediatric: 30-50 mg/kg/day in 4 divided doses x 7 days; may double dose with severe infection; max 100 mg/kg/day; *see* Appendix CC.21: *erythromycin ethylsuccinate* (E.E.S. Suspension, Ery-Ped Drops/Suspension) for dose by weight
EryPed *Oral susp*: 200 mg/5 ml (100, 200 ml) (fruit); 400 mg/5 ml (60, 100, 200 ml) (banana); *Oral drops*: 200, 400 mg/5 ml (50 ml) (fruit); *Chew tab*: 200 mg wafer (fruit)
E.E.S. *Oral susp*: 200, 400 mg/5 ml (100 ml) (fruit)
E.E.S. Granules *Oral susp*: 200 mg/5 ml (100, 200 ml) (cherry)
E.E.S. 400 Tablets *Tab*: 400 mg

➤ *gemifloxacin* (C)(G) 320 mg daily x 5-7 days
Pediatric: <18 years: not recommended; ≥18 years: same as adult
Factive *Tab*: 320*mg

➤ *levofloxacin* (C) *Uncomplicated*: 500 mg daily x 7 days; *Complicated*: 750 mg daily x 7 days
Pediatric: <18 years: not recommended; ≥18 years: same as adult
Levaquin *Tab*: 250, 500, 750 mg

➤ *loracarbef* (B) 200-400 mg bid x 7 days
Pediatric: 15 mg/kg/day in 2 divided doses x 7 days; *see* Appendix CC.27. *loracarbef* (Lorabid Suspension) for dose by weight
Lorabid *Pulvule*: 200, 400 mg; *Oral susp*: 100 mg/5 ml (50, 100 ml); 200 mg/5 ml (50, 75, 100 ml) (strawberry bubble gum)

➤ *ofloxacin* (C)(G) 400 mg bid x 10 days
Pediatric: <18 years: not recommended; ≥18 years: same as adult
Floxin *Tab*: 200, 300, 400 mg

⬤ WRINKLES: FACIAL

TOPICAL RETINOIDS

Comment: Wash the affected area with a soap-free cleanser; pat dry and wait 20 to 30 minutes; then apply topical retinoid sparingly to affected area. Use only once daily in the PM. Avoid eyes, ears, nostrils, and mouth.

▷ *adapalene* (C)(G)
  Pediatric: <12 years: not recommended; ≥12 years: same as adult
    Differin *Crm:* 0.1% (15, 45 gm); *Gel:* 0.1% (15, 45 gm); *Pad:* 0.1% (30/pck)
    (alcohol 30%)
    Differin Solution *Soln:* 0.1% (30 ml; alcohol 30%)
▷ *tazarotene* (X)(G) apply daily at HS
  Pediatric: <12 years: not recommended; ≥12 years: same as adult
    Avage Cream *Crm:* 0.1% (5, 30 gm)
    Tazorac Cream *Crm:* 0.05, 0.1% (15, 30, 60 gm)
    Tazorac Gel *Gel:* 0.05, 0.1% (30, 100 gm)
▷ *tretinoin* (C) apply daily at HS
  Pediatric: <12 years: not recommended; ≥12 years: same as adult
    Atralin Gel *Gel:* 0.05% (45 gm)
    Avita *Crm:* 0.025% (20, 45 gm); *Gel:* 0.025% (20, 45 gm)
    Renova *Crm:* 0.02% (40 gm); 0.05% (40, 60 gm)
    Retin-A Cream *Crm:* 0.025, 0.05, 0.1% (20, 45 gm)
    Retin-A Gel *Gel:* 0.01, 0.025% (15, 45 gm; alcohol 90%)
    Retin-A Liquid *Soln:* 0.05% (alcohol 55%)
    Retin-A Micro Gel *Gel:* 0.04, 0.08, 0.1% (20, 45 gm)
    Tretin-X Cream *Crm:* 0.075% (35 gm) (parabens-free, alcohol-free, propylene
    glycol-free)
    Retin-A Micro *Microspheres:* 0.04, 0.1% (20, 45 gm)
  Comment: topical *tretinoin* is effective for mitigation of fine wrinkles, mottled
  hyperpigmentation, and tactile roughness of skin. No mitigating effect on deep
  wrinkles, skin yellowing, lentigines, telangiectasia, skin laxity, keratinocytic
  atypia, melanocytic atypia, or dermal elastosis. Avoid sun exposure. Cautious use
  of concomitant astringents, alcohol-based products, sulfur-containing products,
  salicylic acid-containing products, soap, and other topical agents.

BOTULISM TOXIN PRODUCT

▷ *prabotulinumtoxina-xvfs Glabellar Lines Administration:* using a 30-33 guage
  needle, 0.1 ml (4 Units) by IM injection into each of 5 sites, for a max total dose
  of 20 Units; consult pkg insert for exact injection sites; must be administered by a
  qualified healthcare provider with knowledge of the relevant neuromuscular and/
  or orbital anatomy of the area involved and any alterations to the anatomy due to
  prior surgical procedures; avoid injection near the levator palpebrae superioris,
  particularly in patients with larger brow depressor complexes; lateral corrugator
  injections should be placed at least 1 cm above the bony supraorbital ridge; ensure
  the injected volume/dose is accurate and where feasible kept to a minimum; avoid
  injecting toxin closer than 1 centimeter above the central eyebrow
    Jeuveau *Vial:* 100 Units vacuum-dried pwdr, single-use, for reconstitution
    with 2.5 ml sterile, preservative-free 0.9% NaCl diluent, to obtain a solution
    concentration of 4 Units/0.1 ml (total 20 Units in 0.5 ml)
    Comment: **Jeuveau** is an acetylcholine release inhibitor and a neuromuscular
    blocking agent indicated for the temporary improvement in the appearance
    of moderate-to-severe glabellar lines ("worry lines" between the brows)
    associated with corrugator and/or procerus muscle activity in adult patients.
    The effects of all botulinum toxin products may spread from the area of
    injection to produce symptoms consistent with botulinum toxin effects. These
    symptoms have been reported hours to weeks after injection. Swallowing and
    breathing difficulties can be life threatening. Adverse event reports have also
    involved the cardiovascular system, some with fatal outcomes. Use caution
    when administering to patients with pre-existing cardiovascular disease.
    Jeuveau is not approved for the treatment of spasticity or any conditions
    other than glabellar lines. Potency Units of **Jeuveau** are not interchangeable

with other preparations of botulinum toxin products. Animal studies have not demonstrated treatment-related effects to the developing fetus when administered intramuscularly during organogenesis at doses up to 12 times the maximum recommended human dose (MRHD). There is no information regarding the presence of *prabotulinumtoxina-xvfs* in human or its effects on the breastfed infant.

XEROSIS

MOISTURIZING AGENTS

Aquaphor Healing Ointment (OTC) *Oint:* 1.75, 3.5, 14 oz (alcohol)
Eucerin Daily Sun Defense (OTC) *Lotn:* 6 oz (fragrance-free)
Comment: **Eucerin Daily Sun Defense** is a moisturizer with SPF 15 sunscreen.
Eucerin Facial Lotion (OTC) *Lotn:* 4 oz
Eucerin Light Lotion (OTC) *Lotn:* 8 oz
Eucerin Lotion (OTC) *Lotn:* 8, 16 oz
Eucerin Original Creme (OTC) *Crm:* 2, 4, 16 oz (alcohol)
Eucerin Plus Creme (OTC) *Crm:* 4 oz
Eucerin Plus Lotion (OTC) *Lotn:* 6, 12 oz
Eucerin Protective Lotion (OTC) *Lotn:* 4 oz (alcohol)
Comment: **Eucerin Protective** is a moisturizer with SPF 25 sunscreen.
Lac-Hydrin Cream (OTC) *Crm:* 280, 385 gm
Lac-Hydrin Lotion (OTC) *Lotn:* 225, 400 gm
Lubriderm Dry Skin Scented (OTC) *Lotn:* 6, 10, 16, 32 oz
Lubriderm Dry Skin Unscented (OTC) *Lotn:* 3.3, 6, 10, 16 oz (fragrance-free)
Lubriderm Sensitive Skin Lotion (OTC) *Lotn:* 3.3, 6, 10, 16 oz (lanolin-free)
Lubriderm Dry Skin (OTC) *Lotn:* 2.5, 6, 10, 16 oz (scented); 1, 2.5, 6, 10, 16 oz (fragrance-free)
Lubriderm Bath & Shower Oil (OTC) 1-2 capfuls in bath or rub onto wet skin as needed, then rinse; *Oil:* 8 oz
Moisturel *Crm:* 4, 16 oz; *Lotn:* 8, 12 oz; *Clnsr:* 8.75 oz

Topical Oil

▷ *fluocinolone acetonide* 0.01% topical oil (C)
Pediatric: <6 years: not recommended; ≥6 years: apply sparingly bid for up to 4 weeks
Derma-Smoothe/FS Topical Oil apply sparingly tid
Topical oil: 0.01% (4 oz; peanut oil)

YELLOW FEVER

Comment: The yellow fever vaccine is recommended for people ≥ 9 months-of-age who are traveling to or living in areas at risk for the yellow fever virus in https://www.cdc.gov/yellowfever/maps/africa.html Africa and South America (www.cdc.gov/yellowfever/maps/africa.html). The vaccine is a live, weakened form of the virus. A single dose provides lifelong protection for most people. Sanofi Pasteur, the manufacturer of the only yellow fever vaccine (**YF-Vax**) licensed in the United States, announced that **YF-Vax** for civilian use is expected to be available from the manufacturer again by mid-2019. However, **YF-VAX** might be available at some clinics, until remaining supplies at those sites are used up. Sanofi Pasteur applied and received approval from the US Food and Drug Administration (FDA) to make another yellow fever vaccine available in the United States under an investigational new drug (IND) program. Although the name of the FDA program is "investigational new drug," **Stamaril** is <u>not</u> investigational <u>or</u> experimental. **Stamaril** has been used in European and other countries for decades but is <u>not</u> licensed in the United States. IND is the mechanism through which FDA gives approval for **Stamaril** to be imported. Manufactured by Sanofi Pasteur in France, this vaccine, **Stamaril**, is registered and distributed in more than 70 countries. It is comparable in safety and efficacy to **YF-Vax**. In order to meet the requirements of the IND program, Sanofi Pasteur can provide **Stamaril** to <u>only</u> a limited number of clinics. Sanofi has identified sites throughout the United States to include in the program so patients can have continued access to yellow fever vaccine. Travelers and health care providers can find locations that can administer **Stamaril**, and those clinics with remaining doses of **YF-VAX**, by visiting the yellow fever vaccination clinic search page. For information about which countries require yellow fever vaccination for entry and which countries the CDC recommends yellow fever vaccination, visit the CDC Traveler's Health website (www.cdc.gov/travel). For more information, contact Sanofi Pasteur at 1-800-VACCINE (1-800-822-2463) <u>or</u> visit https://wwwnc.cdc.gov/travel/news-announcements/yellow-fever-vaccine-access

ZIKA VIRUS

Comment: The Zika virus is transmitted via the bite of an infected mosquito and is associated with severe teratogenicity: a unique and distinct pattern of birth defects, called congenital Zika syndrome, characterized by the following five features: (1) severe microcephaly in which the skull has partially collapsed; (2) decreased brain tissue with a specific pattern of brain damage, including subcortical calcifications; (3) damage to the back of the eye, including macular scarring and focal pigmentary retinal mottling; (4) congenital contractures, such as clubfoot and arthrogryposis; (5) hypertonia restricting body movement. Congenital Zika virus infection has also been associated with other abnormalities, including but <u>not</u> limited to brain atrophy and asymmetry, abnormally formed <u>or</u> absent brain structures, hydrocephalus, and neuronal migration disorders. Other anomalies include excessive and redundant scalp skin. Reported neurologic findings include, hyperreflexia, irritability, tremors, seizures, brainstem dysfunction, and dysphagia. Reported eye abnormalities include, but are <u>not</u> limited to, focal pigmentary mottling and chorioretinal atrophy in the macula, optic nerve hypoplasia, cupping, and atrophy, other retinal lesions, iris colobomas, congenital glaucoma, microphthalmia, lens subluxation, cataracts, and intraocular calcifications. **A synthetic DNA-based preventive vaccine showed promising immune responses with no severe adverse reactions in humans**, an interim analysis of a phase I trial found. Following three doses of vaccine, 100% of patients produced binding antibodies, and 95% of patients produced binding antibodies following two doses of the vaccine, Examining immunogenicity, 41% of participants had detectable binding antibody responses 4 weeks after the first dose, the authors said, with a 74% antibody response at week 6 (2 weeks after the second dose). **The vaccine is not yet available to the public**. The FDA formally approved Roche's cobas Zika molecular test for use on whole donor blood and blood products and living organ donors; it's the first such approval granted.

ZOLLINGER-ELLISON SYNDROME

Comment: Zollinger-Ellison Syndrome is a condition in which a gastrin-secreting tumor <u>or</u> hyperplasia of the islet cells in the pancreas causes overproduction of gastric acid, resulting in recurrent peptic ulcers.

PROTON PUMP INHIBITORS (PPIs)

Comment: If hepatic impairment, or if patient is Asian, consider reducing the PPI dose.

▷ *dexlansoprazole* (B)(G) 30-60 mg daily for up to 4 weeks
　Pediatric: <18 years: not recommended; ≥18 years: same as adult
　　　Dexilant *Cap:* 30, 60 mg ent-coat del-rel granules; may open and sprinkle on
　　　applesauce; do not crush or chew granules
　　　Dexilant SoluTab *Tab:* 30 mg del-rel orally-disint

▷ *esomeprazole* (B)(OTC)(G) 20-40 mg daily; max 8 weeks; take 1 hour before food;
swallow whole or mix granules with food or juice and take immediately; do not crush
or chew granules
　Pediatric: <1 year: not recommended; 1-11 years, <20 kg: 10 mg; ≥20 kg: 10-20
mg once daily; 12-17 years: 20-40 mg once daily; max 8 weeks
　　　Nexium *Cap:* 20, 40 mg ent-coat del-rel pellets
　　　Nexium for Oral Suspension *Oral susp:* 10, 20, 40 mg ent-coat del-rel
　　　granules/pkt; mix in 2 tbsp water and drink immediately; 30 pkt/carton

▷ *esomeprazole+aspirin* (D) take one dose daily; max 8 weeks; take 1 hour before
food
　　　Yosprala
　　　　Tab: **Yosprala 40/81** esom 40 mg+asp 81 mg del-rel
　　　　　　Yosprala 40/325 esom 40 mg+asp 325 mg del-rel

▷ *lansoprazole* (B)(OTC)(G) 15-30 mg daily for up to 8 weeks; may repeat course;
take before eating
　Pediatric: <1 year: not recommended; 1-11 years, <30 kg: 15 mg once daily; >11
years: same as adult
　　　Prevacid *Cap:* 15, 30 mg ent-coat del-rel granules; swallow whole or mix
　　　granules with food or juice and take immediately; do not crush or chew
　　　granules; follow with water
　　　Prevacid for Oral Suspension *Oral susp:* 15, 30 mg ent-coat del-rel granules/
　　　pkt; mix in 2 tbsp water and drink immediately; 30 pkt/carton (strawberry)
　　　Prevacid SoluTab *ODT:* 15, 30 mg (strawberry) (phenylalanine)
　　　Prevacid 24HR *Oral granules:* 15 mg ent-coat del-rel granules; swallow whole
　　　or mix granules with food or juice and take immediately; do not crush or
　　　chew granules; follow with water

▷ *omeprazole* (C)(OTC)(G) 20-40 mg daily; take before eating; swallow whole or
mix granules with applesauce and take immediately; do not crush or chew; follow
with water
　　　Prilosec *Cap:* 10, 20, 40 mg ent-coat del-rel granules
　　　Pediatric: <18 years: not recommended; ≥18 years: same as adult
　　　Prilosec *Tab:* 20 mg del-rel (regular, wild berry)
　　　Pediatric: <1 year: not recommended; 5-<10 kg: 5 mg daily; 10-<20 kg: 10 mg
　　　daily; ≥20 kg: same as adult

▷ *pantoprazole* (B)(G) initially 40 mg bid
　Pediatric: <12 years: not recommended; ≥12 years: same as adult
　　　Protonix *Tab:* 40 mg ent-coat del-rel
　　　Protonix for Oral Suspension *Oral susp:* 40 mg ent-coat del-rel granules/pkt;
　　　mix in 1 tsp apple juice for 5 seconds or sprinkle on 1 tsp apple sauce, and
　　　swallow immediately; do not mix in water or any other liquid or food; take
　　　approximately 30 minutes prior to a meal; 30 pkt/carton any other liquid or
　　　food; take approximately 30 minutes prior to a meal; 30 pkt/carton

▷ *rabeprazole* (B)(OTC)(G) initially 20 mg daily; then titrate; may take 100 mg
daily in divided doses or 60 mg bid
　Pediatric: <12 years: not recommended; ≥12 years: 20 mg once daily; max 8 weeks
　　　AcipHex *Tab:* 20 mg ent-coat del-rel

SECTION II

APPENDICES

*Online only; available at connect.springerpub.com/content/reference-book/978-0-8261-7935-7/section/sectionII/appendix.

---

*Online only; available at connect.springerpub.com/content/reference-book/978-0-8261-7935-7/section/sectionII/appendix.

APPENDIX A. U.S. FDA PREGNANCY CATEGORIES

Comment: For drugs FDA-approved *after June 30, 2015*, the 5-letter categories are no longer used, and there is no replacement (categorical nomenclature) at this time. Rather, information regarding special populations, including pregnant and breastfeeding females, is addressed in a structured narrative format. Prescribers should refer to the drug's FDA labeling (https://www.fda. gov/Drugs/default.htm) or the manufacturer's package insert for this information. Prescription drugs submitted for FDA approval after June 30, 2015, use the new format immediately, while labeling for prescription drugs approved on or after June 30, 2015, are phased in gradually. Labeling for over-the-counter (OTC) medicines will not change, as OTC drugs are not affected by the new FDA pregnancy labeling. For a more detailed explanation of the final rule and new narrative format, **visit** https://www.drugs.com/pregnancy-categories.html

Category	Description
A	Controlled studies in women have failed to demonstrate risk to the fetus in the first trimester of pregnancy, and there is no evidence of risk in later trimesters.
B	Animal reproduction studies have not demonstrated risk to the fetus, but there are no controlled studies in pregnant females, or animal studies have demonstrated an adverse effect, but controlled studies in pregnant females have not documented risk to the fetus in the first trimester of pregnancy and there is no evidence of risk in later trimesters.
C	Risk to the fetus cannot be ruled out. Animal reproduction studies have demonstrated adverse effects on the fetus (i.e., teratogenic or embryocidal effects or other), but there are no controlled studies in pregnant females or controlled studies in women and animals are not available.
D	There is positive evidence of human fetal risk, but benefits from use by pregnant females may be acceptable despite the potential risk (e.g., if the drug is needed in a life-threatening situation or for a serious disease for which safer drugs cannot be used or are ineffective.)
X	Studies in animals or humans have demonstrated fetal abnormalities or there is evidence of fetal risk based on human experience, or both, and the risk of using the drug in pregnant females clearly outweighs any possible benefit. The drug is contraindicated in women who are pregnant or who may become pregnant.

APPENDIX B. U.S. SCHEDULE OF CONTROLLED SUBSTANCES

Schedule	Description
I	High potential for abuse and of no currently accepted medical use. Not obtainable by prescription but may be legally procured for research, study, or instructional use. (e.g., *heroin, LSD, marijuana, mescaline, peyote*).
II	High-abuse potential and high liability for severe psychological or physical dependence potential. Prescription required and cannot be refilled. Prescription must be written in ink or typed and signed. A verbal prescription may be allowed in an emergency by the dispensing pharmacist but must be followed by a written prescription within 72 hours. Includes opium derivatives, other opioids, and short-acting barbiturates.
III	Potential for abuse is less than that for drugs in schedules I and II. Moderate-to-low physical dependence and high psychological dependence potential. Prescription required. May be refilled up to 5 times in 6 months. Prescription may be verbal (telephone) or written. Includes certain stimulants and depressants not included in the above schedules, and preparations containing limited quantities of certain opioids.

(continued)

Appendix B (*continued*)

Schedule	Description
IV	Lower potential for abuse than Schedule III drugs. Prescription required. May be refilled up to 5 times in 6 months. Prescription may be verbal (telephone) or written.
V	Abuse potential less than that for Schedule IV drugs. Preparations contain limited quantities of certain narcotic drugs. Generally intended for antitussive and anti-diarrheal purposes and may be distributed without a prescription provided that • such distribution is made only by a pharmacist; • not more than 240 ml or not more than 48 solid dosage units of any substance containing opium, nor more than 120 ml or not more than 24 solid dosage units of any other controlled substance may be distributed at retail to the same purchaser in any given 48-hour period without a valid prescription order; • the purchaser is at least 18 years old; • the pharmacist knows the purchaser or requests suitable identification; • the pharmacist keeps an official written record of name and address of purchaser, name, and quantity of controlled substance purchased, date of sale, and initials of dispensing pharmacist. This record is to be made available for inspection and copying by the U.S. officers authorized by the Attorney General; • other federal, state, or local law does not require a prescription order. Under jurisdiction of the Federal Controlled Substances Act. Refillable up to 5 times within 6 months.

APPENDIX G. ROUTINE IMMUNIZATION RECOMMENDATIONS

APPENDIX G.6. CHILDHOOD (BIRTH-12 YEARS) IMMUNIZATION SCHEDULE

Type	Birth	1 month	2 months	4 months	6 months	6-18 months	12-15 months	15-18 months	4-6 years	11-12 years
HBV	✔	✔			✔					
DTaP			✔	✔	✔		✔		✔	
IPV			✔	✔		✔			✔	
Hib			✔	✔	✔		✔			
Rotavirus			✔	✔	✔					
MMR							✔		✔	
TDaP										✔
Varicella							✔		✔	
PVC-13			✔	✔	✔		✔			
HAV							✔	✔		
Meningitis										✔
HPV										✔✔✔

Adapted from DHHS CDC 2015.

✔ = immunization due.

✔✔✔ = HPV 3-dose series, months 0, 1, 6.

APPENDIX G.7. CHILDHOOD (BIRTH-12 YEARS) IMMUNIZATION CATCH-UP SCHEDULE

Vaccine	Minimum Interval Between Doses			
	#1 to #2	#2 to #3	#3 to #4	#4 to #5
HBV	4 weeks	8 weeks (16 weeks after #1)		
DTaP	4 weeks	4 weeks	6 months	6 months
IPV	4 weeks	4 weeks	4 weeks	
MMR	4 weeks			
Var	4 weeks			
Rotavirus	4 weeks	4 weeks; do not administer >32 weeks of age		
PCV	2 months	2 months	2 months	6-15 months
HPV	4 weeks	20 weeks (24 weeks after #1		

Adapted from DHHS CDC 2015

APPENDIX G.8. RECOMMENDED ADULT IMMUNIZATION SCHEDULE

Type	19-21 yrs	22-26 yrs	27-49 yrs	50-59 yrs	60-65 yrs	≥65 yrs
Influenza	1 dose annually					
HBV	3 dose series: months 0, 1, 6					
Td/TdaP	Substitute Tdap for Td one time; then continue Td once every 10 years					
MMR*	Born >1957: 2 doses, 4 weeks apart					
Varicella*	Without evidence of immunity: 2 doses, 4 weeks apart					
Herpes zoster*					1 time dose	
PVC-13/ PVC-23					1 time dose	
HAV	Single Antigen, 2 doses: months 0, 6-12 (**Havrix**); 0, 6-18 (**Vaqta**)					
Meningitis	1 or more doses					
HPV (female)*β	3 doses; months 0, 1, 6					
HPV (male)β	3 doses; months 0, 1, 6					

Adapted from ACIP 2021

* Contraindicated in pregnancy

β Only if not previously vaccinated between 11 and 12 years-of-age

APPENDIX H. CONTRACEPTIVES

APPENDIX H.1. NON-HORMONAL VAGINAL CONTRACEPTIVES

▷ *lactic acid, citric acid, and potassium bitartrate vaginal gel* administer 1 pre-filled applicatorful (5 gm) vaginally immediately before or up to 1 hour before each episode of vaginal intercourse; may use during any part of the menstrual cycle

    Phexxi *Pre-filled vaginal applicator:* single-dose, (delivers 5 gm of gel containing lactic acid (1.8%), citric acid (1%), and potassium bitartrate (0.4%)

    Comment: **Phexxi** is a combination of lactic acid, citric acid, and potassium bitartrate, indicated for the prevention of pregnancy in females of reproductive potential for use as an on-demand method of contraception. **Phexxi** is not effective for the prevention of pregnancy when administered after intercourse. The most common adverse reactions (incidence ≥2%) have been vulvovaginal burning sensation, vulvovaginal pruritus, vulvovaginal mycotic infection, urinary tract infection, vulvovaginal discomfort, bacterial vaginosis, vaginal discharge, genital discomfort, dysuria, and vulvovaginal pain. Avoid use in females with a history of recurrent UTI, pyelonephritis, or urinary tract abnormalities. To report suspected adverse reactions, contact Evofem at 1-833-EVFMBIO or FDA at 1-800-FDA-1088 or visit www.fda.gov/medwatch.

APPENDIX H.2. HORMONAL CONTRACEPTIVE CONTRAINDICATIONS AND RECOMMENDATIONS

- All contraceptives are pregnancy category X
- No non-barrier contraceptives protect against STDs
- **Absolute Contraindication**
  - HTN >35 years-of-age
  - DM >35 years-of-age
  - LDL-C >160 or TG >250
  - Known or suspected pregnancy
  - Known or suspected carcinoma of the breast
  - Known or suspected carcinoma of the endometrium
  - Known or suspected estrogen-dependent neoplasia
  - Undiagnosed abnormal genital bleeding
  - Cerebral vascular or coronary artery disease
  - Cholestatic jaundice of pregnancy or jaundice with prior use
  - Hepatic adenoma or carcinoma or benign liver tumor
  - Active or past history of thrombophlebitis or thromboembolic disorder
- **Relative Contraindications**
  - Lactation
  - Asthma
  - Ulcerative colitis
  - Migraine or vascular headache
  - Cardiac or renal dysfunction
  - Gestational diabetes, prediabetes, diabetes mellitus
  - Diastolic BP 90 mmHg or greater or hypertension by any other criteria
  - Psychic depression
  - Varicose veins
  - Smoker >35 years-of-age
  - Sickle-cell or sickle-hemoglobin C disease
  - Cholestatic jaundice during pregnancy, active gallbladder disease
  - Hepatitis or mononucleosis during the preceding year
  - First-order family history of fatal or nonfatal rheumatic CVD or diabetes prior to age 50 years
  - Drug(s) with known interaction(s)
  - Elective surgery or immobilization within 4 weeks
  - Age >50 years

(continued)

Appendix H.2 (*continued*)

- **Recommendations**
  - Start the first pill on the first Sunday after menses begins. Thereafter, each new pill pack will be started on a Sunday.
  - Take each daily pill in the same 3-hour window (e.g., 9A-12N, 12N-3P; a 4-hour window prior to bedtime is not recommended).
  - If 1 pill is missed, take it as soon as possible and the next pill at the regular time.
  - If 2 pills are missed, take both pills as soon as possible and then two pills the following day. A barrier method should be used for the remainder of the pill pack.
  - If 3 pills are missed before 10th cycle day, resume taking OCs on a regular schedule and take precautions.
  - If 3 pills are missed after the 10th cycle day, discard the current pill pack and begin a new one 7 days after the last pill was taken.
  - If very low-dose OCs are used or if combination OCs are begun after the 5th day of the menstrual cycle, an additional method of birth control should be used for the first 7 days of OC use.
  - If nausea occurs as a side effect, select an OC with *lower* **estrogen** content.
  - If breakthrough bleeding occurs during the first half of the cycle, select an OC with *higher* **progesterone** content.
  - Symptoms of a serious nature include loss of vision, diplopia, unilateral numbness, weakness, or tingling, severe chest pain, severe pain in left arm or neck, severe leg pain, slurring of speech, and abdominal tenderness or mass.

APPENDIX H.3. 28-DAY ORAL CONTRACEPTIVES WITH ESTROGEN AND PROGESTERONE CONTENT

Comment: Beyaz, Loryna, Rajani, Syeda, Safyral, Tydemy, Yasmin, and Yaz are contraindicated with renal insufficiency and adrenal insufficiency. Monitor k^+ level during the first cycle if the patient is at risk for hyperkalemia for any reason. If the patient is taking drugs that increase potassium (e.g., ACEIs, ARBS, NSAIDs, K^+ sparing diuretics), the patient is at risk for hyperkalemia.

Combined Oral Contraceptive	Estrogen (mcg)	Progesterone (mg)
Alesse-21, Alesse-28 (X)(G) *ethinyl estradiol+levonorgestrel*	20	0.1
Altavera (X) *ethinyl estradiol+levonorgestrel*	30	0.15
Apri (X)(G) *ethinyl estradiol+desogestrel*	30	0.15
Aranelle (X)(G) *ethinyl estradiol+norethindrone*	35	0.5 1 0.5
Aviane (X)(G) *ethinyl estradiol+levonorgestrel*	20	0.1
Balcoltra (X) *ethinyl estradiol+levonorgestrel* plus *ferrous bisglycinate 36.5 mg*	20	0.1
Balziva (X)(G) *ethinyl estradiol+norethindrone*	35	0.4
Beyaz (X)(G) *ethinyl estradiol+drospirenone* plus levomefolate calcium 0.451 mcg (28 tabs)	20	3

(*continued*)

Appendix H.3 (*continued*)

Combined Oral Contraceptive	Estrogen (mcg)	Progesterone (mg)
Blisovi 24Fe (X)(G) *ethinyl estradiol+norethindrone* plus *ferrous fumarate* 75 mg (4 tabs)	20	1
Brevicon-21, Brevicon-28 (X)(G) *ethinyl estradiol+norethindrone*	35	0.5
Camrese (X) *ethinyl estradiol+levonorgestrel*	30 10	0.15
Camrese Lo (X) *ethinyl estradiol+levonorgestrel*	20 10	0.1
Cesia (X)(G) *ethinyl estradiol+desogestrel*	25 25 25	0.1 0.125 0.15
Cryselle (X)(G) *ethinyl estradiol+norgestrel*	30	0.3
Cyclessa (X)(G) *ethinyl estradiol+desogestrel*	25 25 25	0.1 0.125 0.15
Demulen 1/35-21, Demulen 1/35-28 (X)(G) *ethinyl estradiol+ethynodiol diacetate*	35	1
Demulen 1/50-21, Demulen 1/50-28 (X)(G) *ethinyl estradiol+ethynodiol diacetate*	50	1
Desogen (X)(G) *ethinyl estradiol+desogestrel diacetate*	30	0.15
Enpresse (X)(G) *ethinyl estradiol+levonorgestrel*	30 40 30	0.05 0.075 0.125
Estarylla (X) *ethinyl estradiol+norgestimate*	35	0.25
Estrostep Fe (X) *ethinyl estradiol+norethindrone* plus *ferrous fumarate* 75 mg	20 30 35	1 1 1
Femcon Fe (X)(G) *ethinyl estradiol+norethindrone* plus *ferrous fumarate* 75 mg	35	0.4
Generess Fe Chew tab (X)(G) *ethinyl estradiol+norethindrone* plus *ferrous fumarate* 75 mg	25	0.8
Genora (X)(G) *ethinyl estradiol+norethindrone*	35 35 35	0.5 1 0.5
Gianvi (X)(G) *ethinyl estradiol+drospirenone*	20	3
Gildess 1.5/30 (X)(G) *ethinyl estradiol+norethindrone*	30	1.5

(*continued*)

Appendix H.3 (continued)

Combined Oral Contraceptive	Estrogen (mcg)	Progesterone (mg)
Introvale (X) *ethinyl estradiol+levonorgestrel*	30	0.15
Jenest-28 (X) *ethinyl estradiol+norethindrone*	35 35	0.5 1
Jolessa (X)(G) *ethinyl estradiol+levonorgestrel*	30	0.15
Junel 1/20 (X)(G) *ethinyl estradiol+norethindrone*	20	1
Junel 1.5/30 (X)(G) *ethinyl estradiol+norethindrone*	30	1.5
Junel Fe 1/20 (X)(G) *ethinyl estradiol+norethindrone* plus *ferrous fumarate* 75 mg	20	1
Junel Fe 1.5/30 (X)(G) *ethinyl estradiol+norethindrone* plus *ferrous fumarate* 75 mg	30	1.5
Kaitlib Fe Chew Tab (X)(G) *ethinyl estradiol+norethindrone* plus *ferrous fumarate* 75 mg	25	0.8
Kariva (X)(G) *ethinyl estradiol+desogestrel*	20 10	0.15 0.15
Kelnor 1/35 (X)(G) *ethinyl estradiol+ethynodiol diacetate*	35	1
Kurvelo-28 *ethinyl estradiol/levonorgestrel*	30	0.15
Leena (X) *ethinyl estradiol+norethindrone*	35 35 35	0.5 1 0.5
Lessina 28 (X)(G) *ethinyl estradiol+levonorgestrel*	20	0.1
Levlen 21, Levlen 28 (X)(G) *ethinyl estradiol+levonorgestrel*	30	0.15
Levlite 28 (X)(G) *ethinyl estradiol+levonorgestrel*	20	0.1
Levora-21, Levora-28 (X)(G) *ethinyl estradiol+levonorgestrel*	30	0.15
Loestrin 21 1/20 (X)(G) *ethinyl estradiol+norethindrone*	20	1
Loestrin 21 1.5/30 (X)(G) *ethinyl estradiol+norethindrone*	30	1.5
Loestrin Fe 1/20 (X)(G) *ethinyl estradiol+norethindrone* plus *ferrous fumarate* 75 mg	20	1

(continued)

Appendix H.3 (*continued*)

Combined Oral Contraceptive	Estrogen (mcg)	Progesterone (mg)
Loestrin Fe 1.5/30 (X)(G) *ethinyl estradiol+norethindrone* <u>plus</u> *ferrous fumarate 75 mg (4 tabs)*	30	1.5
Loestrin 24 Fe (X)(G) *ethinyl estradiol+norethindrone* <u>plus</u> *ferrous fumarate 75 mg (4 tabs)*	20	1
Lo Loestrin Fe (X) *ethinyl estradiol+norethindrone* <u>plus</u> *ferrous fumarate 75 mg (2 tabs)*	10	1
Lomedia 24 Fe (X)(G) *ethinyl estradiol+norethindrone* <u>plus</u> *ferrous fumarate 75 mg*	20	1
Lo/Ovral-21, Lo/Ovral-28 (X)(G) *ethinyl estradiol+norgestrel*	30	0.3
Loryna (X) *ethinyl estradiol+drospirenone*	20	3
Low-Ogestrel-21, **Low-Ogestrel-28 (X)(G)** *ethinyl estradiol/norgestrel*	30	0.3
Lutera (X)(G) *ethinyl estradiol+levonorgestrel*	20	0.1
Lybrel (X) *ethinyl estradiol+levonorgestrel*	20	0.09
Mibelas 24 FE (X)(G) *ethinyl estradiol+norethindrone* <u>plus</u> *ferrous fumarate 75 mg*	20	1
Microgestin 1/20 (X)(G) *ethinyl estradiol+norethindrone*	20	1
Microgestin Fe 1/20 (X)(G) *ethinyl estradiol+norethindrone* <u>plus</u> *ferrous fumarate 75 mg*	20	1
Microgestin 1.5/30 (X)(G) *ethinyl estradiol+norethindrone*	30	1.5
Microgestin Fe 1.5/30 (X)(G) *ethinyl estradiol+norethindrone* <u>plus</u> *ferrous fumarate 75 mg*	30	1.5
Mircette (X)(G) *ethinyl estradiol+desogestrel diacetate*	20 10	0.15
Minastrin 24 FE (X)(G) *ethinyl estradiol+norethindrone* <u>plus</u> *ferrous fumarate 75 mg*	20	1
Modicon 0.5/35-28 (X)(G) *ethinyl estradiol+norethindrone*	35	0.5

(continued)

Appendix H.3 *(continued)*

Combined Oral Contraceptive	Estrogen (mcg)	Progesterone (mg)
MonoNessa (X)(G) *ethinyl estradiol+norgestimate*	35	0.25
Natazia (X)(G) *estradiol valerate+dienogest*	30 20 20 10	— 2 3 —
Necon 0.5/35-21, Necon 0.5/35-28 (X)(G) *ethinyl estradiol+norethindrone*	35	0.5
Necon 1/35-21, Necon 1/35-28 (X)(G) *ethinyl estradiol+norethindrone*	35	0.5
Necon 10/11-21, Necon 10/11-28 (X)(G) *ethinyl estradiol+norethindrone*	35 35	0.5 1
Necon 1/50-21, Necon 1/50-28 (X)(G) *mestranol+norethindrone*	50	1
Nelova 0.5/35-21, Nelova 0.5/35-28 (X)(G) *ethinyl estradiol+norethindrone*	35	0.5
Nelova 1/35-21, Nelova 1/35-28 (X)(G) *ethinyl estradiol+norethindrone*	35	1
Nelova 10/11-21, Nelova 10/11-28 (X)(G) *ethinyl estradiol/norethindrone*	35 35	0.5 1
Nelova 1/50-21, Nelova 1/50-28 (X)(G) *mestranol+norethindrone*	50	1
Neocon 7/7/7 (X)(G) *ethinyl estradiol+norethindrone*	35 35 35	0.5 0.75 1
Nextstellis (X) *estetrol+drospirenone* (*estetrol* is plant-derived estrogen)	14,200	3
Nordette-21, Nordette-28 (X)(G) *ethinyl estradiol+levonorgestrel*	30	0.15
Norinyl 1/35-21, Norinyl 1/35-28 (X)(G) *ethinyl estradiol+norethindrone*	35	1
Norinyl 1/50-21, Norinyl 1/50-28 (X)(G) *mestranol+norethindrone*	50	1
Nortrel 0.5/35 (X)(G) *ethinyl estradiol/norethindrone*	35	0.5
Nortrel 1/35-21, Nortrel 1/35-28 (X)(G) *ethinyl estradiol+norethindrone*	35	1
Nortrel 7/7/7-28 (X)(G) *ethinyl estradiol+norethindrone*	35 35 35	0.5 0.75 1
Ocella (X)(G) *ethinyl estradiol+drospirenone*	30	3

(continued)

Appendix H.3 (*continued*)

Combined Oral Contraceptive	Estrogen (mcg)	Progesterone (mg)
Ortho-Cept 28 (X)(G) *ethinyl estradiol+desogestrel*	30	0.15
Ortho-Cyclen 28 (X)(G) *ethinyl estradiol+norgestimate*	35	0.25
Ortho-Novum 1/35-21, Ortho-Novum 1/35-28 (X)(G) *ethinyl estradiol+norethindrone*	35	1
Ortho-Novum 1/50-21, Ortho-Novum 1/50-28 (X)(G) *mestranol+norethindrone*	50	1
Ortho-Novum 7/7/7-28 (X)(G) *ethinyl estradiol+norethindrone*	35 35 35	0.5 0.75 1
Ortho-Novum 10/11-28 (X) *ethinyl estradiol+norethindrone*	35 35	0.5 1
Ortho Tri-Cyclen 21, Ortho Tri-Cyclen 28 (X)(G) *ethinyl estradiol+norgestimate*	35 35 35	0.18 0.215 0.25
Ortho Tri-Cyclen Lo (X)(G) *ethinyl estradiol+norgestimate*	25 25 25	0.18 0.215 0.25
Ovcon 35 Fe (X)(G) *ethinyl estradiol+norethindrone* plus *ferrous fumarate* 75 mg (4 tabs)	35	0.4
Ovcon 50-28, Ovcon 50-28 (X)(G) *ethinyl estradiol+norethindrone*	50	1
Ovral-21, Ovral-28 (X)(G) *ethinyl estradiol+norgestrel*	50	0.5
Portia (X)(G) *ethinyl estradiol+levonorgestrel*	30	0.15
Previfem (X) *ethinyl estradiol+norgestimate*	35	0.25
Quasense (X) *ethinyl estradiol+levonorgestrel*	30	0.15
Rajani *ethinyl estradiol + drospirenone* plus *levomefolate calcium* 0.451 mg	20	3
Reclipsen (X)(G) *ethinyl estradiol+desogestrel* plus *ferrous fumarate* 75 mg (4 tabs)	30	0.15
Safyral (X)(G) *ethinyl estradiol+drospirenone* plus *levomefolate calcium* 0.451 mg	30	3

(*continued*)

Appendix H.3 *(continued)*

Combined Oral Contraceptive	Estrogen (mcg)	Progesterone (mg)
Sprintec 28 (X)(G) *ethinyl estradiol+norgestimate*	35	0.25
Syeda (X) *ethinyl estradiol+drospirenone*	30	3
Tarina Fe 1/20 (X)(G) *ethinyl estradiol+norethindrone* plus *ferrous fumarate* 75 mg (7 tabs)	20	1
Taytulla Fe 1/20 (X)(G) (Softgel caps) *ethinyl estradiol+norethindrone* plus *ferrous fumarate* 75 mg (4 Softgel caps)	20	1
Tilia Fe (X)(G) *ethinyl estradiol+norethindrone* plus *ferrous fumarate* 75 mg (7 tabs)	20 30 35	1 1 1
Tri-Legest 21 (X)(G) *ethinyl estradiol+norethindrone*	20 30 35	1 1 1
Tri-Legest Fe (X)(G) *ethinyl estradiol+norethindrone* plus *ferrous fumarate* 75 mg (7 tabs)	20 30 35	1 1 1
Tri-Levlen 21, Tri-Levlen 28 (X)(G) *ethinyl estradiol+levonorgestrel*	30 40 30	0.05 0.075 0.125
Tri-Lo-Estarylla (X)(G) *ethinyl estradiol+norgestimate*	25 25 25	0.18 0.215 0.25
Tri-Lo-Sprintec (X)(G) *ethinyl estradiol+norgestimate*	25 25 25	0.18 0.215 0.25
TriNessa (X)(G) *ethinyl estradiol+norgestimate*	35 35 35	0.18 0.215 0.25
Tri-Norinyl 21, Tri-Norinyl 28 (X)(G) *ethinyl estradiol+norethindrone*	35 35 35	0.5 1 0.5
Triphasil-21, Triphasil-28 (X)(G) *ethinyl estradiol+levonorgestrel*	30 40 30	0.050 0.075 0.125
Tri-Previfem (X)(G) *ethinyl estradiol+norgestimate*	35 35 35	0.18 0.215 0.25
Tri-Sprintec (X)(G) *ethinyl estradiol+norgestimate*	35 35 35	0.18 0.215 0.25
Trivora (X)(G) *ethinyl estradiol+levonorgestrel*	30 40 30	0.05 0.075 0.125

(continued)

Appendix H.3 (*continued*)

Combined Oral Contraceptive	Estrogen (mcg)	Progesterone (mg)
Tydemy *ethinyl estradiol+drospirenone* plus *levomefolate calcium* 0.451 mg	30	3
Velivet (X)(G) *ethinyl estradiol+desogestrel*	25 25 25	0.1 0.125 0.15
Vienva (X) *ethinyl estradiol+levonorgestrel*	20	0.1
Yasmin (X)(G) *ethinyl estradiol+drospirenone*	30	3
Yaz (X)(G) *ethinyl estradiol+drospirenone*	20	3
Zovia 1/35E-28 (X)(G) *ethinyl estradiol+ethynodiol diacetate*	35	1
Zovia 1/50E-28 (X)(G) *ethinyl estradiol+ethynodiol diacetate*	50	1

APPENDIX H.4. EXTENDED-CYCLE ORAL CONTRACEPTIVES

91 Day

▷ *ethinyl estradiol+levonorgestrel* (X) 1 tab daily x 91 days; repeat (no tablet-free days)

    Ashlyna (G) *Tab:* levonor 15 mcg+eth est 30 mcg (84)+eth est 10 mcg (7)
    (91 tabs/pck)
    Jolessa (G) *Tab:* levonor 15 mcg+eth est 30 mcg (84)+inert tabs (7m91 tabs/pck)
    LoSeasonique *Tab:* levonor 0.1 mcg+eth est 20 mcg (84)+eth est 10 mcg (7) (91 tabs/pck)
    Quartette (G) *Tab:* levonor 15 mcg+eth est 30 mcg (84)+eth est 10 mcg (7) (91 tabs/pck)
    Quasense (G) *Tab:* levonor 15 mcg+eth est 30 mcg (84)+inert tabs (7) (91 tabs/pck)
    Seasonale (G) *Tab:* levonor 15 mcg+eth est 30 mcg (84)+inert tabs (7) (91 tabs/pck)
    Seasonique (G) *Tab:* levonor 15 mcg+eth est 30 mcg (84)+eth est 10 mcg (7) (91 tabs/pck)

365 Day

▷ *ethinyl estradiol+levonorgestrel* (X) 1 tab daily x 28 days; repeat (no tablet-free days)

    Lybrel *Tab:* levonor 0.09 mcg+eth est 20 mcg (28 tabs/pck)

APPENDIX H.5. PROGESTERONE-ONLY ORAL CONTRACEPTIVES ("MINI-PILL")

Brand	Progesterone	mcg
Comment: Take progestin-only pills at the same time each day (within a 3-hour time window). If a pill is missed, another method of contraception should be used for the remainder of the pill pack.		
Camila (X)(G)	*norethindrone*	35
Errin (X)(G)	*norethindrone*	35
Jolivette (X)(G)	*norethindrone*	35
Micronor (X)(G)	*norethindrone*	35
Nora-BE (X)(G)	*norethindrone*	35
Nor-QD (X)(G)	*norethindrone*	35

(*continued*)

Appendix H.5 (*continued*)

Brand	Progesterone	mcg
Ortho Micronor (X)(G)	*norethindrone*	35
Ovrette (X)(G)	*norgestrel*	7.5

APPENDIX H.7. TRANSDERMAL CONTRACEPTIVES

Ethinyl Estradiol+Norelgestromin

Comment: Apply the transdermal patch to the abdomen, buttock, upper-outer arm, or upper torso. Do not apply the transdermal patch to the breast. Rotate the site (however, may use the same anatomical area).

▶ *ethinyl estradiol+levonorgestrel* (X) apply one patch once weekly x 3 weeks; then 1 patch-free week; then, repeat sequence

  Twirla *Trandsermal Patch:* eth est 30 mcg+levo 120 mcg per day (1, 3/pck)

▶ *ethinyl estradiol+norelgestromin* (X)(G) apply one patch once weekly x 3 weeks; then 1 patch-free week; then repeat sequence

  Ortho Evra *Transdermal patch:* eth est 20 mcg+norel 150 mcg per day (1, 3/pck)

APPENDIX H.8. CONTRACEPTIVE VAGINAL RINGS

Ethinyl Estradiol+Etonogestrel

Comment: The vaginal ring should be inserted prior to, or on fifth day, of the menstrual cycle. Use of a backup method is recommended during the first week. When switching from oral contraceptives, the vaginal ring should be inserted anytime within 7 days after the last active tablet and no later than the day a new pill pack would have been started (no back up method is needed). If the ring is accidently expelled for less than 3 hours, it should be rinsed with cool-to-lukewarm water and reinserted promptly. If ring removal lasts for more than 3 hours, an additional contraceptive method should be used. If the ring is lost, a new ring should be inserted and the regimen continued without alteration.

▶ *etonogestrel+ethinyl estradiol* (X) insert 1 ring vaginally and leave in place for 3 weeks; then remove for 1 ring-free week; then repeat

  EluRyng (G) *Vag ring:* eth est 2.7 mg (0.015 mg/day)+etonor 11.7 mg (0.12 mg/day) (1, 3/pck) (polymeric)

  NuvaRing (G) *Vag ring:* eth est 2.7 mg (0.015 mg/day)+*etonor* 11.7 mg (0.12 mg/day) (1, 3/pck) (polymeric)

▶ *segesterone acetate+ethinyl estradiol* (X) insert 1 ring vaginally and leave in place for 3 weeks (21 on-days); then, remove, clean, and store in the compact storage case suppled; after 7 off-days, clean and re-insert for the next 21 on-day/7 off-day cycle; discard the ring after 13 cycles

  Annovera *Vag ring:* eth est 17.4 mg (0.013 mg/day)+segest 103 mg (0.15 mg/day) (1/pck w. compact case)(silicone elastomer)

Comment: Contraindications to **Annovera/NuvaRing** include co-administration with hepatitis C drug combinations containing *ombitasvir+paritaprevir+ritonavir*, with or without *dasabuvir*, age >35 years, smoking, risk of arterial or venous thrombotic diseases, breast cancer or other estrogen or progestin-sensitive cancer, liver tumors or liver disease, acute hepatitis or cirrhosis, undiagnosed abnormal uterine bleeding, and pregnancy. Stop **Annovera/NuvaRing** at least 4 weeks before and through 2 weeks after major surgery. **Annovera/NuvaRing** are not recommended with breastfeeding. Start no earlier than 4 weeks after delivery in females who are not breastfeeding. Drugs or herbal products that induce certain enzymes, including CYP3A4, may decrease the effectiveness of **Annovera/NuvaRing** or increase breakthrough bleeding. Counsel patients to use a back-up or alternative method of contraception when enzyme inducers are used.

(continued)

Appendix H.8 (*continued*)

Comment: NuvaRing is a polymeric vaginal ring containing 11.7 mg *etonogestrel* and 2.7 mg *ethinyl estradiol*, which releases on average 0.12 mg/day of *etonogestrel* and 0.015 mg/day of *ethinyl estradiol*. Do not re-use NuvaRing (discard after 3 weeks in-use and after 7 days, start the next cycle with a new NuvaRing).

Comment: The Annovera vaginal system (ring) is a silicone elastomer vaginal system containing 103 mg *segesterone acetate* and 17.4 mg *ethinyl estradiol*, which releases on average 0.15 mg/day of *segesterone acetate* and 0.013 mg/day of *ethinyl estradiol*. Annovera is the first and only vaginal system/ring that provides contraception for 13 cycles. The removed vaginal system should be cleaned with mild soap and warm water, patted dry with a clean cloth towel or paper towel, and stored in the case provided during the one-week dose-free interval. At the end of the dose-free interval, the vaginal system should be cleaned prior to being placed back in the vagina for the next cycle.

APPENDIX H.9. SUBDERMAL CONTRACEPTIVES

Comment: Implants must be inserted within 7 days of the onset of menses. A complete physical examination is required annually. Remove if pregnancy, thromboembolic disorder including thrombophlebitis, jaundice, and visual disturbances. Not for use by patients with hypertension, diabetes, hyperlipidemia, impaired liver function, epilepsy, asthma, migraine, depression, cardiac or renal insufficiency, thromboembolic disorder including thrombophlebitis, pro-longed immobilization, or who are smokers.

▷ *etonogestrel* (X) implant rod subdermally in the upper inner non-dominant arm; remove and replace at the end of 3 years
    Implanon, Nexplanon
      Implantable rod: 68 mg implant for subdermal insertion (w. insertion device; latex-free)

▷ *levonorgestrel* (X) implant rods subdermally in the upper inner non-dominant arm; remove and replace at the end of 5 years
    Norplant
      Implantable rods: 6-36 mg implants (total 216 mg) for subdermal insertion (1 kit w. sterile supplies)

APPENDIX H.10. INTRAUTERINE CONTRACEPTIVES

Comment: Indicated in women who have had at least one child and who are in a stable, mutually monogamous relationship. Reexamine after menses within 3 months (recommend 4-6 weeks) to check placement.

▷ *levonorgestrel* (X)
    Kyleena *IUD:* 19.5 mg (replace at least every 5 years)
    Liletta *IUD:* 52 mg (replace at least every 5 years)
    Mirena *IUD:* 52 mg (replace at least every 6 years)
    Skyla *IUD:* 13.5 mg (replace at least every 3 years)

APPENDIX H.11. EMERGENCY CONTRACEPTION

Comment: Emergency contraception must be started within 72 hours after unprotected intercourse following a negative urine hCG pregnancy test. If vomiting occurs within 1 hour of taking a dose, repeat the dose.

▷ *ethinyl estradiol+levonorgestrel* (X) 2 tabs as soon as possible after unprotected intercourse or contraceptive failure, then 2 more 12 hours after first dose
Premenarchal: not applicable
    Preven *Tab:* eth est 50 mcg+levonor 250 mcg (4/pck) *plus* Pregnancy test: 1 hCG home pregnancy test
    Yuzpe Regimen *Tab:* eth est 50 mcg+levonor 250 mcg (4/pck)

▷ *levonorgestrel* (X)(OTC)(G) 1 tab as soon as possible, within 72 hours, after unprotected sex or suspected contraceptive failure

(*continued*)

Appendix H.11 (*continued*)

   Premenarchal: not applicable; <17 years (prescription required); ≥17 years (OTC)
      EContra EZ *Tab:* 1.5 mg single-dose
      My Way *Tab:* 1.5 mg single-dose
      Plan B One Step *Tab:* 1.5 mg single-dose
      EContra EZ *Tab:* 1.5 mg single-dose
      Preventeza *Tab:* 1.5 mg single-dose

▷ *ulipristal* (X)(G) take 1 tab as soon as possible within 120 hours (5 days) after unprotected intercourse or contraceptive failure; may repeat dose if vomiting occurs within 3 hours
   Pediatric: premenarchal: not applicable
      ella *Tab:* 30 mg (1/pck)
      Logilia *Tab:* 30 mg (1/pck)

APPENDIX K. TOPICAL CORTICOSTEROIDS BY POTENCY

Comment: All topical, oral, and parenteral corticosteroids are pregnancy category C. Use with caution in infants and children. Steroids should be applied sparingly and for the shortest time necessary. Do not use in the diaper area. Do not use an occlusive dressing. Systemic absorption of topical corticosteroids can induce reversible hypothalamic-pituitary-adrenal (HPA) axis suppression with the potential for clinical glucocorticoid insufficiency.

Potency guide: Face: Low potency
                 Ears/Scalp margin: Intermediate potency
                 Eyelids: Hydrocortisone in ophthalmic ointment base 1%
                 Chest/Back: Intermediate potency
                 Skin folds: Low potency

Generic Name and Pregnancy Category	Brands, Formulation, and Dosing Frequency	Strength and Volume
Low Potency		
alclometasone dipropionate (C)	**Aclovate** Crm bid-tid **Aclovate** Oint bid-tid	0.05% (15,45, 60 gm) 0.05% (15,45, 60 gm)
fluocinolone acetonide (C)	**Synalar** Crm bid-qid	0.025% (15, 60 gm)
hydrocortisone base or *acetate* (C)(G)	**Anusol-HC** Crm bid-qid **Hytone** Crm bid-qid **Hytone** Oint bid-qid **Hytone** Lotn bid-qid	2.5% (30 gm) 1% (1, 2 oz) 1% (1 oz) 1% (2 oz)
	Hytone Crm bid-qid **Hytone** Oint bid-qid **Hytone** Lotn bid-qid **U-cort** Crm bid-qid	2.5% (1, 2 oz) 2.5% (1 oz) 2.5% (1 oz) 1% (7, 28, 35 gm)
triamcinolone acetonide (C)(G)	**Kenalog** Crm bid-qid **Kenalog** Lotn bid-qid **Kenalog** Oint bid-qid	0.025% (15, 80 gm) 0.025% (60 ml) 0.025% (15, 60, 80 gm)
Intermediate Potency		
betamethasone valerate (C)(G)	**Luxiq** Foam bid	0.12% (100 gm)
clocortolone pivalate (C)(G)	**Cloderm** Crm bid	0.1% (30, 45, 75, 90 gm)

(*continued*)

Appendix K (*continued*)

Generic Name and Pregnancy Category	Brands, Formulation, and Dosing Frequency	Strength and Volume
desonide (C)(G)	**Desonate** Gel/Formulation bid-tid	0.05% (15, 60 gm)
	DesOwen Crm bid-tid	0.05% (15, 60 gm)
	DesOwen Lotn bid-tid	0.05% (2, 4 fl oz)
	DesOwen Oint bid-tid	0.05% (15, 60 gm)
	Tridesilon Crm bid-qid	0.05% (15, 60 gm)
	Tridesilon Oint bid-qid	0.05% (15, 60 gm)
	Verdeso Foam	
desoximetasone (C)(G)	**Topicort-LP** Emol Crm bid	0.05% (15, 60 gm; 4 oz)
fluocinolone acetonide (C)(G)	**Capex** Shampoo	0.01% (4 oz)
	Derma-Smoothe/FS Oil tid	0.01% (4 oz)
	Derma-Smoothe/FS Shampoo	0.01% (4 oz)
	Synalar Crm bid-qid	0.025% (15, 30, 60 gm)
	Synalar Oint bid-qid	0.025% (15, 60 gm)
flurandrenolide (C)(G)	**Cordran-SP** Crm bid to tid	0.025% (30, 60 gm)
	Cordran Oint bid-tid	0.025% (30, 60 gm)
	Cordran-SP Crm bid-tid	0.05% (15, 30, 60 gm)
	Cordran Lotn bid-tid	0.05% (15, 60 ml)
	Cordran Oint bid-tid	0.05% (15, 30, 60 gm)
fluticasone propionate (C)(G)	**Cutivate** Oint bid	0.005% (15, 30, 60 gm)
	Cutivate Crm qd-bid	0.05% (15, 30, 60 gm)
	Cutivate Lotn qd-bid	0.05%
hydrocortisone probutate (C)	**Pandel** Crm qd-bid	0.1% (15, 45 gm)
hydrocortisone butyrate (C)(G)	**Locoid** Crm bid-tid	0.1% (15, 45 gm)
	Locoid Oint bid-tid	0.1% (15, 45 gm)
	Locoid Soln bid-tid	0.1% (30, 60 ml)
hydrocortisone valerate (C)(G)	**Westcort** Crm bid-tid	0.2% (15, 45, 60, 120 gm)
	Westcort Oint bid-tid	0.2% (15, 45, 60 gm)
mometasone furoate (C)	**Elocon** Crm qd	0.1% (15, 45 gm)
	Elocon Lotn qd	0.1% (30, 60 ml)
	Elocon Oint qd	0.1% (15, 45 gm)
prednicarbate	**Dermatop** Emol Crm bid	0.1% (15, 60 gm)
	Dermatop Oint bid	
triamcinolone acetonide (C)(G)	**Kenalog** Crm bid-tid	0.1% (15, 60, 80 gm)
	Kenalog Lotn bid-tid	0.1% (60 ml)
	Kenalog Emul Spray bid-tid	0.2% (63, 100 gm)
High Potency		
amcinonide (C)(G)	Crm bid-tid	0.1% (15, 30, 60 gm)
	Lotn bid	0.1% (20, 60 ml)
	Oint bid	0.1% (15, 30, 60 gm)
Betamethasone dipropionate (C)	**Servivo** Spray Emul Spray bid	0.05% (60, 120 ml)

(*continued*)

Appendix K (*continued*)

Generic Name and Pregnancy Category	Brands, Formulation, and Dosing Frequency	Strength and Volume
betamethasone dipropionate, augmented (C)	**Diprolene** AF Emol Crm qd-bid **Diprolene** Lotn qd-bid	0.05% (15, 50 gm) 0.05% (30, 60 ml)
clobetasol propionate (C)(G)	**Bryhali** Lotn bid **Impoyz** Crm bid	0.01% (60, 112 gm) 0.025% (60, 112 gm)
desoximetasone (C)(G)	**Topicort** Gel bid **Topicort** Emol Crm bid **Topicort** Oint bid	0.05% (15, 60 gm) 0.25% (15, 60 gm) 0.25% (15, 60 gm)
diflorasone diacetate (C)	**Psorcon e** Emol Crm bid **Psorcon e** Emol Oint qd-tid	0.05% (15, 30, 60 gm) 0.05% (15, 30, 60 gm)
fluocinonide (C)	**Lidex** Crm bid-qid **Lidex** Gel bid-qid **Lidex** Oint bid-qid **Lidex** Soln bid-qid **Lidex-E** Emol Crm bid-qid	0.05% (15, 30, 60, 120 gm) 0.05% (15, 30, 60 gm) 0.05% (15, 30, 60, 120 gm) 0.05% (20, 60 ml) 0.05% (15, 30, 60 gm)
flurandrenolide (C)	**Cordan** Oint bid-tid **Cordan** Crm bid-tid	0.05% (15, 30, 60 gm) 0.025% (30, 60, 120 gm) 0.05% (15, 30, 60, 120 gm)
halcinonide (C)	**Halog** Crm bid-tid **Halog** Oint bid-tid **Halog** Soln bid-tid **Halog-E** Emol Crm qd-tid	0.1% (15, 30, 60, 240 gm) 0.1% (15, 30, 60, 120 gm) 0.1% (20, 60 ml) 0.1% (15, 30, 60 gm)
triamcinolone acetonide (C)(G)	**Kenalog** Crm bid-tid	0.5% (20 gm)
Super High Potency		
betamethasone dipropionate, augmented (C)(G)	**Diprolene** Oint qd-bid **Diprolene** Gel qd-bid	0.05% (15, 50 gm) 0.05% (15, 50 gm)
clobetasol propionate (C)(G)	**Bryhali** Lotn bid **Clobex** Shampoo daily **Clobex** Spray bid **Cormax** Oint bid **Cormax** Scalp App **Olux** Foam **Olux E** Foam **Temovate** Crm bid **Temovate** Gel bid **Temovate** Oint bid	0.01% (60, 112 gm) 0.05% (4 oz) 0.05% (2, 4.5 oz) 0.05% (15, 45 gm) 0.05% (15, 45 gm) 0.05% (50, 100 gm) 0.05% (50, 100 gm) 0.05% (15, 30, 45, 60 gm) 0.05% (15, 30, 60 gm) 0.05% (15, 30, 45, 60 gm)
	Temovate Scalp App bid **Temovate-E** Emol Crm bid	0.05% (25, 50 ml) 0.05% (15, 30, 60 gm)
fluocinonide (C)(G)	**Vanos** Oint qd-tid	0.1% (30, 60, 120 gm)
flurandrenolide (C)	**Cordran** Tape q 12 hours	4 mcg/sq cm (roll of 3″ x 80″)
halobetasol propionate (C)	**Ultravate** Crm qd-bid **Ultravate** Oint qd to bid	0.05% (15, 45 gm) 0.05% (15, 45 gm)

APPENDIX L. ORAL CORTICOSTEROIDS

Comment: Systemic corticosteroids increase glucose intolerance, reduce the action of insulin and oral hypoglycemic agents, reduce adrenal cortex activity, decrease immunity, mask signs of infection, impair wound healing, suppress growth in children, and promote osteoporosis, fluid retention, and weight gain. Use systemic steroids with caution, using the lowest possible dose to affect clinical response, and withdraw (wean) gradually in tapering doses to avoid adrenal insufficiency. The American Academy of Rheumatology (AAR) recommends the following daily doses for anyone on a chronic systemic corticosteroid regimen: Calcium 1200-1500 mg/day and vitamin D 800-1000 IU/day.

Oral Corticosteroids

▷ *betamethasone* (C)(G) initially 0.6-7.2 mg daily
　　Pediatric: <12 years: not recommended; ≥12 years: same as adult
　　　　Celestone *Tab:* 0.6 mg; *Syr:* 0.6 mg/5 ml (120 ml)

▷ *cortisone* (D)(G) initially 25-300 mg daily or every other day
　　Pediatric: <12 years: not recommended; ≥12 years: same as adult
　　　　Cortone Acetate *Tab:* 25 mg

▷ *dexamethasone* (C)(G) initially 0.75-9 mg/day
　　Pediatric: <12 years: not recommended; ≥12 years: same as adult
　　　　Decadron *Tab:* 0.5*, 0.75*, 4*mg; *Syr:* 0.5 mg/5 ml (100 ml)
　　　　Decadron 5-12 Pak *Tabs:* 0.75*mg (12/pck)

▷ *hydrocortisone* (C)(G) 20-240 mg daily
　　Pediatric: <12 years: 2-8 mg/day; ≥12 years: same as adult
　　　　Cortef *Tab:* 5, 10, 20 mg; *Oral susp:* 10 mg/5 ml
　　　　Hydrocortone *Tab:* 10 mg

▷ *methylprednisolone* (C)(G) 4-48 mg/day
　　Pediatric: <12 years: not recommended; ≥12 years: same as adult
　　　　Medrol *Tab:* 2*, 4*, 8*, 16*, 24*, 32*mg
　　　　Medrol Dosepak *Dosepak:* 4*mg tabs (21/pck)

▷ *prednisolone* (C)(G) initially 5-60 mg/day in 1-2 doses x 3-5 days
　　Pediatric: 0.14-2 mg/kg/day in 3-4 doses x 3-5 days
　　　　Flo-Pred *Susp:* 5, 15 mg/5 ml
　　　　Orapred *Soln:* 15 mg/5 ml (grape) (dye-free, alcohol 2%)
　　　　Orapred ODT *Tab:* 10, 15, 30 mg orally disintegrating (grape)
　　　　Pediapred *Soln:* 5 mg/5 ml (raspberry) (sugar-, alcohol-, dye-free)
　　　　Prelone *Syr:* 15 mg/5 ml
　　　　Comment: Flo-Pred does not require refrigeration or shaking prior to use.

▷ *prednisone* (C)(G) initially 5-60 mg/day in 1-2 doses x 3-5 days
　　Pediatric: 0.14-2 mg/kg/day in 3-4 doses x 3-5 days
　　　　Deltasone *Tab:* 2.5*, 5*, 10*, 20*, 50*mg

▷ *prednisone (delayed release)* (C)(G) initially 5-60 mg/day in 1-2 doses x 3-5 days
　　Pediatric: 0.14-**2 mg**/kg/day in 3-4 doses x 3-5 days
　　　　Rayos *Tab:* 1, 2, 5 mg del-rel

▷ *triamcinolone* (C)(G) initially 4-48 mg/day in 1-2 doses x 3-5 days
　　Pediatric: 0.14-2 mg/kg/day in 3-4 doses x 3-5 days
　　　　Aristocort *Tab:* 4*mg
　　　　Aristocort Forte *Susp:* 40 mg/ml (benzoyl alcohol)
　　　　Aristocort Aristopak *Tab:* 4*mg (16/pck)

 APPENDIX M. PARENTERAL CORTICOSTEROIDS

Comment: Systemic glucocorticosteroids increase glucose intolerance, reduce the action of insulin and oral hypoglycemic agents, reduce adrenal cortex activity, decrease immunity, mask signs of infection, impair wound healing, suppress growth in children, and promote osteoporosis, fluid retention, and weight gain. Use systemic steroids with caution, using the

(continued)

Appendix M. (*continued*)

lowest possible dose to affect clinical response, and withdraw (wean) gradually in tapering doses to avoid adrenal insufficiency. The American Academy of Rheumatology (AAR) recommends the following daily doses for anyone on a chronic systemic corticosteroid regimen: Calcium 1200-1500 mg/day and vitamin D 800-1000 IU/day.

▷ *betamethasone* (C)(G)
    Celestone 0.5-9 mg IM/IV x 1 dose
      Vial: 3 mg/ml (10 ml)
    Celestone Soluspan 0.5-9 mg IM/IV x 1 dose; usual IM dose 6 mg
      Vial: 6 mg/ml (10 ml)

▷ *cortisone* (D)(G) 20-300 mg IM
    Pediatric: <12 years: not recommended; ≥12 years: same as adult
    Cortone Acetate *Vial:* 50 mg/ml (10 ml)

▷ *dexamethasone* (C)(G) initially 0.5-9 mg IM/IV daily
    Pediatric: <12 years: not recommended; ≥12 years: same as adult
    Decadron *Vial:* 4, 24 mg/ml for IM use (5 ml, sulfites)
    Dalalone D.P. *Vial:* 16 mg/ml (1, 5 ml)
    Decadron-LA *Vial:* 8 mg/ml (1, 5 ml)

▷ *hydrocortisone* (C)(G) initially 100-500 mg IM/IV daily
    Pediatric: 2-8 mg/kg loading dose (max 250 mg); then 8 mg/kg/day
    Hydrocortone *Vial:* 50 mg/ml (10 ml)
    Solu-Cortef *Vial:* 100 mg (2 ml); 250 mg (2 ml); 500 mg (4 ml); 1 gm (8 ml)

▷ *hydrocortisone phosphate* (C)(G) for IM, IV, and SC injection
    Pediatric: <12 years: not recommended; ≥12 years: same as adult
    Hydrocortone *Vial:* 50 mg/ml (2 ml)

▷ *methylprednisolone* (C)(G) 40-120 mg IM/week for 1-4 weeks
    Pediatric: <12 years: not recommended; ≥12 years: same as adult
    Depo-Medrol *Vial:* 20 mg/ml (5 ml); 40 mg/ml (5, 10 ml); 80 mg/ml (5 ml)

▷ *methylprednisolone sodium succinate* (C)(G) 10-40 mg IV initially; then, IM or IV
    Pediatric: 1-2 mg/kg loading dose; then 1.6 mg/kg/day in divided doses at least
    6 hours apart
    Solu-Medrol *Vial:* 40 mg (1 ml), 125 mg (2 ml), 500 mg (4 ml); 1 g (8 ml); 2 g (8 ml)

▷ *triamcinolone* (C)(G) 40 mg IM/week
    Pediatric: <12 years: not recommended; ≥12 years: same as adult
    Aristocort *Vial:* 25 mg/ml (5 ml)
    Aristocort Forte *Vial:* 40 mg/ml (1, 5 ml)(*do not administer IV*)
    Aristospan *Vial:* 5 mg/ml (5 ml); 20 mg/ml (1, 5 ml)
    TAC-3 *Vial:* 3 mg/ml (5 ml) for intralesional and intradermal use

Injectable Corticosteroid/Anesthetic

▷ *dexamethasone/lidocaine* (C) 0.1-0.75 ml into painful area
    Decadron Phosphate with Xylocaine *Vial:* dexa 4 mg/lido 10 mg per ml (5 ml)

APPENDIX N. INHALATIONAL CORTICOSTEROIDS

Comment: Inhaled corticosteroids are indicated for the long-term control of asthma. Inhaled corticosteroids are not indicated for exercise-induced asthma or for relief of acute symptoms (i.e., "rescue"). Low doses are indicated for mild persistent asthma, medium doses are indicated for moderate persistent asthma, and high doses are reserved for severe cases. Titrate to lowest effective dose. To reduce the potential for adverse effects with inhalers, the patient should use a spacer or holding chamber and rinse the mouth and spit after every inhalation treatment. Linear growth should be monitored in children. When inhaled doses exceed 1000 mcg/day, consider supplements of calcium (1-1.5 gm/day), vitamin D (400 IU/day).

▷ *beclomethasone* (C)
    Beclovent 2 inhalations tid-qid or 4 inhalations bid; max 20 inhalations/day

(*continued*)

Appendix N. *(continued)*

    Pediatric: <6 years: not recommended; 6-12 years: 1-2 inhalations tid-qid <u>or</u> 4 inhalations bid; max 10 inhalations/day

      Inhaler: 42 mcg/actuation (6.7 g, 80 inh); 16.8 g (200 inh)

Qvar *Previously using <u>only</u> bronchodilators:* initiate 40-80 mcg bid; max 320 mcg/day; *Previously using an inhaled corticosteroid:* initiate 40-160 mcg bid; max 320 mcg/day; Previously taking a systemic corticosteroid: attempt to wean off the systemic drug after approximately 1 week after initiating Qvar

    Pediatric: <12 years: not recommended; ≥12 years: same as adult

      Inhaler: 40, 80 mcg/actuation metered-dose aerosol w. dose counter (8.7 g, 120 inh) (CFC-free)

Vanceril 2 inhalations tid to qid <u>or</u> 4 inhalations bid

    Pediatric: <6 years: not recommended; 6-12 years: 1-2 inhalations tid to qid

      Inhaler: 42 mcg/actuation (16.8 g, 200 inh)

Vanceril Double Strength 2 inhalations bid

    Pediatric: <6 years: not recommended; 6-12 years: 1-2 inhalations bid; >12 years: same as adult

      Inhaler: 84 mcg/actuation (12.2 g, 120 inh)

▶ *budesonide* (B)(G)

Pulmicort Respules use turbuhaler

    Pediatric: <12 months: not recommended; ≥12 months to 8 years: *Previously using <u>only</u> bronchodilators:* initiate 0.5 mg/day once daily <u>or</u> in 2 divided doses; may start at 0.25 mg/day; *Previously using inhaled orticosteroids:* initiate 0.5 mg/day daily <u>or</u> in 2 divided doses; max 1 mg/day; *Previously using oral orticosteroids:* initiate 1 mg/day daily <u>or</u> in 2 divided doses

      Inhal susp: 0.25 mg/2 ml (30/box)

Pulmicort Turbuhaler 1-2 inhalations bid; *Previously on oral corticosteroids:* 2-4 inhalations bid

    Pediatric: <6 years: not recommended; 6-12 years: 1-2 inhalations bid; >12 years: same as adult

      Turbuhaler: 200 mcg/actuation (200 inh)

▶ *flunisolide* (C)(G)

AeroBid, AeroBid M initially 2 inhalations bid; max 8 inhalations/day

    Pediatric: <6 years: not recommended; 6-15 years: 2 inhalations bid; ≥16 years: same as adult

      Inhaler: 250 mcg/actuation (7 gm, 100 inh)

▶ *fluticasone* (C)(G)

Flovent HFA initially 88 mcg bid; if previously using an inhaled corticosteroid, initially 88-220 mcg bid; if previously taking an oral corticosteroid, initially 880 mcg/day

    Pediatric: use **Rotadisk**: initially 50-88 mcg inh bid; <4 years: not recommended; 4-11 years: initially 50-88 mcg bid; >11 years: initially 100 mcg bid; if previously using an inhaled corticosteroid, initially 100-200 mcg bid; *Previously taking an oral corticosteroid;* initially 1000 mcg bid

      Inhaler: 44 mcg/actuation (7.9 g, 60 inh; 13 g, 120 inh); 110 mcg/actuation (13 g, 120 inh); 220 mcg/actuation (13 g, 120 inh)

      Rotadisk 50 mcg/actuation (60 blisters/disk); 100 mcg/actuation (60 blisters/disk); 250 mcg/actuation (60 blisters/disk)

    Pediatric: <12 years: not recommended; ≥12 years: same as adult

▶ *mometasone furoate* (C) *Previously using a bronchodilator <u>or</u> inhaled corticosteroid:* 220 mcg q PM <u>or</u> bid; max 440 mcg q PM <u>or</u> 220 mcg bid; *Previously using an oral corticosteroid:* 440 mcg bid; max 880 mcg/day

    Pediatric: <12 years: not recommended; ≥12 years: same as adult

    Asmanex Twisthaler *Inhaler:* 220 mcg/actuation (6.7 gm, 80 inh); 16.8 gm (200 inh)

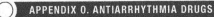

APPENDIX O. ANTIARRHYTHMIA DRUGS

Antiarrhythmics by Classification With Dose Forms		
Brand/Generic and Pregnancy Category	**Class and Indication(s)**	**Dose Form(s)**
Betapace *sotalol* (B)	*Class:* Class II and III Antiarrhythmic *Indications:* Documented life-threatening ventricular arrhythmias	*Tab:* 80*, 120*, 160*, 240*mg
Betapace AF *sotalol* (B)	*Class:* Class II and III Antiarrhythmic *Indications:* Maintenance of normal sinus rhythm in patients with highly symptomatic atrial fibrillation or atrial flutter who are currently in sinus rhythm	*Tab:* 80*, 120*, 160*mg
Calan *verapamil* (C)(G)	*Class:* Calcium Channel Blocker *Indications:* Control (with *digitalis*) of ventricular rate in patients with chronic atrial fibrillation or atrial flutter; prophylaxis of repetitive paroxysmal supraventricular tachycardia	*Tab:* 40, 80*, 120*mg
Cordarone *amiodarone* (D)(G)	*Class:* Class III Antiarrhythmic *Indications:* Documented life-threatening recurrent refractory ventricular fibrillation or hemodynamically unstable ventricular tachycardia	*Tab:* 200*mg
Quinidex *quinidine sulfate* (C) (G)	*Class:* Class I Antiarrhythmic *Indications:* Atrial and ventricular arrhythmias	*Tab:* 300 mg ext-rel
Inderal *propranolol* (C)(G) **Inderal XL** *propranolol* ext-rel (C)(G) **InnoPran XL** *Propranolol* ext-rel (C)	*Class:* Beta-Blocker *Indications:* Atrial and ventricular arrhythmias; tachyarrhythmias due to *digitalis* intoxication; reduce mortality and risk of reinfarction in stabilized patients after myocardial infarction	*Tab:* 10*, 20*, 40*, 60*, 80* mg; *Cap:* 60, 80, 120, 160 mg sust-rel *Cap:* 80, 120 mg ext-rel
Mexitil *mexiletine* (C)	*Class:* Class IB Antiarrhythmic *Indications:* Documented life-threatening ventricular arrhythmias	*Cap:* 150, 200, 250 mg
Multaq *dronedarone* (C)	*Class:* IB Antiarrhythmic *Indications:* Paroxysmal or persistent atrial fibrillation or atrial flutter	*Tab:* 400 mg
Norpace *disopyramide* (C)	*Class:* Class I Antiarrhythmic *Indications:* Documented life-threatening ventricular arrhythmias	*Cap:* 100, 150 mg
Procanbid *procainamide* (C)(G)	*Class:* Class IA Antiarrhythmic *Indications:* Life-threatening ventricular arrhythmias	*Tab:* 500, 1000 mg ext-rel

(continued)

Appendix O (*continued*)

Antiarrhythmics by Classification With Dose Forms		
Brand/Generic and Pregnancy Category	**Class and Indication(s)**	**Dose Form(s)**
Quinaglute *quinidine gluconate* (C)(G)	*Class:* Class I Antiarrhythmic *Indications:* Atrial and ventricular arrhythmias	*Tab:* 324 mg ext-rel
Rythmol *propafenone* (C)(G)	*Class:* Class IC Antiarrhythmic *Indications:* Documented life-threatening ventricular arrhythmias, prolonged recurrence of paroxysmal atrial fibrillation, and/or atrial flutter or paroxysmal supraventricular tachycardia associated with disabling symptoms in patients without structural heart disease	*Tab:* 150*, 225*, 300*mg *Cap:* 225, 325, 425 mg ext-rel
Sectral *acebutolol* (B)(G)	*Class:* Beta-Blocker *Indications:* Ventricular arrhythmias	*Cap:* 200, 400 mg
Sotylize *sotalol* (B)	*Class:* Class II and III Antiarrhythmic *Indications:* Documented life-threatening ventricular arrhythmias, and highly symptomatic A-flutter/A-fib	*Oral soln:* 5 mg/ml
Tambocor *flecainide acetate* (C)(G)	*Class:* Class IC Antiarrhythmic *Indications:* Documented life-threatening ventricular arrhythmias; paroxysmal atrial fibrillation and/or atrial flutter or paroxysmal supraventricular tachycardia in patients without structural heart disease	*Tab:* 50, 100*, 150* mg
Tenormin *atenolol* (C)(G)	*Class:* Beta-Blocker *Indications:* Reduce mortality and in stabilized patients after myocardial infarction	*Tab:* 25, 50, 100 mg *Inj:* 5 mg/ml (10 ml) for IV administration
timolol maleate (C) (G)	*Class:* Beta-Blocker *Indications:* Reduce mortality and in stabilized patients after myocardial infarction	*Tab:* 5, 10*, 20*mg
dofetilide (C)(G)	*Class:* Class III Antiarrhythmic *Indications:* Maintenance of normal sinus rhythm in patients with atrial fibrillation or atrial flutter of >1 week duration who were converted to normal sinus rhythm (only for highly symptomatic patients); conversion to normal sinus rhythm	*Cap:* 125, 250, 500 mcg
Tonocard *tocainide* (C)(G)	*Class:* Class I Antiarrhythmic *Indications:* Documented life-threatening ventricular arrhythmias	*Tab:* 400*, 600*mg
Toprol XL *metoprolol* (C)(G)	*Class:* Beta-Blocker *Indications:* Ischemic, hypertensive, or cardiomyopathic heart failure	*Tab:* 25*, 50*, 100*, 200*mg

APPENDIX P. ANTINEOPLASIA DRUGS

Comment: A new lab test offers potential for early detection of multiple cancer types with a single blood sample. Researchers studied 1005 persons with non-metastatic, clinically detected, stage 2 and 3 cancers of the ovary, liver, stomach, pancreas, esophagus, colorectum, lung, or breast. The blood test, CancerSEEK, accurately identified cancer cases 33%-98% (M = 70%) of the time in the study cohort, with accuracy reportedly 69%-98% for the five cancers that currently have no widely used screening test: ovarian, pancreatic, stomach, liver, and esophageal cancers. CancerSEEK combines tests that look for 16 genes and 10 proteins (mutations in cell-free DNA), linked to cancer. The researchers also tested blood samples from 812 healthy people, to see how often the test gave false-positive results, and were reported to be less than 1%. These findings represent a promising future for screening and early detection of cancer in asymtomatic persons. Optimally, cancers would be detected early enough that they could be cured by surgery alone, but even cancers that are not curable by surgery alone will respond better to systemic therapies when there is less advanced disease.

Anne Marie Lennon, MD, PhD, Johns Hopkins Kimmel Cancer Center, Baltimore, and Len Lichtenfeld, MD, Deputy Chief Medical Officer, American Cancer Society, Atlanta. Online and print announcements, January 2018: PR Newswire, Science, U.S. News & World Report, Los Angeles Times, Forbes, The Guardian, Chicago Tribune

REFERENCE

Cohen, J. D., Li, L., Wang, Y., Thoburn, C., Afsari, B., Danilova, L., . . . Papadopoulos, N. (2018). Detection and localization of surgically resectable cancers with a multi-analyte blood test. *Science, 359*(6378), 926–930. doi:10.1126/science.aar3247

Antineoplastics With Classification and Dose Forms		
Brand, Generic, and Pregnancy Category	**Class and Indications**	**Dose Form(s)**
Adcetris *brentuximab vedotin*	CD30-Directed Antibody-Drug Conjugate	*Vial:* 50 mg single-use, pwdr for reconstitution
Afinitor *everolimus (D)*	Kinase Inhibitor	*Tab:* 2.5, 5, 7.5, 10 mg
Afinitor Disperz *everolimus (D)*	Kinase Inhibitor	*Tab:* 2, 3, 5 mg for oral suspension
Alecensa *alectinib*	Kinase Inhibitor	*Cap:* 150 mg
Alimta *pemetrexel*	Folate Analog Metabolic Inhibitor	*Vial:* 100, 500 mg, single dose, pwdr for reconstitution, dilution, and IV infusion
Aliqopa *copanlisib*	Kinase Inhibitor	*Vial:* 60 mg pwdr for injection, single dose
Alkeran *melphalan (D)(G)*	Alkylating Agent	*Tab:* 2*mg
Alunbrig *brigatinib*	Kinase Inhibitor	*Tab:* 30, 90, 180 mg
Arimidex *anastrozole (D)*	Aromatase Inhibitor	*Tab:* 1 mg
Aromasin *exemestane (D)*	Aromatase Inactivator	*Tab:* 25 mg

(continued)

Appendix P (*continued*)

Antineoplastics With Classification and Dose Forms		
Brand, Generic, and Pregnancy Category	**Class and Indications**	**Dose Form(s)**
Arranon *nelarabine* (D)	Nucleoside Analog	*Vial:* 250 mg/50 ml (5 mg/ml) single-dose, soln for dilution and IV infusion
Asparlas *calaspargase pegol-mknl*	Asparagine-Specific Enzyme	*Vial:* 3750 units/5 ml (750 units/ml, 5 ml) single-dose soln for dilution and IV infusion
Avastin *bevacizumab*	Vascular Endothelial Growth Factor (VEGF) Inhibitor	*Vial:* 100 mg/4 ml (25 mg/ml), 400 mg/16 ml (25 mg/ml), single-dose, soln for dilution and IV infusion
Ayvakit *avapritinib*	Kinase Inhibitor	*Tab:* 100, 200, 300 mg
Azedra *iobenguane I[131]*	Radioactive Therapeutic Agent	*Vial:* 555 MBq/ml (15 mCi/ml), single-dose, soln for dilution and IV infusion
Balversa *erdafitinib*	Kinase Inhibitor	*Tab:* 3, 4, 5 mg
Bavencio *avelumab* (D)	Programmed Death Ligand-1 (PD-L1) Blocking Antibody	*Vial:* 200 mg/10 ml (20 mg/ml), single-dose, soln for dilution and IV infusion
Besponsa *inotuzumab ozogamicin*	CD22-Directed Antibody-Drug Drug Conjugate Mixture of	*Vial:* 0.9 mg single-dose pwdr for reconstitution, dilution, and IV infusion
Bevyxxa *betrixiban*	Factor Xa (FXa) Inhibitor	*Cap:* 40, 80 mg
Blenrep *belantamab mafodotin-blmf*	B-Cell Maturation Antigen (BCMA)-Directed Antibody and Microtubule Inhibitor Conjugate	*Vial:* 100 mg, single-dose pwdr for reconstitution, dilution, and IV infusion
bleomycin sulfate (G)	Cytotoxic Glycopeptide Antibiotics Isolated from a Strain of *Streptomyces verticillus*	*Vial:* 15, 30 units; pwdr for reconstitution and IV, IM, SC, intrapleural administration
Blincyto *blinatumomab*	Bispecific CD19-directed CD3 T-cell Engager	*Vial:* 35 mcg pwdr for reconstitution, dilution, and IV infusion, single-dose
bortizomib	Kinase Inhibitor	*Vial:* 3.5 mg pwdr for reconstitution, dilution, and IV infusion, single-dose
Bosulif *bosutinib*	Kinase Inhibitor	*Tab:* 100, 400, 500 mg
Braftovi *encorafenib*	Kinase Inhibitor	*Cap:* 50, 75 mg

(*continued*)

Appendix P (*continued*)

Antineoplastics With Classification and Dose Forms		
Brand, Generic, and Pregnancy Category	**Class and Indications**	**Dose Form(s)**
Breyanzi *lisocabtagene maraleucel*	Chimeric Antigen Receptor (CAR) T-Cell Therapy	*Vial:* 50 to 110 × 106 CAR-positive viable T cells/5 ml
Brukinsa *zanubrutinib*	Bruton's Tyrosine Kinase (BTK) Inhibitor	*Cap:* 160, 320 mg
Cabometyx *cabozantinib*	Kinase Inhibitor	*Tab:* 20, 40, 60 mg
Calquence *acalabrutinib*	Kinase Inhibitor	*Cap:* 100 mg
Casodex *bicalutamide*	Antiandrogen	*Tab:* 50 mg
Clolar *clofarabine* (**X**)	Purine Nucleoside Metabolic Inhibitor	*Vial:* 20 mg/20 ml (1 mg/ml), single-dose, for dilution and IV infusion
Copiktra *duvelisib*	Dual phosphoinositide-3-kinase (PI3K)-delta/PI3K-gamma Inhibitor	*Cap:* 15, 25 mg
Cytoxan *Cyclophosphamide* (**D**)	Alkylating Agent	*Tab:* 25, 50 mg
Daralex *daratumumab*	Human CD38-directed Monoclonal Antibody	*Vial:* 100 mg/5 ml, (20 mg/ml) 400 mg/20 ml, (20 mg/ml), soln for dilution and IV infusion single-dose
Darzalex Faspro *daratumumab+ hyaluronidase-fihj*	CD38-Directed Cytolytic Antibody+Hyaluronidase	*Vial:* 1800 mg *daratumumab*+30,000 units *hyaluronidase-fihi* (15 ml, 120 mg/2000 units/ ml), single-dose, soln for SC administration
Daurismo *glasdegib*	Hedgehog Pathway Inhibitor	*Tab:* 25, 100 mg
Doxil (**D**) *doxorubicin HCl*	Anthracycline Topoisomerase Inhibitor	Vial: 10 mg/10 ml, 50 mg/30 ml (10 mg/ml) single-use
Eligard *leuprolide acetate* (**X**)	GnRH Analog	*Inj:* 7.5 mg ext-rel per monthly SC injection
Elzonris *tagraxofusp-erzs*	CD123-directed Cytotoxin	*Vial:* 1000 mcg/ml (1 ml) single-dose for IV infusion
Endari *l-glutamine*	Amino Acid	*Oral Pwdr:* 5 gm of L-glutamine pwdr per paper-foil-plastic laminate pkt

(*continued*)

Appendix P (continued)

Antineoplastics With Classification and Dose Forms		
Brand, Generic, and Pregnancy Category	Class and Indications	Dose Form(s)
Enhertu *fam-trastuzumab deruxtecan-nxki*	HER2-directed Antibody and Topoisomerase Conjugate	*Vial:* 100 mg, single-dose, pwdr for reconstitution, dilution, and IV infusion
Eulexin *flutamide* (D)	Antiandrogen	*Cap:* 125 mg
Fareston *toremifene* (D)(G)	Selective Estrogen Receptor Modulator (SERM)	*Tab:* 60 mg
Faslodex *fulvestrant* (D)(G)	Estrogen Receptor Antagonist	*Prefilled syringe for IM inj:* 50 mg/ml (2.5, 5 ml/syringe)
Femara *letrozole* (D)	Aromatase Inhibitor	*Tab:* 2.5 mg
Gavreto *pralsetinib*	RET Kinase Inhibitor	*Cap:* 100 mg
Gleevec *imatinib mesylate* (D)	Signal Transduction Inhibitor	*Cap:* 100 mg
Herceptin *trastuzumab*	HER2/neu Receptor Antagonist	*Vial:* 420 mg multi-dose pwdr for reconstitution, dilution, and IV infusion
Herceptin Hylecta *trastuzumab+ hyaluronidase*	HER2/neu Receptor Antagonist+Endoglycosidase	*trastuzumab* 600 mg+ *hyaluronidase* 10,000 units/5 ml (120 mg/2,000 units per ml), single-dose soln for SC administration
Herzuma *trastuzumab-pkrb*	HER2/neu Receptor Antagonist	*Vial:* 150 mg single-dose, 420 mg multi-dose, pwdr for reconstitution, dilution, and IV infusion
Hydrea *hydroxyurea* (D)(G)	Substituted Urea	*Cap:* 500 mg
Ibrance *palbociclib*	Kinase Inhibitor	*Cap:* 75, 100, 150 mg
Idhifa *enasidenib*	Isocitrate Dehydrogenase-2 (IDH2) Inhibitor	*Tab:* 50, 100 mg
Idhiva *enasidenib*	Isocitrate Dehydrogenase-2 Inhibitor	*Tab:* 50, 100 mg
Imbruvica *imbrutinib*	Kinase Inhibitor	*Tab:* 140 mg
Imfinzi *durvalumab*	Programmed Death Ligand-1 (PD-L1) Blocking Antibody	*Vial:* 120 mg/2.4 ml, (50 mg/ml) 500 mg/10 ml (50 mg/ml), soln for dilution and single-dose

(continued)

Appendix P (*continued*)

Antineoplastics With Classification and Dose Forms		
Brand, Generic, and Pregnancy Category	**Class and Indications**	**Dose Form(s)**
Inqovi *decitabine+ cedazuridine*	Nucleoside Metabolic Inhibitor+Cytidine Deaminase Inhibitor	*Tabs:* 35 mg *decitabine* and 100 mg *cedazuridine*
Iressa *gefitinib* (D)	Epidermal Growth Factor Receptor Tyrosine Kinase Inhibitor	*Tab:* 250 mg
Jakafi *ruxolitinib*	Kinase Inhibitor	*Tab:* 5, 10, 15, 20, 25 mg
Jemperli *dostarlimab-gxly*	Programmed Death Receptor-1 (PD-1)–Blocking Antibody	*Vial:* 500 mg/10 ml (50 mg/ml), single-dose, soln for dilution and IV infusion
Kanjinti *trastuzumab-anns*	HER2/neu Receptor Antagonist	*Vial:* 420 mg (21 mg/ml), multi-dose, pwdr for reconstitution, dilution, and IV infusion
Keytruda *pembrolizumab*	Programmed Death Receptor-1 (PD-1)-Blocking Antibody	*Vial:* 100 mg/4 ml (25 mg/ml) single-dose soln for dilution and IV infusion
Kisquali Femara Co-Pack *ribociclib+letrozole*	Cyclin-dependent Kinase Inhibitor+Aromatase Inhibitor	*Tab:* 600/2.5, 400/2.5, 200/2.5 mg
Kymriah *tisagenlecleucel*	CD19-directed Genetically Modified Autologous T cell Immunotherapy	*IV bag:* frozen suspension for IV infusion after thawing
Kyprolis, *carfilzomib*	Protease Inhibitor	*Vial:* 10, 30, 60 mg, single-dose, pwdr for reconstitution, dilution, and IV infusion
Lartruvo *olaratumab*	Platelet-derived Growth Factor Receptor Alpha (PDGFR-α) Blocking Antibody	*Vial:* 500 mg/50 ml (10 mg/ml), single-dose, soln for dilution and IV infusion
Lemvina *lenvatinib*	Kinase Inhibitor	*Cap:* 4, 10 mg
Leukeran *chlorambucil* (D)(G)	Alkylating Agent	*Tab:* 2 mg
Libtayo *cemiplimab-rwle*	Programmed Death Receptor-1 (PD-1) Blocking Antibody	*Vial:* 350 mg/7 ml (50 mg/ml), single-dose, soln for dilution and IV infusion
Lobrena *lorlatinib*	Kinase Inhibitor	*Tab:* 25, 100 mg
Lumoxiti *moxetumomab pasudotox-tdfk*	Anti-CD22 Recombinant Immunotoxin	*Vial:* 1 mg, single-dose, pwdr for reconstitution, dilution, and IV infusion

(*continued*)

Appendix P (*continued*)

Antineoplastics With Classification and Dose Forms		
Brand, Generic, and Pregnancy Category	**Class and Indications**	**Dose Form(s)**
Lupron *leuprolide* (X)(G)	GnRH Analog	*Vial:* 5 mg/ml (2.8 ml), multi-dose, soln for SC inj: 1 mg (daily); 7.5 mg depot (monthly); 22.5 mg depot (every 3 months); 30 mg depot (every 4 months)
Lynparza *olaparib*	Poly (ADP-ribose) Polymerase (PARP)-Inhibitor	*Tab:* 100, 150 mg
Margenza *margetuximab-cmkb*	HER2/neu Receptor Antagonist	*Vial:* 250 mg/10 ml (25 mg/ml), single-dose, soln for dilution, and IV infusion
Megace, Megace Oral Suspension, Megace ES, *megestrol acetate* (D)(G)	Progestin	*Tab:* 20*, 40*mg; *Susp:* 40 mg/ml; *ES concentrate:* 125 mg/ml, 625 mg/5 ml
Mekinist *trametinib*	Kinase Inhibitor	*Tab:* 0.5, 2 mg
Mektovi *binimetinib*	Kinase Inhibitor	*Tab:* 15 mg
Nerlynx *neratinib*	Tyrosine Kinase Inhibitor (TKI)	*Tab:* 40 mg
Nexavar *sorafenib* (D)(G)	Multikinase Inhibitor	*Tab:* 200 mg
Nilandron *nilutamide*	Nonsteroidal Orally Active Antiandrogen	*Tab:* 150 mg
Nubeqa *darolutamide*	Androgen Receptor Inhibitor (ARi)	*Tab:* 300 mg
Nyvepria *pegfilgrastim-apgf*	Leukocyte Growth Factor	*Prefilled syringe:* 6 mg/0.6 ml, single-dose, soln for SC administration
Ogivri *trastuzumab-dkst*	HER2/NEU Receptor Antagonist	*Vial:* 420 mg, multi-dose, pwdr for reconstitution, dilution, and IV infusion
Ontruzant for Injection *trastuzumab-dttb*	HER2/NEU Receptor Antagonist	*Vial:* 150 mg, single-use; 420 mg pwdr, multi-use; pwdr for reconstitution, dilution, and IV infusion
Onureg *azacitidine*	Nucleoside Metabolic Inhibitor	*Tab:* 200, 300 mg

(continued)

Appendix P (*continued*)

Antineoplastics With Classification and Dose Forms		
Brand, Generic, and Pregnancy Category	**Class and Indications**	**Dose Form(s)**
Opdivo *nivolumab*	Anti-PD1 Monoclonal Antibody	*Vial:* 40 mg/4 ml, 100 mg/10 ml, 240 mg/24 ml (10 mg/ml), single-use, soln for dilution and IV infusion
Orgovyx *relugolix*	Gonadotropin-Releasing Hormone (GnRH) Receptor Antagonist	*Tab:* 120 mg
Padcev *enfortumab vedotin-ejfv*	Nectin-4-directed Antibody and Microtubule Inhibitor Conjugate	*Vial:* 20, 30 mg, single-dose, pwdr for reconstitution, dilution, and IV infusion
Pemazyre *pemigatinib*	Kinase Inhibitor	*Tab:* 4.5, 9, 13.5 mg
Pemfexy *pemetrexed*	Folate Analog Metabolic Inhibitor	*Vial:* 100, 500 mg, single-dose, pwdr for reconstitution, dilution, and IV infusion
Pepaxto *melphalan flufenamide*	Anti-Cancer Peptide-Drug Conjugate	*Vial:* 20 mg, single-dose, pwdr for reconstitution, dilution, and IV infusion
Perjeta *pertuzumab*	HER2/neu Receptor Antagonist	*Vial:* 420 mg/14 ml single-dose
Piqray *alpelisib*	Kinase Inhibitor	*Tab:* 50, 150, 200 mg
Polivy *polatuzumab vedotin-piiq*	CD79b-Directed Antibody-Drug Conjugate	*Vial:* 140 mg, single-dose, pwdr for reconstitution, dilution, and IV infusion
Poteligeo *mogamulizumab*	CC Chemokine Receptor Type 4 (CCR4)-Directed Monoclonal Antibody	*Vial:* 420 mg, multi-dose, pwdr for reconstitution, dilution, and IV infusion
Qinlock *ripretinib*	Kinase Inhibitor	*Tab:* 50 mg
Retevmo *selpercatinib*	Kinase Inhibitor	*Cap:* 40, 80 mg
Revlimid *lenalidomide*	Thalidomide Analogue	*Cap:* 2.5, 5, 10, 15, 20, 25 mg
Riabni *rituximab-arrx*	CD20-Directed Cytolytic Antibody	*Vial:* 100 mg/10 ml (10 mg/ml), 500 mg/50 ml (10 mg/ml), single-dose, soln for dilution and IV infusion

(*continued*)

Appendix P (*continued*)

Antineoplastics With Classification and Dose Forms		
Brand, Generic, and Pregnancy Category	**Class and Indications**	**Dose Form(s)**
Rituxan *rituximab*	CD20-Directed Cytolytic Antibody	*Vial:* 100 mg/10 ml (10 mg/ml), 500 mg/50 ml (10 mg/ml), single-dose, soln for dilution and IV infusion
Rituxan Hycela *rituximab+ hyaluronidase human*	Combination of *rituximab*, a CD20-Directed Cytolytic Antibody and *hyaluronidase human*, an Endoglycosidase	*Vial:* 1400 mg *rituximab* and 23,400 Units *hyaluronidase human* per 11.7 ml (120 mg/2000 Units per ml) single-dose; 1600 mg *rituximab* and 26,800 Units *hyaluronidase human* per 13.4 ml (120 mg/2000 Units per ml), single-dose, soln for SC administration
Rozlytrek *entrectinib*	Selective Tyrosine Kinase Inhibitor	*Cap:* 100, 200 mg
Rubraca *rucaparib*	Poly ADP-ribose Polymerase (PARP)-Inhibitor	*Tab:* 200, 300 mg
Ruxience *rituximab-pvvr*	CD20-directed Cytolytic Antibody	*Vial:* 100 mg/10 ml (10 mg/ml), 500 mg/50 ml (10 mg/ml), single-dose, soln for dilution and IV infusion
Rydapt *midostaurin*	Kinase Inhibitor	*Tab:* 40 mg
Sarclisa *isatuximab-irfc*	CD38-directed Cytolytic Antibody	*Vial:* 100 mg/5 ml (20 mg/ml), 500 mg/20 ml (20/ml), single-dose, soln for dilution and IV infusion
Stivarga *regorafenib*	Kinase Inhibitor	*Tab:* 40 mg
Sutent *sunitinib malate*	Kinase Inhibitor	*Cap:* 12.5, 25, 37.5, 50 mg
Tabrecta *capmatinib*	Kinase Inhibitor	*Tab:* 150, 200 mg
Tagrisso *osimertinib*	Kinase Inhibitor	*Tab:* 40, 80 mg
Talzenna *talazoparib*	Poly (ADP-ribose) (PARP) Inhibitor	*Tab:* 0.5, 1 mg
tamoxifen citrate (G)	Antiestrogen	*Tab:* 10, 20 mg
Tarceva *erlotinib* (D)	Kinase Inhibitor	*Tab:* 25, 100, 150 mg

(*continued*)

Appendix P (*continued*)

Antineoplastics With Classification and Dose Forms		
Brand, Generic, and Pregnancy Category	**Class and Indications**	**Dose Form(s)**
Tasigna *nilotinib*	Kinase Inhibitor	*Cap:* 50, 150, 200 mg
Taxotere *docetaxel* (G)	Microtubule Inhibitor	*Vial:* 20 mg/2 ml (10 mg/ml) single-dose; 80 mg/8 ml (10 mg/ml); 160 mg/16 ml (10 mg/ml) multi-dose
Tazverik *tazemetostat*	Methyltransferase Inhibitor	*Tab:* 200 mg, film-coat
Tecentriq *atezolizumab*	Programmed Death Ligand-1 (PD-L1) Blocking Antibody	*Vial:* 1200 mg/20 ml (60 mg/ml), single-dose, for dilution and IV infusion
Tepmetko *tepotinib*	Kinase Inhibitor	*Tab:* 225 mg
Tibsovo *ivosidenib*	Isocitrate Dehydrogenase-1 (IDH1) Inhibitor	*Tab:* 250 mg
Trazimera *trastuzumab-qyyp*	HER2/neu receptor antagonist	*Vial:* 420 mg, multi-dose, pwdr for reconstitution, dilution, and IV infusion
Treanda *bendamustine*	Alkylating Agent	*Vial:* 45 mg/0.5 ml, 180 mg/2 ml soln, single-dose; 25, 100 mg pwdr, single-dose, for reconstitution, dilution, and IV infusion
Trisenox *arsenic trioxide*	Arsenical	*Vial:* 12 mg/6 ml (2 mg/ml), single-dose, soln for dilution and IV infusion
Trodelvy *sacituzumab govitecan-hziy*	Trop-2-Directed Antibody and Topoisomerase Inhibitor Conjugate	*Vial:* 180 mg, single-dose, pwdr for reconstitution, dilution, and IV infusion
Truxima *rituximab-abbs*	CD20-Directed Cytolytic Antibody	*Vial:* 100 mg/10 ml, 500 mg/50 ml (10 mg/ml), single-use, for dilution and IV infusion
Tukysa *tucatinib*	Kinase Inhibitor	*Tab:* 50 mg
Turalio *pexidartinib*	Kinase Inhibitor	*Cap:* 200 mg
Ukoniq *umbralisib*	Kinase Inhibitor	*Tab:* 200 mg
Uplizna *inebilizumab-cdon*	CD19-Directed Cytolytic Antibody	*Vial:* 100 mg/10 ml (10 mg/ml), single-dose, soln for dilution and IV infusion

(*continued*)

Antineoplastics With Classification and Dose Forms		
Brand, Generic, and Pregnancy Category	Class and Indications	Dose Form(s)
Vectibix	Epidermal Growth Factor Receptor (EGFR) Antagonist	*Vial:* 100 mg/5 ml, 200 mg/10 ml, 400 mg/20 ml (20 mg/ml), single-use, soln for dilution and IV infusion
Velcade *bortezomib* (D)	Proteasome Inhibitor	*Vial:* 3.5 mg, single dose, pwdr for reconstitution, dilution, and IV infusion
Venclexta *venetoclax*	BCL-2 Inhibitor	*Tab:* 10, 50, 100 mg
Verzenio *abemaclclib*	Kinase Inhibitor	*Tab:* 50, 100, 150, 200 mg
Viadur (X) *leuprolide acetate*	GnRH Analog	*SC implant:* 65 mg depot (12 months)
Vitrakvi *larotrectinib*	Selective Tropomyosin Receptor Kinase (TRK) Inhibitor	*Caps:* 25, 100 mg; *Oral soln:* 20 mg/ml (100 ml)
Vizimpro *dacomitib*	Irreversible Pan-Human Epidermal Growth Factor Receptor Tyrosine Kinase Inhibitor (TKI)	*Tab:* 15, 30, 45 mg
Vyxeos *daunorubicin+ cytarabine*	*daunorubicin:* Anthracycline Topoisomerase Inhibitor; *cytarabine:* Nucleoside Metabolic Inhibitor	*Vial: daunorubicin* 44 mg/ *cytarabine* 100 mg, single-dose, pwdr for reconstitution, dilution, and IV infusion
Xalkori *crizotinib*	Kinase Inhibitor	*Cap:* 25, 100 mg
Xeloda (D) *capecitabine*	*Fluoropyrimidine* (prodrug of *5-fluorouracil*)	*Tab:* 150, 500 mg
Xermelo *telotristat*	Tryptophan Hydroxylase Inhibitor (THI)	*Tab:* 150 mg
Xospata *gilteritinib*	Kinase Inhibitor	*Tab:* 40 mg
Xpovio *selinexor*	Selective Inhibitor of Nuclear Export (SINE) XPO1 Antagonist	*Tab:* 20 mg
Yervoy *ipilimumab*	CD19-Directed Genetically Human Cytotoxic T-lymphocyte Antigen 4 (CTLA-4)-Blocking Antibody	*Vial:* 100 mg/5 ml (20 mg/ml), 400 mg/20 ml (20 mg/ml), single-dose, soln for dilution and IV infusion
Yescarta *axicabtagene*	CD19-Directed Genetically Modified Autologous T cell	*Infusion bag:* 68 ml, single autologous use Immunotherapy

(continued)

Appendix P (*continued*)

Antineoplastics With Classification and Dose Forms		
Brand, Generic, and Pregnancy Category	Class and Indications	Dose Form(s)
Zejula *niraparib*	Poly ADP-Ribose Polymerase (PARP)-Inhibitor	*Cap:* 100 mg
Zelboraf *vemurafenib*	Kinase Inhibitor	*Tab:* 240 mg
Zepzelca *lurbinectedin*	Selective Oncogenic Transcription Inhibitor	Vial: 4 mg, single-dose, pwdr for reconstitution, dilution, and IV infusion
Zirabev *bevacizumab-bvzr*	Vascular Endothelial Growth Factor (VEGF) Inhibitor	Vial: 100 mg/4 ml (25 mg/ml), 400 mg/16 ml (25 mg/ml), single-dose, soln for dilution and IV infusion
Zoladex *goserelin acetate*	GnRH Analog	*SC implant:* 3.6 mg depot (28 days), 10.8 mg depot (3-months)
Zometa *zoledronic acid* (D)	Bisphosphonate	Vial: 4 mg, single-dose, pwdr for reconstitution, dilution, and IV infusion
Zydelig *idelaqlisib*	CD79b-Directed Antibody-Drug Conjugate	*Tab:* 100, 150 mg
Zykadia *ceritinib*	Kinase Inhibitor	*Cap:* 150 mg
Zynlonta *loncastuximab tesirine-lpyl*	CD19-Directed Antibody and Alkylating Agent Conjugate	Vial: 10 mg, single-dose, pwdr for reconstitution, dilution, and IV infusion

 APPENDIX Q. ANTIPSYCHOSIS DRUGS

ANTIPSYCHOTICS WITH DOSE FORMS

Comment: Patients receiving an antipsychotic agent should be monitored closely for the following adverse side effects: neuroleptic malignant syndrome, extrapyramidal reactions, tardive dyskinesia, blood dyscrasias, anticholinergic effects, drowsiness, hypotension, photo-sensitivity, retinopathy, and lowered seizure threshold. Use lower doses for elderly or debilitated patients. Prescriptions should be written for the smallest practical amount. Foods and beverages containing alcohol are contraindicated for patients receiving any psychotropic drug. *Neuroleptic Malignant Syndrome* (NMS) and *Tardive Dyskinesia* (TD) are adverse side effects (ASEs), most often associated with the older antipsychotic drugs. Risk is decreased with the newer "atypical" antipsychotic drugs. However, these syndromes can develop, although much less commonly, after relatively brief treatment periods at low doses. Given these considerations, antipsychotic drugs should be prescribed in a manner that is most likely to minimize the occurrence. NMS, a potentially fatal symptom complex, is characterized by hyperpyrexia, muscle rigidity, altered mental status and evidence of autonomic instability (irregular pulse or blood pressure, tachycardia, diaphoresis, and cardiac dysrhythmia). Additional signs may include elevated creatine phosphor-kinase (CPK), myoglobinuria (rhabdomyolysis), and acute renal failure (ARF). TD is a syndrome consisting of potentially irreversible, involuntary, dyskinetic movements that can develop in patients with antipsychotic

(*continued*)

Appendix Q (*continued*)

drugs. Characteristics include repetitive involuntary movements, usually of the jaw, lips, and tongue, such as grimacing, sticking out the tongue, and smacking the lips. Some affected people also experience involuntary movement of the extremities or difficulty breathing. The syndrome may remit, partially or completely, if antipsychotic treatment is withdrawn. If signs and symptoms of NMS and/or TD appear in a patient, management should include immediate discontinuation of antipsychotic drugs and other drugs not essential to concurrent therapy, intensive symptomatic treatment, medical monitoring, and treatment of any concomitant serious medical problems. The risk of developing NMS and/or TD, and the likelihood that either syndrome will become irreversible, is believed to increase as the duration of treatment and the total cumulative dose of antipsychotic drugs administered to the patient increase. The first and only FDA-approved treatment for TD is **valbenazine** (**Ingrezza**) (*see* Tardive Dyskinesia)

ANTIPSYCHOTICS WITH DOSE FORMS

▷ *aripiprazole* (C)(G)

Abilify *Tab:* 2, 5, 10, 15, 20, 30 mg; *Oral soln:* 1 mg/ml (150 ml) (orange crèam; parabens)

Abilify Discmelt *Tab:* 15 mg orally disintegrating (vanilla) (phenylalanine)

Abilify Maintena *Vial:* 300, 400 mg ext-rel pwdr for IM injection after reconstitution; 300, 400 mg single-dose prefilled dual chamber syringes w. supplies

Aristada *Prefilled syringe:* 441, 662, 882, 1064 mg, ext-rel susp for IM injection, single-dose w. safety needle

▷ *aripiprazole lauroxil* (C)

Aristada Prefilled *syringe:* single-use, ext-rel injectable suspension: 441mg (1.6 ml), 662 mg (2.4 ml), 882 mg (3.2 ml), 1064 mg (3.9 ml)

▷ *asenapine* (C)

Saphris *SL tab:* 2.5, 5, 10 mg

Secuado *Trandermal system:* 3.8 mg/24 hours, 5.7 mg/24 hours, 7.6 mg/24 hours

▷ *brexpizole* (C)

Rexulti *Tab:* 0.25, 0.5, 1, 2, 3, 4 mg

▷ *bupropion* (C)

Forfivo XL *Tab:* 450 mg ext-rel

▷ *cariprazine*

Vraylar *Cap:* 1.5, 3, 4.5, 6 mg

▷ *chlorpromazine* (C)(G)

Thorazine *Tab:* 10, 25, 50, 100, 200 mg; *Cap:* 30, 75, 150 mg sust-rel; *Syr:* 10 mg/5 ml (4 oz) (orange-custard); *Vial/Amp:* 25 mg/ml (1, 2 ml) (sulfites)

▷ *clozapine* (B)(G)

Clozapine ODT (G) *ODT:* 150, 200 mg

Clozaril (G) *Tab:* 25*, 100*mg; *ODT:* 150, 200 mg

FazaClo ODT (G) *ODT:* 12.5, 25, 100, 150, 200 mg (phenylalanine)

Versacloz *Oral susp:* 50 mg/ml (100 ml)

▷ *fluphenazine* (C)(G)

Prolixin *Tab:* 1, 2.5, 5*, 10 mg (tartrazine); *Conc:* 5 mg/ml (4 oz w. calib dropper) (alcohol 14%); *Elix:* 5 mg/ml (2 oz w. calib dropper) (alcohol 14%); *Vial:* 25 mg/ml (10 ml)

▷ *fluphenazine decanoate* (C)(G)

Prolixin Decanoate *Vial:* 25 mg/ml (5 ml) (benzyl alcohol)

▷ *fluphenazine* (C)(G)

Prolixin Ethanate *Vial:* 25 mg (5 ml) (benzyl alcohol)

▷ *fluphenazine decanoate* (C)(G)

Prolixin Decanoate *Vial:* 25 mg/ml (5 ml) (benzyl alcohol)

(*continued*)

Appendix Q (*continued*)

▷ **haloperidol** (B)(G)
  Haldol *Tab:* 0.5*, 1*, 2*, 5*, 10*, 20*mg
  Haldol Lactate *Vial:* 5 mg for IM injection, single-dose
  Haldol Decanoate *Vial:* 50, 100 mg for IM injection, single-dose

▷ **iloperidone** (C)
  Fanapt *Tab:* 1, 2, 4, 6, 8, 10, 12 mg

▷ **loxapine** (C)
  Adasuve *Oral inhal pwdr:* 10 mg single-use disposable inhaler (5/box)

▷ **lumateperone**
  Caplyta *Cap:* 42 mg

▷ **lurasidone** (B)(G)
  Latuda *Tab:* 20, 40, 80 mg

▷ **olanzapine fumarate** (C)(G)
  Zyprexa *Tab:* 2.5, 5, 7.5, 10, 15, 20 mg
  Zyprexa Zydis *ODT:* 5, 10, 15, 20 mg (phenylalanine)

▷ **paliperidone palmitate** (C)(G)
  Invega *Tab:* 3, 6, 9 mg ext-rel
  Invega Sustenna *Prefilled syringe:* 39, 78, 117, 156, 234 mg ext-rel suspension w. needle
  Invega Trinza *Prefilled syringe:* 273, 410, 546, 819 mg ext-rel suspension

▷ **pimozide** (C)(G)
  Orap *Tab:* 1, 2 mg

▷ **prochlorperazine** (C)(G)
  Compazine *Tab:* 5, 10 mg; *Cap:* 10, 15 mg sus-rel; *Syr:* 5 mg/5 ml (4 oz) (fruit); *Supp:* 2.5, 5, 25 mg

▷ **quetiapine** (C)(G)
  Seroquel *Tab:* 25, 100, 200, 300 mg
  Seroquel XR *Tab:* 50, 150, 200, 300, 400 mg ext-rel

▷ **risperidone** (C)(G)
  Risperdal *Tab:* 0.25, 0.5, 1, 2, 3, 4 mg; *Soln:* 1 mg/ml (30 ml w. pipette); *Consta Inj:* 25, 37.5, 50 mg
  Risperdal M-Tabs *M-tab:* 0.5, 1, 2, 3, 4 mg orally disint (phenylalanine)

▷ **thioridazine** (C)(G) *Tab:* 10, 25, 50, 100 mg

▷ **trifluoperazine** (C)(G)
  Stelazine *Tab:* 1, 2, 5, 10 mg; *Conc:* 10 mg/ml; 2 oz w. calib dropper (banana-vanilla) (sulfites); *Vial:* 2 mg/ml (10 ml)

▷ **ziprasidone** (C)(G)
  Geodon *Cap:* 20, 40, 60, 80 mg

APPENDIX R. ANTICONVULSANT DRUGS

ANTICONVULSANTS WITH DOSE FORMS

▷ **brivaracetam** (C)
  Briviact *Tab:* 10, 25, 50, 75, 100 mg; *Oral soln:* 10 mg/ml (300 ml); *Vial:* 50 mg/ 5 ml single-dose for IV inj

▷ **carbamazepine** (D)(G)
  Carbatrol *Cap:* 200, 300 mg ext-rel
  Carnexiv *Vial:* 200 mg/20 ml (10 mg/ml) single-dose for IV infusion
  Equetro *Cap:* 100, 200, 300 mg ext-rel
  Tegretol *Tab:* 100*, 200*mg; *Chew tab:* 100*mg
  Tegretol Suspension *Oral susp:* 100 mg/5 ml (450 ml) (citrus vanilla) (sorbitol)
  Tegretol-XR *Tab:* 100, 200, 400 mg ext-rel

(*continued*)

Appendix R (*continued*)

▷ *cenobamate*

    Xcopri *Tab:* 12.5, 25, 50, 100, 150, 200 mg film-coat

▷ *clobazam* (C)(IV)

    Onfi *Tab:* 10*, 20*mg

    Onfi Oral Suspension *Oral susp:* 2.5 mg/ml (120 ml w. 2 dosing syringes) (berry)

▷ *clonazepam* (D)(IV)(G)

    Clonazepam ODT *ODT:* 0.125, 0.25, 0.5, 1, 2, oral-disint

    Klonopin *Tab:* 0.5*, 1, 2 mg

▷ *diazepam* (D)(IV)(G)

    Diastat *Rectal gel delivery system:* 2.5 mg

    Diastat AcuDial *Rectal gel delivery system:* 10, 20 mg

    Valium *Tab:* 2*, 5*, 10*mg

    Valium Injectable *Vial:* 5 mg/ml (10 ml); *Amp:* 5 mg/ml (2 ml); *Prefilled syringe:* 5 mg/ml (5 ml)

    Valium Intensol *Conc oral soln:* 5 mg/ml (30 ml w. dropper) (alcohol 19%)

    Valium Oral Solution *Oral soln:* 5 mg/5 ml (500 ml) (winter green-spice)

▷ *divalproex sodium* (D)(G)

    Depakene *Cap:* 250 mg; *Syr:* 250 mg/5 ml (16 oz)

    Depakote *Tab:* 125, 250, 500 mg

    Depakote ER *Tab:* 250, 500 mg ext-rel

    Depakote Sprinkle *Cap:* 125 mg

▷ *eslicarbazepine* (C)

    Aptiom *Tab:* 200*, 400, 600*, 800*mg

▷ *felbamate* (C)(G)

    Felbatol *Tab:* 400*, 600*mg

    Felbatol Oral Suspension *Oral susp:* 600 mg/5 ml (4, 8, 32 oz)

    Peganone *Tab:* 250, 500 mg

▷ *fosphenytoin sodium*

    Cerebyx *Vial:* 100 mg PE (2 ml); 500 mg PE (10 ml) 50 mg PE/ml, ready-mixed solution in water for Injection

▷ *gabapentin* (C)

    Horizant *Tab:* 300, 600 ext-rel

    Neurontin (G) *Cap:* 100, 300, 400 mg; *Tab:* 600*, 800*mg

    Neurontin Oral Solution *Oral soln:* 250 mg/5 ml (480 ml) (strawberry-anise)

▷ *lacosamide* (C)(V)(G)

    Vimpat *Tab:* 50, 100, 150, 200 mg; *Oral soln:* 10 mg/ml (200, 465 ml); *Vial:* 10 mg/ml soln for IV infusion, single-use (20 ml)

▷ *lamotrigine* (C)(G)

    Lamictal *Tab:* 25*, 100*, 150*, 200*mg

    Lamictal Chewable Dispersible Tab *Chew tab:* 2, 5, 25, 50 mg (black current)

    Lamictal ODT *ODT:* 25, 50, 100, 200 mg oral-disint

    Lamictal XR *Tab:* 25, 50, 100, 200, 250, 300 mg ext-rel

▷ *levetiracetam* (C)(G)

    Elepsia *Tab:* 1000, 1500 mg ext-rel

    Keppra *Tab:* 250*, 500*, 750*, 1000*mg

    Keppra Oral Solution *Oral soln:* 100 mg/ml (16 oz) (grape) (dye-free)

    Keppra XR *Tab:* 500, 750 mg ext-rel

    Levitiracetam IV *Premixed:* 500, 1000, 1500 mg for IV infusion (100 ml)

    Roweepra *Tab:* 250, 500, 750 mg; 1 gm

▷ *mephobarbital* (D)(II)

    Mebaral *Tab:* 32, 50, 100 mg

▷ *methsuximide* (C)

    Celontin Kapseals *Cap:* 150, 300 mg

(*continued*)

Appendix R (*continued*)

▷ *midazolam* (IV)
    Nayzilam Nasal Spray *Nasal Spray:* 5 mg/0.1 ml spray, single-dose

▷ *oxcarbazepine* (C)(G)
    Trileptal *Tab:* 150, 300, 600 mg; *Oral susp:* 300 mg/5 ml (lemon) (alcohol)
    Oxtellar XR *Tab:* 150, 300, 600 mg ext-rel

▷ *perampanel* (C)(III)
    Fycompa *Tab:* 2, 4, 6, 8, 10, 12 mg
    Fycompa Oral Suspension *Oral susp:* 0.5 mg/ml (340 ml w. dosing syringe)

▷ *phenytoin* (D)(G), *primidone* (D)(G)
    Dilantin *Cap:* 30, 100 mg ext-rel
    Dilantin Infatabs *Chew tab:* 50 mg
    Dilantin Oral Suspension *Oral susp:* 125 mg/5 ml (237 ml) (alcohol 6%)
    Phenytek *Cap:* 200, 300 mg ext-rel

▷ *pregabalin* (C)(G)(V)
    Lyrica *Cap:* 25, 50, 75, 100, 200, 225, 300 mg
    Lyrica CR *Tab:* 82.5, 165, 330 mg ext-rel
    Lyrica Oral Solution *Oral soln:* 20 mg/ml

▷ *primidone* (C)
    Mysoline *Tab:* 50*, 250*mg
    Mysoline Oral Solution *Oral susp:* 250 mg/5 ml (8 oz)

▷ *rufinamide* (C)(G)
    Banzel *Tab:* 200*, 400*mg
    Banzel Oral Solution *Susp:* 40 mg/ml (orange) (lactose-free, gluten-free, dye-free)

▷ *stiripentol*
    Diacomit *Cap:* 250, 500 mg; *Pwdr for oral susp:* 250, 500 mg/pkt (60/carton) (fruit)

▷ *tiagabine* (C)(G)
    Gabitril *Tab:* 2, 4, 12, 16 mg

▷ *topiramate* (D)(G)
    Topamax *Tab:* 25, 50, 100, 200 mg
    Topamax Sprinkle Caps *Cap:* 15, 25, 50 mg
    Trokendi XR *Cap:* 25, 50, 100, 200 mg ext-rel
    Qudexy *Tab:* 25, 50, 100, 150, 200 mg ext-rel
    Qudexy XR *Cap:* 25, 50, 100, 150, 200 mg ext-rel

▷ *vigabatrin* (C)(G)
    Sabril *Tab:* 500 mg
    Sabril for Oral Solution 500 mg/pkt pwdr for reconstitution

▷ *zonisamide* (C)
    Zonegran *Cap:* 25, 50, 100 mg

APPENDIX S. ANTI-HIV DRUGS

ANTI-HIV DRUGS WITH DOSE FORMS

▷ Aptivus (C) *tipranavir*
  Gel cap: 250 mg (alcohol); *Oral soln:* 100 mg/ml (95 ml w. dosing syringe) (Vit E 116 IU/ml) (buttermint-butter, toffee)

▷ Atripla (D) *efavirenz+emtricitabine+tenofovir disoproxil*
  Tab: efa 600 mg+emtri 200 mg+teno diso 300 mg

▷ Biktarvy *bictegravir+emtricitabine+tenofovir alafenamide*
  Tab: bict 50 mg+emtri 200 mg+teno alaf 25 mg

(continued)

Appendix S (*continued*)

▷ **Cimduo** *lamivudine+tenofovir disoproxil fumarate*
Tab: lami 300 mg+teno teno diso 300 mg

▷ **Combivir** (C)(G) *lamivudine+zidovudine*
Tab: aba+lami 150+zido 300 mg

▷ **Complera** (B) *emtricitabine+tenofovir disoproxil*
Tab: emtri 200 mg+teno diso 300 mg+rilpiv 25 mg

▷ **Crixivan** (C) *indinavir sulfate*
Cap: 100, 200, 333, 400 mg

▷ **Cytovene** (C)(G) *ganciclovir*
Cap: 250, 500 mg; *Vial:* 50 mg/ml single-dose (500 mg, 10 ml)

▷ **Delstrigo** *doravirine+lamivudine+tenofovir disoproxil fumarate*
Tab: dora 100 mg+lami ala 300 mg+teno dis 300 mg

▷ **Descovy** (D) *emtricitabine+tenofovir alafenamide+rilpivirine*
Tab: emtri 200 mg+teno ala 25 mg

▷ **Dovato** *dolutegravir+lamivudine*
Tab: dolu 50 mg+lami 300 mg film-coat

▷ **Edurant** (B) *rilpivirine*
Tab: 25 mg

▷ **Emtriva** (B)(G) *emtricitabine*
Cap: 200 mg; *Oral soln:* 10 mg/ml (170 ml) (cotton candy)

▷ **Epivir** (C)(G) *lamivudine*
Tab: 150*, 300*mg; *Oral soln:* 10 mg/ml (240 ml) (strawberry-banana) (sucrose
3 gm/15 ml)

▷ **Epzicom** (B) *abacavir sulfate+lamivudine*
Tab: aba 600 mg+lami 300 mg

▷ **Evotaz** (B) *atazanavir+cobicistat*
Tab: ataz 300+cobi 150 mg

▷ **Fortovase** (B) *aquinavir*
Soft gel cap: 200 mg

▷ **Fuzeon** (B) *enfuvirtide*
Vial: 90 mg/ml pwdr for SC inj after reconstitution (1 ml, 60 vials/kit) (preservative-free)

▷ **Genvoya** (B) *elvitegravir+cobicistat+emtricitabine+tenofovir alafenamide (TAF)*
Tab: elv 150 mg+cob 150 mg+emtri 200 mg+teno alafen 10 mg

▷ **Intelence** (C) *etravirine*
Tab: 25*, 100, 200 mg

▷ **Invirase** (B) *saquinavir mesylate*
Hard gel cap: 200 mg

▷ **Isentress** (C) *raltegravir (potassium)*
Tab: 400 mg film-coat; *Chew tab:* 25, 100*mg (orange-banana) (phenylalanine); *Oral susp:*
100 mg/pkt pwdr for oral susp (banana)

▷ **Juluca** *dolutegravir+rilpivirine*
Tab: dolu 50 mg+rilp 25 mg

(*continued*)

Appendix S (*continued*)

▷ **Kaletra (C)** *lopinavir plus ritonavir*
   Cap: lopin 100 mg+riton 25 mg, lopin 200 mg+riton 50 mg; *Oral soln:* lopin 80 mg+riton 20 mg per ml (160 ml w. dose cup) (cotton candy) (alcohol 42%)
   Hard gel cap: 200 mg

▷ **Lexiva (C)(G)** *fosamprenavir*
   Tab: 700 mg; *Oral soln:* 50 mg/ml (grape, bubble gum) (peppermint)

▷ **Norvir (B)** *ritonavir*
   Soft gel cap: 100 mg (alcohol); *Oral soln:* 80 mg/ml (8 oz) (peppermint-caramel) (alcohol)

▷ **Odefsey (D)** *emtricitabine+rilpivirine+tenofovir alafenamide*
   Tab: emtri 200 mg+rilpiv 25 mg+tenof alafen 25 mg

▷ **Pifeltro** *doravirine*
   Tab: 100 mg

▷ **Prezcobix (B)** *darunavir+cobicistat*
   Tab: daru 800+cobi 150 mg

▷ **Prezista (C)(G)** *darunavir*
   Tab: 75, 150, 600, 800 mg; *Oral susp:* 100 mg/ml (200 ml) (strawberry cream)

▷ **Rescriptor (C)** *delavirdine mesylate*
   Tab: 100, 200 mg

▷ **Retrovir (C)(G)** *zidovudine*
   Tab: 300 mg; *Cap:* 100 mg; *Syr:* 50 mg/5 ml (240 ml) (strawberry); *Vial:* 10 mg/ml (20 ml vial for IV infusion) (preservative-free)

▷ **Reyataz (B)** *atazanavir*
   Cap: 100, 150, 200, 300 mg

▷ **Rokubia** *fostemsavir*
   Tab: 600 mg ext-rel

▷ **Selzentry (B)** *maraviroc*
   Tab: 150, 300 mg

▷ **Stribild (B)** *elvitegravir+cobicistat+emtricitabine+tenofovir disoproxil fumarate*
   Tab: elv 150 mg+cob 150 mg+emtri 200 mg+teno diso fumar 300 mg

▷ **Sustiva (C)** *efavirenz*
   Tab: 75, 150, 600, 800 mg; *Cap:* 50, 200 mg

▷ **Symfi** *efavirenz+lamivudine+tenofovir disoproxil fumarate*
   Tab: efav 600 mg+lami 300 mg+teno diso fum 300 mg

▷ **Symfi Lo** *efavirenz+lamivudine+tenofovir disoproxil fumarate*
   Tab: efav 400 mg+lami 300 mg+teno diso fum 300 mg

▷ **Temixys** *lamivudine+tenofovir disoproxil fumarate*
   Tab: lami 300 mg+teno diso fum 300 mg

▷ **Tivicay (B)** *dolutegravir*
   Tab: 50 mg

▷ **Temixys** *lamivudine+tenofovir disoproxil fumarate*
   Tab: lami 300 mg+teno diso fum 300 mg

▷ **Triumeq (C)** *abacavir sulfate+dilutegravir+lamivudine*
   Tab: aba 600 mg+dilu 50 mg+lami 300 mg

▷ **Trizivir (C)(G)** *abacavir sulfate+lamivudine+zidovudine*
   Tab: aba 300 mg+lami 150 mg+zido 300 mg

(*continued*)

Appendix S (continued)

➤ Trogarzo *ibalizumab-uiyk* administer as an IV injection once every 14 days
Vial: 200 mg/1.33 ml (1.33 ml), single-dose

➤ Truvada (B)(G) *emtricitabine+tenofovir disoproxil fumarate*
Tab: emt 100 mg+teno 150 mg, 133 mg+teno 200 mg, emt 167 mg+teno 250 mg, emt 200 mg+teno 300 mg

➤ Valcyte (C)(G) *valganciclovir*
Tab: 450 mg
Comment: *valganciclovir* is indicated for the treatment of AIDS-related cytomegalovirus (CMV) retinitis.

➤ Videx EC (C)(G) *didanosine*
Cap: 125, 200, 250, 400 mg ent-coat del-rel; *Chew tab:* 25, 50, 100, 150, 200 mg (mandarin orange; buffered with calcium carbonate and magnesium hydroxide) (phenylalanine); *Pwdr for oral soln:* 2, 4 gm (120, 240 ml)

➤ Videx Pediatric Pwdr for Oral Solution (C) *didanosine*
Pwdr for oral soln: 2, 4 gm (120, 240 ml)

➤ Viracept (B) *nelfinavir mesylate*
Tab: 250, 625 mg; *Pwdr for oral soln:* 50 mg/gm (144 gm) (phenylalanine)

➤ Viramune (C)(G) *nevirapine*
Tab: 200*mg; *Oral susp:* 50 mg/5 ml (240 ml)

➤ Viramune XR (C) *nevirapine*
Tab: 100, 400 mg ext-rel

➤ Viread (C)(G) *tenofovir disoproxil fumarate*
Tab: 150, 200, 250, 300 mg; *Oral pwdr:* 40 mg/1 gm pwdr (60 gm w. dosing scoop)

➤ Vistide (C) *cidofovir*
Inj: 75 mg/ml (5 ml vials for IV infusion) (preservative free)
Comment: *cidofovir* is indicated for the treatment of AIDS-related *Cytomegalo-virus* (CMV) retinitis.

➤ Vitekta (C) *elvitegravir*
Inj: 75 mg/ml (5 ml vials for IV infusion) (preservative free)

➤ Zerit (C)(G) *stavudine*
Cap: 15, 20, 30, 40 mg; *Oral soln:* 1 mg/ml pwdr for reconstitution (200 ml) (fruit) (dye-free)

➤ Ziagen (C)(G) *abacavir sulfate*
Tab: 300*mg; *Oral soln:* 20 mg/ml (240 ml) (strawberry-banana) (parabens, propylene glycol)

APPENDIX T. ANTICOAGULANTS

APPENDIX T.1. COUMADIN TITRATION AND DOSE FORMS
➤ *warfarin* (X)(G) dosage initially 2-5 mg/day; usual maintenance 2-10 mg/day; adjust dosage to maintain INR in therapeutic range:
Venous thrombosis: 2.0-3.0
Atrial fibrillation: 2.0-3.0
Post MI: 2.5-3.5
Mechanical and bioprosthetic heart valves: 2.0-3.0 for 12 weeks after valve insertion, then 2.5-3.5 long-term
Pediatric: <18 years: not recommended
Coumadin *Tab:* 1*, 2*, 2.5*, 3*, 4*, 5*, 6*, 7.5*, 10*mg
Coumadin for Injection *Vial:* 2 mg/ml (2.5 ml)
Comment: Coumadin for Injection is for peripheral IV administration only.

(continued)

APPENDIX T.2. COUMADIN OVER-ANTICOAGULATION REVERSAL

▷ *phytonadione (vitamin K)*(G) 2.5-10 mg PO or IM; max 25 mg
   AquaMEPHYTON *Vial:* 1 mg/0.5 ml (0.5 ml); 10 mg/ml (1, 2.5, 5 ml)
   Mephyton *Tab:* 5 mg

APPENDIX T.3. AGENTS THAT INHIBIT COUMADIN'S ANTICOAGULATION EFFECTS

Increase Metabolism	Decrease Absorption	Other Mechanism(s)
azathioprine	azathioprine	coenzyme Q10
carbamazepine	cholestyramine	estrogen
dicloxacillin	colestipol	griseofulvin
ethanol	sucralfate	oral contraceptives
griseofulvin		ritonavir
nafcillin		spironolactone
pentobarbital		trazodone
phenobarbital		vitamin C (high dose)
phenytoin		vitamin K
primidone		
rifabutin		
rifampin		

APPENDIX U. LOW MOLECULAR WEIGHT HEPARINS

Comment: Administer by subcutaneous injection *only*, in the abdomen, and rotate sites. Avoid concomitant drugs that affect hemostasis (e.g., oral anti-coagulants and platelet aggregation inhibitors, including *aspirin*, NSAIDs, *dipyridamole*, *sulfinpyrazone*, *ticlopidine*). <18 years: not recommended

Low Molecular Weight Heparins With Dose Forms

▷ *ardeparin* (C)
   Normiflo *Soln for inj:* 5000 anti-Factor Xa U/0.5 ml; 10000 anti-Factor Xa U/0.5 ml (sulfites, parabens)

▷ *dalteparin* (B)
   Fragmin *Prefilled syringe:* 2500 IU/0.2 ml, 5000 IU/0.2 ml (10/box) (preservative-free); *Multi-dose vial:* 1000 IU/ml (95,000 IU, 9.5 ml) (benzyl alcohol)

▷ *danaparoid* (B)
   Orgaran *Amp:* 750 anti-Xa units/0.6 ml (0.6 ml, 10/box); *Prefilled syringe:* 750 anti-Xa units/0.6 ml (0.6 ml, 10/box) (sulfites)

▷ *enoxaparin* (B)(G)
   Lovenox *Prefilled syringe:* 30 mg/0.3 ml, 40 mg/0.4 ml, 60 mg/0.6 ml, 80 mg/0.8 ml (100 mg/ml) (preservative-free); *Vial:* 100 mg/ml (3 ml)

▷ *tinzaparin* (B)
   Innohep *Vial:* 20,000 *anti-Factor Xa* IU/ml (2 ml) (sulfites, benzyl alcohol)

APPENDIX V. FACTOR XA INHIBITORS

Factor XA Inhibitor Dose Forms and Therapy

▷ *apixaban* (C) 5 mg bid; reduce to 2.5 mg bid if any two of the following: ≥80 years, ≤60 kg, serum Cr ≥1.5
   Pediatric: not recommended
   Eliquis *Tab:* 2.5, 5 mg

Comment: Eliquis is indicated to reduce the risk of stroke and systemic embolism in patients with nonvalvular atrial fibrillation (NVAF).

▷ *betrixaban Recommended dose:* is an initial single dose of 160 mg, followed by 80 mg once daily, taken at the same time each day with food;

(continued)

Appendix V (*continued*)

Recommended duration of treatment: 35-42 days; reduce dose with severe renal impairment or with P-glycoprotein (P-gp) inhibitors
Pediatrics: safety and efficacy not established
Bevyxxa *Cap*: 40, 80 mg

Comment: **Bevyxxa** is indicated for the prophylaxis of venous thromboembolism (VTE) in adults who are hospitalized for acute mental illness and at risk for thromboembolic complications due to moderate or severe restricted mobility and other VTE risk factors. There are no data with the use of *betrixaban* in pregnancy, but treatment is likely to increase the risk of hemorrhage during pregnancy and delivery. No data are available regarding the presence of *betrixaban* or its metabolites in human milk or the effects of the drug on the breastfed infant.

▷ *edoxaban* (C) transition to and from **Savaysa**; assess CrCl prior to initiation:
NVAF CrCl >50 ml/min: 60 mg once daily; *CrCl 15-50 ml/min*: 30 mg once daily
DVT/PE CrCl >50 ml/min: 60 mg once daily following initial parental anticoagulant; *CrCl 15-50 ml/min, <60 kg, or concomitant Pgp inhibitors*: 30 mg once daily
Pediatric: safety and efficacy not established
Savaysa *Tab*: 15, 30, 60 mg

Comment: **Savaysa** is indicated to reduce the risk of stroke and systemic embolism in patients with nonvalvular atrial fibrillation (NVAF), treatment of DVT, and pulmonary embolism (PE), following 5-10 days of initial therapy with parenteral anticoagulant. Not for use in persons with NVAF with CrCl >95 ml/min.

▷ *fondaparinux* (B) Administer SC; administer first dose no earlier than 6-8 hours after hemostasis is achieved, start warfarin usually within 72 hours of last dose of *fondaparinux*
Post-op: 2.5 mg once daily x 5-9 days
Hip/Knee Replacement: once daily x 11 days
Hip Fracture: once daily x 32 days
Abdominal Surgery: once daily x 10 days
Prophylaxis: do not use <50 kg
Treatment: once daily for at least 5 days until INR = 2-3 (usually 5-9 days); max 26 days;
<50 kg: 5 mg; 50-100 kg: 7.5 mg; >100 kg: 10 mg
Pediatric: safety and efficacy not established
Arixtra *Soln for SC inj*: 2.5 mg/0.5 ml, 5 mg/0.4 ml, 7.5 mg/0.6 ml, 10 mg/0.8 ml
prefilled syringe (10/box) (preservative-free)

▷ *prasugrel* (B)(G) *Loading dose*: 60 mg once in a single-dose; *Maintenance*: 10 mg once daily;
<60 kg: consider 5 mg once daily; take with aspirin 75-325 mg once daily
Pediatric: safety and efficacy not recommended
Effient *Tab*: 5, 10 mg

Comment: **Effient** is indicated to reduce the risk of thrombotic cardiovascular events in persons with acute coronary syndrome (ACS) who are to be managed with percutaneous coronary intervention (PCI), including unstable angina, non-ST elevation myocardial infarction (NSTEMI), and STEMI. Do not start if active pathological bleeding (e.g., peptic ulcer, intracranial hemorrhage), prior TIA or stroke, or if patient likely to undergo urgent CABG. Discontinue 7 days before surgery and if TIA or stroke occurs.

▷ *rivaroxaban* (C) take with food
Treatment of DVT or PE: 15 mg twice daily for the first 21 days; then 20 mg once daily
Reduction in risk of DVT or PE recurrence: 20 mg once daily with the evening meal; *CrCl <30 ml/min*: avoid
Prophylaxis of DVT: take 6-10 hours after surgery when hemostasis established, then 10-20 mg once daily with the evening meal; *CrCl 30-50 ml/min*: 10 mg; *CrCl <30 ml/min*: avoid; discontinue if acute renal failure develops; monitor closely for blood loss
Hip: treat for 35 days; *Knee*: treat for 12 days
Nonvalvular AF: take once daily with the evening meal; *CrCl >50 ml/min*: 20 mg; *CrCl 15-50 ml/min*: 15 mg; *CrCl >15 ml/min*: avoid
Pediatric: not recommended
Xarelto *Cap*: 10, 15, 20 mg

Comment: **Xarelto** is indicated to reduce the risk of stroke and systemic embolism in nonvalvular atrial fibrillation (AF), to treat deep vein thrombosis (DVT) and pulmonary

(*continued*)

Appendix V (*continued*)

embolism (PE), to reduce the risk of recurrence of DVT and/or PE following 6 months treatment for DVT and/or PE, and prophylaxis of DVT, which may lead to PE in patients undergoing knee or hip replacement surgery. **Xarelto** eliminates the need for bridging with heparin or low molecular heparin; no need for routine monitoring of INR or other coagulation parameters; no need for dose adjustments for age, weight, or gender; no known dietary restrictions. Switching from *warfarin* or other anticoagulant, see mfr pkg insert.

Factor XA Inhibitor Reversal Agent

Comment: **Andexxa** (*coagulation factor Xa [recombinant] inactivated-zhzo*) is indicated to reverse the anticoagulation effects of factor Xa inhibitors (i.e., reversal agent specific to *rivaroxaban* [Xarelto] and *apixaban* [Eliquis]) when needed due to life-threatening or uncontrolled bleeding or emergency surgery). **Andexxa** was approved under the FDA's accelerated approval pathway based on effects in healthy volunteers, and continued approval may be contingent on postmarketing studies to demonstrate an improvement in hemostasis in patients. A clinical trial comparing this agent or usual care is scheduled to start in 2019 and to be reported in 2023.

▷ *coagulation factor Xa [recombinant] inactivated-zhzo* administer as an IV bolus, with a target rate of 30 mg/min, followed by continuous infusion for up to 120 minutes; select a high-dose or low-dose regimen based on the specific FXa inhibitor, dose of FXa inhibitor, and time since the patient's last dose of FXa inhibitor (see pkg insert); resume anticoagulant therapy as soon as medically appropriate following treatment with **Andexxa**.
High Dose Regimen: Initial IV Bolus: 800 mg at a target rate of 30 mg/min; *Follow-on IV infusion:* 8 mg/min for up to 120 min
Low Dose Regimen: Initial IV Bolus: 400 mg at a target rate of 30 mg/min; *Follow-on IV infusion:* 4 mg/min for up to 120 min
Pediatric: >18 years: not studied; ≥18 years: same as adult
     Andexxa *Vial:* 100 mg single dose pwdr for reconstitution and IV infusion
Comment: There are no adequate and well-controlled studies of **Andexxa** in pregnant females to inform patients of associated risks. The safety and effectiveness of **Andexxa** during labor and delivery have not been evaluated. There is no information regarding the presence of **Andexxa** in human milk or effects on the breastfed infant. Safety and efficacy of **Andexxa** in the pediatric population have not been studied. BBW: Treatment with **Andexxa** has been associated with serious and life-threatening adverse events, including arterial and venous thromboembolic events, ischemic events, including myocardial infarction and ischemic stroke, cardiac arrest, and sudden deaths.

◯ APPENDIX W. DIRECT THROMBIN INHIBITORS

Direct Thrombin Inhibitor Dosing and Dose Forms

▷ *aspirin* (D) single dose once daily
Pediatric: safety and efficacy not established
     Durlaza *Cap:* 162.5 mg 24-hour ext-rel (30, 90/bottle)
▷ *dabigatran etexilate mesylate* (C) swallow whole; *CrCl >30 ml/min:* 150 mg bid; *CrCl 15-30 ml/min:* 75 mg twice daily; *CrCl <15 ml/min:* not recommended
Pediatric: not recommended
     Pradaxa *Cap:* 75, 150 mg
     Comment: **Pradaxa** is indicated to reduce the risk of stroke and systemic embolism in nonvalvular AF, DVT prophylaxis, PE prophylaxis in patients who have undergone hip replacement surgery; treat DVT and PE in patients who have been treated with a parenteral anticoagulant for 5-10 days; and reduce the risk of recurrent DVT and PE in patients who have been previously treated. **Pradaxa** is contraindicated in patients with a mechanical prosthetic heart valve and not recommended with a bioprosthetic heart valve. Presently there is only one reversal agent for this drug class. *idarucizumab* (Praxbind) is a specific reversal agent for *dabigatran* (Pradaxa). It is a humanized monoclonal antibody fragment (Fab) that binds to dabigatran and its acylglucuronide metabolites with higher affinity than the binding affinity of dabigatran to thrombin, neutralizing its anticoagulant effects. (See **Pradaxa** reversal agent, *idarucizumab* [Praxbind] at the end of this appendix).

(*continued*)

Appendix W (*continued*)

▷ *desirudin (recombinant hirudin)* **(C)** 15 mg SC every 12 hours, preferably in the abdomen or thigh, starting up to 5-15 minutes before surgery (after induction of regional block anesthesia, if used); may continue for 9-12 days post-op; *CrCl <60 ml/min:* reduce dose (see mfr pkg insert)
    Pediatric: not recommended
      Iprivask *Pwdr for SC inj after reconstitution:* 15 mg/single-use vial (10/box) (preservative-free, diluent contains mannitol)

Comment: Iprivask is indicated for DVT prophylaxis in patients undergoing hip replacement surgery. It is not interchangeable with other hirudins.

Idarucizumab Reversal Agent: Humanized Monoclonal–Antibody Fragment (FAB)

▷ *idarucizumab* administer 5 gm (2 vials) IV drip or push; administer within 1 hour of removal from vial
    Pediatric: safety and efficacy not established
      Praxbind *Vial:* 2.5 g/50 ml, single-use (preservative-free)

Comment: Presently, there is inadequate human and animal data to assess risk of *idarucizumab* (**Praxbind**) use in pregnancy. Risk/benefit should be considered prior to use.

 APPENDIX X. PLATELET AGGREGATION INHIBITORS

Platelet Aggregation Inhibitor Dosing and Dose Forms

▷ *cilostazol* **(B)** 100 mg bid
    Pediatric: not recommended
      Pletal *Tab:* 50, 100 mg

Comment: Pletal is an antiplatelet/vasodilator (PDE III inhibitor).

▷ *clopidogrel* **(B)** 75 mg once daily
    Pediatric: not recommended
      Plavix *Tab:* 75, 300 mg

Comment: Plavix is indicated for the reduction of atherosclerotic events in recent MI or stroke, established PAD, non-ST-segment elevation acute coronary syndrome (unstable angina/non-STEMI), or STEMI.

▷ *dipyridamole* **(B)(G)** 75-100 mg qid
    Pediatric: not recommended
      Persantine *Tab:* 25, 50, 75 mg

Comment: *dipyridamole* is indicated as an adjunct to oral anticoagulants after cardiac valve replacement surgery to prevent thromboembolism.

▷ *dipyridamole+aspirin* **(B)(G)** swallow whole; one cap bid
    Pediatric: not recommended
      Aggrenox *Cap:* dipyr 200 mg+asa 25 mg

▷ *pentoxifylline* **(C)** (hemorrheologic [xanthine])
    Pediatric: not recommended
      Trental *Tab:* 400 mg sust-rel

▷ *prasugrel* **(C)(G)**
    Pediatric: not recommended
      Effient *Tab:* 5, 10 mg

Comment: Effient is indicated to reduce the risk of cardiovascular events in patients with acute coronary syndrome (ACS), who are to be managed with percutaneous coronary intervention (unstable angina or non-STEMI), and STEMI when managed with either primary or delayed PCI.

▷ *ticagrelor* **(C)** initiate 180 mg loading dose once in a single dose with *aspirin* 325 mg loading dose in a single dose; maintenance 90 mg twice daily with *aspirin* 75-100 mg once daily; ACS patients may start *ticagrelor* after a loading dose of *clopidogrel*
    Brilinta *Tab:* 90 mg

Comment: Brilinta is indicated to reduce the risk of cardiovascular events in patients with acute coronary syndrome (ACS) (unstable angina, Non-ST elevation [NSTEMI], myocardial infarction, or STEMI).

(*continued*)

Appendix X (*continued*)

▷ **ticlopidine** (B) 250 mg bid
　　Pediatric: not recommended
　　　　Ticlid *Tab:* 250 mg
Comment: **Ticlid** is indicated to reduce the risk of thrombotic stroke in selected patients. intolerant of ***aspirin***.

 APPENDIX Y. PROTEASE-ACTIVATED RECEPTOR-1 (PAR-1) INHIBITORS

Protease-Activated Receptor-1 (PAR-1) Inhibitor Dosing And Dose Form

▷ **vorapaxar** (B) administer 2.08 mg once daily; use with ***aspirin*** or ***clopidogrel***
　　Pediatric: <12 years: not established; ≥12 years: same as adult
　　　　Zontivity *Tab:* 2.08 mg (equivalent to 2.5 mg vorapaxar sulfate)
Comment: **Zontivity** is indicated to reduce thrombotic cardiovascular events in patients with a history of myocardial infarction or with peripheral arterial disease (PAD). Contraindicated with active pathological bleeding (e.g., peptic ulcer, intra-cranial hemorrhage); prior TIA; or stroke. Not recommended with severe hepatic impairment.

 APPENDIX BB. SYSTEMIC ANTI-INFECTIVES

Comment:
- Adverse effects of aminoglycosides include nephrotoxicity and ototoxicity.
- Use cephalosporins with caution in persons with penicillin allergy due to potential cross allergy.
- Sulfonamides are contraindicated with sulfa allergy and G6PD deficiency. A high fluid intake is indicated during sulfonamide therapy.
- Tetracyclines should be taken on an empty stomach to facilitate absorption. Tetracyclines should not be taken with milk.
- Tetracyclines are contraindicated during pregnancy and breastfeeding, and in children <8 years-of-age, due to the risk of developing tooth enamel discoloration.
- Systemic quinolones and fluoroquinolones are contraindicated in pregnancy and children <18 years-of-age due to the risk of joint dysplasia.

Anti-infectives by Class With Dose Forms		
Generic Name	**Brand Name**	**Dose Form/Volume**
Amebicides		
chloroquine phosphate (C)(G)	**Aralen**	*Tab:* 500 mg
chloroquine phosphate+ primaquine phosphate (C)(G)	Aralen Phosphate+ Primaquine Phosphate	*Tab:* chlor 300 mg+prim 45 mg
iodoquinol (C)	**Yodoxin**	*Tab:* 210, 650 mg
metronidazole (not for use in 1st; B in 2nd, 3rd)(G)	**Flagyl**	*Tab:* 250*, 500*mg
	Flagyl 375	*Cap:* 375 mg
	Flagyl ER	*Tab:* 750 mg ext-rel
tinidazole (C)	**Tindamax**	*Tab:* 250*, 500*mg
Aminoglycosides		
amikacin (C)(G)	**Amikin**	*Vial:* 500 mg, 1 gm (2 ml)
gentamicin (C)(G)	**Garamycin**	*Vial:* 20, 80 mg/2 ml

(*continued*)

Appendix BB (*continued*)

Anti-infectives by Class With Dose Forms		
Generic Name	Brand Name	Dose Form/Volume
streptomycin (D)(G)	Streptomycin	*Amp:* 1 gm/2.5 ml <u>or</u> 400 mg/ml (2.5 ml)
Antifungals		
atovaquone (C)	Mepron	*Susp:* 750 mg/5ml (210 ml)
clotrimazole (B)(G)	Mycelex Troche	10 mg (70, 40/bottle)
fluconazole (C)(G)	Diflucan	*Tab:* 50, 100, 150, 200 mg; *Oral susp:* 10, 40 mg/ml (35 ml) (orange)
griseofulvin, microsize (C)(G)	Grifulvin V	*Tab:* 250, 500 mg; *Oral susp:* 125 mg/ 5 ml (120 ml) (alcohol 0.02%)
griseofulvin, ultramicrosize (C)(G)	Gris-PEG	*Tab:* 125, 250 mg
itraconazole (C)	Sporanox	*Cap:* 100 mg; *Soln:* 10 mg/ml (150 ml); *Pulse Pack:* 100 mg caps (7/pck)
ketoconazole (C)(G)	Nizoral	*Tab:* 200 mg
nystatin (C)(G)	Mycostatin	*Pastille:* 200,000 units/pastille (30 pastilles/pck); *Oral susp:* 100,000 units/ml (60 ml w. dropper)
posaconazole	Noxafil	*Tab:* 100 mg ext-rel; *Oral susp:* 40 mg/ml (105 ml); *Vial:* 300 mg/16.7 ml (18 mg/ ml) soln for IV infusion
terbinafine (B)(G)	Lamisil	*Tab:* 250 mg
voriconazole (D)(G)	Vfend	*Tab:* 50, 200 mg
Antihelmintics		
albendazole (C)(G)	Albenza	*Tab:* 200 mg
ivermectin (C)(G)	Stromectol	*Tab:* 3 mg
mebendazole (C)(G)	Emverm, Vermox	*Chew tab:* 100 mg
pyrantel pamoate (C)(G)	Antiminth Pin-X	*Cap:* 180 mg; *Liq:* 50 mg/ml (30 ml); 144 mg/ml (30 ml); *Oral susp:* 50 mg/ ml (30 ml) (caramel) (sodium benzoate, tartrazine-free)
thiabendazole (C)(G)	Mintezol (currently <u>not</u> available in the United States)	*Chew tab:* 500*mg (orange); *Oral susp:* 500 mg/5 ml (120 ml) (orange)
Antimalarials		
atovaquone (C)	Mepron	*Susp:* 750 mg/5 ml
atovaquone+ proguanil (C)	Malarone	*Tab:* atov 250 mg+proq 100 mg
	Malarone Pediatric	*Tab:* atov 62.5 mg+proq 25 mg
chloroquine (C)(G)	Aralen	*Tab:* 500 mg; *Amp:* 50 mg/ml (5 ml)
doxycycline (D)(G)	Acticlate	*Tab:* 75, 150**mg
	Adoxa	*Tab:* 50, 75, 100, 150 mg ent-coat

(*continued*)

Appendix BB (*continued*)

Anti-infectives by Class With Dose Forms		
Generic Name	**Brand Name**	**Dose Form/Volume**
	Doryx	*Cap:* 100 mg; *Tab:* 50, 75, 100, 150, 200 mg
	Doxsteric	*Tab:* 50 mg del-rel
	Monodox	*Cap:* 50, 75, 100 mg
	Oracea	*Cap:* 40 mg del-rel
	Vibramycin	*Cap:* 50, 100 mg; *Syr:* 50 mg/5 ml (raspberry-apple) (sulfites); *Oral susp:* 25 mg/5 ml (raspberry)
	Vibra-Tab	*Tab:* 100 mg film-coat
	Xerava	*Vial:* 50 mg pwdr for IV infusion
hydroxychloroquine (C)(G)	Plaquenil	*Tab:* 200 mg
mefloquine (C)	Lariam	*Tab:* 250 mg
minocycline (D)(G)	Dynacin	*Cap:* 50, 100 mg
	Minocin	*Cap:* 50, 75, 100 mg; *Oral susp:* 50 mg/5 ml (60 ml) (custard) (sulfites, alcohol 5%)
	Minolira	*Tab:* 105, 135 mg ext-rel
	Solodyn	*Tab:* 55, 65, 80, 105, 115 mg ext-rel
Antiprotozoal/Antibacterials		
quinine sulfate (C)(G)	Qualaquin	*Cap:* 324 mg
metronidazole (**not for use in 1st; B in 2nd, 3rd**)(G)	Flagyl, Protostat	*Tab:* 250*, 500*mg
	Flagyl 375	*Cap:* 375 mg
	Flagyl ER	*Tab:* 750 mg ext-rel
nitazoxanide (C)(G)	Alinia	*Tab:* 500 mg; *Oral susp:* 100 mg/5 ml (60 ml) (strawberry)
tinidazole (C)	Tindamax	*Tab:* 250*, 500*mg
Antituberculars		
ethambutol (EMB) (B)(G)	Myambutol	*Tab:* 100, 400*mg
isoniazid (INH) (C) (G)	generic <u>only</u>	*Tab:* 100, 300*mg; *Syr:* 50 mg/5 ml; *Inj:* 100 mg/ml
pyrazinamide (PZA) (C)	generic <u>only</u>	*Tab:* 500*mg
rifampin (C)(G)	Priftin	*Tab:* 150 mg
	Rifadin	*Cap:* 150, 300 mg
Rifampin+isoniazid (C)	Rifamate	*Cap:* rif 300 mg+iso 150 mg

(*continued*)

Anti-infectives by Class With Dose Forms		
Generic Name	Brand Name	Dose Form/Volume
rifampin+isoniazid+ pyrazinamide (C)	**Rifater**	*Tab:* rif 120 mg+iso 50 mg+pyr 300 mg
Antivirals (for HIV-specific antiviral drugs see page 592)		
acyclovir (C)(G)	**Zovirax**	*Cap:* 200 mg; *Tab:* 400, 800 mg; *Oral susp:* 200 mg/5 ml (banana)
amantadine (C)(G)	**Symmetrel**	*Tab:* 100 mg; *Syr:* 50 mg/5ml (16 oz) (raspberry)
famciclovir (B)	**Famvir**	*Tab:* 125, 250, 500 mg
lamivudine (C)	**Epivir-HBV**	*Tab:* 100 mg; *Oral soln:* 5 mg/ml (240 ml) (strawberry-banana)
oseltamivir (C)	**Tamiflu**	*Cap:* 75 mg
rimantadine (C)	**Flumadine**	*Tab:* 100 mg
valacyclovir (B)	**Valtrex**	*Tab:* 500 mg; 1 gm
zanamivir	**Relenza**	*Tab:* lami 150+zido 300 mg
Cephalosporins		
• 1st-Generation Cephalosporins		
cefadroxil (B)	**Duricef**	*Cap:* 500 mg; *Tab:* 1 gm; *Oral susp:*250 mg/5 ml (100 ml); 500 mg/5 ml (75, 100 ml) (orange-pineapple)
cefazolin (B)	**Ancef, Zolicef**	*Vial:* 500 mg; 1, 10 gm
cephalexin (B)	**Keflex**	*Cap:* 250, 333, 500, 750 mg; *Oral susp:*125, 250 mg/5 ml (100, 200 ml)
• 2nd-Generation Cephalosporins		
cefaclor (B)(G)	generic <u>only</u>	*Tab:* 500 mg; *Cap:* 250, 500 mg; *Susp:* 125 mg/5 ml (75, 150 ml) (strawberry); 187 mg/5 ml (50, 100 ml) (strawberry); 250 mg/5 ml (75, 150 ml) (strawberry); 375 mg/5 ml (50, 100 ml) (strawberry)
cefaclor ext-rel (B)(G)	**Cefaclor Extended Release**	*Tab:* 375, 500 mg ext-rel
cefamandole (B)	**Mandol**	*Vial:* 1, 2 gm
cefotetan (B)	**Cefotan**	*Vial:* 1, 2 gm
cefoxitin (B)	**Mefoxin**	*Vial:* 1, 2 gm
cefprozil (B)	**Cefzil**	*Tab:* 250, 500 mg; *Oral susp:* 125, 250 mg/5 ml (50, 75, 100 ml) (bubble gum) (phenylalanine)
ceftaroline (B)	**Teflaro**	*Vial:* 400, 600 mg

(continued)

Appendix BB (*continued*)

Anti-infectives by Class With Dose Forms		
Generic Name	Brand Name	Dose Form/Volume
cefuroxime sodium (B)(G)	Zinacef	*Vial:* 750 mg; 1.5 gm
loracarbef (B)	Lorabid	*Pulvule:* 200, 400 mg; *Oral susp:* 100 mg/5 ml (50, 100 ml); 200 mg/5 ml (50, 75, 100 ml) (strawberry bubble gum)
• *3rd-Generation Cephalosporins*		
cefoperazone (B)	Cefobid	*Vial:* 1, 2 gm pwdr for reconstitution
cefotaxime (B)	Claforan	*Vial:* 500 mg; 1, 2 gm pwdr for reconstitution
cefpodoxime (B)	Vantin	*Tab:* 100, 200 mg; *Oral susp:* 50, 100 mg/5 ml (50, 75, 100 ml) (lemon creme)
ceftazidime (B)	Ceptaz	*Vial:* 1, 2 gm pwdr for reconstitution
	Fortaz	*Vial:* 500 mg; 1, 2 gm pwdr for reconstitution
	Tazicef	*Vial:* 1, 2 gm pwdr for reconstitution
	Tazidime	*Vial:* 1, 2 gm pwdr for reconstitution
Ceftazidime/ avibactam (B)	Avycaz	*Vial:* 2.5 gm pwdr for reconstitution
ceftibuten (B)	Cedax	*Cap:* 400 mg; *Oral susp:* 90 mg/5 ml (30, 60, 90, 120 ml); 180 mg/5 ml (30, 60, 120 ml) (cherry)
• *3rd/4th-Generation Cephalosporins*		
cefdinir (B)	Omnicef	*Cap:* 300 mg; *Oral susp:* 125 mg/5 ml (60, 100 ml) (strawberry)
cefditoren pivoxil (C)	Spectracef	*Tab:* 200 mg
cefepime (B)	Maxipime	*Vial:* 1 gm pwdr for reconstitution
cefixime (B)(G)	Suprax	*Tab/Cap:* 400 mg; *Oral Susp:* 100 mg/5 ml (50, 75, 100 ml) (strawberry)
ceftaroline (B)	Teflaro	*Vial:* 400, 600 mg
ceftriaxone (B)(G)	Rocephin	*Vial:* 250, 500 mg; 1, 2 gm
cytolozane+ tazobactam (B)	Zerbaxa	*Vial:* 1.5 gm pwdr for reconstitution
Penicillins		
amoxicillin (B)(G)	Amoxil	*Cap:* 250, 500 mg; *Tab:* 500, 875* mg; *Chew tab:* 125, 200, 250, 400 mg (cherry-banana-peppermint) (phenylalanine); *Oral susp:*125, 250 mg/ ml (80, 100, 150 ml) (bubble gum); 200, 400 mg/5 ml (50, 75, 100 ml) (bubble gum); *Oral drops:* 50 mg/ml (30 ml) (bubble gum)

(continued)

Appendix BB (*continued*)

Anti-infectives by Class With Dose Forms		
Generic Name	**Brand Name**	**Dose Form/Volume**
	Moxatag	*Tab:* 775 mg ext-rel
	Trimox	*Cap:* 250, 500 mg; *Oral susp:* 125, 250 mg/5ml (80, 100, 150 ml) (raspberry-strawberry)
amoxicillin+ clavulanate (B)(G)	**Augmentin**	*Tab:* 250, 500, 875 mg; *Chew tab:* 125, 250 mg (lemon lime); 200, 400 mg (cherry-banana; phenylalanine); *Oral susp:* 125 mg/5 ml (banana), 250 mg/5 ml (orange) (75, 100, 150 ml); 200, 400 mg/5 ml (50, 75, 100 ml) (orange)
	Augmentin ES-600	*Oral susp:* 600 mg/5 ml (50, 75, 100, 125, 150, 200 ml) (strawberry cream) (phenylalanine)
	Augmentin XR	*Tab:* 1000*mg ext-rel
ampicillin (B)(G)	**Omnipen**	*Cap:* 250, 500 mg; *Oral susp:* 125, 250 mg/ml (100, 150, 200 ml)
	Principen	*Cap:* 250, 500 mg; *Syr:* 125, 250 mg/5 ml
ampicillin+ sulbactam (B)(G)	**Unasyn**	*Vial:* 1.5, 3 gm
carbenicillin (B)	**Geocillin**	*Tab:* 382 mg film-coat
dicloxacillin (B)(G)	**Dynapen**	*Cap:* 125, 250, 500 mg; *Oral susp:* 62.5 mg/5 ml (80, 100, 200 ml)
ertapenem (B)	**Invanz**	*Vial:* 1 gm pwdr for reconstitution
meropenem (B)(G)	**Merrem**	*Vial:* 500 mg; 1 gm pwdr for reconstitution (sodium 3.92 mEq/gm)
penicillin g benzathine (B)(G)	**Bicillin LA, Bicillin C-R**	*Cartridge-needle unit:* 600,000 million units (1 ml); 1.2 million units (2 ml); 2.4 million units (4 ml)
	Permapen	*Prefilled syringe:* 1.2 million units
penicillin g potassium (B)(G)	generic <u>only</u>	*Vial:* 5, 20 MU pwdr for reconstitution; *Premixed bag:* 1, 2, 3 MU (50 ml)
penicillin g procaine (B)(G)	generic <u>only</u>	*Prefilled syringe:* 1.2 million units
penicillin v potassium (B)(G)	**Pen-Vee K**	*Tab:* 250, 500 mg; *Oral soln:* 125 mg/5 ml (100, 200 ml); 250 mg/5 ml (100, 150, 200 ml)
piperacillin+ tazobactam (B)(G)	**Zosyn**	*Vial:* 2, 3, 4 gm pwdr for reconstitution

(*continued*)

Appendix BB (*continued*)

Anti-infectives by Class With Dose Forms		
Generic Name	Brand Name	Dose Form/Volume
Quinolone and Fluoroquinolones		
• 1st-Generation Quinolone		
enoxacin (C)	Penetrex	*Tab*: 200, 400 mg
• 1st-Generation Fluoroquinolones		
ciprofloxacin (C)(G)	Cipro	*Tab*: 250, 500, 750 mg; *Oral susp*: 250, 500 mg/5 ml (100 ml) (strawberry); *IV conc*: 10 mg/ml after dilution (20, 40 ml); *Premixed bag*: 2 mg/ml (100, 200 ml)
	Cipro XR	*Tab*: 500, 1000 mg ext-rel
	ProQuin XR	*Tab*: 500 mg ext-rel
lomefloxacin (C)	Maxaquin	*Tab*: 400 mg
norfloxacin (C)(G)	Noroxin	*Tab*: 400 mg
ofloxacin (C)(G)	Floxin	*Tab*: 200, 300, 400 mg
lomefloxacin (C)	Floxin	*Tab*: 200, 300, 400 mg
• 3rd-Generation Fluoroquinolone		
levofloxacin (C)(G)	Levaquin	*Tab*: 250, 500, 750 mg
• 4th-Generation Fluoroquinolone		
delafloxacin (C)	Baxdela	*Tab*: 400 mg; *Vial*: 300 mg pwdr for reconstitution
gemifloxacin (C)(G)	Factive	*Tab*: 320*mg
moxifloxacin (C)(G)	Avelox	*Tab*: 400 mg
Ketolide		
telithromycin (C)	Ketek	*Tab*: 300, 400 mg
Macrolides		
azithromycin (B)	Zithromax	*Tab*: 250, 500, 600 mg; *Granules*: 1 gm/pck for reconstitution (cherry-banana)
	ZithPed Syr	*Oral susp*: 100 mg/5 ml, (15 ml); 200 mg/5 ml (15, 22.5, 30 ml) (cherry)
	Zithromax Tri-Pak	*Tab*: 3 x 500 mg tabs/pck
	Zithromax Z-Pak	*Tab*: 6 x 250 mg tabs/pck
	Zmax	*Granules*: 2 gm/pkt for reconstitution (cherry-banana)
clarithromycin (C)(G)	Biaxin	*Tab*: 250, 500 mg; *Oral susp*: 125, 250 mg/5 ml (50, 100 ml) (fruit punch)
	Biaxin XL	*Tab*: 500 mg ext-rel
dirithromycin (C)(G)	*generic only*	*Tab*: 250 mg

(*continued*)

Appendix BB *(continued)*

Anti-infectives by Class With Dose Forms		
Generic Name	Brand Name	Dose Form/Volume
erythromycin base (B)(G)	**Ery-Tab**	*Tab:* 250, 333, 500 mg ent-coat
	PCE	*Tab:* 333, 500 mg
erythromycin estolate (B)(G)	**Ilosone**	*Pulvule:* 250 mg; *Tab:* 500 mg; *Liq:* 125, 250 mg/5 ml (100 ml)
erythromycin ethylsuccinate (B)(G)	**E.E.S.**	*Tab:* 400 mg; *Oral susp:* 200 mg/5 ml (100, 200 ml) (cherry); 200, 400 mg/5 ml (100 ml) (fruit)
erythromycin ethylsuccinate (B)(G)	**EryPed**	*Oral susp:* 200 mg/5 ml (100, 200 ml) (fruit); 400 mg/5 ml (60, 100, 200 ml) (banana); *Oral drops:* 200, 400 mg/5 ml (50 ml) (fruit); *Chew tab:* 200 mg (fruit)
erythromycin stearate (B)(G)	**Erythrocin**	*Film tab:* 250, 500 mg
Macrolide+Sulfonamide		
erythromycin ethylsuccinate+ sulfisoxazole (C)(G)	**Pediazole**	*Oral susp:* eryth 200 mg+sulf 600 mg per 5 ml (100, 150, 200 ml) (strawberry-banana)
Sulfonamides		
sulfamethoxazole (B/D)(G)	**Gantrisin Pediatric**	*Oral susp:* 500 mg/5 ml; *Syr:* 500 mg/5 ml
trimethoprim (C)(G)	**Primsol**	*Oral soln:* 50 mg/5 ml (bubble gum) (dye-free, alcohol-free)
	Trimpex	*Tab:* 100 mg
	Proloprim	*Tab:* 100, 200 mg
trimethoprim+ sulfamethoxazole (C)(G)	**Bactrim, Septra**	*Tab:* trim 80 mg+sulfa 400 mg*
	Bactrim DS, Septra DS	*Tab:* trim 160 mg+sulfa 800 mg*; *Oral susp:* trim 40 mg+sulfa 200 mg per 5 ml (100 ml) (cherry) (alcohol 0.3%)
Tetracyclines		
demeclocycline (D)	**Declomycin**	*Tab:* 300 mg
doxycycline (D)(G)	**Adoxa**	*Tab:* 50, 100 mg ent-coat
	Doryx	*Cap:* 100 mg
	Monodox	*Cap:* 50, 100 mg
doxycycline (D)(G)	**Vibramycin**	*Cap:* 50, 100 mg; *Syr:* 50 mg/5 ml; (raspberry) (sulfites); *Oral susp:* 25 mg/5 ml (raspberry-apple); *IV conc:* doxy 100 mg+asc acid 480 mg after dilution; doxy 200 mg+asc acid 960 mg after dilution

(continued)

Appendix BB (*continued*)

Anti-infectives by Class With Dose Forms		
Generic Name	**Brand Name**	**Dose Form/Volume**
	Vibra-Tab	*Tab:* 100 mg film-coat
	Xerava	*Vial:* 50 mg pwdr for IV infusion
minocycline (D)(G)	**Dynacin**	*Cap:* 50, 100 mg
	Minocin	*Cap:* 50, 100 mg; *Oral susp:* 50 mg/5 ml (60 ml) (custard) (sulfites, alcohol 5%); *Vial:* 100 mg soln for inj
	Minolira	*Tab:* 105, 135 mg ext-rel
tetracycline (D)(G)	**Achromycin V**	*Cap:* 250, 500 mg
	Sumycin	*Tab:* 250, 500 mg; *Oral susp:* 125 mg/5 ml (fruit) (sulfites)
Unclassified/Miscellaneous		
aztreonam (B)	**Cayston**	*Vial:* 75 mg pwdr for reconstitution (preservative-free)
chloramphenicol (C) (G)	**Chloromycetin**	*Vial:* 1 gm
clindamycin (B)(G)	**Cleocin**	*Cap:* 75 (tartrazine), 150 (tartrazine), 300 mg; *Oral susp:* 75 mg/5 ml (100 ml) (cherry); *Vial:* 150 mg/ml (2, 4 ml) (benzyl alcohol)
dalbavancin (C)	**Dalvance**	*Vial:* 500 mg pwdr for reconstitution (preservative-free)
daptomycin (B)(G)	**Cubicin**	*Vial:* 500 mg pwdr for reconstitution
doripenem (B)	**Doribax**	*Vial:* 500 mg pwdr for reconstitution
fosfomycin (B)(G)	**Monurol**	*Sachet:* 3 gm single-dose (mandarin orange; sucrose)
imipenem+ cilastatin (C)(G)	**Primaxin**	*Vial:* imip 500 mg+cila 500 mg; imip 750 mg+cila 750 mg pwdr for reconstitution
lincomycin (B)(G)	**Lincocin**	*Vial:* 300 mg/ml (10 ml)
linezolid (C)(G)	**Zyvox**	*Tab:* 400, 600 mg; *Oral susp:* 100 mg/5 ml (orange) (phenylalanine); *IV:* 2 mg ml (100, 200, 300 ml)
meropenem (B)	**Merrem**	*Vial:* 500 mg; 1 gm (sodium 3.92 mEq/gm)
meropenem+ vaborbactam	**Vabomere**	*Vial:* mero 1 gm+vabor 1 gm pwdr for reconstitution, single-dose
nitrofurantoin (B)(G)	**Furadantin**	*Oral susp:* 25 mg/5 ml (60 ml)
	Macrobid	*Cap:* 100 mg
	Macrodantin	*Cap:* 25, 50, 100 mg

(*continued*)

Appendix BB *(continued)*

Anti-infectives by Class With Dose Forms		
Generic Name	**Brand Name**	**Dose Form/Volume**
quinupristin+ dalfopristin **(B)**	**Synercid**	*Vial:* quin 150 mg+dalfo 350 mg, quin 180 mg+dalfo 420 mg single-dose
tygecycline **(D)(G)**	**Tygacil**	*Vial:* 50 mg pwdr for reconstitution
rifaximin **(C)**	**Xifaxan**	*Tab:* 200, 550 mg
telavancin **(C)**	**Vibativ**	*Vial:* 250, 750 mg pwdr for reconstitution (preservative-free)
vancomycin **(C)(G)**	**Vancocin**	*Cap:* 125, 250 mg; *Vial:* 500 mg, 1 gm pwdr for reconstitution

APPENDIX CC. ANTIBIOTIC DOSING BY WEIGHT FOR LIQUID FORMS

APPENDIX CC.1. *ACYCLOVIR* (ZOVIRAX SUSPENSION)

Weight												
Pounds	15	20	25	30	35	40	45	50	55	60	65	70
Kilograms	6.8	9	11.4	13.6	15.9	18.2	20.5	22.7	25	27.3	29.5	31.8
Single Dose (ml)/Frequency/Strength/5-Day Volume (ml)												
20 mg/kg/d ml/dose qid	3.5	4.5	5.5	6.5	8	9	10	11.5	12.5	13.5	14.5	16
mg/5 ml	200	200	200	200	200	200	200	200	200	200	200	200
Volume (ml)	70	90	110	130	160	180	200	230	250	270	290	320

Zovirax Oral Suspension <2 years: not recommended; >2 years, <40 kg: 20 mg/kg dosed qid x 5 days; ≥2 years, >40 kg: 800 mg dosed qid x 5 days; *Oral susp:* 200 mg/5 ml (banana).

APPENDIX CC.2. *AMANTADINE* (SYMMETREL SYRUP)

Weight												
Pounds	15	20	25	30	35	40	45	50	55	60	65	70
Kilograms	6.8	9	11.4	13.6	15.9	18.2	20.5	22.7	25	27.3	29.5	31.8
Single Dose (ml)/Frequency/Strength/10-Day Volume (ml)												
4 mg/kg/d ml/dose bid	3	4	5	6	7	8	9	10	11	12	13	14
mg/5 ml	50	50	50	50	50	50	50	50	50	50	50	50
Volume (ml)	30	40	50	60	70	80	90	100	110	120	130	140
8 mg/lb/d ml/dose bid	6	8	10	12								
mg/5 ml	50	50	50	50								
Volume (ml)	60	80	100	60								

Symmetrel Suspension (C)(G) Symmetrel <1 year: not recommended; 1-8 years: max 150 mg/day; 9-12 years: 2 tsp bid; >12 years: 100 mg bid <u>or</u> 200 mg once daily; *Syr:* 50 mg/5 ml (raspberry).

APPENDIX CC.3. *AMOXICILLIN* (AMOXIL SUSPENSION, TRIMOX SUSPENSION)

Weight												
Pounds	15	20	25	30	35	40	45	50	55	60	65	70
Kilograms	6.8	9	11.4	13.6	15.9	18.2	20.5	22.7	25	27.3	29.5	31.8
Single Dose (ml)/Frequency/Strength/10-Day Volume (ml)												
20 mg/kg/d ml/dose tid	2	2.5	3	3.5	4	5	5.5	6	7	7.5	8	9
mg/5 ml	125	125	125	125	125	125	125	125	125	125	125	125
Volume (ml)	60	75	90	105	120	150	165	180	210	225	240	270
30 mg/kg/d ml/dose tid	3	3.5	2.5	3	3	3.5	4	4.5	5	5.5	6	6.5
mg/5 ml	125	125	250	250	250	250	250	250	250	250	250	250
Volume (ml)	90	105	75	90	90	105	120	135	150	165	180	195
40 mg/kg/d ml/dose bid	5	7	4.5	5	6	7	8	9	10	11	12	13
mg/5 ml	125	125	250	250	250	250	250	250	250	250	250	250
Volume (ml)	100	140	90	100	120	140	160	180	200	220	240	250
45 mg/kg/d ml/dose bid	4	2.5	3	4	4.5	5	6	6.5	7	7.5	8.5	9
mg/5 ml	200	400	400	400	400	400	400	400	400	400	400	400
Volume (ml)	80	50	60	80	90	100	120	130	140	150	170	180
90 mg/kg/d ml/dose bid	8	5	6	7	9	10	12	13	14	15	17	18
mg/5 ml	200	400	400	400	400	400	400	400	400	400	400	400
Volume (ml)	160	100	120	140	180	200	240	260	280	300	340	360

<40 kg (88 lb): 20-30 mg/kg/day in 3 divided doses or 40-90 mg/kg/day in 2 divided doses; >40 kg: same as adult.

Amoxil Suspension (B)(G) 125, 250 mg/5 ml (80, 100, 150 ml) (strawberry); 200, 400 mg/5 ml (50, 75, 100 ml) (bubble gum).

Trimox Suspension (B)(G) 125, 250 mg/5 ml (80, 100, 150 ml) (raspberry-strawberry).

APPENDIX CC.4. *AMOXICILLIN+CLAVULANATE* (AUGMENTIN SUSPENSION)

Weight												
Pounds	15	20	25	30	35	40	45	50	55	60	65	70
Kilograms	6.8	9	11.4	13.6	15.9	18.2	20.5	22.7	25	27.3	29.5	31.8
Single Dose (ml)/Frequency/Strength/10-Day Volume (ml)												
40 mg/kg/d ml/dose bid	5.5	7	4.5	5.5	6.5	7	8	9	10	11	12	13
mg/5 ml	125	125	250	250	250	250	250	250	250	250	250	250
Volume (ml)	110	140	90	110	130	140	160	180	200	220	240	260

(continued)

Appendix CC.4 (*continued*)

45 mg/kg/d ml/dose bid	3	4	5	6	7	8	9	10	11.5	12.5	13.5	14.5
mg/5 ml	250	250	250	250	250	250	250	250	250	250	250	250
Volume (ml)	60	80	100	120	140	160	180	200	230	250	270	290
45 mg/kg/d ml/dose bid	4	2.5	3	4	4.5	5	6	6.5	7	7.5	8.5	9
mg/5 ml	200	400	400	400	400	400	400	400	400	400	400	400
Volume (ml)	80	50	60	80	90	100	120	130	140	150	170	180
90 mg/kg/d ml/dose bid	4	5	6.5	8	9	10	11.5	13	14	15.5	16.5	18
mg/5 ml	400	400	400	400	400	400	400	400	400	400	400	400
Volume (ml)	80	100	130	160	180	200	240	260	280	300	340	360

Augmentin Suspension (B)(G) 40-45 mg/kg/day divided tid or 90 mg/kg/day divided bid; 125 mg/5 ml (75, 100, 150 ml) (banana), 250 mg/5 ml (75, 100, 150 ml) (orange); 200, 400 mg/5 ml (50, 75, 100 ml) (orange-raspberry) (phenylalanine).

APPENDIX CC.5. *AMOXICILLIN+CLAVULANATE* (AUGMENTIN ES 600 SUSPENSION)

Weight												
Pounds	15	20	25	30	35	40	45	50	55	60	65	70
Kilograms	6.8	9	11.4	13.6	15.9	18.2	20.5	22.7	25	27.3	29.5	31.8
Single Dose (ml)/Frequency/Strength/10-Day Volume (ml)												
40 mg/kg/d ml/dose bid	1	1.5	2	2	2.5	3	3.5	4	4	4.5	5	5
mg/5 ml	600	600	600	600	600	600	600	600	600	600	600	600
Volume (ml)	30	40	40	40	50	60	70	80	80	90	100	100
45 mg/kg/d ml/dose bid	1.25	1.5	2	2.5	3	3.5	4	4.5	5	5	5.5	6
mg/5 ml	600	600	600	600	600	600	600	600	600	600	600	600
Volume (ml)	25	30	40	50	60	70	80	90	100	100	110	120
90 mg/kg/d ml/dose bid	2.5	3.5	4	5	6	7	8	8.5	9.5	10	11	12
mg/5 ml	600	600	600	600	600	600	600	600	600	600	600	600
Volume (ml)	50	70	80	100	120	140	160	170	190	200	220	240

Augmentin ES 600 Suspension (B) <3 months: not recommended; ≥3 months, <40 kg: 90 mg/kg/day in 2 divided doses; ≥40 kg: not recommended; 600 mg/5 ml (50, 75, 100, 125, 150, 200 ml) (strawberry cream) (phenylalanine).

APPENDIX CC.6. *AMPICILLIN* (OMNIPEN SUSPENSION, PRINCIPEN SUSPENSION)

Weight												
Pounds	15	20	25	30	35	40	45	50	55	60	65	70
Kilograms	6.8	9	11.4	13.6	15.9	18.2	20.5	22.7	25	27.3	29.5	31.8

(*continued*)

Appendix CC.6 (*continued*)

Single Dose (ml)/Frequency/Strength/10-Day Volume (ml)						
50 mg/kg/d ml/dose q6h	3.5	4.5	3	3.5	4	4.5
mg/5 ml	125	125	250	250	250	250
Volume (ml)	140	180	120	140	160	180
100 mg/kg/d ml/dose q6h	3.5	4.5	6	7	8	9
mg/5 ml	250	250	250	250	250	250
Volume (ml)	140	180	240	280	320	360

Omnipen Suspension, Principen Suspension (B)(G) >20 kg: 250-500 mg q 6 h 125, 250 mg/5 ml (100, 150, 200 ml) (fruit).

APPENDIX CC.7. *AZITHROMYCIN* (ZITHROMAX SUSPENSION, ZMAX SUSPENSION)

Weight								
Pounds	11	22	33	44	55	66	77	88
Kilograms	5	10	15	20	25	30	35	40
Single Dose (ml)/Frequency/Strength/Volume (ml)								
3 Day Regimen								
10 mg/kg qd	2.5	5	7.5	5	6	7.5	9	10
mg/5 ml	100	100	100	200	200	200	200	200
Volume (ml)	7.5	15	22.5	15	18	22.5	27	30
5 Day Regimen								
10 mg/kg qd								
Day 1	2.5	5	7.5	5	6	7.5	7.5	10
Days 2–5	1.25	2.5	4	2.5	3	4	4	5
Volume (ml)	10	15	23.5	15	18	23.5	23.5	30

Zithromax ES 600 Suspension (B)(G) 100 mg/5 ml (15 ml), 200 mg/5 ml (15, 22.5, 30 ml) (cherry-vanilla-banana).

APPENDIX CC.8. *CEFACLOR* (CECLOR SUSPENSION)

Weight												
Pounds	15	20	25	30	35	40	45	50	55	60	65	70
Kilograms	6.8	9	11.4	13.6	15.9	18.2	20.5	22.7	25	27.3	29.5	31.8
Single Dose (ml)/Frequency/Strength/10-Day Volume (ml)												
20 mg/kg/d ml/dose tid	2	2.5	3	3.5	4	5	5.5	6	7	7.5	8	8.5
mg/5 ml	125	125	125	125	125	125	125	125	125	125	125	125
Volume (ml)	60	75	90	105	120	150	165	180	210	225	240	255
20 mg/kg/d ml/dose tid	1.5	1.5	2	2.5	3	3	4	4	4.5	5	5.5	6

(*continued*)

Appendix CC.8 (*continued*)

mg/5 ml	187	187	187	187	187	187	187	187	187	187	187	187
Volume (ml)	45	45	60	75	90	90	105	120	135	150	165	180
40 mg/kg/d ml/dose tid	2	2.5	3	3.5	4	5	5.5	6	6.5	7	8	8.5
mg/5 ml	250	250	250	250	250	250	250	250	250	250	250	250
Volume (ml)	60	75	90	105	120	150	165	180	195	210	240	255
40 mg/kg/d ml/dose tid	1.5	1.5	2	2.5	3	3	3.5	4	4.5	5	5	5.5
mg/5 ml	375	375	375	375	375	375	375	375	375	375	375	375
Volume (ml)	45	45	60	75	90	90	105	120	135	150	150	165

Ceclor Suspension (B) <6 months: not recommended; 125, 250 mg/5 ml (75, 150 ml) (strawberry); 187, 375 mg/5 ml (50, 100 ml) (strawberry).

APPENDIX CC.9. *CEFADROXIL* (DURICEF SUSPENSION)

Weight												
Pounds	15	20	25	30	35	40	45	50	55	60	65	70
Kilograms	6.8	9	11.4	13.6	15.9	18.2	20.5	22.7	25	27.3	29.5	31.8
Single Dose (ml)/Frequency/Strength/10-Day Volume (ml)												
30 mg/kg/d ml/dose bid	2	3	3.5	4	5	5.5	6	7	7.5	8	9	9.5
mg/5 ml	250	250	250	250	250	250	250	250	250	250	250	250
Volume (ml)	40	60	75	80	100	110	120	140	150	160	180	190
30 mg/kg/d ml/dose qd	2	3	3.5	4	5	5.5	6	7	7.5	8	9	9.5
mg/5 ml	500	500	500	500	500	500	500	500	500	500	500	500
Volume (ml)	20	30	35	40	50	55	60	70	75	80	90	95

Duricef Suspension (B) 250 mg/5 ml (100 ml) (orange-pineapple); 500 mg/5 ml (75, 100 ml) (orange-pineapple).

APPENDIX CC.10. *CEFDINIR* (OMNICEF SUSPENSION)

Weight												
Pounds	15	20	25	30	35	40	45	50	55	60	65	70
Kilograms	6.8	9	11.4	13.6	15.9	18.2	20.5	22.7	25	27.3	29.5	31.8
Single Dose (ml)/Frequency/Strength/10-Day Volume (ml)												
7 mg/kg/d ml/dose bid	2	2.5	3	4	4.5	5	6	6.5	7	7.5	8	9
mg/5 ml	125	125	125	125	125	125	125	125	125	125	125	125
Volume (ml)	40	50	60	80	90	100	120	130	140	150	160	180
14 mg/kg ml/dose bid	4	5	6	8	9	10	12	13	14	15	16	18

(*continued*)

Appendix CC.10 (*continued*)

mg/5 ml	125	125	125	125	125	125	125	125	125	125	125	125
Volume (ml)	40	50	60	80	90	100	120	130	140	150	160	180

Omnicef Suspension (B) <6 months: not recommended; 125 mg/5 ml (60, 100 ml) (strawberry).

APPENDIX CC.11. *CEFIXIME* (SUPRAX ORAL SUSPENSION)

Weight												
Pounds	15	20	25	30	35	40	45	50	55	60	65	70
Kilograms	6.8	9	11.4	13.6	15.9	18.2	20.5	22.7	25	27.3	29.5	31.8
Single Dose (ml)/Frequency/Strength/10-Day Volume (ml)												
8 mg/kg/d ml/dose bid	1.3	1.8	2.2	2.5	3.1	3.5	4	4.5	5	5.5	6	6.5
mg/5 ml	100	100	100	100	100	100	100	100	100	100	100	100
8 mg/kg/d ml/dose qd	2.7	3.6	4.5	5.5	6.3	7.2	8.2	9	10	11	12	13
mg/5 ml	100	100	100	100	100	100	100	100	100	100	100	100
Volume (ml)	27	36	45	55	65	70	80	90	100	110	120	130

Supra Oral Suspension (B)(G) <6 months: not recommended; 100 mg/5 ml (50, 75, 100 ml) (strawberry).

APPENDIX CC.12. *CEFPODOXIME PROXETIL* (VANTIN SUSPENSION)

Weight												
Pounds	15	20	25	30	35	40	45	50	55	60	65	70
Kilograms	6.8	9	11.4	13.6	15.9	18.2	20.5	22.7	25	27.3	29.5	31.8
Single Dose (ml)/Frequency/Strength/10-Day Volume (ml)												
5 mg/kg/d ml/dose bid	3.5	4.5	5.5	7	8	9	10	11	12.5	13.5	15	16
mg/5 ml	50	50	50	50	50	50	50	50	50	50	50	50
Volume (ml)	70	90	110	140	160	180	200	220	250	270	300	320
5 mg/kg/d ml/dose bid	2	2	3	3.5	4	4.5	5	5.5	6	7	7.5	8
mg/5 ml	100	100	100	100	100	100	100	100	100	100	100	100
Volume (ml)	40	40	60	70	80	90	100	110	120	140	150	160

Vantin Suspension (B) <2 months: not recommended; 50, 100 mg/5 ml (50, 75, 100 ml) (lemon-crème).

APPENDIX CC.13. *CEFPROZIL* (CEFZIL SUSPENSION)

Weight												
Pounds	15	20	25	30	35	40	45	50	55	60	65	70
Kilograms	6.8	9	11.4	13.6	15.9	18.2	20.5	22.7	25	27.3	29.5	31.8

(*continued*)

Appendix CC.13 (*continued*)

Single Dose (ml)/Frequency/Strength/10-Day Volume (ml)											
7.5 mg/kg/d ml/dose bid	2	3	3.5	4	5	5.5	6	7	7.5	4	4.5	5
mg/5 ml	125	125	125	125	125	125	125	125	125	250	250	250
Volume (ml)	40	60	70	80	100	110	120	140	150	80	90	100
15 mg/kg/d ml/dose bid	2	3	3.5	4	5	5	6	7	7.5	8	9	9.5
mg/5 ml	250	250	250	250	250	250	250	250	250	250	250	250
Volume (ml)	40	60	70	80	100	100	120	140	150	160	180	190
20 mg/kg/d ml/dose qd	3	3.5	4.5	5.5	6.5	7	8	9	10	11	12	13
mg/5 ml	250	250	250	250	250	250	250	250	250	250	250	250
Volume (ml)	60	70	90	110	130	140	160	180	200	220	240	260

Cefzil Suspension (B) ≤6 months: not recommended; 2-12 years: 7.5-20 mg/kg bid >12 years: same as adult, 250-500 mg bid or 500 mg once daily; 125, 250 mg/5 ml (50, 75, 100 ml) (bubble gum) (phenylalanine).

APPENDIX CC.14. *CEFTIBUTEN* (CEDAX SUSPENSION)

Weight											
Pounds	15	20	25	30	35	40	45	50	55	60	65	70
Kilograms	6.8	9	11.4	13.6	15.9	18.2	20.5	22.7	25	27.3	29.5	31.8
Single Dose (ml)/Frequency/Strength/10-Day Volume (ml)											
9 mg/kg/d ml/dose qd	3.5	4.5	6	7	8	9	10	11.5	12.5	13.5	15	16
mg/5 ml	90	90	90	90	90	90	90	90	90	90	90	90
Volume (ml)	35	45	60	70	80	90	100	115	125	135	150	160
9 mg/kg/d ml/dose qd	1.75	2.3	3	3.5	4	4.5	5	5.4	6.2	6.6	7.5	8
mg/5 ml	180	180	180	180	180	180	180	180	180	180	180	180
Volume (ml)	20	25	30	35	40	45	50	55	60	65	70	80

Cedax Suspension (B) 90 mg/5 ml (30, 60, 90, 120 ml) (cherry); 180 mg/5 ml (30, 60, 120 ml) (cherry).

APPENDIX CC.15. *CEPHALEXIN* (KEFLEX SUSPENSION)

Weight											
Pounds	15	20	25	30	35	40	45	50	55	60	65	70
Kilograms	6.8	9	11.4	13.6	15.9	18.2	20.5	22.7	25	27.3	29.5	31.8
Single Dose (ml)/Frequency/Strength/10-Day Volume (ml)											
25 mg/kg/d ml/dose tid	1	1.5	2	2	3	3	3.5	4	4	4.5	5	5
mg/5 ml	125	125	125	125	125	125	125	125	125	125	125	125

(*continued*)

Appendix CC.15 (*continued*)

Volume (ml)	30	45	60	60	90	90	105	120	120	135	150	150
25 mg/kg/d ml/dose qid	1	1	1.5	2	2	2.5	2.5	3	3	3.5	4	4
mg/5 ml	250	250	250	250	250	250	250	250	250	250	250	250
Volume (ml)	40	40	60	80	80	100	100	120	120	140	160	160
50 mg/kg/d ml/dose tid	2	3	4	4.5	5	6	7	7.5	8	9	10	10.5
mg/5 ml	250	250	250	250	250	250	250	250	250	250	250	250
Volume (ml)	60	90	120	135	150	180	210	225	240	270	300	315
50 mg/kg/d ml/dose qid	2	2	3	3.5	4	4.5	5	6	6	7	7.5	8
mg/5 ml	250	250	250	250	250	250	250	250	250	250	250	250
Volume (ml)	80	80	120	140	160	180	200	240	240	280	300	320

Keflex Suspension (B)(G) <2 months: not recommended; 125, 250 mg/5 ml (100, 200 ml) (strawberry).

APPENDIX CC.16. *CLARITHROMYCIN* (BIAXIN SUSPENSION)

Weight												
Pounds	15	20	25	30	35	40	45	50	55	60	65	70
Kilograms	6.8	9	11.4	13.6	15.9	18.2	20.5	22.7	25	27.3	29.5	31.8
Single Dose (ml)/Frequency/Strength/10-Day Volume (ml)												
7.5 mg/kg/d ml/dose bid	2	3	3.5	4	5	5.5	6	7	7.5	8	9	10
mg/5 ml	125	125	125	125	125	125	125	125	125	125	125	125
Volume (ml)	40	60	70	80	100	110	120	140	150	160	180	200
7.5 mg/kg/d ml/dose bid	1	1.5	2	2	2.5	3	3	3.5	4	4	4.5	5
mg/5 ml	250	250	250	250	250	250	250	250	250	250	250	250
Volume (ml)	20	30	40	40	50	60	60	70	80	80	90	100

Biaxin Suspension (B) <6 months: not recommended; 125, 250 mg/5 ml (50, 100 ml) (fruit-punch).

APPENDIX CC.17. *CLINDAMYCIN* (CLEOCIN PEDIATRIC GRANULES)

Weight												
Pounds	15	20	25	30	35	40	45	50	55	60	65	70
Kilograms	6.8	9	11.4	13.6	15.9	18.2	20.5	22.7	25	27.3	29.5	31.8
Single Dose (ml)/Frequency/Strength/10-Day Volume (ml)												
8 mg/kg/d ml/dose tid	1	1.5	2	2.5	3	3	3.5	4	4.5	5	5	5.5
mg/5 ml	75	75	75	75	75	75	75	75	75	75	75	75
Volume (ml)	30	45	60	75	90	90	105	120	135	150	150	165

(*continued*)

Appendix CC.17 (continued)

16 mg/kg/d ml/dose tid	2.5	3	4	5	5.5	6.5	7	8	9	9.5	10.5	11
mg/5 ml	75	75	75	75	75	75	75	75	75	75	75	75
Volume (ml)	75	90	120	150	165	105	210	240	270	285	315	330

Cleocin Pediatric Granules (B)(G) 75 mg/5 ml (100 ml) (cherry).

APPENDIX CC.18. *DICLOXACILLIN* (DYNAPEN SUSPENSION)

Weight												
Pounds	15	20	25	30	35	40	45	50	55	60	65	70
Kilograms	6.8	9	11.4	13.6	15.9	18.2	20.5	22.7	25	27.3	29.5	31.8
Single Dose (ml)/Frequency/Strength/10-Day Volume (ml)												
12.5 mg/kg/d ml/dose qid	2	2.5	3	3.5	4	4.5	5	6	6	7	7.5	8
mg/5 ml	62.5	62.5	62.5	62.5	62.5	62.5	62.5	62.5	62.5	62.5	62.5	62.5
Volume (ml)	80	100	120	140	160	180	200	240	240	280	300	320
25 mg/kg/d ml/dose qid	3.5	4.5	6	7	8	9	10	11.5	12.5	13.5	15	16
mg/5 ml	62.5	62.5	62.5	62.5	62.5	62.5	62.5	62.5	62.5	62.5	62.5	62.5
Volume (ml)	140	180	240	280	320	360	400	460	500	540	600	640

Dynapen Suspension (B)(G) 6.25 mg/5 ml (80, 100 ml) (raspberry-strawberry).

APPENDIX CC.19. *DOXYCYCLINE* (VIBRAMYCIN SYRUP/SUSPENSION)

Weight												
Pounds	15	20	25	30	35	40	45	50	55	60	65	70
Kilograms	6.8	9	11.4	13.6	15.9	18.2	20.5	22.7	25	27.3	29.5	31.8
Single Dose (ml)/Frequency/Strength/10-Day Volume (ml)												
1 mg/lb/d ml/dose qd	1.5	2	2.5	3	3.5	4	4.5	5	5.5	6	6.5	7
50 mg/5 ml	50	50	50	50	50	50	50	50	50	50	50	50
Volume (ml)	15	20	25	30	35	40	45	50	55	60	65	70
1 mg/lb/d ml/dose qd	3	4	5	6	7	8	9	10	11	12	13	14
25 mg/5 ml	25	25	25	25	25	25	25	25	25	25	25	25
Volume (ml)	30	40	50	60	70	80	90	100	110	120	130	140

Vibramycin Syrup (B)(G) <8 years: not recommended; double dose first day; 50 mg/5 ml (80, 100, ml) (raspberry-apple) (sulfites).

Vibramycin Suspension (B)(G) <8 years: not recommended; double dose first day; 25 mg/5 ml (80, 100, ml) (raspberry).

(continued)

APPENDIX CC.20. *ERYTHROMYCIN ESTOLATE* (ILOSONE SUSPENSION)

Weight												
Pounds	15	20	25	30	35	40	45	50	55	60	65	70
Kilograms	6.8	9	11.4	13.6	15.9	18.2	20.5	22.7	25	27.3	29.5	31.8
Dose/Volume (10 days) in ml												
10 mg/kg/d ml/dose bid	3	3.5	4.5	5.5	6	7	8	9	10	5.5	6	6.5
mg/5 ml	125	125	125	125	125	125	125	125	125	250	250	250
Volume (ml)	60	70	90	110	120	140	160	180	200	110	120	130
15 mg/kg/d ml/dose bid	4	5.5	7	8	9.5	5.5	6	7	7.5	8	9	9.5
mg/5 ml	125	125	125	125	125	250	250	250	250	250	250	250
Volume (ml)	80	110	140	160	190	110	120	140	150	160	180	190
20 mg/kg/d ml/dose bid	3	3.5	4.5	5.5	6.5	7	8	9	10	11	12	13
mg/5 ml	250	250	250	250	250	250	250	250	250	250	250	250
Volume (ml)	60	70	90	110	120	140	160	180	200	220	240	260
25 mg/kg/d ml/dose bid	3.5	4.5	5.5	7	8	9	10	11.5	12.5	13.5	15	16
mg/5 ml	250	250	250	250	250	250	250	250	250	250	250	250
Volume (ml)	70	90	110	140	160	180	200	230	250	280	300	320

Ilosone Suspension (B)(G) 125, 250 mg/5 ml (100 ml).

APPENDIX CC.21. *ERYTHROMYCIN ETHYLSUCCINATE* (E.E.S. SUSPENSION, ERY-PED DROPS/SUSPENSION)

Weight												
Pounds	15	20	25	30	35	40	45	50	55	60	65	70
Kilograms	6.8	9	11.4	13.6	15.9	18.2	20.5	22.7	25	27.3	29.5	31.8
Single Dose (ml)/Frequency/Strength/10-Day Volume (ml)												
30 mg/kg/d ml/dose qid	1.5	2	2	2.5	3	3.5	4	4	4.5	5	5.5	6
mg/5 ml	200	200	200	200	200	200	200	200	200	200	200	200
Volume (ml)	60	80	80	100	120	140	160	160	180	200	220	240
30 mg/kg/d ml/dose qid			1	1.5	1.5	2	2	2	2.5	2.5	3	3
mg/5 ml			400	400	400	400	400	400	400	400	400	
Volume (ml)			60	60	80	80	80	100	100	120	120	
50 mg/kg/d ml/dose qid	2	3	3.5	4.5	5	5.5	6.5	7	8	8.5	9	10

(continued)

Appendix CC.21 (*continued*)

mg/5 ml	200	200	200	200	200	200	200	200	200	200	200	200
Volume (ml)	80	120	140	180	200	220	260	280	320	340	360	400
50 mg/kg/d ml/dose qid	1	1.5	2	2	2.5	3	3	3.5	4	4.5	4.5	5
mg/5 ml	400	400	400	400	400	400	400	400	400	400	400	400
Volume (ml)	40	60	80	80	100	120	140	140	160	180	180	200

Ery-Ped Drops/Suspension (B)(G) 200 mg/5 ml (100, 200 ml) (fruit); 400 mg/5 ml (60, 100, 200 ml) (banana); Oral drops: 200, 400 mg/5 ml (50 ml) (fruit).

E.E.S. Suspension (B)(G) 200 mg/5 ml, 400 mg/5 ml (100 ml) (fruit).

E.E.S. Granules (B)(G) 200 mg/5 ml (100, 200 ml) (cherry).

APPENDIX CC.22. *ERYTHROMYCIN+SULFAMETHOXAZOLE* (ERYZOLE, PEDIAZOLE)

Weight												
Pounds	15	20	25	30	35	40	45	50	55	60	65	70
Kilograms	6.8	9	11.4	13.6	15.9	18.2	20.5	22.7	25	27.3	29.5	31.8
Single Dose (ml)/Frequency/Strength/10-Day Volume (ml)												
10 mg/kg/d ml/dose bid	3	4	5	6	6.5	7.5	8.5	9.5	10	11	12	13.5
mg/5 ml	200	200	200	200	200	200	200	200	200	200	200	200
Volume (ml)	90	120	150	180	200	225	255	285	300	330	360	400

Eryzole (C)(G) <2 months: not recommended; *eryth* 200 mg/*sulf* 600 mg/5 ml (100, 150, 200, 250 ml).

Pediazole (C)(G) <2 months: not recommended; *eryth* 200 mg/*sulf* 600 mg/5 ml (100, 150, 200 ml) (strawberry-banana).

APPENDIX CC.23. *FLUCONAZOLE* (DIFLUCAN SUSPENSION)

Weight												
Pounds	15	20	25	30	35	40	45	50	55	60	65	70
Kilograms	6.8	9	11.4	13.6	15.9	18.2	20.5	22.7	25	27.3	29.5	31.8
Single Dose (ml)/Frequency/Strength/21-Day Volume (ml)												
3 mg/kg/d ml/dose qd	2	3	3.5	4	5	5.5	6	7	7.5	8	9	9.5
mg/ml	10	10	10	10	10	10	10	10	10	10	10	10
Volume (ml)	44	66	77	88	110	121	132	154	165	176	198	209
6 mg/kg/d ml/dose qd	4	5.5	2	2	2.5	3	3	3.5	4	4	4.5	5
mg/ml	10	10	40	40	40	40	40	40	40	40	40	40
Volume (ml)	88	121	44	44	55	66	66	77	88	88	99	110

Diflucan Suspension (B)(G) double-dose first day; 10, 40 mg/5 ml (35 ml) (orange).

APPENDIX CC.24. *FURAZOLIDONE* (FUROXONE LIQUID)

Weight												
Pounds	15	20	25	30	35	40	45	50	55	60	65	70
Kilograms	6.8	9	11.4	13.6	15.9	18.2	20.5	22.7	25	27.3	29.5	31.8
Single Dose (ml)/Frequency/Strength/7-Day Volume (ml)												
5 mg/kg/d ml/dose qid	2.5	3.5	4	5	6	7	8	8.5	9.5	10	11	12
mg/15 ml	50	50	50	50	50	50	50	50	50	50	50	50
Vol	100	140	160	200	240	280	320	340	380	400	440	480

Furoxone Liquid (C)(G) double-dose first day; 50 mg/15 ml (35 ml).

APPENDIX CC.25. *GRISEOFULVIN, MICROSIZE* (GRIFULVIN V SUSPENSION)

Weight												
Pounds	15	20	25	30	35	40	45	50	55	60	65	70
Kilograms	6.8	9	11.4	13.6	15.9	18.2	20.5	22.7	25	27.3	29.5	31.8
Single Dose (ml)/Frequency/Strength/30-Day Volume (ml)												
5 mg/lb/d ml/dose day	3	4	5	6	7	8	9	10	11	12	13	14
mg/5 ml	125	125	125	125	125	125	125	125	125	125	125	125
Volume (ml)	90	120	150	180	210	240	270	300	330	360	390	420

Grifulvin V Suspension (C)(G) double-dose first day; 125 mg/5 ml (120 ml) (orange) (alcohol 0.02%).

APPENDIX CC.26. *ITRACONAZOLE* (SPORANOX SOLUTION)

Weight												
Pounds	15	20	25	30	35	40	45	50	55	60	65	70
Kilograms	6.8	9	11.4	13.6	15.9	18.2	20.5	22.7	25	27.3	29.5	31.8
Single Dose (ml)/Frequency/Strength/7-Day Volume (ml)												
5 mg/kg/d ml/dose qd	3.5	4.5	6	7	8	9	10	11.5	12.5	14	15	16
mg/ml	10	10	10	10	10	10	10	10	10	10	10	10
Volume (ml)	25	32	42	49	56	63	70	71	88	98	105	112

Sporanox V Solution (C)(G) double-dose first day; 10 mg/ml (150 ml) (cherry-caramel).

APPENDIX CC.27. *LORACARBEF* (LORABID SUSPENSION)

Weight												
Pounds	15	20	25	30	35	40	45	50	55	60	65	70
Kilograms	6.8	9	11.4	13.6	15.9	18.2	20.5	22.7	25	27.3	29.5	31.8
Single Dose (ml)/Frequency/Strength/10-Day Volume (ml)												
15 mg/kg/d ml/dose bid	2.5	3.5	4	5	3	3.5	4	4	5	5	5.5	6

Appendix CC.27 (*continued*)

mg/5 ml	100	100	100	100	200	200	200	200	200	200	200	200
Volume (ml)	50	70	80	100	60	70	80	80	100	100	110	120
30 mg/kg/d ml/dose bid	2.5	3.5	4	5	6	7	8	8.5	9.5	10	11	12
mg/5 ml	200	200	200	200	200	200	200	200	200	200	200	200
Volume (ml)	50	70	80	100	120	140	160	170	190	200	220	240

Lorabid Suspension (B) 100 mg/5 ml (50, 100 ml) (strawberry bubble gum); 200 mg/5 ml (50, 75, 100 ml) (strawberry bubble gum).

APPENDIX CC.28. *NITROFURANTOIN* (FURADANTIN SUSPENSION)

Weight												
Pounds	15	20	25	30	35	40	45	50	55	60	65	70
Kilograms	6.8	9	11.4	13.6	15.9	18.2	20.5	22.7	25	27.3	29.5	31.8
Single Dose (ml)/Frequency/Strength/10-Day Volume (ml)												
5 mg/kg ml/dose qid	1.5	2.5	3	3.5	4	4.5	5	5.5	6	7	7.5	8
mg/5 ml	25	25	25	25	25	25	25	25	25	25	25	25
Volume (ml)	60	100	120	140	160	190	200	220	240	280	300	320

Furadantin Suspension (B)(G) 25 mg/5 ml (60 ml).

APPENDIX CC.29. *PENICILLIN V POTASSIUM* (PEN-VEE K SOLUTION, VEETIDS SOLUTION)

Weight												
Pounds	15	20	25	30	35	40	45	50	55	60	65	70
Kilograms	6.8	9	11.4	13.6	15.9	18.2	20.5	22.7	25	27.3	29.5	31.8
Single Dose (ml)/Frequency/Strength/10-Day Volume (ml)												
25 mg/kg/d ml/dose qid	2	2.5	3	3.5	4	4.5	5	5.5	6	7	7.5	8
mg/5 ml	125	125	125	125	125	125	125	125	125	125	125	125
Volume (ml)	80	90	120	140	160	180	200	220	240	280	300	320
25 mg/kg/d ml/dose qid	1	1	1.5	2	2	2.5	2.5	3	3	3.5	4	4
mg/5 ml	250	250	250	250	250	250	250	250	250	250	250	250
Volume (ml)	40	40	60	80	80	100	100	120	120	140	160	160
50 mg/kg/d ml/dose qid	2	2.5	3	3.5	4	4.5	5	6	6.5	7	7.5	8
mg/5 ml	250	250	250	250	250	250	250	250	250	250	250	250
Volume (ml)	80	100	120	140	160	180	200	240	260	280	300	320

Pen-Vee K Solution (B)(G) 125 mg/5 ml (100, 200 ml), 250 mg/5 ml (100, 150, 200 ml).

Veetids Solution (B)(G) 125, 250 mg/5 ml (100, 200 ml).

APPENDIX CC.30. *RIMANTADINE* (FLUMADINE SYRUP)

Weight												
Pounds	15	20	25	30	35	40	45	50	55	60	65	70
Kilograms	6.8	9	11.4	13.6	15.9	18.2	20.5	22.7	25	27.3	29.5	31.8
Single Dose (ml)/Frequency/Strength/10-Day Volume (ml)												
5 mg/kg/d ml/dose qd	3.5	4.5	6	7	8	9	10	11.5	12.5	13.5	15	16
mg/5 ml	50	50	50	50	50	50	50	50	50	50	50	50
Volume (ml)	35	45	60	70	80	90	100	115	125	135	150	160

Flumadine Syrup (B) >10 years: same as adult; 50 mg/5 ml (2, 8, 16 oz) (raspberry).

APPENDIX CC.31. *TETRACYCLINE* (SUMYCIN SUSPENSION)

Weight												
Pounds	15	20	25	30	35	40	45	50	55	60	65	70
Kilograms	6.8	9	11.4	13.6	15.9	18.2	20.5	22.7	25	27.3	29.5	31.8
Single Dose (ml)/Frequency/Strength/10-Day Volume (ml)												
25 mg/kg/d ml/dose qid	1.5	2.5	3	3.5	4	4.5	5	6	6.5	7	7.5	8
mg/5 ml	125	125	125	125	125	125	125	125	125	125	125	125
Volume (ml)	60	100	120	140	160	180	200	240	260	280	300	320
50 mg/kg/d ml/dose qid	3.5	4.5	6	7	8	9	10	11.5	12.5	13.5	15	16
mg/5 ml	125	125	125	125	125	125	125	125	125	125	125	125
Volume (ml)	140	180	240	280	320	360	400	460	500	540	600	640

Sumycin Suspension (D)(G) <8 years: not recommended; 125 mg/5 ml (100, 200 ml) (fruit) (sulfites).

APPENDIX CC.32. *TRIMETHOPRIM* (PRIMSOL SUSPENSION)

Weight												
Pounds	15	20	25	30	35	40	45	50	55	60	65	70
Kilograms	6.8	9	11.4	13.6	15.9	18.2	20.5	22.7	25	27.3	29.5	31.8
Single Dose (ml)/Frequency/Strength/10-Day Volume (ml)												
5 mg/kg/d ml/dose bid	3.5	4.5	6	7	8	9	10	11.5	12.5	13.5	15	16
mg/5 ml	50	50	50	50	50	50	50	50	50	50	50	50
Volume (ml)	70	90	120	140	160	180	200	230	250	270	300	320

Primsol Suspension (C)(G) 50 mg/5 ml (50 mg/5 ml) (bubble gum) (dye-free, alcohol-free).

APPENDIX CC.33. *TRIMETHOPRIM+SULFAMETHOXAZOLE* (BACTRIM SUSPENSION, SEPTRA SUSPENSION)

Weight												
Pounds	15	20	25	30	35	40	45	50	55	60	65	70
Kilograms	6.8	9	11.4	13.6	15.9	18.2	20.5	22.7	25	27.3	29.5	31.8
Single Dose (ml)/Frequency/Strength/10-Day Volume (ml)												
10 mg/kg/d ml/dose bid	2	2	3	3.5	4	4.5	5	5.5	6	7	7.5	8
mg/5 ml	200	200	200	200	200	200	200	200	200	200	200	200
Volume (ml)	40	40	60	70	80	90	100	110	120	140	150	160
20 mg/kg/d ml/dose bid	4	4	6	7	8	9	10	11	12	14	15	16
mg/5 ml	200	200	200	200	200	200	200	200	200	200	200	200
Volume (ml)	80	80	120	140	160	180	200	220	240	280	300	320

Bactrim Pediatric Suspension, Septra Pediatric Suspension (C)(G) trim 40 mg/sulfa 200 mg/5 ml (100 ml) (cherry) (alcohol 0.3%).

APPENDIX CC.34. *VANCOMYCIN* (VANCOCIN SUSPENSION)

Weight												
Pounds	15	20	25	30	35	40	45	50	55	60	65	70
Kilograms	6.8	9	11.4	13.6	15.9	18.2	20.5	22.7	25	27.3	29.5	31.8
Single Dose (ml)/Frequency/Strength/10-Day Volume (ml)												
40 mg/kg/d ml/dose tid	2	2.5	3	3.5	4.5	5	5.5	6	7	7.5	8	8.5
mg/5 ml	250	250	250	250	250	250	250	250	250	250	250	250
Volume (ml)	60	75	90	105	135	150	165	180	210	225	240	255
40 mg/kg/d ml/dose qid	1.5	2	2.5	3	3	3.5	4	4.5	5	5.5	6	6.5
mg/5 ml	250	250	250	250	250	250	250	250	250	250	250	250
Volume (ml)	60	80	100	120	120	140	160	180	200	220	240	260
40 mg/kg/d ml/dose tid	1	1	1.5	2	2	2.5	3	3	3.5	3.5	4	4
mg/6 ml	500	500	500	500	500	500	500	500	500	500	500	500
Volume (ml)	30	30	45	60	60	75	90	90	105	105	120	120
40 mg/kg/d ml/dose qid	1	1	1.5	1.5	1.5	2	2	2.5	2.5	3	3	3.5
mg/6 ml	500	500	500	500	500	500	500	500	500	500	500	500
Volume (ml)	40	40	60	60	60	80	80	100	100	120	120	140

Vancomycin Suspension (C)(G).

ACC/AHA/AAPA/ABC/ACPM/AGS/APhA/ASH/ASPC/NMA/PCNA. (2017). *2017 Guideline for the prevention, detection, evaluation, and management of high blood pressure in adults: A report of the American College of Cardiology/American Heart Association Task Force on clinical practice guidelines.*
http://hyper.ahajournals.org/content/hypertensionaha/early/2017/11/10/HYP.0000000000000065.full.pdf

ACR guidelines on prevention & treatment of glucocorticoid-induced osteoporosis [press release, June 7, 2017]. Atlanta, GA: American College of Rheumatology.
https://www.rheumatology.org/About-Us/Newsroom/Press-Releases/ID/812/ACR-Releases-Guideline-on-Prevention-Treatment-of-Glucocorticoid-Induced-Osteoporosis

Advance for Nurse Practitioners.
http://nurse-practitioners.advanceweb.com

American Academy of Dermatology.
https://www.aad.org/home

American Academy of Pediatrics (AAP).
http://aapexperience.org

American Association of Nurse Practitioners.
www.aanp.org

American College of Cardiology. *Then and now: ATP III vs. IV: Comparison of ATP III and ACC/AHA guidelines.*
http://www.acc.org/latest-in-cardiology/articles/2014/07/18/16/03/then-and-now-atp-iii-vs-iv

American Diabetes Association (ADA), Professional Diabetes Resources Online.
http://professional.diabetes.org/content/clinical-practice-recommendations/?loc=rp-slabnav

American Diabetes Association. (2018). Children and adolescents: Standards of medical care in diabetes—2018. *Diabetes Care, 41*(Suppl 1), S126–S136. doi:10.2337/dc18-S012

American Diabetes Association. (2018). Management of diabetes in pregnancy: Standards of medical care in diabetes—2018. *Diabetes Care, 41*(Suppl 1), S137–S143. doi:10.2337/dc18-S013

American Diabetes Association. (2018). Microvascular complications and foot care: Standards of medical care in diabetes—2018. *Diabetes Care, 41*(Suppl 1), S105–S118. doi:10.2337/dc18-S010

American Diabetes Association. (2018). Older adults: Standards of medical care in diabetes—2018. *Diabetes Care, 41*(Suppl 1), S119–S125. doi:10.2337/dc18-S011

American Diabetes Association. (2018). Pharmacologic approaches to glycemic treatment: Standards of medical care in diabetes—2018. *Diabetes Care, 41*(Suppl 1), S73–S85. doi:10.2337/dc18-S008

American Diabetes Association. (2018). Summary of revisions: Standards of medical care in diabetes—2018. *Diabetes Care, 41*(Suppl 1), S4–S6. doi:10.2337/dc18-Srev01

American Family Physician.
http://www.aafp.org/online/en/home.html

American Geriatrics Society. (2015). Updated Beers Criteria for potentially inappropriate medication use in older adults. *Journal of the American Geriatrics Society, 63*(11), 2227–2246.

American Headache Society.
www.americanheadachesociety.org

American Pain Society.
http://americanpainsociety.org

American Pharmacists Association. (2018). *Pediatric and neonatal dosage handbook: A universal resource for clinicians treating pediatric and neonatal patients* (25th ed.). Hudson, OH: Lexicomp.

American Trypanosomiasis Centers for Disease Control and Prevention. *Parasites—American Trypanosomiasis (also known as Chagas disease).* Resources for health professionals.

Anderson, E., Fantus, R. J., & Haddadin, R. I. (2017). Diagnosis and management of herpes zoster ophthalmicus. *Disease-a-Month, 63*(2), 38–44.

Andorf, S., Purington, N., Block, W. M., Long, A. J., Tupa, D., Brittain, E., . . . Chinthrajah, R. S. (2018). Anti-IgE treatment with oral immunotherapy in multi-food allergic participants: A double-blind, randomised, controlled trial. *Lancet Gastroenterology Hepatology, 3*(2), 85–94. doi:10.1016/S2468-1253(17)30392-8

Antiretroviral Pregnancy Registry at http://www.apregistry.com/index.htm; Research Park, 1011 Ashes Drive, Wilmington, NC 28405; telephone: 800-258-4263; fax: 800-800-1052; e-mail: registies@kendle.com.

Aronow, W. S. *Initiation of antihypertensive therapy.* Presented at: American Heart Association (AHA) Scientific Sessions 2017; November 11–15, 2017; Anaheim, CA. http://www.abstractsonline.com/pp8/-!/4412/presentation/55060

Auron, M., & Raissouni, N. (2015). Adrenal insufficiency. *Pediatric Review, 36*(3), 92–102.

Bosworth, T. (2017). *Testosterone deficiency treatment recommendation.* https://www.medpagetoday.com/resource-center/hypogonadism/treatment-recommendations/a/64511

Bradley, J. S., & Nelson, J. D. (2021). *Nelson's pediatric antimicrobial therapy* (27th ed.). Itasca, IL: American Academy of Pediatrics.

Brunk, D. (2018). Learn 'four Ds' approach to heart failure in diabetes. *Clinician Reviews* [Online]. https://www.mdedge.com/clinicalendocrinologynews/article/157198/diabetes/learn-four-ds-approach-heart-failure-diabetes

Canestaro, W. J., Forrester, S. H., Raghu, G., Ho, L., & Devine, B. E. (2016). Drug treatment of idiopathic pulmonary fibrosis: Systematic review and network meta-analysis. *Chest, 149*, 756–766.

CDC 2015 sexually transmitted diseases treatment guidelines. http://www.cdc.gov/std/tg2015/default.htm

CDC Cases of Public Health Importance (COPHI) Coordinator (for reporting HIV infections in HCP and failures of PEP); telephone 404-639-2050.

CDC guidelines for conception in HIV positive women stress the use of PrEP in sexual partners. https://www.medpagetoday.com/resource-centers/contemporary-hiv-prevention/cdc-guide-lines-conception-hiv-positive-women-stress-use-prep-sexual- partners/775?xid=NL_MPT_MPT_HIV_2017-09-26&eun=g766320d0r

CDC: Morbidity and Mortality Weekly Report (MMWR). http://www.cdc.gov/mmwr/mmwr_wk.html

CDC provider information sheet -PrEP during conception, pregnancy, and breastfeeding information for clinicians counseling patients about PrEP use during conception, pregnancy, and breastfeeding https://www.cdc.gov/hiv/pdf/prep_gl_clinician_factsheet_pregnancy_english.pdf

CDC Traveler's Health. https://wwwnc.cdc.gov/travel/destinations/list

Centers for Disease Control and Prevention. (2016). *Diphtheria, Tetanus, and Pertussis Vaccine Recommendations.*
http://www.cdc.gov/vaccines/vpd/dtap-tdap-td/hcp/recommendations.htm

Centers for Disease Control and Prevention. (2016). *Facts About ADHD.*
www.cdc.gov/ncbddd/adhd/facts.html

Centers for Disease Control and Prevention. (2020). *Update to CDC's treatment guidelines for gonococcal infection, 2020.*
https://www.cdc.gov/mmwr/volumes/69/wr/mm6950a6.htm?s_cid=mm6950a6_w

Chang, A., Martins, K. A. O., Encinales, L., Reid, S. P., Acuña, M., & Encinales, C., ... Firestein, G. S. (2017). A cross-sectional analysis of chikungunya arthritis patients 22 months post-infection demonstrates no detectable viral persistence in synovial fluid. *Arthritis Rheumatology.* doi:10.1002/art.40383

Chang, A., Encinales, L., Porras, A., Pachecho, N., Reid, S. P., Martins, K. A. O., ... Simon, G. L. (2017). Frequency of chronic joint pain following chikungunya infection: A Colombian cohort study. *Arthritis Rheumatology.* doi:10.1002/art.40384

Chow, A. W., Benninger, M. S., Brook, I., Brozek, J. L., Goldstein, E. J., Hicks, L. A., ... Infectious Disease Society of America. (2012). IDSA clinical practice guideline for acute and bacterial rhinosinusitis in children and adults. *Clinical Infectious Diseases, 54*(8), e72–e112.

Chutka, D. S., Takahashi, P. Y., & Hoel, R. W. (2004). Inappropriate medications for elderly patients. *Mayo Clinic Proceedings, 79*(1), 122–139.

Clinician Reviews.
http://www.clinicianreviews.com

Coker, T. J., & Dierfeldt, D. M. (2016). Acute bacterial prostatitis: Diagnosis and management. *American Family Physician, 93*(2), 114–120.

Consultant 360.
http://www.consultant360.com/home

Daily Med: NIH. US Library of Medicine.
https://dailymed.nlm.nih.gov/dailymed/index.cfm

Davis, M. C., Miller, B. J., Kalsi, J. K., Birkner, T., & Mathis, M. V. (2017). Efficient trial design—FDA approval of valbenazine for tardive dyskinesia. *New England Journal of Medicine, 376,* 2503–2506.

Dietrich, E. A., & Davis, K. (2017). Antibiotics for acute bacterial prostatitis: Which agent, and for how long? *Consultant, 57*(9), 564–565.

Domino, F. J., Baldor, R. A., Golding, J., & Stephens, M. B. (2021). *The 5-minute clinical consult.* Philadelphia, PA: Wolters Kluwer.

Dowell, D., Haegerich, T. M., & Chou, R. (2016). CDC guidelines for prescribing opioids for chronic pain. *Journal of the American Medical Association, 315*(15), 1624–1645. doi:10.1001/jama.2016.1464

DRUGS.COM.
www.drugs.com

DRUGS.COM: Drugs Interaction Checker.
https://www.drugs.com/drug_interactions.php

DRUGS at FDA: FDA Approved Drug Products.
http://www.accessdata.fda.gov/scripts/cder/drugsatfda/index.cfm

Durkin, M. J., Jafarzadeh, S. R., Hsueh, K., Sallah, Y. H., Munshi, K. D., Henderson, R. R., & Fraser, V. J. (2018). Outpatient antibiotic prescription trends in the United States: A national cohort study. *Infection Control & Hospital Epidemiology, 39*(05), 584–589. doi:10.1017/ice.2018.26

eMPR: Monthly Prescribing Reference (new FDA approved products, new generics, new drug withdrawals, safety alerts).
http://www.empr.com

Engorn, B., & Flerlage, J. (Eds.). (2021). *The Harriet Lane handbook: A handbook for pediatric house officers* (20th ed.). Philadelphia, PA: Elsevier.

epocrates.
https://online.epocrates.com/drugs

FDA Drug Safety Communication. (2018). *FDA review finds additional data supports the potential for increased long-term risks with antibiotic clarithromycin (Biaxin) in patients with heart disease* [Online].
https://www.fda.gov/downloads/Drugs/DrugSafety/ucm597723.pdf

FDA: News Release: FDA Approves Drug to Treat Duchenne Muscular Dystrophy. (2017).
https://www.fda.gov/NewsEvents/Newsroom/PressAnnouncements/ucm540945.htm

FDA: Recalls, Market Withdrawals, and Safety Alerts.
http://www.fda.gov/Safety/Recalls/default.htm

FDA: Reporting Unusual or Severe Toxicity to Antiretroviral Agents); http://www.fda.gov/medwatch/; telephone: 800-332-1088; address: MedWatch, The FDA Safety Information and Adverse Event Reporting Program, Food and Drug Administration, 5600 Fishers Lane, Rockville, MD 20852.

Fleming, J. E., & Lockwood, S. (2017). Cannabinoid hyperemesis syndrome. *Federal Practitioner, 34*(10), 33–36.

Freedberg, D. E., Kim, L. S., & Yang, Y.-X. (2017). The risks and benefits of long-term use of proton pump inhibitors: Expert review and best practice advice from the American Gastroenterological Association. *Gastroenterology, 152*(4), 706–715. doi:10.1053/j.gastro.2017.01.031

Freedman, M. S., Ault, K., & Bernstein, H. Advisory committee on immunization practices recommended immunization schedule for adults aged 19 years or older—United States, 2021. *MMWR Morbidity and Mortality Weekly Report, 70*, 193–196.
doi:10.15585/mmwr.mm7006a2

Garber, A. J., Abrahamson, M. J., Barzilay, J. I., Blonde, L., Bloomgarden, Z. T., Bush, M. A., . . . Umpierrez, G. E. (2017). Consensus statement by the American Association of Clinical Endocrinologists and American College of Endocrinology on the comprehensive type 2 diabetes management algorithm—2017 executive summary. *Endocrine Practice, 23*(2), 207–238. doi:10.4158/ep161682.cs

Gilbert, D. N., Chambers, H. F., Eliopoulos, G. M., Saag, M. S., & Pavia, A. T. (Eds.). (2020). *The Sanford guide to antimicrobial therapy, 2020* (50th ed.). Sperryville, VA: Antimicrobial Therapy.

Global Initiative for Chronic Obstructive Lung Disease. GOLD Guidelines, 2017. http://goldcopd.org

Gordon, C., Amissah-Arthur, M. B., Gayed, M., Brown, S., Bruce, I. N., D'Cruz D., . . . British Society for Rheumatology Standards, Audit and Guidelines Working Group. (2017). The British Society for Rheumatology guideline for the management of systemic lupus erythematosus in adults: Executive Summary. *Rheumatology (Oxford).* doi:10.1093/rheumatology/kex291 [Epub ahead of print]

Gordon, C., Amissah-Arthur, M. B., Gayed, M., Brown, S., Bruce, I. N., D'Cruz D., . . . British Society for Rheumatology Standards, Audit and Guidelines Working Group. (2017). The British Society for Rheumatology guideline for the management of systemic lupus erythematosus in adults. *Rheumatology (Oxford).* doi:10.1093/rheumatology/kex286

Greenhawt, M., Turner, P. J., & Kelso, J. M. (2018). Allergy experts set the record straight on flu shots for patients with egg sensitivity. *Annals of Allergy, Asthma & Immunology, 120*(1), 49–52. doi:10.1016/j.anai.2017.10.020

Groot, N., de Graaff, N., Avcin, T., Bader-Meunier, B., Brogan, P., Dolezalova, P., . . . Beresford, M. W. (2017). European evidence-based recommendations for diagnosis and treatment of childhood-onset systemic lupus erythematosus [cSLE]: The [Single Hub and Access point for paediatric Rheumatology in Europe] SHARE initiative. *Annals of the Rheumatic Diseases, 76*(11), 1788–1796. doi:10.1136/annrheumdis-2016-210960

Groot, N., de Graeff, N., Marks, S. D., Brogan, P., Avcin, T., Bader-Meunier, B., . . . Kamphuis, S. (2017). European evidence-based recommendations for the diagnosis and treatment of childhood-onset lupus nephritis [cLN]: The SHARE initiative. *Recommendation*. doi:10.1136/annrheumdis-2017-211898

Guidelines updated for thyroid disease in pregnancy and postpartum. (2017). *American Journal of Nursing, 4*(117), 16.

Handbook of antimicrobial therapy (20th ed.). (2015). New Rochelle, NY: The Medical Letter.

Harrison's infectious diseases (3rd ed.). (2016). New York, NY: McGraw Hill Education.

Huang, A. R., Mallet, L., & Rochefort, C. M. (2012). Medication-related falls in the elderly: Causative factors and preventive strategies. *Drugs & Aging, 29*(5), 359–376.

Hughes, H. K., & Kahl, K. (Eds.). (2018). *The Johns Hopkins Hospital: The Harriet Lane handbook for pediatric house officers* (21st ed.). Philadelphia, PA: Elsevier.

International Diabetes Federation (IDF) Clinical Practice Guidelines. http://www.idf.org/guidelines

Jarrett, J. B., & Moss, D. (2017, July). Oral agent offers relief from generalized hyperhidrosis—An inexpensive and well-tolerated anticholinergic reduces sweating in patients with localized—and generalized—hyperhidrosis. *Clinician Reviews*. [Online]. https://www.mdedge.com/sites/default/files/Document/June-2017/CR02707024.PDF

JNC 8 Guideline Summary. *Pharmacist's Letter/Prescriber's Letter*. https://www.scribd.com/doc/290772273/JNC-8-guideline-summary

Journal of the American Academy of Nurse Practitioners. https://www.aanp.org/publications/jaanp

Journal of the American Medical Association (JAMA) Internal Medicine. http://archinte.jamanetwork.com/journal.aspx

Journal of the American Geriatrics Society. http://onlinelibrary.wiley.com/journal/10.1111/(ISSN)1532-5415

Justesen, K., & Prasad, S. (2016). On-demand pill protocol protects against HIV. *Clinician Reviews, 26*(9), 18–19, 22. https://www.mdedge.com/authors/kathryn-justesen-md https://www.mdedge.com/authors/shaliendra-prasad-mbbs-mph

Kasper, D. L., & Fauci, A. S. (2017). Listeria monocytogenes infections. In: *Harrison's infectious diseases* (3rd ed.). New York, NY: McGraw Hill Education.

Khera, M., Adaikan, G., Buvat, J, Carrier, S., El-Meliegy, A., Hatzimouratidis, K., . . . Salonia, A. (2016). Diagnosis and treatment of testosterone deficiency: Recommendations from the Fourth International Consultation for Sexual Medicine (ICSM 2015). *The Journal of Sexual Medicine, 13*, 1787–1804.

Kuhar, D. T., Henderson, D. K., Struble, K. A., Heneine, W., Thomas, V., . . . Cheever, L. W. (2013). Updated US Public Health Service guidelines for the management of occupational exposures to human immunodeficiency virus and recommendations for postexposure prophylaxis. *Infection Control & Hospital Epidemiology, 34*(09), 875–892. doi:10.1086/672271

Kumar, S., Yegneswaran, B., & Pitchumoni, C. S. (2017). Preventing the adverse effects of glucocorticoids: A reminder. *Consultant, 57*(12), 726–728.

Langer, R., Simon, J. A., Pines, A., Lobo, R. A., Hodis, H. N., Pickar, J. H., . . . Utian, W. H. (2017). Menopausal hormone therapy for primary prevention: Why the USPSTF is wrong. *The North American Menopause Society, 24*(10), 1101–1112. doi:10.1097/GME.0000000000000983

Leach, M. Z. (2017, November 7). First UK guidelines for adults with lupus. *Rheumatology Network.* http://www.rheumatologynetwork.com/article/first-uk-guidelines-adults-lupus

Lexicomp. (2021). *Pediatric and neonatal dosage handbook: An extensive resource for clinicians treating pediatric and neonatal patients* (25th ed.). Lexicomp

Lortscher, D., Admani, S., Satur, N., & Eichenfield, L. F. (2016). Hormonal contraceptives and acne: A retrospective analysis of 2147 patients. *Journal of Drugs in Dermatology, 15*(6), 670–674. http://jddonline.com/articles/dermatology/S1545961616P0670X

Manchikanti, L., Kaye, A. M., Knezevic, N. N., McAnally, H., Slavin, K., Trescot, A. M., . . . Hirsch, J. A. (2017). Responsible, safe, and effective prescription of opioids for chronic non-cancer pain: American Society of Interventional Pain Physicians (ASIPP) guidelines. *Pain Physician, 20*(2S), S3–S92.

McDonald, J., & Mattingly, J. (2016). Chagas disease: Creeping into family practice in the United States. *Clinician Reviews, 26*(11), 38–45.

McNeill, C., Sisson, W., & Jarrett, A. (2017). Listerosis: A resurfacing menace. *International Journal of Nursing Practice, 13*(10), 647–654.

MDedge: Family Practice News. https://www.mdedge.com/familypracticenews/

MedlinePlus. https://www.nlm.nih.gov/medlineplus/ency/article/000165.htm

MedPage Today. http://www.medpagetoday.com

Medscape. http://www.medscape.com

Medscape: Drug Interaction Checker. http://reference.medscape.com/drug-interactionchecker?src=wnl_drugguide _170410_mscpref &uac=123859AY&impID=1324737&faf=1

Merel, S. E., & Paauw, D. S. (2017). Common drug side effects and drug-drug interactions in elderly adults in primary care. *Journal of the American Geriatrics Society, 65*(7), 1578–1585.

Miller, G. E., Sarpong, E. M., Davidoff, A. J., Yang, E. Y., Brandt, N. J., & Fick, D. M. (2016). Determinants of potentially inappropriate medication use among community-dwelling older adults. *Health Services Research, 52*(4), 1534–1549.

Molina, J. M., Capitant, C., Spire, B., Pialoux, G., Cotte, L., Charreau, I., . . . ANRS IPERGAY Study Group. (2015). On-demand preexposure prophylaxis in men at high risk for HIV-1 infection. *The New England Journal of Medicine, 373*, 2237–2246.

Monaco, K. (2017). *HRT benefits outweigh risks for certain menopausal women—Menopause Society statement aims to clear up confusion.* https://www.medpagetoday.com/Endocrinology/Menopause/66158?xid=NL_MPT_ IRXHealthWomen_2017-12-27&eun=g766320d0r

Morales, A., Bebb, R. A., Manoo, P., Assimakopoulos, P., Axler, J., Collier, C., . . . Lee, J. (2015). *Appendix 1 (as supplied by the authors): Full-text guidelines Multidisciplinary Canadian Clinical Practice Guideline on the diagnosis and management of testosterone deficiency syndrome in adult males.* http://www.cmaj.ca/content/suppl/2015/10/26/cmaj.150033.DC1/15-0033-1-at.pdf

National Academy of Medicine.
  http://nam.edu

National Center for Emerging and Zoonotic Infectious Diseases (NCEZID).
  https://www.cdc.gov/ncezid/index.html

National Heart Lung and Blood Institute (NHLBI).
  http://www.nhlbi.nih.gov

National Institute of Diabetes and Digestive and Kidney Diseases. *Adrenal insufficiency and Addison's disease.*
  http://www.nidk.nih.gov/health-infromation/health-topics/endocrine/adren [Accessed May 31, 2016]

New England Journal of Medicine (NEJM) Journal Watch General Medicine.
  http://www.jwatch.org/general-medicine

Ní Chróinín, D., Neto, H. M., Xiao, D., Sandhu, A., Brazel, C., Farnham, N., . . . Beveridge, A. (2016). Potentially inappropriate medications (PIMs) in older hospital in-patients: Prevalence, contribution to hospital admission and documentation of rationale for continuation. *Australasian Journal on Ageing, 35*(4), 262–265.

NIH, HIV/AIDS Treatment Information Service.
  http://aidsinfo.nih.gov/

Oliver, S. E., Gargano, J. W., Marin, M., Wallace, M., Curran, K. G., Chamberland, M., . . . Dooling, K. (2020). The Advisory Committee on Immunization Practices' interim recommendation for use of Pfizer-BioNTech COVID-19 vaccine—United States, December 2020. *MMWR Morbidity and Mortality Weekly Report, 69*,1922–1924. doi:10.15585/mmwr.mm6950e2

Oliver, S. E., Gargano, J. W., Marin, M., et al. The Advisory Committee on Immunization Practices' interim recommendation for use of Moderna COVID-19 vaccine—United States, December 2020. *MMWR Morb Mortal Wkly Rep.* 2021;69:1653-1656. doi: 10.15585/mmwr.mm695152e1

Ostergaard, L., Vesikari, T., Absalon, J., Beeslaar, J., Ward, B. J., Senders, S., . . . B1971009 and B1971016 Trial Investigators. (2017). A bivalent meningococcal b vaccine in adolescents and young adults. *The New England Journal of Medicine, 35*(4), 262–265. doi:10.1111/ ajag.12312

PEPline.
  http://www.nccc.ucsf.edu/about_nccc/pepline/; telephone: 888-448-4911

Pharmacist's Letter.
  www.pharmacistsletter.com

Physician's Desk Reference (PDR).
  http://www.pdr.net

Pregnancy and Lactation Labeling Final Rule (PLLR).
  https://www.drugs.com/pregnancy-categories.html

Prescriber's Letter.
  http://prescribersletter.therapeuticresearch.com/pl/sample.
  aspx?cs=&s=PRL&AspxAutoDetectCookieSupport=1

Psychopharmacology.
  http://link.springer.com/journal/213

Reference for Interpretation of Hepatitis C Virus (HCV) Test Results.
www.cdc.gov/hepatitis

Rosenberg, E. S., Doyle, K., Munoz-Jordan, J. L., Klein, L., Adams, L., Lozier, M., Weiss, K., & Sharp, T. M. (2017, November 5–9). *Prevalence and incidence of Zika virus infection among household contacts of Zika patients, Puerto Rico, 2016–2017. ASTMH 2017* . Paper presented at the 66th Annual Meeting of the American Society of Tropical Medicine and Hygiene, Baltimore, MD.

RxLIST.
http://www.rxlist.com/script/main/hp.asp

RxLIST: Drugs A-Z.
http://www.rxlist.com/drugs/alpha_a.htm

Sáez-Llorens, X., Tricou, V., Yu, D., Rivera, L., Jimeno, J., Villarreal, A. C., ... Wallace, D. (2018). Immunogenicity and safety of one versus two doses of tetravalent dengue vaccine in healthy children aged 2–17 years in Asia and Latin America: 18-month interim data from a phase 2, randomised, placebo-controlled study. *The Lancet Infectious Diseases, 18*(2), 162–170. doi:10.1016/s1473-3099(17)30632-1

Sanford Guide Web Edition.
https://webedition.sanfordguide.com

Saunders, K. H., Shukla, A. P., Igel, L. I., & Aronne, L. J. (2017). Obesity: When to consider medication. *The Journal of Family Practice, 66*(10), 608–616.
http://www.mdedge.com/sites/default/files/Document/September-2017/JFP06610608.PDF

Schaeffer, A. J., & Nicolle, L. E. (2016). Urinary tract infections in older men. *The New England Journal of Medicine, 374*(6), 562–571.

Schwartz, S. R., Magit, A. E., Rosenfeld, R. M., Ballachanda, B. B., Hackell, J. M., Krouse, H. J., ... Cunningham, E. R. (2017). Clinical practice guideline (update): Earwax (cerumen impaction). *Otolaryngology Head Neck Surgery, 156*(1S), S1–S29.

Solutions for safer ER/LA opioid prescribing in a new Era of Health Care. *American Nurses Credentialing Center, Post Graduate Institute of Medicine.*
www.cmeuniversity.com

Sterling, T. R., Villarino, M. E., Borisov, A. S., Shang, N., Gordin, F., Bliven-Sizemore, E., ... TB Trials Consortium PREVENT TB Study Team. (2011). Three months of rifapentine and isoniazid for latent tuberculosis infection. *The New England Journal of Medicine, 365*, 2155–2166. doi:10.1056/NEJMoa1104875

Taipale, H., Mittendorfer-Rutz, E., Alexanderson, K., Majak, M., Mehtälä, J., Hoti, F., ... Tiihonen, J. (2017, December 20). Antipsychotics and mortality in a nationwide cohort of 29,823 patients with schizophrenia. *Schizophrenia Research, pii: S0920–9964*(17), 30762–30764. doi:10.1016/j.schres.2017.12.010

Tebas, P., Roberts, C. C., Muthumani, K., Reuschel, E. L., Kudchodkar, S. B., Zaidi, F. I., ... Maslow, J. N. (2017). Safety and immunogenicity of an anti–zika virus DNA vaccine—Preliminary report. *New England Journal of Medicine.* doi:10.1056/nejmoa1708120

The 2017 hormone therapy position statement of The North American Menopause Society. (2017). *Menopause: The North American Menopause Society.* doi:10.1097/GME.0000000000000921

The American Congress of Obstetrics and Gynecology (ACOG).
http://www.acog.org

The American Geriatrics Society.
http://www.americangeriatrics.org

The JAMA Network.com.
www.jamanetwork.com

The Journal for Nurse Practitioners.
www.elsevier.com/locate/tjnp

The Medical Letter on Drugs and Therapeutics.
http://secure.medicalletter.org

The Nurse Practitioner Journal.
www.tnpj.com

Third Report of the National Cholesterol Education Program (NCEP) expert panel on detection, evaluation, and treatment of high blood cholesterol in adults (Adult Treatment Panel III) final report.
http://www.ncbi.nlm.nih.gov/pubmed/12485966

Tomaselli, G. F., Mahaffey, K. W., Cuker, A., Dobesh, P. P., Doherty, J. U., Eikelboom, J. W., ... Wiggins, B. S. (2017). 2017 ACC expert consensus decision pathway on management of bleeding in patients on oral anticoagulants. *Journal of the American College of Cardiology, 70*(24), 3042–3067. doi:10.1016/j.jacc.2017.09.1085

Turner, P. J., Southern, J., Andrews, N. J., Miller, E., Erlewyn-Lajeunesse, M., & Doyle, C. (2015). Safety of live attenuated influenza vaccine in atopic children with egg allergy. *Journal of Allergy and Clinical Immunology, 136*(2), 376–381. doi:10.1016/j.jaci.2014.12.1925

Updated CDC guidance: Superbugs threaten hospital patients. *Medscape Education Clinical Briefs.* (2016, March 31).
http://www.medscape.org/viewarticle/859361?nlid=105320_2713&src=wnl_cmemp_160523_mscpedu_nurs&impID=1106718&faf=1

UpToDate.com.
http://www.uptodate.com

U.S. Pharmacist Weekly Newsletter.
http://www.uspharmacist.com

Vogt, C. (2017, November 14). New AHA/ACC guidelines lower high BP threshold. *Consultant360.*
https://www.consultant360.com/exclusives/new-ahaacc-guidelines-lower- high-bp-threshold

Vrcek, I., Choudhury, E., & Durairaj, V. (2017). Herpes zoster ophthalmicus: A review for the internist. *The American Journal of Medicine, 130*(1), 21–26.

Wald, E. R., Applegate, K. E., Bordley, C., Darrow, D. H., Glode, M. P., Marcy, S. M., ... American Academy of Pediatrics. (2013). Clinical practice guidelines for the diagnosis and management of acute bacterial sinusitis in children 1 to 18 years. *Pediatrics, 132*(1), e262–e280.

Wallace, D. V., Dykewicz, M. S., Oppenheimer, J., Portnoy, J. M., & Lang, D. M. (2017). Pharmacologic treatment of seasonal allergic rhinitis: Synopsis of guidance from the 2017 joint task force on practice parameters. *Annals of Internal Medicine, 167*(12), 876. doi:10.7326/m17-2203

Watkins, S. L., Glantz, S. A., & Chaffee, B. W. (2018). Association of Noncigarette tobacco product use with future cigarette smoking among youth in the population assessment of tobacco and health (PATH) study, 2013–2015. *JAMA Pediatrics, 172*(2), 181. doi:10.1001/jamapediatrics.2017.4173

WebMD: Drugs and Medications A to Z. Latest Drug News.
http://www.webmd.com/drugs

Wimmer, B. C., Cross, A. J., Jokanovic, N., Wiese, M. D., George, J., Johnell, K., ... Bell, J. S. (2016). Clinical outcomes associated with medication regimen complexity in older people: A systematic review. *Journal of the American Geriatrics Society, 65*(4), 747–753. doi:10.1111/jgs.14682

Winkel, P., Hilden, J., Hansen, J. F., Kastrup, J., Kolmos, H. J., Kjøller, E., ... Gluud, C. (2015). Clarithromycin for stable coronary heart disease increases all-cause and cardiovascular mortality and cerebrovascular morbidity over 10years in the CLARICOR randomised, blinded clinical trial. *International Journal of Cardiology, 182*, 459–465. doi:10.1016/j.ijcard.2015.01.020

Wodi, A. P., Ault, K., Hunter, P., McNally, V., Szilagyi, P. G., & Bernstein, H. (2021). Advisory committee on immunization practices—Recommended immunization schedule for children and adolescents aged 18 years or younger—United States, 2021. *MMWR Morbidity and Mortality Weekly Report, 70,* 189–192. doi:10.15585/mmwr.mm7006a1

Wong, J., Marr, P., Kwan, D., Meiyappan, S., & Adcock, L. (2014). Identification of inappropriate medication use in elderly patients with frequent emergency department visits. *Canadian Pharmacists Journal/Revue Des Pharmaciens Du Canada, 147*(4), 248–256. doi:10.1177/1715163514536522

World Health Organization. (2016, August 30.). *Growing antibiotic resistance forces updates to recommended treatments for sexually transmitted infections.* http://www.who.int/mediacentre/news/releases/2016/antibiotics-sexual-infections/en

World Health Organization. (2016). *WHO guidelines for the treatment of Chlamydia trachomatis.* http://www.who.int/reproductivehealth/publications/rtis/chlamydia-treatment-guidelines/en

World Health Organization. (2016). *WHO guidelines for the treatment of Neisseria gonorrhoeae.* http://www.who.int/reproductivehealth/publications/rtis/gonorrhoea-treatment-guidelines/en

World Health Organization. (2016). *WHO guidelines for the treatment of Treponema pallidum (Syphilis).* http://www.who.int/reproductivehealth/publications/rtis/syphilis-treatment-guidelines/en

World Health Organization. (2017, March). *WHO model list of essential medicines* (20th list). Geneva, Switzerland: Author. http://www.who.int/medicines/publications/essentialmedicines/20th_EML2017.pdf?ua=1

World Health Organization. (2017, March). *WHO model list of essential medicines for children* (6th list). Geneva, Switzerland: Author. http://www.who.int/medicines/publications/essentialmedicines/6th_EMLc2017.pdf?ua=1

World Health Organization. (2017, June 6). *WHO updates essential medicines list with new advice on use of antibiotics, and adds medicines for hepatitis C, HIV, tuberculosis and cancer.* Geneva, Switzerland: Author. http://www.who.int/mediacentre/news/releases/2017/essential-medicines-list/en

Xie, Y., Bowe, B., Li, T., Xian, H., Yan, Y., & Al-Aly, Z. (2017, February 22). Long-term kidney outcomes among users of proton pump inhibitors without intervening acute kidney injury. *Kidney International, 91*(6), 1482–1494. doi:10.1016/j.kint.2016.12.021

Yılmaz, D., Heper, Y., & Gözler, L. (2017). Effect of the use of buzzy during phlebotomy on pain and individual satisfaction in blood donors. *Pain Management Nursing, 18*(4), 260–267.

Yoon, I.-K., & Thomas, S. J. (2017). Encouraging results but questions remain for dengue vaccine. *The Lancet Infectious Diseases, 18*(2), 125–126. doi:10.1016/S1473-3099(17)30634-5

Zarrabi, H., Khalkhali, M., Hamidi, A., Ahmadi, R., & Zavarmousavi, P. (2016). Clinical features, course and treatment of methamphetamine-induced psychosis in psychiatric inpatients. *BMC, 44.* doi:10.1186/s12888-016-0745-5

INDEX

NOTE: Generic names are in italics; FDA pregnancy categories and controlled drug categories appear in parentheses after the entry.

Dupixent, *dupilumab* (B)
  allergic rhinitis/sinusitis, 642
  asthma, 49, 50
  atopic dermatitis, 208
  eosinophilia, 51–52
Duratears Naturale, *petrolatum+lanolin+mineral oil*
  dry eye syndrome, 228
Durezol Ophthalmic Solution, *difluprednate* (C)
  eye pain, 258
Duricef, *cefadroxil* (B), 836
  acute exacerbation of chronic bronchitis, 76
  acute tonsillitis, 703
  dose forms, 826
  impetigo contagiosa, 395
  scarlet fever, 650
  wound, 771
Durolane, *sodium hyaluronate* (B)
  osteoarthritis, 502–503
dust mite allergy
  dermatophagoides farinae+dermatophagoides pteronyssinus allergen extract, Odactra, 230
dutasteride, Avodart (X)
  benign prostatic hyperplasia, 65
Dutoprol, *metoprolol succinate+ext-rel hydrochlorothiazide* (C)
  hypertension, 374
Duzallo, *allopurinol+lesinurad*
  gout (hyperuricemia), 284
Dyanavel XR Oral Suspension, *amphetamine, mixed salts of single entity amphetamine* (C)(II)
  attention deficit hyperactivity disorder (ADHD), 55–56
Dyazide, *triamterene+hydrochlorothiazide* (C)
  edema, 244
  hypertension, 366
Dynabac, *dirithromycin* (C)
  acute exacerbation of chronic bronchitis, 77
  acute tonsillitis, 703
  cellulitis, 144
  community acquired pneumonia, 574
  legionella pneumonia, 577
  streptococcal pharyngitis, 561
  wound, 772
Dynacin, *minocycline* (D)
  acne rosacea, 4
  acne vulgaris, 7
  aphthous stomatitis, 39
  Hansen's disease, 294
  Lyme disease, 436
  malaria, 438
Dynapen, *dicloxacillin* (B), 840
  cellulitis, 144
  impetigo contagiosa, 396
  lymphadenitis, 437
  otitis externa, 513
  paronychia, 545
Dyrenium, *triamterene* (B)
  edema, 242
dyshidrosis, 231
dyshidrotic eczema, 143
dyslipidemia
  alirocumab, Praluent (C), 232
  amlodipine+atorvastatin, Caduet (X), 237

  atorvastatin, Lipitor (X), 233
  bempedoic acid, Nexletol, 232–233
  cholestyramine, Questran (C), 235
  colesevelam, WelChol (B), 236
  colestipol, Colestid (C), 236
  evolocumab, Repatha, 232
  ezetimibe, Zetia (C), 232
  ezetimibe+atorvastatin, Liptruzet (X), 234
  ezetimibe+rosuvastatin, Roszet (X), 234
  ezetimibe+simvastatin, Vytorin (X), 234
  fenofibrate, Antara, Fenoglide, FibriCor, TriCor, TriLipix, Lipofen, Lofibra (C), 234–235
  fluvastatin, Lescol, Lescol XL (X), 233
  gemfibrozil, Lopid (X), 234
  icosapent ethyl (omega 3-fatty acid ethyl ester of EPA), Vascepa sgc (C), 231
  lomitapide mesylate, Juxtapid (X), 231
  lovastatin, Mevacor, Altoprev (X), 233
  mipomersen, Kynamro (B), 231–232
  niacin, Niaspan, Slo-Niacin (C), 235
  niacin+lovastatin, Advicor (X), 236
  niacin+simvastatin, Simcor (X), 236–237
  omega 3-acid ethyl esters, Lovaza, Epanova (C), 231
  pitbevacizumabtatin, Livalo, Nikita, Zypitamag (X), 233
  pravastatin, Pravachol (X), 234
  rosuvastatin, Crestor (X), 234
  simvastatin, Zocor (X), 234
dysmenorrhea: primary
  celecoxib, Celebrex (C), 238
  diclofenac, Cataflam, Voltaren, Voltaren-XR (C), 237
  mefenamic acid, Ponstel (C), 237
  meloxicam, Mobic, Vivlodex, Anjeso (C), 238
dyspareunia
  estradiol, Imvexxy (X), 239
  ospemifene, Osphena (X), 239
  prasterone (dehydroepiandrosterone [DHEA]), Intrarosa (X), 238

ebola zaire disease
  ansuvimab-zykl, Ebanga, 241
  atoltivimab+maftivimab+odesivimab, Inmazeb, 240–241
  ebola Zaire vaccine, live, Ervebo, 240
ecallantide, Kalbitor (C)
  hereditary angioedema, 329
echothiophate iodide, Phospholine Iodide (X)
  glaucoma, 277
EC-Naprosyn, *naproxen* (B)
  fever (pyrexia), 260
econazole, Spectazole (C)
  diaper rash, 220
  skin candidiasis, 134
  tinea corporis, 694
  tinea cruris, 696
  tinea pedis, 697
  tinea versicolor, 699
Econopred, Econopred Plus, *prednisolone acetate* (C)
  allergic (vernal) conjunctivitis, 171
EContra EZ, *levonorgestrel* (X), 793
Ecotrin, *aspirin* (D)
  peripheral vascular disease, 557
eculizumab, Soliris (C)

Emflaza, *deflazacort* (B)
  duchenne muscular dystrophy (DMD), 228–229
enfortumab vedotin-ejfv, Padcev, 807
  bladder cancer, 86–87
emicizumab-kxwh, Hemlibra
  hemophilia A, 311–312
Emla Cream, *lidocaine 2.5%+prilocaine 2.5%* (B)
  atopic dermatitis, 208
  burn: minor, 85
  diabetic peripheral neuropathy (DPN), 218
  gouty arthritis, 286
  hemorrhoids, 318
  herpangina, 330
  herpes zoster, 334
  insect bite/sting, 404
  juvenile idiopathic arthritis, 419
  juvenile rheumatoid arthritis, 423
  muscle strain, 466
  pain, 522
  peripheral neuritis, 556
  post-herpetic neuralgia, 589
empagliflozin, Jardiance (C)
  type 2 diabetes mellitus, 730
emphysema
  aclidinium bromide, Tudorza Pressair (C), 245
  dyphylline+guaifenesin, Lufyllin GG (C), 247
  fluticasone furoate+umeclidinium+vilanterol,
      Trelegy Ellipta, 247
  fluticasone furoate/vilanterol, Breo Ellipta (C),
      244
  glycopyrrolate inhalation solution, Lonhala
      Magnair (C), 245
  glycopyrrolate inhalation solution, Seebri
      Neohaler (C), 244
  indacaterol, Arcapta Neohaler (C), 244
  indacaterol+glycopyrrolate, Utibron Neohaler
      (C), 246
  ipratropium, Atrovent (B), 244
  ipratropium/albuterol, Combivent MDI (C), 246
  ipratropium+albuterol, Combivent Respimat
      (C), 246
  olodaterol, Striverdi Respimat (C), 244
  revefenacin inhalation solution, Yupelri, 245–246
  theophylline+potassium
      iodide+ephedrine+phenobarbital,
      Quadrinal (X)(II), 247
  tiotropium (as bromide monohydrate), Spiriva
      HandiHaler, Spiriva Respimat (C), 246
  tiotropium+olodaterol, Stiolto Respimat (C), 246
  umeclidinium, Incruse Ellipta (C), 246
  umeclidinium+vilanterol, Anoro Ellipta (C), 247
Emsam, *selegiline* (C)
  major depressive disorder, 201
  post-traumatic stress disorder, 594
emtricitabine, Emtriva (B)
  human immunodeficiency virus infection, 341
Emverm, *mebendazole* (C)
  hookworm, 337
  pinworm, 565–566
  roundworm, 647
  threadworm, 689
  trichinosis, 705–706
  whipworm, 768
Enablex, *darifenacin* (C)
  urinary overactive bladder, 398

enalapril, Epaned Oral Solution, Vasotec (D)
  heart failure, 304
  hypertension, 367
Enbrel, *etanercept* (B)
  juvenile idiopathic arthritis, 421
  osteoarthritis, 503
  psoriatic arthritis, 613
  rheumatoid arthritis, 634
encopresis
  bisacodyl, Dulcolax (B), 247
  glycerin suppository (A), 247
  mineral oil (C), 154
Endari, *L-glutamine*, 803
  sickle cell disease, 659
endometrial carcinoma
  pembrolizumab, Keytruda, 98
  dostarlimab-gxly, Jemperli, 97–98
endometriosis
  danazol, Danocrine (X), 249
  elagolix, Orlissa (X), 248
  goserelin (GnRH analog), Zoladex (X), 248
  leuprolide acetate (GnRH analog), Lupron Depot
      (X), 248
  medroxyprogesterone acetate, Depo-Provera
      (X), 248
  medroxyprogesterone, Provera (X), 248
  nafarelin acetate, Synarel (X), 249
  norethindrone acetate, Aygestin (X), 248
Enduronyl, Enduronyl Forte,
      methyclothiazide+deserpidine (B)
  edema, 242
  hypertension, 364
enfuvirtide, Fuzeon (B)
  human immunodeficiency virus infection, 345
Engerix-B, *hepatitis B recombinant vaccine* (C)
  hepatitis B, 320
Enhertu *fam-trastuzumab deruxtecan-nxki*, 804
  breast cancer, 93–94
enoxacin, Penetrex (X)
  gonorrhea, 282
  urinary tract infection, 753
enoxaparin, Lovenox, 819
Enpresse (X), *ethinyl estradiol/levonorgestrel* (X)
  estrogen and progesterone, 784
Enstilar, *calcipotriene+betamethasone dipropionate*
      (C)(G)
  psoriasis, 603
entacapone, Comtan (C)
  Parkinson's disease, 544
entecavir, Baraclude (C)
  hepatitis B, 321
Enterereg, *alvimopan* (B)
  bowel resection with primary anastomosis, 74
Entocort EC, *budesonide micronized* (C)
  Crohn's disease, 183
Entresto, *sacubitril+valsartan* (D)
  heart failure, 305
Entyvio, *vedolizumab* (B)
  Crohn's disease, 186
  ulcerative colitis, 744
Envarsus XR, *tacrolimus*
  organ transplant rejection prophylaxis, 498
eosinophilia
  benralizumab, Fasenra, 53–54
  dupilumab, Dupixent, 51–52